ESSENTIALS OF
Family Medicine

Third Edition

D1449291

ESSENTIALS OF
Family Medicine

Third Edition

PHILIP D. SLOANE, M.D.
Professor
Department of Family Medicine
The University of North Carolina at Chapel Hill, School of Medicine
Chapel Hill, North Carolina

LISA M. SLATT, M.Ed.
Research Assistant Professor
Department of Family Medicine
The University of North Carolina at Chapel Hill, School of Medicine
Chapel Hill, North Carolina

PETER CURTIS, M.D.
Professor
Department of Family Medicine
The University of North Carolina at Chapel Hill, School of Medicine
Chapel Hill, North Carolina

MARK H. EBELL, M.D., M.S.
Associate Professor
Department of Family Practice
Michigan State University College of Human Medicine
East Lansing, Michigan

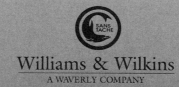

Williams & Wilkins
A WAVERLY COMPANY

BALTIMORE • PHILADELPHIA • LONDON • PARIS • BANGKOK
BUENOS AIRES • HONG KONG • MUNICH • SYDNEY • TOKYO • WROCLAW

Editor: Elizabeth A. Nieginski
Managing Editor: Crystal Taylor
Marketing Manager: Christine Kushner
Production Editor: Bill Cady
Design Coordinator: Mario Fernandez

Copyright © 1998 Williams & Wilkins

351 West Camden Street
Baltimore, Maryland 21201-2436 USA

Rose Tree Corporate Center
1400 North Providence Road
Building II, Suite 5025
Media, Pennsylvania 19063-2043 USA

All rights reserved. This book is protected by copyright. No part of this book may be reproduced in any form or by any means, including photocopying, or utilized by any information storage and retrieval system without written permission from the copyright owner.

The publisher is not responsible (as a matter of product liability, negligence or otherwise) for any injury resulting from any material contained herein. This publication contains information relating to general principles of medical care which should not be construed as specific instructions for individual patients. Manufacturers' product information and package inserts should be reviewed for current information, including contraindications, dosages and precautions.

Printed in the United States of America

First Edition, 1988
Second Edition, 1993

Library of Congress Cataloging-in-Publication Data

Essentials of family medicine   /   editors, Philip D. Sloane . . . [et al.].—3rd ed.
    p.   cm.
    Includes bibliographical references and index.
    ISBN 0-683-30147-0
    1. Family medicine.   I. Sloane, Philip D.
    [DNLM: 1. Family Practice.   WB 110 E78 1998]
  RC46.E88   1998
  616—dc21
  DNLM/DLC
  for Library of Congress   97-42734
                                      CIP

The publishers have made every effort to trace the copyright holders for borrowed material. If they have inadvertently overlooked any, they will be pleased to make the necessary arrangements at the first opportunity.

To purchase additional copies of this book, call our customer service department at **(800) 638-0672** or fax orders to **(800) 447-8438**. For other book services, including chapter reprints and large quantity sales, ask for the Special Sales department.

Canadian customers should call **(800) 665-1148** or fax orders to **(800) 665-0103**. For all other calls originating outside of the United States, please call **(410) 528-4223** or fax us at **(410) 528-8550**.

Visit Williams & Wilkins on the Internet: http://www.wwilkins.com or contact our customer service department at **custserv@wwilkins.com**. Williams & Wilkins customer service representatives are available from 8:30 am to 6:00 pm, EST, Monday through Friday, for telephone access.

98 99 00 01 02
1 2 3 4 5 6 7 8 9 10

To my parents, Allan and Louise Slatt, and

my husband, Alan Spanos

L. M. S.

To my parents, Herbert and Hildegard Ebell,

and my wife, Laura Bierema

M. H. E.

To the many practicing family

physicians who generously give of their

time and expertise to teach our medical

students about the pleasures and

challenges of caring for people

and their families.

Preface

We are pleased and excited about the third edition of *Essentials of Family Medicine*. In this book we have attempted to provide learners with a state-of-the-art guide to the field. *Essentials of Family Medicine* was originally designed to be read cover-to-cover and used as a basic reference by students doing third- and fourth-year clerkships in family medicine. Other professionals, including specialists in other fields, residents in family medicine, physicians' assistants and nurse practitioners, have used it as a comprehensive introduction to the field. The average family medicine clerkship is now longer, and the average student is more knowledgeable than even a few years back, so we feel that it is appropriate to present more information and to be more comprehensive than we were in earlier editions of this book. We hope our readers find it useful and easy to read.

We have endeavored to make this edition a considerable improvement over our second edition. Some of the changes we have made include

- an attempt to communicate basic principles more succinctly and effectively through use of case discussions and an informal writing style.

- far greater use of tables and figures, for easy reference, including algorithms that outline general approaches to common problems.

- increased sophistication to reflect today's learners, who tend to get more family practice instruction earlier in their education than did students a decade ago. In addition to diagnosis, we've placed increased emphasis on management in this edition.

- an evidence-based approach, especially in the prevention and common problems sections.

- general updating to reflect new developments in medicine and in the organization of medical care.

- several new chapters on common problems that had not been covered in the second edition.

As always, we welcome comments, corrections, and suggestions for the next edition. Please address them to Philip Sloane or Lisa Slatt c/o Department of Family Medicine, Aycock Building, CB# 7595, University of North Carolina, Chapel Hill, NC 27599.

Finally, we'd like to thank some of the many people who have helped us put this edition together. The list is long and will, of course, be incomplete, but it must include, first and foremost, our author-colleagues, who drafted chapters while pursuing busy clinical and academic lives. In addition, key assistance has been provided by: Christerlena Singh, Nili Clifford, Roxie Gunter, Jen Hovendon, Tim Ives, Warren Newton, Ken Reeb, Jesse Sloane, Blake Smith, our colleagues in the Examkit Consortium, and our editorial team at Williams & Wilkins, including (but not limited to) Crystal Taylor, Bill Cady, Nancy Evans, Elizabeth Nieginski, and Tim Satterfield.

PHILIP D. SLOANE
LISA M. SLATT
PETER CURTIS
MARK EBELL

Contributors

Dale Alexander, Ph.D., M.S.W.
Clinical Assistant Professor
Department of Family Medicine
Director of Behavioral Sciences
Joint Appointments in Psychiatry
*   Social Work*
The University of North Carolina at Chapel
*   Hill, School of Medicine*
Chapel Hill, North Carolina

B. Lewis Barnett, Jr., M.D.
Walter M. Seward Professor
Department of Family Medicine
University of Virginia School of Medicine
Charlottesville, Virginia

Henry C. Barry, M.D.
Associate Professor
Department of Family Practice
Michigan State University College of Human
*   Medicine*
East Lansing, Michigan

Lorne A. Becker, M.D.
Professor and Chairman
Department of Family Medicine
State University of New York College of
*   Medicine*
Syracuse, New York

George R. Bergus, M.D.
Associate Professor
Department of Family Medicine
University of Iowa College of Medicine
Iowa City, Iowa

J. Kevin Carmichael, M.D.
El Rio Community Health Center
Tucson, Arizona

Alexander W. Chessman, M.D.
Associate Professor
Department of Family Medicine
Medical University of South Carolina
Charleston, South Carolina

Sandra Clark, M.D.
Carrboro Community Health Center
Carrboro, North Carolina

Peter Curtis, M.D.
Professor
Department of Family Medicine
The University of North Carolina at Chapel
*   Hill, School of Medicine*
Chapel Hill, North Carolina

James E. Dunlap, M.D.
Assistant Professor
Department of Family Practice
Michigan State University College of Human
*   Medicine*
East Lansing, Michigan

Paul F. Dunn, M.S.N., F.N.P.
Clinical Assistant Professor
Department of Family Medicine
The University of North Carolina at Chapel
*   Hill, School of Medicine*
Chapel Hill, North Carolina

Mark H. Ebell, M.D., M.S.
Associate Professor
Department of Family Practice
Michigan State University College of Human
*   Medicine*
East Lansing, Michigan

Michael Fisher, M.D., M.P.H.
Clinical Assistant Professor
Department of Family Medicine
The University of North Carolina at Chapel
*   Hill, School of Medicine*
Chapel Hill, North Carolina

John P. Fogarty, M.D.
Professor and Chairman
Department of Family Practice
University of Vermont College of Medicine
Burlington, Vermont

Michael J. Franklin, Jr., M.D.
Department of Family Medicine
University of Iowa College of Medicine
Iowa City, Iowa

John J. Frey, M.D.
Professor and Chair
Department of Family Medicine
University of Wisconsin Medical School
Madison, Wisconsin

Susan Gaylord, Ph.D.
Research Associate
Program on Aging
The University of North Carolina at Chapel Hill
Chapel Hill, North Carolina

Adam O. Goldstein, M.D.
Assistant Professor
Department of Family Medicine
*The University of North Carolina at Chapel
    Hill, School of Medicine*
Chapel Hill, North Carolina

Lee A. Green, M.D., M.P.H.
Associate Professor
Department of Family Practice
University of Michigan Medical School
Ann Arbor, Michigan

Scott H. Grindel, M.D.
Director Sports Medicine
*St. Vincent Family Practice Residency
    Program*
Erie, Pennsylvania

Julie P. Grubb, M.D.
Clinical Assistant Professor
Department of Family Medicine
*The University of North Carolina at Chapel
    Hill, School of Medicine*
Chapel Hill, North Carolina

Robert E. Gwyther, M.D.
Professor
Department of Family Medicine
*The University of North Carolina at Chapel
    Hill, School of Medicine*
Chapel Hill, North Carolina

Wayne A. Hale, M.D.
Assistant Professor
Moses H. Cone Health System
Family Practice Residency
Greensboro, North Carolina

M. Dean Havron, Jr., M.D.
Blue Ridge Family Practice
Winchester, Virginia

Margaret R. Helton, M.D.
Clinical Assistant Professor
Department of Family Medicine
*The University of North Carolina at Chapel
    Hill, School of Medicine*
Chapel Hill, North Carolina

John M. Hickner, M.D., M.S.
Professor
Department of Family Practice
*Michigan State University College of Human
    Medicine*
East Lansing, Michigan

Melissa M. Hicks, M.D.
Adjunct Instructor
*MAHEC Family Practice
    Residency Program*
Asheville, North Carolina

Timothy J. Ives, Pharm.D., M.P.H.
Clinical Associate Professor
Department of Family Medicine
*The University of North Carolina at Chapel
    Hill, School of Medicine*
Chapel Hill, North Carolina

Louis B. Jacques, M.D.
Associate Professor
Department of Family Medicine
*Georgetown University School of
    Medicine*
Washington, D.C.

Joseph M. Keenan, M.D.
Professor
Department of Family Medicine
University of Minnesota Medical School
Minneapolis, Minnesota

David N. Little, M.D.
Associate Professor
Department of Family Practice
*University of Vermont College of
    Medicine*
Burlington, Vermont

Doug McKeag, M.D.
Senior Professor
Department of Orthopedics
University of Pittsburg
Pittsburg, Pennsylvania

Melanie Mintzer, M.D.
Clinical Assistant Professor
Department of Family Medicine
*The University of North Carolina at Chapel
    Hill, School of Medicine*
Chapel Hill, North Carolina

Warren P. Newton, M.D.
Assistant Professor
Department of Family Medicine
The University of North Carolina at Chapel
*   Hill, School of Medicine*
Chapel Hill, North Carolina

Margaret R. H. Nusbaum, D.O., M.P.H.
Clinical Assistant Professor
Department of Family Medicine
The University of North Carolina at Chapel
*   Hill, School of Medicine*
Chapel Hill, North Carolina

Donald Pathman, M.D., M.P.H.
Assistant Professor
Department of Family Medicine
The University of North Carolina at Chapel
*   Hill, School of Medicine*
Chapel Hill, North Carolina

Patricia Ann Payne, C.N.M., M.P.H.
Clinical Assistant Professor
Department of Family Medicine
The University of North Carolina at Chapel
*   Hill, School of Medicine*
Chapel Hill, North Carolina

Richard W. Pretorius, M.D.
Assistant Clinical Professor
Department of Family Medicine
University of Iowa College of Medicine
Iowa City, Iowa

Barbara D. Reed, M.D., M.S.H.
Associate Professor
Department of Family Practice
University of Michigan Medical School
Ann Arbor, Michigan

Mary Jean Schenk, M.D.
Assistant Professor
Department of Family Medicine
Wayne State University School of
*   Medicine*
Detroit, Michigan

Kendra L. Schwartz, M.D., M.S.P.H.
Assistant Professor
Department of Family Medicine
Wayne State University School of Medicine
Detroit, Michigan

Thomas L. Schwenk, M.D.
Professor and Chair
Department of Family Practice
University of Michigan Medical
*   School*
Ann Arbor, Michigan

Philip D. Sloane, M.D.
Professor
Department of Family Medicine
The University of North Carolina at Chapel
*   Hill, School of Medicine*
Chapel Hill, North Carolina

Mindy Smith, M.D., M.S.
Associate Professor
Department of Family Practice
University of Michigan Medical School
Ann Arbor, Michigan

John J. Smucny, M.D.
Assistant Professor
Lafayette Family Medicine Residency
Lafayette, New York

Beat Steiner, M.D., M.P.H.
Clinical Assistant Professor
Department of Family Medicine
The University of North Carolina at Chapel
*   Hill, School of Medicine*
Chapel Hill, North Carolina

Barbara Supanich, R.S.M., M.D.
Associate Chair for Clinical Services
Department of Family Practice
Michigan State University College of Human
*   Medicine*
East Lansing, Michigan

Richard P. Usatine, M.D.
Associate Clinical Professor
Department of Family Medicine
UCLA School of Medicine
Los Angeles, California

Dorothy E. Vura-Weis, M.D.
Assistant Professor
Department of Family Medicine
Loma Linda University School of
*   Medicine*
Loma Linda, California

William C. Wadland, M.D., M.S.
Professor and Chair
Department of Family Practice
Michigan State University College of Human
  Medicine
East Lansing, Michigan

Samuel S. Weir, M.D.
Instructor
Department of Family Medicine
The University of North Carolina at Chapel
  Hill, School of Medicine
Chapel Hill, North Carolina

Contents

Preface | vii
Contributors | ix

I. PRINCIPLES OF FAMILY MEDICINE

1. A Day in a Life / 3
   JOHN J. FREY

2. From Cradle to Rocker: Providing Care Across the Human
   Life Cycle / 11
   B. LEWIS BARNETT, JR.

3. Keeping "The Family" in Focus During
   Patient Care / 25
   DALE ALEXANDER AND SANDRA CLARK

4. Outside the Office Walls / 41
   MARY JEAN SCHENK, JOSEPH M. KEENAN, ADAM O. GOLDSTEIN,
   BEAT STEINER, and DONALD PATHMAN

5. Family Practice in an Era of Rapid Change / 63
   LOUIS B. JACQUES

II. PREVENTIVE CARE

6. Helping Your Patients Stay Healthy / 79
   PETER CURTIS and ADAM O. GOLDSTEIN

7. Pregnancy Prevention and Contraception / 99
   MELANIE MINTZER

8. Prenatal Care / 127
   MARGARET R. HELTON

9. Well Child and Adolescent Care / 141
   BEAT STEINER

10. Well Adult Care / 157
    MELISSA M. HICKS

11. Promoting Health for Women at Menopause / 179
    PATRICIA ANN PAYNE and PETER CURTIS

12. Complementary Therapies in Family Medicine / 191
    SUSAN GAYLORD

III. COMMON PROBLEMS

13. Common Problems: Overview and General Approach / 203
PHILIP D. SLOANE, PETER CURTIS, MARK H. EBELL, MICHAEL FISHER,
TIMOTHY J. IVES, and WARREN P. NEWTON

14. Abdominal Pain / 221
JOHN J. SMUCNY and LORNE A. BECKER

15. Addiction / 243
ROBERT E. GWYTHER

16. Ankle and Knee Pain / 263
JAMES E. DUNLAP and HENRY C. BARRY

17. Anxiety and Depression / 281
THOMAS L. SCHWENK

18. Arthritis and Rheumatism / 291
PETER CURTIS

19. Asthma and Chronic Obstructive Pulmonary
Disease (COPD) / 309
DOROTHY E. VURA-WEIS

20. Breast Problems / 331
KENDRA L. SCHWARTZ

21. Chest Pain / 349
LEE A. GREEN

22. Chronic Cardiac Disease / 367
RICHARD W. PRETORIUS and MICHAEL J. FRANKLIN, JR.

23. Diabetes Mellitus / 381
SAMUEL S. WEIR and TIMOTHY J. IVES

24. Dizziness / 401
ALEXANDER W. CHESSMAN and PHILIP D. SLOANE

25. Dysuria / 411
GEORGE R. BERGUS

26. Fatigue / 425
DAVID N. LITTLE

27. Fever in Infants and Preschool Children / 435
WILLIAM C. WADLAND

28. Headache / 447
JOHN P. FOGARTY

29. HIV Disease / 461
J. KEVIN CARMICHAEL

30. Hypertension / 473
    WARREN P. NEWTON and TIMOTHY J. IVES

31. Low Back Pain / 483
    PHILIP D. SLOANE

32. Menstrual Syndromes / 501
    BARBARA SUPANICH

33. Neck Pain / 519
    PETER CURTIS

34. Prostate Diseases / 527
    JOHN M. HICKNER and JULIE P. GRUBB

35. Respiratory Tract Infections / 543
    PETER CURTIS

36. Sexually Transmitted Diseases / 559
    MARGARET R. H. NUSBAUM

37. Shoulder Pain / 581
    SCOTT H. GRINDEL and DOUG MCKEAG

38. Skin Problems / 597
    RICHARD P. USATINE

39. Skin Wounds: Minor Lacerations, Contusions,
    and Abrasions / 613
    WAYNE A. HALE

40. Sore Throat / 623
    MARK H. EBELL

41. Thyroid Disease / 635
    MINDY SMITH and M. DEAN HAVRON, JR.

42. Vaginitis / 657
    BARBARA D. REED

43. Weight Management and Obesity / 679
    PAUL F. DUNN

    Index / 699

PART I

Principles of Family Medicine

1. A Day in a Life

JOHN J. FREY

STARTING OUT

He has always been an early riser. Up at 5:30 and moving down to the coffee pot in the kitchen. Then with the first cup, to the kitchen table to read. When they were younger, his wife used to get up to make breakfast and talk. When the kids got older and more numerous, she took the time to stay in bed and sleep and he would entertain the children over breakfast. Now that two of the kids have moved away from home, he has the kitchen table to himself.

Being a paperboy trained him well for medicine. He doesn't know too many doctors that sleep in, except after a particularly exhausting night on call. So, he thought, getting up to throw the *Sentinel* was a good way of teaching him to appreciate the silence of the early morning, the changes in seasons, the coming of the birds from the south and then their return. Getting up early back then wasn't easy, never is for a teenager. But he got used to it and, after a while, he took the energy of early mornings for granted and even needed it.

His energy and joyfulness in the morning grates on his wife a bit. But they have worked it out. She pretty much keeps to herself, sometimes with the pillow over her head, and he uses this time, 2 hours, to gather things around him for reading and getting ideas. Some days it is the stack of journals he leafs through; other days it is books or a magazine about furniture that he loves to think about refinishing. But it is all, he thinks, short-loop satisfaction, giving him a bit of pleasure at finding something out about a patient, something to think about that day, something to put into the mix of patients, medicine, and meetings that will nudge his thinking a bit in other directions that day. He likes the Tuesday "Science Section" in the *New York Times*, full of articles about galactic clouds, rain forests, and birds that find their way home. Something to chew on with his toast or cereal!

His wife and daughter slowly move to their own rhythms in the morning. He greets them, then moves out the door to the hospital for rounds. One of the pleasures of solo practice, granted a rare form of medical practice these days of large groups, is that he sets his own time based on what he wants and what his patients need. What he wants most mornings is to be on the floor when the breakfast trays are being collected and the nurses have not yet gotten into their work of passing medicines and tending patients.

At the end of their morning report, the nurses and aides greet him as he moves off to get the patients' versions of what happened in the night. The nurses have come to expect him first, before the other doctors start roaming in clusters to see patients. He spends time in each room, talking, listening, examining. Then he comes to the nurses' station and carries on small conversations with the aides and nurses about each patient—what they seem like, and whether they have been up and about as much as the patients told him they were. Sometimes he feels that it is an interruption for the nurses, but then again, after all these years, they are used to him and seem to look forward to his comments about what he read that morning and what concerns he has, for example, about the 85-year-old woman with pneumonia who lives alone, and whether her family will be able to look after her, stubborn and independent-minded as she is. Although he was taught and learned the concept of *team* when he was a resident, his definition of team includes everyone who has anything to do with his patients. Each staff member has something valuable to offer, even if it is an opinion rather than a urine output, or a weight, or the presence of rales before and after she coughs. All these folks, too, are the patient's neighbors and have ideas about how his patients are doing.

Then he sits and writes out his plans for each patient, changes in their medications, tests to be done. He uses the SOAP (subjective data, objective data, assessment, and plan) method of writing notes, which he learned as a resident years ago. He can't even remember what progress notes were like without problem lists, assessment and plans for each problem, which he uses to organize his thinking about what should be watched for, what should be used as a clinical endpoint. He does remember, though, that when he arrived in town, a few staff commented on his "new" way of writing notes.

3

Soon the morning sounds of the hospital start to increase. His colleagues filter into the ward and pick out charts. He often grabs them, "curb-sides" them, and asks advice—"Jim, would you check Mr. Sandstorm's belly again when you get a chance? I think it's a lot better than yesterday, and his temp is down. I still think it's a flare-up of his diverticulitis, but he is old, and I just want to be sure I am not missing something." "Tony, did you find me anything on anticoagulation and strokes? I am still not sure what I am supposed to do with the 55-year-old who is in atrial fibrilla-tion and is pretty active. Coumadin seems pretty risky."—and so forth and so forth.

When he was younger, he had been con-vinced that the way to stay current—losing touch had been a real fear of his—was to go to continuing medical education conferences. He was aware of the reputation that community doctors had at the medical school as ill informed. Local medical doctors who didn't know the lat-est stuff or even the next-to-latest stuff. He at-tended 3-day meetings, listening to a procession of specialists who presented 20-minute talks on "The Work-up of Fever of Unknown Origin," "Dysmenorrhea," "Immunization Update," and so forth. He would return with a suitcase full of three-ring binders and a headache.

He would organize the binders on his office shelf. They would sit there for years until he had brought so many home and felt so remorseful about not rereading them that he took the whole set to the hospital library where the librarian, without asking him, sent them somewhere, re-lieving him of his guilt. Now, after all these years, he realized that what one of his residency teachers had told him was true—that the best continuing medical education would be from his patients. His colleagues would let him know about things they heard or read, and the infor-mation would have a patient's name attached to it rather than reside in a dusty three-ring binder. "The Management of Melanoma" would be the reprints and National Cancer Institute references on experimental protocols that were filed with Charlie Steptoe's chart, his patient from whom he removed a nevus 5 years ago. He got a tele-phone call from the pathologist telling him that the nevus was a melanoma, Clark's level III. Every time he saw Charlie, who seemed well, he was reminded about the life expectancy charts he had read, and wanted to go back now and then and see if the cure rate had improved.

So, all these early morning conversations with colleagues is a way of doing CME daily, and it makes sense. He realizes the myriad new ways to get information about clinical problems and at times feels overwhelmed by it. He relies on talk-ing and asking and thinking things through with the other community doctors he sees every day. It helps sort out his thinking.

SETTLING IN

When he looked around for a community in which to live, what was clear to him was that he wanted to do full-service family practice. The late 70s was a time when that style of practice was possible in any number of communities. His wife and he sat with a map and a list of things they were looking for in a place to live. They both grew up in smaller communities and felt most comfortable in small towns, but after meeting in college and going to school in Chicago, they had gotten used to the amenities of larger communi-ties. They liked movies, saved up for dinner at a nice restaurant once a month, went to museums and other places that were inexpensive places to spend a day or evening. When it came time to look for residencies, they thought of looking in the Chicago area but settled on a community hospital program in Michigan, in part because they wanted to see what it was like to live in a city whose size was more familiar to them.

Residency didn't give them time to do much of anything. Their first child was born at the hos-pital where he was a resident. His call schedule and the moonlighting he did to earn a little extra money kept him busy. His wife taught as a sub-stitute elementary school teacher until their son was born; then she tried to fill in when it was pos-sible. He always tells medical students who come to his office during their third year of school that they have so much more available, like day care and flexible residency programs and paternity leave, than he and his wife did when he was a resident. He knows this personally, too, since their oldest daughter is a medical student mar-ried to a resident, and expecting a child in 3 months, and she can use community day care and arrange her fourth year so as to spend time with the baby. So much is different; so much is better.

As they got into the third year of residency, he and his wife realized that they had to consider where to live. He liked the Midwest and liked the type of practice he saw other family physicians in the community engaged in. They considered staying in the town where he did his residency but also wanted to look back home. He was torn between going to the town where he was born and another that was like it but was not his home town. All the time when he was growing up and talking about medical school, his grandfather would say, "So, when are you going to come back and take care of us?" and he would answer, "I don't know Grandpa, I have a lot of school ahead of me." He wanted to return home a hero of sorts, but also felt anxiety about being someone else's idea of who he was instead of his own. The pressure worked on him and his wife. They settled on the town where she grew up, partly because it was just like his home town but it wasn't his home town. Also, they realized that, with another child on the way, they would need support from family, and he liked her family. Now, after 20 years, he still does, fortunately.

There were no real group practices in the town, and two of the other doctors asked him to join them. He considered it, but in the end, partly out of a need to try to do things his way and partly out of sheer stubbornness, he decided to go solo. Thankfully, the community hospital agreed to bankroll his practice and to guarantee his income for the first 2 years as an incentive to get him to come to town. The big question was whether the patients would come—they did—and whether the other doctors in the community would work with him to provide cross-coverage at night and weekends—and they did. It seemed almost too easy to get started, and it was, but it wouldn't stay that way.

During his 20 years in town, physicians came and left the community for many reasons. The number of family doctors dwindled dangerously low, until the hospital really put some energy into recruiting and supporting new family doctors in town. At times he resented how easy it was for the new folks, but then he remembered how easy he had thought things were for him at first. Getting started was exciting, stimulating, and something that was a learning experience every day. Staying with it, enduring, thriving, growing, and finding freshness was the real challenge in clinical practice.

THE OFFICE

He tailored the place he worked to his wants and his patients' needs—or was it his needs and his patients' wants? He chose a building near the hospital. He made it bright and warm for his pa-

tients. At first he put his diplomas and certificates on the wall—for his patients. As time went by, he replaced them with pictures of little league teams, his wife and children, sunsets from vacations they took together—for himself. He asked his staff to dress professionally in whites in keeping with his idea of professionalism, then began to dress more comfortably and the staff followed suit, because he thought the patients, many of them farmers, were more at ease with informality. All the reasons he did things became a perplexing mix of what he liked, what he thought his patients and the community liked, and, eventually, after the years, it was just the way he did business. For a time, he was always reading articles in journals about how to run your business better—that was 15 years ago when it was a business, a small business, but a business nevertheless. The articles suggested regular office meetings and business sessions with staff, but he mostly had coffee with them at the start of the day and in 10-minute snatches of time during the day. He had lots of hallway meetings in which he would ask the nurse something about a patient, talk with the front office about a patient's bill or the need to write it off, or lean over the busy receptionist, ignoring her perturbed face as he interrupted her, and leaf through the appointment book looking for a name he had forgotten.

Although he likes the ritual of the office, he realizes that it takes energy for all of them to control the environment around them. He likes now and then to create some unpredictability in the system. When they were younger, his children would sometimes drop over and visit the office after school, sitting next to the laboratory technician and watching the blood tubes go back and forth in the automatic stirrer, or putting bills into envelopes as they sat next to the office manager. He would bring flowers from his garden throughout the summer, carve pumpkins and light them in the waiting room, or sneak out the back door across the street to the coffee shop—later to become a Big Boy—to have a piece of cherry pie with butter pecan ice cream midway through the afternoon when there was a break in patients. He believes that stirring other things into medicine will nudge him to think differently now and then, and the flowers, the pictures, the children's visits, and the cherry pie are all things that remind him of what is important beyond the science of medicine.

He still has an office with a big desk and a couple of comfortable chairs for patients to sit in and talk. He had spent some time during medical school in New England, where doctors still had what they called "consulting rooms," in which they would take the patient's history, and another room, much smaller, on either side for examining patients. His community preceptor said that difficult issues like a pregnancy, a serious illness, or some family crisis were better discussed in the consulting room where everyone was more at ease. So he built in a large office that he used as a consulting room and often talks with families there.

He likes his staff, most of whom had worked with him for many years, and trusts them implicitly. In a small town, patient confidentiality is one of the most important issues, and he would reiterate to his staff that they had to respect confidentiality at all times. Patient trust was essential for their practice to thrive and for them to keep the respect of the community that was such a cornerstone of their success in caring for people. The old World War I warning, "Loose lips sink ships," was one he would remind his staff applied to them, and that it would not be ships, but their practice, that would sink.

The receptionist and the nurses are crucial components of continuity, full of stories that have added to his working knowledge of his community. Their opinions are important, and they make sure that patients are followed up, immunizations updated on everyone, and passed important advice on to patients about what they need to do to stay well. He hired a physician assistant (PA) 5 years ago, and she has added to the thoroughness of his practice by keeping track of the diabetic patients using flow sheets they developed together. She also serves as a preceptor for PA students from the university who spend time in the practice as part of their community training. "Everyone speaks of our practice," and he likes that. He feels more often like the conductor of the orchestra of his office rather than the soloist. They all play music together.

PATIENTS

Tickling Babies

He struggled with whether he could or should deliver babies. For a long time during his training, he was ambivalent, but one night during the second year of his residency he was sitting with a woman during a protracted labor and wondering if he could keep this up when his attending physician came in to help. They sat and watched the fetal heart monitors, checked on the progress of labor, and he found himself sharing his concerns with the attending physician. She had recalled the same feeling about delivering babies years before and told him that she felt that he was a good doctor and gave a great deal of comfort to his patients during this difficult and exciting time in their lives, and she encouraged him to persevere. As the night wore on, they looked up questions about management of the labor together, had many cups of coffee, and, in the end, delivered a very big baby who came into the world reluctantly but, once arrived, made them all smile with relief. Everyone congratulated each other, took pictures with the newborn, had a slice of birthday cake and champagne that had been sitting patiently in the refrigerator, and played the tape of Brazilian birthday music that the parents had wanted their baby to hear as his first experience with song. They gave him the tape and a picture of him with Chico all covered with vernix and red as a beet. The picture still is pinned to the top of the bulletin board of family practice babies in his office. From that time on, he knew that delivering babies would be an important part of doctoring for him.

He always looks forward to well child examinations on his schedule. He has learned to examine children on their parents' laps and has moved over the years to holding children on his lap while he prods their abdomens and listens to their hearts. Some days he tells his wife that he has tickled a lot of babies, and she wonders out loud sometimes if that isn't really why he became a family doctor. He sometimes has to resist the urge to make babies laugh by blowing on their stomachs and making loud noises with his lips. He loved to do that with his own children but realizes that such was a parental noise opportunity, not a doctor's role. But he rubs their heads, pats their fannies, and engages, he realizes, in the high-pitched nonsense noises that babies universally elicit from adults. These moments are like sunshine breaking through the clouds.

He also realizes that he likes to talk with parents, seeing them as a never-ending source of strange and amusing questions about things he has never worried about. He has often thought that a wise, experienced grandparent would probably do as much good with the worried young parents as he does. Parents worry that their child is too thin, too fat, too active, too sleepy. He never remembered learning about "normal" in medical school and not much in residency. But he has learned about "normal" in children by watching his own and those in his practice for over 20 years, so that now he trusts his sense of "abnormal" even though he often can't put his finger on just what it is that is not normal. What he also likes about talking with parents as a family doctor is that he can ask, "So, how are you?" to the mother and see by the tired look in her eyes that she is feeling overburdened and upset. He can then ask her how her husband is, because he knows him, too, and about her work, her parents, and so on. He knows how they were before the baby came and wonders to himself how this little fidgeting person on her lap will turn out. All his patients are like wonderfully interesting novels that have plot twists and nuances that are a source of constant wonder.

Hormones

"Teenagers are tough," a colleague once remarked. "Being one or taking care of one?" he asked with a laugh. "Both," he answered himself.

Teenagers surprise him all the time. They can be the most self-absorbed of humans and then turn around and take your breath away with their passion about righting wrongs. When he went into practice, he felt most uncomfortable with teenagers because he never seemed to connect with them. Teenagers he knew during his residency were strangers. Most came to the clinic irregularly and primarily for injuries; some came for counseling and prescriptions related to family planning or sexually transmitted diseases.

After he had been in practice for many years, he started to see teenagers he had known as children. He remembered one in particular he had counseled about the risk-taking behaviors that threatened to harm so many of them. He felt that he had gotten the boy to confide in him but wondered if the usual banter that he would engage in with young people would actually alter the boy's behavior. Some years later, the boy came in by himself—by that time he was 16 years old—to show him a "rash" that bothered him. The rash turned out to be a hickey, and when he asked the boy about sexual activity, the boy's face lit up in a smile, and he said, "You told me that using a condom was the right thing to do, so I did it." So this young person in front of him actually had listened. That one experience kept him going with advice and understanding for all the teenagers he would see.

Establishing a relationship with teenagers as people independent from their parents is always touchy. He has developed a "rap" to go over with parents when they come in with a son or daughter that emphasizes the young person's right to have what he or she talks about be confidential, as is true for the parents themselves. Most of the time it works. Parents are mostly relieved that teenagers will be able to talk on their own about problems and issues. He always felt that parents turning to their son or daughter and asking if they preferred the parent to stay or leave was a good sign. Teenagers have a right to privacy; indeed they often obsess about it. But the symbolism of a parent leaving the room to wait while a son or daughter continues with the doctor has always touched him. Such a concrete symbol of children leaving the nest, on their own into the world. One older patient once said, "You never stop worrying about them; it's just what you worry about that changes." He remembers one mother who started to cry when he was examining her 4-year-old child. When he asked what was wrong, she looked at him with a smile through her tears and said, "I was just thinking how much I love her and imagining the day she goes off to college, and I realized how much I would miss her. I wish she would never grow up."

Menopause, the female climacteric, the change of life—and many more euphemisms for a biologic phenomenon—is an important event for women and enters into a lot of discussions he has with patients. Some women cry about it as a loss of something, the end of something. Others are anxious to have it over with and get on with the next stage of life. Some women have it brought on operatively. The whole issue of using hormones for perimenopausal women has turned around twice in his clinical lifetime. Early in his practice, studies were published showing an association between hormones and endometrial cancer, and the whole practice of hormonal treatment of menopausal women came to a screeching halt. Then, some years later, studies began to show a protective effect of hormone replacement therapy for women who were at risk for osteoporosis. This meant that, in effect, women in their late 40s and early 50s would be taking medication to decrease their risk of getting something that might happen in their 70s and 80s, and physicians began prescribing hormones again. So for a period of his life, hormones were good, then they were bad, then they were good again. Seeing such reversals happen time and again in therapeutic areas tended to create a sense of disbelief, which he tries to avoid. Often, he has to read the literature and talk with colleagues so that he can interpret "new" findings to his patients for himself.

Pharmaceutical salespersons are always handing him literature about "Dr. so-and-so, from the so-and-so medical school" and how he or she proved conclusively that this is a good drug, better drug, fewer-side-effects drug, and one that will help his patients—all at a cost that is exorbitant. So few real breakthroughs have happened in his lifetime that he has learned to wait a few years for the bugs to be worked out in a "new" drug, sort of like buying a 2-year-old car rather than a new one because the manufacturers are always finding out that new models have "bugs," like the gas tank blowing up, and have to be recalled. He has seen so many promised "whole new treatments" fizzle a few miles up from the launching pad that he became increasingly patient—or skeptical—as time went on.

So as he begins to talk with Betty about starting on hormone replacement therapy, he feels a bit of the old skepticism but ignores it and moves ahead. She is a divorced mother of five children who has had her share of life's burdens but still has a sense of humor. When he asks her to remind him about why she had a hysterectomy years before, she says, "I just left it at the hospital after my last baby." She seems a bit sad; so he asks if she is. She says that she is used to being able to function on her own—indeed has taken pride in it—but now she is needing more things. When he asks her what she means, she says that loneliness is getting to her. With her children growing and moving away, the emotional space they occupied is empty, and she realizes that neither work nor the small social life that she had carved out beyond her family is adequate to make her feel fulfilled. "Will hormones help that feeling?" All of this conversation occurs while he does his usual well woman examination, reenforcing the need for breast self-examination regularly and showing her again how to do it. "So, if you were to find a lump on examination, what would you do next?" he asks. "Cry," she says, "and then call you."

Holding Hands

He prefers to call older patients by their last names—that was a rule he set up for his office—but Mr. Gutbend insists on being called Walter—by him, by his staff, by everyone in town. During medical school, he saw staff calling elderly men and women, many of them poor, by their first names, not, as the staff claimed, out of affection but out of condescension. During his internship, someone asked him about a patient and how he would do things if the patient were his grandmother.

He replies, "First of all, I would not be calling my grandmother 'Dorothy,' because no one except the woman herself ever referred to her as that." Still, Mr. Gutbend always wants to be Walter—"Valter" is how he says it—and so he is. "Been Valter all my life, I have."

Although doctors use laboratory tests and physical examinations to follow the progress of an illness, with Walter the most reliable indicator is donuts. If he feels good, he will bring a dozen donuts for everyone at the office, and if he doesn't, he comes empty handed. "Too tired to stop and get something" he would say, and the staff would do what they could to get him feeling better, in part because the donuts he brings are the filled kind that they all like. He has diabetes and drinks a lot. He is a widower who stubbornly lives alone and whose daughters worry all the time about him falling and breaking his hip—the doctor has begun to call adults in their 50s the "worry-about-your-parents generation," which was the decade after their 40s, when they were the "worry-about-your-teenagers generation." So Walter takes his oral medication for diabetes intermittently, drinks because he misses his wife of 48 years, and has little to look forward to except decline and more visits to the office. The staff often worries whether he is suicidal, and the doctor himself often worries too. But Walter only wants to be listened to, cajoled about not taking his medication, and teased about his garden by the nurse and the receptionist. Thoughts of suicide are less this week, everyone knows, because the flowers are up with the warm spring weather, and it was a two-dozen donut visit.

He thinks of Helene Andrews on days like this. She used to make him laugh in the same way that Walter did. An exotic, long-boned woman, age 75 and more than 6 feet tall, she dressed in wonderful colors and wore lots of bracelets that made noise as she walked down the hallway of the office swinging her arms. He would be coming out of an examining room in his white coat—those were the early, more formal, days—and see Helene coming, and she would throw her arms out like a sandhill crane landing and say, "Doctor, honey" and give him a big hug. At first he didn't know what to do, but after years of hugs he began to expect them, just as she did of him.

She had mysterious tales to tell about her husband who died years before and left her with a fortune. He asked what her husband did, and her face got flat and she said he was a businessman and didn't elaborate.

She got more frail over the 10 years he took care of her, and eventually she felt she had to move to a warmer place, because she hated the winters. Moving to a new place was not easy for anyone, much less a single woman in her 70s with no children. But she was insistent, and he located a family practice residency program in the southern city where she was moving. He felt like he was passing along a family heirloom—something, someone, who was very special—and he wanted a resident to have the chance to take care of this grand, dramatic, whimsical woman who had taught him so much about himself. Before she left she invited him to come to tea at her house, and she gave him five of the beautiful Chinese porcelain plates that she had gotten from her grandmother. "They probably came over with Marco Polo," she said. Then he got up to leave and, for the last time, she threw her arms out, her bright red dress hanging like wings, and said "I'll miss you so much, Doctor, honey." He couldn't say anything just then because, in his Midwestern family, crying was something that you did by yourself and not in public. Later, he copied his records and sent them off to the doctor he had arranged for her to see. He never heard from Helene or her doctor again. He didn't even know if she got to where she was going but, as the Zen saying goes, "It is not the destination that is important, but the journey."

He probably likes older people because all of his grandparents died before he was old enough to know them. He takes great pleasure in hearing his patients talk about their children and grandchildren. He views older people as having things to tell him that might help him along, help him to become wise. He remembered the recommendation of one of his teachers that older people like to be touched. One of the images they have of themselves is that they are not touchable, not attractive. So every time he goes in to see older patients, he takes their hands and pretends to take their pulses, as his teacher had recommended. He carries a toenail clipper with him and, often, when examining his older patients' feet, will clip their toenails. His teacher also said that clipping toenails was increasingly difficult with age, and that clipping an old person's nails was a way of showing that you understood how difficult the little things in their lives were becoming. He also thinks about how

washing others' feet has been a sign of respect and humility in many cultures for thousands of years. Even Christ washed his Apostles' feet.

HOME

The end of the day comes faster than he thought it should; callbacks to patients, checking out with the person from his call group about who is in the hospital and what they may need during the night, and finally the endless dictation from the day.

Sitting with a Dictaphone often makes him reflect not only on the right way to describe what he heard and did with patients that day, but also on the remarkable stories he hears daily. His patients draw him into their lives, carrying along centuries of expectations about the healer. He thinks of himself as an empty vessel into which his patients pour their frequently rambling narratives of what has happened to them—their fears, frustrations, hopes, desires, sadnesses, and dreams. People always want to be forgiven, even if they had no part in what was wrong with them. "I got a cold because I was overtired." "My blood pressure went up because I sneaked some chips watching the game." "I haven't been able to lose weight because I just don't have the will power."

One of the teachers early in his residency once talked to him about being "present with someone." He had spent 20 minutes with a woman who'd had a miscarriage and came in for follow-up, and when he asked how she was, she started crying and was speechless with grief for almost the whole visit. He had felt helpless in the face of her sadness and went out to talk with his preceptor about what to do. The preceptor said that he was doing a lot just by being present, by listening. So he had worked on using body language and touch to let patients know that he was there, but didn't have to say anything. The famous Sir Luke Fildes' picture of the doctor sitting by the side of the bed with the gravely ill child surrounded by the stricken parents is a powerful image of how being with someone can be a central role of the physician. Over the years, he has gotten more and more comfortable with silence and what it really speaks to people.

He has heard today—every day—the things that his patients tell no one else in their lives—not family members, friends, or even spouses—and in that regard he is as much a confessor as a doctor. He realizes that patients often are more picky about whom they choose as their doctor as whom they choose as their confessor. He once told his wife that doctors die with thousands of secrets, big and small.

As he puts a few things in his briefcase to take home, he glances at the schedule for the next day. He is usually the last one out, but tonight is his younger daughter's softball game. She is a wonderful athlete, graceful and strong, and he loves to see her play. Each of their three children is talented in different ways, and the youngest is the athlete. He does the free physicals on the high school sports teams and goes to as many games as he can, sitting on the sidelines as the team doctor. He has spent extra time learning more about common sports injuries and how to handle them acutely. More often, however, his role as team doctor means counseling students with problems and giving advice rather than stabilizing injured knees.

He has always tried to eat dinner with the family and makes it most days that he isn't on call. His father had made a point of having dinner at home with everyone seated. Each person had to tell something that was interesting or difficult about their day, and he has kept that tradition going. He read recently that only about 15% of families have dinner together regularly. He, however, regards dinner as one of the few things he can count on, and "unexcused absences" are frowned upon. His children have kidded him about it, but he knows that they take it as seriously as he and his wife do, because when they bring friends home, they always want to have dinner together with their friends at the table. Easy conversations, old stories, genuine affection always seems easier over mashed potatoes and gravy.

Now it is getting late; his daughter is off to her room to study and, gratefully, to do it with headphones on. His family has gotten into an easy rhythm, he realizes, and what some would call habit he calls "tradition." He and his wife go for a walk before bed now that the springtime seems serious, and they don't have to wrap up in parkas. The idea of walking came when he was talking with a patient about family communication, or the lack of it, and his patient said that he started walking with his wife because they both needed the exercise, and it meant 45 scheduled minutes together when they knew that they would be able to talk. The doctor thought it was a good idea and suggested it to his wife. After their walk, he sits for a while and leafs through magazines and the newspaper, catching up on the news and weather.

So many years in this town, he muses. What has happened to it—what has happened to me? I came

as a young man to do what I wanted to do, and I have been doing it. Hard times, sure, but few regrets. He remembers telling a medical student once that he is not a smarter doctor now than he was 20 years ago, but is a better doctor. The issues that upset him years before, such as patients he couldn't cure, now are simply the reality of taking care of a community. He accepts his failures as sometimes just the way things are. He also learned to trust his own feelings about people—to see when they were ill even before he understood what made them ill—to ask direct questions that he would have hesitated to ask years before. He feels better about his craft, not complacent, just better.

On his way to bed, he passes his study and sees the hand-lettered and framed copy of "Complaint" by William Carlos Williams, the great American physician poet, that first hung on the wall of his office and now hangs above his desk at home (1). The words remind him of how he was then and whom he has to try, every day, to continue to be.

> *They call me and I go.*
> *It is a frozen road*
> *past midnight, a dust*
> *of snow caught*
> *in the rigid wheel tracks.*
> *The door opens.*
> *I smile, enter and*
> *shake off the cold.*
> *Here is a great woman*
> *on her side on the bed.*
> *She is sick*
> *perhaps vomiting,*
> *perhaps laboring*
> *to give birth to*
> *a tenth child. Joy! Joy!*
> *Night is a room*
> *darkened for lovers,*
> *through the jalousies the sun*
> *has sent one gold needle!*
> *I pick the hair from her eyes*
> *and watch her misery*
> *with compassion.*
>
> *William Carlos Williams[1]*

[1]Reprinted with permission from Williams WC. Collected Poems:1909–1939, Vol. 1. New York: New Directions Publishing Corp, 1968.

2. From Cradle to Rocker: Providing Care Across the Human Life Cycle

B. LEWIS BARNETT, JR.

A dedicated family doctor's life, indeed every day of it, is filled with "once in a lifetime" opportunities: occasions to touch patients with one's unique hands and heart. Maybe never again—but today, this time, now—is the time to do something very special for this person. This is because the commonplace experience of the physician often deals with life-shaping issues for the patient. Conception, birth, the first steps, growth and development, starting school, puberty, developing gender identity, dating, marriage, giving birth, parenting, striving to succeed, changes such as climacteric and menopause, accepting the ticking of the clock, coping with acute and chronic illness, loss of dear ones—these are the fabric of family medicine, and the elements that bond family physicians and their patients. Over a lifetime of practice, your experiences with patients will extend across many phases of the life cycle, and your own life will become interwoven with that of your patients, and each will help and learn from the other. In this chapter I will try to provide some guidance, based on almost half a century of practicing family medicine, in approaching patients across the various twists and turns of the cycle of life, from cradle to rocker and beyond.

As we learn from our patients, let me begin with a story. It is about a woman I will call Frieda Mae.

CASE STUDY

On September 26, 1958, I delivered premature twins. The larger one, weighing 2 lb, 15 oz, promptly expired. The second one, weighing only 567 g, refused to die. At birth, Frieda Mae was so small I could hold her lengthwise in my palm and encompass her entire body, a tiny moving collection of bone, organs, and skin, much like a small, wet rat. She remains one of smallest babies to survive; and her birth occurred in the days before neonatal intensive care units and highly trained neonatologists. I remember we discharged her on Christmas Eve; the nurses wrapped her snugly and tied a huge red bow around the little girl—the dearest Christmas gift these parents ever had.

Thirty-six years later, my telephone rang during supper. The unfamiliar voice was loud and clear. "Dr. Barnett, this is Frieda Mae Tucker Jackson. You may not remember me."

"Oh yes, I do!" I interrupted. "You weighed 1 pound, 4 ounces when you were born."

She continued, "I have been trying to find you. I have a 14-year-old son and an 8-year-old daughter." With this, my memory of having held her in my right hand, her arms not hanging over the sides of my palm, almost blocked out her conversation. How tiny her uterus and ovaries must have been! We fed her vegetable formula with an eye dropper rather than animal formula, which would have been harder for her little kidneys to process. Because there was no way to gain access to a vein, we gave her half-strength dextrose in water and laced it with hyaluronidase to make it absorb better, administering it subcutaneously by hypodermoclysis. With a bubble injected over each scapular area and each thigh, she looked like a tike with water wings. As soon as one set of injections had been absorbed, we would give her another aliquot. We had her in an incubator with 1 liter of oxygen. We used 3×3 gauze pads for diapers, not minding when the gauze leaked, because I wanted to know if her kidneys were functioning. So these memories all came back in a rush!

Her main reason for calling was to tell me that she had just had an operation on her eyes. She had cataracts, which are a delayed complication of prematurity. "Now I can see!" she exclaimed. As she was growing, I had feared that her near-blindness was due to retrolental fibroplasia, which can happen if one gives too much oxygen to newborn infants. When caring for Frieda Mae, I had been aware of the possibility and had taken care never to give her more than a liter of oxygen. Still, as I monitored her vision during childhood, I had feared the worst.

"I knew you would want to know," she stated joyfully. She was right; I did want to know!

"Please send me a picture," she said. "I want to see how you look." So I sent her the only recent one I had, knowing full well that it would probably not come up to her memory.

CASE DISCUSSION

This story covers 36 years. What it says is that sometimes it takes patience to see how decisions that we make play out in life. The lilt in Frieda's voice was payment enough for the long wait. Now she has made the doctor feel better. It represents one of the many ways in which the family physician's life seems to balance itself out. Yes, indeed, Frieda, I am happy to know. I will remember always your words, "Now I can see!"

THE SEASONS OF LIFE

Someone once said that the science of medicine has to do with the ways in which all people are alike, and the art of medicine has to do with the ways in which all people are different. When we talk about our patient's individual stories, we are speaking more of the art. Yet there is science here, too, data-based information on normality, basic guidelines, and approaches to care across the human life cycle. The good physician, when conversing with patients, will draw upon learning and experience to provide an informed and humane response, an enlightened interest in the person, and a willingness to try to understand the events and circumstances of that individual.

To help you get an overview of the spectrum of family medicine and to understand the scope of the family physician's work, I like to say that each person goes through stages of development. These stages contain tasks and experiences that are shared by most or all individuals who pass through that stage of life. To simplify, I think in metaphors. The four seasons of life: spring, summer, fall, and winter.

In springtime, growth is fast and furious; nearly every day brings change. Each event, including every doctor visit, is memorable. The doctor shares with parents both expectation and anxiety, which give way to answers as growth unfolds, and school days come. With adolescence, a burst of hormones ushers in the development of womanhood or manhood. Choices, choices; where do we go from here? Almost always with nurturing from parents and teachers, but unfortunately not for some, then we march through the teenage years, some days feeling like a child and some days feeling like an adult, but most days somewhere in between. Good role models are important; sometimes the family doctor is put in this place.

Summer is a time when the gardens of life are growing and beginning to produce. Yet it is a time of thunderstorms, droughts, and plagues, stresses and challenges: acceptance of responsibility, love and heartbreak, demanding function at a level to sustain bread on the table or to provide dependable care for others. Thus, summer brings about fatigue, but also repose, independence, and accomplishment. Some clouds and rain may make us feel inadequate, but the great hope during the summer of life is to learn the secret of coping. Sometimes, the family doctor is important here, too.

Autumn bespeaks maturity. The graying temples, the furrowed brow of one who has known responsibility and succeeded, or has been overwhelmed by it. This season represents the harvested fruits—career success, maturing children, material well-being, realized ambitions, but also broken dreams and new worries. Here there needs to be sensible preparation for winter: lifestyle changes, savings, assurances. One of the most enjoyable parts of life is here, the welcoming of grandchildren. Also, there is more time for understanding and a new dimension of loving others a little more than one's self. At the same time, physical illnesses are more apt to bring one to the doctor more frequently, and quality of life grows vastly more important. There is often little time for the doctor, an impatience at having to take time to see one. Doctors sometimes resent this attitude, but we must try to meet the patients where they are and accept how they are.

When most of us think of winter we think of the cold it brings. However, this time of life need not be bleak. There can be a roaring fire in the hearth and the smell of roasted chestnuts, not to mention a little eggnog for the holidays when the family comes. Strength comes from having family and friends, the camaraderie of others helping us know that we are not alone. But there also can be quietness and silence, reminiscence of youthful thrills on a bobsled, reflective moments that reach deeper into one's spirit. With all these positive things comes the courage to face life as it is and to cope with lessening physical vigor and increasing frailty. Here the family doctor can be helpful as well, to help add crispness to the air so that even its coldness will fill our lungs and lives with a peculiar sort of freshness and peace.

Now we want to take this general philosophy into the daily practice of family medicine. After all, the personhood of your patients will be your stock-in-trade. Meet your patients on their terms, make an effort to understand what they expect, and communicate that you are there for them. And as you do that, you will be a privileged part of this unfolding tapestry of life.

ABOUT CHILDREN

There is a lot of scientific knowledge about normal growth and development during childhood, about the common challenges and problems that arise. Knowing as much as you can about developmental issues in childhood is important. More than half of pediatric visits are for "well child" examinations, and all visits offer opportunities to favorably influence a child's development. Tables 2.1 and 2.2 summarize some of the important points. In Chapter 9, Well Child and Adolescent Care, a description of the well child examination is a valuable complement to this developmental information. Both provide a quick reference about some of the issues you should consider when seeing a child.

Interviewing and Examining Children

Let us approach the first stages of life through the eyes of a child. Imagine that the child awakens with a fever and the worried parent decides to go to the doctor. Can you feel the fear, the tears, the anxiety? Now you make the trip. Soon you arrive at the doctor's office. The child climbs out of the car, legs wobbly and head dizzy. He is picked up in his parent's arms and carried up the big steps to the office (it might be better not to have steps). On arriving in the waiting room the child has to be helped into one of the large chairs (it might be better to have some little ones). Soon a nurse looms over the child and calls his name (mispronouncing it). Down the hall she cannot resist patting the child on the head (a demeaning gesture to some children). Then into the examining room you go, and the child is helped onto the examining table, and waits and waits and waits (children do this very poorly). In comes the doctor, behind schedule and in a hurry. Haste makes for more discomfort; the instruments are cold and obviously not toys. The child feels pain, maybe from an ear that hurts. The tongue blade is a foreign body and the child gags. So many subtle happenings that are unpleasant take place. If we are looking through the eyes of a child, this visit is quite different from the way the doctor plays it out.

Now let's replay the scenario from the physician's point of view. The doctor has been up most of the night seeing other sick patients. Some of them were justifiably in need, others just scared. Nevertheless, she is sleep deprived, and this makes the child's crying and refusal to cooperate especially difficult to accept.

How can the physician cope with such situations? How can we consistently take that extra effort to be calm and loving?

A long list of my own habits come to mind, and I am sure that you have a growing list of your own. Here are the highlights of my own suggestions:

- Always remember that the child is the star of the show. Not the doctor; not the mother; not the father. Maybe the parent is the supporting cast, but not the star. The child usually has something to say; so listen. You may listen to the mother, of course, for the vital parts of the history, but don't listen only to the mother. The child's story may be different. If you talk to children while concentrating in their direction, you'll be more effective. Don't ask the mother, "Did Johnny do this or that?," if you can possibly, ask the child, "Does your throat hurt?" "Does your ear hurt?"

- Make eye contact. It's never good to look down to any patient, especially a child.

Table 2.1.
Selected Milestones of Growth and Development During the Prenatal Period and the First Year of Life

Prenatal Period		
Age from Last Menstrual Period	Milestones	Medical Care Implications
3–4 wk	Implantation occurs	Mild vaginal bleeding can accompany implantation
3–5 wk	Levels of human chorionic gonadotropin begin to rise	Pregnancy tests become positive; symptoms such as nausea and tiredness are noted
4–12 wk	Major organs form	Drug and toxin effects on fetus are greatest
15–20 wk	The fetus grows from about 4.5 inches to 9 inches in length and from about 2.5 oz to 8 oz	First detection of fetal movement by the mother (about 15 wks in multigravidas and 18 wks in primigravidas) is used to date pregnancy
22 wk	Due to circulatory changes of pregnancy, maternal blood pressure reaches its lowest point	Failure of blood pressure to go down in midpregnancy suggests later development of preeclampsia
28 wk	The fetus is about 14 in long and weighs 2-2.5 lb	Fathers can usually feel movement by placing a hand on the mother's abdomen; most fetuses born beyond 28 wks will survive with intensive care
28–40 wk	Rapid growth of fetus and uterus	Increasing maternal discomfort and fatigue; strong desire to prepare home for new baby ("nesting")

First Year of Life		
Age Since Birth	Milestones	Medical Care Implications
0–7 days	Maternal-infant bonding takes place	Hospital and home environment can affect bonding
2–4 wk	Can follow movement with eyes through 10–20°	Early vision screening can take place
2–3 mo	Smiles in response to social stimulation	Parent-infant interaction can be observed
4 mo	Turns head toward sounds	Physician can screen for hearing problems
5–8 mo	Sits unsupported	Sitting represents one common measure of gross motor development
12 mo	Can recognize own name; says a few words (e.g., "mama")	Development of language skills suggests effective hearing, socialization, and brain development
9–14 mo	Learns to walk on own	A period of fussiness often precedes walking; walking itself increases risk of accidental injury or ingestions

Adapted from Sloane PD, Benedict S, Mintzer M. The Complete Pregnancy Workbook. Chapel Hill, NC: Algonquin Books, 1986.

- Try to establish some kind of a common bond between the child and yourself. I can remember noticing such simple things as a new pair of red shoes. "Gee, I like those red shoes." And she liked those red shoes! They were new, and she was proud of them. This common bond can be anything you notice at any given time.

- Have simple little things around to indicate you care about children. In my office, I had a lot of things for children, among which were two clowns I had ordered out of the Sunday supplement of a newspaper for $1. They sat low on a shelf, so that children could reach and handle them. One was called the Bumble Bee clown; the other was called the Fruit Salad clown. These clowns are an example of the fact that simple things, not big productions, are vital. They indicate to children that you want them to be happy.

- Look for nonverbal signals. Try to observe the child, even when you are talking to the mother. Does the child swallow like an ostrich? If so, you can conclude that his throat is probably sore. Did he walk down the hall

Table 2.2.

Parental and Physician Roles in Development, Ages 1–17

Age (Yr)	Developmental Challenges	Parental Role	Family Doctor's Role

1–4	Feeling of security
	Formation of
	  normal attachments
		Be sensitive to cues
		Be available
		Provide a secure
		  environment
		Set appropriate limits
			Observe parenting for poor limits or
			  overprotection
			Inquire sensitively if you suspect
			  problems
			In making recommendations, focus
			  on the family as a single unit
			Give gentle guidance over multiple
			  visits

2–3	Toilet training/
	  autonomy
		Minimize battles
		Learn acceptance
		Learn firmness
		Avoid showdowns
			Help parents to appreciate progress
			  and accept setbacks
			Facilitate parental learning to work
			  through child's autonomy issues
			  as a model for future conflict
			  resolution

	Play and fantasy	Demonstrate respect and
		  interest for the child's
		  inner world
			Encourage and support

	Tantrums	Maintain composure
		  under fire
			Reinforce that this is normal
			  development
			Encourage parents to seek help or
			  respite if needed
			High frequency may merit
			  investigation

2–5	Sexual concerns	Accept curiosity
		Avoid overreacting
			Anticipatory guidance is key when
			  parents may be uncomfortable
			  asking questions

6–12	Separation
	Peer relationships
	Development of
	  conscience
		Allow independence
		Reward achievement and
		  encourage the child's
		  natural industry
		Model adult behavior
			Reinforce the variations of normal
			  development
			Use your long-term relationship to
			  facilitate conflict resolution when
			  appropriate
			Model for parents by addressing
			  children as independent, intelligent
			  people even at a very young age

13–19	Physical changes
	Sexual
	  development
	Identity
	Self-image
	Experimentation
		Maintain own self-esteem
		Nurture and maintain
		  relationship
		Avoid reflecting child's
		  growing pain back to them
		  as frustration
		Deal with waning parental
		  influence gracefully
		Respect the emerging adult
		  but continue to set
		  appropriate limits
		Always listen and try to
		  understand
			Provide information
			Anticipate difficult issues, unasked
			  questions
			Do not condescend; model directness,
			  honesty, and patience
			Help frame specific problems in a
			  family model (it's never one person's
			  problem)
			Distinguish sometimes frightening
			  normal development from truly
			  aberrant behavior
			Remind parents of their still
			  considerable (if unappreciated)
			  influence; adolescents still need
			  parenting
			Encourage limit-setting based on
			  honest, clear expectations
			Always listen and try to understand

Adapted from Waters D, Barnett BL. In: Taylor RB, ed. Family Medicine, Principles and Practice. New York: Springer-Verlag, 1988:19–27.

normally or did he hardly straighten up? This could help you diagnose appendicitis.

- When examining children, do the least intrusive things first. If a child is nervous, sit at the other side of the room, observing as you converse; then gradually approach closer. Listen to the chest and heart before you look at the ears. Learn to examine children while they sit on a parent's lap.

- Modify your behavior so that you communicate comfort and peace. Fast, abrupt, or loud talking often frightens children; if you have a gruff or booming voice, tone it down. I'm not sure that the traditional white coat helps the doctor-child relationship; in my own practice, I finally threw them away.

- Don't rush your visit, even if you are feeling rushed. If you are behind and have to make up time, make it up with somebody else, not a child. Children do not understand assembly lines; they do not understand being shoved around or hurried.

- Explain what you are going to do and what you want from him or her. Alert the child to tell you if you are causing discomfort. Tell the child that you want to know how he or she feels. You don't necessarily want to be screamed at, though; so explain that you have two ears and that the volume does not need to be turned up. Remind the child that you don't really have to hurt, in most cases, but then be honest and say when you might be causing discomfort, and that it is necessary. The doctor, of all people, should be honest and truthful.

- Write down your instructions so that the mother can read them in the peace and quiet of home. It takes no longer to do that than to yell over the confusion.

- If you are worried about a child you have seen recently, never hesitate to make a telephone call to the child (or, in the case of young children, to the mother). Say, "I just wanted to know." You'll sleep better, and it'll be a powerful public relations builder. Sometimes the mother won't want to let you talk to the child, but you should insist. It'll make a lot of difference in your future contacts with the child.

Working with Adolescents

All of us have been there—that time when we did not want to be a child, but were not yet an adult.

We were too big to go to the "baby doctor," yet not ready for the internist. Most of all we didn't really think we needed any doctor. But problems do come and, to the adolescent, no one seems to understand. They often do not know how to talk with their parents or the minister, if they even have one. Sometimes they think about talking to the team doctor, but don't. At any rate, this group of young people often need a confidante, a friend, and adult who will listen and understand. Sometimes the family doctor is there at this time of need.

Life is not in synchrony during adolescence. Everything about adolescents is changing, as is everything around them. They are tempted with all kinds of self-destructive behaviors and peer pressures. This temptation is heightened by a feeling of immortality and invincibility, so that bad things are not supposed to happen to them. Yet sometimes, unexpected things do happen: leukemia, accidents, addictions, depressions, pregnancies, or acquired immunodeficiency syndrome. Adolescents often have a poor self-image. Some, looking in the mirror, do not perceive themselves as others do, and so anorexia or bulimia follows. They perceive life as difficult when most of the time everything is normal.

The most common reasons teenagers visit family physicians are for acute illnesses and physicals for camp or school. Because they visit rarely, any visit should be viewed as an opportunity to make contact about a wide range of health problems and to identify unmet health needs. A visit for acne, for example, can lead to a discussion about self-image, depression, school, peer relationships, dating, sexuality, and the prevention of sexually transmitted diseases. Table 2.2 provides an overview of some of the key issues in adolescent health care; others are provided in Chapter 9.

Here are some tips on approaching your adolescent patients:

- Remember the leading causes of death and disability for adolescents: automobile accidents, depression and suicide, substance abuse, eating disorders, violence, pregnancy, and sexually transmitted disease. These should be major topics of your preventive counseling for adolescents.

- Get the parent(s) out of the room. One technique is to make it an office routine for the nurse to put all patients over a certain age in the examining room alone. Another is to always have an "examination" time when you insist on seeing the adolescent alone; then re-take the history.

- Listen. Allow informal time at the beginning of the visit to talk about relatively impersonal topics such as school or hobbies. Encourage the adolescent to explain what he or she wants to accomplish during the visit. Use those interviewing techniques you learned in medical school, such as open-ended questions, reflection, restatement, summarization, and, most importantly, silence. Some adolescents may not speak easily, and with them you may need to be very directive in your interview.

- Be open with both the parents and the adolescent about confidentiality. Tell them that what either shares with you in confidence will be kept in confidence unless you obtain permission to share it with the other. If possible, have this discussion with both parties present, so that there are no misunderstandings.

CASE STUDY

I remember Danny. He was age 13 when this story took place. He went to a sock hop on a Saturday night, but he did not feel like dancing, so he went home to bed. At 2:00 AM, his alcoholic father came home and started arguing with his mother. Danny heard the noise, as he had many times before. The next morning, he awakened and could not remember his name, where he was, or how old he was.

This happened on one of my weekends off, so he was seen by another physician in town who said, "Oh, this is a conversion-type reaction. He's just upset because his dad came in and started an argument with his mother." He gave Danny diazepam, which made bad things worse. Danny's amnesia continued.

When I got back into town, Danny's mother called me and said that he was still acting strangely and the doctor had said it was nerves. I asked to see him. In taking a history—a common, ordinary, good history—I found out that he'd had a rash the week before but had not been sick enough to come to the doctor. At that time, he had

a fever for a couple of days and complained about tenderness (nodes) behind his ears. He defervesced and felt better, so he went to the dance. As the dance progressed, he began to feel bad again—very dizzy. Danny had felt ill before his parents' argument ever took place! The argument was coincidental with Danny's medical diagnosis!

Danny turned out to have the only case of German measles encephalitis I have ever seen. It was so rare in those days that I sent him to the medical center. I had given him steroids to see if I could do something for the cerebral edema. Apparently, they helped; he was already better by the time he got to the medical center. Anyway, the diagnosis held that he had German measles encephalitis, because the viral study results turned out positive. His memory came back to him, and he seemed normal after that.

When Danny grew up, he joined the Air Force, and I never saw him again, but I heard through others that his life did not go well. While in the service, he started to drink alcohol, then got into drugs. His behavior became intolerable and led to a dishonorable discharge. I am told that afterward he got married, then divorced, and that on one occasion he was arrested and jailed. Furthermore, his father resisted treatment for his alcoholism and, one day, committed suicide. Despite the many visits I'd had with Danny in his early life, I could not overcome the influence of his father.

CASE DISCUSSION

This story, which covers many years, makes a statement about several things. First, it points out that taking a good history often uncovers the truth. Second, it illustrates a sobering fact about primary care: that, although common things do occur commonly, rare diseases happen and must be looked for vigilantly (although not obsessively). Third, tangled family histories sometimes haunt us forever, coming back as recurrent themes over many years. Finally, and this was definitely the case with Danny, you always wish you could have done more. Try to learn from each patient experience so that you can better help your patients in the future. I did my best to provide stability and encouragement to Danny as he grew up; yet, I can't help but wonder if I could have done more to help avert the tragedy his life became.

EARLY ADULTHOOD AND MIDDLE AGE

Development does not stop when growth is complete. Adults continue through a variety of relatively predictable life stages and transitions between or within these stages. Table 2.3 summarizes some of the main tasks and transitions of adulthood; knowing, anticipating, and helping your patients deal with these events is an important part of the physician's role. Of course there are many deviations, and indeed as persons get older they become less uniform (a reason why protocols work better for children than for adults, and especially poorly for the very old). However, one of many services the family physician can perform for his or her adult patients is to help them interpret what is happening to them in the context of the life experience of others. Sometimes it is comforting, for example, to know that many others have faced the same problem, and to learn ways they successfully overcome it. The family physician can help with this.

Health maintenance is a common reason for adults to visit their family physician (see Chapter 10 for information about well adult examinations); however, the majority of visits are for acute and chronic problems.

In times of illness, you will find that vigorous, successful adults often revert to being children at heart. They face the unknown with trepidation and in doing so become smaller and less powerful. And the environment—including the physician with an impending verdict—looms large, dark, and ominous. Their world becomes more lonely, more needful of understanding.

To be in pain and afraid, to be embarrassed by sickness, to lose control of one's fate or destiny—these experiences have a great leveling effect. Even the bank president or the strongest of athletes becomes afraid and wonders what the future holds when he or she is monitored in the intensive care unit.

So, be patient with your patients, even those in the "prime" of life, because at all points along the life cycle our patients view health with anxiety.

When patients are in the most demanding and productive years of their lives, they have to contend with stress as never before. They are trying to maintain a home, keep a job, put back some savings, pay tuition, and they have no time for sickness. They do not have time for us.

Some of the most prevalent problems, such as peptic ulcer disease, angina pectoris, hypertension, adult onset diabetes, prostatism, menopausal symptoms, psychoses, cancer, and stroke, all cause the middle-aged patient to become compromised and vulnerable. These events sometimes bring about changes in personality and make interactions more tedious.

Approximately 95% of patients who walk through the door can be handled by a well-trained family doctor. The others require referral to the proper consultants. Sometimes it is good to attempt to match the personalities of the consultant to the patient. Knowing enough to know when you do not know is important. Diagnosis is key to the ultimate treatment and outcome. It is important to order whatever tests or diagnostic procedures are necessary, but if a test or procedure will not change your treatment, then it is unnecessary. The physician must stay in tune with his or her patient and remain an ally through it all.

CASE STUDY

Lewis Burton is a fellow I delivered. His mother was in her 40s and had an extremely difficult labor. He did not breathe when he was born, and it was only after much resuscitation that he came around. His first breath was mine, because mouth-to-mouth resuscitation was the method employed at that time. After many, many years, I still remember his cry being music to my ears, his mother weeping for joy, and my own tears of relief. Later that day, I told his mother that Lewis was obviously here for some special purpose, such was his will to live.

Little did I know what was to follow. When he was 16, Lewis dove into a lake, not knowing that the level of water was

Table 2.3.
Life Stages and Transitions of Adulthood, Age 17 and Up

Age	Life Stage	Transition	Tasks/Goals/Issues
17–22		Early adult transition	Establishment of independence from family or origin; definition of personal goals and values; career choice; initial attempts at partnering
22–29	Early adulthood		Career launches; early parenting or deferral of reproduction; balancing individual/partnership roles; mentorship relationships can be helpful
28–33		Age-30 transition	Reevaluation of initial choices results in either change or recommitment; lack of perceived choice can lead to depression, alcoholism, marital conflict/abuse
30–39	Settling down		Establishing a place in society through career success, child rearing, or community involvement; nurturance and accommodation to partner and children
33–45		Midlife crisis	Major reassessment of life goals and activities; initial adjustment to early signs of aging; career changes and marital crises are common; completion of childbearing
45–60	Middle adulthood		Movement from career establishment to mentoring others; facilitation of children in obtaining independence; reestablishment of marriage as a dyad after children leave home; interest in individual expression and growth is common among women who have been full-time mothers
47–55		Age-50 transition	Reevaluation of lives; may be particularly traumatic in individuals who changed little during their 30s and 40s; menopause triggers physiologic and psychologic responses in women
58–68		Transition to the early 60s	Anticipation of retirement; greater identification with family and culture; acceptance of one's life
65–79	Young old ("golden years")		High levels of life satisfaction; maintaining connections with family; grandparenting; ability to pursue deferred leisure and community interests; concern about maintaining health and independence
70–84		Transition of physical dependency	Chronic illness and disability reduce independence; help needed with activities of daily living; dependency increases reliance on family
75+	Older old ("frail elderly")		Deaths of partner(s), friends, and siblings; acceptance of physical changes; physical discomfort; considerable social contact with and support from health care providers; desire to share life experiences with others, especially younger persons; readiness for death

dangerously low. He sustained a broken neck, and has since been quadriplegic.

Now, to understand the rest of the story, we must know something about Lewis's family at the time he was injured. Lewis's father was a proud and domineer-ing man. Because Lewis's sister had mar-ried a man her father disapproved of, she and her husband had been forbidden to ever come home again. His older brother had majored in foreign languages (and is now a professor at a major university), but the father thought he should have done something "useful;" so he, too, was estranged from the family.

By then I was living in another town, but one Sunday was back visiting and went to church. Across the auditorium I saw a wheelchair and recognized Lewis Burton. After the service was over, I wondered whether to extend my hand to Lewis. You see, I wasn't sure he could respond with his. As I approached, Lewis made a very difficult effort to offer his hand. So I reached out to him, and an emotional touch took place.

I told him what I had said to his mother when he was born—that he was special, that he had a purpose in life. He stopped me short and said, "I know, I know." His mother had told him. In the course of conversation, he said, "One of my therapists asked me, "If you had it all to do over again, knowing what you know now, would you jump again?" I told her, "Yes, I would." I listened closely to pick up his quiet voice as he continued. "Because it brought my sister home; my brother is part of the family again; and it got my daddy to the front of the church when he rolled me up to thank all of the kind people that showed us their love. Yeah, I'd jump again." With a lump in my throat, I walked out into the bright sunshine, eyes glistening with emotion.

Years later, I learned that Lewis Burton had been chosen "Man of the Year" by his state; and he remains a very productive citizen.

CASE DISCUSSION

Successful adjustment to chronic illness and disability is tremendously difficult, especially for previously vigorous young adults. To change one's goals and expectations so drastically, especially when others don't have to do the same, seems unfair.

And it is unfair. However, the patient who has chronic illness has no choice but to play the hand that was dealt, and the family doctor can play a crucial role in helping that adjustment be successfully made.

Lewis got an unexpected psychologic boost from the way his community and family rallied around his disability. Others are not so fortunate and require more professional help. Still, a host of health care professionals assisted Lewis in his adjustment, most noticeably physical therapists and occupational therapists. His physician, as coordinator of the team, played an important role, too. Lewis had, and continues to have, a variety of medical problems that need constant monitoring and attention. He is at risk for recurrent urinary tract infections, because he requires an indwelling catheter. Also, he has to be watched carefully for aspiration pneumonia and requires a special diet. As with many nonambulatory persons, Lewis is prone to constipation and must maintain a regimen of fiber and stool softeners. He cannot take care of his teeth; so dental hygiene must be maintained by caretakers.

Without careful medical attention to these and other details of his physical care, Lewis would not have been able to be the success that he has become.

CARING FOR OLDER ADULTS

A variety of physiologic, psychologic, and developmental issues are unique to older persons. Tables 2.3 and 2.4 summarize some of them; however, you should anticipate learning about aging from your patients over many years, because it takes a long time to begin to be able to differentiate what should be ignored from what should be watched, and what should be watched from what should be evaluated or treated aggressively. As always, knowing the patient, feeling compassion, and taking a good history are the most crucial elements of good care.

Approach to the Older Patient

The most drastic change you will notice as your patients grow older is that they have time for you now. They do not usually expect miracles. They like to hear about quality of life rather than quantity of life. They resent having to take so many pills and are more prone to adverse effects. So one of the physician's roles is to continuously re-

Table 2.4.
Some Normal Body Changes with Aging

Skin	Elasticity decreases, producing wrinkles. Easy bruising occurs, especially in sun- exposed areas. Thinning occurs, especially on extremities, leading to easy tearing with minimal trauma.
Hair	Graying: >50% of Americans have >50% gray hair by age 50. Distribution: thins on scalp, axilla, pubic area, and on upper and lower extremities Decreased facial hair in men, but women may develop chin and upper lip hair
Nails	Decreased growth rate
Body build	Increase in body fat and decrease in body water. Decrease in height caused by intervertebral space narrowing
Bones	Some demineralization occurs in all elderly, but is greater in women and in whites.
Joints	Range of motion decreases somewhat, although exercise is beneficial. Wearing down of joint surfaces is common, especially in hips, knees, and fingers.
Muscles	Loss of muscle mass and strength is common, but exercise may minimize loss.
Eyes	Thickening of lens (cataracts) is almost universal by the 70s, but may not require removal if vision is not impaired for functions important to patient. Lens accommodation decreases (presbyopia) by age 45. The pupil does not admit as much light. Peripheral vision decreases. Tearing decreases, which may cause easy irritation.
Hearing	Age-related hearing loss (presbycusis) affects the inner ear, leading to loss of high-frequency sounds. About 50% of elderly have enough hearing loss to affect communication abilities.
Teeth	Gum disease is more common than decay, but little dental care and absence of fluoridation in their younger years has led to much tooth loss in today's elderly.
Mental function	Stamina and speed decline with age, but judgment and wisdom increase. Mild memory loss (such as names) is common but only progresses if disease is present. Older persons can learn new information, but more slowly than when younger.
Sleep	Deep (stage 4) sleep is reduced in comparison with younger adults. Spontaneous awakening occurs more frequently, causing many elderly to sleep shorter periods. Total sleep needed in 24 hours is approximately 1 hour less than for younger adults, but older persons spend more time in bed to acquire that sleep.
Cardiovascular system	Systolic blood pressure increases with age, due to increased peripheral vascular resistance. Diastolic blood pressure increases until about age 55, then plateaus or decreases.
Respiratory system	Decreased pulmonary elasticity and increased airway resistance occurs. There is less ventilation at lung bases and more at the apex.
Digestive system	Reduced gastrointestinal motility causes constipation to be more common.
Urinary system	Glomerular filtration decreases with age. Nocturia is common in both men and women. Incontinence becomes more frequent, but is not a part of normal aging.
Reproductive system	Male: prostate enlargement is virtually universal. Testosterone production decreases, leading to decreased testicular size. Phases of sexual arousal are slower, and refractory time is longer. Female: estrogen production decreases at menopause; therefore, the vaginal lining atrophies, and the canal may narrow and shorten. Vaginal secretions become more alkaline.

examine your patient's medication regimens, taking them off drugs whenever possible.

Some doctors talk about "the dwindles." I do not like to use that word because so much symptomatology in older persons is iatrogenic. Our older patients gradually find themselves slipping more and more into the clutches of the physician's care and judgment. Of utmost importance is realizing that it takes longer for them to process what they hear. They may not think as fast as you do, but that doesn't mean they do not deserve to know what you have to say or to state their opinion. So communicate clearly, maybe a little louder and a little slower. Touch them carefully and thoughtfully and with all of the love you know how to give. They will be satisfied.

CASE STUDY

Mrs. Evelyn Hamlin had fallen in her dairy barn as a result of a cardiac arrest. As the full weight of her body struck the hard concrete floor, the jar apparently started her vital functions again. It was later determined that she had suffered a subarachnoid hemorrhage. Leaving an office full of patients, I made a quick trip to her home only to find her unconscious and breathing very irregularly. A neighbor had called the ambulance, but it seemed to take forever to come. While we waited, I made sure that a proper airway was provided and her vital signs were stable. I got into the ambulance with her and away we went, sometimes straddling the median in the split highway. Miraculously, or so it seemed to me, we all arrived at the hospital intact. Mrs. Hamlin was admitted, had several weeks of supportive therapy, recovered, and returned to her farmhouse.

The next landmark with this patient occurred on a Thursday evening, when I had the night off. I had arranged to take my wife and children out to Pete's Restaurant, and everyone was excited and dressed up for the outing. On the way to the restaurant, I decided to run by the hospital for just a minute to check on a patient. As I was exiting out of the emergency room door, two patients were being wheeled in. There had been an automobile accident, and Mrs. Hamlin had gone through the windshield (no seat belt). Her face was bloody, her nose so shredded it was hardly identifiable. She recognized me and said, "Oh, Dr. Barnett!" I froze in my tracks. My family was just outside, full of expectations. The patient was inside, also full of expectations. The urge to be cloned was very strong.

I met briefly with the patient and determined that she really needed a plastic surgeon. But when I told her so, Mrs. Hamlin said in a tone that left no room for negotiation, "I'm not going to a plastic surgeon."

"But Mrs. Hamlin," I replied, "you don't have a nose." Her reply was back in a flash, the old school teacher that she was. "You make me a nose."

I went out to the car and told my family to go back home. For the next several hours, I reconstructed cartilage and skin to come up with a facsimile of the nose I had known before. I reassured her that she could have reconstructive plastic work done if "our nose" didn't suit her.

Time passed, we removed the bandages, and she looked in the mirror. After a silent pensive inspection, she turned to me and said, "I like my new nose. I was kind of tired of the old one anyway. I'd had it a long time."

CASE DISCUSSION

Did I do the wrong thing to abandon my family when I was not on call and treat Mrs. Hamlin? Should I have insisted that Mrs. Hamlin see a plastic surgeon, above her objections?

The tension between an all-demanding profession and one's desire to have a personal life is intense, especially for primary care physicians, and particularly for those who serve in small towns and rural areas. A physician who abandons his or her family regularly is a bad spouse and parent. However, once in a while, when you know that a particular patient really needs you, it is OK to break the rule that time off is time off. Mrs. Hamlin was one of those special patients. I had tended her when she had almost died of her subarachnoid hemorrhage, and because of that I had almost magic healing properties in her mind. I knew that psychologically she would recover much better from her injuries if I attended to her, and she did recover.

The most recent incident with Mrs. Hamlin happened one summer Saturday afternoon, some years after I had left practice in my hometown to teach at the medical school. I was visiting my old town and decided to see my old friend. As had become my custom, I went to the back door—unannounced—and yelled, "Anybody home?" After a few shuffling noises in the house, I heard a voice say, "Why certainly there's somebody at home!" And out came Mrs. Hamlin, arms open and extended, exclaiming with a smile on her face, "How did you know it was my birthday?" I must confess, I did not know it was her birthday, but she thought I remembered everything.

CASE STUDY

I was working in our rural satellite practice at Nellysford, Virginia, when the rescue squad brought in a dear woman who was struggling for breath. We will call her Margaret. She was in extremis from severe heart disease. The next day was her birthday, but her knowing look told me that she did not believe she would make it till then. We gave her oxygen, digoxin, furosemide (Lasix), and meperidine (Demerol).

The rescue squad had been called to take her to the hospital, and the emergency medical technicians were restless. Even though Margaret was considered terminal and was cared for by hospice nurses, they wanted to whisk her off to the emergency room of the university hospital, where she would be among strangers. Their mentality came from structured protocols and the need to be in control. My office staff interfered with all of that; we stopped the usual worldly rush to give her some personal care along with the medications.

I held her hand, gently feeling for a pulse. Finding it to be strong and steady, I leaned over and asked, "If I can do one thing now, what would you wish?" Softly came the words, almost in a whisper, "a sip of water."

I wheeled, ran a cup of water from the tap, and placed it to her parched lips. She took two or three sips between labored breaths, and then burped. "Excuse me," she said.

CASE DISCUSSION

Medicine is much more a matter of little moments than of momentous events. My brief, quiet moment with Margaret embodies the point that I wish to make, and

that point is that tiny, subtle, shared moments between physician and patient make the strongest statements. Just being there when another person needs you will always give you fulfillment and peace about what you are doing, and no change in the health care system can take that away. These little moments define our purpose.

Even so, the rescue squad continued to pace up and down in the hall outside the treatment room. They could not hear Margaret whisper, or see her smile.

CONCLUSION: MAKING THE MOST OF EACH ENCOUNTER WITH YOUR PATIENTS

One of the cornerstones of family medicine is the tenured relationship that develops over time. As you help them through a variety of life and health events, and as they teach you things about yourself and about your own life, your patients become more than clients or customers; they become your friends. Their welfare becomes more significant, and the outcomes of your efforts become more important. The relationship—a combined synergistic energy of patient and doctor—becomes a definite part of healing. Trust evolves; one's words are heeded; and prescriptions are taken according to directions.

How can you, the physician, make the most of your patient encounters, whatever their stage of life? I am reminded of Vince Lombardi, the great former coach of the Green Bay Packers and Washington Redskins. When asked how he got his players "up for each game," he said he always awakened believing that the best game hadn't been played yet, and today just might be the day to play it! I try, as I believe we all can, to walk into each room with that feeling that something special may be about to take place.

When you are with your patient, listen for the story, and wait for that feeling of coupling. It takes no longer to listen intently than it does to ignore; no longer to give 100% of yourself than it does to give 50%. With that approach, your days will be a series of wonderfully interesting short stories, and your life as a physician will be interwoven into the fabric of many other persons' attempts to cope with life. So strive to preserve this spontaneity, this expectation, this excitement and wonder in your approach to the practice of medicine. It will create power and light instead of gloom and doom.

There is a fragile moment when a person (the patient) passes a point of tolerance for his or her problem and reaches out toward the physician for help, and the physician extends the helping hand in return. It contains, among other things, the chance to make a real difference. A difference not only in the life of the patient that affects his or her health, but a difference in our own lives as well.

Looking back on my half century as a family physician, I can say that it has been a most fascinating journey, one that would be hard to match. Would I do it over again? The answer is easy: "Yes." It's been a life full of changes, full of challenges, full of opportunities; yes, a full life.

3. Keeping "The Family" in Focus During Patient Care

DALE ALEXANDER AND SANDRA CLARK

Key Clinical Questions

1. What are the characteristics of a medical practice that provides "family-oriented" medicine?
2. Which family-oriented tools are most frequently used by family physicians, and how are they used in the office setting?
3. What are some "red flags" that might indicate a physician-patient relationship is being negatively affected by the physician's own family background issues?

CASE STUDY

You are caring for a recently diagnosed cancer patient and his family members. Mr. and Mrs. Robert Peterson and their young-adult daughter and son have been your patients for several years. Bob is a 56-year-old tobacco farmer who has smoked for 44 years. Smoking cessation was an area you agreed to not talk about with Bob after his first visit several years ago, as this irritated him. Upon recognizing his irritation and learning he was a tobacco farmer, you both agreed (in a good-natured way) to disagree about this area, as developing a good doctor-patient relationship was the priority. Recently, you diagnosed Bob's lung cancer and referred him to the specialty clinic for radiation treatment.

One day, Bob's wife, Helen, visits your office complaining of a skin rash. While treating the rash, you ask how she and her husband are doing. Helen seems to be holding together fairly well but is anxious about being left alone or having to move off the farm. She also expresses concern that Bob may be depressed. He seems sad much of the time and sits around the house even though he is tolerating his radiation therapy well. You note "possibility of depression" in his medical record and recall a 20% coexistence of depression with cancer.

During your next visit with Bob, you inquire more about his feelings and concerns. He reminds you that both his father and a brother died of cancers. During this discussion, Bob also reminds you he is a religious man who "feels prepared" to face his own death, but is worried about what "I'm going to be able to leave behind" in terms of property and financial resources for his wife and children. He reveals that he has sizable loans, with the farm as security. His son is at college majoring in agriculture and plans to return to work on the family farm after graduation, and his daughter is considering marrying a farmer who's interested in working some acreage on his future father-in-law's farm. The farm is all his wife knows, he says. His local bank has made sizable farm loans in the past to help cover the expenses of planting his tobacco crop and to pay for his son's education.

Bob, who is a second-generation tobacco farmer, complains about "politicians, lawyers and the FDA," who "are going to really screw up tobacco prices this year," along with his government subsidy to not grow as much tobacco as he could. The day of his visit comes just a few days after a verdict by a District Judge in Greensboro that defined tobacco as "an addictive drug" and cigarettes as "a drug delivery device," which the FDA should regulate. Bob also mentions that a heavy windstorm damaged much of his tobacco crop for the year, putting him at considerable financial risk. As he lives in a small town, the local bank loan officer is aware of Bob's "terminal" diagnosis and the crop loss due to the storm, and so is reluctant to carry his debt. He's encouraging Bob to sell the farm to settle the debt.

DISCUSSION

Family issues can overshadow medical issues for many chronically ill patients, and they often involve a variety of systems ranging from the physiologic to the geopolitical. In the case above, Bob is concerned less about his radiation therapy than about the economic well-being of his family, which itself involves a complex interaction of climatic, political, community, and family issues. Although your discussion with Bob confirmed your suspicion of depression, your initial hypothesis—that Bob was depressed because of his disease—was not accurate. Without taking a broad (biopsychosocial) approach to Bob's health, including a major focus on family—as he does in his own life priorities—you would not be providing quality care.

FAMILY-ORIENTED CARE

This chapter focuses on giving you information and tools that will help you provide family-focused care. "Family" means more than the traditional two parents and children. The families you'll encounter in your practice will be more diverse. Family is more broadly defined: persons who are related by blood, marriage, or a strong emotional commitment to each other's physical, emotional, and spiritual well-being.

The Family-Oriented Physician

A family physician or any doctor who uses a family-oriented approach continues to work primarily with individual patients, but does so in significantly different ways than many other physicians. Although the doctor-patient relationship looks like a dyad in the office, in reality it is a therapeutic triangle that also involves the patient's family. Family members influence the patient's choice of physician, expectations about

care, and evaluation of the diagnosis and prescribed treatment. Such influences are observed, even when the family physician has not treated other members of the family.

The family-oriented family physician

- seeks information about the patient's family;

- signals, often at a new patient's first office visit, interest in taking care of other family members;

- has a working understanding of the key relationships the patient has with other family members;

- routinely asks if other family members came to an office visit, and if the patient wants to include them in the encounter;

- uses family-oriented tools, such as the genogram (family tree) and family conference;

- is sensitive to and recognizes when a family-system approach is necessary to understanding or managing a patient's health care problem;

- sometimes suggests to the patient that it would be helpful or necessary to convene the family, or ask other members of the family to come in for a family conference;

- helps the patient and other family members discuss the emotional effects of an illness or disease;

- attempts to intervene in family interaction patterns that impede the patient's well-being;

- engages the patient and family in problem-solving discussions for finding new patterns of coping or for changing maladaptive patterns in more healthy directions;

- may engage the entire family in a number of "family therapy" sessions as an effort to help them work through family issues that are interfering with critical health issues, or may recommend consultation or referral to a family therapist.

All of these family-oriented activities are appropriate for a family physician. They are compatible with the family physician's other daily professional activities and the clinical attributes that define the specialty of family medicine. Because the family physician provides continuous care over the patient's life, he or she has access to the patient and family at various points in the individual and family life-cycle, as well as during major family events and transitions.

The family physician's comprehensive medical role allows for the care of all members of the family, and potentially of the entire family. Much of this family-oriented skill, experience and knowledge operates at an intuitive level—seldom acknowledged, recorded in the chart, or published in the literature. It does exist, however, operating within medical assessment, decision making, and treatment planning. Family-oriented care activities are no more or less important than other professional activities. It is clinically pragmatic for the family physician to pay attention to the family; it saves time, energy and money, and it yields favorable results.

Family-Oriented Care—Rhetoric or Reality?

Family-oriented care is one of the basic principles of family practice; however, it is put into practice to varying degrees. Only a minority of patient visits involve family members, but those visits often involve discussion of family and relationship issues. Table 3.1 summarizes existing qualitative and quantitative evidence supporting the reality of family-oriented care in education and clinical practice.

Little comparison data about family-oriented care are available from other medical specialties. Certainly, there is less of an expectation in other primary care specialties to "care for the whole family," and textbooks and educational programs in other medical specialties contain fewer explicit opportunities for trainees to learn about dealing with family issues. Practice patterns related to family-centered care have not been studied extensively, however. One specialty, pediatrics, involves multiple family members more often during visits, because parents nearly always accompany children to the office. However, only 15% of pediatricians make house calls, as opposed to 47% of general internists and 63% of family physicians (1).

Levels of Providing Family-Centered Care

The family-centered family physician thinks "family" in virtually every encounter, often within the confines of a routine 10- to 15-minute visit. A family-centered approach can involve something as simple as inquiring if the patient is married or single, or asking one of a host of other "family systems" questions. A more formal method could be gathering information to construct a simple family tree (genogram). Occasionally, however, the family physician will become involved more extensively with family issues. This flexibility in the level of involvement to which family is brought into a physician-

Table 3.1.
Are Family Physicians Family Focused? A Review of the Evidence

Indicator of Family-Oriented Care	Actual Application Among Family Physicians
Specialty definition	Family-oriented care is part of the specialty definition of the American Academy of Family Practice and American Board of Family Practice
Residency education	Involved in 3 of 12 "core concepts"
Academic base	All family medicine textbooks contain sections on family care
Expectation regarding "whole-family" care	50–90% of patients attending family practice offices; 62% of family physicians
Patient accompanied by family/ significant other on visit to office	34–50% of all visits
Conduct family conferences	96% of physicians (17% do so weekly, another 20% do so monthly)
Make home visits	63% of family physicians
Perform family therapy	0.5–4% of family physicians

patient encounter is good medical practice, because some medical problems require a more psychosocially-oriented approach than others.

Baird and Doherty (2) and Marvel et al. (3) have described this variation in family-centeredness as occurring in five levels. These levels require increasing degrees of knowledge and skill, as well as time, on the part of the physician. Briefly, they are:

- *Level 1: The physician-centered individual patient encounter.* The physician focuses on gathering biomedical and family information needed to make the correct diagnosis and treatment. Family issues are minimized, and the patient (and family) are largely recipients of care.
- *Level 2: Collaborative information exchange.* The physician solicits patient and family input into diagnostic and treatment planning, and the family is a partner in care.
- *Level 3: Dealing with effect.* The physician goes beyond the "problem" to actively address emotional issues, both in terms of the individual patient and the family.
- *Level 4: Brief counseling.* The physician seeks to work to catalyze change in psychosocial health through encounters with the patient and/or family. This brief counseling, which may occur over one or several visits, is common in practice and can be extremely effective; it generally involves identifying problems and potential solutions; the family then works on its own to carry out the needed changes. Family practice residency training prepares graduates to operate at and below this level.
- *Level 5: Family therapy.* The physician meets with the patient and family regularly for multiple sessions to change unhealthy patterns within the family system. Only family physicians with specific training in family therapy should provide care at this level.

Family-Oriented Tools

All clinical medical specialties struggle with how to integrate basic research, or tools from other disciplines, into direct clinical practice. Family medicine is no different in its struggle to successfully use family-oriented tools and concepts.

Marvel, North, et al. surveyed a random sample of 299 practicing family physicians about the usefulness of 10 family-oriented practice "tools."

Two of these—keeping medical records organized in family folders, and a five-item "Family APGAR"—were rated as not very useful in practice, even by those trained in their use. The remaining eight tools were judged as "useful" by at least 48% of respondents (4, 5). Brief descriptions of these eight family-oriented clinical tools are provided as Table 3.2. In essence, they comprise the key elements that students and residents should learn about family-centered care.

The remainder of this chapter discusses these tools. We do not cover the family context of chemical dependency (covered in Chapter 15) nor family counseling, because this specialized area requires intense training and it is relatively rarely undertaken in family practice (see Table 3.1).

HOW FAMILIES WORK: FAMILY SYSTEMS THEORY

There is a large body of research and theory about how families work. Although we cannot summarize everything known about family dynamics, we will introduce four key concepts that are especially important in physician-family interactions. They are roles, family interaction patterns, boundaries, and triangulation.

Roles

Just as workers in a company have different job descriptions, family members tend to have identified roles within the family. This is true not only of the nuclear family (parents and children), but often of the extended family as well. A common example of family roles in medical practice is the way families approach a chronic illness. Often, different family members will contribute to care in different ways. This is illustrated by the following case.

CASE STUDY

Mrs. Dotters, a 78-year-old widow, suffered a stroke, which left her aphasic and without use of her right arm. While she was hospitalized, her family physician found that different family members were present at different times, and that each

Table 3.2.

Eight Family-Oriented Tools Most Useful in Practice: Results of a Survey of 299 Wisconsin Family Physicians

Family-Oriented Tool	Description	How Often Used (%)
Chemical dependency and families	Identification and management of the effect of chemical dependency on the health of all family members	95
Family conferences	A planned meeting with family members to discuss patient care	96
Family counseling	Meeting with the family for several sessions to address psychosocial and emotional issues	70
Self-awareness of physician's family background	Awareness of how one's own family dynamics can influence patient care	62
Family characteristics of different cultures	Conscious consideration of cultural differences in family structure and how these affect health and illness	68
Family systems theory	The theory of how families function as a social unit	60
Family life cycle	The series of developmental stages that a family undergoes and how this affects health and illness	58
Genograms	A graphical depiction of the patient's family history, used as a component of the medical record	48

Modified from North S, Marvel MK, Hendrichs B, et al. Physicians' usefulness ratings of family-oriented clinical tools. J Fam Pract 1993;37(1):30–34.

seemed to defer to the other on certain issues but not on others. Finally, a family conference was convened. There Mrs. Dotters' niece, Angela, emerged as the family spokesperson. It was decided that Mrs. Dotters would, after a brief nursing home stay, move in with daughter Stephanie, and that her son James would take over her checkbook.

DISCUSSION

Mrs. Dotters' family knew who played what role, but the physician did not. During the family conference, Angela was identified by the family as the person to speak with doctors and make medical decisions, largely because she was a registered nurse. Stephanie's role of caregiver was well established in the family; indeed, she had been looking in on Mrs. Dotters for years, and she had provided the majority of the assistance with personal care

several years ago, when Mr. Dotters had been dying of lung cancer. James, on the other hand, was assigned the role of managing finances, which fit in with his busy schedule as director of marketing for a small company. This division of responsibility is common among families and allows individual members to contribute based on their own available time, interests, and skills.

Interaction Patterns

Family interactions tend to repeat themselves, so an observant physician will often discern patterns. An overt example is the pregnant teenage daughter whose mother becomes angry and insists that she have an abortion. Under the physician's questioning, the mother admits that this very daughter had been the result of an unplanned teenage pregnancy. Mom is especially upset because she felt that her teenage pregnancy prevented her from getting a good education and a good job. Now she is struggling in night school, and she does not want her daughter to do the same.

Repetitive interaction patterns often reflect unstated family rules and can underlie a variety of health issues. For example, chronic headaches may be the result of an underlying family rule that anger cannot be expressed openly. These patterns of interaction and the rules that sustain them are often best observed by an outsider such as a physician.

Boundaries

Boundaries are like fences around the family and its members; they define the rules under which family members interact with and without the family system. Boundaries have a wide range of influences on health behavior. Here are two examples:

- When adult or adolescent members of a family regularly speak for one another in a health care encounter, the boundaries between individuals may be indistinct. In such families, individuality or nonconformity is often not tolerated. This situation can, for example, prevent an adolescent from becoming independent, leading to teenage rebellion.

- When family members communicate little, they become isolated from each other. Such families are termed "disengaged" and are often difficult to treat, because although their problems may involve family issues, they are not used to approaching problems as a family.

Healthy families balance closeness and distance, both within the family and between family members and the outside. Members care about each other and foster each other's individuality.

Triangulation

When tension exists between two family members, someone else can inadvertently get caught in between. This process is called triangulation. It commonly occurs when children live with two parents who are in conflict. To reduce stress between the two adults, attention gets focused on the child. School phobia is a common example of a child's triangulation coming "to the rescue" of two parents who are in conflict. By refusing to go to school, the child shifts the parent's focus from their own issues to distress about the child's fear of leaving home. Triangulation is common in alcoholic families.

Because involving a third person is a natural defense mechanism for couples in conflict, it is not surprising that the family physician can become the object of triangulation. This most commonly occurs when one member of a family tries to enlist the family physician as an ally in a family problem. For example, a wife who calls the family physician asking for treatment for her husband's depression may be attempting to win the physician over to her point of view—that the husband is the problem—when indeed the underlying issue is marital distress or alcoholism.

THE FAMILY LIFE CYCLE

Most families progress through stages just as individuals do. These observable, predictable stages of development constitute the family life cycle. Each stage is characterized by developmental tasks pertinent to that stage and predictable problems associated with the accomplishment of those tasks (6, 7). As families pass through each phase and from one stage to the next, they will go through a number of normal and expected transitions (such as marriage and pregnancy) as well as an occasional unexpected crisis (such as physical disability or an unexpected death). Table 3.3 presents the seven stages of the family life cycle. Each is described briefly below.

Not all families progress in this orderly manner, especially when there is separation, divorce, and remarriage. Most do, however, so the family life cycle model will allow you to approach your patients and families in a more structured manner. It will help you focus your psychosocial interview and to anticipate potential conflicts facing your patients and their loved ones at each stage.

The family life cycle was developed with the two-parent household in mind, but it can be

Table 3.3.
Stages of the Family Life Cycle

I. Family formation
II. Childbearing families
III. Family with preschool-age children (oldest child < 6)
IV. Family with school-age children (oldest child 6–13)
V. Family with teenage children (oldest child 13–18)
VI. Family dispersion (oldest child 18+)
VII. Older couple

adapted to single-parent households and to families in which one or both parents remarry. This often this causes interruption and repetition of some of the cycles. For example, a mother who divorces and remarries will reenter stage one with a new partner while also being in stage two or three with her children by her previous marriage. If the couple then decides to have children of their own, the reconstituted family will then proceed through the childhood stages again.

Family Formation: Setting the Patterns

The formation of a stable union depends upon several factors. These factors include an ability to negotiate and solve problems, economic stability, and common goals, values, and interests. Pathology frequently arises when one of the partners has difficulty separating from his or her family of origin or if one of the partners comes from a dysfunctional family.

Beginning Childbearing: Three's a Crowd

With young families, you should be concerned about how well the parents are adapting to their new roles, how they are sharing the work load, and how they are managing as a couple. Pathology can result when one parent, traditionally the mother, becomes overinvested in her role as parent, leading to feelings of isolation in her partner, who may begin spending more time at work and away from home.

Families with Preschool-Age Children: Busy Times

Families at this stage deal with the emergence of their child's identity, including his or her sexual identity (learning to be a boy or girl). At the same time they face a child who is continuously testing limits and asserting his or her independence. The doctor must counsel parents to set firm boundaries, which are consistently enforced in a nonviolent manner (such as "time out"). Conflict arises when one parent becomes the "good cop," or the permissive partner, while the other parent plays the role of "bad cop," or rule enforcer. This leads to stress between the parents when the child misbehaves. This is also a time when opportunities for intimacy between partners are reduced, and so maintaining closeness is an important feature of healthy couples.

Families with School-Age Children: Growing and Changing

As children begin school they come into contact with a new power structure with different rules and values. It is during these years that children begin experimenting with and testing social norms. It is also a time when children begin defining themselves in relation to others. Prejudice, which children often internalize after observing parents' reactions to different ethnicities and races, becomes apparent. Name calling and social isolation are frequent and painful reminders of children's struggle with identity. Family physicians should ask about school performance and socialization skills. They should help parents anticipate the questions about identity that children may bring home with them.

Within the home, children begin taking on more responsibility in the form of chores, self-care, and homework. In addition, parents take on new roles such as task assignment, discipline, and transportation. These new responsibilities continue and expand through the next phase.

Families with Teenagers: The Launching Years

During this period, the family prepares for the emerging independence and eventual departure of their adolescent. This period is characterized by multiple crises as the teenager and parents define and redefine boundaries and responsibilities within the family. Authority is often questioned and devalued. Experimentation with risky behaviors, such as using illicit drugs, engaging in unprotected sex, and driving recklessly, are common. Coincidentally this usually occurs at a time when the parents are examining their own life decisions and identity (i.e., the "midlife crisis").

Family members frequently react to the demands and crises of adolescents by either distancing themselves from the teenager's behaviors or becoming overinvolved; often, they vacillate between these two extremes. As a family physician, you can play a supportive role, helping parents set reasonable and firm boundaries. You can also be helpful by identifying when a family is having a particularly hard time with this stage, so that referral for family therapy can be made. You should almost always see adolescents alone, to reinforce that the teenager needs to begin taking responsibility for his or her own health and to discuss confidential issues such as sexuality and healthful living.

Family Dispersion: Adjusting to the Emptied Nest

Family dispersion begins when the first child leaves home and continues as subsequent children leave. The tasks for the parents at this time are to adjust to the absence of their children and to redefine their roles within their relationship. Conflict arises when one or both parents become despondent at the departure of their child (the "empty nest syndrome") or if the children continue to stay on in the home beyond acceptable social norms. Conflict can also arise if the parents have neglected to devote time to their relationship during the busy years of parenthood and subsequently have a hard time adjusting to being alone together.

The Older Couple: A Dyad Again

The developmental tasks for the last stage of the family life cycle are facing retirement, facing each other, and facing the issues of aging, disability, and death. This phase of life can also include many good things, such as a feeling of great closeness among couples, relative freedom from the financial worries of earlier adulthood, and time to travel and pursue hobbies. Many older couples find their role as grandparents especially joyful and rewarding.

When working with older couples, you should ask about how the couple has changed since one or both retired, how the couple is spending their time, and how they are sharing the workload in their household. You should invite discussion of reactions to losses, such as the death of a spouse or close friend, movement from a house to an apartment, or declines in function or health. Guidance in end-of-life decisions (e.g., living wills, designating a power of attorney, and estate planning) is very helpful at this stage.

THE GENOGRAM

We all are part of families and, therefore, have meaningful social connections. These social relationships are often crucial in explaining aspects of your patient's behavior and in formulating an effective treatment plan. The genogram provides an easy and convenient method for gathering this information. It can provide a visual representation of the medical and social history of a patient and fam-

ily, communicating it to others as part of the medical record. A common practice is to place it on the left side of the chart, close to or on the same page as the medical problem list. It can also provide a systematic and nonthreatening way of initiating a discussion with the patient about these relationships and their influence on health, well-being, medical complaints, and recovery from illness.

A genogram is a family tree that has been constructed to reflect the relationships of one person. That person is called the "index" family member. Constructing a genogram is an easily learned skill. The genogram can be made over several patient visits and is easily updated as circumstances within the family change. Patients generally enjoy watching the genogram as it evolves and participating in its creation. As you connect the circles and squares that make up a patient's family, you'll find it easy to initiate a discussion of difficult subjects such as alcoholism, depression, and domestic violence, conditions that tend to involve multiple family members.

To begin a genogram, indicate the index patient using a circle (denoting a female) or a square (denoting a male). Put an arrow by this symbol to identify him or her as the index person. Next, identify partners, siblings, parents, and children, representing each by a circle or square. Use horizontal lines to identify siblings and connect couples, and use vertical lines to link generations. Use dotted lines to indicate an unmarried couple and two vertical slashes through a horizontal line to signify a relationship that has broken off. To signify death, blacken in the symbol representing the individual. Write the name, date of birth, medical conditions and relevant social commentary beside the person's symbol on the genogram. Draw a circle around the people with whom the index patient lives. Figure 3.1 illustrates many symbols commonly used in constructing genograms. Figure 3.2 is the genogram for the patient discussed below.

CASE STUDY

A.C. is an 18-year-old college freshman who presents complaining of fatigue to the point that he is missing classes and falling asleep during school examinations. Your

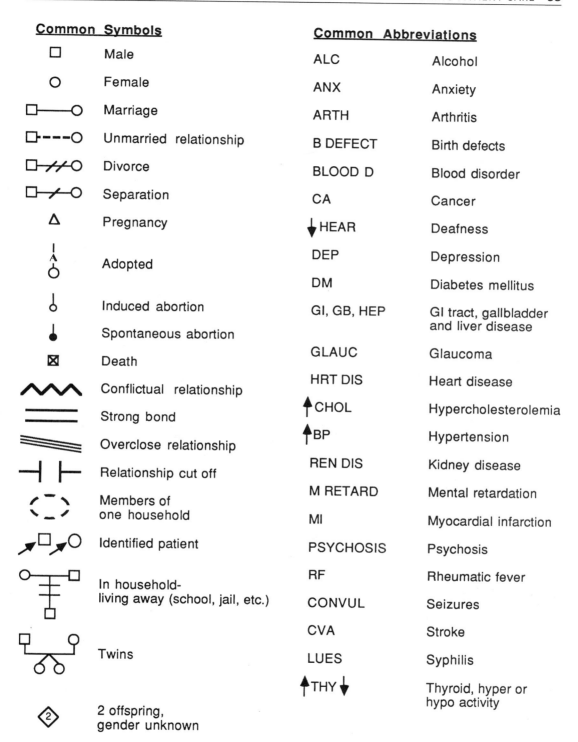

Figure 3.1. *Symbols commonly used in genograms.* (Reprinted with permission from Sloane P, Slatt LM, Curtis P, eds. Essentials of Family Medicine, 2nd ed. Baltimore: Williams & Wilkins, 1993:26.)

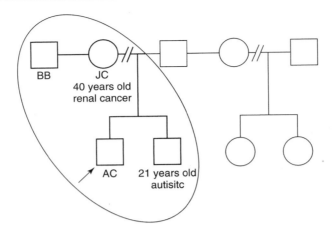

Figure 3.2. *Genogram of A.C.*

physical and laboratory examinations are unremarkable. As part of his psychosocial history, a genogram is constructed.

DISCUSSION

A.C.'s genogram reveals several sources of stress in his life. In addition to the demands of college and living on his own, he is dealing with the stress of his mother's recent illness, his parents' recent divorce and his mother's subsequent remarriage, and the ongoing relationship he has with his autistic older brother, who has recently moved back into the home after performing poorly in college. You advise him to seek out counseling at college and place him on a selective serotonin reuptake inhibitor (SSRI) antidepressant, with good results.

CONDUCTING A FAMILY CONFERENCE

Family conferences are a useful method for implementing family-oriented primary care. A family conference is a meeting, naturally occurring or planned, among the physician, patient, and one or more family members, for the purpose of discussing issues relevant to the patient's medical condition.

Unplanned Family Conferences

Here are the most common settings in which an unplanned family conference occurs:

- When the family physician enters the examining room and finds another family member present with the patient. This often yields a family-initiated family conference.

- When the family physician discovers that a family member is in the waiting room. In such a circumstance, you should decide whether you want to bring the family member into the encounter, first asking the patient for permission.

- When the family physician is making hospital rounds and family are present.

- When the visit involves a child or an older adult with a disability, since family members generally accompany such patients to the doctor's office.

Such conferences offer opportunities for the family physician to become acquainted with other family members and to address direct or indirect concerns about psychosocial issues regarding the patient's problems. Conducting such natural family conferences can occur within the 10 to 15 minutes of a normal office visit, but to do so you will have to focus on identified problems. If broader relationship issues surface, you should defer them for another time, acknowledging that you will be thrown off schedule. The clinical reality is that such unplanned family meetings are often the reasons and bridges for scheduling planned family conferences.

Planned Family Conferences

Planned family conferences are scheduled meetings with the identified patient usually, but not always, present and one or more additional family members or friends. They are usually scheduled at the initiation of the family physician, but may be requested by the family. Common reasons for convening a family conference are to:

- develop a discharge plan for a hospitalized patient;

- make a decision about a treatment issue, such as whether or not to perform surgery on a patient who cannot make his or her own decision;

- help the physician understand the patient's problems and their biopsychosocial context;

- obtain a more thorough assessment of the patient and family system around the specific medical issue;

- involve the family collaboratively to negotiate and develop a comprehensive treatment plan that fits with the family's ability; or

- help family members cope more effectively with a catastrophic health event by providing them information or assisting them in expressing feelings and solving problems.

Planned family conferences require preparation, coordination, a semistructured interview plan, and follow-up. Typically, the agenda or goal is to discuss the family's role in the care of a person with a medical problem, and the result of the conference is a specific plan. Table 3.4 provides a step-by-step guide to conducting a family conference.

DIFFERENCES IN FAMILY BELIEFS AND ROLES IN A MULTICULTURAL SOCIETY

The United States is a multicultural society. In the past three decades, some 20 million immigrants have entered the United States, with the majority coming from Latin America and Asia. African-American, Hispanic, and Native American traditions also contribute to the multicultural nature of American society. Understanding and dealing with patients of differing ethnicity and background demands an open-minded attitude, good

Table 3.4.
How to Conduct a Family Conference

1. Before the conference
   - Set the stage by explaining the rationale for meeting, choosing a family member to help organize, setting the time, and determining who needs to attend.
   - Review the known genogram information and note the family's life cycle stage.
   - Develop tentative hypotheses about the family, their concerns, and your preliminary goals, and set a strategy for conducting the interview.
2. During the conference
   - First, greet the family. Seek to "join" relationally with each member through some personal acknowledgment and brief conversation.
   - Solicit goals from family members. Clarify these goals in realistic terms. Add other goals you consider necessary. Then, prioritize these goals.
   - Start a discussion of the problems or issues. Encourage all family members to express themselves, ask questions, and discuss how they've coped with past problems or the present one.
   - Identify medical and community resources, family strengths, and support systems that may help the family in addressing the problem.
   - With the family's input, establish a plan. Specify what various family and health care team members will do. Clarify next steps to take and solicit final questions from the family.
3. After the conference
   - Reflect on what happened. Adjust your hypotheses about the patient and family in light of new information. Decide how the future treatment plan may be affected by the conference.
   - Revise the genogram with new information obtained, such as past patterns or relationships
   - Write up a conference "report" to include those who did and did not attend, problems addressed, an assessment of the family's functioning, strengths, resources, and the plan for treatment and follow-up. Include the write-up in the medical record.

Adapted from McDaniel S, Campbell TL, Seaburn DB. Family Oriented Primary Care: A Manual for Medical Providers. New York: Springer-Verlag, 1990:73–104.

listening skills, and a willingness to compromise. Barriers to effective communication with persons of different race or ethnicity include language barriers, different cultural norms, and differing expectations of medical care.

When entering into discussions of disease with a patient from a different cultural background, you must take a thorough history, including questions about alternative therapies and home remedies that the patient may have already tried. Practitioners of Western medicine frequently know little about alternative therapies such as acupuncture and yoga, which have a long and successful tradition in other countries. At the least, learning this information will offer insight into the patient's perception of his or her illness. You should also be sensitive to the stress that adjusting to American culture can create. Anxiety and depression are common in foreign-born patients, especially those who do not speak English and those with little education. The following example illustrates some of the key points.

CASE STUDY

Marta is an 18-year-old Hispanic woman who presented complaining of breast engorgement and tenderness a few weeks after giving birth to a healthy boy. She had initially breast-fed her newborn but stopped after witnessing the death of a relative a few days earlier. On further questioning she admitted that she had planned to breast-feed for a year and had been enjoying the feedings with her son. When asked why she had decided to stop, she said "estoy asustada," which is literally translated as "I am frightened."

Her physician discussed the case with a Hispanic colleague and learned that, in parts of Mexico, women believe that strong feelings, especially fear, can poison their milk for several days. Armed with this explanation, the clinician was able to successfully treat Marta by suggesting that she rent a breast pump to relieve her discomfort and keep her milk supply up. The "poisoned" breast milk was to be thrown out and the infant switched to formula feedings for the week. When she felt her milk was no longer bad, Marta resumed breast-feeding.

BEING AWARE OF YOUR OWN FAMILY BACKGROUND AND ISSUES

Physicians are as influenced by their families as are their patients. Your family of origin serves as an internal guide for how you see experiences with patients and their family members. This is unavoidable; as a physician, you should strive to use your family reference map constructively to provide professional care and understanding, and not allow it to compromise your effectiveness with patients.

CASE STUDY

Judy and Kim were residents at a community hospital-based family practice program. Both generally were excellent clinicians, but there was a sharp contrast between the two in their management of alcoholics. Judy attempted to help patients she or others recognized as having problems due to alcoholism or substance abuse, but she often appeared visibly irritated and tended to be preachy in her interactive style. As time went by, she was observed to be increasingly frustrated toward substance abusing patients. On one occasion she expressed cynicism about "putting in clinical time trying to help patients who don't want to change."

Kim, on the other hand, had been active as a medical student in a peer counseling program for students with alcohol problems. As a resident, she sought out supervised work with patients and families with substance abuse problems. Her sensitivity and skill in these areas, particularly in recognizing when the patient and family members are ready to change, were acknowledged by her professional colleagues, who began to seek out her advice for their patients. She also worked within the training program to foster active learning experiences for her peers.

DISCUSSION

Approximately a quarter of medical students report a close family member who has an alcohol problem. These cases illustrate two ways such family experiences can impact professional practice.

When she was 12 years old, Kim's father refused to join her mother in seeking help for his drinking, and so her mother joined Al-Anon and enrolled Kim in Al-A-Teen. Her parents divorced when she was 13; afterward her father began a series of relationships with women, continued to drink, and became increasingly estranged from his family. Two years later, however, under the threat of losing his job, Kim's father entered a treatment program. As part of his recovery, he reconciled emotionally with his daughter and ex-wife. He became a steady and encouraging parent to his teenage daughter and a friend to his ex-wife, although they did not remarry.

Judy's childhood experience was different in that her parents remained married, with escalating conflict, denying that a problem existed. Tension grew and was accompanied by minimization of the role alcohol was playing in their lives. Her mother made excuses for her father's drinking, even calling work to report him as "sick" on some Mondays when he was hung over. Leaving home for college and eventually medical school was a relief for Judy. Trips home were increasingly infrequent, as tension and conflict still characterized her parents' interactions. During college Judy drank little but enjoyed smoking marijuana, which she considered safer than alcohol. During her senior year she married. Her husband continued to smoke marijuana, which became an increasing source of tension as Judy progressed through medical school and residency, as she felt that his drug use was something she needed to hide from her professional colleagues.

Kim's awareness of her family-of-origin experience with alcohol was a characteristic she built upon in her professional growth. Her family system had a more favorable outcome than her colleague's, even though her parents divorced. Unfortunately, Judy's parents' marital conflict continued to revolve around her father's drinking. Her family interactions involved denial, secret "games," and "enabling

roles." This interfered with Judy developing a healthy self-awareness about substance abuse, to the degree that she was unaware of the similar family pattern playing out in her own marriage around her husband's marijuana use. She was not able effectively to help substance-abusing patients until she gained more awareness of these old family patterns and modified her relationship style with patients.

Importance of Awareness of Family-of-Origin Issues

A variety of published studies have demonstrated that a physician's family of origin can contribute to effectiveness or ineffectiveness in patient care, underscoring the need for self-awareness in this area. One such study documents how five physicians were consistently ineffective with their own patients because of "facets of the physician's own family of origin, which the physician carries to all patient care situations." The ineffectiveness was usually the result of the physician "fusing with the patient's system because of certain characteristics resembling the physician's own family-of-origin system." Common patterns involved developing alliances, avoiding conflict, keeping secrets, or assuming unhealthy parental responsibilities toward the patient or within parts of the family system that closely resembled the same troublesome dynamic area(s) in the physician's family of origin. The author speculated that family-of-origin issues may help explain why health professionals are more effective with certain kinds of patients than with others (8).

Hopefully, it's becoming clear why awareness about your own family of origin and current family are important. Some specific reasons for this self-awareness are to help you

- maintain appropriate "neutrality" and objectivity in professional relationships and medical decision making with patients and their families;

- explore and understand patient care situations in which you feel clinically ineffective, in order to minimize the potential hindrance of a family-of-origin issue in patient care; and

- work toward a better understanding of each patient's unique family situation and how it

Table 3.5.
"Red Flags" Suggesting That a Physician's Care May Be Compromised by Family-of-Origin Issues

Red Flag	Example
Overinvolvement with a patient and family	Routinely giving patient/family extra time even when running late
Underinvolvement or distancing	Not wanting to return phone calls from a specific patient and family
Feeling entangled or triangulated	Two sisters entangle you in a "conspiracy" to declare a third sister incompetent
Confusion about confidentiality or secrets	Husband and wife both request confidentiality about extramarital affairs they are engaging in while you are treating them for depression
Feeling pressure that a patient "must" change a specific problem behavior	Insisting that you cannot be a patient's doctor unless he quits smoking
Taking sides in emotionally charged situations	Telling a patient, "If your spouse is having an affair, I'd say leave him"
A strong emotional reaction to a patient	Reluctance to see a terminally ill patient who has the same illness of which your father died
Feeling "stuck" repeatedly with a group of patients who aren't improving	Prescribing the same treatment for obesity over and over even though it isn't working
Repeated dilemmas about providing medical care to one's own family members	Family who insist that you treat them even though you are uncomfortable doing so

may be similar or different from your own unique family-of-origin experiences.

Some general "red flags" suggesting when a patient or their family may be touching upon a sensitive issue in your own family background are listed in Table 3.5.

Gaining Awareness About Your Family of Origin and Current Family

How much self-awareness about your own family background is enough? A good starting point is to appreciate how the type of family structure you grew up in may make it necessary to "stretch" your empathic capacity to understand types of family structures represented by your patients. For example, if you grew up in a "traditional" two-parent, white, Midwestern family, it may not be easy to understand how a divorced, blended, binuclear, multicultural family or a single-parent family is struggling with a health care issue.

You may find it valuable to gain increased self-awareness of your own family of origin by

- constructing your own genogram and presenting it for study and discussion;
- allowing a classmate to construct and conduct an abbreviated genogram interview with you;

- having someone you trust, trained in family systems, conduct a detailed genogram interview and exploration of your family-of-origin issues with you;
- take a course in directed readings on the family with a faculty member, and couple that reading with discussions and exercises about your own family of origin;
- attending a family medicine residency that includes a strong curriculum on family, including exploration of family-of-origin issues; and
- joining a discussion (Balint) group with a family-oriented focus.

Such experiences can benefit your patient care, help your personal life, and also be fun.

REFERENCES

1. Adelman AM, Fredman L, Knight AL. House call practices: a comparison by specialty. J Fam Pract 1994; 39(1):39–44.
2. Baird MA, Doherty WJ. Risks and benefits of a family systems approach to medical care. Fam Med 1990; 22:396–403.
3. Marvel MK, Schilling R, Doherty WJ, Baird MA. Levels of physician involvement with patients and their families. J Fam Pract 1994;39(6):535–544.
4. Marvel MK, Morphew PK. Levels of family involve-

ment by resident and attending physicians. Fam Med 1993;25(1):26–30.

5. North S, Marvel MK, Hendrichs B, et al. Physicians' usefulness ratings of family-oriented clinical tools. J Fam Pract 1993;37(1):30–34.

6. Roberts L. The family life cycle in medical practice. In: Crouch M, Roberts L, eds. The Family in Medical Practice. New York: Springer-Verlag, 1987:74–96.

7. Medalie JH. The family life cycle and its implications for family practice. J Fam Pract 1979;9(1):47–79.

8. Mengel MB. Physician in-effectiveness due to family-of-origin issues. Fam Sys Med 1987;5:(2):176–190.

4. Outside the Office Walls

MARY JEAN SCHENK, JOSEPH M. KEENAN, ADAM O. GOLDSTEIN, BEAT STEINER, AND DONALD PATHMAN

Key Questions

1. How can family physicians promote the health of the communities in which they live and practice?
2. For which patients is home care appropriate? When and how should primary care physicians serve home care patients?
3. What are the most common occupational diseases in the United States? How should the family physician screen for occupational and environmental disease?

The critical factors affecting people's health occur outside of the doctor's office. A person's eating patterns are well established before he is counseled by his primary care clinician to "cut out fatty foods." An adolescent's peers are far more influential on her sexual behavior than the physician's advice presented during a 15-minute visit. The importance of an individual's ethnicity, culture, and family on his or her health are well documented (1). Work-related conditions also play a major role in many patient's lives. Broader issues such as environmental factors (contaminated drinking water, toxic and nuclear wastes in the community, depletion of the ozone, and burning of fossil fuel) can have dramatic effects on people's day-to-day lives.

The episodic, office-based, patient-clinician encounter alone cannot deal effectively with many health problems. Helping those with chronic, debilitating diseases also requires skillful coordination of community resources. Overcoming barriers to care requires increased cultural sensitivity and sometimes even political involvement. Changing the harmful effects of occupational and environmental hazards requires monitoring the community to document adverse events and political activism to push for legislative reform.

This chapter discusses three aspects of care that deal with factors in the community: community medicine, home care, and occupational health.

Community Medicine

When you enter medical practice, you will be serving, and living in, a community. You will have the chance to become involved with your community in different ways. Some of those ways might build upon your role as a physician, some may not. For example, you might choose to become a member of the your child's Parent-Teacher Association (PTA) or to join a local painting society. Indeed, how and why you become involved in your community can influence your personal satisfaction with your community. For example, rural physicians are more likely to leave their work settings if they do not feel appreciated and embraced by their community (2). How you integrate yourself into your community is a personal decision.

Besides becoming involved in your community, there are several other dimensions of community medicine. They are (a) establishing a practice that is aware of, and sensitive to, the cultural diversity in your community; (b) knowing about and coordinating community resources for your patients; and (c) taking a leadership role in your community. Taken together, these dimensions help define community medicine and a community perspective on health care.

CULTURAL DIVERSITY IN THE COMMUNITY

Culture is the sum total of a society's customs, habits, beliefs, and values. Culture has been defined as a way of life that directs people's actions and thoughts, including their health practices (3). The meaning of illness and the ways people respond to it vary greatly among cultural groups. Anglo- Americans view illness as foreign and intrusive and believe the goal of treatment is to fix the problem in the individual (1). Some cultures see illness as a part of a harmony-disharmony pattern for which family members are responsible and in which a kin network may be needed to rid the patient of illness. Other cultures see illness as a form of divine punishment, wherein patients may avoid seeking care to keep their illness hidden (1).

Understanding the cultural norms and patterns that exist in your community is crucial to quality primary care. For example, slight modifications such as increasing privacy for clients and providing greater consistency of health personnel can increase the use of services by African-American families (3). Informal communication networks, such as barber shops, respected elder church members, and social clubs can be used to promote health awareness (3). Open, nonjudgmental inquiries about different ways to understand and respond to illness can encourage dialogue and further lower cultural barriers during patient encounters. It is sometimes necessary to consult with others in the community to clarify cultural nuances or act as translators.

USING COMMUNITY RESOURCES

Chronic illnesses and today's decreasing length of hospitalization require family physicians to have an increased knowledge of community resources in order to provide quality outpatient care. For example, physicians must know when and how to collaborate with hospice programs to provide terminally ill patients with dignified and comfortable lives. They also should know about self-help groups such as Alcoholics Anonymous that can assist those with addictive behaviors (4). Churches and other social networks provide not only spiritual support but also motivation to help people change health behaviors. Our nation's interest in decreasing health care costs makes community agencies such as home health care and Meals on Wheels viable and cost-effective alternatives to institutionalization.

Effectively managing a patient in the community (case management) requires that the clinician know the community resources, so that proper plans, referrals, and follow-up occur (5). When several community resources are involved, the clinician serves a coordinating role. The section on home care later in this chapter describes one aspect of this coordination. Physicians should make every effort to learn about the formal, health-related community resources and also such informal networks as families, neighbors, and churches.

TAKING A LEADERSHIP ROLE IN THE COMMUNITY

As a physician, you can use individual patient education as a powerful tool for helping a patient change an unhealthy behavior. However, the number of people you can influence is relatively limited. For example, one full-time physician may see 2,500 patients a year, 625 of whom may be smokers. If he or she successfully counseled all these patients about smoking cessation, almost 100 of them would quit smoking. Alternatively, a community-wide smoking cessation contest in a city of 100,000, with 25,000 smokers, might get 500 smokers to quit smoking in a single intervention and still reach the other 24,500 smokers with some type of health message.

Community Advocacy

A natural way to have more influence on health is to take a leadership role in one or more health issues. There is a need for clinician leaders who are committed to community advocacy and who want to serve the community in which they live and practice. Our society's respect for physicians gives them real power in this role. Any clinician who wishes to make a contribution as a medical leader in the community should follow three simple rules:

1. Know the leading causes of preventable mortality and morbidity in your community (usually tobacco, alcohol, violence, diabetes, obesity, AIDS, injuries, toxins, and infections);
2. Choose one or two areas on which to concentrate; set specific, focused, achievable goals; and
3. Find like-minded and experienced people in the community with whom you can collaborate (and who will mentor you); form coalitions when appropriate.

The best approach is to unleash your creative talent, combine it with your medical knowledge, and motivate others to become involved. For example, you can devise a campaign that helps you or your group "sell" good health as accessible, fashionable, and most importantly, fun. Learn how to use the media to advocate for health promotion. When sponsoring alcohol prevention or tobacco prevention programs for adolescents, consider developing long-term relationships with a class or school by "adopting" it or by working through the PTA or school administration. Teach teenagers to become "pro-health" advocates toward their peers, helping them devise marketing campaigns that use articles, radio spots, cable TV, and commercials against the noxious products. Alternatively, you can reach the entire community by helping work on a monthly newsletter or a radio talk show.

National organizations well known for their help in supporting leadership development through medical activism include Physicians for Social Responsibility (http://www.PRS.org/index/html), Doctors Ought to Care (DOC) (http://www.bcm.tmc.edu/doc), and Physicians for a National Health Program (http://www.pnhp.org). Professional health organizations such as the American Academy of Family Physicians (AAFP) and the American Medical Association (AMA) have major organizational and financial resources that can help community-wide interventions, particularly at the legislative level. Examples include laws and regulations on food labeling, smoke exposure, use of pesticides, and local toxic waste disposal issues. You can also be an advocate on a topic that you care deeply about and stimulate your professional organization to be more involved.

Do not underestimate what a medical student or physician can accomplish. A published letter to the newspaper, or a featured "op-ed," will be read by potentially thousands of people. You can speak at town or city council meetings and community forums, and, as a medical professional, your motives will be considered altruistic and thus more credible. You can make a great difference, learn a lot, and enjoy the experience.

Community-Oriented Primary Care

Clinicians have the unique ability to become not only effective patient advocates, but also community health promotion specialists. Physicians can become leaders or participate in community health promotion strategies that help pass legislation, implement regulations, or use the mass media. For instance, passage of mandatory seatbelt laws has saved thousands of lives, and most people now "buckle up," thus making the physician's counseling effort much easier. Similarly, comprehensive smoke-free indoor air laws have been far more effective in controlling exposure to environmental tobacco smoke than voluntary restrictions. Public health leaders have used the media to publicize the advantages of testing for lead and cholesterol levels.

Community-oriented primary care (COPC) refers to assessing community needs, developing and implementing appropriate community-based interventions, and evaluating its effects. COPC consists of four steps. First, the "community" of interest must be identified. A community can be defined in several ways. In a sociologic sense, its members share social institutions and common sentiments. Community may also denote populations that are geographically bound, work in the same setting, or are members of the same health plan (6). It is not helpful, however, to define the community simply as the group of "active patients" in a practice.

The second step involves identifying health problems in the community. This second step is often the most difficult because pertinent community-wide data are sometimes unavailable. Useful secondary databases kept by the state or county, such as by the health department, or by schools, private organizations, or other community groups may be identified. Primary data collection also may be carried out, usually through collaboration with academic institutions. At other times, health needs are identified through subjective impressions of clinicians or community members (7). For example, you might realize through your volunteer work at a local elementary school that several children have had bike accidents at the same intersection. Based on available information sources, the clinician (or primary care team) chooses one or more high-priority problems for action.

The third step of COPC involves planning and implementing an intervention tailored to the identified needs. Community participation at this stage is crucial, through community meetings, forming coalitions, and working with opinion leaders in the community. The scope of such interventions must be feasible but need not be limited to the traditional areas of health. Interventions can range from medical interventions such as a cardiovascular risk reduction education program to organizing a thrift shop to raise funds for local schools (8).

As a final step, the tools and skills used to identify the problem can be used to monitor the success of the intervention and develop modifications in the intervention. Statistics such as mortality and major morbidity rates will not adequately reflect the short-term efforts of such a process, so a search must be made for more sensitive indicators such as hospital admissions or high school dropout rates (9). This dimension of community medicine may require substantial efforts by the physician, but the results can be dramatic. By collecting different or more-sensitive measures of health indicators, these type of interventions can be shown to positively affect the health of the community in significant ways (10).

CASE STUDY

While eating out in local restaurants, you notice that only a few have 100% smoke-free areas for employees and patrons. You also know that you are seeing many children with asthma, and a recent newspaper article documented increased cases of asthma among children and adults. Given your knowledge of the effects of environmental tobacco smoke on heart disease, lung cancer, and respiratory infections, including asthma, you believe that a clear air ordinance covering all public places would significantly improve the health of your entire community.

QUESTIONS

1. In getting a local clean air ordinance passed, what steps will be needed?
2. How can the tools of epidemiology help your efforts?
3. What will be the major barriers to success?
4. What resources will you need?

DISCUSSION

This situation is a good example of developing an active community intervention. You must be organized and keep good notes of all activities, meetings, and communications.

- You must become familiar with the current scientific knowledge on the effects of environmental tobacco smoke—(credibility with the public).
- Find some similarly minded people interested in helping you plan and organize your efforts. This can be done through the medical and nursing community, the American Lung Association, friends or the local press—(coalition building).
- Gain knowledge about the legislative decision-making groups and processes, help develop model legislation—(political know-how).
- Develop a data resource of scientific and press articles that have documented the establishment of smoke-free ordinances in other parts of the country or your state.
- Do a local survey (perhaps enlisting a class of high school students for the project) on a sample of community members and restaurant owners on their attitudes—(reinforcing the evidence for your campaign).
- Work out, in advance, possible barriers to implementing the ordinance, including resistance by restaurant owners, lobbyists, and those fearing any loss of tobacco sales. Develop some counter strategies and possible compromises—(identifying problems and solutions).
- Based on the above, develop a media advocacy plan. Contact others who have been successful in such efforts—(contacting experts and resources).
- Establish a rational timeline with flexibility to perform midcourse corrections.
- Evaluate your project afterward to assess accomplishments and difficulties. This will help you improve your approach the next time you get enthusiastic about helping your community.

Homeward Bound: New Directions in Health Care

Until the 1940s, virtually every physician made home visits and, for many, these visits made up the majority of their patient contacts. Most of what physicians could then offer diagnostically and therapeutically in the office could be transported to the home in their "house call bag." However, since World War II, advances in medical technology and services have made the physician home visit less appropriate for the management of most acute illnesses. More recently, physician reluctance to do home visits has increased due to relatively poor reimbursement, the perception of greater medical liability, and the general lack of role models and education in home care (11).

The past decade has seen a renaissance in home care, led largely by the nursing profession. Home health agencies have tripled in number over the past 10 years, and home care is the most rapidly growing segment of the Medicare budget. Medical technology is now quite portable and adaptable to home use: hand-held electrocardiogram (ECG) machines and blood analyzers weigh only a few ounces; finger-tip oximetry units are the size of a walnut; and portable magnetic resonance imaging (MRI), x- ray, and ultrasound machines can fit in a suitcase-sized carrying unit. Two-way video and telephonic communications systems even allow distant assessment of a patient (blood pressure, heart and lung auscultation, etc.) and virtual "hands on" monitoring. Professional services available in the home have also expanded greatly and now include skilled nursing and all of the therapies (physical, respiratory, speech, and occupational), as well as the traditional personal care services. This expanded capacity and capability of home care has resulted in an unprecedented shift of complex and acute patient care to the home setting.

Many patients with illnesses such as congestive heart failure, deep vein thrombophlebitis, and infections requiring intravenous antibiotics can now be managed entirely in the home. The clinical outcomes are similar, but the cost of care is generally about half that of similar care in the hospital. Thus, the renaissance and growth in home care appears to be a sustainable trend.

The major difference in home care versus hospital care is the relative lack of physician involvement. A physician often sees the home care patient initially in the hospital or office to establish the diagnosis and treatment plan. But once the patient is being managed in the home, there is often little further direct physician contact. This has led to the question, "What is the appropriate role for the physician in modern home care?"

PHYSICIAN'S ROLE IN HOME CARE

Physicians have always been responsible for ordering and providing medical oversight of home care, even though now the physicians are rarely directly present in the home. This means that a physician must rely on the assessments and recommendations of other health professionals in home care more than in any other setting of care. In other words, a physician is usually part of a team in the provision of home care. Unlike the hospital or office, the home care team usually involves family members or other lay caregivers as an integral part of the care delivery plan. Frequently, the physician is not the dominant member of the team as in the office or hospital, but is a peer who is respected as the medical authority. The physician often defers to others regarding nursing, social care, or rehabilitative problems. Table 4.1 lists the American Medical Association (AMA) home care guideline for the physician's key roles (12).

Even though the AMA recognizes the importance of the interdisciplinary team and the appropriateness of other health professionals providing the majority of home care, a recent report from the AMA Council on Scientific Affairs strongly urged more direct involvement of physicians in home care (13). The increasing medical complexity and acuity of home care are cited as key reasons indicating the necessity for greater physician involvement. The report acknowledged that financial barriers exist (physician reimbursement, for example, is generally lower than nurse reimbursement), but pointed out that quality of care and patient safety concerns should compel appropriate physician payment reform. Lack of physician experience and training in home care remains another formidable barrier. It is clear that as home care changes, the role of the physician in home care is undergoing redefinition.

Table 4.1.
Role of the Physician in Home Care

Management of medical problems
Identification of home care needs of the patient
Establishment/approval of a plan of treatment with identification of both short- and long-term goals
Evaluation of new, acute, or emergent medical problems based on information supplied by other team members
Provision for continuity of care to and from all settings (institution, home, and community)
Communication with the patient and other team members and with physician consultants
Support for other team members
Participation, as needed, in home care/family conferences
Reassessments of care plan, outcomes of care
Evaluation of quality of care
Documentation in appropriate medical records
Provision for 24-hour on-call coverage by a physician

Adapted from American Medical Association. Role of the Physician. Guidelines for the Medical Management of the Home Care Patient. Chicago: American Medical Association, 1992.

Perhaps it is most appropriate to develop the new definition by examining the issues of selecting and managing the patient in the home.

SELECTION AND MANAGEMENT OF THE HOME CARE PATIENT

Many medical problems can be managed adequately in more than one care setting. The selection of which setting is most appropriate is a function of the cost of care and the intensity of services and resources needed (Fig. 4.1) Physicians must determine not only which setting is best for a given medical problem, but also when to transition from one setting to another as the patient's status changes. The key patient selection criteria for home care are:

- a clinically stable patient

- adequate caregiver support

- availability of necessary professional services

- appropriate home care environment adequate financial support.

In general, patients who need continuous monitoring because of unstable clinical status are not practical candidates for home care. Patients may be seriously and acutely ill, yet still be candidates for home care if they pass the first selection criterion of being clinically stable.

The second criterion for selection of home care for a patient is the availability of a competent and motivated care giver. Care giving for serious or chronic illness can be quite stressful and fatiguing and demands a high level of motivation, so the care giver must be physically and mentally up to the task. Just as the physician must continually assess the setting of care to as-

sure that it is appropriate for the cost and intensity of services, the physician must reassess the adequacy of the care giver with changes in the status of the patient. The astute physician is aware of not only the need for supportive assistance and respite, but also the availability of the many assistive devices and medical equipment that can ease the burden of care giving. Physicians must be aware of the concept of the "prosthetic environment." When a patient has acquired a fixed disability or deficit in function, and physical rehabilitation is no longer effective, prosthetic modification of the environment can often minimize the functional deficit. Lifts, grab bars, ambulation aids, modified eating, cooking, and dressing implements, half-height stairs, a transfer bench, an adjustable bed, and personal hygiene devices, are examples of potentially useful devices for maintaining functional independence and lightening the caregiver's burden.

A third criterion for selection of certain home care patients, given clinical stability and an adequate care giver, is the availability of necessary professional services. Certain types of intravenous infusions (total parenteral nutrition [TPN], chemotherapy), wounds, heart failure, premature labor, deep vein thrombophlebitis, and the various therapy services require the availability of home care professionals with specialized nursing or therapy skills. Most metropolitan and larger urban areas have all of these services available, but a smaller town or rural area may not.

A fourth criterion for selection of home care is a safe and adequate care-giving environment. The home must be evaluated for the usual barriers to function and safety (e.g., throw rugs, poor lighting, loose stair treads, lack of railings or grab bars) and also for reliable heating, cooling, tele-

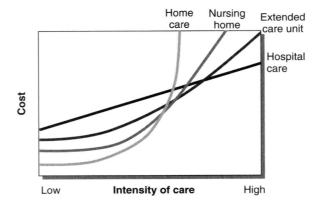

Figure 4.1. *Comparison of settings of care.*

phone, power for electrical devices, and plumbing facilities. Failure of household utilities that would merely inconvenience most people can be life threatening for a frail homebound person. The environmental assessment of the home should include identification of opportunities to improve the home as a functional living space ("prosthetic environment") as well as the elimination of hazards. A look into the refrigerator and the kitchen food shelves provides useful insights into the household eating habits. Likewise, a look into the bathroom medicine cabinet is likely to be more informative than the medication list in your office chart. Environmental assessment should also include barriers to ingress and egress from the house or apartment and a general assessment of the neighborhood safety for home care personnel.

A final criterion for consideration of home care is the financial support needed for provision of adequate home care. When care is shifted from other settings to the home, much of the expense for providing care is shifted to the patient and the family. Medical equipment and supplies, meals, drugs, and personal care services that may be reimbursed in a hospital or a nursing home may not be covered when needed in the patient's home. The cost of remodeling the home to optimize function may be prohibitive. Personal care services under Medicare home health are no longer covered when skilled nursing or therapy is discontinued. The physician should become familiar with community services that can supplement the patient and care giver resources at low or no cost. Area Agencies on Aging are often a good resource for meals, and churches and community groups often have volunteer services. A social worker is a helpful team member in planning this type of support.

UNIQUE ASPECTS OF HOME CARE

Perhaps the most important difference between home care and care in other settings is that you are a guest in the home of your patient and his or her family. This unique circumstance means that you give up much of the control that you have in other settings. You may be forced to respect or at least tolerate ethnic, cultural, and even religious practices that don't comport with your personal or medical science's recommendations and best practices. On the positive side, there are few more appreciative patients and families than those whose doctor has provided the ultimate in care and service by attending them in their own home. Physicians who make house calls have the most loyal of patient followings. It is almost unheard of for a physician to experience a malpractice suit for care rendered in the home.

Another unique aspect of home care is that you must bring with you all of the diagnostic and therapeutic instruments and supplies you anticipate will be necessary for your visit. Table 4.2 lists some of the common items you may want to

Table 4.2.
Equipment for Physician House Calls

Basic	Intermediate	Optional and Advanced
Stethoscope	Audioscope	Portable electrocardiograph machine
Reflex hammer	Nasogastric tube, genitourinary syringe	Pulse oximeter
Sphygmomanometer	Foley and coudé catheter	Portable oxygen
Tuning fork	Phlebotomy equipment	
Oto-opthalmoscope	Intravenous starting kit and fluid	
Cerumen curette	Wound debridement kit	
Tongue depressors	Wound dressing materials	
Cotton tip applicators	Gauze, Kerlix dressing	
Tape measure	4 × 4 gauze	
Gloves	Tape	
Stool guaiac cards and	Scissors	
developer	Saline	
Toenail clippers	Glucometer with lancet and strips	
Snellen chart	Urine dipsticks	
Lubricating jelly	Specimen cups	
Voice amplifier	2-inch, 4-inch Ace wrap	
	Unna Boot dressing	

Adapted from American Geriatrics Society. Geriatrics Review Syllabus: A Core Curriculum in Geriatric Medicine, 3rd ed. New York: American Geriatrics Society, 1996.

carry in a house call bag. Additional items you need for performing minor surgical biopsies or pelvic and Papanicolaou (Pap) examinations are a portable head lamp and speculum, Pap supplies, and fixative.

You may wish to carry some drugs and injection supplies (e.g., epinephrine, lidocaine, and Compazine). However, most physicians have gotten away from carrying much in the way of medications, especially controlled substances. Not only do they want to avoid the invitation for a mugging from drug-seeking individuals, but drug stability and shelf life are often poor when drugs are exposed to the extreme temperatures in a car trunk.

Home care offers many unique aspects, but perhaps none as unique as the professional satisfaction that accompanies the compassionate care of a sick person in his or her own home.

CASE STUDY

A 73-year-old man, previously in good health, presents to the hospital emergency room with shortness of breath. His vital signs are as follows: temperature 38°C, pulse 110, respirations 24, and blood pressure 95/50. He is acutely confused. His skin suggests moderate dehydration; his neck veins are flat; a few rales and rhonchi are heard in the right base; a heart examination shows a grade II systolic murmur at the left sternal border and an S_4 gallop; and the neurologic examination reveals no lateralizing findings, but agitation and confusion were not present 2 days ago by family members' report. The ECG shows sinus tachycardia with occasional PVC, but otherwise is within normal limits. The chest radiograph reveals a right lower lobe pneumonia. Arterial blood gases on room air are: $pO_2 = 80$, $pCO_2 = 35$, pH 7.45, O_2 saturation 80%. Your working diagnosis is (a) right lower lobe pneumonia; (b) moderate dehydration; (c) hypoxemia secondary to (a) with mild respiratory alkalosis; d) delirium secondary to (a), (b), and (c).

QUESTIONS

1. Is this patient a candidate for home care?
2. Under what circumstances?

DISCUSSION

Using the criterion of clinical stability, the answer to the first question is no. Although all of the therapeutic services and monitoring could theoretically be provided in the home, the cost of setting up and staffing a 24-hour home intensive care unit is prohibitive. More importantly, patient safety and quality of care dictate that at least the initial treatment of medical problems occur in the hospital, where potentially serious complications such as dysrhythmias, cardiac failure, shock, or delirious, combative behavior can be managed more effectively. Quite commonly, however, this patient would be ready for discharge after 24 to 48 hours of stabilization in the hospital. Similarly, if the patient had presented to the physician's office earlier in the course of the disease before the delirium and the cardiovascular instability were present, he might well have been managed directly at home.

Occupational Health

Most hazardous exposures occur in the workplace. Family physicians and other primary care physicians are often the first contact for patients with potential exposure-related disease or injury. Thirty-one percent of the medical conditions seen in a primary care practice are related to workplace exposures (14). Work-related factors account for over 10% of all admissions to general internal medicine wards in hospitals, and this proportion is even higher when the primary diagnosis is related to either the respiratory or musculoskeletal system (15). Table 4.3 lists the 10 leading work-related diseases and injuries in the United States. People come to family physicians about work or home environment concerns because they trust and value their advice, and, as a physician, you should remember that many exposure-related illnesses are preventable (16).

Table 4.3.
*Ten Leading Work-Related Diseases
and Injuries in the United States*

1. Occupational lung diseases: asbestosis, byssinosis, silicosis, coal workers' pneumoconiosis, lung cancer, occupational asthma
2. Musculoskeletal injuries: disorders of the back, trunk, upper extremity
3. Occupational cancers (other than lung): leukemia, mesothelioma; cancers of the bladder, nose, liver
4. Amputations, fractures, eye loss, lacerations, traumatic deaths
5. Cardiovascular diseases: hypertension, coronary artery disease, acute myocardial infarction
6. Disorders of reproduction: infertility, spontaneous abortion, teratogenesis
7. Neurotoxic disorders: peripheral neuropathy, toxic encephalitis, psychoses, extreme personality changes (exposure-related)
8. Noise-induced hearing loss
9. Dermatologic conditions, dermatoses, burns (scaldings), contusions (abrasions), chemical injury
10. Psychologic disorders, neuroses, personality disorders, alcoholism, drug dependency

Reprinted with permission from Centers for Disease Control. Leading work-related diseases and injuries in the United States. MMWR 1986;35:613–621.

RECOGNIZING EXPOSURE-RELATED DISEASE AND INJURY

Consider the following four cases:

1. A young woman who worked in a chemical manufacturing plant had numbness and tingling in her hands and feet. Her physician attributed these symptoms to her diabetes.
2. A machinist was noted by his supervisor to have loss of balance and slurred speech on the job. He was sent for evaluation to a local emergency room and was diagnosed as being acutely intoxicated with alcohol. The machinist was suspended and required to undergo alcohol counseling before returning to work.
3. A worker in a poultry plant was told by her physician that her new-onset carpal tunnel syndrome was due to rheumatoid arthritis.
4. A patient with recent onset of headache and fatigue was told by his physician that it was related to the stress of a recent divorce.

In each case, a medically reasonable evaluation was performed and a biologically plausible diagnosis made. However, medical assessment was incorrect because an exposure history was not taken. The first two cases had diseases caused by exposure to chemical agents (solvents, carbon monoxide) at work. The third patient had carpal tunnel syndrome related to the strenuous and forceful repetitive movements she performed with her hands and wrists hundreds of times an hour while processing chickens. The fourth patient was later diagnosed in the emergency room with acute carbon monoxide toxicity as a result of a faulty combustion furnace in his new apartment.

Exposures are either chemical, biologic, or physical. Chemical and biologic agents enter the body through one or more of the following three routes: inhalation, ingestion, and direct skin or bodily contact. Physical agents—repetitive motion, heavy lifting, sustained postures, vibration, temperature, and electrical hazards—mechanically affect the soft tissues, causing trauma to muscles, tendons, joints, and nerves.

Taking an exposure history will identify these and other hazardous agents in the patient's environment. You should routinely take an occupational and environmental exposure history as part of the medical interview, and be knowledgeable enough about exposure-related diseases to know how to advise patients and when to refer patients for further consultation.

OCCUPATIONAL AND ENVIRONMENTAL EXPOSURE HISTORY

The exposure history is often part of the history of present illness and relates to either the chief complaint or the social history. Information about the patient's exposure to potential hazards in the community, home, and occupational setting and the patient's personal habits is collected. Abbreviated as CHOP, this mnemonic should guide your questioning about exposures in the patient's various environments.

An exposure history is collected in two parts. First, ask general questions about exposures, then progress to detailed probing about identified exposures in areas of clinical suspicion. Detailed, probing questions will characterize the exposure and its relation to disease.

An exposure history form (Fig. 4.2) can be filled out by the patient and reviewed by the physician. It is then placed in the patient's medical record for periodic review and updating, much like a medication list. The exposure history

Exposure History Form   Name: Date:

Occupational History: Current

Currently employed? ☐ yes   ☐ no   If yes, approximate date of hire: _____

Name of Employer: _____

Job title: _____

Job description: _____
_____

Hazardous Exposures at Work or Home (check all that apply)

☐ fumes   ☐ arsenic   ☐ silica   ☐ loud noise/mental stress
☐ dusts   ☐ lead   ☐ asbestos   ☐ radiation/vibration
☐ chemicals   ☐ nickel   ☐ isocyanates   ☐ extreme heat/cold
☐ pesticides   ☐ mercury   ☐ cutting oils   ☐ repetitious movement/lifting
☐ solvents   ☐ chromates   ☐ benzene   ☐ cigarette smoke
☐ animals   ☐ gas-powered equipment   ☐ other:_____

Occupational History: Previous

Employer	Dates	Job Title/Description	Known Hazards

Environmental History

Community: Do you live close to any of the following?
        ☐ heavy traffic   ☐ industrial plant / dump   ☐ commercial building

Home: Check all that apply
        ☐ central heat   ☐ septic system   ☐ fireplace/wood stove
        ☐ air humidifier   ☐ air conditioner   ☐ water leaks/moldy area
        ☐ well water   ☐ city water   ☐ purchased water
        ☐ gas stove   ☐ gas space heater   ☐ other:_____

Hobbies: Check all that apply
        ☐ painting   ☐ wood working   ☐ electrical/remodeling
        ☐ photography   ☐ ceramics/pottery   ☐ gardening
        ☐ model making   ☐ autobody repair   ☐ other:_____

Personal: Check all that apply
        ☐ current smoker ____packs/day ____years   ☐ herbal/vitamin supplements
        ☐ alcohol   ____drinks/week   ☐ recreational drugs

Medical Provider Comments:

_____
_____
_____
_____

© 1995 Wayne State University Divison of Occupational and Environmental Medicine.   May copy and distribute freely.
Revised: 4/29/96

Figure 4.2. *Exposure history form.*

gathers information about current and past occupational history, common hazardous exposures, and exposures in the home, community, hobbies, and personal habits.

Current Occupational History

Ask every patient, "What kind of work do you do?" "How is your job performed?" "Please describe a normal work day and any common diversions from that work process." If the patient uses industry-specific jargon, ask him to describe, in detail, what the process is and what types of chemical, physical, or biologic agents are used.

Sometimes, patients will know that they work with chemicals but are unsure of their names. The physician should request information about these chemicals from the patient. If further information is needed, either the patient or the physician can request information about chemicals in the workplace from the employer. Material Safety Data Sheets (MSDS) contain information about the chemical properties of a substance, handling precautions, known health effects, and conditions that might worsen with exposure.

OSHA includes medical surveillance programs for selected chemicals (e.g., lead, arsenic, cadmium, carbon monoxide, and benzene) as part of the regulation of exposure to the chemical. The physicians should ask whether the patient participates in any medical surveillance programs at the workplace.

Ask the patient if personal protective clothing such as boots, coveralls, or gloves are regularly worn at work. If the patient is wearing contaminated clothing home, that environment may become contaminated too. A common example is lead dust-contaminated clothing. If lead dust enters the home, it places any young children at risk for lead toxicity and resultant neurodevelopment delay. The use of personal protective equipment, such as a respirator, should be noted. Asking the patient why they wear the clothing or equipment may lead to identification of a potential hazard.

Past Occupational History

The patient's past occupational history should consist of previous job titles, the duration of previous employment, and information about any known hazardous exposures. Questions about medical surveillance and the use of personal pro-

tective clothing and equipment should be included. In addition, the physician should inquire about any past symptoms or illnesses related to workplace exposures.

Survey of Common Hazardous Exposures

Some well known and common hazardous exposures are listed in Table 4.4. Surveying all patients for these exposures is recommended. Patients need the opportunity to describe any other hazards that may be present in their environment. An open-ended question such as, "Are you aware of any other particular exposures in your workplace, community, or home?" will complete this review. You should also be familiar with the common exposures and their subsequent adverse health effects (Table 4.5).

Home, Hobbies, and Personal Habits Exposure Survey

Finally, ask the patient about sources of water and heat and the location of his or her home near an industrial or community waste site in order to assess potential hazardous agents in drinking water, indoor and outdoor air, or soil. The patient's hobbies or special interests also should be noted, including what the hobby is and where it is performed. Patients with hobbies such as model making, furniture restoration, and stained glass may use hazardous chemicals such as solvents and lead in unventilated basements and garages. This may expose not only the patient, but also family members, to the hazardous chemical.

Obtaining information about personal habits (e.g., smoking, alcohol use, drug use) as part of the exposure history is useful because some interactions between drug use and hazardous, environmental chemical exposures may dramatically increase the risk of disease. Consider the patient who, as a pipe fitter, is exposed to asbestos, and also currently smokes cigarettes. Asbestos and cigarettes are both lung carcinogens. There is a 50-fold risk of lung cancer when asbestos and cigarette exposure are combined. Although the patient cannot modify past asbestos exposure, he or she must be made aware of the additional risk of lung cancer associated with cigarette smoking. This patient must be strongly advised and assisted with his or her efforts to quit smoking.

Table 4.4.

Clues to the Recognition of Exposure-Related Diseases

Classification	Comments	Examples
Exposure-related clues		
Job title or type of industry	Patients may be at high risk or work in hazardous industries in which certain disorders occur at higher than average frequency.	Tuberculosis in health care workers Lead toxicity in radiator-repair shops Asthma in foam manufacturing
Description of work tasks and use of personal protective equipment such as respirators	Job titles are misleading and fail to reflect workplace hazards; a description of a usual day at work and a description of the work process is more helpful.	Asthma in a baker caused by exposure to high-molecular-weight antigens from insect parts in flour dust Chronic upper respiratory complaints in a welder
The most common toxic exposures in local industries and the community	Familiarity of the hazards in local dominant industries should increase the index of suspicion of exposure-related disease.	Latex-induced dermatitis in a local hospital Bladder cancer in rubber-manufacturing workers Cumulative trauma disease such as carpal tunnel syndrome in poultry workers
Coworkers or neighbors who are sick or case clusters noticed in a clinical practice	Clusters of disease are often a helpful clue to both endemic and epidemic exposure-related illness.	Viral hepatitis among workers in a child-care center Hyperkeratosis or peripheral neuropathy in people in a community with arsenic-contaminated drinking water
Past exposure to agents with long latency	Recognizing an important past exposure to toxic compounds helps the physician make the causal link to new symptoms of delayed onset.	Asbestosis, lung cancer, or mesothelioma in a former naval-shipyard worker with exertional dyspnea who has a history of exposure to asbestos
Symptom-related clues		
Pattern of disease onset	The onset of symptoms may be related to a change in (a) employment or personal residence, (b) job duties, (c) the type or use of hazardous materials, or (d) location of a hobby.	New-onset angina after the use of a methylene chloride-containing paint stripper that is metabolized to carbon monoxide in blood
Pattern of aggravation of symptoms	There may be worsening of symptoms during the workday or the workweek or improvement during weekends and vacations. The opposite may occur with home exposures.	Improvement in hand paresthesias and wrist pain in a computer-terminal operator when on vacation, with recurrence on return to work
Unusual combination of multiorgan symptoms and signs	Multiorgan and systemic symptoms usually prompt concern about endocrine, infectious, drug-related, and autoimmune disorders; exposures to toxins should also be considered.	Psychiatric, neurologic, and hematopoietic symptoms and spermatogenetic dysfunction due to the concentration of inhaled or ingested manganese in mitochondrial-rich tissues in workers in welding, mining, and ore extraction
Demographically "wrong" patient	When diseases occur in an unlikely person, one should consider occupational agents that can produce the same symptoms, signs, and pathologic consequences.	Lung cancer in a lifelong nonsmoker due to past asbestos exposure, coke-oven emissions, or arsenic from a smelter

continued

Table 4.4. (*continued*)
Clues to the Recognition of Exposure-Related Diseases

Classification	Comments	Examples
Disease-related clues		
The "usual suspects" are excluded or patient is referred to a specialist for further evaluation	When commonly recognized causes of illness have been eliminated from the differential diagnosis, the likelihood of an occupational and environmental cause increases. Always take a comprehensive exposure history before referring to a specialist.	Hepatitis in a nonalcoholic, nondrug-using patient with no risk factors and negative serologic tests caused by a workplace hepatotoxin. Chronic sinusitis unresponsive to antibiotics from workplace exposure to welding fumes or chlorine-containing cleaning solutions
Idiopathic disease	Before assigning the designation "etiology unknown," one should exclude environmental and occupational causes.	Chronic beryllium disease masquerading as sarcoidosis in a patient who machines metals or ceramics or prepares dental alloys.
Disease that does not respond to conventional medical therapy	In many instances of occupational diseases, the problem has no chance of cure if the patient continues to be exposed.	Asthma in a corticosteroid-dependent patient who works on the line at a car seat manufacturer that could improve or be cured by avoidance of isocyanates
Unusual distribution of disease within an organ	The distribution of pathologic effects in an organ is often related to the area of most direct or intense contact with a hazard.	Rashes selectively involving the face, scalp, neck, and hands but sparing nonexposed parts of the body due to contact dermatitis to a toxin in the workplace.

Modified from Newman LS. Occupational illness. N Engl J Med 1995;333:17, 1128–1134.

After identifying exposures in the patient's environment, the relationship between exposure and illness or injury must be determined.

IS THE HAZARDOUS EXPOSURE A POTENTIAL THREAT TO THE PATIENT'S HEALTH?

Consider these two cases:

1. A woman working as a nurse anesthetist is concerned about the possible relationship between the anesthetic gases she handles and her recent miscarriage. Her physician tells her that miscarriages are not uncommon in the first 12 weeks of pregnancy, and reassures her that her job exposures are not related to this miscarriage. Further, her physician encourages her to "try again."
2. A family who lives in a rural area is concerned about contamination of their drinking water with arsenic and asks their family physician to examine them for any arsenic-related diseases. The physician performs a standard medical examination and assures them that they are all healthy.

Exposure to environmental hazards, such as anesthetic gases in the first case and arsenic in drinking water in the second case, does not mean that illness will follow. Asking probing questions that characterize the exposure and link it to a health effect is required. An exposure assessment evaluates the extent of human exposure to hazardous agents. This assessment includes the route, concentration, frequency, and duration of the exposure. This information is used to estimate the amount of internal dose acquired by the patient.

In both cases, the physician provided inappropriate reassurance because of lack of knowledge about exposure-related diseases. In the case of the nurse anesthetist, further questioning would have revealed that the patient worked in an antiquated operating room and was exposed to anesthetic gases on a regular basis. Anesthetic gases have been implicated as a risk factor of miscarriage, and the patient could be advised of this additional risk. The physician could also refer this patient to an occupational/environmental medicine (OEM) specialist for further review of the workplace and to determine the advisability of the patient's return to it.

Table 4.5.

Examples of Environmental Causes of Medical Problems

Medical Problem	Agent	Potential Exposures
Immediate or short-term effects		
Dermatoses (allergic or irritant)	Metals (chromium, nickel), fibrous glass, epoxy resins, cutting oils, solvents, caustic alkali, soaps	Electroplating, metal cleaning, machining, tanning, housekeeping, plastics, leather
Headache	Carbon monoxide, solvents; methylene chloride metabolizes to carbon monoxide	Firefighting, inhaling automobile exhaust, working in a foundry, dry cleaning, wood finishing
Acute psychoses	Mercury (especially organic), lead, carbon disulfide	Handling gasoline, seed handling, fungicide, wood preserving, viscose rayon industry
Asthma or dry cough	Formaldehyde, toluene diisocyanate, animal dander	Textiles, plastics, polyurethane kits, lacquer, handling animals
Pulmonary edema, pneumonitis	Nitrogen oxides, ozone, phosgene, halogen gases, cadmium	Welding, farming ("silo filler's disease"), chemical operations, smelting
Cardiac arrhythmias	Solvents, fluorocarbons	Metal cleaning, solvent use, refrigerator maintenance
Angina	Carbon monoxide, methylene chloride	Car repair, traffic exhaust, incomplete combustion in furnace or wood-burning stove, foundry, wood finishing
Abdominal pain	Lead	Battery making, enameling, smelting, painting, welding, ceramics, plumbing, stained glasswork
Tuberculosis infection	airborne *Mycobacterium tuberculosis*	Health care workers, jail personnel
Hepatitis	Halogenated hydrocarbons, e.g., carbon tetrachloride, virus	Solvent use, lacquer use, heath care workers
Latent or long-term effects		
Chronic dyspnea		
Pulmonary fibrosis	Asbestos, silica, beryllium, coal, aluminum	Mining, insulation, pipe fitting, sandblasting, quarrying, metal alloy work, aircraft or electrical parts
Chronic bronchitis emphysema	Cotton dust, cadmium coal dust, organic solvents, cigarettes	Textile industry, battery production, soldering, mining, solvent use
Lung cancer	Asbestos, arsenic, uranium, coke oven emissions, radon	Insulation, pipefitting, smelting, coke ovens, shipyard workers, nickel refining, uranium mining, residential radon exposure
Bladder cancer	β-Naphthylamine, benzidine dyes, arsenic	Dye industry, leather, rubber-workers, chemists, contaminated water or soil
Peripheral neuropathy	Lead, arsenic, *n*-hexane, methyl butylketone, acrylamide	Battery production, plumbing, smelting, painting, shoemaking, solvent use, pesticides
Behavioral changes	Lead, carbon disulfide, solvents, mercury, manganese	Battery makers, smelting, viscose rayon industry, degreasing, manufacturing/repair of scientific instruments, dental amalgam workers
Extrapyramidal syndrome	Carbon disulfide, manganese	Viscose rayon industry, steel production, battery production, foundry

continued

Table 4.5. (*continued*)
Examples of Environmental Causes of Medical Problems

Medical Problem	Agent	Potential Exposures
Aplastic anemia, leukemia	Benzene, ionizing radiation	Chemists, furniture refinishing, cleaning, degreasing, radiation workers

Modified from Goldman RH, Peters JM. The occupational and environmental health history. JAMA 1981;246:2831.

The second case, evaluating family members exposed to arsenic in drinking water, is an opportunity to provide information about the exposure and its relation to a potential health risk. Although the family members have no acute arsenic-related illness, evaluation of the amount of arsenic in the drinking water, the amount absorbed and excreted by the individual patient, and the subsequent risk of a chronic condition such as cancer could be evaluated. The physician may recognize a potentially hazardous exposure but be unsure about evaluating the potential health threat. The physician can consult and work with the local health department or an OEM specialist.

Some chemical and biologic agents have associated biomarkers of exposure that can be measured in blood (e.g., blood lead) and/or urine (e.g., urine arsenic levels). Patient-related factors such as young or old age, pregnancy, renal or liver dysfunction, or preexisting disease may increase the risk. Understanding exposure assessment, internal dose estimation, and awareness of patient-related factors is similar to the laws of pharmacology—i.e., knowledge about entry, absorption, metabolic transformation, distribution, storage, and excretion of drugs is applicable to chemical and biologic agents. Ultimately, your goal is to determine if an environmental agent poses a health risk to the patient. Further, for symptomatic patients, you want to determine if the environmental agent is causing or contributing to the patient's illness.

The following criteria are used to evaluate whether an environmental agent is associated with a health effect:

- Temporal association of the exposure to the health effect
- Route, duration, and biologic pathway of the agent
- Estimated dose of the agent and the subsequent health effect
- The complex of symptoms associated with the exposure

- Whether other people with similar exposure are similarly affected
- Whether a better medical explanation is found for the medical condition.

The most important criterion is *temporal association*. The exposure must precede the patient's symptoms, and there must also be biologic plausibility. For example, if a physician suspects that a patient's leukemia is caused by a workplace exposure to the well-known leukogenic agent benzene, the physician should verify that the patient was exposed to this chemical a minimum of 5 years before the date of diagnosis.

Temporal association is particularly true for skin and respiratory allergens. For example, a worker must be in contact with formaldehyde for several weeks before symptoms of red, irritated, and itching skin appear over the hands and forearms. The physician may not realize that the formaldehyde is the inciting agent because the patient will give a history of working with the chemical for weeks without any apparent problem. The timing and location of the rash should influence the clinician to consider the work-relatedness and chemical causation of the skin rash.

Patients with exposure-related illness or injury often present with common, undifferentiated symptoms such as itchy skin, back pain, shortness of breath, abdominal pain, cough, and fatigue. Workplace and other environmental exposures to hazardous agents cause common diseases such as dermatitis, lumbar strain, asthma, hepatitis, tuberculosis, and cancer. Table 4.5 lists examples of diseases, associated agents, and jobs or uses of the agent that may place the patient at risk for exposure.

By identifying hazardous exposures early, timely diagnosis and treatment or referral can occur. The treatment plan must include reduction or removal of the hazard from the patient's environment or vice versa, in order to prevent further disease and/or dysfunction. If the patient

Business Identity _____

Date_____

Employee's Name _____

Job Title_____

Employer _____

DIAGNOSIS (work-related only, otherwise note "private medical condition"): _____

_____

CARE PROVIDED ❑ Physician Exam   ❑ X-ray   ❑ Physical Therapy   ❑ Medication

  ❑ Other _____

WORK STATUS

❑ No restrictions

❑ Return to work on _____ with the following restrictions:

  ❑ No exposure to cold, heat, water dampness,   ❑ No repetitive shoveling

  chemicals, paint, dust, welding (circle)   ❑ No lifting over ___ lbs.

  ❑ Keep affected area clean and dry   ❑ No reaching above shoulder level

  ❑ No climbing of stairs or ladders   ❑ No kneeling or squatting

  ❑ No work around high speed or moving machinery

  ❑ No operating of mobile equipment

  ❑ Should be sitting _____ % of time

  ❑ No work requiring repetitive bending of _____

❑ Should be considered permanent

❑ No use of _____

❑ Limited use of _____

❑ Unable to work _____

❑ Expected return to full-duty _____

FOLLOW-UP CARE

❑ Scheduled for physician appointment **Date** _____   **Time** _____

❑ Recommended treatment includes_____

_____

_____

_____   _____
Physician's printed name   Physician's signature/date

Figure 4.3. Report-to-work form. (Modified from Welter ES. The role of the primary care physician in occupational medicine. In: Zenz C, ed. Occupational Medicine. St. Louis: CV Mosby, 1994:19.)

identifies coworkers, neighbors, or family members as being at risk, the physician should encourage further investigation by the employer or health department.

The family physician can determine the patient's ability to return to restricted work during the course of evaluation and treatment. Figure 4.3 is an example of a return-to-work form that will effectively communicate the patient's ability to work to the employer. You must identify that the diagnosis may be work-related; clearly delineate the patient's restrictions; provide an estimated date of return to full duty; and, communicate whether an evaluation of the work process or agents is necessary. An OEM specialist can give the family physician a comprehensive evaluation of whether an occupational or environmental exposure is related to an illness or injury and provide guidance regarding the patient's ability to return to the work or home environment.

ETHICAL ISSUES RELATED TO OCCUPATIONAL AND ENVIRONMENTAL HEALTH

Worker's compensation is the major financial resource available to individuals who cannot work because of a work-related illness or injury. This compensation is a legal mechanism and is based on a no-fault principle. Because each state is responsible for worker's compensation, the type and extent of coverage varies. Coverage usually includes all medical expenses, prescriptions related to diagnosis and treatment of a work-related illness or injury, and partial payment of wages. The physician's responsibility is to inform the patient whether or not the medical condition is work- related, briefly explain the state worker's compensation law, treat the illness, or refer the patient to an OEM specialist. The family physician should have an honest and forthright discussion with the patient regarding his or her opinion about the level of impairment related to the patient's medical condition rather than making a broad statement about disability. The physician should provide objective information in support of the patient's disability claim, but the physician does not determine whether the patient is eligible for disability benefits. Often the patient experiences a lengthy administrative process regarding eligibility for benefits and is frustrated and angry with the process and, therefore, may be frustrated and angry with the physician. Continued dialog with the patient and filling out all the necessary forms in a timely manner will promote a continued positive relationship between the patient and the physician.

Family physicians are often asked to provide medical services on behalf of employers. The most-often-requested services include (a) employment preplacement examinations, (b) employee injury care, and (c) return-to-work examinations. In addition, the family physician may also be the employee's personal physician. This occurs most often in smaller communities in which there are a limited number of industries and a limited number of primary care physicians. Three issues should be considered when working with the employer and the individual patient. These include (a) accountability (to whom does a physician respond, and to whom is the physician accountable); (b) confidentiality (who should have access to what medical information about the patient); and (c) reporting responsibility (to whom should suspected or known work-related and environmentally related hazards or illnesses be reported).

In all patient-physician relationships, it is the duty of the physician to advocate and be accountable for the health of the patient. The American College of Occupational and Environmental Medicine stresses that (a) the highest priority is to be given to the health and safety of the individual; (b) the physician must practice on the scientific basis of objectivity and integrity, and; (c) the physician must give an honest opinion and avoid having his or her medical judgment influenced by any conflict of interest. Consultation from a health and safety specialist, an industrial hygienist, or an OEM specialist regarding potential workplace hazards can be requested from the employer to further facilitate the family physician's ability to promote the health and well-being of the employees.

Who should have access to what medical information about the patient has been decided by OSHA and other legal opinions. The courts have ruled that, with respect to employment preplacement examinations, the patient has waived his or her rights to confidentiality, and the information obtained during this medical evaluation is the property of the employer. Further, employees and their designated representatives have the right of access to relevant exposure and medical records kept by the employer. Patients must authorize the release of their medical information before the medical record is disclosed to another third party. These confidentiality rules apply to oral communication as well as written information. Often, the physician is called on the telephone by another health care provider or case manager, such as when the patient's personal physician is called by the employer's nurse or doctor, for medical information. The physician should secure a signed release from the patient before disclosing private medical information. It is important to always be guided by the principle of what is best for the health and welfare of the patient.

In addition to the physician's responsibility to insure the health of the patient, the physician is also obligated to protect the health of the patient's fellow workers, neighbors, and family. Many states require physician reporting of occupational illnesses. Always discuss disclosure of the hazardous environment with the patient employee, and document and abide by any agreed-upon decision. Do not enter into a binding agreement with a patient if there is an overriding public health concern.

RESOURCES

Many resources are available to assist the family physician with obtaining additional knowledge and skill related to hazardous exposures and subsequent health risk or disease and injury. Consultation on specific cases of suspected exposure-related illness is also available through both local and national resources. Table 4.6 lists some of these resources.

CASE STUDY 1

Mr. Sean Mulligan is a 38-year-old man who presents with sharp pain in his right wrist and numbness in his right hand. The pain is intermittent, sharp, and localized to the wrist. The numbness is in the middle finger, thumb, and dorsum of his right hand. The problem started approximately 2 years ago; however, it has been worsening over the past 8 months, during which he has frequently awakened at night with the pain and numbness. All over-the-counter anti-inflammatory medication only slightly relieved the pain. He does not perform many tasks at home with his hand because resting the hand provides some relief. He presents today because the pain and numbness is beginning to interfere with his work and his ability to grip and turn the steering wheel of his car.

QUESTION

1. What additional questions should you ask Mr. Mulligan about how he uses his hands?

DISCUSSION

You acquire more information about Mr. Mulligan's job. He is a machinist in an aircraft engine plant, where he has worked 5 years. Two years ago he was moved into a job that involves repetitive turning of set screws in an engine part using an Allen wrench. He describes having to use quite a bit of force in order to adjust the screw to the appropriate position. He has had to work a 12-hour shift many times; one of these periods of increased work time coincided with the onset of his hand problem. At first, the hand problem resolved overnight. Mr. Mulligan works very quickly because he is paid based on a "piecework" rate, such that the more pieces he finishes, the higher his pay. He has no hobbies and he lives in a newer home that requires little maintenance.

QUESTIONS

1. What is your differential diagnosis?
2. What steps do you take next?

DISCUSSION

The symptoms described—the pain in his wrist and the numb feeling in the middle finger, thumb, and dorsum of the palm of his hand—suggest carpal tunnel syndrome (CTS). Symptoms of CTS usually begin gradually and tend to be most severe at night as a result of wrist flexion during sleep. The symptoms may progress to sensations of swelling and hand grip weakness owing to loss of nerve function. Advanced cases may include wasting of the muscles at the base of the thumb (thenar atrophy). You suspect that the patient's job is either causing the medical problem or aggravating an underlying medical condition. You recall that diabetes mellitus, rheumatoid arthritis, and thyroid disease can cause CTS and so inquire

Table 4.6.

Resources for Information and Assistance in the
Clinical Evaluation of Exposure-Related Illness and Injury

Government agencies

Occupational Safety and Health Administration (OSHA), (202) 219-9148 (general information), (202) 219-4667 (publications), Internet: http://www.osha-slc.gov/	OSHA sets and enforces workplace health and safety standards. OSHA distributes fact sheets about engineering controls and work practices to limit exposures to selected hazardous exposures.
National Institute for Occupational Safety and Health (NIOSH), (800) 356-4674, Internet: http://www.cdc.gov/niosh/homepage.html	NIOSH provides information about substance toxicity and workplace hazards. The health hazard evaluation program can investigate worksites at which physicians, employers, or employees suspect work-related illness and injury to have occurred.
Agency for Toxic Substances and Disease Registry (ATSDR), (404) 639-6000 (toxicology) and (404) 639-6206 (health education)	ATSDR provides toxicologic profiles and clinically 26 useful case studies in environmental medicine with CME credits.
Environmental Protection Agency (EPA), (202) 554-1404, Internet: http://www.epa.gov	Assesses and controls environmental problems such as air and water pollution and hazardous waste.

National organizations

American College of Occupational and Environmental Medicine (ACOEM), (847) 228-6850 (general information), (800) 226-3626 (ACOEM INSTA-facts), Internet: http://www.acoem.org	A list of board certified occupational and environmental medicine specialists can be obtained through INSTA-facts.
Association of Occupational and Environmental Clinics (AOEC), (202) 347-4976, Kathy Kirkland, Executive Director	A list of a clinics affiliated with medical schools throughout the country can be obtained. Member clinics provide professional training, community education, and clinical evaluations/consultations. Clinicians can contact the AOEC office for the nearest geographically located site. Clinical and other OEM information that is reviewed and updated by AOEC member Gary Greenberg, MD, can also be viewed at internet address http://occ-env-med.mc.duke.edu/oem

Local resources

Poison Control Centers; contact your local health department for the nearest poison control center.	These centers have medical toxicologists on staff.
University-based programs in occupational health, industrial hygiene, or toxicology; contact your local university.	Schools of public health, medical schools, universities, and comprehensive cancer centers function as resources to local communities.
Hospital-based occupational health service programs; contact your local hospital.	Some hospitals have occupational and environmental medicine specialists on staff.

Suggested textbooks for reference

Preventing Occupational Disease and Injury	Weeks JL, Berry SL, Wagner GR, eds. American Public Health Association, 1991. ISBN 0-87533-172-5
Occupational Health: Recognizing and Preventing Work-Related Disease, 3rd ed.	Levy BS, Wegman DH. Little, Brown and Co., 1995. ISBN 0-316-52271-6
Principles and Practice of Environmental Medicine	Tarcher AB. Plenum Publishing, 1992. ISBN 0-306-42893-8
Occupational and Environmental Reproductive Hazards: A Guide for Clinicians	Paul M. Williams & Wilkins, 1993. ISBN 0-683-06801-6
The Workplace Walk-Through	Kornberg J. Lewis Publishers, 1992. ISBN 0-87371-620-5 (vol.1)
Guides to the Evaluation of Permanent Impairment, 4th ed.	American Medical Association, 1993. ISBN 0-89970-553-7
Morbidity and Mortality Weekly Report	Massachusetts Medical Society, PO Box 9120, Waltham, MA 02254-9120. ISSN 0149-2195
State-specific workers compensation manual. Example: Worker's Compensation in Michigan: Law and Practice	Welch EM. Institute of Continuing Legal Education, (313) 764-0533.

about these; his medical history is negative. Your differential diagnosis includes de Quervain's tenosynovitis, which affects primarily the thumb.

The physical examination reveals callused skin over his fingers on the right hand, which correlates with his repetitive grasping of the Allen wrench. No swelling, erythema, or muscle atrophy is observed. There is no visible evidence of arthritic changes, and there is minimal pain to palpation. Finklestein's test (for de Quervain's tenosynovitis) and Phalen's test (for CTS) are both positive. There is no decreased sensation to pinprick. The patient's right-hand grip is considerably less strong than his left-hand grip (he is right-handed).

Based on your history and physical examination, you suspect Mr. Mulligan has CTS or de Quervain's tenosynovitis. Blood tests confirm that Mr. Mulligan does not have diabetes, thyroid disease, or rheumatoid arthritis. You order nerve conduction velocity studies (NCV) and electromyography studies (EMG) to confirm CTS. You are concerned that the job-related risk factors for CTS/CTD (carpal tunnel syndrome/decompression), such as repetitive motions, forceful gripping of the hand and fingers, awkward joint positions, and prolonged posture of the hand, are the cause of his hand problems. You share your suspicion with Mr. Mulligan, and he agrees with your assessment of the work-relatedness of his condition.

You decide to take Mr. Mulligan off work for the next 2 weeks as a trial of rest for the hand. He is visibly alarmed at your recommendation and tells you that he cannot afford to take this time off, and, further, he is concerned that he might lose his job if you contact the employer with your suspicions that his condition is work-related. He reminds you that you care for his special-needs son who requires extensive medical care covered by employer-provided medical insurance.

QUESTION

1. Rather than taking Mr. Mulligan off work, what job modifications can you recommend?

DISCUSSION

If work-related actions that cause or aggravate the illness can be identified, suggestions for job modifications become a crucial part of the therapeutic plan. Practical approaches to job modification include (a) identification of the job-related risk factors causing the medical problem, (b) assessment by the employee and the employer of the risk factors that can be modified, and (c) assessment of options that modify the exposure to the risk factors by changing the work process, using alternate tools, reducing the time spent on a high-risk task by job rotation or transfer, or using protective equipment.

After some discussion, you and Mr. Mulligan decide to notify his employer of Mr. Mulligan's work-related CTS/CTD. You recommend work modifications based upon information provided by Mr. Mulligan.

After 2 weeks, Mr. Mulligan returns for his follow-up visit. Rest, splinting, and anti-inflammatory medication have not substantially reduced his pain or numbness. He did file a workers' compensation claim, which has yet to be accepted. He is scheduled to see a workers' compensation physician to review his claim in 2 weeks and is requesting a copy of his complete medical record. There was no modified work available for him at the plant; therefore, he has been at home, taking it easy. His income loss is covered by sick benefits.

You review the results of the NCV/EMG tests, which show prolongation of the distal latency of the right median nerve, absence of the right median nerve sensory amplitudes, and early pattern of right median nerve enervation. These results are consistent with right CTS. You recommend that he see a specialist for surgical release of the right median nerve. You provide him with a copy of his medical record, including the results of the NCV/EMG studies.

He proceeds with the surgery, which is uneventful, undergoes hand-strengthening rehabilitation, and is returned to unrestricted work by the medical specialist in approximately 6 weeks. Workers' compensation accepts his claim and pays for your professional services rendered to Mr. Mulligan. You report Mr. Mulligan's work-related CTS to the proper state agency.

QUESTION

1. Will Mr. Mulligan return to you in the future with the same medical condition?

DISCUSSION

Without permanent job modifications, his condition will likely recur.

CASE STUDY 2

You see a patient in the office for the first time. He is a 26-year-old, healthy-appearing white man who complains of headaches, irritability, breathing problems, a ready loss of temper, stinging eyes, a chronic rash, and difficulty keeping his balance. He admits to occasional alcohol use and to being under stress at work. When you ask him about his employment, he tells you that he is an incinerator operator in a waste treatment facility in the town where you practice. He claims that several other people at work have similar symptoms—headaches, irritability, and rashes—and that he has a friend who lives in the neighborhood who also is ill.

Physical examination reveals a healthy-appearing man. You notice a reddish eczematoid rash on his extremities and face. On neurologic examination, he cannot do tandem gait, and the Romberg is questionable. Otherwise the physical and neurologic examinations are unremarkable.

QUESTIONS

1. Given this information, what diagnostic hypotheses come to mind?
2. How can you differentiate stress-related symptoms from those induced by occupational exposure to hazardous substances?
3. If you felt that an occupational ideology were likely, what steps would you take to help this patient?

DISCUSSION

This case scenario presented in the mid-1980s to Dr. Mark Guerra, a family physician in a small town in North Carolina. He had seen a couple of other patients with a similar story, but it was not until a friend challenged him to go to the incinerator that he began to appreciate the severity of the complaints. On site near the incinerator at 1:00 o'clock in the morning, a time when the incinerator managed especially toxic substances, he noted severe burning of his eyes and face and development of dyspnea. Spurred by direct observation and concern for his patients, Dr. Guerra began a long series of inquires and advocacy. Through working with his patient, who operated the incinerator during the daytime and, therefore, was aware of what chemicals were shipped into the facility, Dr. Guerra found that the facility was managing a wide variety of toxic solvents, including tetrachlorethylene (which turns into phosgene and hydrochloric acid upon incineration), heavy metals such as lead and cadmium, and benzodioxin. He reported his findings to the County Health Department and the State Department of Human Resources, but neither took action. Over the next 6 months, as other individuals in the community learned of Dr. Guerra's interest, over 14 patients came forth concerned about their health, with stories of headaches, nausea, vomiting, rashes, personality changes, memory problems, and balance disorders.

As time went by, Dr. Guerra became increasingly involved in the impact of the incinerator on the health of his patients and their community. Unsatisfied with the response from local and state authorities, he contacted and worked with his Congressman, who got him in touch with the Environmental Protection Agency (EPA) and the Federal Agency for Toxic Substance and Disease Registry. He sent his patients to specialists with expertise in occupationally induced reactive airway syndrome and solvent-induced neurologic disorders.

One patient went to San Francisco to be evaluated by a world expert in the field. Federal investigators from the EPA documented that symptoms were most severe immediately around the incinerator and downwind from the facility. They documented that the facility was operating at more than twice the maximum feed rate recommended by the incinerator manufacturer and that employees were paid on a productivity basis.

Eventually, the facility was closed, and Dr. Guerra was able to get a number of his patients financial support through workers' compensation for their disabilities. In addition, his work through the EPA was considered a model for practicing physicians, and it resulted in the development of national protocols to enhance the EPA's responsiveness to physician inquires. Dr. Guerra was asked to testify before Congress in support of the Worker Family Protection Act, which subsequently passed. In 1995, an international conference on hazardous waste met in Atlanta; six of the 20 papers presented there involved Dr. Guerra's patients.

REFERENCES

1. Ahmann E. "Chunky stew:" Appreciating cultural diversity while providing health care for children. Pediatr Nurs 1994;20:320–324.
2. Pathman DE, Konard TR, Ricketts TC. The national Health Service Corps experience for rural physicians in the late 1980s. JAMA 1994;272(17):1341–1348.
3. Russell K, Jewell N. Cultural impact of health-care access: challenges for improving the health of African Americans. J Community Health Nurs 1992;9:161–169.
4. Health and Public Policy Committee American College of Physicians. Chemical dependence. Ann Intern Med 1985;102:405–408.
5. Liptak GS, Revell GM. Community physician's role in case management of children with chronic illnesses. Pediatrics 1989;84:465–471.
6. Abramson JH. Community-oriented primary care-strategy, approaches, and practice: A review. Public Health Rep 1988;16:35–98.
7. Nutting PA. Community-oriented primary care: researchable questions for family practice. J Fam Pract 1990;30:633–635.
8. Gold MR, Franks P. A community-oriented primary care project in a rural population: reducing cardiovascular risk. J Fam Pract 1990;30:639–644.
9. Rogers DE. Community-oriented primary care. JAMA 1982;248:1622–1625.
10. Mullan F. Sounding board—Community oriented primary care: an agenda for the '80s. N Engl J Med 1982;307(17):1076–1078.
11. Keenan JM. Home care: past and present, problems and potential. J Am Geriatr Soc 1989;37(11):1076–1083.
12. American Medical Association. Role of the Physician. Guidelines for the Medical Management of the Home Care Patient. Chicago: American Medical Association, 1992.
13. Physician involvement in home care: a report of the AMA Council on Scientific Affairs. American Medical Association House of Delegates meeting, December 1996.
14. Discher DP, Kleinman GD, Foster FJ. National Occupational Hazard Survey: Pilot Study for Development of an Occupational Disease Surveillance Method. Washington, DC: National Institute for Occupational Safety and Health, 1975.
15. Gennart JP, Hoet P, Lison D, Lauwerys R, Coche E, Lambert M. Importance of accurate employment histories of patients admitted to units of internal medicine. Scand J Work Environ Health 1991;17:386–391.
16. McCallum DB, Covello VT. What the public thinks about environmental data. EPAJ 1989;May/June:22–23.

5. Family Practice in an Era of Rapid Change

LOUIS B. JACQUES

Key Questions

1. What are the main organizational and administrative characteristics of today's family practice?
2. What employment opportunities exist in family practice?
3. What forces are shaping the medical practice environment that you will enter when you finish your training?

If you are beginning a medical career, you can anticipate a lifetime during which medical practice will evolve markedly. This chapter provides an overview of the state of medical practice in the United States today, focusing on issues relevant to family medicine. It is designed to guide your observations and aid your interpretation of the business aspects of medicine as a student and resident. Just as reading about low back pain or sore throat provides a framework for you to see patients with these conditions, this material will help you to understand the operation of medical practices within which you work.

CHOOSING A CAREER AND FINDING A JOB

Specialty Choice

Specialty choice is an individualized process that depends on personal, professional, and financial priorities. Although many students enter medical school with specific career goals, research shows that many will change their minds at some point during the 4 years (1). Most students firm up their decision during the third-year clinical clerkships, in preparation for the fourth year task of residency application and "the match." Factors important in career choice have been studied extensively, with sometimes contradictory results (2). The easiest way to determine the current demand for the specialties you are considering is to examine the classified advertising sections in relevant journals, noting employment opportunities by geographic location and field of interest.

Residency

Residency training is crucial for future employability, since employers and insurers generally favor physicians who are board certified. Many physicians who initially entered practice after 1 or 2 years of postgraduate training have returned to complete residency training because of their difficulty in obtaining hospital privileges and insurance reimbursement without board certification.

By 1996, there were 452 accredited family practice programs in the United States, training a total of 10,102 residents (3). Most programs (268) were in community hospitals and affiliated with medical schools. The American Academy of Family Physicians publishes a yearly directory of the civilian and military residency programs in family medicine. Your school's department of family medicine can provide a copy. Some students apply to as few as two or three programs; others consider as many as 40. Most students seem to focus seriously on between five and 10. Approximately 90% of family practice positions are filled during the match; postmatch activity fills another 8% (4).

Residency training in family practice lasts 3 years; 6% of graduates pursue additional fellowship training in fields such as geriatrics and sports medicine. A key characteristic of training is continuity care for a personal panel of patients over 3 years. First-year residents usually spend 1 half-day per week in the Family Practice Center seeing their own patients. This increases to 3 half-days in the second year and 5 half-days in the third year. Behavioral science is taught longitudinally in each year. The majority of programs follow a traditional block month schedule for other subjects. A typical first-year resident experiences surgery; pediatrics, including neonatology; obstetrics; inpatient medicine (including intensive care and coronary care); inpatient family practice; and emergency care. Second-year residents rotate in medical and surgical subspecialty areas such as orthopedics, ophthalmology, otolaryngology, cardiology, and urology. Third-year residents manage the inpatient family practice service and take additional required and elective experiences such as geriatrics, dermatology, community medicine, and gynecology. There is some flexibility in the timing and elective options of these experiences, especially in years two and three.

Job Hunting

Finding a job becomes a priority for family practice residents during the middle of the second year, as they receive an increasing volume of mail from physician placement firms and inquiries from local physicians and medical groups. Approximately half of new residency graduates initially practice in or near the community of their residency program. Of the almost 3,000 residents who graduated from family practice programs in 1996, 46% entered single-specialty groups. Twelve percent joined multispecialty groups, and less than 5% chose solo practice. Thirty percent opted for small town (2,500 to 10,000) locations greater than 25 miles from a large city (5).

OFFICE PRACTICE

Practice Types

Your initial interest in medicine may have been fostered by a childhood role model, possibly your own personal physician. The image of the kindly doctor in solo practice is part of the lore of American medicine. Before World War II, physician groups were very rare; the Mayo Clinic began in the 1890s, and Kaiser in 1938. Over the past 30 years, group practice has steadily grown, from 10% in 1965 to 33% in 1995 (6).

Group practice offers competitive advantages for physicians. Medical groups reduce expenses through the sharing of resources and achievement of economies of scale. Given an oversupply and maldistribution of physicians in many locales, especially in large metropolitan areas, insurance companies have powerful leverage to limit payment to physicians. By serving a larger market share and offering a comprehensive array of services at lower cost, groups can be more competitive. Rapid growth of managed care with

its emphasis on cost control and shared risk has hastened this movement. A large medical group can accept more risk because of its financial strength, being better able to absorb the cost of a few sick patients.

Larger multispecialty groups are able to offer services that are integrated both vertically and horizontally. Vertical integration (or depth) refers to the provision of services at many locations and levels of intensity to individual patients and populations. For example, a vertically integrated health system includes hospital care, professional physician services, medical equipment, home care, and health insurance. In contrast, providers that are not vertically integrated provide services at one or a few levels and depend on referrals to outside providers for other services. Horizontal integration (or breadth) refers to the delivery of services by many providers within a level of care. A solo physician practice would have no horizontal integration compared to a multispecialty physician group, which offers a wide variety of physician services within the same organization. Integration, both vertical and horizontal, increases with organizational size.

Group practice offers the individual physician a wealth of other benefits, as well as some significant liabilities. The "culture" of the group, with its camaraderie and security, can be reassuring. Physicians generally spend less time performing administrative practice management duties because these are assumed by the officers of the group. On-call coverage is shared, although the physician is responsible for a larger number of patients while on-call. Consultation is readily available, often informally at the "curbside," and a shared medical record allows the primary care physician and the consultant easy access to the same patient information. In general, primary care physicians receive higher salaries in group practice than they would otherwise generate by patient care alone. Recognizing the value of affiliation with a large pool of referring physicians, subspecialists accept a lower salary in order to ensure a steady source of referrals. This practice is called cross-subsidization.

For some physicians, the loss of autonomy in group practice is a significant drawback. Medical groups generally have a formal utilization review process, and may have "cookbook" practice guidelines and restricted prescribing practices. With shared responsibility comes shared risk; all of the partners are accountable for the acts of a single member. Equitable compensation across specialty lines continues to be a problem.

Managed Care

Managed care is based on the principle of capitation (payment per assigned patient). Utilization (and thus cost) is controlled through the prepayment of a fixed fee for each "covered life" (the technical term for a person enrolled in the insurance plan). This is commonly expressed as payment per member per month. Correspondingly, the expense generated by the care of a panel of patients is expressed as cost per member per month. By paying a fixed fee up front (prepayment) for physician services, the third-party payer (insurance company, health maintenance organization [HMO], Medicare, etc.) hopes to limit the physician's incentive to provide expensive services. A portion of the capitation fee, called a withhold, is kept until the end of the year to encourage the physician to be frugal. Thus, the physician shares the risk for the health of the patient, in effect becoming a co-insurer. Plainly, this can create a real or perceived conflict between the patient's interests and the physician's need to control costs and maximize practice income.

In contrast, fee-for-service insurance, such as traditional Blue Cross/Blue Shield, reimburses the physician for each service performed. Simply put, do more to make more. Most fee-for-service insurance requires that the patient pay a portion of the bill (co-pay) for some outpatient services.

It is convenient to think of these insurance options as falling upon a managed care continuum, or spectrum. On one end is care that is totally managed, exemplified by an HMO; at the opposite end is traditional fee-for-service. HMOs are characterized by lower costs, fewer choices, and more covered services. In contrast, fee-for-service offers greater choice but with increased cost and fewer covered services. Other compromise options, such as a PPO (preferred provider organization) or an IPA (independent practice association), share some characteristics of each extreme. As the number of patients enrolled in managed care plans has expanded, exceeding the number enrolled in traditional fee-for-service plans in 1993, market consolidation has decreased the number of managed care insurers. Between 1976 and 1994, managed care enrollment rose from 6 million to 51 million covered lives (7).

Physician utilization varies by age and sex. Average patients who are less than a year old make about four visits annually in outpatient settings, and those who are over 65 make about seven visits annually (8). From young adulthood until middle age, women make more visits than men, largely for reproductive care. For small practice populations, age and sex become inadequate predictors. Historical data from prior years can provide estimates of future needs.

Utilization Review

Utilization review (UR) evaluates the delivery of health care by physicians and hospitals. There are two types of UR—retrospective and prospective:

- Retrospective UR involves selected individual patient charts being audited according to criteria that may serve as a proxy for quality. These include issues of documentation, such as timely and complete progress notes, substantive issues of care, such as the prescription of appropriate medication or testing, and outcomes such as morbidity, mortality, and total monetary cost. From these individual pieces of information, assumptions are made about the physician practice as a whole.

- Prospective UR requires the physician to call the insurer to obtain *prior authorization* before ordering certain tests or referring the patient to a consultant. Nonauthorized procedures may still be performed, but will not be reimbursed.

For utilization review to affect behavior, the data must be made available to individual physicians. This is accomplished in a variety of ways. If the auditing process generates questions about an individual case, the physician is required to provide documentation to support the care given. Summary data are provided on a monthly, quarterly, or yearly basis. These reports generally include charts or graphs that compare the physician to other physicians on the insurance plan panel, national average data, or Medicare guidelines. Examples are shown in Figure 5.1 and Table 5.1. Although not explicitly stated in the letters that accompany the data, many physicians interpret these reports as incentives to lower utilization and cost.

Establishing and Running a Practice

The tasks of establishing and running a practice are similar whether it is a solo private practice or a large multispecialty group. In group practices, these duties are generally handled by an

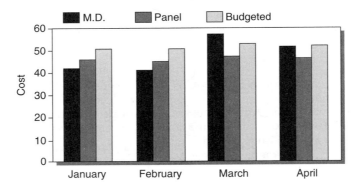

Figure 5.1. *Sample HMO cost report.* This sample report compares the cost per member per month (PMPM) of a physician to that of peers on the HMO staff panel and to a budget prediction. For each month, the individual physician's data have been summarized to show an average cost. Reasons for the variation between quarters might include variations in patient diagnoses and severity of illness, number of tests done, and an increase in the number of patient visits due to, for example, an outbreak of viral diarrhea in the community. The ability of the physician to control some of these factors may be minimal.

administrative staff; for a solo practitioner, these are the physician's responsibilities.

Office Location and Space

An obvious question that is too often overlooked is, "Are there enough potential patients to support my practice?" Because of the nature of the services they provide, generalists can practice successfully with a patient population as small as 2,000. In contrast, a neurosurgeon may need to draw from a population of 100,000 in order to have enough patients. Intuitively, this is obvious: the proportion of people needing basic primary care is larger than the proportion of people needing brain surgery. If you are thinking of practicing in a certain community, data from the U.S.

census can provide a snapshot view of the characteristics of your potential patients by age, sex, and household income. An aging community in the sunbelt may be ideal for an internist but disastrous for a pediatrician. When you have established that there are enough suitable potential patients for your practice, the next step is to make sure that there is enough demand for another physician (you) in this community.

Where can you find patients? How can they find you? Patients come to you from four sources: capitated members of insurance plans, referrals from other satisfied patients, self-referrals from your marketing efforts, and professional referrals from your colleagues. If you start a practice in the same city as your residency training, many of your patients will follow you to your new

Table 5.1.
Sample Data for an HMO Physician[a]

Month	No. of Enrolled Patients	No. of Visits	Hospital Days	Lab and X-ray $	Pharmacy $	Total $ PMPM
January	1,609	387	15	$457	$7,566	$42
February	1,634	371	17	$870	$6,989	$41
March	1,701	453	24	$1,543	$8,807	$57
April	1,721	414	18	$514	$7,005	$51

[a]The chart shown in Figure 5.1 was derived from data in this table, which summarizes the utilization over the past 4 months for a sample physician's panel of enrolled patients. In any given month, most patients were not seen in the office. The practice is growing, shown by the steady increase in the number of enrolled patients. A disproportionately high number of patient visits occurred in March, possibly due to an outbreak of influenza in the community. This caused a rise in the number of days spent in the hospital by the patients in the panel and contributed to an increase in laboratory, radiograph, and drug costs. Total pharmacy costs include chronic medications, such as antihypertensive drugs that are taken by patients who were not actually seen during the month, and acute medications, such as antibiotics and analgesics.

practice. Physician advertising is still relatively rare. Commonly, a small advertisement describing your new practice will be run in the local newspaper for a period of weeks. If you are new to a small town, your arrival may even be the topic of a newspaper article. Colleagues can be a valuable referral source. Thus, it is important to participate in hospital staff meetings and professional society activities. Unattached patients from the hospital emergency department may be referred to you for follow-up care.

A solo family physician needs a minimum of 1,000 to 1,200 square feet of office space (9). Many options exist. An office within an existing medical building may provide convenient parking, proximity to laboratory x-ray, pharmacy, and consultants, and access to a pool of potential patients. An office in a commercial development, such as a strip mall or business district, may be more convenient for patients who come from work or who are running errands. A site in a residential area, possibly even in your home, may promote a sense of belonging to the community. While this arrangement can be very convenient for seeing the occasional after-hours patient, it will make it difficult to protect your privacy and family time.

New offices must comply with the 1991 Americans With Disabilities Act (ADA), which requires accessibility for disabled individuals. For example, hallways must be wide enough to permit two wheelchairs to pass, doors must permit easy entry and egress, rest rooms must be wheelchair accessible, and stairs should be avoided if possible. These measures also make it easier for emergency personnel to treat and transport critically ill patients in your office.

For efficiency, examination rooms should have a standardized layout, which will increase the ease of finding and stocking supplies. Floors should not be carpeted, as carpeting prevents easy detection and cleanup of potentially hazardous spills. Examination tables should be positioned to assure patient privacy from hallway traffic when doors are opened and from windows. Toxic chemicals, hazardous waste products, and "sharps", such as drugs, cleaners, and needles must be out of reach of young children. Personal protective equipment and waste disposal containers should be readily accessible in every room. The overall flow of patients from waiting room to checkout and billing is enhanced by a logical floor plan that accounts for traffic patterns between related and sequential activities.

Personnel

Staffing needs depend on the services you provide, but the following functions should be covered in any office: telephone answering and appointment scheduling; greeting and registration; escort to the examination areas and triage; assistance with physical examination (including chaperoning, collecting specimens, and performing laboratory tests and x-rays); billing; collection and checkout; medical record keeping; ordering and stocking of supplies; housekeeping; and hazardous waste disposal.

Personnel (human resources) issues are quite complex and have legal and tax implications. Most offices find it helpful to have a personnel manual or employee handbook. Great care must be taken to maintain the confidentiality of personnel records, and they should be stored in a secure area with strictly limited access. Adherence to proper administrative procedures for hiring and disciplining employees must be well-documented. As with patient charts, all supporting material should be included. State and federal law govern the disposal of these records. For example, the Occupational Safety and Health Administration (OSHA) regulations on employee exposure to bloodborne pathogens requires employers to maintain employee medical records for the duration of the employee's employment *plus 30 years* (10). If the employer goes out of business, these records must be sent to the government.

Increasingly, physicians work with nonphysician providers. Collaborative relationships exist in many practices between physicians and physician assistants, nurse practitioners, and nurse midwives. There are many reasons for this. Nonphysicians are paid significantly less than physicians, allowing some health care services to be provided with less expense. In 1996, the average salary for a physician assistant employed by a family physician was $58,547 (11). The professional nature of these relationships is governed by state law. Many states restrict the practice and prescribing authority of nonphysicians, requiring a supervisory role for the physician.

Equipment and Supplies

Before rushing out to purchase or lease equipment, it is important to be realistic about what procedures you will be performing on a regular basis. You do not need to replicate your residency site; because of their teaching function, many residency sites have pieces of equipment that may be appropriate for a larger, multiphysician office but inappropriate for a solo practitioner. To the extent that a piece of equipment must be paid for whether you use it or not, it makes little sense to fill your office with tools (aside from some emergency supplies) that will be largely unused. Instead, it may be more efficient for you to concentrate on a few procedures that you will do on a frequent basis, and refer other seldom-performed procedures to a trusted colleague.

Medical Records

The components of the record seem endless: flow sheets, databases, problem lists, genograms, family charts, insurance information, consent forms, advance directives, test reports, consultants' letters, and progress notes. There are paper records, electronic records, and combinations of the two. The availability of so many possibilities suggests that no single system satisfies everyone's needs.

A central question can be posed, "Who will use this record, and what will they use it for?" Beside you and your staff, other legitimate users of the record include other health care providers, reviewers from insurance companies, attorneys representing your patient in disability or malpractice claims, attorneys defending you against a malpractice claim, medical investigators conducting practice-based research, governmental auditors examining your billing practices, and the patient himself.

A good medical record fulfills three criteria:

- It is a comprehensive, lasting record of relevant information about the patient. Imagine reviewing the chart with your patient's attorney or with an insurance auditor. Do the history and physical findings support your diagnostic plan and treatment? Does the record contain embarrassing or inappropriate statements about the patient or other physicians? Does the service you provided justify the fee you charged? Have you documented informed consent for the procedures you performed? Have abnormal results been communicated to the patient and appropriate follow-up provided? If you or your partners have provided after-hours telephone advice to your patient, is there a supporting note in the chart?

- Data entry and retrieval should be easy. When faced with a patient who has the proverbial "chart as thick as a telephone book," can you quickly find an old x-ray report or ECG? For patients with chronic illnesses like hypertension, can you monitor their progress over time with a flow sheet, or do you flip pages looking for old blood pressure readings? When the patient calls for a medication refill, are the dose and amount legibly documented, or do you have to call the patient to find out what she's taking? Is the timing of appropriate screening tests or immunizations recorded in a manner that allows you to quickly see when your patient is due for her next Papanicolaou (Pap) smear or tetanus toxoid booster, or do you waste time hunting for this information? Is progress note entry efficient and easy?

- Confidentiality must be easily maintained. Storage and release of the information contained in a medical record to authorized parties is governed by state and federal law. Although the physician practice owns the physical chart (i.e., the papers, etc.), the patient is acknowledged as the owner of the information, and may request its release.

Finances

Few new physicians have financial resources to cover the start-up expenses of a new practice; this generally requires a loan from a bank or similar institution. Table 5.2 shows representative costs of common practice expenses. Those entering an existing partnership often have these costs covered by the practice in exchange for a lower starting salary. After a specified period of time depending on the contract provisions, the new physician may be given the opportunity to become a practice partner. This can involve an additional monetary payment to the practice. The need for sound financial and legal advice is apparent.

Physician reimbursement is tied to diagnosis; thus, a common terminology of "diagnostic codes" was needed to describe medical conditions and physician services. The clinical modification of the tenth revision of the World Health Organization's *International Classification of Diseases and Related Health Problems* (ICD-10) is generally used in family practice; it lists three- to five-digit alphanumeric codes for virtually every conceivable medical diagnosis in minute detail. Picking the correct code is vital because payment varies significantly between seemingly related codes. Some codes are not reimbursed at all.

In addition to a diagnosis code, every bill requires an E & M (evaluation and management)

Table 5.2.
Median Practice Spending in Major Categories, Per Physician

	Office Payroll	Office Space	Malpractice Premiums	Business Supplies	Drugs and Medical Supplies	Laboratory
Family practice	$59,000	$15,350	$6,800	$5,850	$7,290	$6,410
General practice	$44,680	$13,690	$7,330	$3,320	$4,140	$5,320
Internal medicine	$52,600	$15,920	$7,020	$4,970	$3,580	$5,000
OB/GYN	$58,540	$24,720	$34,390	$7,000	$5,760	$8,160
Pediatrics	$56,930	$18,360	$7,130	$6,390	$23,520	$2,000
All nonsurgery	$49,590	$15,210	$7,230	$4,880	$5,590	$4,760
All fields	$52,680	$17,320	$10,220	$5,180	$5,500	$5,030

The source for all data is the *Medical Economics* Continuing Survey, 1991 and 1996. Spending figures are based on 1995 expenses. Office payroll includes salaries, bonuses, and retirement-plan contributions for nonphysician employees. Office space includes rent or mortgage payments. Medical supplies include small instruments that are not depreciated. (Reprinted with permission from Rice B. Winning times for primary care physicians. Med Econ 1997:88–99.)

code and a code for any procedures performed. Five levels of E & M coding are used for most ambulatory services, with allowance made for new patients versus established patients.

Billing and reimbursement are based on the complexity of the medical decision making needed to address the patient's problems. This is classified into four levels: straightforward, low, moderate, and high. Except in cases in which the major purpose of the encounter is counseling, complexity is not explicitly linked with time. In other words, a 45-minute visit is not necessarily more complex than a 20-minute visit. Procedures are described with Current Procedural Terminology (CPT) codes. It is important to remember that every CPT code must be supported by an appropriate ICD-10 code. For example, a CPT code for incision and drainage would be rejected without an ICD-10 code for a condition requiring incision and drainage, such as an abscess. If a patient is seen for multiple problems, each problem must be accounted for by separate codes.

You should be familiar with a few basic accounting terms commonly used in medical practice:

- *Accounts payable:* bills that you owe but have not yet paid

- *Accounts receivable:* money owed to you that has not been collected. This is reported in 30-day increments, which tell you how much time has passed since the bill was sent

- *Collection ratio:* the ratio of the dollar amount collected over the dollar amount billed

- *Depreciation:* adjustment for the diminished value of a capital asset, such as an ECG machine, over time

Consults and Referrals

Although the terms are often and erroneously used interchangeably, consults and referrals are not the same.

- A consult is a request for assistance with a specific question, with the understanding that the consulting physician will provide an expert opinion and return the patient back to his primary physician. In general, the primary physician will discuss the consultant's findings and recommendations with the patient and proceed with a mutually agreeable diagnostic and treatment plan.

- In a referral, the primary physician sends the patient to the referral physician for the diagnosis and follow-up treatment of a specified condition. Although the primary physician expects to be kept informed of the patient's progress, the referral physician keeps the patient for the duration of the treatment period for the original condition. The patient continues to see his primary physician for other problems and for health maintenance.

The optimal care of the patient depends on a coordination of services, which is one of the strengths of a primary physician who knows the patient's overall health history. No physician wants to be caught off guard by a patient who is asking for results of a test that the physician did not know had been performed. By following the guidelines below, physicians can coordinate their efforts and provide better service to patients.

Primary care doctors should:

- Choose consultants who are professionally competent, and build a long-term relationship with them.
- Explain to the patient why they are being asked to see another doctor and what that doctor is likely to do.
- Provide clear instructions as to whether this is a consultation or a referral.
- Give a specific question or problem that the consultant or referral physician is to address.
- Send background history, physical examination, and test results to the consultant so that they are available when the patient arrives.
- Describe any treatments that have already been tried and their effectiveness.
- Provide feedback to the consultant about the patient's progress.

Physicians receiving consults and referrals should:

- Keep the primary physician informed about the status of the patient.
- Have copies of all reports, operative notes, laboratory tests, and pathology results sent to the primary physician.
- Call the primary physician personally with results that are ominous and unexpected.
- Never, except in a true emergency, send the patient on to another physician without the approval of the primary physician. If necessary in an emergency, the primary physician should be contacted as soon as reasonably possible and informed of the reasons for the action.
- Never make remarks that may be interpreted by the patient as disparaging to the primary physician such as, "This is a very straightforward case; I don't know why he asked me to see you." Such concerns should be discussed privately between the two involved physicians.
- Always return the patient to the primary doctor.

Ethical Issues

In addition to the traditional principles of medical ethics such as nonmaleficence (do no harm) and patient confidentiality, office practice mandates the consideration of practical points that may raise ethical dilemmas for some physicians.

- Do you treat members of your own family? If yes, what are the boundaries of that relationship? Do you prescribe controlled drugs to family and acquaintances?
- Do you treat your employees? Is there a conflict of interest if one of your employees seeks treatment for an occupational illness?
- Do you provide professional courtesy for physicians, residents, and medical students?
- If you teach, do you treat your students? How might your grading be influenced by information that you uncover during the evaluation and treatment of a medical condition?
- What is your policy on seeing pharmaceutical representatives and accepting pharmaceutical samples? Do office staff use samples for themselves?
- Do you see patients who cannot pay? At what point do you refer unpaid bills to a collection agency?
- Are you able to balance patient care with financial disincentive in a managed care environment?

HEALTH CARE FINANCING

Current total U.S. expenditure for health care is approximately 1 trillion dollars per year. By comparison, this figure was 27.1 billion in 1960 and 250.1 billion in 1980. Care to individuals accounts for almost 90%; the remainder is spent on administration, construction, public health, and research. The proportion paid by the Federal government has grown steadily to about one-third of this total. Figure 5.2 illustrates the breakdown of health care costs by major category.

Medicare

Medicare provides health insurance for persons over 65 years old and those under age 65 with

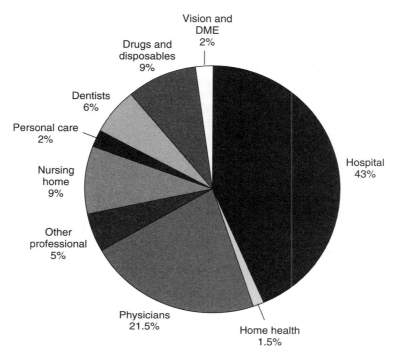

Figure 5.2. *Spending on personal health demonstrated by major category.* DME refers to durable medical equipment, such as wheelchairs and oxygen concentrators. It is likely that the proportion of expense attributable to home health has increased since these data were analyzed, as a result of cost pressures that are decreasing average hospital length of stay, thereby increasing home care. (Reprinted with permission from Congressional Research Service based on National Health Expenditure. Office of the Actuary, Health Care Finance Administration.)

chronic disabilities and end-stage renal disease (ESRD) (Table 5.3). It is administered nationally by the federal Health Care Financing Administration (HCFA) through contracts with over 70 local and regional insurance managers. Of the almost 40 million persons covered by Medicare; approximately three-quarters have annual incomes below $25,000 (12). Medicare is divided into two separate plans.

- Part A covers hospital services, home health services, hospice care, and short stays in skilled nursing facilities and is financed by a 1.45% payroll tax (each) on all employees and employers. Eligibility for Medicare Part A is automatic at age 65 for those who also meet the eligibility requirements for Social Security.

- Part B covers physician services and some outpatient laboratory and x-ray tests, and is funded by general tax revenues and a supplemental insurance premium paid by recipients. Participation in Part B is not automatic; the patient must enroll.

Medicare pays for 80% of the allowable physician charge. The patient pays the remaining 20% and an annual deductible personally or through the purchase of supplemental *Medigap* coverage from private insurers. Ninety percent of Medicare recipients have supplemental insurance coverage. Physicians who participate in Medicare (accept assignment) are paid the 80% directly by Medicare and are required to bill the patient for the remainder. Nonparticipating physicians can still see Medicare patients, but must bill the patient directly, who is then reimbursed by Medicare. The incentive for the physician to participate is to simplify the billing process; but nonparticipating physicians may be able to collect more money.

Because of its market share and governmental stature, Medicare has unique influence. This allows Medicare to affect major changes in the health care arena that a private insurer would be hard pressed to accomplish. It is not uncommon for other insurers to follow Medicare's footsteps.

Table 5.3.
Medicare and Medicaid[a]

	Medicare Part A	Medicare Part B	Medicaid
Financed by	2.9% payroll tax on current workers	General tax revenue and monthly premiums paid by beneficiaries	Federal and state taxes
Eligibility	• Automatic at age 65 for those eligible for Social Security • Permanently disabled and end-stage renal disease	Voluntary enrollment over age 65 or eligible for Part A	Poor who meet one of the following: • AFDC recipients • SSI beneficiaries (disabled) • Pregnant women and children with low family incomes
Coverage	Inpatient hospital, short-term skilled nursing facilities, home health care, hospice	Physician services, outpatient hospital services, laboratory, x-ray	Inpatient hospital, nursing home, home health care, physician services, laboratory, x-ray, prenatal care, medically necessary transportation (benefits may vary by state)

[a]By 1995, Medicare provided coverage for 33 million persons who had reached the age of 65 and an additional 4.5 million younger patients with disabilities or end-stage renal disease (ESRD). Hospital services account for 44% of Medicare expenditures, and physician services make up an additional 18.5%. In 1996, the monthly premium for Part B coverage was $42.50, with an annual deductible of $100.00

Medicaid

Medicaid is a federal and state insurance program for the eligible poor, financed by tax revenues and administered individually by the states. As such, there are almost as many different programs as there are states. States have broad discretion beyond the basic requirement to cover hospital and nursing home care, physician services, prenatal and preventive care, and some ancillary services. Trends in Medicaid include the enrollment of recipients in managed care plans and restrictions on services.

HEALTH CARE REGULATION

Antitrust

As groups have grown and consolidated, public concern has grown about the loss of competition in the marketplace and the threat of medical monopolies. Legislative initiatives, such as the "Stark" rules, have placed limits on self-referrals. Briefly, these regulations prohibit physicians from referring patients to facilities in which the physician or his or her relatives have a financial interest. An example would be a doctor who sends a patient to have a computed tomography scan at a radiologic center of which the doctor is a part owner. The potential for confusion and

conflict is self-evident when these rules are applied to physician groups and joint ventures between physicians and hospitals.

Professional Liability

Professional liability (malpractice) insurance protects the physician from claims arising from the provision of medical care. For primary care practice, the average cost is about $7,000 annually (13). There are two basic types of malpractice insurance: *claims made* and *occurrence*. These are best illustrated by a case example.

CASE STUDY

A physician buys an insurance policy from Company A for the calendar year 1997. On March 10, 1997, he treats a patient for apparent "heartburn" symptoms. On April 2, the patient suffers a massive myocardial infarction and becomes permanently disabled. The physician moves to a new practice on December 31, 1997, and does not renew his policy with Company A. Eventually the patient contacts an attorney and files a claim on February 3, 1998. If the physician has a claims-made policy, he is *not* protected, since the actual claim was not filed during the period of coverage. (If the patient had instead filed suit on November 4, 1997, the physician would be covered.) If the physician has an occurrence policy he *is* protected, since the act took place during the period of coverage.

During the medical malpractice crisis of the 1970s, many commercial insurance companies stopped offering insurance to physicians, and the remaining companies stopped offering occurrence coverage. By offering greater protection to the physician, occurrence policies pose greater risk for the insurer. Protection in later years is addressed through the purchase of supplemental *tail* coverage, which covers the physician for claims arising after the policy period.

The National Practitioner Data Bank (NPDB) became operational in 1990 as a repository for disciplinary and malpractice claim information about individual physicians. Four categories of adverse actions must be reported to the data bank by the party making the payment or imposing the sanction: malpractice insurance claim payments made by or on behalf of physicians; disciplinary actions by a state licensing board; reduction or termination of hospital privileges secondary to disciplinary review; and violations of health care fraud and abuse statutes. Hospitals are required to request information about their staff physicians when they initially apply for privileges and every 2 years thereafter. State licensing boards and prospective employers may request reports, as may plaintiffs' attorneys in some cases. Reports are not available to the general public, although some states are considering legislation that would make state board disciplinary information available to the public. Individual physicians may obtain a copy of their own files. There are almost 6,000 queries to the NPDB on every working day. Nationally about 14% of physicians have been reported to the data bank (14).

Practice Regulation

Some regulations create physician responsibilities as employers; others create physician rights as

employees. Two examples of recent legislation on the national level are the Clinical Laboratory Improvement Amendment (CLIA 88) and the Bloodborne Pathogens regulations from the Occupational Safety and Health Administration (OSHA).

Laboratory Services

CLIA 88 establishes and enforces quality standards for laboratory services provided in physician offices. It established minimum standards for laboratory technicians and required that each laboratory have a clinical director, a technical director, and an overall director. Some of these roles could be filled by a primary care physician; others required formal laboratory training. Individual tests were classified into four categories, based on the technical characteristics of the test protocol and the apparent level of expertise needed to perform it. These categories were "waivered," "physician waivered," "moderate complexity," and "high complexity." Physician reaction to CLIA 88 was mixed. Although many had recognized the need for improvement, the rules proved burdensome for many busy practitioners, who simply stopped offering laboratory services. This loss was more significant in isolated rural areas, where alternative testing sites were distant. Physician lobbying has brought about significant compromise from the original regulation.

Occupational Exposure

OSHA's Bloodborne Pathogens regulations created certain protections for physicians as employees and greater responsibilities for physicians as employers. Designed to minimize exposure to HIV and hepatitis B, the OSHA guidelines mandate the use of personal protective equipment, such as gloves and masks, the location of "sharps" containers in clinical areas, and the regulation of biohazardous waste disposal. Employers are required to provide education, vaccination, and treatment if needed for employees whose jobs involved significant risk of contact with bloodborne pathogens.

Professional Qualifications

The American Board of Family Practice certifies family physicians as specialists. It requires applicants to have a valid and unrestricted state medical license and to have completed a family practice residency before they can take the board certification examination. Practicing physicians must obtain licensure in each state of practice, plus state and federal permits to prescribe controlled substances such as narcotics and amphetamines.

Hospital admitting privileges are obtained through the medical staff or the medical affairs office of the hospital. The request for privileges will list specific diagnoses and procedures that are available to you. Depending on the hospital and its policies, you may be asked to provide documentation of your competency to perform specific procedures. Therefore, it pays to keep detailed records of your residency training experience.

Once you have a license and hospital privileges, you will need to apply for credentials from insurance companies, if you want to see their enrolled patients, and to register as a provider for Medicare and Medicaid. You will receive a Unique Provider Identification Number (UPIN), which identifies you to the various insurance plans. Although you can practice without insurance credentialing, you will have to bill your patients directly, which will discourage them from seeing you.

THE FUTURE OF PRIMARY HEALTH CARE IN THE UNITED STATES

Nationally, the demand for primary care physicians (family practice, general internal medicine, and general pediatrics) has increased greatly in the last 10 years, in part due to the needs of managed care organizations (15). This is in marked contrast to the previous 50 years, which saw a

Table 5.4.

Five-Year Growth in Median Net Incomes for Office-Based Primary Care Physicians

	1990 Net	1995 Net	% Change
Family practice	$99,030	$123,620	+24.8
General practice	$84,490	$97,440	+12.7
Internal medicine	$110,740	$122,440	+10.6
OB/GYN	$198,720	$197,260	− 0.7
Pediatrics	$107,380	$126,980	+18.3
All nonsurgery	$129,890	$133,380	+2.7
All fields	$140,460	$153,480	+9.3

The source for all data is the *Medical Economics* Continuing Survey, 1991 and 1996. For unincorporated physicians, net is individual practice income minus tax-deductible professional expenses before income taxes. For incorporated physicians, net is total compensation from practice (salary, bonuses, and retirement set-asides) before income taxes. Doctors of Osteopathy are included in the 1995 data but were not included in the 1990 data. (Reprinted with permission from Rice B. Winning times for primary care physicians. Med Econ 1997:88–99.)

steady decrease in the supply of primary care physicians relative to the supply of subspecialists. Whereas more than 80% of physicians were generalists in 1931, by the late 80s only 24% of graduating U.S. medical school seniors were considering generalist careers in primary care specialties (16). In 1997, 56% of graduating U.S. medical students entered primary care residencies. Comparative practice data are provided in Tables 5.4, 5.5, and 5.6.

Table 5.5.

Managed Care and Primary Care Physicians

	Participation (% of Physicians Participating (1996))		Revenue (% of 1995 Gross Income from)		Patient Volume (% of Total 1996 Patient Visits from)	
	In any HMOs/PPOs	In Capitation	All HMOs/PPOs	Capitation	All HMOs/PPOs	Capitation
Family practice	86	54	46	20	41	20
General practice	69	61	41	15	37	15
Internal medicine	84	57	45	20	42	25
OB/GYN	91	25	62	15	59	15
Pediatrics	92	68	63	17	64	24
All nonsurgery	81	46	45	15	41	20
All fields	84	38	44	15	41	20

The source for all data is the *Medical Economics* Continuing Survey, 1991 and 1996. Percentages are medians. Revenue and patient visit figures exclude respondents reporting no HMO/PPO participation or capitation. Patient visits are total physician-patient visits in any medical setting during a typical week in spring 1996. (Reprinted with permission from Rice B. Winning times for primary care physicians. Med Econ 1997:88–99.)

Table 5.6.
Median Workload for Primary Care Physicians

	Hours Worked per Week		Patient Visits per Week	
	1991	1996	1991	1996
Family practice	60	52	138	125
General practice	51	50	119	100
Internal medicine	60	60	107	105
OB/GYN	61	60	108	100
Pediatrics	60	52	155	128
All nonsurgery	60	55	105	102
All fields	60	57	104	95

The source for all data is the *Medical Economics* Continuing Survey, 1991 and 1996. For family physicians, hours worked per week decreased by 13% and patient visits per week decreased by 9%. (Reprinted with permission from Rice B. Winning times for primary care physicians. Med Econ 1997:88–99.)

Evidence-Based Practice

Cost containment has encouraged the growth of medical practice guidelines to reduce the variability of clinical care. Guidelines can be based on many factors such as cost, common practice, and expert opinion. As proponents of prevention, primary care physicians have taken leadership roles in the development of guidelines based on reviews of the scientific literature. In 1989 the U.S. Preventive Services Task Force published the first edition of its *Guide to Clinical Preventive Services*, which examined the scientific evidence supporting age-group specific screening and prevention. Revised in 1996 as a second edition, this resource promotes effective strategies, discourages ineffective ones, and notes areas of continuing debate and uncertainty. More details on evidence-based approaches to practice are provided in Chapter 19.

Health Care Restructuring

Rising health care costs have become the driving force behind revolutionary changes in the organization and operation of American medical practice. Managed care continues to grow in the public and private sectors, although consumer backlash about issues such as same-day mastectomy and 1-day postpartum discharges has been prominent. In this regard, the federal and some state governments have considered legislation to require coverage for minimum hospital stays. As physicians have gained more experience with managed care, and more clout through political activism and professional association, a movement to reassert physician influence has grown.

Nationally, health care reform resurfaces periodically as a "hot topic." Common areas of conflict include public versus private payment, universal coverage, access to care, rationing of services, definition of basic services, and physician reimbursement. The waves of public sentiment rise and fall on an ocean of inertia. Changes are made in small increments, which reflect the difficulty of achieving broad consensus.

REFERENCES

1. Babbott D, Baldwin DC, Jolly P, Williams DJ. The stability of early specialty preferences among medical school graduates in 1983. JAMA 1988;258:1970–1975.
2. Bland CJ, Meurer LN, Maldonado G. Determinants of primary care specialty choice: a non- statistical meta-analysis of the literature. Acad Med 1995;70(7): 620–641.
3. American Academy of Family Physicians Residency Census Survey. Reprint no. 150. Kansas City, MO: American Academy of Family Physicians, August 1, 1996.
4. Kahn NB, Garner JG, Schmittling GT, Ostergaard DJ, Graham R. Results of the 1996 National Resident Matching Program: Family Practice. Fam Med 1996; 28(8):548–552.
5. American Academy of Family Physicians Report on Survey of 1996 Graduating Family Practice Residents. Reprint no. 155-V. Kansas City, MO: American Academy of Family Physicians, 1996.
6. Bodenheimer TS, Grumbach K. Understanding Health Policy. Norwalk, CT: Appleton & Lange, 1995.
7. Group Health Association of America. 1995 National Directory of HMOs. Washington, DC: Group Health Association of America, 1995.
8. GHAA 1990 Pilot Utilization Data Supplement to the Annual HMO Industry Survey. Washington, DC: Group Health Association of America, 1990.
9. Ramsey CN, Durett JP, eds. Practice Management for Family Practice Residents. Kansas City, MO: American Academy of Family Physicians. 1992.
10. Rules and Regulations 64175–81. Federal Register December 6, 1991;56(235).
11. American Academy of Physician Assistants. Health Workforce Newslink 1996;3(1):16.
12. Office of the Actuary. Health Care Financing Administration. Kansas City, MO: American Academy of Family Physicians, 1992.
13. Rice B. Winning times for primary care physicians. Med Econ March 24, 1997:88–99.
14. Oshel RE, Croft T, Rodak J. The National Practitioner Data Bank: the first 4 years. Public Health Rep 1995; 110(4):383–394.
15. Seifer SD, Troupin B, Rubenfield GD. Changes in marketplace demand for physicians. JAMA 1996;276(9): 695–699.
16. Primary Care Physician Supply. HRSA Fact Sheet, March, 1992.

PART II

Preventive Care

6. Helping Your Patients Stay Healthy

PETER CURTIS AND ADAM O. GOLDSTEIN

Key Clinical Questions

1. What is the role of disease prevention and health promotion in primary care?
2. What are the characteristics of a good screening test?
3. How can patients be persuaded/encouraged to improve their health through lifestyle changes?

Approach to Prevention of Illness

PREVENTION AND SCREENING: BACKGROUND

Good health is a state of physical and mental well-being that involves far more than the absence of disease. Building skills in health promotion and disease prevention will help you help your patients achieve good health.

In many countries of the world, disease, poverty, accidents, conflicts, and natural disasters batter the health of populations, from newborn to the aged. Individuals and families have difficulty in taking measures to prevent disease and improve their health without the underlying safety nets of sanitation, clean water, food, housing, and insect vector eradication. The chapters in this section are written in the context of the wealthier cultures that have broader access to public health, primary care, and specialist services as part of the infrastructure of the social system. With these assumptions in mind, we describe the interventions that primary care health professionals can undertake to help their patients stay healthy.

Historically, physicians have advocated for prevention, primarily by encouraging and providing immunizations. It is common knowledge that the epidemics of poliomyelitis, pertussis, and diphtheria that caused so many deaths and disabilities in the 19th Century were greatly decreased by immunization. In 1964, before the introduction of rubella vaccine in the United States

(1969), the disease caused 11,000 fetal deaths and 20,000 infants to be born with congenital defects (1). Since then, rubella has been almost eliminated through widespread vaccination.

In the past 30 years, preventive care has developed beyond immunization to screening for risk factors or asymptomatic disease such as cervical cancer, hypertension, and lipid disorders (2). Several decades ago, enthusiasm for preventive care, combined with the rewards of fee-for-service medicine, led to tremendous growth in "health maintenance" programs, culminating in the "annual physical," in which a broad array of laboratory tests and procedures were offered to individuals and industry as an insurance against falling ill later in life. In 1983, the American Medical Association withdrew its recommendation of the annual physical examination for adults (originally suggested by the same organization 60 years earlier), because of the lack of evidence that this approach had any clinical effectiveness.

Since that time, there has been growing interest in emphasizing preventive measures that (a) show scientific evidence that they reduce the burden of suffering, and (b) eliminate interventions that are ineffective. In addition, it is increasingly clear that many chronic and costly diseases prevalent in society result from lifestyle behaviors (violence, accidents, smoking, obesity, and lack of exercise), so that changing the way people live, eat, and interact in society may be more important than patching them up with costly medications after the damage is done. Political, legislative, and community-level interventions (e.g., school-based programs or seat belt regulations) can also lead to major changes in societal behavior. Individual clinicians can play an important role in all such efforts, given their often intimate knowledge of the patient, family, and community.

Relationships among patient, clinician, and public health factors are shown in Figure 6.1. For the patient, healthy behaviors derive from the learned norms of family and culture. For example, is washing the hands after going to the bathroom taught and modeled for children? Do parents exercise regularly and use preventive services

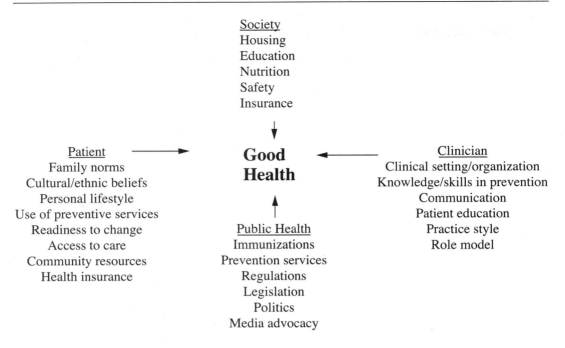

Figure 6.1. *Factors in promoting good health and preventing illness.*

appropriately? Does your patient have access and financial resources to take advantage of health services—and a readiness to change unhealthy behaviors? The clinician must have the knowledge and skills to apply and implement preventive services efficiently, to understand how to communicate and promote change in health behavior, and to provide a personal example to the office staff and patients. Finally, the state or federal government provides a limited safety net of services through the public health service in terms of immunization programs, preventive care (i.e., prenatal care), and sanitation services.

The purpose of this and following chapters on preventive health care is to help the student:

- Define the three levels of prevention with examples of each one
- Assess the major preventable causes of morbidity and death for different populations, in terms of gender, age and ethnicity
- Know the criteria for an effective screening test
- Define the major components of effective health education/communication
- Apply an evidence-based approach to counseling patients about health behavior

- Understand the use of behavior change theory in modifying lifestyle behaviors.

SCOPE OF PREVENTION IN FAMILY PRACTICE

A principal objective of prevention and health promotion is to reduce the burden of suffering for the major preventable diseases. The U.S. Preventive Services Task Force, begun in 1984, has identified 70 leading and preventable causes of death and disability in the United States and ranked them by severity, prevalence, incidence, and potential for improvement. Table 6.1 summarizes the burden of suffering for the most common problems.

We define "disease prevention" as the method of avoiding target diseases through specific interventions. There are three levels of preventive care:

- *Primary prevention* consists of those interventions, such as immunizations, that can completely prevent the disease in individuals at risk.
- *Secondary prevention* identifies established risk factors for disease. Blood pressure, serum cholesterol, and cervical cancer screening are

Table 6.1.

Leading Actual and Reported Causes of Death in the United States, 1990

Leading Actual Causes	Deaths	Leading Reported Causes	Deaths
Tobacco	400,000	Coronary heart disease	720,000
Diet (obesity, cholesterol, etc.) and inactivity	300,000	Cancer	505,000
Alcohol	100,000	Strokes	144,000
Infections/immunizations	90,000	Accidents	92,000
Toxins	60,000	COPD	87,000
Firearms and motor vehicles	60,000	Pneumonia/influenza	80,000
Sexual behavior	30,000	Diabetes	48,000
Illicit drug use	20,000	Suicide	31,000

Modified from McGinnis JM, Foege WH. Actual causes of death in the United States. JAMA 1993;270:2207–2212.

examples in which identifying abnormal results can lead to effective interventions that prevent serious disease developing (3).

- *Tertiary prevention* is a process for optimizing health after disease is present. Examples include programs to rehabilitate athletes after injuries or to prevent a second heart attack. Tertiary prevention will not be specifically addressed in this section of the book, but the chapters in Section Three covering common problems contain much information about its application in specific disease states. *Students should know that tertiary prevention is an integral part of all patient education.*

Preventive screening measures are performed for all patients using either screening tests (e.g., Papanicolaou [Pap] smear or sigmoidoscopy), immunizations (e.g., poliomyelitis, diphtheria, pertussis, etc.), chemoprophylaxis (e.g., fluoride to prevent tooth decay in children), or counseling

to improve healthy behavior (e.g., exercise, smoking cessation) (Table 6.2). These efforts may occur in the physician's office, public health clinic, community health center, hospital, or out in the community.

Because the widespread application of these measures costs time, dollars, and other resources, it is essential that preventive measures are effective. Five criteria are necessary to justify the use of a screening or preventive intervention by the clinician:

1. The prevalence of the disease and the burden of suffering caused by the disease must be high enough to justify widespread screening (3).
2. The condition must have an asymptomatic period during which treatment will significantly reduce morbidity or mortality.
3. Acceptable methods of treatment must be available at a reasonable cost.

Table 6.2.

Types of Preventive Interventions

Type of Activity	Maneuver	Effectiveness Criteria
Screening test	Physical examination Physiologic measure (i.e., blood pressure) Laboratory test/procedure	Sensitivity/specificity of maneuver/test (false positive and false negative) Value of early detection
Immunization	Injection—active (modified live vaccine) Injection—passive	Biologic efficacy Adverse effects
Chemoprophylaxis	Giving medication (i.e., aspirin for heart disease)	Biologic efficacy Cooperation of patient Adverse effects
Counseling health promotion	Giving advice/information before and during health problem	Efficacy of risk reduction Efficacy of counseling

4. The screening test and/or intervention must be effective with few adverse effects.

5. The screening test must have a high sensitivity.

To pick up all cases of a disease, a good screening test must have a high "sensitivity," which is the likelihood that someone with the disease will test positive. The test should also have a high "specificity," or the likelihood that someone without the disease will test negative (to reduce the number of false-positive tests) (4). False-positive tests cause patients anxiety and lead to expensive or harmful medical evaluation. For example, elevated prostate-specific antigen (screening for prostate cancer) has low specificity in men below 60 years, so that abnormal results are frequently "false positives," often leading to referral for unnecessary ultrasound and biopsy.

The approach used by the U.S. Preventive Services Task Force to develop its recommendations was based on an extensive literature review (over 6,000 articles). The quality of evidence from the literature was carefully rated and then used to make final recommendations to clinicians (Table 6.3). The strength of these recommendations also varied depending on a mix of evidence, burden of suffering, prevalence, adverse effects, and costs of each intervention. Despite this body of evidence, the bias toward accepting new and unproven pre-ventive technologies into routine practice without considering the effects on patients is clearly illus-trated by the introduction in the late 1980s of the prostate-specific antigen test for prostate cancer (PSA). The PSA test was rapidly introduced into practice because it was innovative and heavily publicized and because the fear and prevalence of prostate cancer was high enough to persuade many patients that the test promised a diagnosis. These factors created a new demand for medical services, and the medical profession, despite the evidence, was willing to incorporate the test into standard practice. Its value in screening is still not clear, and the U.S. Preventive Services Task Force does not recommend it (evidence rating: D) (see Chapter 34, Prostate Diseases).

IMPLEMENTING PREVENTION IN THE OFFICE

Because the family physician cares for people of all ages and does so in a longitudinal and com-prehensive style, there are unique opportunities to identify problems early on or to guide patients and families over time. A typical example is the role played by the physician who first delivered and cared for a young boy who is now 13 years old and develops risk-taking behaviors. The un-derstanding and relationship between the physi-

Table 6.3.
Evidence Used to Substantiate Disease Prevention and Health Promotion Strategies

Evidence→	Analysis→	Clinical Practice Recommendations/Ratings
Literature review	U.S. Preventive Services Task Force 1989, 1996	A. Good evidence for routine use of this preventive activity
Burden of suffering		B. Fair evidence for routine use
Costs, savings, benefits		C. Lack of evidence but can be recommended on other grounds
Adverse effects		D. Fair evidence to *not* routinely do this activity
Characteristics of intervention		E. Good evidence to *not* routinely do this

Quality of Evidence		
High	I.	Based on at least one good randomized controlled trial
	II-1.	Based on well-designed controlled studies (no randomization)
↕	II-2.	Based on well-designed cohort/case control studies
	II-3.	Based on many time-series studies, with or without intervention
Low	III.	Opinions of respected authorities

Adapted from US Preventive Services Task Force. Guide to Clinical Preventive Services: A Report of the US Preventive Services Task Force, 2nd ed. Baltimore: Williams & Wilkins, 1996.

cian and the family may be powerful tools in helping them through difficult times and preventing unhealthy and even dangerous behaviors. At the other end of the spectrum, the family physician is often the despairing observer of significant illness and misery that come from inability to prevent long-standing problems such as alcoholism or violence, which never received attention early enough (see Chapter 2).

Effective preventive practice involves being familiar with current recommendations, knowing your individual patient, and applying your knowledge and skills in a manner that is efficient and individualized. Putting prevention into practice requires use of the clinical history and physical examination, appropriate priority setting, spending time educating and counseling patients, and using a prevention-friendly charting system.

Clinical History

Historical data pertinent to preventive care include:

- Dates and results of previous preventive procedures (such as prior immunizations, Pap tests, tuberculosis [TB] skin tests, mammograms, cholesterol determinations, and blood pressures)

- A careful family history for common and unusual diseases that have a hereditary component (gout, diabetes, hypertension, etc.)

- A past medical history (coronary artery disease, diabetes, etc.)

- Information about the workplace, leisure, and living conditions at home

- Habits such as alcohol abuse, smoking, exercise, sexual practices, and seat belt use

- Information about normal body functions such as eating, sleep, urination, vision, hearing, and bowel function

Physical Examination

Physical examination should be limited or more extensive depending on the time available. At each patient age, a relatively small number of problems are epidemiologically of highest priority, and the clinical evaluation should also be perceived as a screening test to be used efficiently (2). Therefore, before beginning a physical you should ask yourself, "What part of physical examination should be done, and in what way?"

Just as important is the realization that the precision and accuracy of physical findings (e.g., sensitivity and specificity) are variable for different maneuvers and between clinicians. Physical diagnosis skills are most effective in identifying disease in patients who already have symptoms, but they are often of little use in asymptomatic patients. In other words, maneuvers that do a good job of diagnosing disease often make poor screening tests, because the predictive value of a positive physical finding is low when the prevalence of disease is low (4). For example, hearing rales on auscultation of the chest provides valuable diagnostic information in a patient with fever and shortness of breath. But in a healthy, vigorous elderly patient, rales usually represent benign conditions, either a prior chest infection or simply that the patient has not taken a deep breath recently. Similarly, the neurologic examination has many false-positive results in asymptomatic patients and rarely screens for diseases in which early treatment improves outcomes; therefore, a detailed neurologic examination may be omitted in the well-person visit.

A physical examination of a well older man should consist of items that identify "preclinical" signs of disease, including:

- Vital signs of weight, blood pressure, and tobacco use

- Vision and hearing

- Cardiovascular examination (for bruits, diminished peripheral pulses, atrial fibrillation, cardiomegaly, aortic stenosis, and peripheral vascular disease)

- Abdominal examination (hepatomegaly, abdominal bruits)

- Rectal and prostate examination (for anorectal cancer and prostatic hypertrophy)

- Skin (for premalignant and malignant tumors)

In a well older woman, the physical examination would also include breast and pelvic assessments.

Setting Priorities

Often, physicians become so engaged in the routine care of unwell patients that they find little time to reflect as a practice on the prevention and health promotion activities they are delivering. The U.S. Preventive Services Task Force has developed age-specific charts for periodic health screening for the general population with interventions for high-risk populations (2). Age-specific recommendations are reported in the chapters on well child and adult care.

One crucial aspect of preventive primary care practice is how to incorporate selected prevention and promotion practices into the office visit, the length of which varies from 15 to 45 minutes. Even short visits for acute problems, when patients are expecting management of their immediate problem, provide an easy opportunity to check on smoking, the last Pap smear status, or one or two other preventive measures. For example, when you notice that a patient is overweight, just asking how much he or she is exercising and then giving brief advice takes only a few seconds (5).

To select the most important topics for preventive counseling during an office visit, consider the most common causes of morbidity and death for that particular patient (see Table 6.1). For example, a preparticipation sports examination for a high-school football player might productively include vision and hearing screening, testicular examination (with instruction on self-examination), a diphtheria-tetanus booster, questions about depression and seat belt use, and counseling about substance abuse and safe sex. These particular concerns are based on knowledge of cost-effective screening and causes of death (accidents, suicide, and homicide) for that age group.

Systematic Preventive Services and Office Systems

Better office-based routines can help raise adherence to recommendations above the current level of 20 to 70% (7). Preventive services can be routinized in several ways. A flow sheet on the chart will display, at each visit, the needed schedule for health maintenance. This can be checked by the nurse before the patient is shown into the examination room and a note written for the physician. Computer tracking and reminder systems can prompt the appropriate test or intervention at the appropriate time and then print out results on a personalized letter sent to the patient. Even simple monthly "tickler" card files can be used to send reminders to patients to return for their immunization or Pap smear. Delegation of certain tasks to nurses and office staff is effective, provided they are given the time and training. The fact that blood pressure measurements are almost universally performed in ambulatory care settings underscores how effective prevention can be if it becomes an office routine. Smoking status has now become a new recommended "vital sign" to be noted at each visit. The frequency with which office systems and resources are used in prevention and counseling is shown in Table 6.4.

Table 6.4.
Frequency of Routine[a] Use of Preventive Care "Tools" in Family Physicians' Offices

Tool	% Physicians Using Tool
TRACKING/PROMPTING PREVENTIVE SERVICES	
Minirecord (kept by patient, i.e., immunization card)	80
Flow sheet in chart	73
Patient reminders	46
Chart reminders	43
Card file ticklers	32
Computer-based preventive programs	14
PROVIDING HEALTH EDUCATION	
Pamphlets	92
Posters in waiting areas	76
Nurse counseling	69
Video/slide presentations	26

Adapted from Dickey LL, Kamerow DB. Primary care physician's use of office resources in the provision of preventive care. Arch Fam Med 1996;5:399–404.

[a]Incorporated into daily patient care activities

In 1994, the U.S. Public Health Service developed and disseminated the "Put Prevention into Practice" (PPIP) program to improve the delivery of clinical preventive services in private practice. The program contains many of the tools and office systems to improve the rate of preventive care. However, there is no clear evidence that this program actually improves the performance of preventive services, demonstrating the difficulty of changing physician behavior (7).

The growth of managed care has had a favorable effect on the performance of preventive services in office practice. The benefits a patient receives from a health insurance plan or health maintenance organization (HMO) include specified preventive services. A family practice office holding contracts with several managed care companies will, however, need to adhere to different preventive protocols depending on the company. This adds to the complexity of organizing services. Organized office systems can clearly help with documentation.

The final factor in setting priorities for preventive services is physician compensation. In managed care, fees are folded into the contractual payments, and the clinician is required to perform the services. Health insurance will reimburse for some but not all services. Preventive care reimbursement by Medicaid and Medicare is often so low that it does not even cover the practice overhead for the visit. Thus, the physician will have to balance the desire to do the best job for the patient with a recognition of the patient's options and ability to pay.

Counseling Patients

PATIENT EDUCATION AND COUNSELING

A growing literature demonstrates the effectiveness of physician counseling of patients about lifestyle-related diseases, including discussions of the risks of AIDS, the use of tobacco and alcohol, weight loss, and improving adherence to medical regimens. To be successful in helping patients change their health behaviors, you should know the epidemiology of medical problems among different sociodemographic and gender groups and be aware of the scientific evidence that supports the interventions chosen. Clinicians must also understand the nature of effective health communication and practice counseling skills to ultimately facilitate lifestyle changes for patients.

Ten important aspects to maximizing successful patient education and behavior change are summarized in Table 6.5 and discussed below.

- Because of their expertise and the respect given to them, physicians have enormous power to motivate patients toward behavior change. This power comes with the responsibility to use it appropriately and not to give out wanton or inaccurate advice. For instance, when counseling about alcohol use, physicians must be alert to any signs of abuse, but they may also have an obligation to inform their adult patients who drink one to two beers a day that such behavior actually decreases the risk of a fatal heart attack by 30%, whereas drinking more than four beers a day will increase such risk.

- Clinicians must be patient-centered and understand how patients perceive their lifestyle, illness, or unhealthy behavior. This includes using language and information that considers age, educational level, cultural background, and patient or family values. Patients who are satisfied with their physicians are three times more likely to follow a prescribed medical regimen (8), so the best therapeutic plan is to build a solid doctor-patient relationship. For instance, some patients who smoke will not be

Table 6.5.
10 Steps to Maximizing Patient Education for Behavioral Change

1. Understand the power of physician's expertise as a motivator toward behavior change
2. Be patient-centered and patient-responsive (understand the patient's perceptions of their illness/behavior, their readiness to change their behavior, and their self-efficacy for behavior change)
3. Choose one or at most two behavior goals for changing at any one time
4. Be specific in giving advice
5. Obtain a firm commitment from the patient for change
6. Use positive reinforcement and short-term rewards
7. Use multiple educational modalities when possible
8. Use social support when possible
9. Assure appropriate follow-up
10. Be realistic

persuaded, for any reason, to quit. In this case, it makes little sense to spend much time teaching the patient how to quit smoking. Rather, you could ask what it would take to get the patient to want to quit smoking.

A useful theoretic action model, developed by Prochaska and DiClimente (Readiness to Change), can help you tailor your counseling message to the individual patient (9). In this model (Fig. 6.2), a patient's ability and willingness to change an unhealthy behavior ranges across a spectrum and is often circular:

Precontemplation—the patient has not yet thought seriously about changing his or her unhealthy behavior;

Contemplation—the patient has thought about changing, but no active or particular plans have been made to change;

Preparation and action—the patient is ready to change and, if encouraged, will undertake a behavior modification;

Maintenance—the patient continues behavior change, supported by the physician;

Relapse—the patient returns to the unhealthy behavior if not successful in his or her efforts to change and thus must recycle again through these stages.

In using the model, clinicians are constantly seeking to move patients to the next stage, e.g., from contemplation to taking and maintaining action. To be effective, you must give the patient understandable and clear information, explore potential barriers, and collaborate in finding possible solutions. Offer specific suggestions with confidence and with good follow-up to monitor progress. Avoid threats and blame if there is no initial success. Patients with higher self-confidence are more likely to succeed; those with low self-efficacy need more assistance and encouragement.

- Do not try to persuade patients to change all their unhealthy behaviors at the same time.

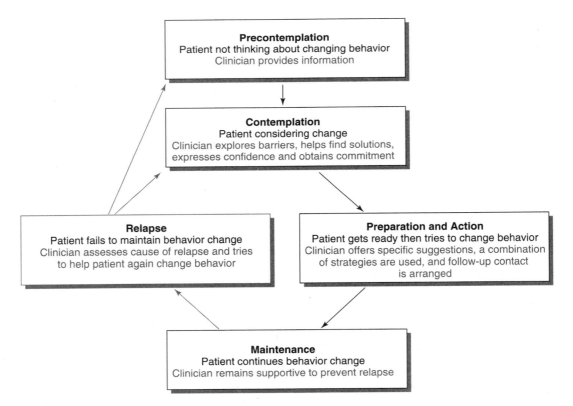

Figure 6.2. *Patient readiness to change model.* (Adapted from Prochaska JO, DiClemente CC, Norcross JC. In search of how people change. Applications to addictive behaviors. Am Psychol 1992;47:1102–1114.)

Someone who smokes cigarettes, is overweight, does not exercise, and has a high cholesterol clearly would benefit from major lifestyle modification, but the chances for success are greater if you and the patient agree to focus initially on one or two behaviors.

- When giving advice in health education, be specific and set targets (10). If you want a patient to exercise, specify the type of exercise, how often to perform it, where it will be performed, the short-term outcomes that are to be expected, and the potential side effects to expect.

- Write your instructions down, since studies show that patients remember less than one-half of what physicians tell them in the clinical encounter (11). Written instructions are particularly effective in increasing adherence to medications. On the medication instruction list, indicate the purpose for each medication (i.e., diuretic or "water pill" for heart failure). A wise strategy is to go through dosage instructions, ask the patient to read the written directions, and then repeat them back to you. Remember, making more than two to three medication changes at any one office visit will likely lead to nonadherence or to mistakes. For example, if you tell a patient to increase their Coumadin (warfarin) dose (an anticoagulant) from 5 mg a day to alternating 5 mg and 7.5 mg, it is easy for the patient to think that you want them to take 12.5 mg a day; the consequences of such a mistake could be life-threatening for the patient.

Appropriate and specific education is known to improve blood pressure reduction in hypertensive patients, lead to better blood glucose control in diabetic patients, reduce hospitalization rates for patients with congestive heart failure, and reduce mortality from melanoma and breast cancer (12). Strategies to increase patient adherence with medications are shown in Table 6.6.

- Obtain a firm commitment from the patient for specific behavior change. Patients who are undertaking a serious behavior change should prepare for the change with at least the same degree of planning as they would for a long vacation or a new job. Such preparation will include agreement on a start date for the process of change and making plans for how to accomplish the goal. Often, patients can sign a written contract on a blank prescription

Table 6.6.
Ways to Optimize Patient Adherence with Medications

- Give clear, concise, and written-down instructions on drug, names, dosage, reason for medication, duration of use, and instructions for use with foods or other medications
- Explain the main adverse effects clearly and in writing
- Use medications that can be given once or twice a day whenever possible compared to three or four times a day
- Use the less expensive medication whenever two medications have equal therapeutic effect
- Assess comprehension, such as having patients repeat back to you the directions for medication usage

pad as a form of a "behavioral prescription," and the patient keeps a copy of the contract as a reminder of the goal (Fig. 6.3). This technique can use the power of the symbolic exchange of the prescription that has epitomized the healing relationship for centuries.

- During the process of helping patients improve their health behaviors, it is important to acknowledge when they are making progress. Clinicians can use various forms of positive reinforcement and build in short-term rewards for behavior change. For instance, when a patient first decides on undertaking a change, the physician should immediately say, "Congratulations on wanting to make a positive choice to improve your health." A specific reward can also increase the positive motivation, such as saying, "One month after you have lost 4 pounds, what do you plan on doing for yourself to acknowledge this accomplishment," or, "What will you do with the $30 you saved from not smoking this month?"

- People vary greatly in the ways they best acquire and understand information. This may be through verbal, visual, or auditory pathways, so multiple targeting is the most efficient way to get the message across (13). Give written patient education materials to augment your counseling message. Use the behavioral prescriptions mentioned earlier. Books, videos, or audiotapes, reminders and

A

UNC Hospitals

**UNIVERSITY OF
NORTH CAROLINA HOSPITALS**

UNIVERSITY OF NORTH CAROLINA
Chapel Hill, N.C. 27514 • (919) 966-4131

ATTENTION PHARMACIST:
See Reverse Side Before Filling.

Imprint

Yellow Duplicate for UNC Hospitals Use Only.

PATIENT'S NAME __Elizabeth Appal__   UNIT NO. _____

ADDRESS _____   DATE __6/8/97__

DATE OF NEXT UNC Hospitals CLINIC VISIT _____   1 month   2 month   3 month
(enter date or circle interval)

Rx
1. Quit smoking on Monday 6/12.
2. Practice 5 stress reduction activities
3. Reward for quitting after one month __Book__

Do Not Refill   Refill 1 2 3 4 5 Times

HD 882 Rev 1/93

N.C. law requires that this area be completed for ALL
prescriptions.

PRINT _____ M.D.

Signed _____ M.D.
Product Selection Permitted

UPIN _____

DEA Number _____

Signed __Elizabeth Appel__ M.D.
Dispense As Written

B

UNC Hospitals

**UNIVERSITY OF
NORTH CAROLINA HOSPITALS**

UNIVERSITY OF NORTH CAROLINA
Chapel Hill, N.C. 27514 • (919) 966-4131

ATTENTION PHARMACIST:
See Reverse Side Before Filling.

Imprint

Yellow Duplicate for UNC Hospitals Use Only.

PATIENT'S NAME __Jonathen Smiley__   UNIT NO. _____

ADDRESS _____   DATE __6/20/97__

DATE OF NEXT UNC Hospitals CLINIC VISIT _____   1 month   2 month   3 month
(enter date or circle interval)

Rx
(1) Eat less than 2200 calories a day
(2) Eat no more than 20% saturated fats a day
(3) Eat less than 200mg of cholesterol a day

Do Not Refill   Refill 1 2 3 4 5 Times

HD 882 Rev 1/93

N.C. law requires that this area be completed for ALL
prescriptions.

PRINT _____ M.D.

Signed _____ M.D.
Product Selection Permitted

UPIN _____

DEA Number _____

Signed _____ M.D.
Dispense As Written

Figure 6.3. *Behavioral prescription slip.* A. Sample smoking cessation prescription. **B.** Sample diet prescription.

follow-up telephone calls can reinforce understanding.

- Help your patient contact a local support group or national organization, which will often publish a regular newsletter about a certain problem or disease (i.e., American Cancer Society). The Internet is becoming a great health resource for patients with computers.

- Have patients share their upcoming behavior change with coworkers, sympathetic friends, and family members (including children). Social support clearly increases positive outcomes (14). A husband and wife who quit smoking together are more likely to stay off cigarettes than if one tries to quit while the other continues to smoke.

- Arrange appropriate follow-up by the physician or nurse. Depending on the intervention, follow-up may occur as soon as a few days after a change is made. Patients who know that their physician is actively interested in their condition by making a follow-up appointment or telephone call are more likely to follow-through on change plans (15).

- Lastly, despite the best of intentions, it is equally important to be realistic in your expectations. Changing unhealthy behaviors is hard work, and the initial success rate rarely rises above 30%. Remember that a .300 batting average will get most baseball players into the Hall of Fame, and if all U.S. physicians could get 30% of their patients to change unhealthy behaviors, thousands of lives and millions of dollars would be saved.

SPECIFIC STRATEGIES FOR HEALTH PROMOTION

Preventing Tobacco Use

Counseling to get patients to change their smoking habits has received a high effectiveness rating (A). Cessation counseling is recommended for all persons who use tobacco products (cigarettes, cigars, chewing tobacco, etc.). Physicians also must advocate that children and nonsmoking adults not be exposed to environmental tobacco smoke.

Tobacco use is the greatest cause of preventable death and disease in the United States, killing more people than alcohol, AIDS, suicide, homicide and toxins combined. The U.S. Federal Agency for Health Care Policy and Research has published tobacco cessation guidelines for physicians that summarize data on counseling interventions (16). A simplified algorithm to help in the counseling process is shown in Figure 6.4.

As with blood pressure, tobacco-use status should be a vital sign, taken and recorded in the chart at all clinical encounters. If a patient uses tobacco, the single most important questions to ask are, "Do you want to quit using tobacco?," "Can we set a quit date in the next 2 weeks?," "Name 10 things you will do instead of smoking," and "When will you follow-up with me?"

Transition from nicotine dependence can be facilitated by a range of products (nicotine gum and patches—over-the-counter, nicotine inhalers, nasal spray, and sustained release bupropion hydrochloride—by prescription) to help those who must have a cigarette upon awakening, or cannot go through the day without smoking. Physicians who are good at counseling should be able to get 20 to 30% of their patients to quit over a year's duration (compared to a spontaneous quit rate of 2.5%) (16).

Promoting Physical Activity

The evidence that physical activity reduces the risk of heart disease, hypertension, osteoporosis, mental health disorders, obesity, and diabetes is strong enough to receive an "A" recommendation. Almost two-thirds of U.S. adults lead a sedentary life. Physical inactivity is more common in women, African-Americans, older adults, those with lower incomes, and those with less education. Recently, the U.S. Surgeon General released a landmark publication on the effects of exercise (17). The report demonstrates that physical activity does not need to be strenuous for health benefits; people who are inactive can improve health by moderate, regular exercise; benefits increase with greater duration, frequency, and intensity of exercise; men and women of all ages benefit from moderate amounts of physical activity; there are equal benefits to longer sessions of moderate intensity as in shorter sessions of higher intensity; and previously sedentary individuals should start slowly.

The evidence is less strong (effectiveness rating "C"), however, that physician counseling of asymptomatic patients increases physical activity. Yet, given the success reported in other lifestyle interventions and the potential benefits, counseling should be strongly considered in the office visit. Before giving a behavioral prescription to

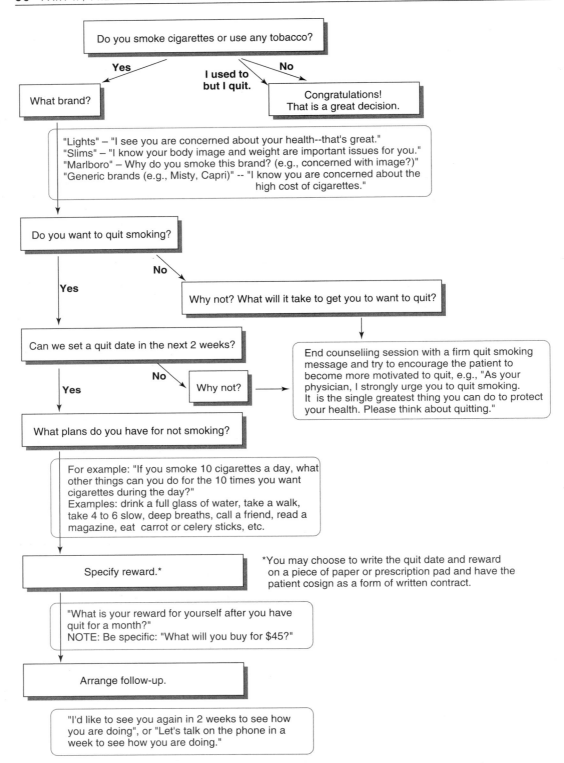

Figure 6.4. *Algorithm for smoking cessation counseling.*

increase physical activity, first ascertain current activity and potential barriers and discuss the benefits of exercise. Emphasize incorporating daily activities into the patient's daily routine, such as walking more briskly, parking further away from work, taking stairs instead of the elevator, and setting aside daily but brief time for exercising. Both stretching and aerobic conditioning are important components of an effective exercise prescription (Table 6.7).

Promoting a Healthy Diet

Levels of evidence for effectiveness are:

- "A" recommendation to limit intake of saturated fats

- "B" recommendation to limit intake of cholesterol

- "B" recommendation to emphasize a diet high in fruits, vegetables, grains, and fiber

- "B" recommendation for women to maintain an adequate calcium intake

- "C" recommendation for most vitamin supplements

- "C" physicians are effective in changing dietary habits of patients

Poor eating patterns and obesity are exceedingly common among adolescents and adults (see Chapter 43, Weight Management and Obesity), but eating habits are difficult to change. Yet, elevated cholesterol levels affect over one-third of the adult population, and hypercholesterolemia is a causal factor in cardiovascular disease; obesity and high animal fat intake are linked to lung, breast, colon, rectal, and prostate cancer; and certain antioxidants (found in fruits and vegetables) and selenium protect against cancer (18). A healthy diet plan and the recommended daily dose of certain vitamins and minerals are shown in Tables 6.8 and 6.9. More and more patients expect their physicians to know basic information about common vitamins, minerals, and even herbal preparations.

Preventing Injuries

Levels of evidence for effectiveness are:

- "A" recommendation for patients to wear seatbelts in automobiles

- "A" recommendation for motorcyclists and child cyclists to wear helmets

- "B" recommendation on counseling children's parents about the dangers of fires, hot tap water, drowning, poisoning, bicycles, firearms, and falls

- "B" seatbelt counseling increases seatbelt use

- "C" counseling increases helmet use

- "C" counseling helps prevent pedestrian injuries

Table 6.7.
Sample Patient Exercise Prescription

Pick an aerobic exercise

- Exercise three to five times a week for 10–20 minutes at a time
- Exercise at a pace that will allow you to maintain a conversation without undue stress
- Stop exercising or slow down if you get very tired or begin to have pain

Perform stretching and build up your regimen slowly

- Stretch your muscles for 5 minutes every morning and evening, and before and after exercise
- Increase activity levels slowly over 3 months

Incorporate exercise into your daily routines

- Park farther away at work or when shopping
- Use stairs instead of the elevator
- Walk faster wherever you go
- Most outdoor activities (mowing lawn, raking, gardening) provide aerobic benefits

Table 6.8.
Tips for a Healthier Diet

Assess

- Patient's ideal body weight (IBW)[a]
- Any family history of a lipid disorder
- Patient's perception about ideal body weight and diet
- Use of supplements, herbal products, or special diets

Counseling Advice

- Keep total fat to less than 30% of total calories
- Use monounsaturated fats (olive or peanut oil) or polyunsaturated fats (sunflower or safflower) instead of hydrogenated or saturated fats (coconut, palm, cottonseed)
- Get at least 30 g of fiber a day by eating fruits, vegetables, cereals, and grains
- Eat less meat and animal-based products

[a] To calculate IBW for men: to 106 lbs for the first 60 inches of height, add 6 lbs for each additional inch. For women, to 100 lbs for the first 60 inches, add 5 lbs for each additional inch. Subtract or add 10% for those with small or large body frames, respectively.

- "C" recommendation for screening/counseling for youth on violence prevention; women for domestic violence prevention

Homicide is the leading cause of death among African-American males between the ages of 15 and 34. Almost one-half of all violent crimes and unintentional injuries take place under the influence of alcohol and other drugs. Violent acts, including physical and sexual assault, suicides, and child, spouse, and elder abuse occur at alarmingly high rates (19). Based on the evidence, physicians should clearly raise issues of violence prevention with many, if not all, of their patients. Depending on the patient and encounter, appropriate questions and counseling may focus on poison prevention, and seat-belt and helmet use. Some clinicians are increasingly asking patients whether or not there is a gun in the home, because research demonstrates that the presence of a gun in the home, rather than conferring protection, increases the chance of homicide to the homeowner two to three times (20, 21).

Family violence is pervasive. For instance, child abuse affects all sociodemographic groups. Teenage and college women have an increased risk of "date rape." Women presenting to the emergency room or office with any traumatic injury have a 25% chance of being in an abusive relationship. Asking such patients about exposure to physical or sexual violence may initially feel awkward for some clinicians. In addition, some patients are reluctant to disclose such information for fear of being judged because of lack of trust, denial, or fear of "recrimination" from the clinician. The physician must also ask questions in ways that are not offensive and do not seem to invade the patient's privacy. Thus, a physician must become comfortable with asking about the occurrence of violence, injuries, or risk factors, and counseling patients and their families on ways to prevent intentional or unintentional injuries.

With a trusting relationship and sensitive and clear communication, you can use certain questions (SAFE) to screen for family violence (22):

- **Stress/Safety:** What kind of stress exists in your relationships? How safe do you feel in your relationships/marriage? Should I have any concerns for your safety?

- **Afraid/Abused:** Have there been situations in relationships in which you have felt afraid? Have you ever had a partner threaten or abuse you or your children? Have you been physically hurt or threatened before or now? Have you had to engage in sexual intercourse against your will?

- **Fight/Friends/Family:** People in relationships/marriages sometimes fight. What happens when you and your partner disagree? Are any friends or family members aware that you ever have been hurt? Do you think you could tell them, and do you think they would be able to give you support?

Table 6.9.

Vitamins and Minerals: Sources, Benefits, and Recommended Adult (Nonpregnant) Daily Allowances

Vitamin/Mineral	Sources	Benefits	Deficiency	Recommended Dietary Allowance (RDA)
Vitamin A[a]	Sweet potatoes, carrots, milk	Improved skin resistance to infection; good eyesight	Night blindness, xerophthalmia	1000 µg retinol equivalents (5000 IU)
Vitamin D[a]	Sunlight, dairy products	Strengthens bone development	Rickets	5–10 µg (1000–1200 IU)
Vitamin E[a]	Green leafy vegetables, nuts, whole grains, wheat germ	Oxidative protection of red blood cells	Anemia	8–10 mg (30 IU)
Vitamin K[a]	Green leafy vegetables, tomatoes	Blood clotting cascade	Bleeding diathesis	70–140 µg
Vitamin B$_1$[b] (thiamine)	Whole grains, vegetables, nuts, wheat germ	Carbohydrate metabolism	Beriberi	1–1.5 mg
Vitamin B$_2$[b] (riboflavin)	Animal products, mushrooms, broccoli	Protein metabolism, skin and eye protectant	Angular stomatitis/ blepharitis	1.2–1.5 mg
Vitamin B$_6$[b] (pyridoxine)	Brewers yeast, whole grains, nuts, meat	Helps regulate central nervous system	Peripheral neuropathy	1.7–2 mg
Vitamin B$_{12}$[b]	Animal products, fish, soybeans	Red blood cell formation	Mental status changes	3 µg
Vitamin C[b]	Broccoli, tomatoes, brussel sprouts, citrus fruits	Resistance to stress; oral hygiene; wound healing	Scurvy	60 mg
Niacin[b]	Nuts, poultry, fish	Cholesterol-lowering agent, coenzyme oxidation reductions	Pellagra	13–16 mg
Calcium	Dairy products	Bone growth	Rickets, osteomalacia	800 mg
Potassium	Tomatoes, citrus fruits	Cellular function	Ileus, muscle weakness	1.8–6 g
Sodium	Most foods	Cellular function	Weakness, confusion	1–3.3 g
Phosphorus	Cereals, dairy products	Cellular function	Mental status changes, osteomalacia	800 mg
Iron	Green leafy vegetables, dried fruits, meat, wheat germ	Red blood cell formation	Anemia	10–18 mg

Reprinted with permission from Sloane P, Slatt L, Curtis P, eds. Essentials of Family Medicine. Baltimore: Williams & Wilkins, 1993:169.

[a]Fat soluble.

[b]Water soluble.

- Emergency plan: Do you have a safe place to go and the resources you (and your children) need for any emergency? If you are in danger now, would you like help in locating a shelter? Would you like to talk with a social worker, a counselor, or me to develop an emergency plan?

Improving Mental Health

Level of evidence for screening effectiveness is:

- "C" recommendation for screening for depression or suicide risk in asymptomatic patients.

Good mental health includes not only freedom from depression and psychiatric illness, but more importantly, the ability to cope effectively with life's daily stresses and feel good about one's overall physical and social well-being. This is closely linked with a sense of responsibility to oneself and others and the maintenance of meaningful relationships. Unfortunately, at least one in five adults has some mental dysfunction annually, and suicides destroy as many Americans as homicides (19). Thus, good mental health describes the ability to both cope with daily stresses and feel good about the many aspects and challenges of life.

For many mental health issues, such as sleep disorders, stress management, and spirituality, groups such as the U.S. Preventive Services Task Force have not systematically reviewed the effectiveness of certain treatments. However, there is an increasing amount of interest on the part of patients and clinicians about these issues, and there is a growing research body for those interested in the scientific basis for certain treatments. For example, there is good evidence that certain practices (e.g., relaxation, hypnosis, biofeedback) can significantly improve mental health conditions such as insomnia and chronic pain (23).

At every office visit, ask about mental health stressors and any family or interpersonal problems by using simple questions about family functioning, sleep, satisfaction with work, major recent life events, stress, and anxiety. A nice lead-off question is, "Are you content or happy with your life?"

Adequate sleep is part of good general and mental health. Most people function best when they average between 7 and 8 hours of sleep, although the elderly may only need 5 to 6 hours. Insomnia resulting from stress, anxiety, depression, alcohol abuse, or physical illness is the most common sleep disorder. Poor sleep habits on top of heavy workloads and family and financial responsibilities often lead to poor mental health.

After ruling out medical causes of sleep disturbances, such as sleep apnea, research suggests that behavioral approaches can help patients redevelop good habits (24). If a patient cannot get to sleep after 15 to 30 minutes, advise them to get out of bed and pursue some relaxing activity for half an hour and then go back to bed. Another approach is to have the patient learn progressive relaxation and imaging techniques. Other simple advice includes:

- Avoid caffeinated beverages and alcohol within 4 hours of bedtime
- Go to bed at the same time each night

- Do regular daily exercise, but not after dinner
- Avoid using the bed for watching TV or eating
- Eliminate noise and pets from the bedroom.

Some people with insomnia believe they derive sleep benefits from a tryptophan drink (Ovaltine) or from valerian or melatonin (herbal remedies). The evidence for their effectiveness is at best inconclusive (25). Hypnotics, such as benzodiazepines, should be reserved for short-term management or acutely stressful situations.

Stress Management

Although not routinely taught in medical education, stress management techniques may be useful for both the clinician and patient (23). Incorporating two or three techniques into practice is a valuable skill and can be acquired by taking short courses or reading texts. The following methods are commonly used:

- Biofeedback—helpful in some conditions, but costly
- Exercise—underused and low cost
- Hypnosis—usually needs referral; costly
- Massage—good for muscle tension. Can be done at home and self-massage an option
- Meditation—inexpensive, effective, easily taught
- Prayer—works well for some patients
- Progressive muscular relaxation—easy to teach and learn
- Reading, music, pets—can be incorporated into routine daily use.

Spirituality

For many people, religion and spirituality play an important role in coping with stress, uncertainty, and illness. Again, medical training rarely addresses spiritual aspects of well-being and illness, yet there is increasing research about the importance of spirituality in the clinical encounter (26). For instance, frequent attendance at religious services is associated with lowered mortality (27). You may initially feel uncomfortable asking patients about their faith, but questions such as, "Where do you turn for support in times of trouble?" or, "Do you ever attend a religious institution?" will usually lead to responses that clarify core values and how these are used in health. For patients with social and medical problems, religious leaders offer a valuable source of referral and consultation. Acknowledging and supporting your patient's spiritual values will strengthen the doctor-patient relationship and add to your understanding of the whole person.

CASE STUDY 1

A 43-year-old female clerk comes into your office for a cough of 2 weeks' duration. She has had no fever or weight loss but coughs up a thick green sputum. She has smoked one pack of Marlboros per day for the last 25 years but has no history of chronic medical problems. She is afebrile, has a blood pressure of 140/94, weighs 206 pounds, and has a normal lung examination. You diagnose bronchitis, and place her on a 1-week course of antibiotics.

QUESTIONS

1. Which health promotion issues should you address at this initial visit?
2. In what context will you bring up your concerns?
3. How will you deliver a succinct and effective counseling message?
4. Which issues would you address at a follow-up visit?

DISCUSSION

At this visit, you have the chance to link the acute episode of bronchitis to her history of smoking. You decide to evaluate her motivation to quit smoking, and give a short but firm smoking cessation message, when you discover that she is not interested in quitting at the moment. Because smoking is often associated with alcohol use, you also perform a quick assessment for underlying alcohol-use problems using the CAGE questionnaire (see Chapter 15). You also mention that her blood pressure is slightly elevated. You ask to see her back in 1 week to check recovery from the bronchitis, but mainly to repeat the blood pressure and discuss lifestyle issues. At the follow-up visit, you plan to explore her health beliefs and priorities in depth, while being alert for any signs of mental or family dysfunction. To assist her with smoking cessation when she is ready to quit, you know she will need to learn alternative ways of relieving stress in her life.

CASE STUDY 2

A 16-year-old black male student comes into your office for a sports physical. He has no history of prior injuries or other medical problems. His weight is 146 lbs; he is 5'10" tall and has a normal physical examination. During your examination, you ask about health habits and discover that he is a nonsmoker but does drink beer with friends on weekends, that he has had intercourse within the last month without using a condom, and that there is at least one gun in his household.

QUESTIONS

1. What are the three top causes of death for this patient?
2. How do you bring up the issues of health promotion that enable you to ask sensitive health questions with a teenager?
3. How comfortable are you in asking these questions?

DISCUSSION

The three leading causes of death for 16- to 25-year-old African-American males are homicide, accidents, and AIDS. While examining this patient and then signing the forms for sports participation, you ask several questions: (a) Has he been exposed to any health education programs at school or in the community? (b) Does he have any concerns about his body or development? (c) Does he know details about the gun in the house, i.e., its location and whether it is loaded, locked up, or accessible to younger children? Comment in a nonjudgmental way that many teenagers are concerned with problems associated with drinking alcohol, particularly those related to sports performance and driving with anyone who has been drinking. Check on his knowledge of sexually transmitted diseases (STDs), condoms, and pregnancy prevention, and offer him an educational brochure on the prevention of AIDS. Finally, inform him of his higher risk for being involved in a firearm injury and some ways to cut down on that risk.

CASE STUDY 3

A 55-year-old man presents to the office with tennis elbow. He has an asymptomatic blood pressure elevation of 200/110. After addressing his elbow problem, you learn through careful questioning that the patient was diagnosed as having hypertension 2 years ago and started on β-blocker therapy. He developed symptoms of fatigue and sexual dysfunction, so he stopped the medication. He believes that all blood pressure medications cause impotence and does not want to take any more.

QUESTION

1. What is the best approach to bringing the patient's hypertension under control?

DISCUSSION

Although the office nurse detected the patient's elevated blood pressure on routine screening before the doctor entered the room, the physician dealt first with the patient's presenting complaint. Later in the visit, the patient's experiences with hypertension were reviewed. The history of adverse effects, and his health belief that all such medications cause impotence, are

important data in reconsidering the management of his hypertension. A plan that addresses these issues will be effective in developing a new therapeutic alliance between you and the patient to improve long-term outcome. In addition, understanding the patient's spiritual beliefs about life, death, and disability, as well as looking for any other signs of mental distress, may be critical to a successful long-term, doctor-patient therapeutic relationship.

REFERENCES

1. Orenstein WA, Bart KJ, Hinman AR, et al. The opportunity and obligation to eliminate rubella from the United States. JAMA 1984;251:1988–1994.
2. US Preventive Services Task Force. Guide to Clinical Preventive Services: A Report of the US Preventive Services Task Force, 2nd ed. Baltimore: Williams & Wilkins, 1996.
3. Frame PS. A critical review of adult health maintenance. Part 1. Prevention of atherosclerotic diseases. J Fam Pract 1986;22:341–348.
4. Sackett DL. A primer on the precision and accuracy of the clinical examination. JAMA 1992;267:2638–2644.
5. Jaen CR, Stange KC, Nutting PA. Competing demands of primary care: a model for delivery of clinical preventive services. J Fam Pract 1994;38:166–171.
6. Leininger LS, Finn L, Dickey L, et al. An office system for organizing preventive services. A report by the American Cancer Society Advisory Group on Preventive Health Care Reminder Systems. Arch Fam Med 1996;5:108–115.
7. McVea K, Crabtree BF, Medder JD, et al. An ounce of prevention? Evaluation of the "Put Prevention into Practice" program. J Fam Pract 1996;43:361–369.
8. Rosenberg EE, Lussier MT, Beaudoin C. Lessons for clinicians from physician-patient communication literature. Arch Fam Med 1997;6:279–283.
9. Prochaska JO, DiClemente CC, Norcross JC. In search of how people change. Applications to addictive behaviors. Am Psychol 1992;47:1102–1114.
10. Jones TF, Eaton CB. Exercise prescription. Am Fam Physician 1995;52:543–555.
11. Ley P. Doctor-patient communication: some quantitative estimates of the role of cognitive factors in noncompliance. J Hypertens 1985;3:S51–S55.
12. Spiegel D, Bloom JR, Kraemer HC, et al. Effects of psychosocial treatment on survival of patients with metastatic breast cancer. Lancet 1989;2:888–891.
13. Bennett SE, Lawrence RS, Angiolillo DF, et al. Effectiveness of methods used to teach breast self-examination. Am J Prev Med 1990;6:208–217.
14. Cameron C. Patient compliance: recognition of factors involved and suggestions for promoting compliance with therapeutic regimens. J Adv Nurs 1996;24:244–250.

15. Law M, Tang JL. An analysis of the effectiveness of interventions intended to help people stop smoking. Arch Intern Med 1995;155:1933–1941.
16. Smoking Cessation—Clinical Practice Guidelines. USDHHS publication no. 96–0692, US Department of Health and Human Services, Public Health Service, Agency for Health Care Policy and Research, 1996.
17. Physical Activity and Health: A Report of the Surgeon General. Atlanta: US Department of Health and Human Services, Centers for Disease Control and Prevention, 1996.
18. American Cancer Society. 1996 Advisory Committee on Diet, Nutrition and Cancer Prevention. CA Cancer J Clin 1996;46:325–341.
19. Rosenberg ML, Fenley MA, eds. Violence in America—A Public Health Approach. New York: Oxford University Press, 1991.
20. McVea K, Crabtree BF, Medder, et al. An ounce of prevention? Evaluation of the "Put Prevention into Practice" program. J Fam Pract 1996;43:361–369.
21. Kellermann AL, Rivara FP, Rushforth NB, et al. Gun ownership as a risk factor for homicide in the home. N Engl J Med 1993;329:1084–1091.
22. Neufeld B. SAFE questions: overcoming barriers to the detection of domestic violence. Am Fam Physician 1996;53:2575–2582.
23. NIH Technology Assessment Panel on Integration of Behavioral and Relaxation Approaches into the Treatment of Chronic Pain and Insomnia. Integration of behavioral and relaxation approaches into the treatment of chronic pain and insomnia. NIH, Consensus Development Conference. JAMA 1996;276:313–318.
24. Jacobs GD, Benson H, Friedman R. Perceived benefits in a behavioral-medicine insomnia program: a clinical report. Am J Med 1996;100:212–216.
25. DeVries MW, Peeters FP. Melatonin as a therapeutic agent in the treatment of sleep disturbance in depression. J Nerv Ment Dis 1997;185:201–202.
26. Leetun MC. Wellness spirituality in the older adult. Assessment and intervention protocol. Nurse Pract 1996;21:65–70.
27. Strawbridge WJ, Cohen RD, Sherman SJ, Kaplan GA. Frequent attendance at religious services and mortality over 28 years. Am J Public Health 1997;87:957–961.

7. Pregnancy Prevention and Contraception

MELANIE MINTZER

Key Clinical Questions

1. What are the effects of unintended pregnancy in the United States?
2. What are the common methods of contraception?
3. How should you counsel patients on the choice of a contraceptive method?
4. What resources are available to adolescents who seek contraceptive methods and counseling? Which contraceptive methods are particularly appropriate for this age group?
5. Which methods are particularly appropriate for women with common medical conditions such as hypertension, migraine headaches, gallbladder disease, or breast cancer?

PROBLEM OF UNINTENDED PREGNANCY

No other technologic advance has so profoundly affected women as the ability to control fertility through the use of effective contraception. This has changed American social structure by helping women enter and remain in the work force. For many women, however, successful contraception and planned parenthood remain an unrealized dream. An estimated 65% of all pregnancies are unintended (i.e., either mistimed or unwanted) (1). Most Americans wish to control family size and maximize their incomes, yet we are less successful at preventing unintended pregnancy than any other developed country (2). Because of the high rate of unintended pregnancy and abortion, large numbers of women do not complete their education and become single parents who bear the burden of financial and psychologic stress (3). Unintended pregnancy affects women from all levels of society. In 1987, among all women be-tween 20 and 34 years, 57% of pregnancies were unintended; for women 40 years or older, (married or unmarried), over 75% of all pregnancies were unintended (4).

The National Survey on Family Growth (NSFG) uses specific definitions to classify pregnancies:

- *Intended* at conception—wanted at the time of conception or sooner, regardless of whether or not contraception was used
- *Unintended* at conception—pregnancy not wanted at the time the conception occurred, regardless of whether contraception was used
- *Mistimed* conception—pregnancy wanted by the woman some time, but which occurred sooner than desired
- *Unwanted* conceptions—those occurring when the woman did want not any more pregnancies (5)

These definitions and distinctions carry important implications. For example, unintended pregnancies are more likely to end in abortion than intended or mistimed pregnancies, and births resulting from unwanted conceptions appear to carry particular risks for both mother and child (1).

Population at Risk

The 1990 NSFG survey estimated that, based on 1988 data, there were 31 million women of childbearing age (age 15 to 44 years) at risk for unintended pregnancy (6, 7). Analysis of socioeconomic characteristics shows that the majority of unintended pregnancies occur in women who are married, white, and not very poor. Figure 7.1 illustrates the outcome of all pregnancies in the United States.

Teenagers, poor women, African-American women, poorly educated women, and unmarried women, however, are more likely to report that a birth was unwanted or mistimed rather than unintended. The determinants of these unwanted births have not changed over the past 25

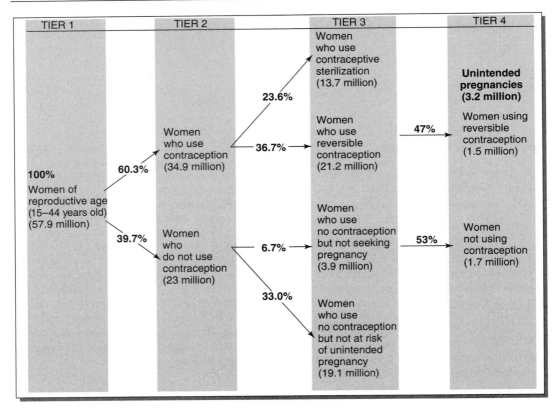

Figure 7.1. *Outcome of all pregnancies in the United States, 1988.* A breakdown of women of reproductive age in relation to contraception and pregnancy. (Sources: Harlap S, Kost K, Forrest JD. Preventing Pregnancy, Protecting Health: A New Look at Birth Control Choices in the United States. New York: Alan Guttmacher Institute, 1991; Mosher WD. Contraceptive practice in the US, 1982–1988. Fam Plann Perspect 1990;22:198–205.)

years, with low education, low income, older age, and black race all increasing the probability of an unwanted birth (4).

EFFECT OF UNINTENDED PREGNANCY ON SOCIETY

During the 25 years referred to previously, there were an estimated 3.5 million unintended pregnancies (4). At an estimated cost of $3,800 (in a managed-care setting) for each pregnancy, the cost is about $13 billion annually for medical care alone (8). Births to unmarried women accounted for 80% of the 1.1 million growth in the welfare rolls over the past 12 years.

From 1970 to 1990, births to unmarried teens rose 150% (9). The estimated annual cost of adolescent childbearing together with the cost of other disadvantages by adolescent mothers was between $13 and $19 billion per year (10). This amount could be saved if an effective pregnancy prevention policy could be introduced. Teenage parenthood is linked to long-term poverty and reliance on the welfare system. Approximately half of teen mothers go on the welfare roles within 5 years, and 53% of all Aid to Families with Dependent Children (AFDC) funds go to families that began with a teenage birth (11).

Adolescent mothers are at high risk for dropping out of school, never receiving a high school diploma, being unemployed or underemployed, and being a single parent (11–13). There is a high likelihood that a teen mother will have a second child within 2 years, thus locking the mother and children into a life of poverty and dependency on public assistance (11).

The adolescent mother is at risk for physical abuse and abandonment by her partner. Both the teenage mother and father suffer economic hardships and often fail to realize their educational and career goals. The children of teenage parents are at extreme risk for exposure to tobacco and alcohol in utero, premature delivery, dying in the first year of life, being abused, developmental delays, and school problems (14). It is clear to many that welfare reform without parallel initiatives to prevent or postpone unintended pregnancy will not solve these overwhelming societal problems, which deplete governmental resources and affect the quality of life of a significant number of young children born to unmarried teen parents.

Causes of Unintended Pregnancy

Contraceptive use and unintended pregnancy are influenced by multiple factors, such as general knowledge, family attitudes about contraceptive methods, ability to use the method correctly, personal feelings, varying patterns of sexual behavior, and access to care. The following are explanations for the increasing rate of unintended pregnancy in the United States:

- Early age of sexual activity and increased sexual activity

- Controversy over abortion

- Decreased access for minors to contraceptive services

- Delayed marriage

- Unwed cohabitation

- Changing sexual values

- Peer pressure

- Increased risk-taking behavior

- Cultural acceptance of early pregnancy

- Conscious decision by some female adolescents to have children despite youth, poverty, and absences of marriage or a committed partner (13, 15, 16)

Unintended pregnancy is caused by failed contraception use or the lack of use of contraception. Organizational and system issues also contribute to failure of contraception. Effective contraceptive use in Western countries is strongly influenced by public policies and programs related to reproduction and family planning. Authors of a 1992 study noted that "the U.S. system for delivering family planning services differs among systems in other Western countries in ways that makes it less conducive, on the whole, to the promotion of highly effective contraceptive methods" (14).

In other countries, contraceptive care is integrated into the primary health services, thus making it available at many convenient and familiar locations. Contraceptive care is generally delivered by primary care physicians and nurse practitioners, usually not obstetrician-gynecologists. In addition, family planning clinics are highly regarded, and they offer services that address contraceptive needs of women at high risk (3). In contrast, the American family planning clinics are designed for low-income women who are too poor to purchase contraceptive methods or services from the private sector. The public view of the family planning clinics is that they are inferior and should be avoided (3).

Fewer contraceptive methods are available in the United States compared to other Western countries, and access to many effective methods is limited by legal issues such as the fear of litigation by both providers and manufacturers of instruments such as the intrauterine device (IUD). Except for the United States, most developed countries provide contraceptive methods at little or no cost to everyone, without restriction to minors (3).

PREVENTING UNINTENDED PREGNANCY: FAMILY PLANNING SERVICES

The controversy over changing sexual mores is palpable in any examination of the American political system. It is reflected in public debate over the legality of abortion and whether sex education should be included in the public school curriculum. The current struggle among U.S. political, religious, and medical establishments is whether the primary intervention against unintended pregnancy should be abstinence or increased contraceptive use. This polarization of opinions obstructs the organization of programs to limit the number of unintended births. Abstinence, as the primary preventive method for all women at risk, cannot be counted on as adequate in reducing unintended pregnancy. Solutions to these controversies are critical if cost-effective family planning programs are to be successful (17).

Family planning and reproductive health care services are delivered by a variety of health care professionals, working in the private and public sector. Funding comes mainly from the federal government, (about 20%) through Title X of the Public Health Service Act, the first nationally funded family planning program, and Medicaid.

Title X provides comprehensive family planning and reproductive health services for most poor and low-income women who do not qualify for Medicaid and has helped correct inequalities in health care services across the nation (18). State funds contribute about 23%, and the remaining dollars come from private funds from such diverse organizations as church-based charities, United Way, Planned Parenthood Federation of America, and other nonprofit organizations (19).

How effective are publicly funded family planning services? In 1994, it was estimated that 1.5 million unplanned pregnancies were averted among 6.5 million women who obtained contraceptive services from family planning clinics, with nearly one million of these women receiving care from Title X-funded sites (20).

In the past decade, public funding for family planning services has shifted from the federal government to the states, and regular cuts in state budgets have resulted in decreased services. Publicly funded clinics often cannot afford to offer routine preventive testing and counseling. For poorer women seeking these services, many of whom must leave the welfare rolls, decreased resources present significant obstacles to care, and the number of unintended pregnancies and births may increase (18, 19).

The need for low-cost reproductive services provided by publicly funded family planning clinics is vital, as a high proportion of the women at risk are uninsured (20). Even for women with some health care coverage, publicly funded clinics are needed to provide certain types of contraceptive methods and services because of patients' concerns over confidentiality and fear of cancellation of covered services.

CONTRACEPTION

Regular contraceptive counseling for all men and women at risk for unintended pregnancy is a key component of comprehensive preventive health. Thus, the primary care physician must become expert at giving his or her patient the latest information about efficacy, risk factors, and benefits of a variety of contraceptive methods. Patients need guidance in choosing the right method and are entitled to be given information in their own language, with consideration of their ability to actively participate in the counseling sessions. The challenge is to provide information in an environment of informed consent, yet still understand how a patient is clearly influenced by the clinician's preferences and attitudes about contraceptive methods. To depend on one's own anecdotal experience violates the principles of expert counseling.

Sixty percent of women use some form of contraception. The primary method used is the oral contraceptive pill (OCP) (28%), followed by female sterilization (25%), condoms (13%), and male sterilization (11%) (21) (Fig. 7.2). Women

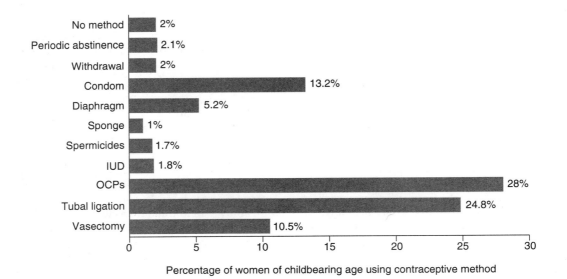

Percentage of women of childbearing age using contraceptive method

Figure 7.2. *Methods of contraception most commonly used by American couples.*

generally prefer coitus-independent methods of contraception, such as sterilization or oral contraceptive use, which provide protection over longer periods of time. Use of oral contraceptives is highest in women aged 15 to 30 years and lower in women aged 30 to 44 years (21). Condom use is significantly higher in adolescent women than in older women (22). However, there are still significant delays in obtaining medical assistance for contraception (17), so health care systems and providers need to improve their counseling and diagnostic skills and services.

CONTRACEPTIVE COUNSELING

Prescribing the appropriate contraceptive method for a woman requires the integration of clinical skills with an understanding of endocrinology and human behavior. The choice of a contraceptive method depends on the level of sexual activity, the timing of childbearing and childspacing, the risks of acquiring sexually transmitted diseases (STDs), and past experiences with contraceptive methods.

The office visit for contraception often represents the entry of a young woman into the health care system and provides an opportunity to address important health concerns—menses, sexual activity, pregnancy prevention or planning, infertility, and the avoidance of STDs. A family physician who is concerned, trusted, and knowledgeable is in an excellent position to counsel individuals and couples about contraceptive methods through the course of their lives. For example, the single female college student may choose a different contraceptive method than a married woman who has completed her childbearing. In some instances, the male takes contraceptive responsibility by using condoms or having a vasectomy.

Remember to individualize the contraceptive method to the patient or couple. Evaluate each contraceptive method in relation to the patient's age, marital status, childbearing potential, lifestyle, income, religion, and medical history. Expect the patient to change methods depending on personal circumstances. Previous contraceptive experiences, successful or otherwise, also color a woman's choice of birth control methods. A method failure in a conscientious patient usually precludes the use of the same method. After the birth of a child, a contraceptive method change will often be requested, and the intent of the contraceptive counseling session will likely

shift to address issues of child spacing and breast-feeding. As all methods carry with them measurable, technical failure rates as well as fairly accurate estimated failure rates due to misuses, understanding this information is critical in helping the patient decide which contraceptive method to use.

Anticipatory guidance must include a discussion of sexual behaviors that place the patient at increased risk for STDs. A history of prior STDs requires screening for asymptomatic infections and counseling about the use of safe sexual practices and condoms. Certain contraceptive devices can foster or inhibit transmission of STDs. For all patients who are uncertain of their partner's human immunodeficiency virus (HIV) status, and for patients with multiple sexual partners, the use of condoms in addition to other contraceptive methods is recommended.

A contraceptive counseling session has three purposes: (a) to provide the patient with information in a nonjudgmental way; (b) to explain the risks, benefits, and side effects of available methods (Tables 7.1 and 7.2); and (c) to answer questions. These questions can include concerns about sexuality, fears about pregnancy and childbearing, or previous problematic sexual encounters. Components of an effective counseling session include the following:

- Have a face-to-face discussion with the dressed patient either before or after the physical examination is performed. This allows a more respectful and focused communication on the main questions and issues. Choose terms the patient understands and do not use medical jargon (e.g., "STDs"). If this is the patient's first contraceptive counseling session, begin with a simple review of reproductive anatomy and physiology, using visual aids that show the menstrual cycle and male and female anatomy. Even well-educated patients may have questions about the reproductive cycle.

- Ask about the patient's concerns about pregnancy and whether or not she understands its medical side effects. Also inquire about the patient's need for spontaneity in sex, the frequency of intercourse, prior episodes of STDs, comfort with touching one's own or a partner's genitals, and the quality of communication between partners. Responses to these questions can help you decide which contraceptive methods are most appropriate for your patient.

Table 7.1.
Contraceptive Methods and Their Failure Rates[a]

Method (1)	% of Women Experiencing an Accidental Pregnancy Within the First Year of Use		% of Women Continuing Use at 1 Year (4)
	Typical Use (2)	Perfect Use (3)	
Chance	85	85	
Spermicides	21	6	43
Periodic abstinence	20		67
Calendar		9	
Ovulation method		3	
Sympto-thermal		2	
Postovulation		1	
Withdrawal	19	4	
Cap			
Parous women	36	26	45
Nulliparous women	18	9	58
Sponge			
Parous women	36	20	45
Nulliparous women	18	9	58
Diaphragm	18	6	58
Condom			
Female (reality)	21	5	56
Male	12	3	63
Pill	3		72
Progestin only		0.5	
Combined		0.1	
IUD			
Progesterone T	2.0	1.5	81
Copper T 380A	0.8	0.6	78
LNg 20	0.1	0.1	81
Depo-Provera	0.3	0.3	70
Norplant (six capsules)	0.09	0.09	85
Female sterilization	0.4	0.4	100
Male sterilization	0.15	0.10	100

Reprinted with permission from Hatcher RJ, et al. Contraceptive Technology Update, 16th rev. ed. New York: Irvington Publishers, 1994:113.

[a]**Emergency contraceptive pills:** Treatment initiated within 72 hours after unprotected intercourse reduces the risk of pregnancy by at least 75%. **Lactational amenorrhea method:** LAM is a highly effective, *temporary* method of contraception.

- Describe each contraceptive method, using a pictorial chart. Explain the side effects and minor complications that may arise from each method. Just handing out reading material is not sufficient to assure the patient's understanding. Discuss the patient's personal experiences and her knowledge of various methods. Check that the patient understands and can read the materials, which should be written at the 8th grade level.

- When a method has been selected, reiterate its advantages and disadvantages in relation to the patient's history. Once the medical history and physical examination have been performed, if appropriate, prescribe, insert, fit, or inject the method or explain instructions for its use.

- Make plans for a return visit, reminding the patient about the warning signs or problems that might warrant an earlier contact. Make sure the patient understands who to contact should questions and problems with the contraceptive method arise.

For the adolescent, a discussion of the teen's needs and desires helps build trust between patient and the physician. By assessing the frequency of intercourse and estimating the number of partners, adherence with the chosen method can be significantly improved. For instance, if

Table 7.2.

Major Methods of Contraception and Related Safety Concerns, Side Effects, and Noncontraceptive Benefits

Method	Dangers	Side Effects	Noncontraceptive Benefits
Pill	Cardiovascular complications (stroke, heart attack, blood clots, high blood pressure, hepatic adenomas)	Nausea, headaches, dizziness, spotting, weight gain, breast tenderness, chloasma	Protects against pelvic inflammatory disease (PID), some cancers (ovarian, endometrial), some benign tumors (leiomyomata, benign breast masses) and ovarian cysts; decreases menstrual blood loss and pain
IUD	PID, uterine perforation, anemia	Menstrual cramping, spotting, increased bleeding	None known except progestin-releasing IUDs, which may decrease menstrual blood loss and pain
Male condom	None known	Decreased sensation, allergy to latex, loss of spontaneity	Protects against sexually transmitted diseases, including AIDS; delays premature ejaculation
Female condom	None known	Aesthetically unappealing and awkward to use for some	Protects against sexually transmitted diseases, including on the vulva
Implant	Infection at implant site	Tenderness at site, menstrual changes	May protect against PID; lactation not disturbed; may decrease menstrual cramps, pains, and blood loss
Injectable	None definitely proven	Menstrual changes, weight gain, headaches	May protect against PID; lactation not disturbed; may have protective effects against ovarian and endometrial cancers
Sterilization	Infection	Pain at surgical site, psychologic reactions, subsequent regret that the procedure was performed	None known; may have beneficial effects *vis à vis* PID
Abstinence	None known	Psychologic reactions	Prevents infections including AIDS
Abortion	Infection, pain, perforation, psychologic trauma	Cramping	None known
Barriers: diaphragm, cap, sponge	Mechanical irritation, vaginal infections, toxic shock syndrome	Pelvic pressure, cervical erosion, vaginal discharges if left in too long	Protects somewhat against sexually transmitted diseases
Spermicides	None known	Tissue irritation	Protects against many sexually transmitted diseases
Lactational amenorrhea method (LAM)	None known	Mastitis from staphylococcal infection	Provides excellent nutrition for infants under 6 months old

Reprinted with permission from Hatcher RJ, et al. Contraceptive Technology Update, 16th rev. ed. New York: Irvington Publishers, 1994:129.

your patient feels that taking a pill every night will be difficult, the combined use of an injectable progestin or a barrier method and condoms may prove a wiser choice. Regardless of what other method is used, routine use of a condom by the male partner is recommended to prevent possible transmission of HIV disease.

Consent and Confidentiality

Confidentiality is a relatively straightforward task when counseling adults. It becomes more complicated with adolescents because you must determine if the adolescent can provide informed consent for the intervention. Informed consent means that "an individual can understand the risks and benefits of the proposed treatment and its treatment alternatives, and decide voluntarily whether to proceed with the physician's recommendations" (24).

In counseling and treating teenagers, confidentiality is of utmost importance. Confidentiality refers to "the privileged and private nature of information during the health care transaction" (25). Ideally, one would like to have obtained parental consent before providing contraceptive services to teens, however, that situation is unusual.

Many clinicians allow mature or emancipated minors to give informed consent for general health services including the diagnosis of pregnancy and prenatal care, contraceptive services, diagnosis and treatment of STDs, and alcohol and drug treatment (26). Emancipated minors include adolescents under legal age who are married, serving in the military, or living away from home and managing their own financial affairs. Mature minors include those adolescents under the age of 21 still living at home who demonstrate the cognitive maturity to understand the risks and benefits of a proposed medical treatment and its alternatives and who can voluntarily decide whether to undergo treatment (27). There have been no cases in which a physician has been successfully sued for providing adequate treatment to an adolescent over the age of 14 without parental consent (26).

It is prudent to ask adolescents if they have discussed their decision to seek contraceptive services with their parents, understanding that most will answer, "No." Be aware of your personal feelings about prescribing contraceptives for minors. Reassure the teen that your interactions are confidential. If you feel you cannot maintain confidentiality, or the insurance billing system used will inevitably compromise confidentiality, you can refer the patient to a free or low-cost family planning clinic where confidentiality can be better ensured.

When faced with the situation of providing a contraceptive method to minors, especially those under the age of 14 or cases in which the possibility of sexual abuse, assault, coercion, or incest is identified, it is vital to take a complete, detailed history to assess the circumstances specific to that adolescent. Sexual abuse is defined as "the involvement of dependent, developmentally immature children and adolescents in sexual activities that they do not understand, to which they are unable to give informed consent, or that are inappropriate for family roles" (25). In sexual abuse, the perpetrator is a relative; in sexual assault, (i.e., molestation, rape, etc.) the offender is a stranger or an acquaintance (28). If abuse is suspected, additional evaluation is needed to determine the circumstances surrounding the abuse and the degree to sequelae, i.e., suicidal ideation, involvement in risky behaviors such as alcohol and drug use, or unsafe sexual practices. A careful history will clarify and identify the presence of physical, emotional, and psychologic factors, untoward consequences, and the patient's need for further evaluation and treatment. In all states, abuse is an offense that must be reported to the appropriate child protective authorities. Because reporting of abuse breaches confidentiality, physicians must ensure that their adolescent patients are counseled on the procedures and actions that follow disclosure. Because of the sensitive nature of this issue, inquiries about abuse should be made while the clinician is alone with the adolescent patient. Appropriate follow-up for this complicated situation includes the monitoring of the patient's situation by the clinician that identified the abuse and a determination that the patient is being protected from the abusive conditions (28).

CLINICAL EVALUATION

All women need a history and physical examination before being prescribed a contraceptive method. Taking the history and performing the physical examination provides a natural structure to discuss issues of sexuality, and allows the patient to bring up other medical problems or share anxieties about personal or family medical problems. In most cases, given the devastating statistics about the incidence of unintended pregnancy in women ages 18 and younger, it is entirely safe to prescribe low-dose birth control pills before actually performing a physical examination (29). The health benefits of preventing pregnancy in an adolescent far outweigh any of the risks and effects of unplanned pregnancy.

Most women are anxious about having a pelvic examination, especially a first examination or an examination with a new clinician. This is especially true for adolescents. The first pelvic examination is somewhat awkward for both the patient and the health care provider and can influence a patient's attitudes about physicians for the rest of their lives. You can create a positive atmosphere by (30)

- Interviewing the patient privately in a comfortable environment

- Reiterating confidentiality of doctor-patient communication

- Being aware of the fears the patient might have about the first pelvic examination, and listening rather than lecturing when providing information

- Addressing the misconceptions and worries that women often have regarding pain, loss of virginity, embarrassment about body odors, loss of control, or anxiety over feeling that their anatomy is abnormal

- Being aware of your own concerns about performing a pelvic examination such as competency, loss of trust or confidence by the patient in your ability, and anxiety about causing pain

History

No one set of questions will be ideal for all of your patients, and the items below are presented to guide you and facilitate the subsequent performance of the physical examination. Elements of the history, taken in a confidential setting, are as follows (30, 31):

- Identify the reason for coming or the presenting complaint.

- Take a menstrual history including the age at menarche, duration of menses, interval between periods, and regularity of cycles, characteristics and changes in flow date of the last period and the presence or absence of dysmenorrhea.

- Obtain relevant past history of vaginitis, STDs, urinary tract infections (UTIs), pregnancies, or sexual activity causing other diseases.

- Take a sexual history knowing that the most important question to ask of each patient is what they are doing to protect themselves from acquiring AIDS. Include an exploration of gender preferences, i.e., homosexuality, heterosexuality, bisexuality, which might put the patient at more or less risk; the number of partners in the past year; any history of sharing needles or injection equipment with another person; or whether the patient has had sexual contact with a high-risk partner (31).

- Identify and explore whether the patient has used any methods of contraception and how comfortable she was with that method.

- Ask questions about relationships, substance abuse, sexual dysfunction, or other concerns if there is adequate time.

Physical Examination

The physical examination should include the following:

- Vital signs, height and weight, blood pressure, and temperature if the patient has other concurrent medical complaints.

- An examination of the thyroid, breasts, chest, heart, abdomen, and extremities.

- Examination of the pelvis, including inspection of the external genitalia, clitoris, urethra, Bartholin's glands, vulva, and hymeneal ring, if still present. Perform a speculum examination of the vagina, cervix, and fornix, noting signs of estrogenization, inflammation, or tumors.

- If the patient is symptomatic or if you suspect the presence of an STD, obtain a gonorrhea culture, chlamydia specimen, and swabs for examination of vaginal secretions for presence of yeast, bacteria, or trichomonads.

- Perform a Papanicolaou (Pap) smear of the endocervix using an Ayres spatula and a nylon Cytobrush or Cytobroom to collect cells from the squamocolumnar junction, the site of most cervical cancer lesions.

- Perform a bimanual examination, palpating the cervix, checking for cervical motion tenderness to exclude infection, noting the size and position of the uterus and any masses or tenderness. Explore the posterior fornix and the retrouterine pouch for masses, fullness, fluctuance, or sensitivity. Palpate the adnexa, noting the presence of masses, size, tenderness or abnormalities of the ovaries, and thickening or abnormalities of the fallopian tubes. In large women, one often cannot palpate ovaries due to tissue redundancy.

- A rectal examination may be necessary to complete the evaluation of the adnexa or uterus as well as the rectum, anus, and posterior cul-de-sac. In younger women, especially adolescents, the rectovaginal examination can be deferred.

- Remember to review and discuss the results of the physical examination with the adolescent patient, addressing her concerns about the normalcy of her anatomy and physiology and sexual practices (30).

CHOOSING A CONTRACEPTIVE METHOD

The effectiveness of any contraceptive method is measured by perfect use and typical use. "Perfect use" is the annual rate of pregnancy among couples who use the method correctly at each intercourse; "typical use" is the pregnancy rate measured in clinical trials or clinical studies. You should know the safety and effectiveness rates of each contraceptive method. Quote "actual" rather than "theoretical" failure rates. Table 7.1 outlines the different contraceptive methods and their relative failure rates (31).

All contraceptive methods involve risk to the user. Some are safer than others (barrier methods versus oral contraceptives); some can have significant untoward complications (such as IUDs); and some can result in minor but uncomfortable side effects, such as contraceptive gels or spermicides, which can cause a chemical vaginitis. When assessing the efficacy of various methods, remember to think about relative risk of a particular method as compared to the risks of unwanted pregnancy (31). Figure 7.3 outlines the steps in contraceptive counseling.

The costs and availability of the various contraceptive methods are important factors in patient compliance and should always be considered carefully by physicians. For patients without insurance, a referral can be made to a local health department family planning clinic that provides contraceptive services and examinations at no charge or on a sliding fee scale. If the patient qualifies for the federally funded Title X family planning funds, she can receive a year's supply of free birth control pills, contraceptive jelly, or condoms. In most states, Medicaid will pay for Norplant insertion and removal, IUD insertion, diaphragm or cervical cap fitting and supplies, four Depo-Provera shots/year or 12-months' supply of oral contraceptive pills (18). Table 7.3 lists available contraceptive methods, efficacy, and annual costs.

See patients at least once a year to review the effectiveness of the contraceptive method and risks for STD and to repeat the Pap smear. At that time, a problem that precludes using a specific method also may be discovered, e.g., hypertension in an oral contraceptive pill user or pelvic inflammatory disease with an IUD. It is always prudent to review the patient's views on pregnancy. Should the patient wish to become pregnant, the visit can include the opportunity to do preconception counseling and begin vitamin supplementation with folic acid.

Because many women use family planning visits as their yearly general health care examination, many family physicians will perform other screening tests. There is good evidence to support screening for cervical cancer (Pap smear), STDs in high-risk populations, and lipids in women over 45 (or with strong family history of cardiovascular [CV] disease) (32). HIV antibody screening tests are now a routine part of yearly family planning visits for high-risk women, those anticipating a new sexual relationship, or those with multiple partners.

ORAL CONTRACEPTIVES

Oral contraceptive pills (OCPs) provide women with a reliable, nonsurgical, reversible method of contraception that has an extremely low failure rate (0.1 to 3 failures per 100 woman-years) (31). Consisting of estrogen and progesterone components, the combined oral contraceptive pill is given daily for 3 out of every 4 weeks; it prevents ovulation by acting on the hypothalamic and pituitary centers to inhibit gonadotropin secretion. Estrogen prevents the production of follicle-stimulating hormone (FSH), which inhibits development of a dominant follicle. Progesterone suppresses the production of luteinizing hormone (LH), which is necessary for ovulation. Estrogen also increases the transit time of the ovum through the fallopian tubes, thus reducing the available time for fertilization. The progestin component of the combined pill makes the cervical mucus more viscous, thus hampering the transport of sperm. Progestins also inhibit endometrial proliferation, making it less hospitable

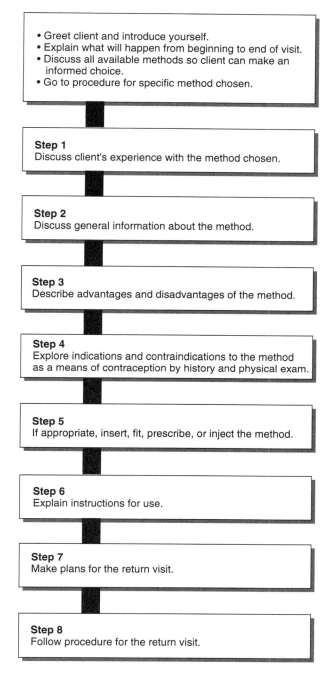

- Greet client and introduce yourself.
- Explain what will happen from beginning to end of visit.
- Discuss all available methods so client can make an informed choice.
- Go to procedure for specific method chosen.

Step 1
Discuss client's experience with the method chosen.

Step 2
Discuss general information about the method.

Step 3
Describe advantages and disadvantages of the method.

Step 4
Explore indications and contraindications to the method as a means of contraception by history and physical exam.

Step 5
If appropriate, insert, fit, prescribe, or inject the method.

Step 6
Explain instructions for use.

Step 7
Make plans for the return visit.

Step 8
Follow procedure for the return visit.

Figure 7.3. *Algorithm for contraceptive counseling.*

to implantation by a fertilized ovum. Figure 7.4 outlines an algorithm for selecting an OCP.

There are two types of estrogen used in the United States: ethinyl estradiol and mestranol. Ethinyl estradiol (EE) (dose: 20 to 100 μg) is an active compound, whereas mestranol (ME) (50 μg) must be converted by the liver to an active compound.

The Federal Drug Administration (FDA) has approved the use of many different progestins,

Table 7.3.
Currently Available Contraceptive Methods' Yearly Cost and Efficacy

Contraceptive Method	Unit Cost ($)	Annual Cost ($)	% of Women Experiencing Accidental Pregnancy Within First Year Assuming Typical Use
Combined oral contraceptive pills	10–20/cycle	130–270	3.0
Progesterone-only pills	10–20/cycle	100–300	3.0
Norplant implant in place for 5 yrs	350/kit plus 150–200 for insertion/removal	130–170 if retained 5 yrs; 5-yr cost 650–850	0.2
Depo-Provera injection	35/injection	140	0.3
Copper T 380A intrauterine device (IUD)	120 plus 50 for insertion/lab tests	20 for CuT 380A if retained for 8 yrs	0.8
Diaphragm and spermicide, twice weekly use	20 plus 50–150 for fitting	Cost of spermicide: 85	18
Condoms (male), twice weekly use	.50–3.00	100–300	12
Condoms (female), twice weekly use	2.50–3.00	250–300	21
Sponge, parous	4/pack of 3	133	36
Cervical cap, twice weekly use	20 plus 50–150 for fitting	Cost of spermicide: 85	36
Spermicide alone, twice weekly use	.85/application	85	21

Modified from Hatcher RJ, et al. Contraceptive Technology Update, 16th rev. ed. New York: Irvington Publishers, 1994:133.

which include norethindrone, norethindrone acetate, ethynodiol diacetate, levonorgestrel, norethynodrel, desogestrel, and norgestimate. Currently available only in Western Europe, gestodene will most likely be approved in the United States in the near future. The newer progestins, desogestrel and norgestimate and gestodene, have three benefits currently being marketed by their manufacturers: greater protection against cardiovascular disease, reduced testosterone effect, and less frequent amenorrhea (33).

Advantages and Indications for Use

The OCP is safe and can be used as a contraceptive method throughout the reproductive years without a rest period. It is safer for women under age 35 and for nonsmokers to use OCPs than to have a baby. The OCP is a reversible method that does not affect the ability to become pregnant, although some women experience a delay of 2 to 3 months in becoming pregnant (31, 33).

All OCP formulations provide equivalent contraceptive efficacy as long as no pills are missed. They have few side effects or complications when used by healthy women under 45 years of age. The noncontraceptive benefits of oral contraceptives are numerous and provide many women with significant relief from menstrual disorders, such as:

- Reduction of menstrual cramps and pain (34)

- Decreased menstrual flow and blood loss

- Increased iron stores in those women with iron deficiency anemia secondary to menorrhagia (35)

- Regulation of menstrual cycles and elimination of the midcycle pain some women experience with ovulation (35)

- Reduction in hirsutism by suppressing androgens (35)

- Reduction in the incidence of functional ovarian cysts by up to 80% (36)

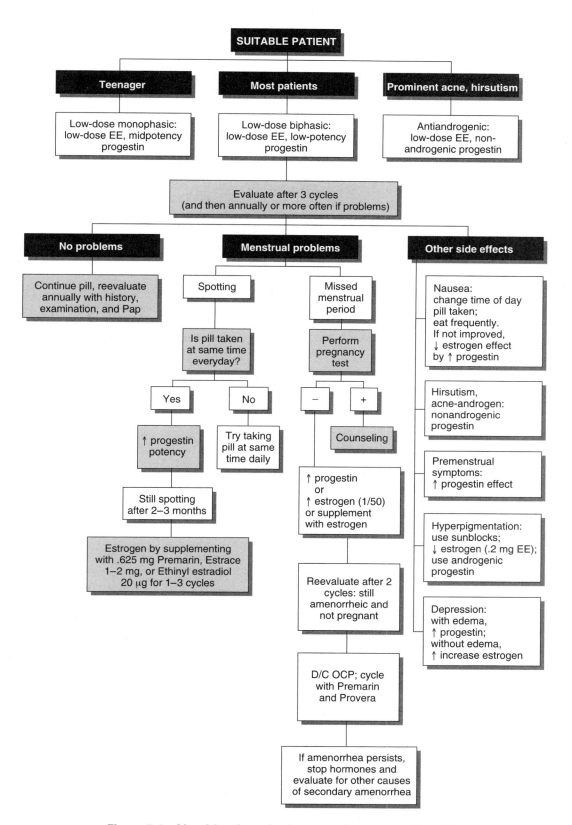

Figure 7.4. *Algorithm for selecting an oral contraceptive pill.*

- Management of menstrual cycling to improve hygiene (for example, in mentally impaired women)

- Symptomatic treatment of premenstrual syndrome (PMS) (37).

Other noncontraceptive benefits include decreased risk for benign breast disease; decreased risk of ovarian and endometrial cancer, and protection against pelvic inflammatory disease and ectopic pregnancy.

Another benefit of combined oral contraceptives is their use as immediate postcoital contraceptives. Widespread availability of OCPs for use as postcoital therapy could prevent as many as 2.3 million unintended pregnancies and 1 million induced abortions annually in the United States (38).

Contraindications and Disadvantages

Absolute and relative contraindications to oral contraceptions are outlined in Table 7.4. In women who have relative contraindications to OCPs, it is important to review risks and benefits of this method before prescribing. Despite contraindications, there may be situations in which the OCP presents the overall lowest risk to the patient.

Disadvantages of using the OCP include:

- There is no protection from STDs, so concurrent use of condoms must be recommended.

- The incidence of chlamydia infections is increased in pill users, as the cervix can develop an ectropion, which is more vulnerable to infection (37).

- Pills must be taken about the same time every day to prevent method failures. Adherence to this schedule can be a problem for some women, especially teenagers.

- Pills are relatively expensive, and cost is often the reason that women discontinue contraception.

- Pills can cause missed periods, breakthrough bleeding, scanty bleeding, or spotting. Combined OCPs can precipitate headaches and

Table 7.4.
Absolute and Relative Contraindications to Birth Control Pills

Absolute contraindications
- Thromboembolic disorder (or history thereof)
- Cerebrovascular accident (or history thereof)
- Coronary artery disease (or history thereof)
- Known or suspected carcinoma of the breast (or history thereof)
- Known or suspected estrogen-dependent neoplasia (or history thereof)
- Pregnancy
- Benign or malignant liver tumor (or history thereof)
- Impaired liver function at time of prescribing

Strong relative contraindications
- Vascular or migraine headaches that start after the initiation of oral contraceptives
- Hypertension with resting diastolic BP of 90 or greater; a resting systolic BP of 140 or greater on three or more separate visits; or an accurate measurement of 110 diastolic or more on a single visit
- Diabetes mellitus
- Active gallbladder disease
- Impaired liver function as in mononucleosis, acute phase
- Lactation
- Sickle cell disease (SS) or sickle C disease (SC)
- Elective major surgery planned in next 4 weeks or major surgery requiring immobilization
- Long-leg cast or major injury to lower leg
- 50 years of age or older, accompanied by a second risk factor for the development of cardiovascular disease
- 35 years of age or older and currently a heavy smoker (15 or more cigarettes a day)
- Unexplained (abnormal) vaginal or uterine bleeding
- Completion of term pregnancy within the past 10–14 days
- Cardiac or renal disease or history thereof

Adapted from Hatcher RA, Trussell J, Stewart F, Stewart GK, Kowal K, Guest F, Cates W, Policar M. Contraceptive Technology, 16th rev. ed. New York: Irvington Publishers, 1996:242–248.

induce depression, mood changes, and decreased libido (34, 35, 37).

Cardiovascular Effects

Women who are smokers, sedentary, overweight, over 50 years old, hypertensive, diabetic, or have elevated lipids are at increased risk for cardiovascular disease (CVD) and its complications. OCP therapy produces dose-related hypercoagulability of the blood; therefore, use of the OCP modestly increases a woman's risk of developing myocardial infarction (MI), subarachnoid hemorrhage, nonhemorrhagic stroke, and venous thrombosis, especially in older smokers (39).

Smoking combined with OCP use increases the risk of venous thrombosis and embolism threefold (40). The adverse effects of the pill on hypercoagulability and on the incidence of cardiovascular disease disappear within a month if a woman discontinues medication (33).

It is recommended that women discontinue the pill or switch to a progesterone-only method at least 1 month before elective surgery. Women with polycythemia or other conditions that would promote a hypercoagulable state should not use OCPs (41, 42). Those who have bleeding disorders or are anticoagulated can use OCPs as a method without concern.

Hypertension is a documented adverse effect of OCPs; however, the elevation is usually mild and reversible with discontinuation of the pill. Clinically significant hypertension has been associated with both the estrogen and progestin in pills but is rare in women using low-dose combinations. Periodic blood pressure measurements in women using OCPs is critically important. Persistent diastolic elevation above 90 mm Hg is a sign that the pills should be changed to a lower dose, discontinued, or switched to a progestin-only pill, which may help to normalize blood pressure (33, 37).

Combined OCP use is associated with numerous other physiologic effects, including minor changes in glucose tolerance (norgestrel being the most diabetogenic of the progestins), acceleration of the development of gallstones predisposed in patients, and in rare cases the development of benign liver tumors (34, 35).

Today's low-dose OCPs have no adverse effect on lipid profiles except a slight increase in triglyceride levels that reverses with discontinuation. For those women with known hypertriglyceridemia > 350 mg/dL, OCPs are con-

traindicated. For women under age 40 without a family history of lipid disorder, diabetes, or coronary artery disease, obtaining a fasting lipid profile is not indicated (29, 31).

Breast Cancer

Many epidemiologic studies have explored the relationship between oral contraceptives and breast cancer, and the findings are not consistent. There appears to be an increased risk in the diagnosis of breast cancer in women under the age of 35, but this is balanced by a decreased risk after age 45, when the disease is more prevalent. These data are taken from studies of women on higher dose OCPs (43–45). Although data indicate that it is safe to prescribe OCPs to women with a family history of breast cancer, women with strong family histories are now electing to use nonhormonal methods of contraception to counter any, as yet unproven, effects (45).

All women, regardless of age, should be counseled to stop smoking when taking OCPs. For young women who are persistent smokers, many experts advise using a low-dose estrogen formula (less than 50 μg). After age 35, oral contraceptive use in smokers is definitely contraindicated (34, 35).

Choosing the Right Contraceptive Pill for Your Patients

Combined estrogen and progesterone oral contraceptives contain one of two estrogens (mestranol or ethinyl estradiol) and one of seven progestins (norethindrone, ethynodiol diacetate, norethynodrel, norethindrone acetate, norgestrel, norgestimate, or desogestrel). Combinations of these two hormones account for all types of oral contraceptives on the market, each of which has a predictable, specific profile of adverse effects. Consequently, it is more helpful to think about the characteristics of each pill combination in terms of its estrogen or progestin potency rather than actual microgram or milligram amounts of a drug. Table 7.5 illustrates the relative potencies of estrogens and progestins in currently available OCPs.

When comparing the relative merits of OCPs, keep these points in mind:

- The potency of estrogens in OCPs cannot be compared on a microgram or milligram basis.

- Total estrogenic effect reflects both endogenous production in the ovaries and adipose

Table 7.5.
Composition of Oral Contraception

Type	Name	Estrogen	µg	Progestin	mg
Low androgenic activity of progestin component					
Monophasic	Modicon	EE	35	norethindrone	0.5
	Brevicon	EE	35	norethindrone	0.5
	Ovcon 35	EE	35	norethindrone	0.4
	Ortho-Cyclen	EE	35	norgestimate	0.25
	Ortho-Cept	EE	30	desogestrel	0.15
	Desogen	EE	30	desogestrel	0.15
	Alesse	EE	20	levonorgestrel	0.1
Triphasic	Ortho Tri-Cyclen	EE	35/35/35	norgestimate	0.18/0.215/0.25
Medium androgenic activity of progestin component					
Monophasic	Ovcon 50	EE	50	norethindrone	1.0
	Ortho-Novum 1/50	mestranol	50	norethindrone	1.0
	Demulen 1/35	EE	35	ethynodiol diacetate	1.0
	Demulen	EE	50	ethynodiol diacetate	1.0
	Mestranol		50	norethindrone	1.0
	Norinyl 1 + 50	EE	50	ethynodiol diacetate	1.0
	Ortho-Novum 1/35	EE	35	norethindrone	1.0
	Norinyl 1+ 35	EE	35	norethindrone	1.0
Triphasic	Ortho Novum 7/7/7	EE	35/35/35	norethindrone	0.5/0.75/1.0
	Tri-Norinyl	EE	35/35/35	norethindrone	0.5/1.0/0.5
	Triphasil	EE	30/40/30	levonorgestrel	0.05/0.075/0.125
	Tri-Levlen	EE	30/40/30	levonorgestrel	0.05/0.075/0.125
High androgenic activity of progestin component					
Monophasic	Ovral	EE	20	norgestrel	0.5
	Loestrin 1.5/30	EE	30	norethindrone acetate	1.5
	Lo/Ovral	EE	30	norgestrel	0.3
	Nordette	EE	30	levonorgestrel	0.15
	Levlen	EE	30	levonorgestrel	0.15
Composition of progestin-only OCs					
Monophasic	Micronor	None	N/A	norethindrone	0.35
	Nor-QD	None	N/A	norethindrone	0.35
	Ovrette	None	N/A	norgestrel	0.075

Modified from Health Learning Systems. Risks and Benefits of Oral Contraceptive Pills. University of Minnesota Monograph. Little Falls, NJ: Health Learning Systems, 1997:39.

tissue and exogenous intake. Because of individual variation, pills will cause less suppression of endogenous estrogen production in some women than in others.

- Estrogens produce different side effects in different women.

- Progestins have both estrogenic and androgenic effects. Some progestins are quite estrogenic (ethynodiol diacetate), and some are very androgenic (norgestrel).

- Progestins also have antiestrogenic effects.

- Estrogens are responsible for most major pill-associated complications, such as cerebrovascular accidents and thrombosis, as well as for many minor side effects.

- Progestins are responsible for some minor side effects and contribute to some major estrogen-induced complications, such as increased HDL levels from norethindrone and norgestrel.

There are three types of OCPs: monophasic, biphasic, and triphasic pills. The monophasic pills (e.g., Ortho-Novum 1/35) deliver the same amount of estrogen and progesterone for each of 21 days. Biphasic pills (e.g., Ortho-Novum 7/7/7, Tri-Norinyl, Ortho Tri-Cyclen) vary the amount of progesterone through the menstrual cycle, raising the concentration around the time of ovulation. The triphasic pills (e.g., Triphasil) alter the levels of both the estrogen and progestin throughout the menstrual cycle, simulating more closely what happens to normal hormone levels. Advantages to prescribing triphasic pills include lower total dosages of both estrogen and progestin components and fewer metabolic effects on lipids, blood pressure, and carbohydrate metabolism. The main disadvantages of triphasic OCPs are confusion when a patient misses a pill and then does not know which pill to make up (because the pills are different colors and potencies) and more breakthrough bleeding.

You should generally start the patient on a low-dose estrogen/progestin combination and observe for adverse effects over the first three to four menstrual cycles. Many common adverse effects, such as nausea and breakthrough bleeding (spotting), often resolve within the first three cycles of use. If adverse effects continue, choose an alternative pill that is hormonally structured to treat the adverse effect(s). It is common for a woman who has taken Ortho-Novum 1/35 or Brevicon for 15 months to report secondary amenorrhea. Often by switching the patient to a more progestin-dominant pill, such as Ortho-Cyclen/Ortho Tri-Cyclen, Nordette, or Lo/Ovral, you can produce more adequate withdrawal bleeding. Figure 7.4 is an algorithm for selecting and changing oral contraceptives. Table 7.6 lists OCP formulations for women with medical conditions.

General instructions on prescribing follow:

1. Begin with a low-dose estrogen/progestin combination (Ortho 7/7/7, Brevicon, Loestrin 1/20 or 1/35, Ortho-Novum 1/35, or Norinyl 1/35, Ortho-Cyclen), with 35 μg or less of estrogen and a progestin dose of about 1 mg of norethindrone. Advise the woman that breakthrough bleeding is common and usually resolves within three cycles. If a patient has severe acne or is very hirsute, start her on an antiandrogenic pill such as Demulen 1/35, Ortho-Cyclen, Ortho-Cept, or Ortho Tri-Cyclen.

2. Have the patient start medication on the Sunday closest to the first day of her next period or on the first day of menses. Advise the patient to take the pills at the same time each day. If the pills are prescribed after an abortion, the pill can be started immediately to prevent ovulation. After a pregnancy or surgery, allow 2 weeks before starting, because of the risk of thromboembolism.

3. Any newly menstruating, sexually active adolescent should have three to six regular menstrual cycles before taking the pill. This insures that primary amenorrhea is not a problem.

4. Evaluate the choice of pill after four cycles in adult women, because most minor adverse effects resolve after three cycles of use. Reevaluate adolescents after one cycle. Some teens will discontinue taking OCPs during the first cycle because of minor side effects. If significant side effects are present after three cycles, change the pill prescription.

5. If spotting occurs during the 21 days the patient is taking hormones, inquire whether the pill is being taken at the same time each day. If bleeding is heavy, changing the prescription to a pill with a stronger progestin usually stops the spotting. If that fails, change to one with more estrogen.

6. If a missed menses occurs, check if any pills have been missed. Perform a pregnancy test. If the pregnancy test result is

Table 7.6.
Formulation Selections in Women with Medical Conditions[a]

Patient Characteristic	Progestin Androgenic Activity		
	Low	Medium	High
	• norgestimate • desogestrel • norethindrone 0.4–0.5 mg monophasic	• levonorgestrel triphasic • norethindrone 1.0 mg monophasic or triphasic • norethindrone acetate 1.0 mg • ethynodiol diacetate 1.0 mg	• norgestrel 0.3 mg • norethindrone acetate 1.5–2.5 mg • levonorgestrel 0.15 mg
Acne/hirsutism	1	2	
Obesity	1	2	
Hypertension (controlled or history of pregnancy-induced)	1	2	
Hypercholesterolemia	1	2	
Smoker 30–35 years of age	1	1 (less than 50 μg estrogen)	
Heavy smoker less than 30 years of age	1	1 (less than 50 μg estrogen)	
Family history of coronary heart disease	1	2	
Common migraine	1	2	
Depression	1	2	
Family history breast cancer	1	2	
Benign breast disease	1	2	
Diabetes/gestational diabetes	1	2	
Antiepileptic drug user	Formulation containing 50 μg estrogen may be preferable		
Family history of ovarian cancer	1	2	
Sickle cell disease	1	2	
Prosthetic heart valve	1	2	
Anticoagulant user	1	2	
Mitral valve prolapse	1	2	
Ovulatory dysfunctional uterine bleeding	1	1	
Persistent anovulation	1	2	
Premature ovarian failure	1	2	
Dysmenorrhea	1	1	
Functional ovarian cysts	1 (monophasic only)		2 (monophasic only)
Mittelschmerz	1	2	
Endometriosis (pain)	1 (monophasic continuous)	2 (monophasic continuous)	
Bleeding with blood dyscrasias	1 (continuous)	2 (continuous)	

continued

Table 7.6.   (*continued*)
Formulation Selections in Women with Medical Conditions[a]

Oral Contraceptives Are Generally Contraindicated for These conditions	Comments
History of vascular disease (e.g., thromboembolism, CAS)	
Hypertension (uncontrolled)	
Hypertriglyceridemia	OCs contraindicated above 350–600 mg/dL, depending on panel member's view and presence/absence of other factors (e.g., low HDL); with mild elevations, a norgestimate-containing OC may be preferred
Smoker older than 35 years	
Classic migraine	
Personal history breast cancer	

Modified from Health Learning Systems. Risks and Benefits of Oral Contraceptive Pills. University of Minnesota Monograph. Little Falls, NJ: Health Learning Systems, 1997.

[a]1, first choice; combination formulations containing 30 to 35 μg of ethinyl estradiol (EE) except where noted. 2, second choice; combination formulations containing 30 to 35 μg of ethinyl estradiol (EE) except where noted. In some instances, there are two first two choices.

negative, have the patient take another month of pills. If a second missed menses occurs, change the pill to one with more progestin, and if that fails to produce withdrawal bleeding, increase the estrogen dose.

7. If nausea persists, try changing the time of day the pill is taken (e.g., switching to evening) or have the patient take the pill with food. If that fails, decrease the dose of estrogen or prescribe a pill with the same estrogen dose but a more antiestrogenic progesterone.

8. If hyperpigmentation occurs, decrease the estrogen dose and advise the patient to stay out of direct sunlight and use sun block. Some patients must discontinue the pill to eliminate hyperpigmentation.

9. If depression or premenstrual syndrome symptoms occur, increasing the progestin dose or changing to a progestin-dominant pill may help.

10. Oral contraceptives cost about $16.00 to $22.00 per monthly cycle if purchased in a pharmacy. Most are supplied either in 21-day packages (with instructions to the patient to wait 1 week before beginning the next cycle) or 28-day packages (with 7 days of placebo).

Table 7.7 lists common problems associated with OCPs and possible solutions.

The Minipill or Progesterone-Only Pills

Progesterone-only or minipills contain a microdose of progestin. They are indicated for women who are lactating or in whom estrogen-containing pills are contraindicated (women with hypertension or with estrogen-receptor positive breast cancer). Progesterone modifies cervical mucus, tubal motility, and endometrial lining, thus making it difficult for the fertilized egg to implant. In some women, the minipill also prevents ovulation.

The actual-use failure rate, two pregnancies per 100 woman-years, is higher than that of other oral contraceptives (31). The adverse effect of breakthrough bleeding (10 to 30%) can be troublesome. Other adverse effects include an increased risk of ectopic pregnancy, amenorrhea, and fluid retention. This pill must be taken daily at the same time without a pill-free interval, and no regular menstrual cycle is established with its use. Many women find it upsetting not to know whether they might be pregnant, and prefer to use other methods of contraception, usually barrier methods, while lactating.

Advantages of this method include:

• No estrogen-related adverse effects: safe for women with progesterone-negative breast cancers;

Table 7.7.
Common Problems Associated with Oral Contraceptive Pills (OCPs) and Solutions

Problem	Solution
Acne or oily skin	Try newer progestin pills or increase estrogen component of OCP.
Amenorrhea	Usually a result of inadequate endometrial buildup or lack of estrogen. Always check for pregnancy. Increase the estrogen potency in a low-dose pill or switch to one of the newer progestin pills if problem persists past two cycles.
Breast tenderness	Rule out other causes such as caffeine use, pregnancy. Try switching to a low estrogen pill or a progestin-only pill, or try decreasing the amount of progestin
Chloasma (facial hyperpigmentation)	May be permanent. Consider stopping the pill.
Depression	Difficult to assess. If temporary or related to onset of OCP use, discontinue for three to six cycles and observe. Supplement with pyridoxine (vitamin B_6), increasing physical activity, or lowering both the estrogen and the progestin component of the pill.
Eye problems	Pill use can dry out the eyes, requiring supplementation of liquid tears in contact lens users. More serious complications cause inflammation of the optic nerve and predispose women to transient or partial visual loss accompanying migraine headaches. If this occurs, discontinue the pill use immediately.
Galactorrhea	Check for pregnancy; if negative, draw prolactin level at a time when the breast has not been stimulated. If due to OCPs, nipple discharge will occur on the week off the OCPs.
Decreased libido	Perhaps due to decreased androgen production by the ovary. Try using a more androgenic progestin such as levonorgestrel, contained in Nordette or Triphasil pills.
Weight gain	Usually minimal and unrelated to pill use, but some women gain up to 10 lbs. or more. May be due to fluid retention (estrogen or progestin), increased fat deposition (estrogen) or increased appetite (androgenic effect).
Timing of menstruation	If a woman wishes to postpone a period, she may begin a new pack of pills on day 21 of her pack, skipping the week-off pills. Some spotting may occur, but after 3 to 4 days, most spotting resolves.
Drug interactions	Numerous and somewhat unpredictable. The following drugs may cause decreased contraceptive potency by altering liver metabolism: rifampin, phenobarbital, phenytoin, primidone, carbamazepine, ethosuximide and griseofulvin. Vitamin C, when taken in greater than 1-g dosages within 4 hours of ingestion of an OCP, can cause 50% higher concentration of the serum hormones.

- Reversibility: contraceptive effect stops within hours of missing a dose or discontinuing pills;

- Decreased bleeding: no menses resulting in less anemia;

- Decreased menstrual cramps and pain and suppression of ovulation-related pain (mittelschmerz);

- Easier use for some women who prefer to take a pill every day rather than in a cyclic fashion.

This method is not recommended for women who have had unexplained vaginal bleeding during the past 3 months or for those women with functional ovarian cysts. Concomitant use of certain antibiotics such as rifampin or most anticonvulsant medications is discouraged, as these medications decrease efficacy. Also, there is a higher incidence of ectopic pregnancies in pill failures.

INJECTABLE AND SUBDERMAL PROGESTINS

Depomedroxyprogesterone acetate (DMPA or Depo-Provera) and norethindrone enanthate have been used in the Third World for the past 20 years and are both effective and safe. This method was approved by the FDA in 1993, and it has been approved with some reservations by England, Sweden, Canada, and over 100 developing nations. This method acts by inhibiting ovulation, most probably at the level of the hypothalamus, resulting in a reduction of follicle-stimulating hormone (FSH) and luteinizing hormone (LH) (33). There also are effects on peripheral organs, making cervical mucus thick, making the endometrium unsuitable for implantation, and possibly inhibiting ovum transport through the fallopian tubes. The progestin is delivered as microcrystals suspended in an aqueous solution, which dissolve slowly. The effect lasts for 14 weeks, so there is a margin of safety for those patients who cannot have their next injection at the scheduled 12-week interval. Progestin is given as a deep intramuscular injection into the deltoid or gluteus muscles.

DMPA has the highest efficacy rate of a reversible contraceptive—0.3 pregnancies in 100 woman-years—and one injection provides protection for 3 months. Both DMPA and norethindrone enanthate interfere with the normal menstrual cycle, and their effects are unpredictable. Typically, serum levels take a week to peak, and effectiveness lasts for 2 to 4 months. Many women experience intermittent spotting, but at the end of 1 year of use, approximately 50% of users will become amenorrheic. A small percentage of users will have episodes of heavy vaginal bleeding, although treatment of this is not usually required.

Troublesome side effects include irregular menses, bloating, fluid retention, mood changes, headache, dizziness, and weight gain (13 lbs. over 17 years). Carpal tunnel syndrome and alopecia have also been noted. Most studies do not reveal serious changes in blood pressure or liver function. This method is not rapidly reversible, with average time to conception being 9 months after the last shot if more than three have been given. There is no overall alteration of the pregnancy rate.

Advantages of this method include its superb efficacy without use of an estrogen, it is long acting with a decrease in incidence of ectopic pregnancy, and it is associated with decreased blood loss, anemia, and dysmenorrhea, and has no significant drug interactions. It provides better seizure control in epileptic patients, may inhibit sickling and increase red cell survival in sickle cell disease patients, and increases the quantity and protein content of breast milk (46). This method is recommended for women who are very fertile, have failed other contraceptive methods, have poor success with barrier methods, are not good IUD candidates, or those with risk factors (such as hypertension or migraine headaches) that preclude using combined OCPs who want short-term contraception. A 150-mg injection costs approximately $25 to $28 every 3 months.

SUBDERMAL PROGESTINS

Norplant, a nonbiodegradable subdermal implant, consists of six 2.4-mm wide, 34-mm long flexible capsules that release 36 mg of levonorgestrel over 5 years. These capsules are inserted subdermally, using local anesthesia, inside the upper arm and can be removed at any time, with rapid return of fertility. This method is extremely effective, with failure rates averaging 0.04 per 100 users per year. Failure rates increase over the subsequent 4 years, with the average failure rate being 1.1% during the fifth year of use. Norplant is more effective than other reversible methods, with a documented pregnancy rate of 0.2 pregnancies per 100 women in a study of over 12,000 women (47). Insertion and removal requires special training, and the implants may show.

Advantages include its reliability, reversibility, continuous effect for up to 5 years, and the fact that the user does not need to worry about remembering to use the method. It contains no estrogen, which is an advantage for women in whom estrogen therapy is contraindicated. It is an excellent method for adolescents. It is the method of choice for women with a history of ectopic pregnancy, with the incidence being lower than among women using no contraception at all. It produces amenorrhea, thus decreasing the risk of endometrial cancer, ovarian cancer, pelvic inflammatory disease, and possibly breast cancer (31).

The major disadvantage of Norplant is the effect on menses. Altered bleeding patterns, including prolonged bleeding and spotting, and absent or scanty menses, are common. Other side effects are similar to those of injectable progestins.

Menstrual disturbances can be managed with short courses of oral estrogen such as 0.35 mg ethinyl estradiol, 1.25 conjugated estrogens, 2 mg estradiol daily for 7 days (31). Breast tenderness can be treated with vitamin E (600 mg/day), danazol (200 mg/day) bromocriptine (2.5 mg/day) or tamoxifen (20 µg/day) once pregnancy has been ruled out (31). Acne can usually be treated with topical antibiotics. Ovarian cysts are more common in Norplant users and need only be followed clinically, because most regress spontaneously with one month of detection.

Contraindications to Norplant use include antiseizure medications, acute liver disease, jaundice, unexplained vaginal bleeding, pregnancy, and a history of thrombophlebitis, pulmonary embolism, stroke, or myocardial infarction. The device costs approximately $350, in addition to approximately $200 for insertion and removal. If the cost is averaged over 5 years, however, it is lower than that of OCPs.

Intrauterine Devices

The intrauterine device (IUD), when properly used and carefully inserted into a monogamous, parous woman, is one of the most effective forms of contraception available. In the past decade, the IUD has received considerable negative publicity. A. H. Robins, which produced the Dalkon shield in 1970, declared bankruptcy after multiple malpractice suits were filed by users and their families. That intrauterine device had a multifilament tail that facilitated entry of bacteria into the uterus, resulting in infection, abscess, sepsis, and some deaths. Several other intrauterine devices have also been removed from the market for fear of legal suits, even though many women are at low risk for these complications.

The IUDs' theoretical failure rate and the actual failure rate are quite similar (three pregnancies in 100 women), since the patient has little to do with its use except check that the IUD string is present. IUDs are made of flexible plastic, some with copper wrapped around the device (Copper-7, Copper T 380, and ParaGard). Others contain progesterone (Progestasert), which is slowly released into the woman's system. Both copper- and hormone-containing devices lose their effectiveness and must be replaced. Plastic IUDs (Lippes loops), now off the market in the United States only, were designed to be left inside the uterus indefinitely, although the manufacturers suggested replacing them every 5 years to prevent actinomycoses. Most types of IUDs, except for the Progestasert and CuT 380 (ParaGard), are unavailable in the United States. In the next 2 years, a levonorgestrel-containing IUD (LNG IUD) will be marketed (31). Levonorgestrel will be released directly into the uterus at a constant rate of 20 µg/day for up to 5 years.

Nonhormone-containing devices prevent pregnancy by setting up a local inflammatory response that lyses the blastocyst and sperm, and prevents implantation by increasing local production of prostaglandins. In addition to this inflammatory response, copper-containing devices alter carbonic anhydrase and alkaline phosphatase activity and probably interfere with estrogen effects on the endometrium, and progesterone devices provide a microdose of the hormone that prevents implantation. Copper-containing devices are the most common method of contraception in many third-world countries.

The Progestasert is particularly suited for women who have dysmenorrhea and heavy periods, as the progesterone in the IUD decreases these two troublesome occurrences. It also seems to help women with significant premenstrual symptoms. It requires yearly reinsertion and often causes breakthrough bleeding.

The IUD is inserted into the patient's uterus during menses, when slight cervical dilation makes insertion easier. The IUD string, which is connected to the end of the device, is cut to leave 2 to 4 cm protruding from the external cervical os. Most women tolerate the insertion procedure well. A preinsertion dose of naproxen 500 mg or ibuprofen 800 mg relieves cramps caused by insertion. A few women have several days of bleeding, cramping, or backache after insertion; time and prostaglandin-inhibiting drugs lessen these symptoms. During the first few months, spotting between periods can occur, and the period itself may become heavier. The position of the device is checked at a 1-month follow-up visit. At this time, most major side effects will have subsided.

IUDs do have some problems. Careful patient selection will minimize complications. IUD recipients should have no evidence of genital infection, unexplained bleeding, or genital cancer. Other contraindications include subacute bacterial endocarditis, glomerulonephritis, renal failure, mitral valve prolapse, or immunosuppression. Ideally, IUD patients should not have any of the following risk factors: multiple sexual partners, previous history of pelvic inflammatory disease (PID), risk of gonorrhea or chlamydia exposure, nulliparity, history of infertility, heavy menstrual cramps, or heavy menstrual periods. They should be mentally capable of noting and reporting any IUD-associated infection, the expulsion of the IUD, the possibility of pregnancy, or the occurrence of unusually heavy menstrual periods. Women who have large uteri or who have had children and who have one sexual partner are ideal IUD candidates, as the IUD can be inserted with little or no difficulty, the expulsion rate is low, and pelvic infections are unlikely (33, 48).

The most common problems of IUD use are spotting (10 to 15% of users), heavy menstrual bleeding, and bleeding between cycles, which can cause iron deficiency anemia. Other problems include expulsion of the device (5 to 20% of users in the first year, rarely thereafter), the IUD shifting location in the uterus or becoming embedded in the endometrium, and uterine perforation.

The IUD increases the risk of pelvic infections, which begin slowly and may progress to endometritis, myometritis, and occasionally tubo-ovarian abscess. This illness can present as menstrual syndrome (bloating, backache, or spotting), as a foul-smelling vaginal discharge, as fever, chills, anorexia, and severe lower abdominal pain, or as infertility. PID can be treated in its early stages as an outpatient illness with ceftriaxone, doxycycline, azithromycin and metronidazole, or with an intravenous cephalosporin and doxycycline in more serious cases. If PID is suspected in an IUD user, the device must be removed immediately.

As with other methods of contraception, the risks and benefits of this method need to be reviewed with the patient before insertion. Careful follow-up of all problems can usually prevent a pelvic infection and its complications.

The costs of the IUD insertion and device vary between $125 and $300. The Progestasert device itself is good for 1 year and costs about $125; the ParaGard costs about $200 and can remain in place for up to 8 years.

BARRIER METHODS

Barrier contraceptives (male and female condoms, spermicides, diaphragms, cervical caps, and contraceptive sponges) all function to kill sperm or block their entry into the cervical os. They are readily available to both adolescents and adults, and rarely produce side effects. The theoretical and actual use effectiveness rates vary because effectiveness depends on proper use by the patient. Diaphragms and cervical caps must be fitted to the individual patient, but the other barrier methods can be used by anyone. All barrier methods are reversible. When used in combination, they are almost 100% effective.

Condoms are the oldest, most reliable method of contraception for men. They are now becoming more popular because rubber condoms inhibit spread of the HIV virus. Condoms are made of rubber or processed collagen's animal tissue and fit over the erect penis. They are easy to apply. The differences among brands involve slight modifications in shape, color, texture, the presence or absence of lubricant, and the presence or absence of spermicide on the inside or outside of the condom. The more expensive condoms are more comfortable and more flexible.

The female condom is a thin plastic sheath in the form of a double-ringed tube with a blunt end that covers the cervix. It is inserted like a tampon and, when opened up in the vaginal vault, creates a plastic canal into which the penis is placed. An outer ring lies outside the vagina,

covering the perineum and protecting them from contact with possible skin lesions, and the internal ring holds the plastic around the cervix to create a fitted cover. Another type of female condom is a latex condom pouch worn as a panty. The pouch is pushed up into the vagina when the penis first enters the vaginal vault. This type of condom also provides protection of the labia and perineum from contact with possible skin lesions that can transmit STDs. Thus, both devices provide contraceptive protection and STD protection for the female.

The actual use effectiveness rate is about 10 pregnancies per woman-year, whereas the theoretic rate is about three pregnancies per 100 woman-years. Three large British studies found the failure rate to be one pregnancy in 10,000 uses. Condoms are contraindicated in men that cannot maintain an erection, as the condom can slip off. Allergy to the rubber or spermicide used in condoms can occur; natural lambskin condoms can be used by these men but provide no protection against HIV.

There are many noncontraceptive benefits of condoms, the most important being the prevention of many sexually transmitted bacterial or parasitic infections and inhibition of HIV transmission. Male condoms enhance sexual pleasure in men with premature ejaculation, as they reduce glans sensitivity. Although the use of condoms requires the interruption of lovemaking, applying the condom can be incorporated into the lovemaking. The cost ranges from 35 cents to about $5 each. Anyone of any age and either sex can purchase condoms in drugstores.

Spermicides require neither a prescription nor a pelvic examination and rarely cause side effects. Some come in a single-application form, such as preloaded vaginal applicators of jelly or foam, or vaginal suppositories. The convenience and ease of application make them popular with adolescents. Used in combination with condoms, spermicides provide excellent protection from pregnancy. All spermicides act to prevent conception by immobilizing or killing sperm. They are made up of an inert base that holds the spermicide, usually nonoxynol-9.

Foam spermicides are more effective than jellies or suppositories, because foam disperses in the vagina more readily. All spermicides must be applied 30 minutes or less before intercourse. In addition to its contraceptive benefit, nonoxynol-9 provides some protection against gonorrhea and chlamydia and may provide some protection against viral disease. The only known contraindication is allergy to the spermicidal chemical. A foam kit costs approximately $10 to $12 for 20 applications. A tube of contraceptive jelly (15 applications) costs about $7. They can be purchased in the feminine hygiene section of most major supermarkets or pharmacies. Adverse effects include allergy and local irritation.

Diaphragms and cervical caps are somewhat more difficult to use than other barrier methods because their efficacy depends on both correct placement over the cervix and an effective spermicide. The appliance must be left in place for at least 6 hours. The rubber cup or cap serves as a reservoir to hold the spermicide against the cervix, preventing conception by acting as both a physical and a chemical barrier to sperm from the cervical os.

A diaphragm must be fitted by a clinician so that it covers the cervix and wedges snugly behind the pelvic bone. Then, the patient must be taught to properly insert and remove the device. Its actual effectiveness rate varies between 6 and 18%, with the more experienced users having greater success than the younger users (31). Contraceptive failures result from lack of use with every intercourse, improper insertion, improper fit of the appliance, displacement during coitus (most common in the female superior position), a hole in the diaphragm, and failure to use additional spermicide with each additional intercourse. Both the diaphragm and the cervical cap can be used during menses to hold back menstrual flow during intercourse. The major disadvantage of the diaphragm is that it increases the incidence of urinary tract infections in some women.

The cervical cap, which snugly fits over the cervix, is smaller than the diaphragm and somewhat more difficult to insert. Failure rates may be slightly higher than those of the diaphragm. Major advantages are that it can be kept in place for 24 hours and is less likely to cause urinary tract infections that the diaphragm.

A diaphragm costs about $15, and the contraceptive jelly or cream used with it costs about $7 for a tube with 15 applications. The cervical cap costs about $70 and does not require the user to place extra spermicide in the vagina with additional intercourse.

The contraceptive sponge is a round, flexible synthetic material that contains 1 g of nonoxynol-9 spermicide, which provides 24-hour contraceptive effect. It is currently not available in the United States. There is a slight dimple in the circle, which fits over the cervix. A polyester loop on the bottom of the sponge is used to remove it from the vagina after 24 hours. As with all other barrier methods, there is no need to wait after insertion before having intercourse. Its effectiveness rate is similar to that of foam alone. It is less messy to use than foam or jelly and is a more spontaneous method because no additional spermicide is necessary with repeated intercourse. It can sometimes be difficult to remove and may be forgotten, resulting in vaginal infection.

POSTCOITAL CONTRACEPTION

This is usually reserved for emergency/accidental situations (i.e., condom rupture, expelled or removed IUD, missed OCPs, unprotected intercourse), and there is strong evidence for its effectiveness (75% efficacy). In the United States, the FDA has approved the use of oral contraceptives as postcoital contraceptives (31).

A common and effective postcoital contraceptive is two Ovral tablets taken within 72 hours (preferably as soon as possible) after intercourse. Twelve hours later, two additional tablets are taken. The total dose is 2.0 mg of norgestrel and 200 μg of estrogen. Other combinations of drugs include 4 Lo/Ovral or Ovral, Nordette or Levlen, Triphasil or Tri-Levlen yellow pills only taken twice, 12 hours apart. The mechanism of action is to induce a menstrual period within 21 days of administration. It is thought that the failure rate is approximately 2% with this method. Most women feel quite nauseated after taking the tablets; one can counter these symptoms with promethazine (Phenergan) suppositories or tablets (31).

Insertion of an intrauterine device up to 7 days after intercourse is also an effective postcoital method, as it prevents implantation of a fertilized ovum. It has been essentially eliminated as a method because of the loss of the availability of Copper-7 and the Tatum T devices. It is contraindicated in the event of a possible STD.

FERTILITY AWARENESS OR NATURAL FAMILY PLANNING

Fertility awareness methods include the "rhythm" or calendar method in combination with the basal body temperature (BBT) method and the mucus method (Billings) of predicting ovulation. Fertility awareness is now very popular, being used both to predict fertility and to prevent pregnancy. It is the only method sanctioned by the Catholic Church. This method requires significant motivation by the couple. Success with this method depends on the couple's ability to pinpoint the days when another method of contraception (or abstinence) needs to be used as a backup, i.e., when the woman is most fertile and conception is most likely.

Couples who choose this method must become facile with all the signs of fertility, such as temperature rise, change in cervical mucus, and pain of ovulation. Family planning experts feel that this method is generally ineffective, with fertility awareness advocates identifying actual failure rates around 25 pregnancies per 100 woman-years). Courses to learn fertility awareness, taught by various family planning and state agencies and by planned parenthood clinics, usually cost between $30 and $75 per couple.

Sterilization

For men and women requesting a permanent method, sterilization is the only option. It is the most common method of contraception for married women in the United States today. The most important issue is informed consent. The patient should fully understand that sterilization must be considered irreversible. Although a slight possibility of pregnancy exists, sterilization is nearly 100% effective.

Vasectomy is a surgical operation that permanently blocks sperm passage by cutting out, ligating, and cauterizing the vas deferens. The sperm are then absorbed in the testes and epididymis, leaving the semen sterile. Vasectomy can safely be performed under local anesthesia as an outpatient procedure costing $300 to $500. It is often performed by family physicians. Tubal ligation is a similar procedure on the fallopian tubes. It too can be performed as an outpatient procedure, but spinal, epidural, or general anesthesia is required. It can be done using a laparoscope. The cost of these procedures varies, depending on whether they are performed in an outpatient facility or in the hospital. The average cost is $600. Many states provide funding for eligible women over 21 years of age.

FUTURE METHODS

Research is being done in the following areas: (a) female-controlled methods to prevent against pregnancy and STDs; (b) disposable diaphragms with antiviral spermicide; (c) a one-size-fits-all diaphragm with a one-way valve to allow air to escape during placement, but improving retention against the cervix; and (d) chemical barriers that improve spermicide delivery systems to protect against HIV and other pathogens as well as sperm.

New hormonal methods include Implanon, a single implant containing 3-ketodesogestrel that is effective for 2 to 3 years, a new improved NORPLANT II, and newer biodegradable implants that will be injected subcutaneously, dissolve spontaneously, and be effective over a 2-year period. New male hormonal methods show little promise, as there is an unpredictable return to normal sperm count when the method is discontinued.

CASE STUDY 1

A 35-year-old woman who has successfully used Ortho-Novum 7/7/7 for many years without problems comes in to your office for her yearly well woman physical examination. She asks you what she should use for birth control now that she is older. She has two children and is in a stable marital relationship. She is mildly obese, a non-smoker and her father had a myocardial infarction at age 52.

QUESTIONS

1. What is the optimal method of contraception for a 35-year-old woman who has successfully used oral contraceptive pills (OCPs)?
2. What factors would preclude the use of OCPs in this patient?
3. Does obesity put this patient at risk for any complications that present with pill use?

DISCUSSION

Once a contraindication to continuing pill use, age is no longer the primary factor that limits oral contraceptive use in women.

Studies have shown that women up to age 45 with normal lipid values and no history of thrombosis or vascular disease can use the oral contraceptive pill safely. This patient has used this method successfully without complications and would have little difficulty continuing use of this method. An important question to ask this patient would be whether she had completed her childbearing. If so, suggesting use of a permanent method of contraception, such as tubal ligation or vasectomy, would be in order, understanding that sterilization carries with it psychologic issues for every person. If she is undecided, continuing the use of OCPs is appropriate.

Factors that would preclude the use of OCPs in a woman over 35 are elevated blood pressure, elevated lipid values, diabetes, smoking, or previous history of thromboembolism. Appropriate screening of women ages 35 and over who desire to use the pill should include a fasting lipid screen, fasting blood sugar, and clear documentation of normal blood pressures. A strong family history of cardiovascular disease is a relative contraindication in women who are normotensive, have normal weights and normal lipid values, and does not preclude the use of this method.

There is no evidence to show that obese women have more complications with use of OCPs unless they have any of the other risk factors such as smoking, known breast or endometrial cancer, hepatic adenoma or cancer, cholestatic jaundice of pregnancy, or, with previous OCP use, hypertension, diabetes, or thromboembolism, which preclude the use of oral contraceptives in general. Obese women tend to be more physically inactive and have a higher overall incidence of developing hypertension or adult onset diabetes, but these factors are not linked to pill usage.

CASE STUDY 2

A 24-year old, unmarried, G4P2–0-2–2, with her last child born 10 months ago, presents to your office for a new patient visit. She had one therapeutic abortion, two unplanned pregnancies, and a spontaneous abortion, and she thinks that one of the pregnancies occurred while she was using the pill. She is now in a new relationship, has been using no method of contraception, and would like to start back on the pill. She does not remember which pill she used before. She smokes one-half to one pack of cigarettes a day.

QUESTIONS

1. What is the optimal method of contraception for a young woman who smokes and has had method failures resulting in unwanted or unplanned pregnancies?
2. Which contraceptive method would provide her with the best protection against contracting STDs?
3. Is there a relationship between pill use and spontaneous miscarriage, therapeutic abortion, and spontaneous miscarriage and between smoking and miscarriage?

DISCUSSION

This woman has had four pregnancies in her life, possibly all of them unplanned. She states that she has at least one time become pregnant using an effective method of contraception. Given her history, the use of a method that required less attention for maximal compliance, i.e., a long-acting injectable or implantable contraceptive such as Depo-Provera or Norplant, or an IUD would be good choices. Her smoking history puts her at some risk for use of an estrogen-containing method, so a progestin-only methods or barrier methods would obviate this complication.

Except for condoms, NO contraceptive method provides protection against transmission of STDs. There is evidence that use of a spermicide decreases the risk of acquiring chlamydia; however, this method does not protect against transmission of the AIDS virus. Unless your patients are absolutely sure that they are at no risk for acquiring an STD, condom use is recommended for every sexual encounter.

There is no epidemiologic evidence that use of OCPs is causally related to the incidence of spontaneous miscarriage. There also is no evidence that therapeutic abortions increase one's risk of spontaneous miscarriage unless there has been anatomic damage such as a uterine perforation. There is a relationship between smoking and spontaneous miscarriage, although the actual pathophysiologic mechanism is not well understood.

REFERENCES

1. Brown SS, Eisenberg L. The Best Intentions: Unintended Pregnancy and the Well-being of Children and Families. Washington, DC: National Academy Press, 1995.
2. Moore K, et al. Beginning Too Soon: Adolescent Sexual Behavior, Pregnancy, and Parenthood. A Review of Research and Interventions. Report prepared for the Office of the Assistant Secretary for Planning and Evaluation, US Department of Health and Human Services. Washington, DC: US Department of Health and Human Services, 1995.
3. Jones EF, Forrest JD, Henshaw SK, Silverman J, Torres A. Pregnancy, Contraception, and Family Planning Services in Industrialized Countries. New Haven, CT: Yale University Press, 1989.
4. Forrest JD. Epidemiology of unintended pregnancy and contraceptive use. Am J Obstet Gynecol 1994;170: 1485–1488.
5. Centers for Disease Control, National Center for Health Statistics. National Survey of Family Growth, 1982 and 1988. Telephone Reinterview, 1990 (preliminary data).
6. Henshaw SK, Forrest JD. Women at Risk of Unintended Pregnancy, 1990 Estimates: The Need for Family Planning Services, Each State and County. New York: Alan Guttmacher Institute, 1993.
7. Mosher WD, Bachrach CA. Understanding U.S. fertility: continuity and change in the national survey of family growth. Fam Plann Perspect 1996; 28:4–12.
8. Forrest JD, Singh S. The sexual and reproductive behavior of American women 1982–88. Fam Plann Perspect 1990; 22:206–214.
9. Family Planning Councils of America. The Role of a Pregnancy Prevention Outreach Initiative in Welfare Reform. A Special Task Force Report. Des Moines, IA: Family Planning Councils of America, February, 1995.
10. Lee PR, Stewart FH. Failing to prevent unintended pregnancy is costly. Am J Public Health 1995;85(4):479–480.
11. Moore KA. Bivariate analysis: age at first birth and well-being at ages 23, 27, and 35. In: The Consequences of Early Childbearing in the 1980s. Final Report to National Institute of Child Health and Human Development. Bethesda, MD: National Institute of Child Health and Human Development, 1992.
12. Bacon L. Early motherhood, accelerated role transition, and social pathologies. Social Forces 1974;52: 333–341.
13. Alan Guttmacher Institute. Sex and America's Teenagers. New York: Alan Guttmacher Institute, 1994.
14. National Institute of Child Health and Human Development. Summary of a conference. Outcomes of early childbearing: an appraisal of recent evidence. Bethesda, MD: National Institute of Child Health and Development, May, 1992.
15. Trussell J. Teenage pregnancy in the United States. Fam Plann Perspect 1988;20(6):262–272.
16. Dash L. When Children Want Children: The Urban Crisis of Teenage Childbearing. New York: William Morrow, 1989.
17. DaVanzo J, Rajman MO. American Families: Trends and Policy Issues. Santa Monica, CA: RAND Corporation, 1993.
18. Sollom T, Gold RB, Saul R. Public funding for contraceptive, sterilization, and abortion services, 1994. Fam Plann Perspect 1996;28:166–173.
19. Family Planning Councils of America. The Role of a Pregnancy Prevention Outreach Initiative in Welfare Reform: A Report to the National Family Planning and Reproductive Health Association. Des Moines, IA: Family Planning Councils of America, February, 1995.
20. Forrest JD, Samura R. Impact of publicly funded contraceptive services on unintended pregnancies and implications for Medicaid expenditures. Fam Plann Perspect 1996;28:188–195.
21. Alan Guttmacher Institute. Preventing Pregnancy, Protecting Health. New York: Alan Guttmacher Institute, 1991.
22. Goldsheider C, Mosher WD. Patterns of contraceptive use in the United States: the importance of religious factors. Stud Fam Plann 1991;22:102–115.
23. Mosher WD. Contraceptive practice in the US, 1982-1988. Fam Plann Perspect 1990;2:198–205.
24. Hoffman AD. A rational policy toward consent and confidentiality in adolescent health care. J Adolesc Health Care 1980;1:9–17.
25. Elster AB, Kuznets NJ. AMA Guidelines for Adolescent Preventive Services GAPS. Chicago: American Medical Association, 1994.
26. Holder AR. Disclosure and consent problems in pediatrics. Law Med Health Care 1988;16:219–228.
27. Morrissey JM, Hoffmann AD, Thorpe JC. Consent and Confidentiality in the Health Care of Children and Adolescents: A Legal Guide. New York: The Free Press, 1986.
28. Hibbard RA. Sexual abuse. In: McArney ER, Kreipe R, Orr R, Comerci G, eds. Textbook of Adolescent Medicine. Philadelphia: WB Saunders, 1992.
29. Planned Parenthood Federation of America. Manual of Medical Standards and Guidelines. Section III-A. New York: Planned Parenthood Federation of America, 1995.
30. Neinstein L. Adolescent Health Care: A Practical Guide, 3rd ed. Baltimore: Williams & Wilkins, 1996: 755–761.
31. Hatcher RJ, et al. Contraceptive Technology Update, 16th rev. ed. New York: Irvington Publishers, 1994.
32. US Preventive Services Task Force. Guide to Clinical Preventive Services. Report of the US Preventive Services Task Force, 2nd ed. Baltimore: Williams & Wilkins, 1996.
33. Darney P, Speroff L. A Clinical Guide of Contraception. Baltimore: Williams & Wilkins, 1989.

34. American College of Obstetrics and Gynecology. Hormonal contraception. ACOG Tech Bull no. 198, October, 1994.
35. Speroff L, Glass RH, Kase NG. Clinical Gynecologic Endocrinology and Infertility, 5th ed. Baltimore: Williams & Wilkins, 1994.
36. Lanes SF, Birmann B, Walker AM, et al. Oral contraceptive type and functional ovarian cysts. Am J Obstet Gynecol 1992;166:956–961.
37. Guillebaud J. The pill and other hormones for contraception, 14th ed. Oxford: Oxford University Press, 1991.
38. Trussell J, Stewart F, Guest F, Hatcher RA. Emergency contraception pills (ECPs): a simple proposal to reduce unintended pregnancies. Fam Plann Perspect 1992; 24(6):269–273.
39. Harlap S, Kost K, Forrest JD. Preventing Pregnancy, Protecting Health. New York: Alan Guttmacher Institute, 1991.
40. Fruzzetti F, Ricci C, Fioretti P. Hemostasis profile in smoking and nonsmoking women taking low-dose oral contraceptives. Contraception 1994;49:579.
41. Vessey MP, Mant D, Smith A, et al. Oral contraceptives and venous thromboembolism: findings in a large prospective study. Br Med J 1986;292;526.
42. Gerstman BB, Piper JM, Tomita DK, et al. Oral contraceptive estrogen dose and the risk of deep venous thromboembolic disease. Am J Epidemiol 1991;133:32.
43. Centers for Disease Control and Prevention. Oral contraceptive use and the risk of breast cancer. The Centers for Disease Control Cancer and Steroid Hormone Study. N Engl J Med 1986;315:405.
44. Wingo PA, Lee NC, Ory HW, et al. Age-specific differences in the relationship between oral contraceptive use and breast cancer. Obstet Gynecol 1991;78:161.
45. Murray P, Stadel BV, Schlesslman JJ, et al. Oral contraceptive use in women with a family history of breast cancer. Obstet Gynecol 1989;73:977.
46. Liskin L , Blackburn R. Hormonal contraception: new long-acting methods. Popul Rep 1987; Series K(3).
47. Population Council. Norplant levonorgestrel implants: a summary of scientific data. Monograph. New York: Population Council, 1990.
48. Chi I-c, Farr G. Postpartum IUD contraception—a review of an international experience. Adv Contracept 1989;5(3):127–146.

8. Prenatal Care

MARGARET R. HELTON

Key Clinical Questions

1. What are the most important risk factors in the prenatal phase of pregnancy?
2. What screening tests are useful in the first trimester of pregnancy?
3. What psychosocial issues affect pregnant women and their families?

The prenatal period offers a unique opportunity for practicing health promotion. At no other time in the human life cycle do patients in good health visit the physician so frequently. It is a time when many women (and couples) are particularly receptive to changing their own health behaviors. Furthermore, the entire process of prenatal care revolves around preventive measures: the identification and management of risk factors, the early detection of potential problems, and health education.

For many physicians, prenatal care is one of the most rewarding aspects of family practice because it is a time during which strong doctor-patient bonds often develop. The continuity of care provided by family physicians allows these bonds to continue postpartum, since the family physician provides ongoing care of the infant and mother after delivery. Continuing to care for the woman, other family members, and the new baby are gratifying aspects of the comprehensive care provided by family physicians. This chapter explores some of the medical and social issues facing family physicians who deliver prenatal care.

PRENATAL CARE IN PERSPECTIVE

In the United States, the maternal mortality rate has decreased from 582 per 100,000 live births in 1935 to 7.5 per 100,000 live births in 1993 (1). Most of this decrease is due to innovations in the management of labor and delivery, such as the use of antibiotics, safer blood transfusion capabilities, and the development of safer methods of anesthesia. The independent contribution of prenatal care to this decline in maternal mortality is difficult to assess because many of the modern advances responsible for better outcomes relate to the delivery. However, among the aspects of prenatal care that reduce maternal morbidity and mortality are the prevention of pyelonephritis through screening for bacteriuria, better control of diabetes mellitus, and improved detection and control of preeclampsia.

Several lines of evidence link proper prenatal care with reduced infant mortality rates. In 1940, the infant mortality rate in the United States was 47 per 1000 live births (2). By 1994, that rate had fallen to 8.0 infant deaths per 1000 live births (1). Although this is an impressive decline, 20 countries had 1994 infant mortality rates lower than that of the United States, led by Japan and Sweden at 4 per 1000 live births (3). In every country with an infant mortality rate below the United States', essentially all pregnant women receive early and adequate prenatal care. In contrast, women in the United States with the highest infant mortality rates are those who receive little or no prenatal care.

In the United States, twice as many African-American mothers receive no or inadequate prenatal care as whites, and the mortality of black infants is twice that of white infants (1). In settings where access to prenatal care is equally available to black and white persons, such as in the military, the difference between black and white infant mortality is markedly reduced. Thus, prenatal care seems to contribute to better pregnancy outcomes. The U.S. Public Health Service goal for the year 2000 is for at least 90% of American women to begin prenatal care in the first trimester (4).

Unfortunately, there have been times when prenatal care, rather than enhancing the pregnancy, brought about just the opposite effect. This occurred when harmful drugs were prescribed for nausea or fluid retention, inappropriate dietary restrictions were advised, or undue anxiety was caused by misguided patient education. *Primum non nocere* (first do no harm), the credo taught to all practitioners of medicine, is aptly applied to prenatal care, especially since most pregnancies will have a healthy outcome anyway. Pregnancy and childbirth are natural processes, not disease states, and should represent joyful and enriching experiences for the woman and her family. The new paradigm for medical practice, known as evidence-based medicine, must be applied and no intervention accepted into the course of prenatal care unless it has been critically appraised and proven to be effective (5). The U.S. Preventive Services Task Force *Guide to Clinical Preventive Services* is an established source for evidence-based recommendations, which cover many components of prenatal care (6). The Cochrane Database is a computer-based collaborative effort that critically reviews aspects of prenatal and maternal care and is updated quarterly (7).

PLANNING THE PREGNANCY AND RISK ASSESSMENT

Ideally a pregnancy is planned or at least wanted, and the prospective mother visits her health care provider before conception has occurred. At the time of such a visit, you should explore and clarify the motives for pregnancy, help the patient maximize her health in anticipation of pregnancy, and provide counseling about behaviors and exposures that might jeopardize the health of her or the fetus. The reality is that in most cases you will be reviewing these issues when the woman is already pregnant.

The points that should be covered before or in early prenatal care are listed in Table 8.1. Any conditions or behaviors that increase the likelihood of poor outcome, including medical complications, premature delivery, stillbirth, and neonatal mortality, should be identified. Maternal health should be reviewed, and women with significant medical illnesses will require closer surveillance. All medications used by the patient should be noted, including over-the-counter preparations. The woman's previous obstetric and gynecologic history should be reviewed. Nu-

Table 8.1.
Areas to Assess Early in Maternal Care

Maternal health	Medical diseases such as diabetes, hypertension, anemia, epilepsy, or cardiopulmonary disease Medications
Previous obstetric and gynecologic history	Number of previous deliveries, including method of delivery, or abortions (induced or spontaneous) Previous poor pregnancy outcome such as fetal or neonatal death, hemorrhage, preeclampsia, small or large-for-gestational age infant, cervical incompetence Cervical dysplasia or surgery
Nutrition	Obesity Folic acid supplementation
Genetic counseling	Familial genetic diseases or malformations Parental age Ethnic risks (e.g., Tay-Sachs, sickle cell, cystic fibrosis, and thalassemia)
Behaviors	Tobacco, alcohol, cocaine, or other drug abuse Promiscuity
Infectious diseases	Sexually transmitted diseases Tuberculosis Hepatitis Toxoplasmosis Rubella immunity
Environmental exposures	Toxins Radiation Physical stress
Psychosocial status	Marital status Personal support systems Medically significant religious beliefs Housing Education Work situation and income

trition should be assessed and obese patients should be encouraged to lose weight before or restrict weight gain during pregnancy. All women planning pregnancy or in the early phase of pregnancy should supplement their diet with 0.4 to 1 mg of folic acid per day, as this has been shown to reduce the risk of neural tube defects (8). A history of familial genetic diseases or malformations should be taken. The age of the parents should be assessed, as the risk of chromosomal defects increases with parental age. Ethnic risks (e.g., Tay-Sachs disease in Jews, sickle cell disease in African-Americans, and thalassemia in persons of Mediterranean or Asian descent) need to be identified.

The patient's behaviors should be assessed. Promiscuity increases the risk of sexually transmitted diseases. Smoking increases the risk of premature delivery, low birth weight babies, and perinatal death (9, 10). Alcohol abuse causes miscarriage and fetal alcohol syndrome (mental retardation, microcephaly, growth retardation, and facial deformities) (11). Cocaine use can cause placental abruption (12); other drugs can cause fetal withdrawal.

Certain occupations (e.g., those that involve exposure to toxic substances) pose significant health risks to the mother because of exposure to either toxins or physical stress, so these risk factors should be identified and minimized. Psychosocial factors, such as marital status, personal support systems, medically significant religious beliefs, poor housing, low education, and limited income, should be assessed. The woman's attitude toward the pregnancy and any psychosocial stresses should be evaluated; they can adversely affect pregnancy outcomes and contribute to a family's inability to care for the new baby.

Even though many risk factors associated with pregnancy are recognized, they are not reliably predictive of maternal and fetal morbidity and mortality. Just as perplexing is the fact that half of adverse pregnancy outcomes cannot be identified before labor.

DIAGNOSING AND DATING THE PREGNANCY

Pregnancy tests used today are very accurate, with a 98% sensitivity and 99% specificity at the time of the first missed menstrual period (13). Signs that the woman herself notices include a missed period, breast tenderness and enlargement, fatigue, and nausea. The clinician should look for uterine enlargement (an accurate method of dating the pregnancy during the first trimester) and dark bluish coloring to the vaginal mucosa and cervix (Chadwick's sign).

Establishing a reliable expected date of confinement (EDC), or "due date," is important because effective detection and management of such problems as intrauterine growth retardation, premature labor, multiple gestation, and postdate pregnancy depend on accurate dating. The simplest method estimates the EDC as being 280 days from the date of the last menstrual period, taking into account the reliability of the patient's recall and the length and predictability of her cycles. Nägele's rule (14) estimates the EDC by adding 7 days to the first day of the last normal menstrual period and counting back 3 months. This same principle is embodied in pregnancy wheels (such as those provided by pharmaceutical companies), which are commonly used in office practice to calculate the EDC. Inaccurate dating can result from failure to consider menstrual irregularities, unusual cycle lengths, recent use of oral contraceptives, and the possibility that the presumed last menstrual cycle was really first-trimester or implantation bleeding.

Uterine size, which changes proportionately more from week to week in the first months than at any other time, is another helpful parameter to use in estimating the EDC. During the first trimester, uterine size is detected by bimanual pelvic examination. At 7 weeks, the uterus is the size of a large hen's egg. At 10 weeks, the uterus has grown to the size of an orange. After 12 weeks, the uterus is the size of a grapefruit, and the upper portion can be felt abdominally above the pelvic symphysis. The fetal heartbeat can first be heard with an ultrasonic Doppler at between 10 and 12 weeks and with a fetoscope (a specially adapted stethoscope) at 18 to 20 weeks. These milestones should be recorded to add support to other evidence dating the pregnancy.

If there is still doubt about the EDC, ultrasonography performed in the first or second trimester can be helpful. Third-trimester sonography is an unreliable predictor of gestational age.

PRENATAL CARE IN THE OFFICE

Prenatal care aims for three outcomes: a smooth labor and delivery, a healthy baby and mother, and a smooth adjustment of the mother and family to this life event. Prenatal care must emphasize clinical surveillance of both the mother and her fetus. This aspect of the care is usually provided by a clinician such as a family physician, obstetrician, midwife, or nurse practitioner. Other important health care team members may include a nurse, nutritionist, and social worker. Expectant mothers and their partners should receive psychosocial support and patient education. They should be encouraged to write a birth plan detailing their expectations and hopes regarding the labor and delivery. The value of a prepared patient and support person in reducing complications of labor cannot be overemphasized. Companion support during childbirth has been shown to decrease the use of anesthesia, shorten the length of labor, and lower the rate of cesarean section (15). Thus, the time spent educating the patient and her support person(s) during prenatal care and the techniques they have learned in any prenatal education will generally pay great dividends during the stress of labor and delivery (16).

Pregnancies are conventionally split into three trimesters, each with unique medical and emotional issues. By convention, gestational age is stated as the number of weeks since the last menstrual period, even though conception does not occur until approximately 2 weeks after that date. Delivery occurs on average at 40 weeks. In the United States, women average 14 prenatal visits, a much higher number than most countries. The visit schedule is typically one visit per month during the first 32 weeks of pregnancy, biweekly visits between 32 and 36 weeks, and weekly visits thereafter until delivery. The U.S. Public Health Service's Expert Panel on the Content of Prenatal Care recommends fewer visits for most women and more resources directed toward higher-risk pregnancies (17). For women with low-risk pregnancies, good perinatal outcomes and patient satisfaction were maintained when the visit schedule was reduced by an average of 2.7 visits (18).

First-Trimester Prenatal Care

The first trimester (weeks 0 to 13) is in many ways the most crucial for the developing child. Nearly all organogenesis takes place during these early weeks, making this the period of greatest susceptibility to embryotoxic and teratogenic substances. For the mother, these weeks are often characterized by fatigue, nausea, and the emotional changes that accompany learning of, and adjusting to, the pregnancy. For the physician or

other health care provider, initial contacts during the first trimester should help set the stage for a healthy pregnancy.

History and Risk Assessment

If the patient did not have a preconception visit, you should conduct a thorough evaluation of the mother's general health, health behaviors, genetic assessment, and so forth (see Table 8.1) at the initial visit. The number of previous pregnancies should be determined and noted using the $G_N P_{FPAL}$ shorthand method:

- G, gravidity, how many times (N) the patient has been pregnant, including the current pregnancy
- P, parity (results of previous pregnancies), designated:
  - F, number of full-term births
  - P, number of premature births
  - A, number of abortions, elected or spontaneous
  - L, number of living children

For example, a pregnant woman who has had five previous pregnancies that resulted in two full-term deliveries, one premature delivery, two miscarriages, and three living children would be designated $G_6 P_{2\text{-}1\text{-}2\text{-}3}$. Use this common mnemonic to remember the parity notation: "Florida **P**ower **A**nd **L**ight," or invent your own.

An obstetric history must include details of all previous pregnancies—the route of delivery, weight and gestation of the newborn, and any complications, especially those that resulted in morbidity or fetal mortality. From this historical information, patients requiring closer surveillance can often be identified. A history of premature delivery, for example, should alert you to the risk of recurrence of this outcome. A history of second-trimester losses due to early cervical dilation can signify cervical incompetence, a condition in which the patient may benefit from early placement of a purse-string suture (cerclage). It should also be remembered that women of high parity have an increased risk of placenta previa, puerperal hemorrhage, and multiple gestation.

Physical Examination

On the first prenatal visit, you should conduct a thorough physical examination, paying special attention to blood pressure, the size and shape of the uterus and adnexal areas, and the configuration of the bony pelvis. On subsequent visits, your examination will generally be limited to blood pressure checks, verifying fetal cardiac activity, and watching for edema. At each visit in the second and third trimester, measure fundal height in centimeters from the pubic symphysis; fundal height when above 20 cm and below 36 cm corresponds to gestational age within 2 weeks (19). Figure 8.1 is a sample flowchart for recording prenatal visits.

Laboratory Testing

Table 8.2 lists the laboratory tests that are routinely performed in prenatal care, along with the sensitivity, specificity, and level of evidence of the test.

Maternal blood type and an antibody screen identify which women might develop ABO, D (formerly Rh), or other antigen incompatibility with the fetal blood cells. Approximately 15% of persons are D (Rh)-antigen-negative. If a mother is D-negative and the father is D-positive, the fetus has a 50% chance of inheriting the father's D antigen on the fetal red blood cells. The mother could develop an antibody to the D antigen that can cross the placenta into the fetal circulation and hemolyze the fetal red blood cells, causing hemolytic anemia that leads to hyperbilirubinemia or fetal hydrops, also known as erythroblastosis fetalis. The incidence of this problem has dropped dramatically in the past 30 years since the introduction of D immunoglobulin (RhoGAM), which is given to a D-negative pregnant woman at 28 weeks and within 72 hours of delivery, as well as at other times when there might be a maternal-fetal transfusion, such as with a miscarriage or at the time of amniocentesis.

Iron deficiency anemia (e.g., Hct < 30% or Hgb < 9 g/dL) is screened for because it is associated with poor outcomes (20, 21). Women at risk for hemoglobinopathies such as sickle cell disease and certain thalassemias (women of African, Middle Eastern, Mediterranean, Latin American, or Southeast Asian descent) should have hemoglobin electrophoresis performed.

Several blood tests will detect infectious diseases that could be transmitted to the fetus. Rubella immunity should be determined, since rubella contracted by the mother during early pregnancy is devastating to the fetus. Ideally, if the mother is not immune, she should be immu-nized at least 3 months before attempting pregnancy. If she is already pregnant, she should be immunized after delivery, so that at least the next pregnancy will be protected. A screening test should be done to detect maternal active (acute or chronic) hepatitis B infection, since infants born to these mothers will need hepatitis B immune globulin and vaccine at birth (22). If the mother has syphilis, disease in the baby can be prevented with prenatal antibiotic therapy (23). Testing for human immunodeficiency virus (HIV) is strongly encouraged, since transmission of HIV to the baby can be significantly reduced by prenatal treatment with zidovudine (azidothymidine, or AZT) starting at 14 weeks' gestation (24, 25).

Other prenatal screening tests are aimed at reducing the risk of delivering a premature baby. A urine culture is recommended to detect asymptomatic bacteriuria, which increases the risk of maternal pyelonephritis, premature delivery, and low-birth-weight. Treatment with antibiotics significantly lowers this risk (26). Gonorrhea infection increases the risk of premature delivery, stillbirth, and low birth weight babies. Infants exposed to gonorrhea during birth can develop gonococcal conjunctivitis, which can cause blindness. Similarly, *Chlamydia* infection increases the risk of endometritis, premature delivery, and neonatal infection. Treatment reduces these risks, so screening is recommended. Gonorrhea screening is done by culturing a cervical swab sample, whereas *Chlamydia* screening can be done with culture, enzyme immunoassay, or direct fluorescent antibody.

If the woman has not had a Papanicolaou (Pap) test in the past year, early pregnancy is an opportune time to screen for cervical disease, although the sampling process is not as effective in the pregnant cervix as in the nonpregnant.

Patient Education and Psychosocial Support

First-trimester visits usually occur about once a month and help establish the doctor-patient relationship. In routine visits, ask about symptoms and milestones. Discuss the rapid physical and emotional adjustments that will be demanded of the mother, and educate the mother about fatigue, nausea, work, nutrition, and sexuality. Signs of miscarriage should be discussed at the earliest visit because nearly all miscarriages occur during the first trimester.

Encourage good nutrition, and advise patients that a total pregnancy weight gain should

Last Menses __8/7/97__ EDC __5/15/98__ (Circle if reliable)

Date	Week Gest.	Fundal Ht.	Fetal Heart	Presen-tation	Edema	BP	Urine pro/sug	Weight (lbs)	Next Visit	Comments	Resident/Attending
10/2	8	8 to 10	—	—	0	110/70	N/N	129	4 wk	Nausea Care plan reviewed	JF/CD
10/30	12	12	+$_{DT}$	—	0	110/78	N/N	131	4 wk	Excited to hear heart	JF/MN
11/30	16	16	+$_{DT}$	—	0	108/70	Tr/N	135	4 wk	UTI symptoms resolved	JF/TP
12/27	20	21	+$_{DT}$	—	0	112/68	N/N	139	4 wk	+ Fetal movement	JF/JG
1/23	24	24	+$_{FS}$	—	0	120/60	N/N	143	4 wk	Active fetus. Husband here today. Prenatal classes.	JF/DS
2/20	28	29	+$_{FS}$	VTX	0	120/68	N/N	146	4 wk	Occasional Braxton-Hicks contrac.	JF/AD
3/16	31	31	+$_{FS}$	VTX	Tr	130/72	N/N	151	2 wk	Reviewed birth plan	SKF/MF
4/3	34	33	+$_{FS}$	VTX	Tr	130/76	N/Tr	153	2 wk	Traveling home next week, doing well	SKF/MM
4/19	36	36	+$_{FS}$	VTX	0	120/70	N/N	154	2 wk	Active fetus, again reviewed pain management plans	SKF/WN
4/24	37	37	+$_{FS}$	VTX	Tr	120/80	N/N	155	1 wk	No complaints x back pain	JF/BG

Figure 8.1. Sample flowchart for prenatal care. *BP*, blood pressure; *DT*, Doppler tones; *FS*, fetoscope; *pro*, protein; *sug*, sugar; *Tr*, trace; *VTX*, vertex.

Table 8.2.
Routine Laboratory Testing in Prenatal Care

Test	Purpose	Sensitivity[a] (%)	Specificity[a] (%)	Level of Evidence for Effectiveness[b]
First trimester				
Blood type and antibody screen	Determine likelihood of blood antigen incompatibility	99–100	99–100	A
Hepatitis B surface antigen	Screen for maternal infection, acute or chronic	98	98	A
Syphilis test (VDRL or RPR)	Screen for maternal syphilis infection	62–100	75–99	A
HIV	Screen for maternal infection	95	99.5	A
Urine culture	Screen for asymptomatic bacteriuria	98	94	A
Pap smear	Screen for cervical cancer	60–80	90–99	A
Hematocrit or hemoglobin	Screen for maternal anemia	90	44	B
Hemoglobin electrophoresis	Screen for hemoglobinopathies	99–100	99–100	B
Rubella titer	Determine maternity immunity status	92–100	71–100	B
Gonorrhea culture	Screen for maternal infection	80–95	99–100	B
Chlamydia	Screen for maternal infection	70–90	97–99	B
Second trimester				
Serum multiscreen	Screening for congenital malformations	48–91	—	B
Third trimester				
Repeat gonorrhea, syphilis, chlamydia, hepatitis, and HIV tests	Repeat in women with behaviors that place them at high risk for acquiring these diseases.	—	—	A
Group B strep culture	Identify carriers	70	90	B
Diabetes testing	Identify mothers with gestational diabetes	71–83	78–87	C

VDRL, Venereal Disease Research Laboratory; RPR, rapid plasma reagin; HIV, human immunodeficiency virus.

[a]Modified from US Preventive Services Task Force. Guide to Clinical Preventive Services. Report of the US Preventive Services Task Force, 2nd ed. Baltimore: Williams & Wilkins, 1996.

[b]Level of evidence for effectiveness: A, strong or moderate research-based evidence (consistent across several studies, including at least two randomized controlled trials); B, limited research-based evidence (less consistent or extensive evidence, but preponderance of evidence supports use of treatment); C, common practice with little or no research-based evidence.

be between 20 and 30 lbs. Calcium intake of 1200 to 1500 mg/d is important and should be supplemented if the patient is unable to take in three to four servings of dairy products daily.

Many patients and their partners wonder about sexual relations during pregnancy. Unless contraindicated by bleeding or premature labor, sexual intercourse can continue through the entire pregnancy. In fact, many couples find this period of time to be especially pleasurable.

Other psychosocial issues for the woman include a changing body image, a sense of loss of control, fears and fantasies, the father's adjustment, and financial concerns. Advice regarding work and pregnancy (whether it is safe, how long during pregnancy to continue working, and what plans to make for time off after delivery) is usually sought.

Ultrasound

Ultrasound has had a great positive impact on prenatal care. When clinically indicated, it helps in monitoring pregnancies with uncertain dating, multiple gestations, or malformations, or in assessing fetal growth. An ultrasound in the early second trimester is particularly helpful, as it can date the pregnancy to an accuracy of within 2 weeks (27). Other appropriate indications for ultrasound include evaluation of suspected fetal growth retardation, assessment of vaginal bleeding, and reassurance of fetal health in late pregnancy.

Many women have come to expect that an ultrasound will be performed routinely, and indeed in many practices it is, although when critically appraised, the routine use of ultrasound has not been shown to affect outcomes (28). The U.S. Preventive Services Task Force (6), the American College of Obstetricians and Gynecologists (29), and the National Institutes of Health (30) have all taken the position that ultrasound should only be used when clinically indicated. Assessment of the importance of its use will continue to be an issue, especially in this era of cost containment. However, it is widely desired and accepted by patients and physicians.

Second-Trimester Prenatal Care

Between 14 and 26 weeks' gestation, a woman really begins to feel pregnant. The common experience of disbelief in early pregnancy is supplanted by an obviously pregnant body and an awareness of fetal movements. Women are socially recognized as being pregnant and start to notice reactions by others. The risk of miscarriage is largely past, nausea has faded, and the uterus is beginning to "show," but it is not yet large enough to significantly reduce mobility. Energy and spirits are often high. The blood pressure drops modestly, a phenomenon that can lead to patient complaints of lightheadedness or fainting.

For the physician, this is an ideal time to get to know the couple better, laying a solid groundwork for working together during labor and delivery. It is an excellent time to schedule a longer visit with both the mother and father, to obtain a genogram, and to discuss family and individual expectations about parenting.

Visits to the doctor normally occur at monthly intervals throughout the second trimester. During these visits, you should continue to follow the various parameters of pregnancy, as described previously. Assess uterine size from symphysis to fundus at every visit. Between the 18th and 34th week, the uterine height in centimeters approximates the gestational age in weeks. Discrepancies of several centimeters merit further investigation. At approximately 20 weeks, the uterus is at the umbilicus and fetal heart tones can usually be heard with a fetoscope.

Ask the patient when she first detected fetal movements. This is known as "quickening" and usually occurs between 16 and 20 weeks. The timing of this sign is too variable to really contribute to the dating of the pregnancy; however, it is a milestone to the woman and should be noted. These first flickerings of detectable life inside a woman can generate great excitement, as the pregnancy is made real by these movements and by the ever-growing belly. With the belly not yet large enough to interfere with sex, and birth control not an issue, many couples find this to be a time of great intimacy and satisfaction. The second trimester can be a high point psychologically and physically for the expectant mother.

Prenatal Diagnosis

Congenital malformations occur in approximately 3% of newborns. Although most of those malformations are minor and do not threaten life, congenital anomalies are now the leading cause of infant mortality in the United States. The most common defects that can be detected through antenatal screening are those caused by neural tube defects, such as anencephaly, and those caused by chromosomal abnormalities, such as Down's syndrome (trisomy 21). You should begin your assessment of genetic risks during the preconception visit or the first prenatal visit, but most of the effort toward early detection of congenital birth defects occurs during the second trimester, during which prenatal testing is routinely offered to pregnant women.

Screening for neural tube defects such as spina bifida, anencephaly, and encephalocele is one of the tests offered. These defects occur in 4 per 10,000 live births (31). The test involves measuring the maternal serum α-fetoprotein (MSAFP) between 16 and 18 weeks' gestation with an elevated level being a good predictor of a neural tube defect (32). Approximately 1 to 5% of women will have an elevated MSAFP level; however, 90 to 95% of these test results will be false-positives, due to underestimated gestational age, multiple gestation, or other anomalies. For this reason, you should not unduly alarm the parents, but should proceed to perform an ultrasound to assess gestational age and look for twins or other anomalies. Amniocentesis should be offered to women who are still without an explanation for the elevated MSAFP (33).

Screening for trisomy 21, or Down's syndrome, is focused primarily on mothers who will be over the age of 35 when they deliver, because the risk of having a baby with a chromosomal abnormality increases with age (34). Amniocentesis (done at 15 to 19 weeks' gestation) or chorionic villus sampling (done at 10 to 12 weeks' gestation) with karyotyping is routinely offered to these women. The age of 35 is the threshold for routine testing because that is when the risk of the chromosomal abnormalities first approximates the iatrogenic fetal loss rate of amniocentesis (0.5 to 1%) (35). However, the majority of pregnancies are in younger women; so—although the risk of trisomy 21 is highest in older mothers—most children with trisomy 21 are born to mothers under age 35. In an effort to detect these younger mothers whose fetuses have trisomy 21, all women are routinely offered a screening blood test for trisomy 21 that involves measuring maternal serum α-fetoprotein, unconjugated estriol levels, and human chorionic gonadotropin levels. Reduced levels of MSAFP and estriol, with elevated levels of human chorionic gonadotropin, have been associated with trisomy 21, and it is estimated that this method of screening will identify 62% of cases, with a false-positive rate of 5% (36). A definite diagnosis via amniocentesis is then offered to women who have a positive screening result.

Genetic screening remains controversial. Some physicians are concerned that the unnecessary amnioscenteses and parental anxiety associated with screening do not justify the relatively small number of abnormal fetuses detected. Many parents-to-be, for personal or religious reasons, would not choose to terminate a pregnancy even if a fetal abnormality were detected. For these reasons, parents should be carefully counseled regarding the benefits and limitations of these screening tests and allowed to make their own decision whether to proceed with testing. The discussion and decision should be documented in the chart.

Third-Trimester Prenatal Care

For the expectant mother, the third trimester (weeks 27 to 40) often seems to pass in slow motion. Her enlarging abdomen and loosening pelvic synostoses cause increasing discomfort, sleep problems, shortness of breath, urinary frequency, and fatigue. For the physician, this is a time of more intensive medical monitoring, as the incidence of complications (e.g., preeclampsia, maternal hypertension, malposition of the fetus) increases as the due date approaches.

An important parameter to follow is the patient's blood pressure. A blood pressure greater than 140 mm Hg systolic or 90 mm Hg diastolic or a rise of 30 mm Hg systolic or 15 mm Hg diastolic heralds the onset of a hypertensive disorder of pregnancy, which is a potentially life-threatening complication. Edema and proteinuria in addition to the blood pressure rise confirms a diagnosis of preeclampsia and warrants intensive surveillance, bed rest, hospitalization, and timely delivery of the endangered fetus.

Fetal growth is still assessed by measuring the distance in centimeters from the top of the pubic symphysis to the top of the uterine fundus. Fetal position should be determined using abdominal palpation. Most babies are vertex (head down) by the final month of pregnancy. If a breech (or other) presentation is detected, version (an attempt to turn the baby to vertex) should be offered to the mother. Versions are usually successful and increase the likelihood of the mother having a vaginal delivery.

If the woman has D (Rh)-negative blood, she should receive a RhoGAM shot at 28 weeks and again within 72 hours of delivery in an effort to prevent isoimmunization from fetal-maternal bleeds. This immune globulin will prevent D sensitization if the baby is D-positive. Such sensitization could seriously affect subsequent pregnancies.

Women at risk for gestational diabetes should be screened with a 1-hour 50-g glucose challenge at 26 to 28 weeks' gestation. This includes women with a previous poor pregnancy outcome, obesity, hypertension, or strong family history of diabetes. A positive screening test result should lead to a 3-hour, 100-g glucose tolerance test that, if its results are positive, is diagnostic for gestational diabetes. These women should then receive dietary counseling and glucose monitoring. Neither the U.S. Preventive Services Task Force (6) nor the American College of Obstetrics and Gynecology (37) recommend routine screening of all pregnant women for diabetes.

Women at high risk for sexually transmitted diseases should have a repeat gonorrhea culture, syphilis serology, and hepatitis B screen, so the need for treatment can be recognized before birth. If the patient has a past history of genital herpes, the patient should be questioned as to whether she believes she has an outbreak of the infection. If so, the perineal, vaginal, and cervical region must be carefully inspected, as neonatal herpes can be acquired by the baby during the birth process and is usually devastating to the neonate, causing neurologic impairment or death (38). Although the risk of transmission for recurrent disease is probably less than 1%, the consequences are so catastrophic that delivery by cesarean section is the standard of care in most settings.

Another serious neonatal problem is group B streptococcal (GBS) infection, which is also usually acquired by the baby during childbirth. In the United States, GBS sepsis occurs in 1.8 of 1000 live births, with a case-fatality rate of 5 to 20%, which leads to approximately 310 newborn deaths per year. It is now routine practice to screen pregnant women at 35 to 37 weeks with a rectovaginal culture to identify those women who are carriers of GBS (39). These women are offered prophylactic treatment with antibiotics during labor. An alternative strategy is to omit the prenatal screening but treat with antibiotics during labor any women who develop a fever, have ruptured membranes for more than 18 hours, deliver before 37 weeks' gestation, showed GBS bacteriuria during the pregnancy, or had a previous infant with significant GBS disease.

Once the medical assessment is complete, your attention should turn to the patient and her family's eager anticipation of labor and delivery. Be sure to discuss experiences that warrant calling the doctor: ruptured membranes, bleeding, and regular contractions. Allow time to talk about the myriad of sensations of late pregnancy, such as heartburn, leg cramps, backache, and false labor.

In addition to preparing for the delivery itself, patient education should focus on caring for the new baby. Breast-feeding should be encouraged through discussion and recommended readings. In fact, promotion of breast-feeding should start early in pregnancy. Preparations for the new baby should be reviewed as well, particularly if your patient is having her first child.

Postdate Pregnancy

It is difficult to find a more weary and exasperated patient than a woman who has seen her due date come and go. Often, she will come to her appointment expecting her physician to "do something" to get labor started. Hopefully, the physician has educated her earlier in the course of prenatal care that delivering up to 2 weeks past her due date is still within the normal range.

Postdate pregnancy is defined as one that extends more than 42 weeks beyond the last menstrual period. The most common explanation for a postdate pregnancy is incorrect dating of the gestation. The concern with these extended pregnancies is development of oligohydramnios with umbilical cord compression and uteroplacental insufficiency, leading to fetal compromise during labor. Also significant is the fact that many postdate babies weigh more than 4000 g, resulting in a greater incidence of birth trauma, shoulder dystocia, and cesarean section.

Ideally, the due date will have been accurately established as part of your earlier prenatal care. Still, these data should be reviewed. In addition, you should verify fetal health through frequent monitoring as the woman approaches 42 weeks. This monitoring can include (a) an ultrasound study of the baby, to assess fetal movement and the amount of amniotic fluid present; and (b) a nonstress test on the fetal monitor, to verify the baby's cardiac rate and reactivity. Findings of concern may mandate labor induction.

FAMILY PHYSICIAN'S APPROACH TO MATERNAL CARE

The care of families throughout the life cycle enables family physicians and their patients to view prenatal care as part of an ongoing relationship. This view more closely matches how patients experience their own pregnancies, without artificial punctuation of their lives imposed by a health care system that recognizes pregnancy, newborn care, and adult health as belonging to different specialties.

The provision of prenatal care is itself very rewarding to family physicians, but the benefits to the physician extend beyond the joy of childbirth. Family physicians who deliver babies, as compared with those who do not, report higher incomes, are more psychologically satisfied with their work, tend to perform more procedures, and serve a more diverse patient population, including more children (40). The same study found that despite the fact that these family physicians pay higher malpractice premiums, they rarely experience malpractice claims.

There has been a dramatic increase in childbirth technology over the past two decades. With this has come the assumption that the technologic approach should constitute the standard of care. The value of "high-tech" labor management in uncomplicated pregnancy has not been demonstrated. Thus, although high-risk pregnancies should receive appropriate intervention and technology, routinely applying these techniques to normal pregnancies is misguided. Heightened patient awareness and the emergence of evidence-based medicine have increased the demand for a "low-tech" approach to labor and delivery management.

One might hypothesize that family physicians practice a type of care that is somewhere between the more intensive practice style adopted by obstetricians and the less technologic approach practiced by midwives. Some studies have suggested this is true (41), whereas others have found that family physicians practice a similar style to obstetricians, with midwives standing out as using fewer interventions (42). Most practitioners claim that their approach is best, again underscoring the importance of critical appraisal regarding outcomes and resource use. Among family physicians, there is a broad range of practice styles, depending on the training received and the environment in which they practice.

The family physician should promote personalized care for the woman and her family, even in large institutions with many rules. Above all, any practitioner delivering babies must learn patience, patience, patience.

FAMILY PHYSICIANS AND OBSTETRIC CONSULTANTS

As generalists, family physicians at times serve their patients best by working with colleagues who have a greater depth of knowledge in a spe-

cialized field. Perinatal medicine, like most medical disciplines, has continued to grow and become more specialized. Family physicians are trained to provide independent prenatal and delivery care to women, identifying and managing emergencies and risk factors as they occur. In the care of complicated patients, family physicians work closely with obstetric colleagues, turning to them for expert opinion about patient management and technical skill for some operative maneuvers or deliveries. To clarify their shared responsibility for such patients, family practice and obstetric departments in many hospitals have negotiated a list of high-risk conditions appearing during prenatal care or labor and delivery, which constitute situations in which the family physician should consider involvement of obstetric colleagues in the care of the patient. Table 8.3 contains one such list of consultation guidelines,

Table 8.3.
Guidelines for Obstetric Consultation[a]

Prenatal Indications
Amniocentesis or chorionic villus sampling desired
Blood group antibodies
Cervical incompetence (by history)
Cervical cancer or CIN III
Deep venous thrombosis
Diabetes mellitus
DES exposure in utero
Intrauterine growth retardation
Significant medical disease (autoimmune, cardiac, endocrine, gastrointestinal, hematologic, neurologic, pulmonary, renal)
Multiple gestation
Preeclampsia, severe
Presentation nonvertex > 35 weeks
Placenta previa > 24 weeks
Premature labor < 35 weeks unresponsive to hydration and oral tocolysis
Uterine abnormality
Vaginal bleeding > 20 weeks, significant

Intrapartum Indications
Eclampsia
Fetal distress, significant
Labor abnormality, significant
Malpresentation
Operative vaginal delivery from above outlet
Placental abruption
Placental previa
Preeclampsia, severe
Vaginal bleeding, significant

CIN, cervical intraepithelial neoplasia; DES, diethylstilbestrol.

[a]The threshold for consultation will vary with the comfort level and experience of individual physicians.

which was developed at the University of North Carolina.

When the consultation process works well, the patient benefits from incorporation of specialty expertise while maintaining the trusted continuity relationship with her primary doctor. For such a collaborative effort to benefit the patient, the family physician must be aware of personal limitations, be committed to consultation agreements, communicate the needs and expectations of the consultation directly and clearly, and trust the consultant. The consultant must be responsive to the request for consultation or technical assistance, value the ongoing primary role of the family physician, respect the long-standing doctor-patient relationship, and be open and direct in negotiating the details of sharing responsibility for patient care.

CASE STUDY

Tonya is a 24-year-old $G_3P_{1-0-1-1}$ who comes to your office with a positive pregnancy test. This was an unplanned pregnancy; she had been taking birth control pills but admits to missing several doses. Her menstrual bleeding has been erratic, and she last bled 6 weeks ago. She lives in an apartment with her husband of 2 years and 5-year-old son; the father of her son was a former boyfriend with whom she now has minimal involvement. She works as a secretary, and her husband is a fireman. They are hoping to save money to buy a house. Tonya is interested in prenatal classes, but her husband thinks they are a "waste of time" and says that she will be "knocked out" at the time of delivery anyway.

General observation reveals a healthy-appearing woman. She complains of nausea and fatigue. On examination, she is average height but slightly underweight. Her uterus is the size of a grapefruit, and fetal heart tones are heard with Doppler ultrasonography.

QUESTIONS

1. Based on the aforementioned information, how would you estimate her EDC?

2. What information is important to elicit about her previous pregnancy?
3. What education will you provide on this visit?
4. Are there psychosocial concerns raised by this case? If so, how would you approach them?

DISCUSSION

Tonya's recent use of birth control pills and the uncertain timing of her last menstrual period lead to uncertainty regarding the dating of this pregnancy. If the bleeding 6 weeks ago was a menstrual period, then she is 6 weeks pregnant, but her uterine size is consistent with 12 weeks. The bleeding 6 weeks ago might have been bleeding during early pregnancy, which is very common. Twin gestation might also explain a larger than expected uterus. An ultrasound would be helpful because it can predict the EDC within 2 weeks of reliability and detect multiple gestations.

You'll want to take a thorough history of the previous pregnancy. In this case, Tonya explains that her previous pregnancy was without complications, but delivery was by cesarean section due to a breech presentation. This requires you to obtain the operative report from the previous delivery, to confirm that she received a low-transverse uterine incision, meaning she can be cleared for attempted vaginal birth after cesarean section.

Because she is slightly underweight, you'll want to review nutritional guidelines and encourage her to gain at least 25 lbs. She should be taking folic acid supplements. You should assess her interest in breast-feeding and address this repeatedly throughout the course of the pregnancy.

Your other patient education should focus on recommendations regarding her nausea and vomiting and assurance that these symptoms are usually self-limited. In addition, explain that you will be discussing many issues throughout the pregnancy. Among the topics you'll emphasize are: encouraging childbirth classes, empowering the patient to feel like she has some control over her labor and delivery, encouraging her by suggesting that the odds are favorable that she can successfully deliver vaginally, and inviting her husband to as many prenatal visits as possible (and encouraging him to attend childbirth classes).

Psychosocial issues include addressing any substance abuse in either parent and assessing for significant marriage and family issues. The status of the 5-year-old sibling should be addressed. If you do not already have a relationship with this patient, you can better familiarize yourself with her situation during the pregnancy. She, in turn, is likely to develop a sense of trust in you.

REFERENCES

1. Gardner P, Hudson BL. Advanced report of final mortality statistics 1993. Monthly Vital Statistics Rep 1996; 44 (suppl).
2. Dunn HL. Vital Statistics of the United States, 1941, Part 1. Washington, DC: US Department of Commerce Bureau of Vital Statistics, 1943:27.
3. UNICEF. The State of the World's Children 1996. New York: Oxford University Press for UNICEF, 1996:81.
4. Public Health Service. Healthy People 2000, National Health Promotion and Disease Prevention Objectives. Washington, DC: US Department of Health and Human Services, Public Health Service, 1992:381.
5. Guyatt G, Cairn SJ, Churchill D, et al. Evidenced-based medicine: a new approach to teaching the practice of medicine. JAMA 1992;268:2420–2425.
6. US Preventive Services Task Force. Guide to Clinical Preventive Services. Report of the US Preventive Services Task Force, 2nd ed. Baltimore: Williams & Wilkins, 1996.
7. The Cochrane Database of Systematic Reviews (available in the Cochrane Library). The Cochrane Collaboration, Issue 1. Oxford: Update Software, 1997.
8. Milinski A, Jick H, Jick SS, et al. Multivitamin/folic acid supplementation in early pregnancy reduces the prevalence of neural tube defects. JAMA 1989;262: 2847–2852.
9. Department of Health and Human Services. Reducing the Health Consequences of Smoking: 25 years of Progress. A Report of the Surgeon General. Publication no. DHHS (CDC) 89–8411. Rockville, MD: Department of Health and Human Services, 1989.
10. Department of Health and Human Services. The Health Benefits of Smoking Cessation: A Report of the Surgeon General. Publication no. DHHS (CDC) 90–8416. Rockville, MD: Department of Health and Human Services, 1990.
11. Rosett HL, Weiner L, Edelin KC. Treatment experience with pregnant problem drinkers. JAMA 1983;249: 2029–2033.
12. Volpe JJ. Effect of cocaine use on the fetus. N Engl J Med 1992;327:399–407.
13. Chard T. Pregnancy tests: a review. Hum Reprod 1992;7:701–710.
14. Cunningham FG, MacDonald PC, Gant NF, Leveno KJ, Gilstrap LC III. Prenatal care. In: Williams Obstetrics, 19th ed. Norwalk, CT: Appleton & Lange, 1993:249.
15. Kennell J, Klaus M, McGrath S, et al. Continuous emotional support during labor in a US hospital. JAMA 1991;265:2197–2201.
16. Simkin P, Enkin M. Antenatal classes. In: Chalmers I, Enkin M, Keirse M, eds. Effective Care in Pregnancy and Childbirth. New York: Oxford University Press, 1989:318–334.
17. Public Health Service Expert Panel on Prenatal Care. Caring for Our Future: The Content of Prenatal Care. NIH publication no. 90–3182. Washington, DC: Public Health Services, US Department of Health and Human Services, 1989.
18. McDuffie RS, Beck A, Bischoff K, et al. Effect of frequency of prenatal care visits on perinatal outcome among low-risk women. JAMA 1996;275:847–851.
19. Kochenour NK: Normal pregnancy and prenatal care. In: Scott JR, DiSaia PJ, Hammond CB, et al, eds. Danforth's Obstetrics and Gynecology, 7th ed. Philadelphia: JB Lippincott, 1994:67–104.
20. Murphy JR, O'Riordan J, Newcombe RG, et al. Relation of haemoglobin levels in first and second trimester to outcome of pregnancy. Lancet 1986;1:992–994.
21. Scholl TO, Hediger ML. Anemia and iron-deficiency. Compilation of data on pregnancy outcome. Am J Clin Nutr 1994;59:492S–501S.
22. Wong VCW, Ip HMH, Reesink HW, et al. Prevention of the HBsAg carrier state in newborn infants of mothers who are chronic carriers of HBsAg and HBeAg by administration of hepatitis-B vaccine and hepatitis-B immunoglobulin: double-blind randomized placebo controlled study. Lancet 1984;1:921–926.
23. Marx R, Aral SG, Rolfs RT, Sterk CE, Kahn JG. Congenital syphilis, United States, 1983–1985. MMWR 1986; 35:625–628.
24. Connor EM, Sperling RS, Gelber R, et al. Reduction of maternal-infant transmission of HIV-1 with zidovudine treatment. N Engl J Med 1994;331:1173–1180.
25. Fiscus SA, Adaora A, Schoenbach VJ, et al. Perinatal HIV infection and the effect of zidovudine therapy on transmission in rural and urban counties. JAMA 1996; 275:1483–1488.
26. Romero R, Oyarzun E, Mazor M, et al. Meta-analysis of the relationship between symptomatic bacteriuria and preterm delivery/low birth weight. Obstet Gynecol 1989;73:576–582.
27. Campbell S, Warsof SL, Little D, et al. Routine ultrasound screening for the prediction of gestational age. Obstet Gynecol 1985;65:613–620.
28. Ewigman BD, Craine JP, Figoletto FD, et al. Effect of prenatal ultrasound screening on perinatal outcome. The RADIUS Study Group. N Engl J Med 1993;329: 821–827.
29. American College of Obstetricians and Gynecologists. Ultrasonography in pregnancy. Tech Bull 1993;187: 1–9.
30. National Institutes of Health Consensus Development Conference. The use of diagnostic ultrasound imaging during pregnancy. JAMA 1984;252:669–672.
31. Flood T, Brewster M, Harris J, et al. Spina bifida

incidence at birth—United States, 1983–1990. MMWR 1992; 41:497–500.

32. Maternal serum alpha-fetoprotein screening for neural tube defects: results of a consensus meeting. Prenatal Diagn 1985;5:77–83.

33. American College of Obstetricians and Gynecologists. Maternal serum screening. Tech Bull 1996;228:1–9.

34. Hansen JP. Older maternal age and pregnancy outcome: a review of the literature. Obstet Gynecol 1986; 41:726–742.

35. NICHD National Registry for Amniocentesis Study Group. Midtrimester amniocentesis for prenatal diagnosis: safety and accuracy. JAMA 1976;236: 1471– 1476.

36. Haddow JE, Palomaki GE, Knight GJ, et al. Prenatal screening for Down's syndrome with use of maternal serum markers. N Engl J Med 1992;327:588–593.

37. American College of Obstetricians and Gynecologists. Diabetes and pregnancy. Tech Bull 1994;200:1–8.

38. Whitley R, Arvin A, Prober C, et al. Predictors of morbidity and mortality in neonates with herpes simplex virus infections. The National Institute of Allergy and Infectious Disease Collaborative Antiviral Study Group. N Engl J Med 1991;324:450–454.

39. Centers for Disease Control and Prevention. Prevention of perinatal group B streptococcal disease: a public health perspective. MMWR 1996;45(RR-7):1–24.

40. Larimore WL, Sapolsky BS. Maternity care in family medicine: economics and malpractice. J Fam Pract 1995;40:153–160.

41. Rosenberg EE, Klein M. Is maternity care different in family practice? A pilot matched pair study. J Fam Pract 1987;25:237–242.

42. Rosenblatt RA, Dobie SA, Hart LG, Schneeweiss RS, et al. Interspecialty differences in the obstetric care of low-risk women. Am J Public Health 1997; 87: 344–351.

9. Well Child and Adolescent Care

BEAT STEINER

Key Clinical Questions

1. What screening tests are recommended for a 4-year-old child who comes for a "well child" visit?
2. What information should be provided to patients and parents when discussing the risks and benefits of the immunizations that are given to a 6-month-old child?
3. What health-related behavior can physicians expect to influence most when seeing adolescent patients in the office?

BACKGROUND

Well care for children and adolescents can be one of the most interesting parts of family practice because it provides an ideal opportunity to offer preventive services that not only prevent or postpone serious illness during childhood but have positive effects on health into late adulthood. Despite the proven benefits of many preventive services, they are frequently not put into practice. Hindrances to implementation include: poor reimbursement for preventive services, insufficient time, lack of reminder systems, and even disinterest and insufficient knowledge on the part of both clinicians and patients or parents (1). To overcome these obstacles and provide effective well child care, clinicians should be familiar with effective preventive services, find efficient ways to incorporate prevention into the routine of a busy day, and meet the needs and expectations of children and families.

Preventive strategies will fall on deaf ears if the parent is primarily concerned about the child's recent cough. However, if the acute concern is effectively addressed, it is frequently possible, and even necessary, to incorporate certain aspects of "well child care" into such acute care visits. Many patients, especially adolescents and others with limited access to health care, rarely come in specifically for preventive care appointments, only asking for help when there is a problem.

In the family practice office, well child visits are scheduled alongside adult care, usually for 15 to 20 minutes. By contrast, health departments in some parts of the country have clinics exclusively devoted to providing well child care. Such clinics are frequently more successful at incorporating preventive services, including formal developmental and nutritional assessments, and detailed anticipatory guidance. Visits in such clinics generally last longer and involve a more multidisciplinary approach. In both settings, however, practitioners must be familiar with a clinical approach to children and adolescents, which frequently differs from that used with adults.

For young children, parents are the primary source for the clinical history and the important decision makers in accepting treatment plans. However, it is important to establish a trusting relationship with the child to facilitate the clinical examination. Spending a minute interacting with the child when first coming into the examination room is the first step to building trust. In older children it is important to find an appropriate balance between recognizing the increased independence of the child while still respecting the role of the parent. With the parent present, a 6-year-old child can give much of the history. A 9- or 10-year-old child should be offered the opportunity to be alone with the physician for at least part of the visit. With adolescents, most of the visit will occur without the parent, but if possible, the concerns of the parents should still be elicited. Many children have anxiety about strangers, particularly those wearing white coats. Physically approaching the child too quickly may also cause fear. To build confidence and allay fears, the least invasive (or painful) parts of the examination should be done first. Let the child touch the stethoscope, maybe even listen to the parent's heart first. Give the child permission to explore the examination room. Find toys that the child or other siblings can play with. Attention to such details can facilitate a smooth visit and result in satisfied parents.

In addition to addressing any specific concerns of the patient and the family, the well child visit should address three major areas of preventive care: screening, immunizations, and counseling. This chapter examines each of these three areas as they apply to children and adolescents, emphasizing services that have been found to be effective.

SCREENING

Screening tests are used to identify asymptomatic patients requiring special interventions. The criteria for an effective screening test are discussed in Chapter 6. Although medical, family and social history questions (e.g., well water versus city water? number of sexual partners?) are not considered formal screening tests, such questions can identify risk factors so that specific screening measures can then be chosen (e.g., measuring fluoride content of drinking water; testing for sexually transmitted diseases). As previously mentioned, such an approach increases the pretest prevalence of the condition and the predictive value of the screening test.

Recommended screening tests for children and adolescents are listed in Table 9.1. Supporting evidence for those recommendations is taken from the Guide to Clinical Preventive Services unless otherwise referenced (2). The relative lack of proven effectiveness of the physical examination as a screening tool becomes obvious from this table and speaks to the importance of obtaining historical data from patients or parents during well child care visits. A clinician should also remain alert for conditions listed in Table 9.2, but realize that no effective screening tests

Table 9.1.
Screening Recommendations for Children and Adolescents

Age	Screening Test	Comments	Level of Evidence for Effectiveness[a]
Newborn	PKU, TSH, hemoglobin electrophoresis	Repeat TSH, PKU at 2 weeks of age if tested before 24 hours of life	A
6–12 mo	Hemoglobin or hematocrit	Screen only high-risk groups	B
	Blood-lead concentration	Screen only high-risk groups	B
3–5 yr	Vision screening for amblyopia and strabismus	Use cover-uncover test or Random Dot E; screening before age 3 difficult, but consider red reflex	B
All children	Height, weight, head circumference, developmental screen	The optimal frequency has not been defined.	B
	Blood pressure, auscultation of heart (in children) and palpation of femoral pulses (in newborns)	The optimal frequency has not been defined; accurate blood pressure measurements are particularly difficult in children < 3 years of age	B
	Mantoux test (using PPD) for TB	Screen only high-risk groups; start screening at 12–15 months of age	B
Adolescents	Culture for gonorrhea, fluorescent antibody assay for *Chlamydia*, ELISA for HIV, VDRL or RPR for syphilis	Screen high-risk group as defined in text	B
Adolescent females	Pap smear	Screen if sexually active or older than 18 years	A

Data from US Preventive Services Task Force. Guide to Clinical Preventive Services. Report of the US Preventive Services Task Force, 2nd ed. Baltimore: Williams & Wilkins, 1996.

PKU, phenylketonuria; TSH, thyroid-stimulating hormone; PPD, purified protein derivative; ELISA, enzyme-linked immunosorbent assay; HIV, human immunodeficiency virus; VDRL, Venereal Disease Research Laboratory; RPR, rapid plasma reagin.

[a]Level of evidence for effectiveness: A, strong or moderate research-based evidence (consistent across several studies, including at least two randomized controlled trials); B, limited research-based evidence (less consistent or extensive evidence, but preponderance of evidence supports use of treatment); C, common practice with little or no research-based evidence; X, moderate or strong evidence suggesting that this intervention is not effective.

Table 9.2.
Conditions for Which Screening Is Not Recommended but Clinicians Should Remain Alert

Age	Condition
Children less than 3 years of age	Symptoms and signs of hip instability or dislocation
	Congenital heart disease
	Undescended testes
	Signs of ocular misalignment
	Symptoms and signs of hearing impairment
All children	Evidence of early childhood caries
	Dental crowding or misalignment
Children and adolescents	Family violence
	Hyperlipidemia
	Exercise-induced asthma
	Visual acuity
Adolescents	Depressive symptoms
	Large spinal curvatures

exist to discover these conditions in asymptomatic individuals.

Screening for Newborns

The Newborn Period

Most states have laws that require neonates to be screened for a number of conditions. The profound, irreversible effects of unrecognized hypothyroidism and phenylketonuria, as well as the documented benefits of early treatment, have led to the requirement of screening all term newborns for these disorders before discharge from the hospital. Other conditions are included in mandatory newborn screening on a state-by-state basis, depending on the resources, the regional prevalence of such disorders, and input from state advisory committees. Some states screen for as few as three disorders and others for as many as nine, so you should become familiar with the characteristics of the screening tests that are used in the state in which you practice. Remember, too, that infants discharged at less than 24 hours of age should have the test repeated by 1 week of age, because of the possibility of false-negative results in the immediate postpartum period.

Screening Children

Iron Deficiency Anemia (Hemoglobin or Hematocrit)

Iron deficiency anemia in low-income populations, immigrants from developing countries, and low-birth-weight and premature infants is substantially higher than in the general population (10 to 30% vs. < 3%). Iron deficiency anemia in infancy and early childhood has been associated with delayed growth and development and is reversible with adequate supplementation (note that the criteria for anemia in children are age dependent) (3). In children with significant anemia, the effects of treatment are dramatic. The clinical benefits of reversing mild anemia remain less well proven. High-risk infants (as defined previously) should be screened with a hematocrit or hemoglobin between the ages of 6 to 12 months. Mass screening of low-risk infants and older children is not justified due to the cost of screening and low prevalence of clinically significant anemia.

Lead Toxicity (Blood Lead Concentration)

Low-level lead exposure (corresponding to serum levels of 10 to 25 µg/dL) can lead to subtle effects on behavior, cognition, sleep patterns, and growth rate. Higher exposures cause anemia, abdominal cramping, acute encephalopathy, and even death. The highest mean blood lead levels in the United States occur in children between the ages of 1 and 2, primarily because of more lead paint and lead dust ingestion and higher lead-absorption rates compared with older children and adults. In a recent national survey, 9% of children between the ages of 1 and 5 had lead levels between 10 and 25 µg/dL. Such elevated levels were particularly common in children living: (a) in communities where prevalence of elevated lead levels is high, (b) in houses built before 1950 with dilapidated paint or undergoing recent renovation, (c) near industrial lead facilities, and (d) with someone whose hobby involves lead exposure. Chelation therapy and environmental lead abatement programs are effective in reducing blood lead levels, but it remains controversial how well this reduction correlates with improved behavior and cognition. Nevertheless, children belonging to high-risk subgroups should be screened at approximately 12 months of age, because identifying children with elevated lead levels can also lead to interventions that prevent other children from being exposed.

Vision Screening (Red Reflex, Cover-Uncover Test, Random Dot E)

Undetected vision problems are present in 5 to 10% of preschool children. Undetected congenital cataracts, strabismus and amblyopia may result in irreversible visual deficits. In contrast, refractive errors generally manifest themselves during school age, and there appears to be little benefit from earlier detection.

The eye examination of the newborn and infant less than 4 months of age concentrates on detection of congenital cataracts and ocular tumors such as retinoblastoma. A normal red reflex test should reveal identical, simultaneous red images; asymmetry indicates either a problem with light transmission through the eye or a retinal defect. In children older than 6 months, the aim should be to identify children with strabismus. However, the use of screening tests to detect occult visual abnormalities in children less than 3 years of age has generally been unsuccessful.

In children between ages 3 and 5, stereograms such as the Random Dot E can be used to detect strabismus and amblyopia (sensitivity of 54 to 64%, specificity 87 to 90%). This test is easy and quick to perform but involves a set of stereo-optic glasses and special cards. The cover-uncover test requires no special equipment, but the sensitivity and specificity of this test are not known. In this test the child is asked to focus on a distant object. While the clinician covers one eye of the child, he or she observes the other eye. If the uncovered eye jumps to fix on the object, strabismus is detected. Next the clinician uncovers the eye, now observing the eye that was previously covered. If that eye jumps to fix on the object, latent strabismus is detected.

Because refractive errors can be easily corrected when they produce symptoms, and because there is no clear evidence that uncorrected

refractive errors that would be detected by screening programs have any adverse effect on school performance, screening for visual acuity is not included in Table 9.1. As pointed out in Table 9.2, however, clinicians must remain alert for early symptoms of refractive errors, and for this reason, parents and children should be asked if they have concerns about vision. Can the child see letters on the blackboard or read billboards when in the car? Does the child have trouble reading or drawing?

Screening Children and Adolescents

Growth and Development

Poor growth may be the presenting feature of a variety of disorders, such as poor psychosocial support, family dysfunction, endocrinopathies, as well as cardiac and renal disorders. Height, weight, and head circumference should be measured during all routine office visits during the first 2 years of life (head circumference is 90% complete by 2 years of age) and plotted on a standardized growth chart. Significant deviations should give cause for concern. Subsequently, height and weight should be measured on all well child visits through adolescence to screen for obesity. Studies suggest that as many as 25% of children in the United States are overweight and that many of these children suffer socially and have increased mortality as adults. Early detection and culturally sensitive counseling to promote physical activity and a healthy diet may reverse this morbidity and mortality.

Development can be monitored by following up on age-appropriate milestones of intellectual, motor, and social skills. The most common method of assessing development is the Denver Developmental Screening Test (DDST). The DDST identifies children who are developing at an unusually slow rate, so that appropriate investigation and intervention can be undertaken. Items from the DDST can be integrated with other screening tests, immunizations, and educational reminders to form a health maintenance flowchart.

Sexual development should also be assessed using Tanner staging (stages 1 to 5). Boys are rated based on pubic hair and genital development; girls are rated based on pubic hair and breast development. Tanner stage 1 represents an absence of secondary sex characteristics, whereas secondary sex characteristics in Tanner stage 5 are fully adult. Recently published results suggest that the onset of puberty, at least in girls, occurs earlier than previously published norms. The first signs of pubertal development in girls occur at a mean age of 8.8 years in African-Americans and 9.9 years in whites (4).

Hypertension and Heart Disease

Hypertension is much less common in children than in adults. However, a relatively high proportion of children with hypertension have secondary, potentially curable forms; thus, there is a general consensus that blood pressure should be measured periodically in children and adolescents. No good evidence exists for when measurement should first occur and at what intervals it should be repeated. Guided by how well children can cooperate and the tradition of the annual examination, many clinicians first check blood pressure when a child is 3 years old and repeat these measurements annually. Blood pressure measurements should be taken with the correct cuff width (two thirds of upper arm length). An undersized cuff will give a falsely elevated reading. Criteria of hypertension in children vary with age, but in general a blood pressure greater than 95% for that age group defines hypertension (5). As in adults, elevated blood pressure should be confirmed on at least three separate occasions.

Congenital heart disease has an incidence of approximately 1% and accounts for half of all deaths due to congenital defects. Most cases can be detected in the first 6 months of life. Although not specifically evaluated by the Guide to Clinical Preventive Services as a screening test, most clinicians advise auscultation of the heart and palpation of pulses (including femoral pulses) during the newborn period and at least twice in the first 6 months to detect asymptomatic septal defects and aortic coarctation. As discussed in a later section, currently there also is insufficient evidence to recommend routine screening for hyperlipidemia.

Tuberculosis

Reported tuberculosis cases in the general population increased by 20% from 1985 to 1992. Newborns and infants suffer considerable morbidity from the disease, whereas untreated older children and adolescents may remain asymptomatic carriers for prolonged periods of time. Detection of asymptomatic infection is performed with the Mantoux test in which purified protein derivative (PPD) is injected intradermally. When administered properly, the sensitivity of the test is between 90 and 95%. Induration of 10 mm constitutes a positive test for high-risk individuals (see later text) and children less than 4 years of age, and induration of 15 mm for low-risk individuals is assumed to be specific for tuberculous infection (remember to measure induration, not erythema!). If the test is positive, chemoprophylaxis with isoniazid (INH) is an effective means of preventing the subsequent development of active tuberculosis. The true specificity of the test, however, remains poorly defined because there is no reliable "gold standard" for latent infection. False-positive reactions do occur with atypical mycobacteria infection, prior bacille Calmette-Guérin (BCG) vaccine, and hypersensitivity reaction. For this reason combined with the potential toxicity, cost, and inconvenience of INH, many recommend the routine use of the Mantoux test only in high-risk populations, including persons infected with human immunodeficiency virus (HIV), close contacts of persons with known or suspected tuberculosis, immigrants from countries with high tuberculosis prevalence, and medically underserved populations including the homeless. Screening should begin at 12 to 15 months of age and be repeated annually or biannually if the child or adolescent remains in a high-risk group. Any child or adolescent found to have active tuberculosis should also be tested for HIV infection.

Screening Adolescents

Screening for Venereal Disease and Cervical Dysplasia

More than 1 million cases of infections with *Neisseria gonorrhoeae* and 4 million cases of infection with *Chlamydia trachomatis* are reported annually. The majority of these cases occur in men and women under 25 years of age. The asymptomatic carrier state is common in both infections and may persist for months or even years. These infections are associated with significant morbidity, especially in females, causing infertility, ectopic pregnancies and chronic pelvic pain. Infection may also be a cofactor in the heterosexual transmission of HIV. Detection is simple and relatively inexpensive with the direct fluorescent antibody assays for chlamydia and culture media for gonococci. Samples must be obtained from the cervical canal in females and the urethra in males. The fastidiousness of both organisms makes proper collection techniques crucial. Treatment for both infections is available using short courses of antibiotics.

Adolescents who are sexually active with two or more sexual partners over the past year, who have sexual partners with multiple other partners, who exchange sex for money or drugs, or who have a history of prior sexually transmitted diseases should be screened for chlamydial and gonococcal infections. Although screening of low-risk adolescents may be less cost effective, communities with a high prevalence of gonorrhea and chlamydial infection should consider universal screening of sexually active adolescents.

This high-risk group of adolescents should also be screened for syphilis, a continued major infection in the United States, resulting in severe complications if left untreated. Nontreponemal tests, such as the Venereal Disease Research Laboratory (VDRL) or rapid plasma reagin (RPR), are used to screen patients. Although the sensitivity of these tests is only 62 to 76% for primary syphilis, it is close to 100% for secondary syphilis. Specificity can be lowered (75 to 85%) in patients who have collagen vascular diseases, injection drug use, malignancy, and pregnancy, but is close to 100% in patients without such conditions.

With appropriate consent, this same high-risk group of adolescents, as well as those admitting to intravenous drug use, men who have had sex with men, and those who received blood transfusions before 1985 should also be screened for HIV. Patients who wish anonymous testing for HIV should be advised of appropriate options. Although no cure currently exists for this disease, available therapies clearly prolong life and reduce morbidity. Clinicians should also remember that adolescent females who are sexually active or older than 18 years of age should have routine Papanicolaou (Pap) smears (See Chapter 10, Well Adult Care).

Substance Abuse

Among young adolescents, 73% have tried alcohol at least once. Among 12th graders, 45% of males and 33% of females reported binge drinking (five or more drinks on one occasion) in the past (6). In addition to the long-term medical and social consequences of problem drinking, alcohol is also involved in half of all adolescent deaths due to motor vehicle accidents, other unintentional injuries, suicides, and homicides. The burden of suffering of alcohol abuse, the sensitivity of simple screening questions such as the CAGE questionnaire (see Chapter 13), and the availability of substance abuse treatment resources makes this an important topic to address with all adolescents. The effectiveness of screening for drug use with short standardized questionnaires has been less well proven, but because of the multiple problems associated with drug use among adolescents, this topic should probably be incorporated into the care of adolescents as well.

Suicide and Youth Violence

Although suicide among adolescents has increased substantially over the last several years and is the third leading cause of death in persons 15 to 24 years old, there is insufficient evidence for or against routinely screening asymptomatic adolescents for suicide risk. Youth violence is also increasingly recognized as a major health problem, but again the effectiveness of screening remains unproven. Clinicians should, however, remain keenly alert for signs and symptoms of depression, problems with drugs or alcohol, a history of violent or criminal behavior, and availability of weapons in the home.

Screening Examinations and Laboratory Tests for Which Insufficient Evidence Exists

Some physical examination maneuvers and laboratory tests are commonly used in well child visits but have not been mentioned previously because they do not meet the strict criteria for effective screening tools. A thorough abdominal examination is performed by many clinicians in children less than 5 years of age to pick up occult abdominal tumors such as neuroblastomas (annual incidence: 7 to 10 cases per million) or Wilms' tumor (annual incidence: 7 cases per million). No evidence exists that such routine examinations result in improved outcomes for these rare tumors. A similar situation is found for developmental dysplasia of the hip (1.5 per thousand births), cryptorchidism (1% of toddlers), and scoliosis (5% of adolescents). Untreated developmental dysplasia of the hip is associated with permanent limitations of movement, and surgery does appear to be an effective treatment. However, the screening tool used, the Ortolani-Barlow maneuver, has poor test characteristics, even when performed by experienced clinicians (sensitivity 26%, specificity 84%) (7). Ultrasound may prove to be a more cost-effective screening tool. Cryptorchidism is associated with oligospermia and increased risk of testicular cancer, and it is hoped but unproven that early corrective surgery can reduce these risks (8). Specific testing for curvatures of the spine is also not a useful screening test in asymptomatic children and adolescents. Although large curvatures should prompt referral, smaller curves picked up by the forward-bending test have not led to interventions that improve clinical outcome.

These statistics should not dissuade clinicians from performing a thorough physical examination during well child care. Patients and families expect a thorough examination; thus, the "laying on of hands" may have a therapeutic benefit. Also, an abnormality that later presents itself may damage the doctor-patient relationship if, on an earlier visit, a thorough examination had not been performed. The successful clinician will continue to balance evidence-based medicine with the art of caring for patients.

Many clinicians order a number of laboratory tests, including urinalysis and cholesterol levels, during well child visits. Routine urine dipstick testing of school-aged children is not recommended owing to the low prevalence of asymptomatic disease and the high proportion of false-positive tests. Routine cholesterol screening is not currently recommended because of the lack of clear evidence that therapy is beneficial and the unknown toxicities of cholesterol-lowering medications in children. Regardless of cholesterol level, all children and adolescents should receive periodic counseling regarding dietary fat intake.

IMMUNIZATIONS

Providing immunizations is the second major type of preventive service. Immunization against infectious diseases has largely been responsible for the significant reduction in illnesses such as measles, poliomyelitis, and congenital rubella syndrome over the past decades. Despite such evidence, a recent study estimated that less than 70% of children between ages 19 to 35 months are adequately immunized (9). In addition to the general barriers to implementing prevention already mentioned, withholding immunizations for inappropriate contraindications is another important cause of inadequate immunization rates (Table 9.3). Clinicians should withhold immunizations only for true contraindications, implement office systems to effectively track immunization status of patients, obtain appropriate informed consent from the patient or the family, use every visit to provide indicated immunizations, and stay up to date on current immunization recommendations (1). The immunization schedule recommended as of 1996 by most major authorities, including the U.S. Preventive Services Task Force, the American Academy of Family Physicians, and the American Academy of Pediatricians, is shown in Table 9.4. Clinicians should, however, be aware that this schedule has changed a number of times during the past decade and is likely to continue to change as new and more effective vaccines are introduced.

When obtaining informed consent from par-

Table 9.3.
Contraindications and Precautions for Childhood Immunizations

True Contraindications and Precautions	Not True Contraindications (Vaccines May Be Given)

Anaphylactic reaction to vaccine
Moderate or severe acute illness
  with or without fever
	Mild-to-moderate local reactions (soreness, redness, swelling)
	  following a dose of an injectable vaccine
	Mild acute illness with or without low-grade fever
	Current antimicrobial therapy
	Convalescent phase of illness
	Prematurity (same schedule and indications as full-term infants)
	Recent exposure to an infectious agent
	History of penicillin or other nonspecific allergies in child or any
	  allergy in a relative

Adapted from National Coordinating Committee on Clinical Preventive Services. Clinician's Handbook for Preventive Services: Put Prevention into Family Practice. Washington, DC: US Department of Health and Human Services, 1994.

Table 9.4.
Routine Child Immunization Schedule[a]

Age	Diphtheria Pertussis Tetanus[b,c]	Polio[d]	Measles Mumps Rubella	Hepatitis B	*H. influenzae* B[e]	Varicella
Birth				x		
2 mo	x	x		x	x	
4 mo	x	x			x	
6 mo	x	x		x	x	
12–15 mo	x		x		x	x
4–6 yr	x	x	x			
Every 10 yr	x					

Adapted from National Coordinating Committee on Clinical Preventive Services. Clinician's Handbook for Preventive Services: Put Prevention into Family Practice. Washington, DC: US Department of Health and Human Services, 1994.

[a]Because of rapid advances in vaccine technology, clinicians should also consult updated recommendations of the Advisory Committee on Immunization Practices, the American Academy of Pediatrics, and the American Academy of Family Physicians.

[b]After booster at age 4 to 6 years, booster every 10 years should include only vaccination against diphtheria and tetanus and not pertussis (DT).

[c]Acellular pertussis component (DaPT) appears equally effective and with less side effects than cellular vaccine for all age groups.

[d]Inactivated polio vaccine may replace oral polio vaccine (see text).

[e]Haemophilus influenzae vaccine can be purchased in a premixed form with the diphtheria acellular pertussis, tetanus vaccine (Hib-DaPT).

ents, discuss the benefits as well as the small but definite risks of immunizations. Reactions can range from a mild fever and irritability to anaphylaxis and even death. The pertussis vaccine (**P in diphtheria, pertussis, tetanus [DPT]**), in particular, has received some notoriety for adverse reactions (encephalopathy: 2.7 cases per million doses; hyporesponsive/hypotonic episodes: 3.5 to 291 cases per 100,000 doses; febrile seizures: 57 cases per 100,000 doses). The recently developed acellular pertussis vaccine (**aP in DaPT**) appears to be equally effective and associated with even fewer side effects. Thus, the pertussis vaccine's benefits should outweigh its risks in most cases. The live oral polio vaccine (**OPV**) is highly effective against the poliovirus, but one of 2.5 million vaccines does result in a case of vaccine-induced paralytic polio. For this reason, some authorities have started to advocate replacing OPV with the inactivated polio virus, which must be injected but has no documented serious adverse effects. The hepatitis B vaccine is produced by recombinant DNA technology and to date has no known serious adverse effect.

In counseling about potential adverse effects, tell patients that reactions to toxoid vaccines such as DPT and *Haemophilus influenzae* B oligosaccharide conjugate occur within 48 hours, whereas reactions to live vaccines occur later. Warn parents whose children have received the measles,

mumps, rubella (MMR) immunization that the child is likely to experience mild rash, arthralgias, and a low-grade fever 8 to 12 days later. Patients who have received the live varicella vaccine may also develop varicella-like rashes and fever. In general, the use of live virus immunizations during pregnancy or in an immunocompromised host carries increased risk for causing clinical disease. Susceptible immunocompromised hosts and pregnant women can also acquire these infections when a close contact is immunized with a live vaccine. Before taking responsibility for immunizing anyone in this litigious society, the health care provider should be familiar with the current relevant vaccine information and be willing and able to convey such information completely, yet understandably, to the child's caretaker. Ideally, this should include written material to take home.

Although most clinicians believe that the benefits of immunization to individual patients and society as a whole outweigh the potential risks, families have the legal and ethical right to refuse vaccinations. In most states, however, a physician's signature is required to allow an nonimmunized child to attend school. Negotiations between clinicians and families opposed to immunizations should take available scientific evidence as well as sociocultural issues into careful consideration.

COUNSELING

Screening identifies asymptomatic conditions that need to be addressed. Immunization has reduced the prevalence of vaccine-preventable infections to a point at which even nonimmunized children are relatively rarely infected. The third component of well child care—counseling—has the powerful potential for changing behavior and improving the long-term health of the patients. Certain behaviors can lead to adverse outcomes in the short term, such as motor vehicle deaths because a car seat or seat belt was not used or sexually transmitted diseases from unprotected sexual intercourse. Other health-risk behaviors increase the risk for chronic adult illnesses, such as lung cancer from cigarette smoking and heart disease associated with poor diet. Unfortunately, counseling interventions are often perceived as time intensive and ineffective. To help clinicians prioritize their counseling services, this chapter cites the magnitude of the problem and presents the available evidence that examines the effectiveness of individual counseling messages. Remember, however, that the effectiveness of many of these interventions remains unknown. A summary of counseling topics is presented in Table 9.5.

A key principle of preventive counseling is that it must be patient centered. This means using language and information that considers the age, educational level, cultural background, and values of the patient. An adolescent may see little personal relevance to the fact that cigarette smoking can cause lung cancer but may be very concerned about the cost of cigarettes and that they make the breath smell bad. The Readiness to Change Model developed by Prochaska and DiClimente (see Chapter 6, Helping Your Patients Stay Healthy) will help you tailor your counseling message appropriately. A parent who does not perceive his or her 6 year old as overweight despite the fact that the child is in the 90th percentile for weight but only in the 20th percentile for height is in the *precontemplation phase* and may need to be told that the child is overweight and given some information about the potential ill effects of obesity. That parent may need time to study this material before making a commitment to help change the child's diet or exercise pattern. In the *contemplation phase,* your counseling should focus on exploring the barriers that make changing the child's diet difficult, and working together to find possible solutions. You should express confidence that dietary changes will be successful and seek explicit commitment from the parent and the child to work on improving the diet. In the *preparation and action phase,* you should offer specific suggestions to improve the diet and exercise. Review meal plans with parents or offer suggestions for exercising, such as walking around the block each afternoon after school or joining the YMCA for swim classes. A combination of strategies, such as giving verbal instructions, providing audiovisual aides, and referring to community resources has proven to be the most effective at promoting behavior change. Follow-up will help monitor progress. In the event of *relapse,* the difficulty of changing behaviors should be acknowledged. You may want to emphasize that it can take several attempts to achieve a desired behavior change.

Counseling to Reassure and Guide

Counseling during infancy and early childhood is aimed mainly at informing parents what to expect and reassure them about the wide ranges of normal development. Such counseling also teaches parents what is abnormal and what may require further evaluation. Ideally, child care education should begin during the parents' prenatal visits and continue during the newborn hospital stay. The most frequently raised topics during infancy involve "routine care" items such as infant stimulation, feeding, sleeping, crying, skin care, and bowel habits.

Infant Stimulation

Parents will agree intuitively that stimulation is important to an alert and curious infant. As their physician, you can play a pivotal role in providing ideas and encouragement. Examples of ways to stimulate the child include talking (and later reading), creating a brightly colored environment, periodically changing the location of the bed, rearranging the toys in the crib, hanging attractive mobiles over the crib, dancing and singing with the baby, and taking frequent walks.

Feeding

There are well-proven benefits to breast-feeding, including better digestibility, improved absorption of calcium, lower risk of allergies, less susceptibility to infections, reduced cost, quicker

Table 9.5.
Counseling for Children and Adolescents

Age	Counseling Message	Does Health Improve if Behavior Is Changed?[a]	Does Counseling Help Change Behavior?[a]
Newborns	Counseling to prevent sudden infant death syndrome	A	C
	Place infant on back to sleep		
	Counseling to promote a healthy diet and breast-feeding	A	C
Children	Counseling to prevent household injuries		
	Smoke detectors	B	B
	Flame-retardant sleepwear	A	B
	Hot water heaters set < 120–130°F	A	B
	Childproof containers for medication	A	B
	Approved bicycle helmets	A	B
	Safe storage of firearms	B	C
	Counseling to prevent dental disease		
	Fluoride supplementation if inadequate in water	A	C
	Regular visits to dentist	B	C
	Regular brushing and flossing	B	C
	Counseling to prevent tobacco use		
	Effects of passive smoking	A	A
Children and adolescents	Counseling to prevent motor vehicle injuries		
	Use child safety seats, lap/shoulder belts	A	B
	Counseling to promote a healthy diet and physical activity		
	Limiting intake of dietary fat	A	C
	Emphasizing products containing fiber	B	C
	Regular physical exercise	A	C
Adolescents	Counseling to prevent tobacco use	A	C
	Counseling to prevent alcohol use	B	C
	Counseling to prevent drug use	B	C
	Counseling to prevent sexually transmitted diseases		
	Abstinence	A	C
	Regular use of condoms	A	C
	Regular use of female barrier methods	B	C
	Counseling to prevent unintended pregnancies		
	Abstinence or regular use of contraceptives	A	B
	Counseling to prevent youth violence		
	Acquisition of problem-solving skills	C	C
	Reduction of heavy or problem drinking	B	C

Data from US Preventive Services Task Force. Guide to Clinical Preventive Services. Report of the US Preventive Services Task Force, 2nd ed. Baltimore: Williams & Wilkins, 1996.

[a]Level of evidence for effectiveness: A, strong or moderate research-based evidence (consistent across several studies, including at least two randomized controlled trials); B, limited research- based evidence (less consistent or extensive evidence, but preponderance of evidence supports use of treatment); C, common practice with little or no research-based evidence; X, moderate or strong evidence suggesting that this treatment is not effective.

recovery from pregnancy, and stronger mother-baby relationship. With some important exceptions (certain maternal infections or medications), breast-feeding should be encouraged. At the same time it is important to respect the preferences of parents. A baby who is fed with love and care is likely to develop normally, regardless if breast or bottle milk is used. In most situations, breast or bottle milk should remain the sole source of intake until age 4 to 6 months, when swallowing reflexes and digestive processes are developed enough to begin to handle simple nonliquids such as infant cereal and purified vegetables. Introduce these one at a time so that parents will know which food is responsible if an allergy or intolerance develops.

Sleeping

Infant sleeping patterns vary, with the amount of sleep time generally decreasing from birth through the preschool years. To prevent dental caries, a baby should never be put to bed with a bottle of milk or juice. Sleep location (a crib versus the parents' bed, a separate room versus the parents' room) is controversial, with arguments in favor of all arrangements. The most reasonable option is to be flexible in the advice given. In the first few months of life a child will sleep according to his or her own schedule, but providing external cues as early as possible will help the child establish a routine closer to the routine of the parents. When the child wakes in the middle of the night, light and noise should be kept low and stimulation minimal. During the day, by contrast, the household members should follow their normal routine and provide lots of stimulation when the baby is awake.

Crying

All babies cry as their primary way of communicating. Crying may signal hunger, a wet diaper, fever, frustration, anger, pain, or the desire for physical contact. Labeling the child as a "bad baby" or the caretaker as a "bad parent" because the baby is fussy is inappropriate. Daily periods of irritability and crying, usually in the afternoon or early evening, are common. It sometimes reassures parents to point out that the average 6-week-old infant cries 2 to 3 hours a day and that crying may be the baby's only way to "get exercise." However, it is also important to point out that unusual patterns of crying and irritability can signify an illness that may require medical attention.

Repeated crying and irritability during much of the baby's waking hours is often referred to as colic. The cause of this syndrome is unknown, but family turmoil or stress, parental misinterpretation of the baby's crying pattern, heightened sensitivity to natural bowel distention, gastroesophageal reflux, and cow milk intolerance have been incriminated in what is surely a multifactorial process. Holding the crying baby closely, holding the baby more frequently during noncrying times, rubbing and applying gentle warmth to the abdomen, burping more frequently during feeding, relieving stress at home, going for a stroll or ride, swinging the baby in a mechanical device, and attempting a dietary intervention (avoiding cow milk formula in a bottle-fed baby or a trial of maternal milk-free diet in a breast-fed baby) are all techniques that merit individual trials in the colicky infant. Large doses of your empathy and support, combined with a tincture of time, are usually sufficient in this self-limiting process. Colic usually resolves or improves by 4 months of age.

When the child is somewhat older, episodes of fussiness and crying are often attributed to teething. Teething usually begins from 5 to 8 months of age and may cause local discomfort and fussiness, especially when the molars are erupting. Local treatment of the gums with cool liquids, chilled teething rings, and acetaminophen for analgesia should be sufficient symptomatic care. Do not use paregoric for teething, because of its high toxic-to-therapeutic ratio. High fever and profuse diarrhea should not be attributed to teething.

Skin Care

A sponge bath is advised until separation of the umbilical cord (average, 10 to 14 days), after which a tub bath using mild nondetergent soap is acceptable. To prevent dry skin, bathing is recommended every other day for babies, rather than daily. Washing the scalp, including the anterior fontanel area, once or twice a week with a shampoo such as Sebulex can effectively treat the very common seborrhea or "cradle cap." Oils and powders should be avoided to prevent contact dermatitis and ingestion or inhalation of potentially harmful substances. Eucerin cream applied sparingly after bathing treats excessively dry skin.

Bowel Habits

The most common concern regarding bowel habits is one of frequency and consistency. In most situations, reassurance will be appropriate. Frequencies in normal children can vary from one bowel movement every few days to several bowel movements per day. Consistency can vary from very loose and yellow in breast-fed babies to more well formed in bottle-fed infants. Further exploration may be warranted if the stool has a very foul odor or is very voluminous.

Choice of diapers is the other frequently raised concern of parents. Parents currently have a choice of many types of diapers, such as reusable cloth or disposable paper/plastic products. Cost and environmental impact are two important factors for parents to consider when choosing diapers for their child. Cloth diapers are now available with Velcro fasteners instead of safety pins. Frequent diaper changes to assure good perineal hygiene are essential to prevent diaper rash. Contact dermatitis may occur due to fragrances or chemicals in disposable diapers or residual ammonia or detergent in cloth diapers. Clinicians should consider these irritants as possible offenders when a diaper rash occurs. Leaving the perineum open to air is excellent therapy for almost all types of diaper rash; other therapies include barriers such as zinc oxide and medications such as nystatin.

Counseling About Healthy Behaviors

Although much of well child counseling, especially in the early years, consists of addressing the types of parental concerns discussed previously, there are also a number of relatively well-studied behavior changes that parents should be encouraged to adopt if they have not already done so (see Table 9.5) (10).

Prevention of Sudden Infant Death Syndrome (SIDS)

Although the pathophysiology of SIDS remains largely unknown, a number of associations in studies have helped clinicians provide advice on how to reduce the chance of this devastating event. A modifiable association between SIDS and the sleeping position of the child has been found in repeated studies. Children who slept on their stomachs had roughly twice the incidence of SIDS, an association that has prompted multiple organizations to call on parents to put healthy children to sleep on their backs (11).

Injury Prevention

Injuries remain the leading cause of mortality in children. Motor vehicle injuries are the principal cause during most of childhood and adolescence, accounting for one third of all deaths in persons between the ages of 15 and 24. Drowning, fires, asphyxiation, unintentional shootings, poisoning and falls (in that order) are the cause of many of the remaining deaths in ages 0 to 19. Although it remains unclear how often clinician counseling convinces parents to modify hazards that can lead to such injuries, the number of children in-

jured by these hazards, the health benefits of such modifications, and the ease with which many of these hazards can be modified, likely make brief counseling on these topics (e.g., the use of car seats) an effective use of clinician time.

Dental Health

Dental caries and periodontal disease are significant health problems for children, and evidence suggests that people of low socioeconomic status are especially lacking in the knowledge of oral disease prevention. Counseling all children and adolescents to brush their teeth daily and floss between the teeth is recommended because of the proven efficacy of brushing and flossing. The effectiveness of such counseling is unknown. Brushing should start soon after the child has teeth, but toothpaste should not be added until the child is old enough to not swallow the toothpaste. For children living in an area with inadequate water fluoridation, daily fluoride drops are recommended (Table 9.6). Advice about baby-bottle tooth decay should be given to all parents of children using bottles. Routine visits to a dentist have also been shown to improve dental health, although the optimal frequency remains unknown and economic barriers may prevent children from receiving such care.

Table 9.6.
Daily Fluoride Dosage (mg) According to Age and Water Supply Content[a]

Age	Fluoride Concentration in Local Water Supply (ppm)		
	< 0.3	0.3–0.6	> 0.6
0–6 mo	0	0	0
6 mo–3 yr	0.25	0	0
3–6 yr	0.5	0.25	0
6–16 yr	1.0	0.5	0

Adapted from American Academy of Pediatrics. Fluoride supplementation for children: interim policy recommendations. Pediatrics 1995;95(5):777. ppm, parts per million.

[a]Water can often be tested for fluoride concentration by the local health department. Although canned or bottled fluids (i.e., ready-to-feed formula or sodas) are generally not fluoridated, fluoride supplementation should be adjusted according to other sources of fluoride that the child is receiving (i.e., drinking fluoridated water while out of the home, fluoride supplementation programs at school, and so forth). All breast-fed babies over the age of 6 months should receive supplementation as well, because fluoride does not enter breast milk in appreciable amounts.

Diet and Exercise

Although routine screening for iron deficiency anemia is not recommended in the general population of children, evidence does show that parents should be advised to include iron-enriched foods in the diet of infants and young children. In children and adolescents, counseling should focus on limiting dietary intake of fat ($<$ 30% of total calories) and cholesterol ($<$ 300 g/d), and increasing the intake of fruits, vegetables ($>$ 5 servings), and grain products containing fiber ($>$ 6 servings). Children and adolescents should also be strongly encouraged to participate in regular physical exercise. As with counseling on injury prevention, these recommendations rest largely on the proven efficacy of dietary modifications and regular physical exercise. How successfully clinicians can promote such behavior in the office remains less well studied.

Tobacco, Alcohol, and Drug Use

Tobacco use is the behavior for which evidence is the strongest that brief counseling messages by clinicians can motivate behavior changes. This evidence should be used to urge parents of children to stop smoking because of the documented ill effects on health of second hand smoke. Clinicians should also give antitobacco messages to adolescents who smoke. Although the evidence is less strong with alcohol and other drugs, most guidelines urge clinicians to discuss these topics with adolescents because of the short- and long-term health burdens of these behaviors. Although a discussion around drugs and alcohol may not change the adolescent's behavior on that visit, it may give the adolescent permission to ask questions or raise concerns on that topic on future visits (12).

Sexual Behavior

The effectiveness of counseling about sexuality remains uncertain. Discussions should be based on a careful sexual history and tailored according to the needs of individuals. Effective risk-reducing measures to discuss with the adolescent include abstaining from sex, maintaining a mutually faithful monogamous relationship with an uninfected partner, regularly using latex condoms, and avoiding sexual contact with casual partners. Other forms of contraception for prevention of unintended pregnancies should be discussed, but clinicians must emphasize that only latex condoms have been shown to effectively prevent transmission of most forms of sexually transmitted diseases.

Youth Violence

Violence is a major health problem, especially among adolescents. Interpersonal, violence-related injuries are highest for young males, people with a history of delinquent behavior, and people living in poor urban communities. The etiology of youth violence is a complex interaction between personal, family, and community factors. The effect of any one intervention by a clinician in an office is probably limited, and no well-designed studies show that such counseling has effect. Still, several factors may be amenable to interventions in the office setting and should be incorporated into well adolescent care, especially a discussion of the association between injury and the availability of firearms and the use of drugs and alcohol, and nonviolent approaches to conflict resolution.

Community Interventions

Clinicians interested in addressing child health problems can become valuable contributors by working closely with the communities in which they practice. They can serve as a school team physician, help collect data to identify pressing community health concerns, participate in a community-based health intervention, or become politically active in health-related issues.

CASE STUDY

Travis is a 15 year old who comes to the office complaining of a sore throat. He is accompanied by his mother who is concerned that he has strep throat. He has no significant medical history and in fact has not been seen in the office since he was 12 years old. A "rapid strep" test is positive, and he gets a prescription for penicillin.

QUESTION

1. How can you work prevention into this acute visit?

DISCUSSION

This is perhaps the only opportunity to address some important prevention issues with Travis. Although it may be tempting, for the sake of time efficiency, to address only the acute complaint, an important opportunity to affect his future health may be lost.

When a parent or guardian accompanies an adolescent into the examination room, most clinicians will take an opportunity early in the visit to make it clear that they prefer to see adolescents alone for most of the visit. Most parents or guardians readily agree when clinicians emphasize that they are trying to teach adult ways of using the health care system, and indeed Travis's mother agreed for him to be seen alone by the physician.

The reason for coming to the office, in this case a sore throat, can often be used as a natural transition to topics of preventive health. With practice, incorporating prevention can be done smoothly and effectively, with little additional time. Statements such as, "Because exposure to cigarette smoke can lead to sore throats, I am going to ask you some questions about smoking," will help the adolescent understand the reason for subsequent questions and discussion. Transitioning to topics that are less directly related to the current complaint may be more difficult but can also be accomplished with introductory statements such as, "Generally, healthy people like yourself don't come to the doctor very often, so I like to take advantage of the times that you are here to talk about areas of health that are very important to adolescents . . . would that be OK with you?"

A statement regarding the confidentiality of conversations between doctors and patients may also help reassure the adolescent. As much as possible, such conversations should actively engage the adolescent and should touch on the areas of health mentioned in this chapter. Questions such as, "If this were a 'pop' test at school, and you were asked what health topics doctors talk to adolescents about . . . what would you answer? Why?" can help put the patient at ease, provide valuable insights into how much the adolescent already knows, and lead to an opportunity to discuss important health-risk behaviors.

Sequencing questions from less to more private topics can also help draw the adolescent into the conversation. For an example, you might first ask, "Some people your age drink alcohol. Do you know any such people?" If the answer is "yes," the follow-up question might be, "Are any of them close friends of yours?," and finally, "Have you yourself tried alcohol?" When risk behaviors are identified, short counseling messages tailored to the receptiveness of the adolescent are appropriate. When significant concerns are uncovered (e.g., very high-risk sexual behavior, drug abuse), follow-up visits or even acute interventions may be needed. If the adolescent does not disclose any health-risk behaviors, perhaps the most important component of the visit is to make it clear that these topics are a legitimate reason for seeking care in the future.

As a footnote, one of the most common preventive health services forgotten in adolescents is immunizations. Travis is due for a tetanus-diphtheria booster if his last booster was before kindergarten. He should also get the hepatitis B series, if he has not received it already.

REFERENCES

1. National Coordinating Committee on Clinical Preventive Services. Clinician's Handbook for Preventive Services: Put Prevention into Family Practice. Washington, DC: US Department of Health and Human Services, 1994.
2. US Preventive Services Task Force. Guide to Clinical Preventive Services. Report of the US Preventive Services Task Force, 2nd ed. Baltimore: Williams & Wilkins, 1996.
3. Johnson BK. The Harriet Lane Handbook, 13th ed. Philadelphia: Mosby-Year Book, 1993:231.
4. Herman-Giddens ME, Slora EJ, Wasserman RC, et al. Secondary sexual characteristics and menses in young girls seen in office practice: a study from the Pediatric Research in Office Settings network. Pediatrics 1997; 99(4):505–512.

5. Task Force on Blood Pressure Control in Children. Report of the Second Task Force on Blood Pressure Control in Children—1987. Pediatrics 1987;79:1–25.
6. Centers for Disease Control and Prevention. Youth risk behavior surveillance—United States, 1993. MMWR 1995;44(SS-1):1–56.
7. Jimenez C, Delgado-Rodriguez M, Lopez-Moratalla M, Sillero M, Galvez-Vargas R. Validity and diagnostic bias in the clinical screening for congenital dysplasia of the hip. Acta Orthop Belg 1994;60(3): 315–321.
8. Oski F, ed. Principles and Practice of Pediatrics, 2nd ed. Philadelphia: JB Lippincott, 1994.
9. Steiner J, Lowery E, Siegel CD, Barton PL, Goodspeed JR. Immunization services in rural settings. J Fam Pract 1996;43(4):326–328.
10. Green M, ed. Bright Futures: Guidelines for Health Supervision of Infants, Children, and Adolescents. Arlington, VA: National Center for Education in Maternal and Child Health, 1994.
11. Freed G, Steinschneider A, Glassman M, Winn K. Sudden infant death syndrome prevention and an understanding of selected clinical issues. Pediatr Clin North Am 1995;41(5):967–989.
12. Steiner B, Gest KL. Do adolescents want to hear preventive counseling messages in outpatient settings? J Fam Pract 1996;43(4):375–381.

10. Well Adult Care

MELISSA M. HICKS

Key Clinical Questions

1. How does preventive health care fit into a busy primary care practice?
2. What issues should be addressed with a 67-year-old woman who comes into the office for a physical examination?
3. What are the opportunities for preventive care and education during an acute visit by an 18-year-old woman with an ankle sprain?

Preventive care for adults (over the age of 17 years) relies heavily on personal and family history. The clinician must therefore be a skilled interviewer and keep accurate records of identified risk factors. The clinician and his or her staff must also be good educators and able to explain the rationale and evidence for their recommendations.

RATIONALE FOR PREVENTIVE CARE

Preventive care, as outlined in the overview (Chapter 6), combines preventing disease by primary action (immunizations), screening for early detection of common and devastating diseases, and educating about the lifestyle changes needed for primary or secondary prevention of disease. Practices that offer frequent acute, as well as wellness, care to patients are in a position to provide excellent preventive care.

In order for preventive care to be valued and effective, the services must be applicable for large groups of people and meet certain evidence-based criteria (see Chapter 6). This applies to all types of preventive services, whether screening tests, immunizations or chemoprophylaxis, or education and counseling efforts. There must be a need for the screening or intervention (prevalence of the condition), and the tests must meet two important criteria:

- They must be able to detect the target population earlier than without screening and with sufficient accuracy to avoid producing large numbers of false positive and false negative results.
- Screening for and treating persons with early disease should improve the likelihood of favorable health outcomes compared to treating persons when they present with signs or symptoms of the disease (1).

Information on the leading causes of morbidity and mortality in the populations receiving preventive care should be a guide to rational and efficient preventive efforts designed to target the individual as well as the general public. This information is generally broken down into age-related and gender-related information (1). Figure 10.1 shows these data for adults (2–4). Rational use of preventive care requires the periodic examination to be tailored to the individual, based on the person's age, gender, and specific history-related risks (using family history, drug history, sexual history, etc.). Consequently, the history and risk assessment are vital parts of the periodic preventive examination.

Equally important is the patient's willingness to modify risks that are identified in a clinical encounter. Consequently, education becomes a key to the successful visit. The primary care provider has the ideal opportunity to help the patient manage his or her own health care, as there is already an element of trust based on the provider-patient relationship. In settings in which the same provider can see the patient for acute and preventive care, a presenting clinical problem can leverage open a window of opportunity—for example, responsible sexuality can be discussed with a college student during a visit for a sports physical or in the follow-up after an acute ankle sprain.

Using knowledge of the most common causes of morbidity and mortality for various age groups facilitates more effective specific screening and education, even in a 15- to 20-minute encounter. In the above example of the student attending for a sports physical, questions can be asked specifically about physical activity, tobacco, alcohol and driving, and sexual activity. The clinician should be sensitive to the possibility of diverse practices

Rank	All races, both sexes, all ages	Number
...	All causes	2,312132
1	Diseases of heart	737,563
2	Malignant neoplasms	538,455
3	Cerebrovascular diseases	157,991
4	Chronic obstructive pulmonary diseases	102,899
5	Accidents and adverse effects	93,320
6	Pneumonia and influenza	82,923
7	Diabetes mellitus	59,254
8	HIV infection	43,115
9	Suicide	31,284
10	Chronic liver disease and cirrhosis	25,222
...	All other causes	440,106

Rank	All races, male, 25–44 years	Number
...	All causes	111,957
1	HIV infection	25,615
2	Accidents and adverse effects	21,096
3	Diseases of heart	12,268
4	Suicide	10,314
5	Malignant neoplasms	10,069
6	Homicide and legal intervention	7,910
7	Chronic liver disease and cirrhosis	3,119
8	Cerebrovascular diseases	1,863
9	Diabetes mellitus	1,421
10	Pneumonia and influenza	1,302
...	All other causes	16,980

Rank	All races, female, 25–44 years	Number
...	All causes	48,058
1	Malignant neoplasms	11,916
2	Accidents and adverse effects	6,564
3	HIV infection	5,139
4	Diseases of heart	4,796
5	Suicide	2,445
6	Homicide and legal intervention	2,370
7	Cerebrovascular diseases	1,629
8	Chronic liver disease and cirrhosis	1,190
9	Diabetes mellitus	1,037
10	Pneumonia and influenza	800
...	All other causes	10,172

Rank	All races, male, 45–64 years	Number
...	All causes	233,212
1	Diseases of heart	72,337
2	Malignant neoplasms	70,077
3	Accidents and adverse effects	11,429
4	HIV infection	9,119
5	Cerebrovascular diseases	8,365
6	Chronic liver disease and cirrhosis	7,557
7	Chronic obstructive pulmonary diseases	6,673
8	Diabetes mellitus	6,462
9	Suicide	5,679
10	Pneumonia and influenza	3,400
...	All other causes	32,114

Rank	All races, female, 45–64 years	Number
...	All causes	145,300
1	Malignant neoplasms	62,007
2	Diseases of heart	30,401
3	Cerebrovascular diseases	6,843
4	Chronic obstructive pulmonary diseases	6,071
5	Diabetes mellitus	5,722
6	Accidents and adverse effects	4,575
7	Chronic liver disease and cirrhosis	3,046
8	Pneumonia and influenza	2,137
9	Suicide	1,657
10	HIV infection	1,380
...	All other causes	21,461

Figure 10.1. *Causes and ranking of death in the United States, 1995.* (Adapted from Anderson RN, Kochanek KD, Murphy SL. Report of final mortality statistics, 1995; Monthly Vital Statistics Report 1997;45(11)(suppl 2); and Centers for Disease Control and Prevention, National Center for Health Statistics. Frequently asked questions: deaths. www.cdc.gov/faq/deaths. July, 1997.)

or alternative sexual orientation. Guidelines for a sexual history are outlined in Table 10.1. If the ankle injury had occurred during a sports-related endeavor, a gentle reminder of safety measures (helmets with bicycles, pads and wrist protectors with in-line skates, etc.) can be offered as part of the discussion. An element of praise for the pursuit of physical activity is also in order!

RISE Format

In approaching prevention, the RISE mnemonic, using history and education as its cornerstone, is a useful tool. *R* is for risk identification, *I* is for immunizations or chemoprophylaxis, *S* is for screening (primary and secondary), and *E* is for education.

Table 10.1.
Sexual History Taking and Ethics[a]

An Approach to the Sexual History

1. Are you sexually active (having sexual encounters with a partner)?
2. If not, have you ever been sexually active? Did you have any problems with that (those) experience(s)? How old were you at your first sexual encounter?
3. When you have sex with a partner, are your partners men, women, or both?
4. How many partners have you had?
5. Do you use a barrier (condom, female condom, foam) to protect yourself from infections? If having sex with someone of the opposite sex, are birth control measures used?
6. Do you have a current partner? One or more than one? Does your partner have other sex partners at present?
7. Is sex satisfying for you?
8. Do you or your partner have any concerns about your sexual relationship?
9. Are drugs and/or alcohol an important part of your sexual experiences?
10. Do you have sex with persons you do not know? Do you ever pay for sex?
11. Do you and a partner share sex toys (dildos, etc.)?
12. What types of sexual experiences do you share: e.g., oral-genital, anal, oral-anal (rimming), vaginal, digital?
13. Have you ever had diseases from sex partners, such as chlamydia, herpes, gonorrhea, syphilis, warts, etc.?

[a]A careful, matter-of-fact sexual history can identify STD risks, domestic violence risks, and sexual dysfunction. For persons who report same-sex encounters, questions about opposite sex encounters must also be asked; many lesbian-identified patients may have had male partners, for example.

Risk Assessment

Focusing on the age- and gender-related information will expedite your questioning and screening for risk factors. We know, from Figure 10.1, that a 28-year-old man has the highest risk of dying from AIDS, unintentional injuries (accidents of all kinds), heart disease, cancer, or homicide (violence). Screening questionnaires about sexual history and careful questions about exposure to violence or personal violent behaviors help focus on relevant information. You should also know that a male's lifetime risk of dying is greatest from heart disease, stroke, cancer, and accidents (see Fig. 10.1); therefore, questions for primary prevention

would concentrate on identifying behaviors or family or genetic factors that increase risk—e.g., tobacco use, a positive family history of early heart disease or hypertension, the use of seat belts and other safety measures, the presence of firearms in the home, etc. The information you gather will help tailor the education efforts, and can be used in the continuum of prevention. Specific risk factors or behaviors may point to specific high-risk categories that require further screening; for example, a young man or woman who identifies as a gay male or lesbian, particularly one without good family support, has an increased risk for suicide over a heterosexual of the same age group (5).

Standard health surveys or history questionnaires can be used to obtain a general history. Specific screening based on initial risk assessment may also be implemented by questionnaire instruments as shown in Figures 10.2 (diet), 10.3 (depression), and 10.4 (mental status) (6). Using properly trained office staff such as a nurse, nurse practitioner, physician assistant, or trained educator to conduct these screening efforts can increase office efficiency, enhance the patient's education and satisfaction, and save the physician time.

Immunizations and Chemoprophylaxis

Immunizations have cut the incidence of diseases such as measles, rubella, mumps, tetanus, and polio by a 100-fold, or even a 1000-fold in some cases (1). Adults are less likely than children to be up-to-date with recommended vaccinations. For example, most adults don't know their tetanus immunization status, and most cases of tetanus in this country now occur in inadequately immunized older adults.

The recommended routine immunizations for adults include a diphtheria-tetanus (DT) booster every 10 years. For persons with other underlying diseases, who are asplenic, or who are over 65 years of age, yearly influenza vaccines and a one-time pneumococcal vaccine (Pneumovax) are recommended. Health care workers should consider a yearly influenza (flu) vaccine and also the hepatitis B vaccine series (three injections) (7, 8). Men who have sex with men, IV drug users, and others with high-risk behaviors also should be considered candidates for the hepatitis vaccine.

Traveling to another country requires an awareness of local health risks. The most common risk of any travel is accidental injury, but there are preventable causes of morbidity as well (1). In counseling patients about travel outside the

Diet History

Date					Name	

Food or Drink		Time	Where	Alone or With Whom	Paired With	Mood Bored Worried Sad Happy Mad Tired Other
How Much	What Kind					

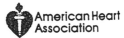

© 1986, American Heart Association

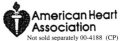

Not sold separately 00-4188 (CP)

Figure 10.2. *American Heart Association diet history.* (Reproduced with permission. ©AHA Diet History, 1986, Copyright American Heart Association.)

Diet History
Instructions

Hi!

Thanks for caring enough about your diet to complete this diet history. The information you put down on the forms your doctor or dietitian gave you will help him/her design an eating program to meet your special needs. These instructions will help you get the most value out of doing a complete diet history.

First, there are some basic rules to remember:

Write down everything: Keep your form with you all day and write down everything you eat or drink. A piece of candy here, a handful of pretzels there, a can of pop, or a small donut may not seem like much at the time, but over a week these calories add up!

Do it now: Do not depend on your memory at the end of the day. Record your eating as you go.

Be specific: If you ate a burger with cheese, write that down. Make sure to mention gravy on your meat or cheese sauce on your vegetables. If you had french fries, don't say potatoes. The fact that they are fried makes a difference.

Estimate amounts: If you had a piece of cake, estimate the size (2″ × 1″ × 2 ″). If you had a vegetable, was it 1/2 cup or 2 cups? When eating meat, record the size or the estimated weight. If the steak said 1 1/2 pounds on the label and you had half of it, say 3/4 pound.

Now let's look at the sample form attached to these directions and go over how to fill it out.

The "how much" column: In this space you want to indicate the amount of the particular food item. Estimate the size (in inches), the volume (1/2 cup), the weight (2 ounces), and/or the number of items (12) of that type of food.

What kind: In this column write down the type of food as specifically as you can. Mention sauces and gravies. Don't forget to put down salad dressing, mayonnaise, butter, sour cream, sugar and catsup.

Time: Indicate the time of day you ate that food.

Where: When you eat, indicate what room or part of the house you were in. Also list restaurants, fast food chains or your car.

Alone or with someone: If you ate by yourself, put down "alone." If you were with friends or family members, list them.

Paired with: In this column list any activities you were involved in while you were eating (working, watching TV, ironing, watching a football game, etc.).

Mood: How were you feeling at the time you were eating (sad, happy, depressed, etc.).

Helpful Tips

1. Don't change your eating habits from normal, unless your doctor or dietitian has given you specific instructions.

2. Tell the truth. There is nothing to be gained by trying to look good on these forms. Your doctor can only help if he/she knows how you typically eat.

3. Do it for all days your doctor recommends.

4. **Be sure to bring the completed forms back with you at your next appointment.**

If you have any questions, call us at _____.

Thank You!

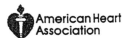
©1986, American Heart Association

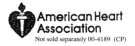
Not sold separately 00-4189 (CP)

Figure 10.2. (*continued*) *American Heart Association diet history.* (Reproduced with permission. ©AHA Diet History, 1986, Copyright American Heart Association.)

PATIENT NAME _____

AGE _____ SEX _____ DATE _____

Please check a response for each of the 20 items.	None OR a Little of the Time	Some of the Time	Good Part of the Time	Most OR All of the Time	
1. I FEEL DOWNHEARTED, BLUE, AND SAD	○ 1	○ 2	○ 3	○ 4	
2. MORNING IS WHEN I FEEL THE BEST*	○ 4	○ 3	○ 2	○ 1	
3. I HAVE CRYING SPELLS OR FEEL LIKE IT	○ 1	○ 2	○ 3	○ 4	
4. I HAVE TROUBLE SLEEPING THROUGH THE NIGHT	○ 1	○ 2	○ 3	○ 4	
5. I EAT AS MUCH AS I USED TO*	○ 4	○ 3	○ 2	○ 1	
6. I ENJOY LOOKING AT, TALKING TO, AND BEING WITH ATTRACTIVE WOMEN/MEN*	○ 4	○ 3	○ 2	○ 1	
7. I NOTICE THAT I AM LOSING WEIGHT	○ 1	○ 2	○ 3	○ 4	
8. I HAVE TROUBLE WITH CONSTIPATION	○ 1	○ 2	○ 3	○ 4	
9. MY HEART BEATS FASTER THAN USUAL	○ 1	○ 2	○ 3	○ 4	
10. I GET TIRED FOR NO REASON	○ 1	○ 2	○ 3	○ 4	
11. MY MIND IS AS CLEAR AS IT USED TO BE*	○ 4	○ 3	○ 2	○ 1	
12. I FIND IT EASY TO DO THE THINGS I USED TO DO*	○ 4	○ 3	○ 2	○ 1	
13. I AM RESTLESS AND CAN'T KEEP STILL	○ 1	○ 2	○ 3	○ 4	
14. I FEEL HOPEFUL ABOUT THE FUTURE*	○ 4	○ 3	○ 2	○ 1	
15. I AM MORE IRRITABLE THAN USUAL	○ 1	○ 2	○ 3	○ 4	
16. I FIND IT EASY TO MAKE DECISIONS*	○ 4	○ 3	○ 2	○ 1	
17. I FEEL THAT I AM USEFUL AND NEEDED*	○ 4	○ 3	○ 2	○ 1	
18. MY LIFE IS PRETTY FULL*	○ 4	○ 3	○ 2	○ 1	
19. I FEEL THAT OTHERS WOULD BE BETTER OFF IF I WERE DEAD	○ 1	○ 2	○ 3	○ 4	
20. I STILL ENJOY THE THINGS I USED TO DO*	○ 4	○ 3	○ 2	○ 1	
				RAW SCORE	
				SDS INDEX	

SDS Index	Equivalent Clinical Global Impressions
Below–50	Within normal range, no psychopathology
50–59	Presence of minimal to mild depression
60–69	Presence of moderate to marked depression
70 and over	Presence of severe to extreme depression

Conversion of Raw Scores to the SDS Index									
Raw Score	SDS Index	Raw Score	SDS Index	Raw Score	SDS Index	Raw Score	SDS Index	Raw Score	SDS Index
20	25	32	40	44	55	56	70	68	85
21	26	33	41	45	56	57	71	69	86
22	28	34	43	46	58	58	73	70	88
23	29	35	44	47	59	59	74	71	89
24	30	36	45	48	60	60	75	72	90
25	31	37	46	49	61	61	76	73	91
26	33	38	48	50	63	62	78	74	92
27	34	39	49	51	64	63	79	75	94
28	35	40	50	52	65	64	80	76	95
29	36	41	51	53	66	65	81	77	96
30	38	42	53	54	68	66	83	78	98
31	39	43	54	55	69	67	84	79	99
								80	100

Figure 10.3. *Zung self-rating depression scale.* (Reprinted with permission from Zung WWK. A self-rating depression scale. Arch Gen Psychiatry 1965;12:63–70.)

United States, it is useful to know where to access information about communicable disease risks, immunization recommendations, and food and water precautions, advice on the prevention and treatment of traveler's diarrhea, and other health information. Local health departments have immunization clinics that usually include overseas travel information. One can also access pertinent information from travel guidebooks or from the Centers for Disease Control and Prevention (CDC)

Mini-Mental State Examination

Maximum score	Patient's score	Questions
5		"What is the (year) (season) (date) (day) (month)?"
5		"Where are we?" Name of (state) (county) (city or town) (place, such as hospital or clinic) (specific location, such as floor or room)
3		The examiner names three unrelated objects clearly and slowly, then asks the patient to name all three of them. The patient's response is used for scoring. The examiner repeats them until patient learns all of them, if possible.
5		"Begin with 100 and count backwards by subtracting seven." Stop at 65. (five responses)
3		If the patient learned the three objects above, ask the patient to recall them now.
2		The examiner shows the patient two simple objects, such as a wrist watch and a pencil, and asks the patient to name them.
1		"Repeat the phrase, 'No ifs, ands or buts.'"
3		The examiner gives the patient a piece of blank paper and asks him or her to follow the three-step command: "Take the paper in your right hand, fold it in half, and put it on the floor."
1		On a blank piece of paper the examiner prints the command "Close your eyes," in letters large enough for the patient to see clearly, then asks the patient to read it and follow the command.
1		"Make up and write a sentence about anything." This sentence must contain a noun and verb.
1		The examiner gives the patient a blank piece of paper and asks him or her to draw this symbol. All 10 angles must be present and two must intersect. 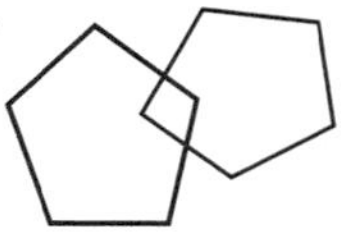
Total possible = 30	Patient's total =	If total score is 23 or below, further evaluation may be indicated

Instructions: Score one point for each correct response within each question or activity.

Figure 10.4. *Mini-Mental State Examination*. (Adapted from Folstein MF, Folstein SE, McHugh PR. "Mini-mental state". A practice method for grading the cognitive state of patients for the clinician. J Psychiatr Res 1975;12:189–198.)

directly (Internet http://www.cdc.gov, or phone the 24-hour information line, 404-332-4555) (9).

The main prevention targets for travelers include malaria, cholera, and traveler's diarrhea, which is caused by many different types of bacteria and protozoa. Most countries expect travelers to have received the basic childhood immu-nizations, and an updated tetanus toxoid booster injection is also important. Some countries may also recommend the following:

- Hepatitis A vaccine or γ-globulin

- Malaria chemoprophylaxis: different drugs are recommended for different countries, depending on the type of malaria and the prevalence of primaquine-resistant strains in that area

- Cholera vaccine: despite the fact that healthy travelers rarely have major problems and the disease does respond to treatment

- Yellow fever vaccine (now a shot or a tablet series)

- Typhoid vaccine

Prophylaxis for traveler's diarrhea can include avoidance of unpurified water, peeling local fruit rather than just washing it, and avoiding natively prepared foods as much as possible. The use of bismuth salicylate (Pepto-Bismol) tablets or liquid every day may also prevent diarrhea. There also are some antibiotics that can be taken as needed for the symptoms of traveler's diarrhea. Bactericidal pills to sterilize water can be obtained from drugstores or outfitters stores. Portable water filters do not have guaranteed efficacy.

Equatorial countries, in particular, are prone to malaria, and African and Caribbean areas are also prone to yellow fever. The range and the spread of these diseases are changing quite rapidly because of fast international travel. Malaria is now occurring in Texas and Louisiana (9).

Screening for Asymptomatic Disease

A large part of the public's perception of the "routine physical" is that it involves screening for disease that might be present but not yet symptomatic (secondary prevention). A large number of tests and examinations are available with little agreement on who should receive which measures, and how often the screens should be done. Tables 10.2 and 10.3 are derived from the U.S. Preventive Services Task Force (USPSTF) recommendations (1). They should be applied to individual patients based on the consideration of other priorities, such as your location, the availability of testing, and the probability of disease in this patient (risk factor assessment). For example, not all men are at high risk for HIV, but only careful questioning will ascertain the risks of an individual.

Although the recommendations are based on expert opinion and available data, many are still controversial, and the intervals for some of the screening procedures are unclear. The recommendation for blood pressure screening has strong support, with testing every 2 years recommended in an adult with a normal baseline blood pressure (systolic <140, diastolic <85), and more often if the reading is borderline (diastolic between 85 and 90) (2).

Any screening effort is perceived and justified based on the concept of *burden of suffering*. The disease being screened for must be prevalent in the population; knowledge of its long-term effects should be cited; and positive interventions must be stated. In the case of hypertension, for example, the screen is simple and standardized (using a sphygmomanometer), treatment is available, end-organ effects are severe, and treatment does decrease lifetime risk of endpoint diseases (stroke, heart disease, etc.), thus demonstrating the potential effectiveness of the preventive measures.

Many of the available screening tests have less valid recommendations, and the controversy continues as more data are gathered. Prime examples include prostate-specific antigen (PSA), which screens for prostate cancer, and fecal occult blood test (FOBT) and other screens for colon cancer (see Tables 10.2 and 10.3).

If a test is available to screen for a disease that can affect large numbers of people, why should there be any controversy? Remember the terms *sensitivity* and *specificity*, and the *positive predictive value* in Chapter 6? If a test has *low specificity*, but *high sensitivity*, the number of false positives increases. A positive screening test almost always leads to another, more expensive, or more invasive test. In the case of colon cancer screening, a positive FOBT usually leads to a sigmoidoscopy (up to 60 cm) or colonoscopy (examination of the full colon) with biopsies (10, 11). The risks of these tests, although fairly low, include perforation, bleeding from the biopsy site or irritation, and for some, metabolic disorders due to the medicated preparation, with significant pain or discomfort. If FOBT screening were conducted annually on a person between the ages of 50 and 75, that individual would have a 45% probability of a false positive result at some point, leading to another test, usually a colonoscopy (11). The preparation and trepidation, along with the cost and risk for the one false positive, adds up quickly in a population in which the average risk of having colon cancer is about 5 to 6% (or 1 in 19 persons). This "snowball effect" of screening is a definite factor in terms of morbidity and cost.

A major issue in screening is, *Who pays the bill?* For example, Medicare covers mammography

Table 10.2.
Well Adult Female Screening Recommendations

R—Risk Factor Identification (History)

Risk Factor	When to Begin	Interval	Tools	Level of Evidence for Effectiveness[a]
Sexual history, if sexually active	First visit—include sexual satisfaction, sexual orientation	Periodically	Sexual history (see Table 10.1)	B/C
STD/HIV risk	With above; also with drug history, number of sexual partners	As needed	Discuss risk, use of condoms, etc.; testing for *Chlamydia*, HIV; (risk reduction)	Education for risk reduction: B/C
Pregnancy/contraception	Before the onset of sexual activity (or by age 18)	Every 1–2 years		B
Drugs/alcohol/tobacco	First visit	Ongoing	MAST/CAGE; smoking cessation	B
CHD risk—family history of cardiac disease, diabetes mellitus	First visit	Update each year	Genogram	A/B
Cancer risk—family history (colon, breast, ovarian, lung)	First visit	Update each year	Genogram	B
Situational/emotional stressors (depression, anxiety)	First visit	Ongoing, as needed	Genogram, family circle; Zung or other depression scale	B

I—Immunizations (Primary Prevention)

Immunization	When to Begin	Interval	Tools/Special Concerns	Level of Evidence for Effectiveness[a]
Obtain history of childhood immunizations and illnesses (e.g., chickenpox)	First visit	—	Health record, computerized flow sheet	—
Td boosters (tetanus, diphtheria)	10 years after last one	Every 10 years	Health record, computerized chart, patient card	B
Hepatitis B	Now, or in infancy	At 1 month, at 6 months (series of three shots)	Health record	A
Rubella or MMR for reproductive age group	Check status; repeat if no known immunity or no known second MMR (could also do a rubella titer)	None. (Children 1 year and 5 years of age.) Check rubella status for preconception/pregnancy.	Health record. Do not give during pregnancy.	A

continued

Table 10.2. *(continued)*
Well Adult Female Screening Recommendations

I—Immunizations (Primary Prevention)

Immunization	When to Begin	Interval	Tools/Special Concerns	Level of Evidence for Effectiveness[a]
Pneumococcal vaccine	Age 65, or after splenectomy, or HIV + or other chronic illness	One time	Health record	A
Influenza	Same as above; also health care workers	Yearly, just before flu season	Health record; need to know allergy status	A
Hepatitis A; cholera, yellow fever, typhoid, etc. (See text and references)	For travel (check with local health department)	See text. Check with local health department.	Immunization record	A

S—Screening for Disease

Screen	When to Begin	Interval	Tools/Special Concerns	Level of Evidence for Effectiveness[a]
Weight	First visit (childhood)	Each visit	Use comparison tables, patient trends	—
Blood pressure	First visit (childhood)	Every 1–2 years (or each visit; no optimum interval has been determined (at least every 2 years if ≥ 140/84; if on medication, screen two to three times a year).	Chart record, flow sheet. If family history, more frequently.	A
Cholesterol	Age 45–65; sooner if family history. Some advocate childhood plus young adult screening as well.	Perhaps every 5 years; more often if abnormal or history changes.		B
Colon cancer screening	US PSTF recommends fecal occult blood test (FOBT) and/or sigmoidoscopy. American	Yearly		B

continued

Table 10.2. *(continued)*
Well Adult Female Screening Recommendations

S—Screening for Disease

Screen	When to Begin	Interval	Tools/Special Concerns	Level of Evidence for Effectiveness[a]
Fecal occult blood test (rehydrated)	Cancer Society recommends digital rectal examination (DRE) ≥ age 40; two examinations (DRE+) ≥ age 50, with sigmoidoscopy every 3–5 years; and FOBT every year ≥ Age 50	Yearly	High false positive rate; better if patient follows diet guidelines for the testing	B
Digital rectal examination	≥ Age 40 (ACS) ≥ Age 50 (World Health Organization)	Yearly	Some task forces do not recommend, including US PSTF	C
Sigmoidoscopy (colonoscopy for high-risk populations, every 3–5 years)	≥ Age 50	Every 3–5 years	May be combined with barium enema	B
Pap smear	Age 19, or onset of sexual activity	ACOG recommends yearly, US PSTF recommends every 1–3 years; other sources recommend every 2 years after ≥ 2 normal Pap smears	Controversy about interval, also no need for "routine" Pap smears after hysterectomy for benign reasons. There is a question as to what age to stop.	A, B
Pelvic examination	With Pap smears	With Pap smears	—	C
Self breast examination (SBE)	Teach at first health check with Pap smear	Recommended monthly by ACS	Efficacy questioned; many groups are unsure of its worth as a screen	C/X
Clinician breast examination (CBE)	≥ Age 50. Many advocate for beginning with first Pap smear.	Yearly	Should one stop CBE after age 69?	B/C
Mammogram	≥ Age 50. Earlier if high risk: family history ≥ age 40, less sensitive in younger persons.	Yearly. Some insurers may only pay every 2 years.	Should one not do mammograms after age 69–70? Studies are looking at earlier screens to examine efficacy.	A

continued

Table 10.2. (continued)
Well Adult Female Screening Recommendations

Screen	When to Begin	Interval	Tools/Special Concerns	Level of Evidence for Effectiveness[a]
S—Screening for Disease				
Visual acuity/glaucoma screen	Childhood testing; then ≥ age 40 if HTN or DM; ≥ 65 otherwise.	Recommendations are unclear	Snellen's chart ≥ age 65	B/C
Dental screening	Childhood	Regular visits (not defined). Commonly recommended yearly.	Regular at-home care; intervals left to recommendation of the dental provider	A

Screen	When to Begin	Interval	Tools/Special Concerns	Level of Evidence for Effectiveness[a]
E—Education				
Sexual activity, risk of STDs, HIV risk, pregnancy	At or before onset of sexual activity (teens)	Every periodic visit	Education flowsheet would be useful; computerized education form	A/B
Preconception counseling (age appropriate; e.g., birth control, family planning, fertility, age)	Early adult/adolescence	Any contraceptive or preventive health visit	Review fertility issues if patient desires; look at medications, toxin exposures, family/genetic history	B/C
Estrogen replacement therapy (ERT) for osteoporosis and cardiac prevention and symptom relief. Combination or single drug (combined with progesterone if uterus present).	Discuss and review *before* menopause, or as soon as possible during/thereafter (natural or surgical menopause)	Review each routine or preventive visit	Combine with discussion of diet (calcium) and exercise; bone densitometry may be useful for high-risk patients (osteoporosis)	A
Diet/nutrition	As soon as possible	Discuss at each visit; significant review with major body habitus change	Iron, calcium; food pyramid; decrease fat intake, increase fiber	A
Exercise	Early	Each visit	Benefits of regular exercise for cardiac and overall health	A/B
Injury prevention (e.g., seat belts, bicycle helmets, no drinking and driving)	Early (see risk factor identification in Tables 10.2 and 10.3 for age groups)	Each visit, particularly health maintenance visits	Review occupation risks, recreation risks, etc.	B

continued

Table 10.2. *(continued)*
Well Adult Female Screening Recommendations

E—Education

Screen	When to Begin	Interval	Tools/Special Concerns	Level of Evidence for Effectiveness[a]
Skin examination and review use of sunscreen, clothing	By age 20–30, early if history of melanoma in family	At periodic examinations	Examination by clinician if history significant or self examination is positive	A
Stressors, losses; depression; relaxation techniques	Early	Review every 2–4 years or at each visit	Genogram, periodic family circles, depression scale (see Fig. 10.3), relaxation strategies, referrals for stress management	B

Data are from US Preventive Services Task Force. Guide to Clinical Preventive Services. Report of the US Preventive Services Task Force, 2nd ed. Baltimore: Williams & Wilkins, 1996; American Academy of Family Physicians. Summary of Recommendations for Periodic Health Examination. http://www.aafp.org/members/pracguid/html. June, 1997; Mulrow CD, et al. Case-finding instruments for depression in primary care settings. Ann Intern Med 1995;122:913–921; Neufeld B. SAFE questions: Overcoming barriers to the detection of family violence. Am Fam Physician 1996;53:2575–2580; Dominitz, et al. Colorectal cancer: Latest approaches to prevention and screening. Patient Care 1996;3:124–145; Kerlikowske K, et al. Likelihood ratios for modern screening mammography. JAMA 1996;276:39–43; American Heart Association. Patient Education: Diet History. 1986; Frame PS. A critical review of adult health maintenance. Part I: Prevention of atherosclerotic diseases. J Fam Pract 1986;22:341–346; Thompson DC, et al. Effectiveness of bicycle safety helmets in preventing head injuries. A case-control study. JAMA 1996;276:1968–1973; Schieber RA, Branche-Dorsey CM, Ryan GW, Rutherford GW Jr, Stevens JA, O'Neil J. Risk factors for injuries from in-line skating and the effectiveness of safety gear. N Engl J Med 1996;335:1630–1635; Lui S, Siegel PZ, Brewer RD, Mokdad AH, Sleet DA, Serdula M. Prevalence of alcohol-impaired driving. Results from a national self-reported survey of health behaviors. JAMA 1997;277:122–125; Fleming MF, et al. Brief physician advice for problem alcohol drinkers. JAMA 1997;277:1039–1045.

[a]Level of evidence for effectiveness: A, strong or moderate research-based evidence (consistent across several studies, including at least 2 randomized controlled trials); B, limited research-based evidence (less consistent or extensive evidence, but preponderance of evidence supports use of treatment); C, common practice with little or no research-based evidence; X, moderate or strong evidence suggesting that this treatment is not effective.

Table 10.3.
Well Adult Male Screening Recommendations

R—Risk Factor Identification (History)

Risk Factor	When to begin	Interval	Tools	Level of Evidence for Effectiveness[a]
Sexual history, if sexually active	First visit (include sexual satisfaction, sexual orientation)	Periodically	Sexual history (see Table 10.1)	B/C
Contraceptive responsibility and STD/HIV risk	Early adolescence	Each visit; periodically	—	C
Drugs/alcohol/tobacco	First visit	Ongoing	MAST/CAGE; smoking cessation	B
CHD risk—family history of cardiac disease, diabetes mellitus	First visit	Update each year	Genogram	B
Cancer risk—family history (colon, lung, prostate)	First visit	Ongoing, as needed	—	—
Situational/stressors (depression, anxiety)	First visit	Periodically	Genogram, family circle; depression/anxiety screening	B

I—Immunizations (Primary Prevention)

Immunization	When to Begin	Interval	Tools/Special Concerns	Level of Evidence for Effectiveness[a]
Obtain record of childhood immunizations and illnesses (e.g., chickenpox)	First visit	—	Health record, computerized flow sheet	—
Td boosters (tetanus, diphtheria)	Ten years after last one	Every 10 years	Health record, computerized chart, patient card	B
Hepatitis B	Now, or in infancy	At 1 month, at 6 months (series of three shots)	Health record	—
Pneumococcal vaccine	Age 65, or after splenectomy, or HIV+ or other chronic illness	One time	Health record	A
Influenza	Same as above; also health care workers	Yearly	Health record; need to know allergy status	A
Hepatitis A; cholera, yellow fever, typhoid, etc. (See text and references)	For travel (check with local health department)	See text. Check with local health department.	Immunization record	A

continued

Table 10.3. *(continued)*
Well Adult Male Screening Recommendations

S—Screening for Disease

Screen	When to Begin	Interval	Tools/Special Concerns	Level of Evidence for Effectiveness[a]
Weight	First visit (childhood)	Each visit	Compare to national norms	A
Blood pressure	First visit (childhood)	Every 1–2 years (or each visit; no optimum interval has been determined (at least every 2 years if ≥ 140/84); if on medication, screen two to three times a year.	Chart record, flow sheet. If family history, more frequently.	A
Cholesterol	Age 35–64; sooner if family history. Some advocate childhood plus young adult screening as well.	Perhaps every 5 years; more often if abnormal or history changes.	Laboratory flow sheet. Men with early MI in family history are at greater risk.	A
Colon cancer screening	US PSTF recommends fecal occult blood test (FOBT) and/or sigmoidoscopy. American Cancer Society recommends digital rectal examination (DRE) ≥ age 40, two tests (sigmoidoscopy & FOBT) ≥ age 50; US PSTF recommends sigmoidoscopy every 3–5 years, FOBT every year.	—	Family genogram	B
Fecal occult blood test (rehydrated)	≥ Age 50	Yearly	High false positive rate; better if patient follows diet guidelines for the testing	C
Digital rectal examination	≥ Age 40 (ACS) ≥ Age 50 (World Health Organization)	Yearly	Some task forces do not recommend, including US PSTF	C
Sigmoidoscopy (colonoscopy for high-risk populations, every 3–5 years)	≥ Age 50	Every 3–5 years	May be combined with barium enema	B

continued

Table 10.3. *(continued)*
Well Adult Male Screening Recommendations

S—Screening for Disease

Screen	When to Begin	Interval	Tools/Special Concerns	Level of Evidence for Effectiveness[a]
Prostate screening DRE	ACS ≥ age 40	Annually	—	B/C
PSA	ACS ≥ age 50	Annually	See text; not recommended, but controversial	C
Visual acuity/glaucoma screen	Childhood testing; then ≥ age 40 if HTN or DM; ≥ 65 otherwise.	Recommendations are unclear	Snellen's chart ≥ age 65	B/C
Dental screening	Childhood	Regular visits (not defined). Commonly recommended yearly.	Regular at-home care; flossing; fluoride if needed; intervals left to recommendation of the dental provider	A/B

E—Education

Screen	When to Begin	Interval	Tools/Special Concerns	Level of Evidence for Effectiveness[a]
Sexual activity, risk of STDs, HIV risk, pregnancy responsibility	At or before onset of sexual activity (teens)	Every periodic visit	Education flowsheet would be useful; computerized education form	B
Preconception counseling (planned pregnancy, responsibility, etc.)	Early adult/adolescence	Any contraceptive or preventive health visit	Periodically	B/C
Diet/nutrition	First visit	Discuss at each visit; review family history risk (DM, heart disease, etc.)	Iron, calcium; food pyramid; decrease fat intake, increase fiber	A
Exercise	Early; history at first visit	Periodically	Primary and secondary prevention	B
Injury prevention (e.g., seat belts, bicycle helmets, no drinking and driving)	Early (see risk factor identification in Tables 10.2 and 10.3 for age groups)	Each visit, particularly health maintenance visits	Review occupation risks, recreation risks, etc.	B
Skin examination and review use of sunscreen, clothing	By age 20–30, early if history of melanoma in family	At periodic examinations	Examination by clinician if history significant or self examination positive	A/B

continued

Table 10.3. *(continued)*
Well Adult Male Screening Recommendations

Screen	When to Begin	**E**—Education Interval	Tools/Special Concerns	Level of Evidence for Effectiveness[a]
Stressors, grief, depression, relaxation techniques	Early	Review every 2–4 years or at each visit	Genogram, periodic family circles, depression scale (Fig. 10.3), relaxation strategies, referrals for stress management	Unknown

Data are from US Preventive Services Task Force. Guide to Clinical Preventive Services. Report of the US Preventive Services Task Force, 2nd ed. Baltimore: Williams & Wilkins, 1996; American Academy of Family Physicians. Summary of Recommendations for Periodic Health Examination. http://www.aafp.org/members/pracguid/html. June, 1997; Mulrow CD, et al. Case-finding instruments for depression in primary care settings. Ann Intern Med 1995;122:913–921; Neufeld B. SAFE questions: Overcoming barriers to the detection of family violence. Am Fam Physician 1996;53:2575–2580; Dominitz, et al. Colorectal cancer: Latest approaches to prevention and screening. Patient Care 1996;3:124–145; American Heart Association. Patient Education: Diet History. 1986; Frame PS. A critical review of adult health maintenance. Part I: Prevention of atherosclerotic diseases. J Fam Pract 1986;22:341–346; Thompson DC, et al. Effectiveness of bicycle safety helmets in preventing head injuries. A case-control study. JAMA 1996;276:1968–1973; Schieber RA, Branche-Dorsey CM, Ryan GW, Rutherford GW Jr, Stevens JA, O'Neil J. Risk factors for injuries from in-line skating and the effectiveness of safety gear. N Engl Med 1996;335:1630–1635; Lui S, Siegel PZ, Brewer RD, Mokdad AH, Sleet DA, Serdula M. Prevalence of alcohol-impaired driving. Results from a national self-reported survey of health behaviors. JAMA 1997;277:122–125; Fleming MF, et al. Brief physician advice for problem alcohol drinkers. JAMA 1997;277:1039–1045.

[a]Level of evidence for effectiveness: A, strong or moderate research-based evidence (consistent across several studies, including at least two randomized controlled trials); B, limited research-based evidence (less consistent or extensive evidence, but preponderance of evidence supports use of treatment); C, common practice with little or no research-based evidence; X, moderate or strong evidence suggesting that this treatment is not effective.

every 2 years, but does not pay for routine checkups in healthy older adults. Preventive care can be expensive. Because many insurance plans do not cover preventive care, the patient is responsible for the cost. Needless to say, if one has limited resources, a flexible sigmoidoscopy may not be a high priority. One advantage of some prepaid (HMO, PPO-type) health insurance plans is that some preventive care is valued and the patient does not directly pay for these services. In fact, over time, such plans may benefit financially by preventing illness or reducing its severity.

Educating Patients

The last section of the RISE mnemonic is education of patients. This aspect of prevention uses risk factor identification to tailor educational messages about lifestyle changes. Both public and one-to-one programs have been shown to be effective (1). For example, recent reductions in coronary heart mortality have resulted from public education and individual counseling about diet and exercise, as well as from better control of hypertension (12). The value of an individual physician in guiding patients to make lifestyle changes is considerable. Recommendations should be individualized and include community resources such as a weight-loss group or a smoking cessation class.

Some students and practitioners develop a certain fatalism about patient education. This attitude results from seeing many patients who do not make lifestyle changes that would obviously benefit their health. When this occurs, remember that education is only one element needed to produce change. The crucial element is motivation, which comes largely from within the individual, the family, and the social support network. This means that the physician, while responsible for providing the best preventive and educational care possible, is only one factor in determining behavior change. From this perspective, it is often better to be content with partial results and to be encouraged by the patients who do follow your recommendations.

SPECIAL CONSIDERATIONS IN PREVENTION

Some topics deserve further mention in the area of adult preventive care, particularly the topics of aging and violence, especially family violence.

Each of these raises difficult issues for both the patient and the care provider.

Aging issues affect not only the patient, but also the persons closest to him or her. Many older adults are active and continue to work, travel, and maintain a home for the remainder of their lives, but for some, aging proves a challenge in day-to-day physical and cognitive activities. All older adults need routine care as shown in Tables 10.2 and 10.3. The American College of Physicians recommends screening each older adult for functioning in basic activities of daily living (ADLs) and mental status (13). The Mini-Mental Status Examination is a tool that is useful for cognitive screening (Fig. 10.4).

It is important to remember that older adults can also be affected by alcoholism, depression, drug abuse, and violence. These problems may not be evident unless the questions are asked. Loneliness and depression can manifest as a dementia-like illness.

Family violence is a difficult and often avoided issue. The victims are generally women and children, but men and the elderly are also at risk in some settings. Persons encountering violence rarely reveal this to the physician as their chief complaint. Often, they present symptoms of chronic pain, anxiety, insomnia, drug use, or depression (14, 15). The patient may not be willing bring up the subject, but may be relieved to be asked. The American College of Obstetrics and Gynecology (ACOG), American Medical Association (AMA), and American Academy of Family Physicians (AAFP) all have recently published statements stressing the importance of screening patients (women in particular) about violence (14, 15). A set of questions known as the SAFE screen has been advocated by some, even though its validity as a screen has not yet been proven (Table 10.4).

Another special consideration in adult well care is the use of a sexual history, as discussed earlier. The questions in Table 10.2, or another format, may help as a tool in becoming accustomed to seeking out this sensitive information as part of a comprehensive well adult periodic examination. If the questions are presented in a calm and matter-of-fact way, most persons will not be offended, and honest answers will be obtained. Part of the difficulty is overcoming one's own qualms about asking direct questions about sex and sexuality. Practicing these questions on yourself or others may help demystify the process.

Table 10.4.
SAFE Questions

Stress/safety
  What stress do you experience in your relationship?
  Do you feel safe in your relationship (marriage)?
  Should I be concerned for your safety?
Afraid/abused
  Are there situations in your relationships in which you have felt afraid?
  Has your partner ever threatened or abused you or your children?
  Have you been physically hurt or threatened by your partner?
  Has your partner ever forced you to have sexual intercourse that you did not want?
Friends/family
  If you have been hurt, are your friends or family aware of it?
  Do you think you could tell them if it did happen?
  Would they be able to give you support?
Emergency plan
  Do you have a safe place to go and the resources you (and your children) need in an emergency situation?
  If you are in danger now, would you like help locating a shelter?
  Would you like to talk with a social worker, a counselor, or me to develop an emergency plan?

Reprinted with permission from Neufield B. SAFE questions: overcoming barriers to the detection of domestic violence. Am Fam Physician 1996;53:2575–2580.

IMPLEMENTING PREVENTIVE CARE

Successful implementation requires using every teachable moment and maintaining documentation of preventive health areas as they are addressed. Acute visits offer a chance to review safety issues, to update immunization records, or to recommend future preventive screening, if warranted. Mammograms can be recommended, for example, during a routine follow-up visit for hypertension. Prevention is often forgotten while attending to other diagnoses, but if given the right emphasis, preventive care can be done even in an acute setting. For example, emergency rooms generally do an excellent job of updating tetanus immunizations. Along the same lines, each history and physical examination for hospital admission should include a section on health maintenance issues. Preventive care data must be updated by physicians during each visit, whether or not the stated purpose of the visit is preventive care; otherwise, most patients will not have these issues addressed.

CHALLENGES IN PROVIDING PREVENTIVE CARE

A significant challenge in preventive care involves motivating both patients and physicians. From a patient's point of view, there are several impediments to using preventive care. Preventive care may not be offered or available. Even if it is, patients may refuse it. They may not accept the risks associated with certain procedures. Often patients know of others who experienced adverse reactions to immunizations or other procedures, such as flexible sigmoidoscopy, rectal examination, and mammography.

What are the impediments to screening from a physician's perspective? Preventive care standards are constantly changing (1, 16, 17). Various organizations provide recommendations that frequently conflict with each other; for example, published recommendations regarding Papanicolaou (Pap) smears for a specific patient may range from every 6 months to every 5 years depending upon the authority. Furthermore, the "right" answer also depends on individual patient risk factors and personal preferences.

Some physicians feel that there are insufficient data to show that preventive care has a positive effect on morbidity or mortality or that it even saves money. For many practitioners, the problem is one of inertia. We all know that flossing our teeth daily is important and probably prevents periodontal disease, but how many of us do it? Preventive medical care is much the same: it is difficult to perform tasks when the benefits are not readily apparent.

As with most of medicine, preventive care cannot be learned from one article or one chart. It takes experience in providing preventive care to patients to learn that this approach is as important as much of modern "curative and high technology" medicine.

CASE STUDY 1

A 40-year-old white man comes to your office requesting a physical examination. The only remarkable item in his history is a myocardial infarction in his father at age 50.

QUESTION

1. How would you plan for this patient's preventive care?

DISCUSSION

Using the RISE format, you can focus on each element of preventive care for this man.

R: Risk factors need to be identified. Does he abuse tobacco, alcohol, or drugs? Is there a family history of cancer or a personal history of problems such as elevated cholesterol or blood pressure? Are there sexual or occupational risk factors?

I: Immunizations must be updated. When was his last diphtheria-tetanus vaccination? Is he in a special risk group that needs the hepatitis vaccine? Is he a health care provider or an asplenic who should have a flu shot?

S: He can then be screened by physical examination and laboratory tests, as indicated in Table 10.3 and by your assessment of risk factors.

E: A large part of this patient's encounter will focus on education, centered on his risk factors and what he can do to minimize them. The family history of early coronary artery disease is an indication and likely a motivator for learning about diet, exercise, and weight control (see Table 10.3) (12).

Obviously this may be too much to discuss effectively in a routine 15-minute office visit. In a family practice setting, these issues and others are usually covered over several visits, often over many years. Scheduling a visit to interpret laboratory data presents another opportunity to discuss preventive health issues.

CASE STUDY 2

A 67-year-old African-American woman comes to your office complaining of shoulder pain. A focused history and physical examination reveals fibromyositis with one tender trigger point, which you inject with local anesthetic to relieve pain and spasm.

QUESTION

1. How would you address prevention in this acute visit?

DISCUSSION

As a physician, you have two choices with this patient. You can treat the acute problem and spend 5 minutes discussing preventive health, or you can recommend a return visit for preventive care. By managing an acute problem, the physician gains trust and can proceed with caring for the total person. At the same time, you can raise some important issues and follow them up when the patient returns to reassess her shoulder problem. Discussing immunizations and cancer screening at the first visit can help prepare the patient for these interventions during the next visit.

REFERENCES

1. US Preventive Services Task Force. Guide to Clinical Preventive Services. Report of the US Preventive Services Task Force, 2nd ed. Baltimore: Williams & Wilkins, 1996.
2. Centers for Disease Control. HIV is now the leading cause of death among young US men. MMWR 1993; 42:869–872.
3. Centers for Disease Control. Mortality patterns—United States, 1993. MMWR 1996;45:161–163.
4. National Center for Health Statistics. Home page. http://www.cdc.gov. July, 1997.

5. D'Augelli AR. Preventing mental health problems among lesbian and gay college students. J Primary Prevention 1993;13:245–261.

6. Mulrow CD, Williams JW Jr, Gerety MB, Ramirez G, Montiel OM, Kerber C. Case-finding instruments for depression in primary care settings. Ann Intern Med 1995;122:913–921.

7. Potter J, Stott DJ, Roberts MA, Elder AG, O'Donnell B, Knight PV, Carman WF. Influenza vaccination of health care workers in long-term-care hospitals reduces the mortality of elderly patients. J Infect Dis 1997;175:1–6.

8. Mustin HD. Pneumococcal vaccine: a preventive care winner. J Am Board Fam Pract 1996;9:461–462.

9. Centers for Disease Control and Prevention. Health Information for International Travel, 1996–97. Atlanta, GA: Department of Health and Human Services, 1997.

10. Dominitz JA, McCormick LH, Rex DK. Colorectal cancer: latest approaches to prevention and screening. Patient Care April 15, 1996;124–145.

11. Lewis SF, Jensen NM. Screening sigmoidoscopy: factors associated with utilization. J Gen Intern Med 1996;11:542–544.

12. Frame PS. A critical review of adult health maintenance. Part I: prevention of atherosclerotic diseases. J Fam Pract 1986;22:341–346.

13. US Public Health Services. Cognitive and functional impairment. Am Fam Physician 1995;51:633–636.

14. Family violence: an AAFP white paper. Am Fam Physician 1995;50:1636–1640, 1644–1646.

15. Neufield B. SAFE questions: Overcoming barriers to the detection of domestic violence. Am Fam Physician 1996;53:2575–2580.

16. American Academy of Family Physicians. HELP: Health education lifetime plan. http://www.aafp.org/members/patient/pol-care.html. June, 1997.

17. American Academy of Family Physicians. Summary of recommendations for periodic health examination. http://www.aafp.org/members/pracguid/html. June, 1997.

11. Promoting Health for Women at Menopause

PATRICIA ANN PAYNE AND PETER CURTIS

Key Clinical Questions

1. What issues should be discussed when a 45-year-old woman comes in for an office visit complaining of hot flashes and irregular menses?
2. What is known about the benefits and drawbacks of hormone replacement therapy (HRT)?

INTRODUCTION

Menopause is a normal event in women's lives. Unfortunately, many women learn to dread menopause rather than look forward to it. Menopause marks the end of reproductive capability; however, the perimenopausal process begins long before the diagnosis is made. The average age of menopause for women in the United States is 51 years, which means that women can expect to spend one third of their lives after menopause. As women approach menopause and seek care, the family physician has an opportunity to provide anticipatory guidance and care that can affect the severity of heart disease and osteoporosis that may occur in later years.

NATURAL HISTORY OF MENOPAUSE

Menopause is a retrospective diagnosis defined by amenorrhea for 1 year or amenorrhea of short duration, with an elevated serum level of follicle stimulating hormone (FSH). Women who smoke or who have had chemotherapy are likely to experience an earlier menopause. There is also a familial tendency toward similarity in age of onset of the menopause. The decline in estrogen production that occurs in natural menopause may be rapid, but it more commonly progresses over several years. The change in hormonal levels is more dramatic for women undergoing oophorectomy, particularly those at a young age.

The ovary produces most of the body's circulating estrogen, which consists of three types: estriol, estradiol, and estrone. Estrogen decreases by 60% after menopause with the major reduction in estradiol, whereas the proportion of estrone, which is primarily metabolized in fat cells, increases. This is why obese women tend to have fewer symptoms of menopause. Women experiencing natural menopause may notice short, more irregular periods before stopping menstruation completely. Once the ovaries have ceased producing sufficient amounts of estrogen to trigger the normal rise and fall of reproductive hormones, the anterior pituitary acts more intensively to maintain hormone production, causing a rise in FSH greater than 40 mIU/mL. Accurate levels of FSH to check on menopausal status can be obtained at any time in women who are not taking some form of estrogen (e.g., oral contraceptives). Women using oral contraceptives should have their FSH level drawn during the week they are off hormone therapy.

Besides the menopause, there are other changes that affect women in the middle years. These include personal issues of sexuality and aging, the "empty nest" response generated by children becoming fledgling adults, aging parents who may be ill or disabled, and health problems of friends and spouses. These developmental life changes can provoke symptoms similar to those of menopause or aggravate ones that already exist. For example, a woman who is having menstrual changes and at the same time is caring for a dying parent may have symptoms of depression and menopause simultaneously. On the other hand, there are many women who find "menopausal zest." Their children are out of the home, financial security may be reached, and there no longer is a fear of pregnancy.

CLINICAL EVALUATION

History

The symptoms of menopause are due to declining levels of estrogen, progesterone, and androgens (Table 11.1). These symptoms can start 8 to 10

Table 11.1.
Symptoms of Perimenopause/Menopause

Vasomotor symptoms	Hot flash/flushes
Activity levels	Insomnia, fatigue
Menstrual changes	Irregularity, menorrhagia
Urogenital symptoms	Enlarged fibroids
	Vaginal dryness/itching/discharge
	Urinary urgency, frequency, dysuria, or stress incontinence
	Dyspareunia
Changes in affect	Nervousness, irritability
	Depression
	Emotional lability
Other physical symptoms described by women	Headaches
	Breast tenderness
	Musculoskeletal aching/joint pain
	Constipation
	Weight gain
Sexuality	Increased/decreased libido
	Dyspareunia

years prior to the physiologic state of menopause. This means that women in their forties may begin to notice subtle changes in their menstrual cycles as well as a variety of symptoms. The most common symptom of estrogen decline is hot flashes (reported by 60 to 80% of women), which often cause women to seek medical advice. Hot flashes occur most commonly during the first 2 years after other symptoms begin, but may continue for up to several years after menopause. Estrogen affects the thermoregulatory part of the brain so that women become highly sensitive to temperature changes. They may experience mild symptoms or have up to 20 to 30 hot flashes per day. Hot flashes can be triggered by a variety of factors such as alcohol, caffeine, or stress.

Women experience wide variations in symptoms during perimenopause/menopause, and factors such as culture, race, and socioeconomic status can influence the significance and perception of symptoms (Table 11.2). Although a majority of women experience symptoms, less than a third find them problematic (1). Hot flashes do not last forever.

The patient-centered medical history can be divided into three areas: menstrual, urogenital, and general symptoms. Key items include:

- Menstrual history—LMP, LNMP (last normal menstrual period), length of cycles, regularity of cycles, amount of bleeding, associated symptoms such as dysmenorrhea, premenstrual symptoms, breast tenderness, break-

through bleeding or spotting, and contraception (past and current)

- Urogenital—change in sexual activity/libido, dyspareunia, urinary frequency/incontinence, cystitis, vaginitis

- General—hot flashes: frequency, timing, triggering stimuli, successful relief measures; mood; weight and appetite; sleep patterns; skin and hair texture; changes in bowels, bloating, gas

- Health maintenance issues—exercise, appetite, sleep, recreation, alcohol, smoking, drug habits, diet and vitamin supplements, Papanicolaou (Pap) smear and mammogram, social support

- Relevant family history—familial history of menopause and current health status of family members, risk factors for osteoporosis, heart disease, cancer, and diabetes

Physical Examination

The physical examination focuses on evaluation of general appearance and breast and pelvic examinations.

- General appearance—evidence of dry skin or fatigue; condition of hair and nails; affect, redistribution of fat

- Height and spine—change in height; kyphosis or cervical hump

Table 11.2.

Menopausal Women's Experience of Symptoms over 6 Months

Symptoms	% Experiencing Symptom (n = 6084)	% Experiencing as Problem (n = 6084)
Classic		
Hot flashes	57	22
Night sweats	55	24
Sleep problems	66	33
Dry/sore vagina	34	14
Somatic		
Aching/painful joints	67	29
Headaches	60	23
Sore breasts	51	14
Nocturia	48	16
Palpitations	37	13
Dizziness	35	11
Psychologic		
Irritability	72	25
Concentration/memory problems	64	30
Anxiety	58	26
Depression	51	22
Feeling unable to cope	43	19

Modified from Porter M, Penny GC, Russell D. A population-based survey of women's experience of the menopause. Br J Obstet Gynaecol 1996;103:1025–1028.

- Breast tenderness—check lymph nodes and thyroid

- Pelvic examination—genitalia, urethra, vagina, (atrophy, discharge), cervix (friability, discharge)

- Uterus—size, mobility; adnexa (should not be palpable in postmenopausal women)

Differential Diagnosis

The clinician should minimize the use of costly and unnecessary tests by following an algorithm for making the diagnosis of menopause (Fig. 11.1). An FSH over 40 mIU/mL confirms the diagnosis. Patients with borderline results, or those who may still have significant endogenous estrogen production, should be retested within 3 to 6 months. A thyroid-stimulating hormone and complete blood count are useful in all patients since hypothyroidism and anemia commonly develop at this age and can coexist with menopausal symptoms (see Fig. 11.1).

THERAPEUTIC CONSIDERATIONS

There are two clinical objectives in treating women at menopause:

- Improve their quality of life by relieving perimenopausal/menopausal symptoms

- Prevent morbidity and prolong life for women at risk for heart disease and osteoporosis

Therapies for menopause include hormonal and complementary therapies.

Hormonal Therapy

The Report of the U.S. Preventive Services Task Force recommends that all perimenopausal and postmenopausal women receive counseling regarding the use of hormone replacement therapy (HRT), including risks and potential preventive benefits (2). Patients should receive adequate information in order to make an informed decision about the use of hormonal therapy including the contraindications, risks, benefits, and adverse effects of each hormone. The majority of women who initiate HRT do so in an effort to decrease symptoms of menopause. They may not be receptive to a lengthy discussion of the long-term risks and benefits of HRT until these symptoms are addressed. In spite of the publicity surrounding estrogen use, more than half of the eligible women in the United States have not taken HRT, and of those who have, many discontinue

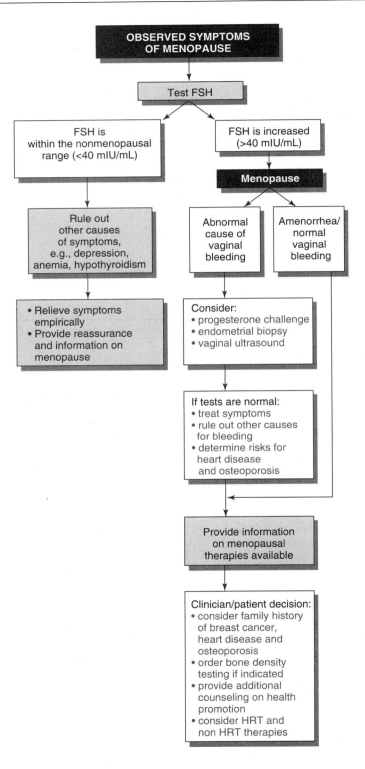

Figure 11.1. *Algorithm for evaluating and managing menopause.*

therapy during the first year. The most common reasons for stopping therapy are fears about potential or real adverse effects. However, many women never start therapy because their primary provider has not discussed the risks, benefits, and multiple options for therapy (3).

There is general agreement among health professionals that estrogen has a positive effect on the prevention of heart disease and osteoporosis, particularly in those women with risk factors; however, the limits of this effect will not be known until the large clinical trials, such as the Women's Health Initiative, are completed (4). An example of the relative risks of selected diseases with long-term HRT is shown in Table 11.3.

Estrogen Replacement Therapy

Estrogen replacement therapy (ERT) is provided through several delivery systems and preparations (Table 11.4). The decision to use a particular formulation is dependent on the severity of symptoms, age, and other medical concerns. Dosages may need to be adjusted as women age, in order to maximize the physiologic effect and minimize adverse effects. In general, younger women or women who experience menopause from premature ovarian failure or oophorectomy require higher doses of estrogen to compensate for the rapid decline in estrogen levels. Premarin, or equine estrogen, is the most commonly prescribed hormone in the United States, and most of the research has used this product.

There are some women who refuse therapy because they object to the conditions under which the product is obtained from horses. Alternative preparations that contain varying ratios of estra-diol, estrone, and estriol exist. A "natural" form of estrogen that contains a higher percentage of estriol compared to estrone or estradiol also is available from compounding pharmacists. Most women who are prescribed ERT have had hysterectomies and take estrogen daily since there is no need to cycle them with progesterone to protect the uterus from cancer.

Hormone Replacement Therapy

Hormone replacement therapy (HRT) involves taking estrogen with progesterone and/or androgens (see Table 11.4). Progesterone will block estrogenic effects on the endometrium and lessen the added risk of endometrial cancer to almost zero. There are several progestogens available. However, medroxyprogesterone is the most common product used in the United States. Oral hormones can be given cyclically or continuously. Cyclic therapy includes several options. These are:

- Take an estrogen pill on days 1 to 25 and add a progestin from days 14 to 25, then stop both medications for days 25 to 30.
- Take estrogen daily with progestin 10 to 14 days out of each month.
- Take estrogen and progesterone for 5 days of each week and skip them both for 2 days.
- Take estrogen and progesterone daily for 3 months, then stop both for 2 weeks.
- Take a low-dose progestin pill (2.5 mg) with each estrogen pill on a continuous basis.

Bleeding should occur after the progesterone is finished—i.e., on or after day 10 of progesterone therapy. For continuous estrogen/progesterone

Table 11.3.
Relative Risk of Selected Disease for a 50-Year-Old White Woman Treated with Long-Term HRT

Disease	Relative Risk[a] Estrogen Therapy	Nonuser	Relative Risk[a] Estrogen plus Progestin	Nonuser
Coronary heart disease	0.65	1.0	0.65–0.80	1.0
Stroke	0.96	1.0	0.96	1.0
Hip fracture	0.75	1.0	0.75	1.0
Breast cancer	1.25	1.0	1.25–2.00	1.0
Endometrial cancer	8.22	1.0	1.00	1.0

Modified from Grady D, Rubin SM, Petitti DB, et al. Hormone replacement therapy to prevent disease and prolong life. Ann Intern Med 1992;117(12):1016–1037.

[a]"Best" estimates of the relative risk for developing each disease in long-term hormone users compared with nonusers.

Table 11.4.
Common Formulations for Estrogen and Hormone Replacement Therapy

Hormone	Brand Name/Type	Dosage
Estrogens	Conjugate equine estrogen • Brand name: Premarin	33% equine estrogen/60% estrone sulfate Oral Premarin: 0.3 mg, 0.625 mg, 0.9 mg, 1.25 mg, 2.5 mg Vaginal cream: (2–4 g/day to start, 1 g one to three times weekly for maintenance)
	Esterified estrogens • Brand name: Estratab	85% equine estrogens/15% estrone sulfate Oral: 0.3 mg, 0.625 mg, 1.25 mg, 2.5 mg
	Estropipate • Brand name: Ogen	Estrone sulfate with piperazine from pregnant mare urine Oral: 0.625 mg, 1.25 mg, 2.5 mg, 5.0 mg Vaginal: use as vaginal cream above

	Estradiol
	• Brand names: Estrace,
	   Estraderm, Climara,
	   Vivelle
		Micronized E2
		Oral: 1 mg, 2 mg
		Vaginal: 0.1 mg/g (use daily 5–10 days, then
		   every 2–3 days)
		Transdermal patch: 0.05 mg or 0.1 mg; Climara one time
		   weekly, or Estraderm two times weekly

Progestogens	Medroxyprogesterone acetate • Brand names: Provera, Amen, Cycrin	10 mg/day for last 12–14 days of estrogen Oral: 2.5–5 mg daily with estrogen for continuous therapy

	Norethindrone acetate
	• Brand name: Aygestin
		Natural progesterone: produced from the wild
		   yam, chemically identical to human progesterone
		Micronized progesterone:
		   Oral: 100–400 mg
		   Vaginal suppository: 200 mg

Testosterone		Oral: 2.5–10 mg/day
		Testosterone cream 1–2%: apply sparingly to the clitoris
		   and the inner labia (small pea-sized dab of cream, use daily
		   for 1 week and then two to three times a week as
		   needed); must be made to order by pharmacist

Estrogen and
   testosterone
	Esterified estrogens (ee) and
	   methyltestosterone (mt)
	• Brand name: Estratest,
	   Estratest HS
		Oral: 1.25 mg (ee) and 1.25 mg (mt)
		
		Oral: 1.25 mg (ee) and 1.25 mg (mt) (3 weeks on, 1 week off)

therapy for 25 days, bleeding should occur after day 25. For women who take continuous estrogen and progesterone 365 days a year, breakthrough bleeding is common during the first 6 months of therapy, but amenorrhea will occur in about 40% of women within the first 3 months of therapy (5). Once amenorrhea has occurred, any subsequent irregular bleeding should be evaluated to exclude cancer.

Specific Health Considerations

Heart Disease

Estrogen has a direct effect in reducing risk factors for cardiovascular disease by increasing high-density lipoprotein and reducing low-density lipoprotein, as well as promoting degradation of lipids in the liver and peripheral blood flow. If a 50-year-old white woman takes long-term HRT, she still has a 46% lifetime probability of developing coronary heart disease and a 31% probability of dying of heart disease, but with an average life expectancy increase of 1.6 years (6). A maximal benefit for cardiovascular disease is achieved with conjugated estrogen (0.625 mg) and micronized progesterone as compared with other forms of progesterone (7).

Osteoporosis

Approximately one-third of all women in their seventies develop osteoporosis as a result of a variety of factors (Table 11.5). Long-term estrogen re-

Table 11.5.
Risk Factors for Osteoporosis

Family history of osteoporosis or early menopause

Ancestors from the British Isles, northern Europe, China, or Japan

Fair skin, small bone structure

Menstrual dysfunction
- Late menarche/early menopause
- Amenorrhea (exercise, eating disorder, breast-feeding)
- Oophorectomy or early menopause

Gastric surgery

Chronic health problems
- Chronic liver disease
- Chronic liver failure
- Endocrinopathies (i.e., diabetes, hyperthyroidism)
- Malabsorption syndromes
- Rheumatoid arthritis

Medications
- Anticonvulsants
- Antacids containing aluminum
- Thyroxine formulations
- Cholestyramine (lowers cholesterol)
- Heparin
- Methotrexate
- Steroids

Stress, smoking, excessive amount of alcohol, sedentary lifestyle

Diet high in caffeine, phosphorus, or protein, low in calcium

---

Table 11.6.
Preventive Therapy for Osteoporosis

Exercise
- Rationale: Exercise of the long bones results in increased calcium deposition.

Vitamin D
- Rationale: It is a key factor in calcium absorption.
- Common sources are sunlight, milk products, eggs, fish, and beef. Current RDA is 200 IU/day; up to 800 IU/day may be required for older women; amounts > than 1,000 IU/day can be toxic.

Phamacotherapy
A. Antiresorptive therapy sources
   1. Calcium supplementation (1500 mg of elemental calcium) with vitamin D
   2. Diuretics
   3. Vitamin D
   4. Hormone therapy (HRT/ERT, testosterone) promotes bone anabolism
   5. Estrogen agonists (tamoxifen, droloxifene)
   6. Oral contraceptives
   7. Calcitonin (Calcimar, Miacalcin) injections or nasal spray: positive analgesic effects for advanced osteoporosis and fractures[a]
   8. Biphosphonates: Alendronate (Fosamax) interferes with breakdown by osteoclasts; gastrointestinal (GI) symptoms: use with caution for women with low serum calcium, renal disease, or upper GI disorders. Etidronate cannot be given continuously owing to inhibition of bone mineralization, GI symptoms.
B. Bone production stimulation
   1. Sodium fluoride: should be taken with calcium citrate
   2. Androgens
      - Nandrolone
      - Stanozolol

---

[a]Sewell KL. Calcitonin. J Clin Rheumatol 1997;3:540–545.

placement therapy (ERT) can reduce the risk of osteoporotic hip fractures by 60%. Unfortunately, compliance rates with long-term therapy are uniformly low (around 10%) (8). Estrogen started later in the postmenopausal phase will reduce the rate of bone loss but does not restore previously lost bone mass. Osteoporosis can recur after ERT has been stopped because the benefits of hormone therapy for bone protection are lost after 7 years from the time it is stopped. This means that women at high risk for osteoporosis should take hormones at the menopause and continue for the rest of their lives (9). Some clinicians recommend that women begin ERT in their seventies if they are at high risk for osteoporosis and were not previously offered ERT (10). There are other approaches to preventing and treating osteoporosis should a woman not be able to take ERT (Table 11.6).

Cancer

Most women are particularly concerned about the risk of breast cancer associated with HRT.

There is no doubt that unopposed estrogen therapy increases risk of uterine cancer. What remains less clear is the degree of risk of breast cancer and, more importantly, how to weigh the increased risk with potential benefits of ERT. Retrospective studies suggest that women who have taken ERT for 20 years have a 30 to 40% increase in the risk of breast cancer when compared with women who never used ERT (6). The Nurses Health Study showed a relative risk of 1.4 to 1.7. In contrast, Stanford et al. described no increased risk (11, 12). These data are confounded by the aging process in which the incidence of breast cancer increases steadily and the limitations of retrospective studies prevent clinicians from providing clear data on this subject. It will be several years before information from the large Women's Health Initiative project will provide prospective data on women randomized to hormone or nonhormone therapy (4). The majority opinion in the United States is that the benefits of HRT therapy considerably outweigh the risks, and that HRT can play a major role in preventing heart disease and osteoporosis (13).

The question of hormone therapy for breast cancer survivors is controversial. A major concern is that a second breast cancer will arise from activation of dormant tumor cells by estrogen. There is, however, no clear evidence to suggest that this is more likely (14). Quality-of-life issues are important to this population of women and should be given careful consideration before excluding them from HRT.

In addition to the more researched issues above, recent observational studies have suggested that a decreased risk of Alzheimer's disease and colorectal cancer is associated with hormonal therapy combined with vitamin E and aspirin.

COMPLEMENTARY THERAPIES FOR SYMPTOMS OF MENOPAUSE

There are several alternative approaches to managing the common discomforts of menopause. These include behavioral changes, pharmacotherapy, acupuncture, herbal medicines, vitamins, and other pharmacologic agents (Table 11.7). Although the National Institutes of Health (NIH) is supporting studies of the effectiveness of alternative therapies, there is little evidence available at this time to support their use other than observational studies and personal anecdotes. Some herbal preparations have been used to treat menopausal symptoms for hundreds of years; however, there currently are no pharmacologic standards for herbal preparations, and it is impossible to guarantee bioavailability, purity, or side effects related to the estrogenic qualities of these preparations.

Diet therapy is an area of great interest. There is preliminary evidence suggesting that phytoestrogens (foods with estrogenic qualities) can modify the severity of menopausal symptoms (15). The Japanese consume large quantities of soy in their diet and coincidentally have very low rates of breast cancer, and, in fact, have no word for the term hot flash in their language. Soy beans contain chemicals known as isoflavones, which are plant forms of estrogen. Preliminary randomized studies of menopausal symptoms have shown a positive effect for women receiving a soy protein supplement versus those who did not. This may be one alternative therapy that women can use with little concern for adverse effects. Phytoestrogens are far less potent than estrogens. Soy is more potent than other phytoestrogens such as vegetables, but the use of either would be beneficial as an alternative to red meats or high-fat foods.

There is no debate about the benefit of lifestyle changes for women of all ages. All women, regardless of their use of ERT/HRT, should be given information about exercise, diet, alcohol and caffeine intake, and calcium/vitamin D requirements. Many of these topics can be discussed well before menopause, thus contributing to risk reduction prior to menopause.

When taking vitamins, patients should be instructed to start out slowly and avoid excessive amounts of A, D, and E, which are fat soluble and can build up to toxic levels in the body. Herbs and herbal preparations with estrogenic qualities should be used with caution in women who have a history of breast cancer or have been advised not to take estrogen.

SPECIAL CONSIDERATIONS

Although the rate of fertility declines with age, women who have not experienced menopause should be offered counseling on the use of contraception if they are sexually active and do not want to become pregnant. Age is no longer a contraindication to oral contraceptives with the exception of women over 35 who smoke. Oral contraceptives are often used for women with metromenorrhagia in order to suppress their bleeding. Other options include those available for women of all ages, including the IUD, progesterone-only contraception, and barrier methods (see Chapter 7, Pregnancy Prevention and Contraception).

ANTICIPATORY GUIDANCE AND PATIENT EDUCATION

Many women read magazines and books and talk to friends for information about menopause. It is a challenge to clinicians to discuss this topic adequately during brief office visits. Preprinted questionnaires may assist clinicians in reviewing symptoms and concerns in a more efficient manner. Patients may need to come in several times in order to address symptoms, HRT, and personal issues related to menopause. This can also be a challenging subject for patients and

Table 11. 7.
Summary of Traditional, Alternative, and Behavioral Approaches for Symptoms of Menopause

Symptoms	Behavioral Change	Alternative Therapies	Medications
Hot flash/flush	• Keep a diary to determine what specific activities cause hot flashes • Wear layered clothing; avoid activities associated with hot flashes: vigorous exercise on hot days, ingesting spicy foods, caffeine, hot beverages, alcohol. • Practice low, deep breathing • At night, wear cotton clothing and sleep on cotton sheets; keep room cool; keep a thermos of water by the bed; splash cool water on your face, drink ice water, or take a cool shower if warm	• Vitamin E: 100–600 IU (international units) daily (do not take more than 100 IU if you have high blood pressure, diabetes, or rheumatic heart disease). Start with 100 IU and increase over 6–8 weeks to 600 IU maximum, or less if symptoms have improved. • Diet sources: Wheat germ, whole grains, vegetable oils, soybeans, peanuts, spinach, cold-pressed oils, dark green leafy vegetables. • Bioflavonoids (500 mg to 1 g) combined with vitamin C • Ginseng tea—take on an empty stomach before or between meals (don't take with vitamin C; it has a component closely resembling digitoxin; avoid if you have diabetes or cardiac problems; watch in combination with other drugs; may also be associated with postmenopausal bleeding) • Herbs: Bee pollen, Don Quai, Cohosh, vitamin B complex (one/two daily; dietary sources include whole grains, wheat germ; yogurt, brewer's yeast, milk)	• ERT/HRT • Belladonna (inhibits parasympathetic nervous system); adverse effects include dry mouth, dilated pupils, constipation, rapid pulse • Clonidine (Catapres) inhibits release of norepinephrine in brain; adverse effects: sleepiness, dry mouth, decreased blood pressure • Megace (megestrol acetate) used in women with breast cancer • Methyldopa 500–1000 mg/day; may affect adrenoreceptors • Propranolol • Veralipride 100 mg/day, dopamine antagonist active in the hypothalamus
Insomnia	• Take steps to avoid hot flashes while sleeping • Avoid caffeine, alcohol, tobacco, and liquids in the evening • Exercise regularly during the day • Develop a bedtime routine —Identify a regular bedtime —Drink warm milk —Take a hot bath —Use your bed only for sleeping or sex —If you can't sleep, get up and do something until you feel tired —Avoid naps during the day	• Herbs: Valerian (strong sedative)/chamomile tea (weak sedative effect, avoid if allergic to ragweed/ chrysanthemums) • Peppermint, catnip, hops, passion flower, lavender oil on pillow • Warm milk before bed (tryptophan) • Natural diuretics	• ERT/HRT • Progesterone can have a sedative effect; take in PM to help sleep

continued

Table 11. 7. *(continued)*
Summary of Traditional, Alternative, and Behavioral Approaches for Symptoms of Menopause

Symptoms	Behavioral Change	Alternative Therapies	Medications
Headaches (usually decrease with menopause)	• May occur on days that estrogen is not taken; some women find that estrogen increases headaches • Avoid stress and get adequate rest	• Herbs: Chasteberry, peppermint oil, feverfew, royal jelly products	• Diuretics may be used when estrogen is not taken • Androgen therapy or continuous estrogen therapy may improve symptoms
Urogenital symptoms	• Drink lots of water and empty your bladder frequently and after intercourse • Practice Kegel exercises daily • Continue sexual activity to maintain elasticity of vagina • For vaginal dryness, use water-soluble lubricant (not petroleum jelly) or vegetable oil, or use saliva for added lubrication (commercial lubricants include Replens, Astroglide, KY Jelly)	• For vaginal dryness/itch: vitamin E 400–600 IU/day or vitamin E oil on skin • Herbs: Evening primrose oil, Aloe Vera/ slippery elm paste • Dip pads in witch hazel and glycerin for itching	• ERT/HRT vaginal cream
Nervousness, irritability	• Relaxation/deep breathing exercises	• Yoga • Vitamin B_6 5–25 mg daily • Diet sources: brewer's yeast, bran, wheat germ, organ meats, molasses, walnuts, peanuts, brown rice	

providers, as matters of sexuality, relationships, and physical complaints may not be recognized as symptoms of the perimenopausal period. Partners should be included in discussions whenever possible. Many practices identify a nurse who provides support for postmenopausal women by answering questions and running an ongoing support group.

There are many good books written about the menopause. Some are related to a positive attitude in midlife such as Gail Sheehy's book, *Silent Passages;* others, such as *Menopause Naturally* by Sadja Greenwood, MD, a family physician, provide objective information about pharmacotherapy and nonpharmacotherapy options. It is important that women be provided with objective educational materials and not those written by a pharmaceutical company attempting to advertise their hormonal preparation between the lines. The decision to initiate HRT/ERT requires information and understanding of the risks and benefits for each individual. There are several formats for presentation of this information, such as pamphlets from the North American Menopause Society, the American College of Obstetricians/Gynecologists, or the American Academy of Family Physicians; an informed-decision video; or a computer program used to calculate the specific risk for individuals based on identified variables (Table 11.8).

Table 11.8.
Resources/Patient Education Materials

- *Hormone Replacement Therapy, A Shared Decision-making Program Videotape.* Foundation for Informed Medical Decision Making. Hanover, NH, 1995. Excellent discussion of relative risks of ERT/HRT based on individual's health status. Based on meta-analysis by Deborah Grady and colleagues.
- *Menopause Naturally* by Sadja Greenwood, MD. Volcano Press, Volcano, CA, 1996. Easy reading with options for hormonal and nonhormonal therapies objectively presented.
- *Menopause Self-Help Book* by Dr. Susan Lark. Westchester Publishing Co, Los Altos, CA, 1993. Heavy emphasis on diet, exercise, herbal, and nontraditional therapies for menopausal symptoms.
- Mid-life Women's Network, 5129 Logan Ave. South, Minneapolis, MN 55419–1019. Monthly newsletter that objectively explores one topic related to women's midlife concerns per issue.
- LISTSERV@PSHUHMC.HMC.PSU.EDU. Write in the body of the message: SUB MENOPAUS, your first name; your last name.

The topic of menopause is best initiated as part of a routine visit for all women over 40. This allows the physician the opportunity to find out if there are familial trends for early or late menopause, present the option of HRT, distribute educational materials, and provide anticipatory guidance about concerns women face during this midlife transition.

CASE STUDY

Mrs. R.A. comes in for a routine physical examination. She is 44 years old, married, and works full-time as a secretary. Her periods are regular but have changed during the last year. They are now 25 days apart and quite heavy with clots and cramping. She reports that she is not sleeping well, finds herself irritable, and is concerned that she has no interest in sex. She believes her change in behavior is causing difficulty in her marriage. Her 17-year old daughter is having academic problems at school and her 70-year old mother was recently institutionalized for Alzheimer's Disease. She is tired all the time and wonders if something is wrong with her.

QUESTIONS

1. Is this patient going through menopause?
2. What laboratory tests would you order?
3. How would you counsel this patient?

DISCUSSION

Many women experience symptoms several years prior to menopause. Heavy bleeding in this age group is commonly caused by hormonal changes or fibroids. Fibroids may be felt on examination, causing the uterus to be irregular/globular in shape. It is important to rule out a tumor if an irregularly shaped uterus is noted on examination. It is common for women to be fatigued if they have heavy periods and anemia. Laboratory testing with a CBC, FSH, or TSH can evaluate possible anemia, menopause vs. perimenopause, and/or thyroid dysfunction as a cause of fatigue. An in-depth discussion of family issues may reveal an underlying depression as a cause or exacerbating factor in her symptoms. Evaluation of menopause should also include patient education about the physiology of reproductive decline, options for therapy including HRT/ERT, complementary therapies, and health promotion. Some women prefer a pharmacotherapy, which might include oral contraceptives for perimenopausal symptoms, rather than a nonpharmacologic approach, which might include diet, exercise, stress reduction, and adequate rest.

REFERENCES

1. Porter M, Penny GC, Russell D. A population-based survey of women's experience of the menopause. Br J Obstet Gynaecol 1996;103:1025–1028.
2. US Preventive Services Task Force. Guide to Clinical Preventive Services. A Report of the US Preventive Services Task Force, 2nd ed. Baltimore: Williams & Wilkins, 1996.
3. Mayeaux EJ, Johnson C. Current concepts in postmenopausal hormone replacement therapy. J Fam Pract 1996;43:69–75.
4. Prentice RL, Rosou WJE, Johnson R, et al. The role of randomized controlled trials in assessing the benefits and risks of long-term hormone replacement therapy: example of the Women's Health Initiative. Menopause 1996:3(2):71–76.
5. Rosenfeld J. Update on continuous estrogen-progestin replacement therapy. Am Fam Phys 1994;50:1519–1523.
6. Grady D, Rubin SM, Petitti DB, et al. Hormone replacement therapy to prevent disease and prolong life. Ann Intern Med 1992;117(12):1016–1037.
7. Writing Group for the PEPI Trial. Effects of estrogen or estrogen/progestin regimens on heart disease risk prevention in postmenopausal women. The Postmenopausal Estrogen/Progestin Interventions (PEPI) Trial. JAMA 1995;273(3):199–208.
8. Battistini M. Estrogen and the prevention of osteoporosis. J Clin Rheumatol 1997;3:528–533.
9. Cauley JA, Seeley DG, Ensrud D, et al. Estrogen replacement therapy and fractures in older women. Ann Intern Med 1995;122(1):9–16.
10. Kiel DP, et al. Hip fractures and the use of estrogens in postmenopausal women: the Framingham study. N Engl J Med 1987;817:1169–1174.
11. Colditz GA, Hankinson SE, Hunter DJ, et al. The use of estrogens and progestins and the risk of breast cancer in postmenopausal women. N Engl J Med 1995;332:1589–1593.
12. Stanford JL, Weiss NC, Voight LF, et al. Combined estrogen and progestin hormone replacement therapy in relation to risk of breast cancer in middle age women. JAMA 1995;274:137–142.
13. Colditz GA. Hormone replacement therapy—the benefits of hormone replacement therapy do not outweigh the increased risk of breast cancer. J NIH Res 1996;8:41–44.
14. Smith HO, Kammerer-Doak DN, Barbo DM, et al. Hormone replacement therapy in the menopause: a pro opinion. CA Cancer J Clin 1996;46(6):343–363.
15. Murkies AL, Lombard C, Strauss BJ, et al. Dietary flour supplementation decreases postmenopausal hot flushes: effect of soy and wheat. Maturitas 1995;21:189–195.

12. Complementary Therapies in Family Medicine

SUSAN GAYLORD

Key Clinical Questions

1. What is the role of complementary medicine in primary care?
2. What are the most frequently used therapies?
3. What are the theoretical or scientific bases for these therapies?

BACKGROUND

Complementary medicine, also called unconventional, alternative, or holistic medicine, has been defined as "those medical interventions not taught widely at U.S. medical schools or generally available at U.S. hospitals" (1). They include such practices as acupuncture, homeopathy, chiropractic, herbal medicine, energy healing, and mind-body therapies. Although these therapies are "complementary" to conventional Western medicine, most have existed for hundreds or even thousands of years, and are used widely throughout the world. In the last decade, the striking growth in public awareness and use of complementary therapies has caught the attention of the medical profession. Increasingly, physicians are discovering the value of being familiar with these therapies, both to enhance communication with their patients who use them and to improve clinical practice. This chapter describes some of the more widely used alternative and complementary therapies and their applications.

Prevalence of Complementary Therapy Use in the United States

A recent national survey found that one third of U.S. adults used complementary therapies (1). In 1990, Americans made an estimated 425 million visits to providers of unconventional therapies, compared with an estimated 388 million visits to all primary care physicians, and spent approximately $13.7 billion dollars, of which $10.3 billion was paid out of pocket. Patients who sought complementary versus conventional treatment were generally younger, of higher socioeconomic status, and female.

Particular population groups regularly using complementary medicine include those with limited access to health services, those suffering from chronic or incurable diseases, and those whose beliefs about illness and healing differ from that of mainstream medicine. One aspect of complementary medicine is folk medicine, a diverse body of unofficial health practices that shows no sign of dying out (2). Cultural minorities and rural people are among those who use folk systems of healing in addition to available medical services. For example, one study found that 76% of patients attending rural primary care clinics (and 70% attending urban clinics) in West Virginia used folk remedies (3). In particular, treatment is sought for ailments for which biomedicine has no real cure, including chronic problems such as arthritis, headaches, and depression. One study found that 55% of caregivers of Alzheimer's patients tried one or more complementary treatments in efforts to improve patients' memories, of which 40% perceived the remedy to be helpful (4).

Religious beliefs and complementary health practices may go hand in hand, as in the example of faith healing, often practiced in the context of religious services. In one study of patients attending a family practice clinic in rural North Carolina, 21% reported attending a faith healing service, and 6% reported being cured by faith healers.

One factor enhancing the popularity of alternative forms of health care is dissatisfaction with the high cost and often disappointing outcomes of technologic medicine. Increasingly, patients realize that powerful pharmaceuticals are not without a price, chronic diseases can be controlled but not cured, and no magic potion has yet been developed that can eradicate heart disease or prevent cancer. In addition, there is growing disenchantment with a medical system that dehumanizes the physician-patient relationship.

Complaints that the doctor doesn't listen well, spend enough time with the patient, or resolve problems are heard more often in this era of consumer consciousness. Increased global awareness, respect for other cultural traditions, and patient activism have combined to enhance the desire to explore new ways of healing.

In 1992, the U.S. Congress established the Office of Alternative Medicine (OAM) at the National Institutes of Health, in response to the recognized growth in the public's use of these therapies. The mission of the OAM is to evaluate the effectiveness of alternative medical treatment and to integrate effective treatments into mainstream medical practice. According to the OAM, a medical practice or intervention is "alternative" if it (a) does not have sufficient documentation in the United States to show that it is safe and effective against specific diseases and conditions, (b) is not generally taught in medical schools, and (c) is not generally reimbursable for third-party insurance billing.

All the elements of this definition are now being challenged. Research is documenting the effectiveness of some of these therapies for particular conditions; many medical schools now offer courses in complementary medicine; and many managed care organizations and other third-party insurance carriers are beginning to pay for certain complementary therapies.

Learning About Complementary Health Care Practices

Learning about the philosophies, practitioners, and techniques of these therapies can benefit the patient and the family physician in the following ways:

- Enhancing communication with patients who favor nonbiomedical approaches to treatment.

- Coordinating care: Increasingly, family physicians are placed in the role of gatekeeper for other health care professionals or services. Continuity and quality of care are enhanced when the primary care physician can communicate knowledgeably with other members of the patient's health care team.

- Improving patients' well-being through the appropriate use of, and referral to, complementary medical therapies: Many complementary therapies offer health promotion/disease preventive strategies not available in the allopathic medical repertoire. In addition, they offer a variety of generally safe, and often effective, therapeutic tools that can be used in place of, or as complementary to, existing treatments.

One of the important differences between complementary approaches and allopathic medicine is the time commitment of the health professional. Whereas a primary care physician may spend about 15 minutes per visit with a patient, alternative practitioners may take up to 2 hours. This reflects the different emphases of allopathic medicine (using powerful, rapid interventions to reduce symptoms and control diseases) and complementary medicine (using multifaceted, individualized healing processes).

Cultural Context of Alternative Health Beliefs and Practices

Patients using complementary therapies may have different explanatory models of health and illness (6). For example, root work, a coherent medical tradition still prevalent among subcultures of African-Americans in the American South, involves the belief that supernatural forces can be controlled and manipulated by humans to heal or harm. For a patient who subscribes to this belief system, illness that is unresponsive to conventional treatment may have arisen because an enemy has placed a root on or near the individual. The cure involves removal of the root by expert root doctors with counteracting potions. Similarly, faith healing involves the belief that some illnesses represent a punishment from God, with cure requiring belief in, and surrender to, God's power.

In many alternative systems, including traditional Chinese medicine, homeopathy, and many mind-body therapies, underlying explanations involve the concepts of balance and imbalance, the body as a self-healing system, the inseparability of mind and body, and the importance of spiritual development in the course of healing.

Those who seek complementary therapies tend to be more skeptical of the efficacy of modern medicine, to have greater belief in treatment of the whole person versus a particular disease, and to have suffered longer from their complaints (7, 8). Often they are active managers of their own "team" of health professionals, which may include one or more alternative care providers, often unbeknownst to their physician. One study found, for example, that 72% of patients visited the offices of alternative care providers without informing their primary care physician (1).

Conflicts in explanatory models of health and illness between patients and health care professionals can lead to distrust, conflicting expectations, reduced compliance, and discontinuity of care. Respect for patients' explanatory models builds mutual trust and cooperation. Recognizing and using the powerful role that beliefs play in illness and health can help patients manage their own medical problems.

SURVEY OF COMPLEMENTARY THERAPIES

Many complementary therapies emphasize the following principles to a greater extent than allopathic medicine:

- Using the therapy to stimulate the body's own healing abilities

- Preventing illness by strengthening homeostatic balance and remaining in harmony with the psychosocial and physical environment

- Individualizing treatment to the particular patient, rather than to the disease condition

- Addressing the mental, emotional, or environmental factors in disease, rather than simply eliminating (suppressing) physical manifestations

- Using natural nonpharmaceutical substances or techniques, while avoiding use of prescription medications (particularly those that might suppress symptoms, thus compromising the body's ability to heal itself)

- Enhancing wellness with optimal diet, exercise, and stress-reducing regimens

Some of the most popular therapies are summarized in the following paragraphs. One caveat is that there is a wide variety in the quality and quantity of evidence available to support the use of these therapies. In many cases, only clinical case reports or long-standing tradition serve to bolster the claim to effectiveness. In other cases, there are excellent research studies, including double-blind, placebo-controlled experimental trials. The latter are expensive and often challenging in terms of experimental design.

Mind-Body Therapies

These interventions are based on the concept of the inseparability and interaction of cognitive and emotional processes with the body's organ systems. These include hypnosis, biofeedback, guided imagery, relaxation therapies, mindfulness meditation, and mindful exercise. Research demonstrating the psychobiologic mechanisms by which regulation of physiologic processes occurs, including immune and neurotransmitter substances, provides evidence that these approaches may have some validity (9).

Biofeedback

This training is based on the realization that a person can learn to modify his or her own vital functions such as breathing, skin temperature, or heart rate, to prevent, control, and treat a range of dysfunctions. Sleep disorders, incontinence, back pain, temporomandibular joint (TMJ) syndrome, heart dysfunction, gastrointestinal disorders, difficulty swallowing, ringing of the ears, migraine and tension headaches, asthma, and hypertension are conditions that have been ameliorated with biofeedback. Biofeedback training is particularly useful in treating patients whose problems have a psychosocial component (10).

Hypnosis

This technique uses the power of suggestion to induce trance-like states to access deep, often unconscious levels of the mind to effect positive behavioral change and treat a range of health problems. Hypnotic techniques have been used effectively to overcome ulcers, warts, migraine and tension headaches, sleep disorders, anxiety, phobias, depression, eating disorders, cigarette smoking, and alcohol and substance abuse. Hypnosis and guided imagery are increasingly being used to reduce the need for anesthesia during surgery and to control pain (11).

Meditation

This technique keeps the attention pleasantly anchored in the present moment, so that the mind is not preoccupied with thoughts and feelings of the past and future. Concentrative meditation techniques focus on an image or sound, or simply on breathing. Mindfulness meditation involves expanding the attention to include awareness of thoughts and emotions without being distracted by them. Both techniques have been shown to modify markers of stress such as heart rate, pulse rate, and plasma cortisol levels, and enhance electroencephalogram alpha states.

Meditation also has been used effectively to enhance immune function in patients who have cancer, acquired immunodeficiency syndrome, and autoimmune disorders, as well as to decrease anxiety, hypertension, and chronic pain (12).

Mindful Exercise

This modality includes such activities as yoga, tai chi, Alexander technique, and Feldenkrais. Research has shown that *mindful* exercise is more beneficial in many respects than simply exercise, in terms of certain physiologic responses. Some of these exercises are suitable for all ages. For example, tai chi was found to reduce frailty and falls in older people (13,14).

Chiropractic

Chiropractic is the third largest independent health profession in the Western world, following allopathic medicine and dentistry, with about 52,000 licensed practitioners in the United States. These practitioners are trained in 4-year postbaccalaureate programs and see approximately 20 million patients per year. Chiropractic is based on the understanding that structural distortions can cause functional abnormalities. Vertebral subluxation of the spine is an important structural distortion that disturbs body function primarily through neurologic pathways. Chiropractic adjustment is a specific and definitive system for correcting vertebral subluxation, harmonizing neuronal function, and stimulating the body's innate healing potential (15).

Chiropractic therapy focuses primarily on manual adjustment or manipulation of the spine. Patients visit chiropractic physicians most frequently for the prevention and treatment of low back pain, neck pain, and headache—conditions for which spinal manual therapy has been shown to be safe and effective (16–18).

The Agency for Health Care Policy and Research has concluded that spinal manual therapy hastens recovery from acute low back pain and recommends it either in combination or as a replacement for nonsteroidal anti-inflammatory drugs, cautioning against other pharmaceutical approaches and lumbar surgery except in the most severe cases (19). Chiropractic has been shown to be more effective than amitriptyline for long-term relief of pain from muscle tension, and it is also claimed to be useful for lowering blood pressure, decreasing infant colic,

reducing vertigo, and alleviating TMJ syndrome (20, 21).

Bodywork

Bodywork can maintain good health by decreasing tension, stress, and structural imbalances. Techniques include traditional massage as well as a variety of contemporary and energy-based systems, examples of which are described in the following paragraphs.

Therapeutic Massage

This therapy is beneficial in relieving muscle spasm, pain and soreness, headache, whiplash, TMJ syndrome, and tension-related respiratory syndromes such as bronchial asthma and emphysema. Massage is reported to produce relaxation, alleviate swelling, correct poor posture, and improve circulation. It can alleviate chronic inflammatory conditions by increasing lymphatic circulation. in treatment of cardiovascular, neurologic and gynecologic disorders, it can be used as adjunctive therapy. Massage can also be used to (a) break up scar tissue and lessen fibrous adhesions resulting from injury or immobilization, (b) increase peristaltic action in the intestines to promote fecal elimination, and (c) loosen mucus and promote drainage of sinus fluids via percussive and vibratory techniques (22).

Reflexology

Introduced to the United States in the 1940s by Dr. William Fitzgerald and further developed by physiotherapist Eunice Ingham, this therapy involves application of precise pressure to points of the hands and feet that are believed to correspond to organs, glands, and other parts of the body, to relieve tension, stimulate deep relaxation, increase circulation, and modify nerve impulses so as to balance the entire body. Little research has been performed to evaluate the efficacy of this therapy. It is widely used for self-care.

Applied Kinesiology

This modality is a diagnostic system developed recently by George Goodheart, a chiropractic physician, and involves determining imbalances in the body's organs and glands by identifying weaknesses in specific muscles. Once imbalances are identified, various techniques may be used to strengthen the muscles involved in the underlying dysfunction.

Therapeutic Touch

This modality, an energy-based healing system that is now used widely in U.S. hospitals, was developed by Dolores Krieger, Ph.D., R.N., and Dora Kunz, a healer. It is based on the philosophy that the practitioner, using the hands combined with loving intention, can consciously direct healing energy to and modulate the patient's energy field. The energy field is described as a felt or seen force or heat radiating from the body. Studies suggest that therapeutic touch can decrease anxiety, reduce pain, and promote wound healing. Physiologic changes include altered enzyme activity and increased hemoglobin levels (20, 21, 23).

Other Bodywork Techniques

The Alexander technique was pioneered by Frederick Matthias Alexander and uses awareness, movement, and touch to change habitual movement patterns that interfere with proper body functioning. The Feldenkrais method, founded by Moshe Feldenkrais, involves altering the self-image along with corresponding negative habitual patterns of movement. Group exercise programs called "Awareness Through Movement" guide participants through slow, gentle sequences of movement designed to replace old patterns with new ones. "Functional integration" involves individualized hands-on touch and movement, in which the practitioner directs the client's body through movements tailored to the client's needs. Structural integration, commonly called rolfing, is based on the philosophy that proper alignment of body segments (head, torso, pelvis, legs, feet) via manual manipulation and stretching of the body's fascial tissues, improves body movement and function. Some research on rolfing points toward a role in reducing chronic stress, promoting change in body function, and enhancing neurologic function (20).

Acupuncture

Acupuncture developed as part of Chinese traditional medicine, over a period of at least 3000 years. It is based on the belief that health is dependent on the balanced flow of "chi," the vital life energy, throughout the body. Illness is due to a disturbance of chi within the body. Acupuncture treatment involves balancing the chi by inserting needles at specific points on the body where the chi flows.

Acupuncture is used to treat a wide variety of symptoms and diseases. Studies assessing its usefulness have often suffered from flaws in research design. Nevertheless, evidence is accumulating that acupuncture can be effective in the treatment of menstrual pain, migraines, back pain, knee pain, nausea and vomiting, withdrawal from substance abuse, bronchial asthma, and chronic bronchitis (20, 21, 24–28). Some physicians are now undertaking courses in acupuncture and incorporating it into their practices.

Dietary Therapies

Conventional and complementary medicine agree on the preventive and healing properties of diets that are low in saturated fat and animal protein, high in fiber and complex carbohydrates, and high in proportions of fresh fruits and vegetables. Research has validated the protective antioxidative effects of vitamins E and C. Cancer-protective substances, known as phytochemicals, occur in fruits, vegetables, and whole grains.

Alternative medicine has always emphasized the importance of whole, organic foods and the elimination from food products of such chemical substances as pesticides, antibiotics, hormones, and food additives such as preservatives, dyes, and artificial flavors. Although data are unavailable on the long-term consequences of humans' ingesting these substances, there is evidence, particularly from animal studies, that they may play a role in decreased immune function, increased food allergies, increased chemical sensitivities, and other disorders.

Dietary therapies are based on a variety of nutritional prescriptions. The simplest is the introduction of an organic, plant-based, whole-foods diet, which decreases the body's burden of chemical additives, maximizes natural vitamin and mineral intake, decreases fat and sugar, and increases fiber. Other dietary therapies include:

- Macrobiotics—a dietary prescription formulated by Michio Kushi based on the ancient Chinese philosophy of balancing "yin and yang" and emphasizing whole foods;

- Vegetarian diet—the elimination of all meat;

- Vegan diet—eliminates all animal products, including milk and eggs.

- Juice therapies—used to provide supplementary nutrients, particularly vitamins and minerals, both for prevention of illness (i.e., during times of stress) and to restore the body to health (e.g., an unproven but popular alternative cancer therapy involves drinking high quantities of carrot juice).

- Fasting—used to enhance immune function and to purge the body of toxic substances, as well as to increase spiritual awareness (fasts may involve drinking only pure water or may be modified to include vegetable juices).

Other dietary therapies are used to treat specific disease states, particularly cancer. Although clinical evidence exists for the usefulness of some of these therapies, more rigorous research is needed to establish efficacy (20).

Herbal Medicine

Until the late 19th century, physicians prescribed herbal preparations extensively, but with the growth of manufactured drugs, knowledge and use of herbs declined and practically ceased in the United States. The recent spread in popularity of self-prescribed herbal preparations has caught the medical community unprepared in terms of knowledge of these agents' properties, uses, and drug interactions. Raw herbs and preparations can be purchased over the counter in health food stores and some pharmacies.

The use of many herbal preparations is based on tradition rather than scientific study. There are, however, a growing number of controlled clinical trials validating the efficacy of herbal preparations for specific conditions (29–31). Table 12.1 describes commonly purchased over-the-counter herbal medicines, their uses, and available research.

Aromatherapy

Aromatic molecules interacting with the cells of the nasal mucosa transmit signals to the limbic system through which they connect with parts of the brain controlling heart rate, blood pressure, breathing, memory, and hormone balance. Research has shown that inhalation of particular essential oils can have either a calming or a stimulatory effect on brain waves. In France, use of aromatherapy is widespread among laypersons and prescribed by physicians, who have developed a system of aromatherapeutic medicine (20, 21).

Homeopathy

The fundamental principle of homeopathy is the law of similars: "like is cured by like," that is, a remedy can cure a disease if it produces in a healthy person symptoms similar to those of the disease. In the late 19th century, Samuel Hahnemann formally tested this principle and established it as the basis of a system of medicine. Although the mechanism by which the similar remedy acts is unknown, homeopathic theory maintains that in some way it stimulates the organism's own innate healing capacities. Illness is viewed as a disturbance of the vital force, manifested in physical, mental, and emotional responses that are unique to each patient. A symptom is viewed as the organism's expression of its life energy. Thus, symptoms should not be suppressed, but used in the cure of the whole person.

Central to homeopathic therapeutics is the infinitesimal dose. Through experimenting with lower and lower doses of drugs in efforts to minimize adverse effects, Hahnemann developed a technique called potentization, in which the original substance is repeatedly diluted to produce a medicinal substance so dilute that, in many cases, there is unlikely to be a single original molecule left. The nonmolecular dose has remained a fundamental obstacle to the acceptance of homeopathy by the scientific community, because there is no acceptable explanatory model for therapeutic action within the framework of present biomedical theory.

Patients seek homeopathic consultation for both acute conditions (e.g., a cold, influenza, poison ivy rash) and chronic illnesses (e.g., a lingering cough or fever, chronic fatigue, long-lasting depression, or anxiety or phobias). Homeopathic treatment involves selection of a preparation that produces symptoms similar to that of the patient's complete symptom picture. Even for acute conditions, prescribing takes into account the individualized response to illness. In chronic conditions, treatment may incorporate the person's entire symptomatology not only with regard to the present complaint, but over the course of a lifetime. The latter is termed constitutional prescribing.

Homeopathy is now used widely in Europe, India, and South America by both physicians and laypersons: in Germany, 25% of all physicians prescribe homeopathic remedies; in France, it is taught in medical schools and prescribed by 32% of general practice physicians; and in Great

Table 12.1.
Herbal Medicines in Common Use

Herb	Common Uses	Level of Evidence for Effectiveness[a]
Chamomile (*Matricaria recutita*)	Digestive aid, mild sedative	B[a]
	Anti-inflammatory	B[a]
Echinacea (*Echinacea augustifolia*)	Immunostimulant	A[b]
	Treatment of viral infections	B[a,c]
Feverfew (*Tanacetum parthenium*)	Migraine prevention	B[d]
	Premenstrual syndrome	B[e]
	Fever reduction	B[e]
Garlic (*Allium sativum*)	Prevention and treatment of viral and bacterial infections and flu	A[f]
	Antihypertensive, cholesterol lowering	A[g–i]
Ginger (*Zingiber officinalis*)	Prevention and treatment of nausea and motion sickness	A[j–m]
Ginkgo (*Ginkgo biloba*)	Memory enhancement	A[n–p]
	Treatment of cardiovascular insufficiency	A[q]
	Treatment of peripheral vascular conditions	A[r–u]
Ginseng (*Panax ginseng/ Panax quinquefolius*)	Adaptogen; antioxidant	A[v–y]
	Antihepatotoxic	
	Immunostimulant	
Goldenseal (*Hydrastis canadensis*)	Immunostimulant	B[a]
	Antimicrobial (against bacteria, protozoa, and fungi)	B[a]
Milk thistle (*Silybum marianum*)	Prevention, treatment of liver disorders	A[z, aa]
Saint-John's-wort (*Hypericum perforatum*)	Treatment of depression; sleep aid	A[bb, cc]
	Externally, speeds wound healing; anti-inflammatory	B[dd]
Saw palmetto (*Serenoa repens*)	Tones and strengthens male reproductive system	A[ee]
Senna (*Cassia augustifolia*)	Laxative	A[ff–jj]
Siberian ginseng (*Eleutherococcus senticosus*)	Adaptogen	B[kk–nn]
Valerian (*Valeriana officinalis*)	Sedative, sleep aid	A[oo–qq]

[a]Level of evidence for effectiveness: A, strong or moderate research-based evidence (consistent across several studies, including at least two randomized controlled trials); B, limited research-based evidence (less consistent or extensive evidence, but preponderance of evidence supports use of treatment.

REFERENCES

Chamomile (*Matricaria recutita*)

a.   Mowrey DB. The Scientific Validation of Herbal Medicine. New Canaan, CT: Keats Publishing, 1986.

Echinacea (*Echinacea augustifolia*)

b.   Melchart D, Linde K, Worku F, Bauer R, Wagner H. Immunomodulation with echinacea: a systematic review of controlled clinical trials. Phytomedicine 1994;1:245–254.
c.   Bauer R. Echinacea drugs—effects and active ingredients. Z Arztl Fortbild 1996;90:117–122.

Feverfew (*Tanacetum parthenium*)

d.   Murphy JJ, Heptinstall S, Mitchell JR. Randomised double-blind placebo-controlled trial of feverfew in migraine prevention. Lancet 1988;2:189–192.
e.   Heptinstall S, White A, Williamson L. Mitchell JR. Feverfew. Lancet 1985;1(8437):1071–1074.

continued

Table 12.1. (continued)
Herbal Medicines in Common Use

Garlic (*Allium sativum*)

f. Adetumbi MA, Lau BH. *Allium sativum* (garlic)—a natural antibiotic. Med Hypotheses 1983;12:227–237.
g. Silagy CA, Neil HA. Garlic as a lipid-lowering agent—A meta-analysis. J R Coll Physicians 1994;28:39–45.
h. Silagy CA, Neil HA. A meta-analysis of the effect of garlic on blood pressure. J Hypertension 1994;12:463–468.
i. Warshafsky S, Kamer RS, Sivak SL. Effect of garlic on total serum cholesterol. A meta-analysis. Ann Intern Med 1993;119:599–605.

Ginger (*Zingiber officinalis*)

j. Bone ME, Wilkinson DJ, Young JR, McNeil J, Charlton S. Ginger too—A new antiemetic. Anaesthesia 1990;45:669–671.
k. Fischer-Rasmussen W, Kjaer SK, Dahl C, Asping U. Ginger treatment of hyperemesis gravidarum. Eur J Obstet Gynecol Reprod Biol 1991;38:19–24.
l. Mowrey DB, Clayson DE. Motion sickness, ginger, and psychophysics. Lancet 1982;1(8273): 655–657.
m. Grontved A, Brask T, Kambskard J, Hentzer E. Ginger root against seasickness. A controlled trial on the open sea. Acta Otolaryngolog 1988;105:45–49.

Ginkgo (*Ginkgo biloba*)

n. Winter E. Effects of an extract of *Ginkgo biloba* on learning and memory in mice. Pharmacol Biochem Behav 1991;38:109–114.
o. Gessner B, Voelp A, Klasser M. Study of the long-term action of a *Ginkgo biloba* extract on vigilance and mental performance as determined by means of quantitative pharmaco-EEG and psychometric measurements. Arzneimittelforschung 1985;35:1459–1465.
p. Rai G, Shovlin C, Wesnes K. A double-blind, placebo controlled study of *Ginkgo biloba* extract (tanakan) in elderly out-patients with mild to moderate memory impairment. Curr Med Res Opin 1991;12:350–355.
q. Kleijnen J, Knipschild P. Ginkgo biloba for cerebral insufficiency. Br J Clin Pharmacol 1992;34:352–358.
r. Raabe A, Raabe M, Ihm P, et al. Therapeutic follow-up using automatic perimetry in chronic cerebroretinal ischemia in elderly patients: prospective double-blind study with graduated dose *Ginkgo biloba* treatment. Klin Monatsbl Augenheilkd 1991;199:432–438.
s. Meyer B. Multicenter randomized double-blind drug vs. placebo study of the treatment of tinnitus with *Ginkgo biloba* extract. Presse Med 1986;15:1562–1564.
t. Haguenauer JP, Cantenot F, Koskas H, Pierart H. Treatment of equilibrium disorders with *Ginkgo biloba* extract. A multicenter double-blind drug vs. placebo study. Presse Med 1986;15:1569–1572.
u. Dubreuil C. Therapeutic trial in acute cochlear deafness. A comparative study of *Ginkgo biloba* extract and nicergoline. Presse Med 1986;15:1559–1561.

Ginseng (*Panax ginseng*)

v. Scaglione F, Ferrara F, Dugnani S, et al. Immunomodulatory effects of *Panax ginseng*. Drugs Exp Clin Res 1990;16:537–542.
w. Bol'shakova IV, Lozovskaia EL, Sapezhinskii II. Antioxidant properties of a series of extracts from medicinal plants. Biofizika 1997;42:480–483.
x. Martinez B, Staba EJ. The physiological effects of *Aralia, Panax* and *Eleutherococcus* on exercised rats. Jpn J Pharmacol 1984;35 (2):79–85.
y. Ben-Hur E, Fulder S. Effect of *Panax ginseng* saponins and *Eleutherococcus senticosus* on survival of cultured mammalian cells after ionizing radiation. Am J Chin Med 1981;9(1):48–56.

Milk Thistle (*Silybum marianum*)

z. Muriel P, Carciniapina T, Perez-Alvarez V, et al. Silymarin protects against paracetamol-induced lipid peroxidation and liver damage. J Appl Toxicol 1992;12:439–442.
aa. Ferenci R. Dragorisics B, et al. Randomized controlled trial of silymarin treatment in patients with cirrhosis of the liver. J Hepatol 1989;9:105–113.

Saint-John's-wort (*Hypericum perforatum*)

bb. Linde K, Ramirez G, Mulrow CD, et al. St John's wort for depression—An overview and meta-analysis of randomized clinical trials. Br Med J 1996;313:253–258.
cc. Schulz H, Jobert M. Effects of *Hypericum* extract on the sleep EEG of older volunteers. J Geriatr Psychiatr Neurol 1994;7(suppl 1):S39–43.
dd. Diwu Z. Novel therapeutic and diagnostic applications of hypocrellins and hypericins. Photochem Photobiol 1995;61:529–539.

Saw palmetto (*Serenoa repens*)

ee. Champault G, Patel JC, Bonnard AM. A double-blind trial of an extract of the plant *Serenoa repens* in benign prostatic hyperplasia. Br J Clin Pharmacol 1984;18:461–462.

Senna (*Cassia augustifolia*)

ff. Ashraf W, Lof J, Jin G, Quigley EM. Comparative effects of intraduodenal psyllium and senna on canine small bowel motility. Aliment Pharmacol Ther 1994;8:329–336.
gg. Kinnunen O, Winblad I, Koistinen P, Salokannel J. Safety and efficacy of a bulk laxative containing senna versus lactulose in the treatment of chronic constipation in geriatric patients. Pharmacology 1993;47(1):253–255.
hh. Passmore AP, Davies KW, Flanagan PG, Stoker C, Scott MG. A comparison of Agiolax and lactulose in elderly patients with chronic constipation. Pharmacology 1993;47(1):249–252.
ii. Ewe K, Ueberschaer B, Press AG. Influence of senna, fibre, and fibre + senna on colonic transit in loperamide-induced constipation. Pharmacology 1993;47(1):242–248.
jj. Passmore AP, Wilson-Davies K, Stoker C, Scott ME. Chronic constipation in long-stay elderly patients: a comparison of lactulose and a senna-fibre combination. Br Med J 1993;307:769–771.

continued

Table 12.1. (*continued*)
Herbal Medicines in Common Use

Siberian ginseng (*Eleutherococcus senticosus*)

kk. Farnsworth NR, Kinghorn AD, Soejarto DD, Waller DP. Siberian ginseng (*Eleutherococcus senticosus*): current status as an adaptogen. Econ Med Plant Res 1985;1:156–215.

ll. Hallstrom C, Fulder S, Carruthers M. Effect of ginseng on the performance of nurses on night duty. Complement Med East West 1982;6:277–282.

mm. Bohn B, Nebe CT, Birr C. Flow-cytometric studies with *Eleutherococcus senticosus* extract as an immunomodulatory agent. Arzneimittelforschung 1987;37:1193–1196.

nn. Kupin VI, Polevaia EB. Stimulation of the immunological reactivity of cancer patients by *Eleutherococcus* extract. Voprosy Onkologii 1986;32:21–26.

Valerian (*Valeriana officinalis*)

oo. Leathwood PD, Chauffard F, Heck E, Munoz-Box R. Aqueous extract of valerian root improves sleep quality in man. Pharmacol Biochem Behav 1982;17:65–71.

pp. Leathwood PD, Chauffard F. Aqueous extract of valerian reduces latency to fall asleep in man. Planta Med 1985;54:144–148.

qq. Lindahl O, Lindwall L. Double blind study of a valerian preparation. Pharmacol Biochem Behav 1989;32:1065–1066.

Britain, 42% of physicians refer patients to homeopaths. In the United States, Eisenberg's national survey found that 1% of the U.S. population had used homeopathy within 1 year (11).

Homeopathy has been shown to be effective in rheumatoid arthritis, allergies, fibrosis, influenza, asthma, and acute childhood diarrhea (32, 33). A meta-analysis in the *British Medical Journal* found that 15 of 22 well-designed studies showed positive results (34). Case reports have suggested that homeopathy may be useful in a range of psychologic disorders, including anxiety, depression, agoraphobia, and posttraumatic stress and personality disorders.

CONCLUSION

Physicians often look askance at the use of complementary therapies. Their own limited knowledge base or strongly directed beliefs in the biomedical model may frequently prevent them from being open to other approaches to healing. A more positive approach is to become knowledgeable about the range of therapies, the evidence that supports their use, and any possible adverse effects. It is important to appreciate the healing effects of patients' efforts to help themselves and recognize that the power of belief in a particular therapy in itself has a healing benefit. A skillful physician should, when possible, attempt to incorporate patients' beliefs and practices into any health intervention.

To be a well-rounded physician, you should learn about the use and efficacy of complementary medicines and develop skill in communicating with patients of diverse belief systems. Take the time to visit alternative health care providers.

Developing a personal relationship with these providers, who may include the local root doctor, chiropractic physicians, herbalists, and faith healers, could provide the basis for understanding and collaborative involvement in patient care.

REFERENCES

1. Eisenberg DM, Kessler RC, Foster C, et al. Unconventional medicine in the United States. Prevalence, costs, and patterns of use. N Engl J Med 1993;328:246–252.
2. Hufford DJ. Folk medicine in contemporary America. In: Kirkland J, Mathews H, Sullivan CW III, Baldwin K, eds. Herbal and Magical Medicine. Traditional Healing Today. Durham, NC: Duke University Press, 1992: 14–31.
3. Cook C, Baisen D. Ancillary use of folk medicine by patients in primary care clinics in Southwestern West Virginia. South Med J 1986;79:1098–1101.
4. Coleman LM, Fowler LB, Williams ME. Use of unproven therapies by people with Alzheimer's disease. J Am Geriatr Soc 1995;43:747–750.
5. King DE, Sobal J, DeForge BR. Family practice patients' experience and beliefs in faith healing. J Fam Pract 1988;27:505–508.
6. Kleinman A. Concepts and a model for the comparison of medical systems as cultural systems. Soc Sci Med 1978;12:85–93.
7. Furnham A, Rawlinson A. Beliefs about the efficacy of complementary medicine: a vignette study. Complement Ther Med 1996;4:85–89.
8. Furnham A, Smith C. Choosing alternative medicine: a comparison of the beliefs of patients visiting a general practitioner and a homeopath. Soc Sci Med 1988; 26:685–689.
9. Rossi EL. The Psychobiology of Mind-Body Healing: New Concepts of Therapeutic Hypnosis. New York: Norton, 1993.
10. Hatch JP, Fisher JG, Rugh JD. Biofeedback: Studies in Clinical Efficacy. New York: Plenum Press, 1987.
11. Lang EV, Joyce JS, Spiegel D, Hamilton D, Lee KK. Self-hypnotic relaxation during interventional radiological

procedures: effects on pain perception and intravenous drug use. Int J Clin Exp Hypnosis 1996;44:106–119.

12. Kabat-Zinn J, Lipworth L, Burney R. The clinical use of mindfulness meditation for the self- regulation of chronic pain. J Behav Med 1985;8(2):163–190.

13. Wolf SL, Huiman XB, Kutner NG, et al (Atlanta FICSIT Group). Reducing frailty and falls in older persons: an investigation of tai chi and computerized balance training. J Am Geriatr Soc 1996;44:489–497.

14. Wolfson L, Whipple R, Derby C, et al. Balance and strength training in older adults: intervention gains and tai chi maintenance. J Am Geriatr Soc 1996;44:498–506.

15. Strang VV. The Essential Principles of Chiropractic. Davenport, IA: Palmer College of Chiropractic, 1984.

16. Aker PD, Gross AR, Goldsmith CH, Peloso P. Conservative management of mechanical neck pain: systematic overview and meta-analysis. Br Med J 1996;313:1291–1296.

17. Assendelft WJJ, Bouter LM, Knipschild PG. Complications of spinal manipulation: a comprehensive review of the literature. J Fam Pract 1996;42:475–480.

18. Mootz RD. Art, science and philosophy: enthusiasm and the untestable. J Manip Physiol Ther 1992;15:542–545.

19. Agency for Health Care Policy and Research. Clinical Practice Guidelines for Acute Low Back Problems in Adults. Agency for Health Care Policy and Research publication no. 95-0642. Rockville, MD: US Department of Health and Human Services, Public Health Service, Agency for Health Care Policy and Research, 1994.

20. Burton Goldberg Group, eds. Alternative Medicine. The Definitive Guide. Fife, WA: Future Medicine Publishing, 1994.

21. Micozzi MS, ed. Fundamentals of Complementary and Alternative Medicine. New York: Churchill Livingstone, 1996.

22. Van Why R. The Body Work Database. Evanston, IL: American Massage Therapy Foundation, 1997.

23. Wirth DP. The effect of noncontact therapeutic touch on the healing rate of full thickness dermal wounds. Subtle Energies 1990;1:1–19.

24. al-Sadi M, Newman B, Julious SA. Acupuncture in the prevention of postoperative nausea and vomiting. Anesthesia 1997;52:658–661.

25. Ernst E, White AR. Acupuncture as an adjuvant therapy in stroke rehabilitation? Wien Med Wochenschr 1996;146:556–558.

26. Lewith GT, Watkins AD. Unconventional therapies in asthma: an overview. Allergy 1196;51:761–769.

27. Gurevich MI, Duchworth D, Imhof JE, Katz JL. Is auricular acupuncture beneficial in the inpatient treatment of substance-abusing patients? A pilot study. J Subst Abuse Treat 1996;12:165–171.

28. Peterson JR. Acupuncture in the 1990s. A review for the primary care physician. Arch Fam Med 1996;5:237–240.

29. Mowrey DB. The Scientific Validation of Herbal Medicine. New Canaan, CT: Keats Publishing, 1986.

30. Murray MT. Natural Alternatives to Prozac. New York: William Morrow, 1996.

31. Linde K, Ramirez G, Mulrow CD, et al. St. John's Wort for depression—an overview and meta-analysis of randomised clinical trials. Br Med J 1996;313:253–258.

32. Reilly DT, Taylor MA, McSharry C, Atchison T. Is homeopathy a placebo response? Controlled trial of homeopathic potencies with pollen in hayfever as a model. Lancet 1986;2:881–886.

33. Jacobs J, Jimenez M, Lloyd S, Gale JL, Crothers D. Treatment of acute childhood diarrhea with homeopathic medicine: a randomized clinical trial in Nicaragua. Pediatrics, 1994;93:719–725.

34. Kleijnen J, Knipschild P, Riet G. Clinical trials of homeopathy. Br Med J 1991;302:316–323.

Common Problems

13. Common Problems: Overview and General Approach

PHILIP D. SLOANE, PETER CURTIS, MARK H. EBELL, MICHAEL FISHER, TIMOTHY J. IVES, AND WARREN P. NEWTON

"Common problems" constitute the bulk of a family physician's work. They are varied, present often as symptoms rather than diagnoses, and frequently have a psychosocial component. The remainder of this book consists of chapters about these common problems. This introductory chapter provides background material to give you a general understanding and approach to both reading the chapters and approaching common problems in the office. We'll begin by discussing what we mean by common problems.

WHAT IS COMMON IN FAMILY MEDICINE?

The Broad Range of Problems in Family Medicine

People who claim that family medicine is humdrum and repetitive have never spent a day in a family physician's office. Indeed, family physicians deal with a broader range of patients and problems than any other medical specialty. The majority of visits to a family physician involve complaints that are relatively rare, occurring in fewer than 1 in 50 patients. In contrast, over half of a pediatrician's practice consists of one (admittedly complex) problem: well child care. Similarly, a urologist sees a few common problems over and over, most notably prostatic hyperplasia, urinary tract infections, and men who have elevated prostate-specific antigen tests.

The most common reason patients come to family physicians is for well person examinations. These include "routine" physicals, prenatal care, well child examinations, well adult examinations, and visits for administrative purposes such as to fill out a form for work or school. These preventive visits, which constitute approximately one third of family practice visits, have been covered in section two of this book.

The majority of office visits are for medical conditions, and those that occur most frequently are called common problems.

Symptoms and Diagnoses

One aspect that differentiates family medicine (and other primary care disciplines) from the medical and surgical subspecialties is that patients more often come in without established distinguishable diagnoses. Instead, they come with symptoms, and it is up to the physician to make the diagnosis (Fig. 13.1). Most patients who present with symptoms leave with a (sometimes imprecise and often tentative) diagnosis. The process by which family physicians solve these undifferentiated problems is one of the most interesting and, at the same time, challenging aspects of family medicine.

Thus, common problems can be defined in two ways: what is bothering the patient (i.e., the symptoms) or how the physician defines the problem (i.e., the diagnosis). Table 13.1 lists some of the most common symptoms and diagnoses seen in family practice offices.

Uncovering the Psychosocial Issues Behind the Symptoms

Why does one patient with a cold come to see a physician when others do not? It is because the runny nose, sneezing, and sore throat may not be the patient's actual reason for coming (ARC). Thus, in the patient with a cold, the ARC could be concern that it might develop into pneumonia, because this happened in the past. Or perhaps it's because he is a smoker and wants reassurance that he does not have cancer, or because he is going out of town in a few days and believes that an antibiotic will help him get better quicker. Or perhaps his son was killed in an auto accident 1 year ago and he is having an "anniversary reaction," is feeling depressed, and wants to talk.

Thus, common problems frequently are accompanied by a "hidden agenda" (the ARC), which is usually psychosocial rather than biomedical. Thus, it is the family physician's job to discover the psychosocial issues behind the visit,

203

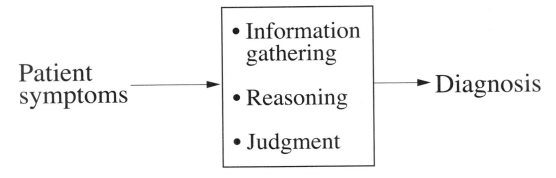

Figure 13.1. *Patients generally come in with symptoms and leave with diagnoses.*

so that the patient can receive the treatment, education, or reassurance that he or she needs.

Consider the following example (1):

CASE STUDY 1

A 54-year-old man returns to the office before his first scheduled appointment after hospitalization. In the hospital, he was treated for an acute myocardial infarction, which was accompanied by congestive heart failure. Now he comes to the office complaining of headache and backache, but these symptoms are vague and have no obvious medical diagnosis. So the physician asks directly, "How do you think we can help you today?" (which is often a good way of eliciting the ARC).

"Well, I was hoping you could tell me if being on all of these pills means that I had a 'specially bad attack or whether everyone gets treated like this," says the man, who was discharged with prescriptions for a β-adrenergic blocker, an angiotensin converting enzyme inhibitor, and aspirin. "I never took so much as an aspirin in my life, and now I'm eating pills day and night. And at work I used to carry heavy boxes around, and now I'm not even allowed to walk to the corner for the paper."

The physician then points out that the patient is still wearing his plastic identifi-

cation bracelet from the hospitalization. "They forgot to cut it off me," the patient replies, "and I didn't get around to cutting if off. Besides, maybe I'll flop over again, and with the bracelet they'll know to bring me right here."

DISCUSSION

In this example, the patient has used somatic complaints—headache and backache—to gain entry to the physician's office. However, his ARC involved fears of death and disability; so appropriate management involved allowing the patient to further express his fears, providing information about prognosis, and reassuring him that he is expected to make a full recovery.

It has been estimated that more than half of family practice office visits have a significant psychosocial component. Sometimes the psychosocial concern is related to a medical condition, as in the case presented previously; in other cases the ARC is unrelated to the presenting problem, and uncovering it takes patience and good interviewing technique. Some of these psychosocial issues include life stress, emotional distress, psychiatric disorders, social isolation, or the need for information.

Overemphasizing the latent psychosocial origin of a visit can be just as damaging, however, as illustrated in the following case:

Table 13.1.

The 12 Most Common Symptoms and Diagnoses Seen in Ambulatory Care[a]

Most Common Symptoms	Most Common Diagnoses
1. Cough	1. Hypertension
2. Sore throat	2. Otitis media
3. Earache or ear infection	3. Acute upper respiratory tract infection
4. Back pain	4. Diabetes mellitus
5. Skin rash	5. Allergic rhinitis
6. Abdominal pain	6. Bronchitis
7. Fever	7. Pharyngitis
8. Vision problems	8. Sinusitis
9. Knee pain	9. Anxiety/depression
10. Headache	10. Acne and related conditions
11. Runny/congested nose	11. Back strain/sprain
12. Chest pain	12. Asthma

Reprinted with permission from DeLozier JE, Gagnon RD. Summary: National Ambulatory Medical Care Survey, 1989. Advance Data from Vital and Health Statistics. Publication no. 203. Hyattsville, MD: National Center for Health Statistics, 1991.

[a]Excluding well person examinations.

CASE STUDY 2

A 29-year-old school librarian has a several-week history of fatigue and lack of energy. She had been seen 2 weeks earlier for a sore throat, which was believed to be viral. At that time several psychosocial issues were elicited. She had broken up with her boyfriend 5 months earlier and spent a couple of months in counseling because she was quite "low" after the breakup, and she had recently changed jobs because of a conflict with her boss at work. She felt isolated and did not spend much time with friends. Her chart was rather thick and included a number of visits for trivial medical complaints. Physical examination findings were normal. The physician told her that her symptoms appeared psychologically based, due to the separation from her boyfriend. The patient seemed upset, required extensive explanation, and left unconvinced.

After the visit, the results of a mononucleosis test drawn at the visit came back positive. The physician called the patient,

informing her of the diagnosis and apologizing for assuming that her symptoms were purely psychological. The patient returned twice in the next 3 weeks, and was allowed to vent her frustration with the misdiagnosis.

DISCUSSION

In this case the physician made a premature declaration of the symptom etiology. He should have emphasized that the diagnosis was tentative, and that he was considering other possibilities. Fortunately, he had ordered the appropriate test and was able to correct his error. Although overtesting can be as harmful as undertesting, patients often need to be told that a diagnosis is tentative and that only with time will it become certain.

Dealing with mistakes in clinical diagnosis can be difficult. A simple apology without extensive explanation is always helpful. Identifying and verbalizing to the patient his/her emotion can be helpful, like "you seem angry" or "this must have been frustrating for you," and just listening. Most patients need permission to express negative feelings to their doctor. These lessons are some of our most important educational experiences.

CLINICAL REASONING IN FAMILY PRACTICE

Medical students often feel quite confused as they begin to observe a busy, private medical practice. Many patients have problems that seem to defy classification, and the causes of illness are often multifactorial. Patient management proceeds at an unfamiliarly fast pace, and apparently without need of detailed histories or comprehensive examinations. The physician seems to be cutting corners much of the time. Decisions are made that often have a social rather than medical context. Outcomes of care are mostly good, and the patients seem satisfied. Why and how is this done?

The answer is, partly, because the physician is experienced and well trained. But just as important is the fact that decision making in primary care differs in certain respects from what the student has been taught in hospital settings. Traditional medical education, which focuses on mechanisms of disease, teaches that symptoms result from disease, and that treatment of the disease heals the symptoms. In primary care, this concept is often reversed. Symptoms are often quite likely to get better on their own, and making a specific diagnosis may not be necessary or even beneficial to the patient. Thus, clinical reasoning and decision-making styles learned in medical school are often not appropriate for primary care.

Decision making develops from three main activities: gathering information, analyzing the information (the reasoning process) and making judgments about the data. Figure 13.2 diagrams this concept. Information consists of the history, physical examination findings and results of tests. It is enriched by previous knowledge of the patient and their environment—the context of the decision. After accumulating data and creating hypotheses or differential diagnoses, the physician makes a judgment about what the problem is, and how it should be managed. This is communicated to the patient, and the decision is confirmed or rethought, with the patient ideally being a partner in management decisions.

Gathering Information

In primary care, effective clinical reasoning depends on good communication and understanding the biopsychosocial model of disease. Developed by Engel, this model affirms the close relationship of mind, body, and environment in promoting health and causing illness (2). The family physician evaluates the patient using two paths: (1) the biomedical path of symptoms and objective findings and (2) the psychosocial path of assessing stressors, family factors, and resources.

Getting a history that addresses both pathways simultaneously takes skill and experience. The patient needs to be made comfortable and initially asked open-ended questions that address his or her concerns. In other words, what the patient wants to express, know, and decide is as important as what you want to find out. Only through open-ended communication techniques will adequate and accurate data be collected as the basis for the clinical reasoning process.

Assembling Information

With the exception of some "routine physicals," most patients come to see the family physician because of a problem. They want the problem addressed and solved. However, this "presenting problem" may be complex, have multiple components, and more confusingly, may not be a "medical" problem at all. In fact, the stated problem may not be the ARC. The process of helping the patient with his or her problem involves a number of steps, which constitute a framework for the doctor-patient interaction in the office setting. This framework organizes not only the per-

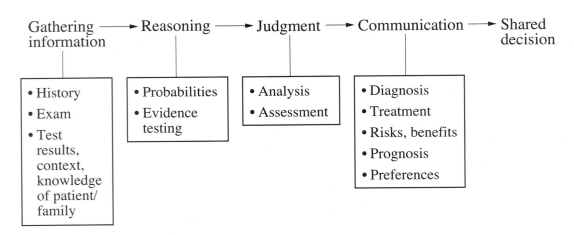

Figure 13.2. *Decision making in family practice.*

sonal encounter, but also the physician's data collection and decision making.

Organizing the Patient Encounter

For the first step, define in your own mind why the patient is making this visit. The reason or reasons may be physical, emotional, or social. The patient may have a symptom, but the problem may be that the patient or family group may no longer be able to cope with the symptom, with the anxiety it causes, or both. The patient is looking for answers to questions such as: What has happened? What's wrong? Why to me? Why has it happened? Why now? What can be done about it? What if we did nothing? What are my options? What are you going to do? and What will happen in the future? Getting at the patient's ARC may be difficult, but usually a simple question such as, "What made you decide to come to see me today?" is effective.

Your next task is to obtain enough data from the history and examination (and possibly laboratory tests) to enable you to make a good management decision. A diagnosis may not necessarily figure in this process: good management decisions can be made when the diagnosis is not yet known. The accuracy and value of data from the history, physical examination, and tests are being increasingly studied in primary care and are an essential part of evidence-based decision making.

This process of assembling information is fairly complex. From the first moment of the encounter, the history and then the physical examination provide cues that trigger hypotheses in your mind. Each cue from the history influences the questions to be asked next, and each finding in the examination may affect the next step in that examination. Usually, initial hypotheses are based on the recognition of patterns, helped by recall of patients with similar patterns. You assemble more data to confirm or rule out these patterns, and each new piece of data may alter the pattern that you are hypothesizing. In addition, immediate and past information about the patient's personal life, illness behavior patterns, beliefs, and family all contribute to the working diagnosis.

This process can proceed quite rapidly in primary care; indeed initial hypothesis are generally identified within 30 to 60 seconds, and on average about five hypotheses are considered per encounter. Approximately 75% of the critical information to test the hypotheses is obtained in the first half of the encounter; the remaining time is spent building rapport, and negotiating and agreeing on a management plan with the patient (3).

Clinical Reasoning Styles

Primary care physicians use four distinct clinical reasoning styles to develop working diagnoses: "algorithmic," "exhaustive," "heuristic," and "hypotheticodeductive." These are not mutually exclusive; a particular piece of reasoning may involve more than one of the styles. We will briefly describe these four reasoning styles:

- *Algorithmic* clinical reasoning proceeds systematically along a series of branching decision paths, using objective data to choose one pathway or another. The method is thorough, time-consuming, and costly. It is most useful when the data required to move through the algorithm are relatively discrete (i.e., black and white) and accurate, because one wrong path will lead to misdiagnosis. The evaluation of anemia can be managed using this reasoning style.

- *Exhaustive* methods gather very comprehensive history and physical examination data and pursue intensive laboratory testing to cover all possibilities. The data are then sifted for abnormal findings. This reasoning style is often the model taught and used in medical schools for inpatient care. It is useful for some unusual and complex medical problems, but it is inefficient, time-consuming, and too expensive for most problems seen in the office. Personal clinical experience and prior knowledge of the patient do not play a major role in this reasoning process. More importantly, this method may be hazardous for patients, because it poses real risks of laboratory errors and adverse effects of invasive tests. It is rarely used in office practice. An example of its legitimate use might be the assessment of a new elderly patient with multisystem disease.

- *Heuristic* reasoning (pattern recognition) seeks to fit the patient's clinical presentation to previously learned patterns of disease using any combination of data from the history and examination. Usually, this quickly limits the working diagnosis to one or two diseases. This method is quick, efficient, and inexpensive, but it requires considerable clinical experience to be successful. It is used extensively by office-based clinicians but has the drawback that some visits may be closed prematurely, missing important problems or cues. Conditions that are often diagnosed using this method include those that rely largely on physical findings, such as rashes or bursitis, and common diseases with distinctive clinical patterns, such as otitis media, depression, and cystitis.

- *Hypotheticodeductive* reasoning involves generating and testing hypotheses during the interview, using information from the patient to modify the hypotheses. This process eventually yields a diagnosis (or differential diagnosis). In a typical clinical encounter, expert clinicians generate likely diagnoses, on average, within 30 seconds and correct hypotheses within 6 minutes. This is an efficient and low-cost reasoning process, widely applied in office practice. Examples of problems effectively addressed with this reasoning style are fatigue, abdominal pain, and dizziness.

A physician may vary clinical reasoning styles, depending on the environment, the presenting problem, and patient needs.

Developing a Differential Diagnosis

Complex clinical cases often require the physician to consider multiple diagnoses. In these situations it helps, as part of the hypothesis-generating process, to think more broadly, so that you consider all the possibilities. One strategy is to use the mnemonic VINDICATE to develop a differential diagnosis: V, vascular; I, inflammatory; N, neoplasm; D, degenerative/deficiency; I, intoxication/idiopathic; C, congenital; A, autoimmune; T, trauma; and E, endocrine.

To this should be added the checklist BEEFS, which you can use to develop hypotheses about the psychosocial aspects of the specific illness: B, beliefs; E, experiences; E, emotions; F, function; and S, supports.

CASE STUDY 3

This example involves a 3-minute telephone call made to Dr. Jordan by Ms. An-

drews about her 1-year-old son, Johnny. He is running a low-grade fever, sniffling and coughing, and his mother says he has swollen lymph nodes in his neck. Instead of proceeding to a detailed screen of the different systems involved, Dr. Jordan immediately asks if Johnny is active. He is generating a key hypothesis that will predict further questioning as well as promoting efficiency. If Johnny is playing and eating normally, and is not fussy; then the first hypothesis is "mild, self-limited upper respiratory tract infection." Questioning will then be directed to confirming this diagnosis and eliminating other possibilities. Knowing that Ms. Andrews is a reliable mother, Dr. Jordan decides that Johnny does not need to be seen at this point, and home observation with symptomatic management with analgesics and good fluid intake over the next 2 days is a reasonable plan.

DISCUSSION

Dr. Jordan first identified a pattern: that of a 1-year-old with swollen neck glands who is feverish, congested, and coughing. The pattern resembles that of a mild viral syndrome. Other hypotheses included reactive airway disease, streptococcal disease, and otitis media. Having used the heuristic process to generate a working hypothesis, the doctor then uses a hypotheticodeductive style in asking questions to rule out alternative hypotheses, including life-threatening disease. The answers help confirm that the pattern originally posited is correct, and this confirmation justifies the resultant management decisions.

If the algorithmic style had been used for this telephone call, it would have taken much longer, perhaps 10 to 15 minutes. This style might be used by a novice clinician, or if the physician did not already know the patient and his family. The exhaustive style could not have been applied at all, because it depends on a comprehensive database, not just a history.

DIAGNOSIS

Epidemiology: "Think Horses, Not Zebras"

In office practice, hypotheses are modified by data from the patient's personal characteristics, family, and community. These modifiers have a very powerful influence on diagnostic strategies. For example, the familiar injunction about horses and zebras would be appropriate almost anywhere except when on safari in Africa where zebras dot the landscape.

Within the United States, certain diseases, although rare in many areas, are relatively common in others. Examples include Rocky Mountain spotted fever in North Carolina (fever and headache); lead poisoning in the inner cities (exhaustion, muscle cramps); and Lyme disease in New England (fever, rash, arthritis). Epidemiology provides the background data for developing hypotheses and making diagnoses. The physician must therefore be aware of the incidence and prevalence of illness in the community when making diagnostic and treatment decisions. For instance, if 10% of the population in your town has depression, and human immunodeficiency virus (HIV) infection is rare in the community, then patients who have weight loss and fatigue are far more likely to have depression than acquired immunodeficiency syndrome. The reverse may be true in some other communities.

Judgment: Using Probabilities to Make Decisions

After analyzing the data and developing a working diagnosis, you should make a judgment about further testing. The usefulness of a test in confirming the diagnosis depends on how accurate the test is and how well it performs in a given population with a certain prevalence of the disease being considered. For some well-researched fields, (e.g., coronary artery disease), these probabilities are reasonably well known, based on numerous epidemiologic studies of risk factors, outcomes of treatment, effectiveness of tests, and so on. But for many other important problems in primary care, there are few data available on which to base decisions for patients. This is one of the great challenges and opportunities for research by generalists (4). Evidence-based medicine, which is discussed later in this chapter, provides specific data on tests, which can be used to evaluate their usefulness in clinical situations.

Evidence-based knowledge of the properties of tests and treatments is not enough, however. Other factors should influence your judgments; these include cost, time, convenience for the patient, and any potential adverse effects of the testing or therapy. Finally, and most importantly, the patient's personality, anxieties, and social situation may all bear on your clinical decision. Is this patient well known in the practice for "crying wolf" over minor symptoms? Is the patient the family breadwinner who will lose income while submitting to hospital tests? How high is the patient's need for reassurance that he is not seriously ill? How far does he or she trust the doctor (unaided by laboratory tests) to provide this reassurance?

"Knowledge" of the patient (as in the telephone call, when the doctor knew that Johnny's mother was "reliable") is relevant data accumulated from past experience. Long-term continuity with an individual and family helps the physician learn how they deal with stress, what they believe about their health, how they take their medications, and how responsible they are in managing their own problems. All of these factors enter the melting pot of clinical decision making.

Clinical Uncertainty

In primary care practice, uncertainty "goes with the territory" (5). Diagnostic uncertainty comes from three sources:

- Cognitive uncertainty, which is related to the physician's perception of the clinical problem;

- The feeling state (anxiety, usually) of the physician; and

- The variability of the patient's response to communication and therapy.

In many cases, the physician is not able to make a specific diagnosis or will need to wait a period of time before the diagnosis becomes clear or the patient gets better. It is not uncommon for physicians to identify and treat symptoms, realizing that they may resolve spontaneously before a diagnosis is made; examples include diarrhea and abdominal pain, both of which typically resolve without a specific, laboratory-confirmed diagnosis.

In resolving uncertainty, *time* is a very powerful diagnostic tool. Its effective use requires considerable skill, however. The physician who is too anxious to await the evolution of a symptom may order unnecessary tests and have the patient return too frequently, at considerable cost. On the other hand, the physician who does not consider more than one hypothesis or who does not ask the patient to return is likely to miss the diagnosis.

Methods of managing uncertainty include:

- Sharing your uncertainty with colleagues and patients
- Educating patients about possible outcomes
- Reassuring them that you will continue to observe them for diagnostic clues

The degree of uncertainty faced by primary care clinicians is greater than that faced by other providers because of the larger numbers of undifferentiated problems and relative lack of research data. As a result, good communication and follow-up between doctor and patient is essential. Management of clinical uncertainty is one of the keys to the craft and science of primary care.

Writing a Problem-Oriented Progress Note

When you see a patient in the family practice office, we recommend that you write problem-oriented progress notes. Each progress note should be organized as follows:

Problem No. 1: (here name the primary problem addressed—for example, fever and cough, or well person examination)

    S (for subjective): (all relevant historical data)
    O (for objective): (physical examination and laboratory data)
    A (for assessment): (your clinical impression)
    P (for plans): (plans for therapy, additional testing, and patient education)

Organize the next progress note the same way.

Problem No. 2: (name the second problem)

    S:
    O:
    A:
    P:

Progress in a similar manner for however many problems you actually address in the visit (on average, a family physician addresses either one and two problems per encounter).

Prescription Writing

The prescription is your formal communication of therapeutic plans regarding a medication. It should be legible and complete. Figure 13.3 provides a model prescription, with labels discussing its components.

EVIDENCE-BASED MEDICINE (EBM)

In evidence-based medicine, the physician makes diagnostic and therapeutic decisions based on an exhaustive review of the relevant medical literature. For example, if you practiced EBM when you saw a patient with a sore throat, you would:

- Think in terms of the probability of certain diagnoses.
- Ask questions, perform physical examination maneuvers, and choose laboratory tests based on knowledge of their sensitivity, specificity, and ability to effectively narrow a differential diagnosis.
- Once a diagnosis is reached, select the treatment whose ability to affect important patient outcomes is supported by the highest level of evidence.

To practice in an evidence-based manner, you must have ready access to objective, exhaustive, up-to-date reviews of research findings about the properties of available testing or treatment options. Citing a reference is not practicing EBM; all too often single references reflect research that is methodologically weak or not relevant to the patient the physician is treating. Because the literature is vast, such reviews must be performed by others and then made readily available to the physician. Admittedly, the current state of medicine is that EBM can only be practiced partially, because the needed data are either not available or not readily accessible. However, medical research is increasingly generating relevant data, and improvements in information science are making it more readily accessible to practitioners. Thus, EBM can be expected to have an increasingly prominent role in all medical practice over the coming decades.

There are many sources of evidence-based medical information. A helpful framework for evaluating the usefulness of data is to use the following equation:

$$\text{Usefulness of medical information} = \frac{(\text{Relevance} \times \text{Validity})}{\text{Work}}$$

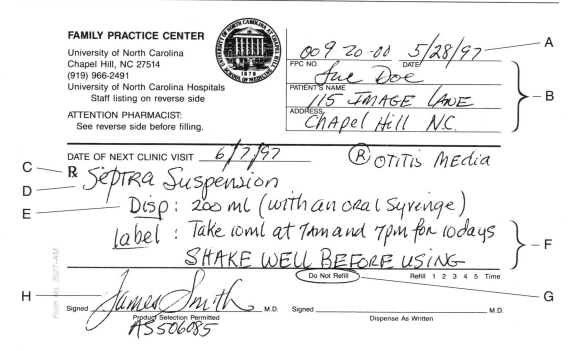

Figure 13.3. *Standard prescription form.* A. Date: Schedule II medication prescriptions must be filled within 72 hours after writing. Schedule III and IV prescriptions cannot be filled or refilled 6 months after writing. **B.** Patient's name and address: Required on schedule II prescriptions. **C.** Superscription: designated as the symbol Rx, the abbreviation for recipe (Latin for "take thou"). **D.** Inscription. The body of the prescription, containing the name and strength of the drug. **E.** Subscription. The direction(s) to the pharmacist, detailing the amount of the drug to be dispensed, such as "dispense 30 tablets," "dispense 3 months (of oral contraceptives)," or "dispense 120 mL with an oral syringe." **F.** Transcription: The directions for the patient. Latin abbreviations (e.g., bid, ac, qhs) should not be used. The directions cover the amount of drug to be taken, the timing and frequency of dosing, route of administration, and duration of therapy. Directions for use should always begin with a verb such as "take," "apply," or "insert." Use directions that remind the patient of the purpose of the prescription, such as "for pain relief" or "to relieve itching." **G.** Refill information: Schedule II drugs cannot be refilled and Schedule III and IV prescriptions cannot be refilled more than five times within the 6-month duration. Unless refills are specified, always circle or write "Do Not Refill" to prevent forgeries for extra refills. **H.** Signature. The physician's personal signature, Drug Enforcement Agency registry number, and practice address.

Thus, valid information that is relevant to your practice but doesn't take much work to access is the most useful. Although the information in a journal article may be highly valid because the authors used a strong design, it may be hard to find this particular article (high work) and the patients studied may not be representative of those in your practice (low relevance). Similarly, although the advice from a colleague may be quick to access (low work) and relevant to primary care practice (high relevance), the validity may be low if it is based on anecdote rather than objective research. These sources, rated for relevance, validity, and work, are summarized in Table 13.2.

In this textbook, we have incorporated evidence-based approaches whenever feasible. To best utilize that information, you'll need some background.

Evaluating the Evidence: "Critical Appraisal" of the Literature

Critical appraisal of the literature is the application of clinical epidemiology to published human research. Its principles include:

- An emphasis on the clinicians' perspective. Whereas traditional epidemiology has a population focus and studies the causation of

Table 13.2.
Sources of Medical Information, Ranked by Their Usefulness[a]

Information Source	Relevance	Validity	Work Required	Usefulness
Evidence-based textbook	High	High	Low	High
Systematic review (evidence-based)	High	High	Low	High
Portable summary of systematic reviews	High	High	Low	High
Internet in 10 years	High	High	Low	High
Drug reference book *(PDR)*	High	Mod	Low	High-mod
JFP journal club, ACP journal club, evidence-based medicine	Moderate	High	Low	High-mod
Colleagues	High	Mod	Low	High-mod
Practice guidelines (evidence-based)	Mod	High	Low	High-mod
Cochrane Database of Systematic Reviews	Mod-High	High	Mod-High	High-mod
Standard textbook	High	Low	Low	Mod
Standard journal review	High	Mod	Mod	Mod
Free medical newspapers	High	Low	Low	Mod
CME lectures	Mod	Mod	Low	Mod
CME small groups	High	Mod	Mod	Mod
Consensus statements	Mod	Mod	Low	Mod
Practice guidelines (consensus)	Mod	Mod	Low	Mod
Online searching	Mod	High	High	Mod
Journal articles	Low	High	Mod	Low
Drug advertising	Mod	Low	Low	Low
Drug company representatives	High	Low	Low	Low
Mass media	Low	Low	Low	Low
Internet now	Low	Low	High	Low

Adapted from Smith R. What clinical information do doctors need? Br Med J 1996;313:1062–1068.

ACP, American College of Physicians; CME, continuing medical education.

[a] Usefulness is (relevance × validity)/work.

disease, clinical epidemiology emphasizes the fundamental questions physicians face: diagnosis, prognosis, and treatment.

- Application of a set of guidelines derived from epidemiology to specific articles. The particular set of guidelines depends on the clinical question being addressed: diagnosis, prognosis, treatment, or causation.

- A focus on the internal validity of studies. Concerns of internal validity revolve around whether the design is randomized, the outcomes are appropriate, there are confounding effects, and so on.

- Evaluation of the external validity of studies. Concerns of external validity deal with whether or not the subjects in a study were similar to the patients you see in your practice.

Evidence-Based Approaches to Diagnosis

To make a diagnosis, physicians apply a variety of "diagnostic tests," including:

- Items from the history, such as whether and where chest pain radiates

- Questionnaires, such as the Michigan Alcoholism Screening Test (MAST)

- Elements of the physical examination, such as a Homan's sign in suspected thrombophlebitis

- Laboratory tests, such as the rapid strep test

When you use a test, you expect it to provide information that will help you decide whether or not your patient has a certain diagnosis (such as angina pectoris) or category of diagnoses (such as heart disease).

To evaluate its usefulness in clinical practice, a diagnostic test should have information available about its performance against a "gold standard," (i.e., the best single test or combination of tests for a particular diagnosis). Articles on a diagnostic test should, based on the test's performance against the gold standard, report the sensitivity, specificity, positive predictive value, and negative predictive value of the test. In addition, many studies now report the positive and negative likelihood ratios.

Sensitivity, Specificity, Predictive Value, and Likelihood Ratios

Traditionally, the ability of a test to distinguish between diseased and healthy patients has been described using the terms sensitivity and specificity. These terms are defined as follows:

- Sensitivity is the likelihood of a positive/abnormal test result among patients who have the disease.

- Specificity is the likelihood of a negative/normal test result among patients who do not have the disease.

Sensitivity and specificity are characteristics of a test, and do not vary from setting to setting or when the overall prevalence of disease changes. The major limitation of sensitivity and specificity is that when we order the test, we don't know if the patient has disease; that is why we are ordering the test in the first place!

Determining the likelihood of disease given a positive or negative test result, which is much more useful clinically, requires a complicated transformation called "Bayes' theorem." Physicians are not very good at making this transformation, as the following example will demonstrate:

QUESTION

Based on her age and risk factors, assume your patient has a 1% probability of breast cancer when you order her screening mammogram. Further, assume that the mammogram is 90% sensitive and 90% specific. If your patient has a positive mammogram, what is the likelihood that she has cancer?

DISCUSSION

When given this scenario, most physicians and students estimate that the likelihood of cancer is between 50 and 90%. However, the actual answer is only 8.3%! How can this be? Consider a group of 1000 women identical to your patient. Only 10 will have

---

cancer (1% probability), and 9 of the 10 will have their cancer detected by the mammogram (90% sensitivity). Of the 990 without cancer, 90% (891 women) will have a normal mammogram (90% specific). The remaining 99 healthy women will have a false-positive mammogram. Therefore, of the 108 positive mammograms (9 true positives + 99 false positives), only 9 will represent a malignancy (8.3%).

The figure of 8.3% quoted in the previous paragraph is the positive predictive value, and tells you the likelihood that a patient with a positive test has the disease in question. Conversely, the negative predictive value is the likelihood that a patient with a negative or normal test does not have the disease in question (99.9% in the above example). Positive and negative predictive values vary from setting to setting and will depend on the prevalence of the disease in the population, which is not always easy to estimate in clinical practice. Two useful clinical pearls emerge from an understanding of positive and negative predictive values and their relationship to the prevalence of disease:

- If a disease is rare, a positive test result probably represents a false positive, and should be confirmed or repeated.

- If the disease is common, a negative test result may well represent a false negative, and should not overly reassure you.

Likelihood ratios are another useful way to interpret information about diagnostic tests. They integrate the sensitivity and specificity into a more clinically relevant measure that reflects the way clinicians think diagnostically about ruling in or ruling out disease. Often a test has two possible outcomes, positive or negative, and therefore has two likelihood ratios:

$$\text{Positive likelihood ratio (LR+)} = \text{sensitivity}/(100 - \text{specificity})$$

$$\text{Negative likelihood ratio (LR-)} = (100 - \text{sensitivity})/\text{specificity}$$

where sensitivity and specificity are expressed as percentages from 0 to 100.

Some sample likelihood ratios are shown in Table 13.3. Interpreting the LR+ and LR- is easy:

Table 13.3.
Sample Likelihood Ratios for Various Tests

Diagnosis	Test	LR+	LR−
Streptococcal pharyngitis	Rapid antigen screen	9	0.1
Sarcoidosis	Bilateral hilar adenopathy on chest radiograph	76	0.25
Pancreatitis	Abnormal serum lipase level	24	0.06
Systemic lupus erythematosus	Antinuclear antibody	5	0.013
Systemic lupus erythematosus	anti-ds-DNA	25	0.25
Pelvic inflammatory disease	Cervical motion tenderness	2.3	0.70
Appendicitis	Psoas sign	3.2	0.88
Acute cholecystitis (young patients)	Murphy's sign	1.9	.06

LR+, positive likelihood ratio; LR−, negative likelihood ratio.

the higher the LR+, the more likely disease is, and the lower the LR−, the less likely disease is. Values of LR+ above 10 to 20 are generally believed to rule a disease "in" without further testing, whereas values of the LR− below 0.1 rule it out. Therefore, from Table 13.3, it is clear that the presence of bilateral hilar adenopathy is valuable in ruling "in" suspected sarcoidosis, but its absence is not as valuable in ruling it out. On the other hand, Murphy's sign is especially useful when absent in ruling out acute cholecystitis in young patients. However, it is relatively nonspecific; so its presence is not as good at ruling in disease.

Using Likelihood Ratios in Clinical Practice (See Nomogram on Inside Cover of This Book)

It is possible to estimate changes in the likelihood of disease based on the results of a test. Begin with an estimate of how likely you think disease is before any test results are available. For example, say that you estimate the likelihood of streptococcal pharyngitis among patients with sore throat in your practice to be approximately 20%. You see a patient, administer a rapid strep antigen test, and get a positive result. Next, refer to the nomogram in the inside cover of this book, and find 20% along the left axis. Then, draw a line from 20% through 9 on the middle axis (the LR+ for a rapid antigen screen is 9), and extend the line until you hit the right-hand axis. You should cross that line at approximately 70%; this is the probability of strep if the rapid antigen screen result is positive.

What if the test result is negative? Draw a line from 20% on the left axis through 0.1 on the mid-

dle axis (the LR− for a rapid antigen screen is 0.1), and extend the line until you hit the right-hand axis. You will cross that line at approximately 2.5%; this is your revised probability of strep given that the rapid antigen screen result is negative.

It is also possible to estimate the likelihood of disease using the LR+ and LR− without the nomogram. It requires that you be able to convert probability to odds, and back again. With a little practice, this can be done very rapidly at the bedside. A probability of 1% is the same as odds of 1:99; 10% = 1:9; 20% = 1:4; 50% = 1:1; 80% = 4:1; 90% = 9:1; 99% = 99:1, and so on.

Taking our strep example again, a 20% probability of strep is the same as odds of 1:4. To calculate the odds of disease with a positive test, multiply 1:4 by the LR+2 of 9. The result, 9:4, is the odds of streptococcal pharyngitis in patients with a positive test. Odds of 9:4 are the same as a probability of 9/13, or approximately 70%. If the test result is negative, multiply 1:4 by the LR− of 0.1. The result is 0.1:4, which is equivalent to a probability of 0.1/4.1, or approximately 2.5%.

It is important to remember, especially when the "test" being evaluated is an element of the history or physical examination, that it be performed in a standardized way. Careful attention to detail, practice, and preference for simpler, more reproducible maneuvers and questions are all-important.

Clinical Prediction Rules

When physicians see a patient, they typically apply multiple diagnostic tests in rapid succession. Doing an evaluation of someone with chest pain, for example, may involve gathering dozens of pieces of information from the history, physical, and laboratory. It's not reasonable to expect the physician to mentally keep altering probabilities formally during this process; yet some guidance needs to be provided on the overall diagnostic process. This is especially important because we know that personal experience with a few patients may be misleading. Indeed, the practice of educating medical students exclusively in tertiary care hospitals, which fortunately is changing, has contributed to this problem. Other forms of information-gathering that can over-influence the physician include a recent journal article (especially about a rare or bizarre outcome) and opinions from colleagues or experts that are based on anecdote rather than actual data.

Clinical prediction rules are tools that take the experience of a group of physicians with hundreds or even thousands of patients and distill that into a simple score or scale. Hundreds of clinical prediction rules have been developed, and many have been well validated. Examples include

- The Ottawa Ankle Rules, which help clinicians determine which patients with ankle pain need a radiograph.

- A strep score, which estimates the probability a patient has streptococcal pharyngitis based on key items from the history and physical examination.

- The CAGE questions, which screen for alcoholism (see Table 15.3, Screening Questions for Alcohol Abuse).

- A treadmill score, which estimates the likelihood of a cardiac event in the next 4 years among patients who have had an exercise electrocardiogram, based on elements of the history and the test results.

Evidence-Based Approaches to Prognosis

Prognosis is an important element of family medicine. It is often the most useful advice the physician can give a patient. In addition, it is part of the decision-making process in virtually every patient encounter. Consider the example of a 4-year-old child who has diarrhea. If you could determine, based on his activity level, ability to take oral fluids well, amount of fever, and absence of blood in the stool, that he had a greater than 95% chance of spontaneous recovery within 2 weeks

without antibiotics, you could be reassuring to the mother and would not launch into a laboratory evaluation.

Often, information about prognosis is based on experience, and indeed an experienced family physician's assessment of prognosis is generally very good. For students and for rare conditions, but indeed for even the most common conditions, access to good, relevant data can sharpen the clinician's prognostic ability.

For most studies of prognosis, a randomized design is not possible; one cannot, for example, randomize hazardous exposures like tobacco use or hyperbilirubinemia. The next strongest design is a cohort study, in which subjects are identified and followed up over years. A well-designed cohort study identifies the people at the beginning (an inception cohort), which allows better measurements of exposures and better tracking of the group, and is stronger methodologically than identifying a group retrospectively. For example, a well-designed study of prognosis for children with neonatal hyperbilirubinemia should have the following characteristics:

- Subjects in the study are similar to those seen in primary care offices.

- Subjects are followed up for enough years to ensure that the clinically relevant outcomes have an opportunity to occur.

- The study is large enough to identify rare outcomes and track and adjust for possible confounding variables.

- The study does not lose more than 20% of subjects to follow-up.

This kind of "ideal study" is not often done; however, the summarization of multiple studies, with an emphasis of those with good design from primary care settings, can help guide the physician in an evidence-based manner.

Evidence-Based Approaches to Therapy

Therapy is any intervention made by a clinician to prevent, cure, or ameliorate disease. It includes not only prescription drugs and surgery, but other kinds of interventions as well, such as an exercise program to lower cholesterol, physician advice about screening mammograms, or over-the-counter medication for allergies. In evaluating the literature on a therapy, the following must be considered:

- Whether or not there was a control group. Although controlling sounds basic, it is surprising how often new technologies or drugs are promoted on the basis of uncontrolled studies.

- How similar the experimental and control groups were at the beginning of the trial. Randomization is the best way to make the control and experimental groups similar.

- Whether the outcomes that were measured are the ones you and your patients care about.

- Whether outcomes were measured objectively, using (if possible) persons who were unaware of whether a subject was in the treatment or control group.

- Whether the results, if statistically significant, are clinically meaningful. Studies with large numbers of subjects can yield results that are statistically significant but clinically unimportant, and studies with small numbers of subjects can yield results that would be clinically important if, with larger numbers, statistical significance were achieved.

- Whether the study results are likely to generalize to your population. The more dissimilar the study population was from your patients, and the more dissimilar the study conditions were from the office and community settings, the more concern you should have about whether a study really is applicable to your population.

To learn more about EBM concepts presented previously, please visit the Mount Sinai School of Medicine, Levy Library web site: http://academic.mssm.edu/library/resources/ebm.htm. It's practical, well-organized, links to other important EBM sources, and is easy to use.

Nomenclature Used in This Book to Evaluate Therapies

In this book, many of the chapters evaluate the available literature on therapies, and to some extent on diagnostic procedures, using a system adapted from the Canadian Task Force on the Periodic Examination and the United States Preventive Services Task Force to evaluate the level of evidence. Letter grades are assigned that correspond to the strength of the evidence supporting the specific therapeutic maneuver: A, good evidence exists to support the use of the treatment; B, fair evidence exists to support the treatment; C, insufficient evidence exists to recommend for or against the treatment, although it may be recommended for other reasons, such as clinical tradition; X, existing evidence supports excluding the treatment from usual practice.

The emphasis is on the quality of the evidence. Higher weight is given to study designs that are less subject to bias and inferential error, include important patient-oriented outcomes, and that studied populations similar to those in primary care. In evaluating specific therapeutic maneuvers, we looked for well-done, randomized-controlled trials in primary care settings, with an A grade corresponding roughly to more than one randomized controlled trial and a B grade corresponding to the presence of multiple controlled trials. Well-designed and well-conducted meta-analyses are graded according the quality of the pooled studies.

The purpose of this grading system is not to censure current clinical practice, but rather to provide a current assessment of the scientific basis of clinical practice. Much of what we do as clinicians merits a C recommendation, because very few of our common practices have been examined rigorously. Indeed, a lot of medical practice is based on the fact that we have always done it a certain way or because authorities say we should do it that way.

How then should clinicians use the grading system to improve their practice? We know that every clinical encounter includes countless elements, most of which have a grade of C. As much as possible, however, the clinician should strive to include interventions graded A or B and exclude the X recommendations from routine practice. Furthermore, because most of what physicians do lacks evidence of effectiveness, clinicians should maintain an attitude of continuing self-examination, constantly submitting what they do to investigation, and asking, "Does this diagnostic or therapeutic maneuver improve my patients' outcomes?"

Practice Guidelines

One application of evidence-based methods has been the development of practice guidelines. The process of making guidelines has been pioneered by the U.S. Agency for Health Care Policy and Research (AHCPR), which has convened panels of experts to conduct evidence-based literature reviews, from which they make practical recommendations for clinicians. Over 18 guidelines have been produced by the AHCPR, including such primary care-focused issues as the management of low back pain, the early detection of Alzhheimer's disease, and the management of otitis media. A variety of other organizations have issued their own guidelines, which generally represent some degree of synthesis and some degree of the application of evidence-based principles.

Guidelines have become popular in part because of the growth of health systems and managed care, who find guidelines helpful in standardizing care and in developing definitions of "quality" care. The reason for this change in perspective is that clinical decision making is the key factor in generating health care costs, and primary care is one of the main gateways to controlling complex and expensive medicine (6). Consumer guides on the same topics are also offered by these agencies. Information on guidelines can be obtained from the following:

- American Academy of Family Physicians: (816) 333–9700, http://www.aafp.org/;

- American Academy of Pediatrics: (847) 228–5005, http://www.aap.org/;

- American Medical Association: (312) 464–5000, http://www.ama-assn.org/;

- American College of Physicians: (800) 523–1546, http://www.acponline.org/;

- Agency for Health Care Policy and Research: (800) 358–9295, http://www.ahcpr.gov/.

CLINICAL DECISIONS IN FAMILY PRACTICE

The final part of the decision-making process is the point at which the physician makes the judgment of what and how to inform the patient of the possible diagnosis, further testing options, referral or treatment and prognosis of the problem. This involves discussing benefits and risks of a range of plans, including the value and dangers of tests or effects and reactions to medications.

We now realize that shared decision making between patient and physician offers the most ethical and satisfactory approach to providing care, but it is not easy (7, 8). First, there is a natural deference by patients toward "experts," which makes it easy for the physician's opinion to dominate the process. Second, there may be cultural or social barriers that make the patient feel inadequate or vulnerable. Third, it is hard for

physicians to realize that they may not always know what is best for the patient. Finally, it is difficult to genuinely attain a full understanding of patient preferences in a short office visit.

In hospital settings, the majority of clinical decisions fall into only three categories: ordering a treatment; ordering a test; or obtaining a consultation. By contrast, in family practice, the variety of potential decisions is much richer (9). In addition to the three just cited, others include:

- Giving reassurance without treatment

- Dealing with a problem other than the presenting one

- Rechecking the patient at a return visit

- Counseling the patient and/or family

- Collecting data from other sources (family, other physicians, psychotherapists, physical therapists, and so forth)

- A therapeutic trial

- Arranging community resources (e.g., home nursing)

It is this wealth of alternatives, presenting themselves in almost every encounter in family practice, that gives this specialty much of its challenge as well as much of its fascination. These decisions lead to specific plans that may or may not address the patient's original "problem." Plans are made in the context of the potential positive actions that can occur at each visit:

- Management of the presenting problem

- Enhancement of the doctor-patient relationship

- Modification of help-seeking behaviors by patients

- Management of continuing problems

- Opportunistic health promotion

- Enlargement of the patient's database

In situations in which you may be observing experienced office-based physicians in action, try to identify their clinical reasoning styles and discuss the process with them. They will give you insight into your own.

THE "PROBLEM" PATIENT

Family physicians and their office staff groan when they see certain names on the schedule. These "problem" patients take extra time, are emotionally draining, and often do not respond well to treatment. They are also twice as likely to have a psychiatric diagnosis than the remainder of family practice patients (10), the most common of which are somatoform disorder, panic disorder, dysthymia, generalized anxiety, major depression, and alcohol abuse or dependence. Compared with "nonproblem" patients, these patients have more functional impairment, higher health care utilization, and lower satisfaction with care. Underlying mental disorders account for a substantial proportion of the excess functional impairment and dissatisfaction that problem patients have over nonproblem patients.

When you have a "bad" interaction with a patient, chances are that one or more of the following has occurred:

- Personality clash between the patient and the physician
- Stress and/or fatigue on the part of the patient or physician
- Lack of understanding
- Lack of common goals
- Battle for control
- Transference and countertransference
- Patient borderline personality disorder

The last two processes are common situations that "push the doctor's 'buttons'" (e.g., a substance-abusing patient presents to a physician who has not worked through his/her own parent's addiction).

If you have negative feelings toward a patient, acknowledge them (but, in most cases, not to the patient). Examine them and try to understand why and how they developed, and how you can overcome them. Talking about such a patient with one or more colleagues is the best method of working through such feelings; a spouse or office staff member can also serve this role. Many family physicians have found it extremely useful to get together regularly to discuss problem patients in so-called Balint groups (11).

With experience, physicians learn to recognize the challenging personality patterns and interaction styles of problem patients and to handle such encounters more successfully. Indeed, learning to manage problem patients is one of the goals of family practice residency training, for the fact that a patient is a "problem" suggests that there are solutions. Successful management strategies with such patients often involve:

- Getting to know the patient better—personality, life circumstances, hopes, fears, values, and personal support system
- Involving the patient in therapeutic decisions
- Setting limited goals (e.g., fewer emergency department visits, or accepting a partial rather than a complete cure)
- Developing a strong physician-patient relationship (and having the same physician manage all calls and encounters with the patient, except in emergency situations)
- Defining behavioral limits (e.g., only one narcotic injection a week), but providing the patient with some control
- Frequent, regular office visits (e.g., once a week) until problems are less acute

CASE STUDY 4

A family practice resident was seeing a patient who was not his regular patient. She was a 32-year-old woman with long-standing systemic lupus erythematosus and a seizure disorder, who had come to the clinic because of a slowly growing tumor on her right thigh. She had a history of thromboembolic events and was convinced the lump was a "blood clot." The physical examination was consistent with a lipoma (a benign tumor), but when offered that explanation, she replied, "Wrong!" in a sarcastic manner, excluding it based on her earlier experiences with blood clots and information gained from the Internet. "I don't like this patient," the resident later stated to his faculty preceptor.

DISCUSSION

This patient-physician encounter involved a battle for control and possibly a hidden agenda. In situations like this, when the patient appears to have a great deal invested in being "right" and in control (with a disease that is quite hard to control), questions like "Where do we go from here?" or "What would you like me to do?" may help the patient and physician join forces instead of being at odds with each other. Open-ended questions about other problems or concerns, such as the frequency of her seizures, may also be helpful.

In fact, this patient has probably been exposed to many providers (including this resident) who did not know as much about her signs and symptoms as she does. So it might make her more comfortable if you relinquish a little control, by saying something like, "I know that someone with a complex disease like yours learns more about it and takes more responsibility as time goes on; tell me more about your experiences," or to have the patient bring in her information so that you both can learn from it. Acknowledging her expertise and not threatening the patient is important in this instance.

HOW THE COMMON PROBLEM CHAPTERS ARE ORGANIZED IN THIS BOOK

The remainder of this book consists of chapters on one or a group of related common problems. Each begins with several questions that highlight key learning points of the chapter. Next, the chapters proceed to sections that mirror the typical flow of a physician-patient encounter: background (including clinical epidemiology and pathophysiology), clinical evaluation, and management. Special considerations are then covered. Finally, case studies, often with questions and discussion, are presented.

Most visits for common problems fall into two categories, each of which demands a somewhat different approach:

- Visits in which the patient comes in with one or more symptoms (e.g., abdominal pain or dizziness), and the job of the physician involves making a tentative diagnosis, from which a management plan is developed; and

- Visits in which the patient already has a diagnosis (e.g., hypertension or HIV disease), and the majority of the physician's work involves optimal management of the disease and its complications.

This being the case, the organization of our chapters varies somewhat so as to focus on the type of

decision making that you are most likely to need to manage a specific common problem.

Whenever it is relevant, we have tried to summarize key information in quick-access tables and figures. These are standardized across the chapters. Like the text, the series of tables and figures for each topic models clinical thinking. These standard tables and figures include:

- Differential diagnosis (symptom chapters only)

- Key elements of the clinical evaluation

- Red flags suggesting serious and/or emergent problems

- Diagnostic testing

- General approach to the patient (a flowchart)

- Management

- Drug therapy

We have incorporated evidence-based approaches into the chapters in several ways. We have, whenever possible, drawn from and/or conducted our own evidence-based reviews of the literature, and used existing clinical guidelines to help inform our writing. In discussing areas of the clinical evaluation (the history, physical examination, and laboratory testing), we have tried to locate and provide information on sensitivity, specificity and positive and negative likelihood ratios, and at the front of the book we provide a nomogram for interpreting likelihood ratios. Finally, in discussing therapies, we have attempted to provide information on levels of evidence using a standard nomenclature (A, strong supportive evidence for effectiveness; B, limited research-based evidence; C, common practice with little or no evidence; and X, evidence against effectiveness).

REFERENCES

1. Barsky AJ. Hidden reasons some patients visit doctors. Ann Intern Med 1981;94:492–498.
2. Engel GL. The clinical application of the psychosocial model. Am J Psych 1980;137:535–544.
3. Barrows HS, Norman GR, Neufeld VR, Feightner JW. The clinical reasoning process of randomly selected physicians in general medical practice. Clin Invest Med 1982;5:49–55.
4. Marley DS, Mengel MB. Clinical decision making. In: Mengel M, ed. Principles of Clinical Practice, vol. 11. New York: Plenum, 1991:99–123.
5. Mushlin AI. Uncertain decision making in primary care: causes and solutions. Primary Care Research: Theory and Methods Conference. US

Department of Health and Human Services Agency for Health Care Policy and Research, September 1991:153–166.

6. Eddy DM. Clinical Decision Making: From Theory to Practice: A Collection of Essays from the Journal of the American Medical Association. Sudbury, MA: Jones and Bartlett Publishers, 1996.

7. Helman CG. Culture, Health and Illness, 2nd ed. London: Wright, 1990.

8. Stewart M, Brown JB, Weston WW, et al. Patient-centered Medicine. Transforming the Clinical Method. Thousand Oaks, CA: Sage Publications, 1995.

9. Stott NCH, Davis RH. The exceptional potential in each primary care consultation. J R Coll Gen Pract 1979; 29:201–205.

10. Kahn S, Kronke K, Spitzer R, et al. The difficult patient: prevalence, psychopathology, and functional impairment. J Gen Intern Med 1996;11:1–8.

11. Balint M. The Doctor, His Patient, and the Illness. New York: International Universities Press, 1972.

14. Abdominal Pain

JOHN J. SMUCNY AND LORNE A. BECKER

Key Clinical Questions

1. Does the patient have a surgical (acute) abdomen?
2. Is the pain acute or chronic?
3. Is the pain due to an intra-abdominal or an extra-abdominal condition?
4. Are diagnostic tests or a specialty consultation necessary?

More than 25% of adults and 75% of adolescents report abdominal pain during the preceding year, and for most, the pain is recurrent (1, 2). Although only a minority seek medical attention, this complaint is still one of the most commonly presenting symptoms in primary care (1). Conditions that cause abdominal pain range from the urgently life-threatening to the benign and self-limited, and may result from intra-abdominal or extra-abdominal pathology. Although no specific diagnosis can be determined in one-half of patients who present to family physicians with abdominal pain, a logical and comprehensive approach will allow you to formulate an accurate differential diagnosis and appropriate management plan (3).

The most important determination in evaluating a patient with abdominal pain is whether the patient has a "surgical" abdomen; these patients require immediate referral to a surgeon for further evaluation. Next, decide whether the patient's pain is acute or chronic; this allows you to determine the pace of further evaluation. Patients with acute pain may require more prompt evaluation and treatment than those with chronic pain. However, some of the conditions that cause chronic pain may be serious in their own right (e.g., pancreatic cancer), and others can develop very acute and life-threatening complications (e.g., perforation of a duodenal ulcer).

Many patients who complain of abdominal pain do not need diagnostic workups. Some conditions can be treated empirically, whereas others are self-limited and will resolve without specific therapy. Regardless of whether any tests are ordered, appropriate follow-up must be arranged. Depending on your differential diagnosis, options can include admission to the hospital for serial observations, a scheduled follow-up visit, or a reassessment at the patient's discretion if the condition does not resolve.

PATHOPHYSIOLOGY AND DIFFERENTIAL DIAGNOSIS

Intra-abdominal Conditions

Intra-abdominal conditions cause pain that is either visceral or parietal. Visceral pain is due to spasm or stretching of the muscle wall of a hollow viscus, distention of the capsule of a solid organ, or ischemia or inflammation of a visceral structure. The pain is typically deep, dull, and diffusely located in the epigastric, periumbilical, or hypogastric regions (see Fig. 14.1 for a diagram of the anatomic regions of the abdomen). The pain is midline because the innervation to most intra-abdominal viscera is bilateral, and pain is transmitted to the spinal cord and brain by bilateral autonomic sensory nerves. Epigastric visceral pain is mediated by both the celiac plexus and some of the parasympathetic nerves from the thorax; this type of pain can therefore be due to pathology in either the thoracic organs (heart, lungs, esophagus, mediastinum) or abdominal organs (stomach, duodenum, pancreas, liver, biliary system). Periumbilical visceral pain is mediated by the celiac and superior mesenteric ganglia and generally is due to disorders of the small intestine, cecum, or appendix. Hypogastric pain is mediated by the inferior mesenteric ganglion and pelvic parasympathetic nerves, and it results from disease in the colon, rectum, or pelvis.

Parietal pain is caused by irritation of the parietal peritoneum from a contiguous, diseased intra-abdominal organ. This type of pain (also called somatic or peritoneal) is sharper and more localized than visceral pain because the parietal peritoneum is innervated unilaterally by peripheral nerves that travel to the spinal cord at segmental levels. The pain is located directly over the

221

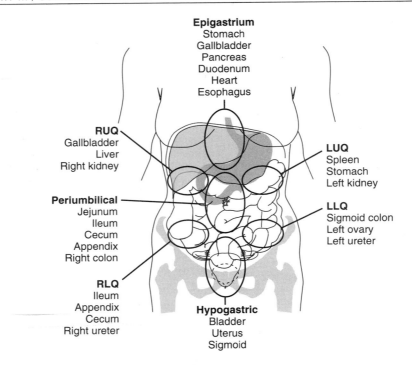

Epigastrium
Stomach
Gallbladder
Pancreas
Duodenum
Heart
Esophagus

RUQ
Gallbladder
Liver
Right kidney

LUQ
Spleen
Stomach
Left kidney

Periumbilical
Jejunum
Ileum
Cecum
Appendix
Right colon

LLQ
Sigmoid colon
Left ovary
Left ureter

RLQ
Ileum
Appendix
Cecum
Right ureter

Hypogastric
Bladder
Uterus
Sigmoid

Figure 14.1 *Structures that commonly cause abdominal pain, grouped by type and site of pain.*
LLQ, left lower quadrant; *LUQ,* left upper quadrant; *RLQ,* right lower quadrant; *RUQ,* right upper quadrant.
(Redrawn from Currie DJ. Abdominal Pain. Washington, DC: Hemisphere Publishing, 1979.)

anatomic location of the diseased organ and usually worsens with movement. Although parietal pain can be located anywhere in the abdomen, it most commonly lateralizes to the quadrant corresponding to the location of the diseased organ (see Fig. 14.1). Diffuse parietal pain represents generalized peritonitis, which occurs with perforation or rupture of an organ.

A few conditions characteristically progress from visceral to parietal pain. Appendicitis begins with periumbilical visceral pain and proceeds to right lower quadrant parietal pain; diverticulitis begins in the hypogastrium and lateralizes to the left lower quadrant; and pain from acute cholecystitis proceeds from the epigastrium to the right upper quadrant. Pain may also radiate from one location to another, depending on the innervation of the affected organ. For example, pancreatic pain often radiates from the epigastrium to the middle of the back, whereas pain in cholecystitis may radiate to the right subscapular area. Finally, some diseases cause referred pain in extra-abdominal locations, such as subphrenic abscesses, which can present with ipsilateral shoulder pain.

Extra-abdominal Conditions

Pain from extra-abdominal disease may be referred or radiate to the abdomen. For example, myocardial infarction (see Chapter 21) can present with epigastric pain; pneumonia (see Chapter 35) can cause ipsilateral upper quadrant pain; and testicular torsion or epididymitis can refer pain upward to the lower abdomen. Pain may radiate to the abdomen from the back as a result of any condition that causes spinal nerve root irritation, such as compression fractures (see Chapter 31), arthritis (see Chapter 18), or herpes zoster (see Chapter 36). Abdominal wall conditions, such as muscle strains and rectus sheath hematomas, cause pain directly due to inflammation of the associated tissues; this pain is usually constant and aching and increases with voluntary tightening of the abdominal wall. Renal diseases, such as pyelonephritis (see Chapter 25) or calculi, usually cause flank pain; the pain from calculi may radiate through the abdomen to the ipsilateral groin.

A wide variety of systemic and toxic conditions can cause abdominal pain, but most of these are uncommon. Some of the more common include sickle cell disease, diabetes mellitus, and uremia. Of course, patients with these medical problems may develop any other intra-abdominal disease as well. Rare causes of systemic or toxic conditions include porphyria, cholinesterase deficiency, black widow spider bites, and lead poisoning.

Finally, psychologic conditions can lead patients to complain of abdominal pain. Patients who have underlying stress or psychologic illness are more likely to present with conditions such as irritable bowel syndrome and nonulcer dyspepsia. Women with chronic pelvic pain may be survivors of physical or sexual abuse. In addition, patients who complain of abdominal pain may

actually have another reason for their visit, which can only be determined by appropriate history-taking. Therefore, in all but the most urgent situations, you should inquire into psychosocial issues.

Differential Diagnosis

Studies characterizing the most common causes of abdominal pain in primary care and emergency settings show that a relatively limited number of conditions cause the great majority of cases of abdominal pain, and a considerable number of patients will not be given a specific diagnosis (Table 14.1). The proportion of patients who need emergent referral to a surgeon is smaller in primary care clinics than in emergency

Table 14.1.
Differential Diagnosis in Adults with Abdominal Pain

Diagnosis	% of Total Visits for Abdominal Pain	
	Family Practice Office[a] (N = 556; age > 18)	Emergency Department[b] (N = 1000; age > 15)
Nonspecific abdominal pain	50.4	41.3
Acute gastroenteritis	9.2	6.9
Urinary tract infection/pyelonephritis	6.7	6.9
Irritable bowel syndrome	5.8	
Pelvic inflammatory disease	3.8	6.7
Hiatal hernia or reflux	2.3	
Diverticulosis	2.2	
Diarrhea, cause undetermined	1.6	
Cholelithiasis/cholecystitis	1.6	3.7
Tumor, benign	1.4	
Duodenal ulcer	1.4	2
Urolithiasis	1.3	4.3
Appendicitis	1.1	4.3
Ulcerative colitis	0.9	
Muscle strain	0.9	
Intestinal obstruction		2.5
Constipation		2.3
Dysmenorrhea		1.8
Simple pregnancy		1.8
Gastritis		1.4
Ovarian cyst		1.0
Incomplete abortion		0.9
Pancreatitis		0.9
Abdominal aneurysm		0.7
Epididymitis		0.7
Percent admitted	9.2	27.4
Percent undergoing surgery	4.7	15

[a]Adapted from Adelman A. Abdominal pain in the primary care setting. J Fam Pract 1987;25:27–32.

[b]Adapted from Brewer RJ, Golden GT, Hitch DC, Rudolf LE, Wangensteen SL. Abdominal pain—an analysis of 1,000 consecutive cases in a university hospital emergency room. Am J Surg 1976; 131:219–223.

departments. The prevalence of various conditions is also related to age; older adults with pain are more likely to have specific diagnoses and require urgent management (see Table 14.2).

Nonspecific abdominal pain (NSAP; or abdominal pain, etiology undetermined) is the most common diagnosis recorded in patients who present with abdominal pain. Half of the patients who present to family physicians (and over 40% who present to emergency departments or are admitted with acute abdominal pain) are given this diagnosis (3–5). These patients likely have a variety of specific causes for their pain and, in general, a good prognosis. When diagnostic coding for insurance purposes was compared with the medical record, 60% of patients coded as having NSAP did have a specific diagnosis listed in the physician's note (6); the most common were irritable bowel syndrome, infectious diarrhea, gastritis, muscle strains, ovarian cysts, and peptic ulcer disease. Most patients with NSAP have improvement or resolution of pain within days to months of presentation (5, 7, 8).

CLINICAL EVALUATION

The number of potential causes of abdominal pain can be narrowed by first considering the acuity and severity of the patient's condition. For acute or acutely worsening pain, "red flags" for emergent intervention are of primary importance (Table 14. 3). If the patient does not have any "red flags," you

Table 14.2.
Differential Diagnosis of Acute Abdominal Pain by Patient Age

	% of Total Patients with Acute Abdominal Pain	
Diagnosis	Age <50 (n = 6317)	Age >50 (n = 2406)
Nonspecific abdominal pain	39.5	15.7
Appendicitis	32	15.2
Cholecystitis	6.3	20.9
Bowel obstruction	2.5	12.3
Pancreatitis	1.6	7.3
Diverticular disease	<0.1	5.5
Cancer	<0.1	4.1
Hernia	<0.1	3.1
Vascular	<0.1	2.3

Adapted from Telfer S, Fenyo G, Holt PR, de Dombal FT. Acute abdominal pain in patients over 50 years of age. Scand J Gastroenterol 1988;23(suppl 144):42–50.

Table 14.3.
Red Flags Suggesting Life-Threatening Disease in Patients with Abdominal Pain

History	Diagnoses Suggested
Abrupt onset of pain	Perforation or rupture (ulcer, appendix, gallbladder, colon, ectopic pregnancy, spleen, abdominal aortic aneurysm) Acute vascular event (mesenteric infarction, aortic dissection, myocardial infarction, pulmonary embolus) Volvulus, strangulated hernia, ovarian torsion, pancreatitis

Examination	Diagnoses Suggested
Shock	Perforation or rupture (see above) with intra-abdominal hemorrhage or peritonitis, severe pancreatitis, acute vascular event (see above), gastrointestinal hemorrhage
Distention	Bowel obstruction, ileus, volvulus, toxic megacolon, bowel ischemia, intra-abdominal hemorrhage, abdominal aortic aneurysm, ascites
Peritoneal signs (diffuse)	Perforation or rupture (see above), severe pancreatitis, mesenteric infarction
Peritoneal signs (focal)	Appendicitis, diverticulitis, cholecystitis, cholangitis, abscess, pelvic inflammatory disease, pancreatitis

should determine whether the pain is visceral or parietal and the location of the pain. This process will narrow your differential diagnosis to a small number of likely causes of the patient's abdominal pain. For chronic or recurrent pain, the location of the pain and its associated symptoms help to refine the differential diagnosis. Diagnostic tests are then used, if needed, to confirm the most likely diagnoses or to exclude other potentially serious conditions (see Fig. 14.2 for an algorithmic approach to the diagnosis of abdominal pain).

History

The location, quality, timing, and severity of pain are the most important elements of the history (9). The location and quality of the pain can help you determine whether the pain is due to a visceral (deep, dull, diffuse, and midline), parietal

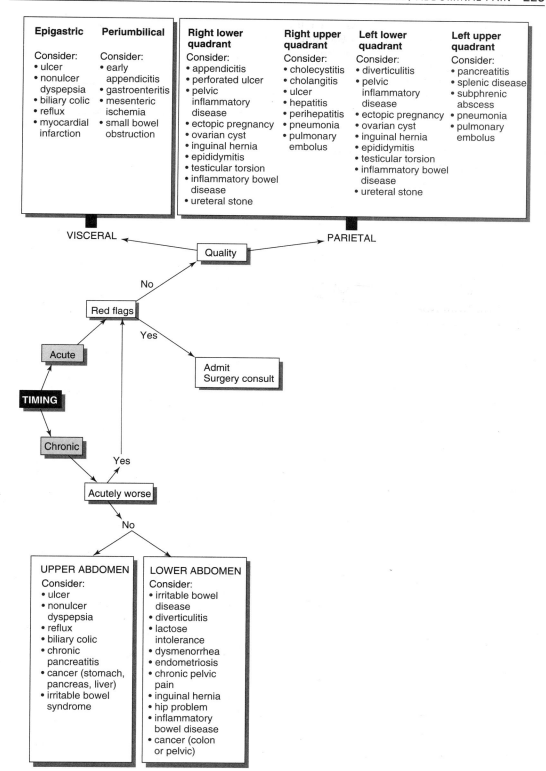

Figure 14.2. *Algorithmic approach to diagnosing nontraumatic abdominal pain in adults.*

(sharper, more localized, and usually lateralized to a quadrant), or extra-abdominal source. Timing and severity are important because the abrupt onset of severe pain often signifies a serious condition, such as perforation of a viscus (e.g., duodenal or gastric ulcer) or pelvic organ (e.g., ruptured ectopic pregnancy), obstruction of a nonintestinal viscus (e.g., ureter), or an acute vascular event (e.g., bowel infarct or leaking aortic aneurysm). Gradual onset of pain over a few hours to a few days is more likely to represent an inflammatory process (e.g., appendicitis or diverticulitis) or intestinal obstruction. The abrupt worsening of such pain may signify the perforation of the inflamed or obstructed organ. The temporal progression of pain is also helpful. Progression from visceral to parietal pain is characteristic of certain conditions, including appendicitis, cholecystitis, and diverticulitis. Colicky pain that comes and goes often represents gastroenteritis, a partial bowel obstruction, or irritable bowel syndrome (biliary "colic" is a misnomer, as this pain is generally steady). Additional items in the history you should obtain include associated symptoms, precipitating and/or alleviating factors, underlying medical conditions, and potentially toxic, infectious, or drug exposures. A menstrual history should be taken in all women of childbearing age (see Table 14.3) for a summary of "red flags" in the history that suggest life-threatening disease).

Physical Examination

The physical examination should be thorough and directed to determining first the need for urgent referral and then the most likely diagnoses. Urgent conditions usually manifest in one or more of three ways: shock, abdominal distention, or peritonitis (see Table 14.3). Shock may result from intra-abdominal hemorrhage or fluid sequestration, sepsis, or nonabdominal disease (e.g., acute myocardial infarction). Remember that patients in shock do not have to be overtly hypotensive; orthostatic hypotension is more sensitive in early cases. Potentially serious causes of abdominal distention include obstruction, intra-abdominal masses, and ascites. Peritonitis can be either diffuse or focal. Diffuse peritonitis is usually caused by perforation or hemorrhage of intra-abdominal organs; patients generally are in severe pain, lie motionless, and have absent bowel sounds, diffuse tenderness, guarding, and rigidity. Focal peritonitis results from inflammation that is local-

ized to a single structure in contact with the peritoneum (e.g., appendicitis); patients may be in as much pain as with diffuse peritonitis, but on examination tenderness, guarding and rigidity are usually localized to one area. Two specific clinical maneuvers useful in diagnosing peritonitis are the rebound tenderness test (LR+ 1.6, LR− 0.4) and the cough test, in which pain is worse with coughing (LR+ 3.7, LR− 0.3).

The physical examination of patients with abdominal pain (particularly if acute) should also include a brief examination of the back and thorax, palpation of all potential hernia orifices, a pelvic examination for females, a genital examination for males, and a rectal examination. Patients with severe disease may present with more subtle findings from the history and physical examination than described above. This is particularly true in the elderly and the immunocompromised; for these patients, you should have a lower threshold for more aggressive evaluation and referral.

Laboratory Tests

Because of the large number of conditions that can lead to abdominal pain, there are no specific diagnostic tests recommended for all patients. You should base your test selection on an assessment of the most likely diagnoses, and, if appropriate, the serious conditions that must be excluded (e.g., a pregnancy test should be checked in women of childbearing age to exclude ectopic pregnancy). Some patients, such as those with mild symptoms and normal examinations, may require no testing at all. "Watchful waiting" is a particularly useful diagnostic tool in the primary care setting, where patients often present early in the course of an illness and have an established relationship with their physician. Furthermore, the ability to rapidly obtain information from tests is usually more limited in office practice compared to emergency departments; therefore, direct referral prior to ordering tests may be appropriate in urgent situations. Diagnostic tests to consider in various circumstances are included in the discussion of specific conditions that follows.

Specific Conditions

The remainder of this chapter discusses the clinical evaluation of common conditions that present primarily as abdominal pain in adolescents and adults. Abdominal pain in the setting of trauma or pregnancy is beyond the scope of this chapter. Diseases that may include abdominal pain as part of the symptom complex, but generally have other more distinguishing characteristics, are also excluded. Examples of the latter (with their typical presentations) include gastroesophageal reflux (heartburn; see Chapter 20), hepatitis (jaundice), gastroenteritis (vomiting or diarrhea), inflammatory bowel disease (diarrhea), pyelonephritis (flank pain; see Chapter 25), renal calculi (flank pain radiating to the groin), cystitis (dysuria; see Chapter 25), and hernias (symptomatic bulge). These common conditions should be considered in the differential diagnosis of abdominal pain, when appropriate.

Biliary Tract Disease

Although 10% of men and 20% of women have gallstones, most are asymptomatic (10). Complications from gallstones include acute cholecystitis, choledocholithiasis (stones in the common bile duct), cholangitis, pancreatitis, gallstone ileus, and gallbladder cancer. The most common manifestation of gallstones is biliary pain (or "colic"). This is characterized by recurrent episodes of steady, severe pain in the epigastrium or right upper quadrant that typically lasts from 1 to 5 hours and often awakens the patient. The pain may radiate to the back or right scapular area, be precipitated by meals, and be associated with nausea and emesis, but these characteristics are only marginally helpful in diagnosing gallstones. The physical examination between episodes (when patients typically present) is usually unremarkable. The best imaging study for detecting gallstones is real-time ultrasonography (LR+ 19.4, LR− 0.03). In those rare cases in which an ultrasound is technically inadequate, an oral cholecystogram (LR+ 18.0, LR− 0.11) is helpful.

Acute calculous cholecystitis (inflammation of the gallbladder secondary to persistent obstruction of the cystic duct) occurs in less than 2% of individuals with gallstones per year (11). Most have had prior episodes of typical biliary colic. This condition usually begins as biliary colic, but the pain persists for more than 5 hours. On physical examination, most patients have right upper quadrant (RUQ) tenderness and Murphy's sign (cessation of inspiration because of pain with palpation of the RUQ). Absence of Murphy's sign would tend to rule out acute cholecystitis in younger patients (LR− 0.06), but is less useful in the elderly (LR− 0.66). Fever, RUQ guarding or rebound, and jaundice are present in a minority

of patients; because they are highly specific signs, their presence helps rule in acute cholecystitis (Table 14.4). Laboratory tests may show leukocytosis and mild elevations of alkaline phosphatase, transaminases, and bilirubin (12). Absence of gallstones on ultrasound helps rule out acute cholecystitis (LR− 0.10). The presence of gallstones alone is relatively nonspecific, so a positive test does not necessarily rule in acute cholecystitis (LR+ 3.4). Adding other criteria, such as gallbladder wall thickening or an ultrasonographic Murphy's sign, increases specificity and makes the test more useful for ruling in cholecystitis (LR+ 11.1) (14). Cholescintigrams are more accurate than ultrasound, but are also more time-consuming and expensive (Table 14.5).

Common bile duct stones are present in 10 to 20% patients who have cholelithiasis (13). Although most of these pass asymptomatically into the duodenum, obstruction of the common bile duct may occur, which can lead to acute cholangitis. This condition develops in less than 1% of patients with cholelithiasis and may also be caused by obstruction due to tumor (11). Cholangitis is potentially lethal, particularly if not treated urgently. The classic presentation of acute cholangitis (Charcot's triad of pain, fever, and jaundice) occurs in 50 to 60% of patients; right upper quadrant tenderness with peritoneal signs is present in 67% (13). Laboratory studies commonly show leukocytosis and elevations of transaminases, alkaline phosphatase, and bilirubin; amylase is also elevated in 33%. Ultrasonography is not sensitive for the detection of common bile duct stones (sensitivity < 55%). If suspicion for common bile duct stones is high, endoscopic retrograde cholangiopancreatography (ERCP) should be considered. Patients with typical biliary colic but without gallstones may have recurrent pain due to biliary dyskinesia. This condition is diagnosed by an abnormally low (< 35 to 40%) gallbladder ejection fraction on cholecystokinin-stimulated cholescintigraphy.

Dyspepsia

Dyspepsia is a symptom complex of recurrent upper abdominal discomfort or pain that is variably related to meals and may be associated with nausea, vomiting, fullness, early satiety, bloating, and belching. This common condition has a community prevalence of 30%. Among dyspeptic patients referred for endoscopy, 13% generally have duodenal ulcers, 10% have gastric ulcers,

Table 14.4.
Key Elements of the History and Physical Examination for Abdominal Pain

Diagnosis	Maneuver	Sensitivity[a]	Specificity[a]	LR+	LR−	Reference
Peritonitis (focal or diffuse) in patients with acute abdominal pain	Cough test	0.78	0.79	3.71	0.28	a
	Rebound tenderness	0.81	0.50	1.62	0.38	b
Acute cholecystitis (among emergency department (ER) patients with acute upper abdominal pain)	History of fever	0.15	0.99	15.00	0.86	c
	History of chills	0.13	0.95	2.60	0.92	c
	History of jaundice	0.02	0.99	2.00	0.99	c
	Palpable gallbladder	0.02	0.99	2.00	0.99	c
	Murphy's sign	0.97	0.48	1.87	0.06	c
	History of gallstones	0.35	0.77	1.52	0.84	c
	Jaundice on examination	0.02	0.98	1.00	1.00	c
	Rebound/guarding	0.02	0.85	0.13	1.15	c
Acute cholecystitis (vs. biliary colic in patients with upper abdominal pain)	Oral temperature >37.7°C (100°F)	0.33	0.73	1.22	0.92	d
Acute cholecystitis (elderly patients)	Murphy's sign	0.48	0.79	2.29	0.66	e
Peptic ulcer disease (vs. nonulcer dyspepsia in patients with dyspepsia)	Vomiting	0.38	0.86	2.71	0.72	f
	Night pain	0.75	0.58	1.79	0.43	f
	Weight loss	0.31	0.82	1.72	0.84	f
	Anorexia	0.40	0.70	1.33	0.86	f
	Pain relieved by food, milk, or antacids	0.89	0.27	1.22	0.41	f
	Postprandial pain	0.55	0.50	1.10	0.90	f
	Pain aggravated by food/milk	0.29	0.59	0.71	1.20	f
	Epigastric tenderness					
	To deep palpation	0.52	0.27	0.71	1.78	g
	To light palpation	0.04	0.75	0.16	1.28	g
Any organic esophagogastro-duodenal disease (vs. nonulcer dyspepsia in patients with dyspepsia)	Epigastric tenderness					
	To deep palpation	0.64	0.30	0.91	1.20	g
	To light palpation	0.12	0.71	0.41	1.24	g
Small bowel obstruction (in patients with abdominal pain)	Abdominal distension	0.67	0.96	16.7	0.34	h
	Abnormal bowel sounds	0.76	0.88	6.33	0.27	h
	Previous abdominal surgery	0.85	0.78	3.86	0.19	h
	Abdominal scar	0.85	0.77	3.70	0.19	h
	Constipation	0.37	0.90	3.70	0.70	h
	Relieved by vomiting	0.19	0.93	2.71	0.87	h
Appendicitis (in hospital or ER patients with abdominal pain)	Migration	0.64	0.82	3.56	0.44	i
	Psoas sign	0.16	0.95	3.20	0.88	i
	Fever	0.67	0.79	3.19	0.42	i
	Pain precedes vomiting	0.99	0.64	2.75	0.02	i
	Rigidity	0.27	0.87	2.08	0.84	i
	Rebound	0.63	0.69	2.03	0.54	i
	Rectal tenderness	0.41	0.77	1.78	0.77	i
	Guarding	0.74	0.57	1.72	0.46	i
	RLQ Pain	0.81	0.53	1.72	0.36	i
	No previous similar pain	0.81	0.41	1.37	0.46	i
	Anorexia	0.68	0.36	1.06	0.89	i
	Nausea	0.58	0.37	0.92	1.14	i
	Surgeon's clinical impression	0.63	0.82	3.50	0.45	j

continued

Table 14.4. *(continued)*
Key Elements of the History and Physical Examination for Abdominal Pain

Diagnosis	Maneuver	Sensitivity[a]	Specificity[a]	LR+	LR−	Reference
Irritable bowel syndrome (vs. organic disease in patients with abdominal pain, constipation, or diarrhea)	# Manning's criteria present					
	Four or more	0.5	0.88	4.17	0.57	k
	Three or more	0.84	0.76	3.50	0.21	k
	Two or more	0.93	0.55	2.07	0.13	k
Ectopic pregnancy (in pregnant ER patients with abdominal pain or bleeding)	Cervical motion tenderness	0.43	0.81	2.26	0.70	l
	Vaginal bleeding	0.76	0.64	2.11	0.38	l
	Adnexal tenderness	0.64	0.51	1.31	0.71	l
	Clinical examination	0.185	0.99	18.5	0.82	m
PID (in women with lower abdominal pain)	Temperature > 38°C	0.33	0.82	1.83	0.82	n
	Pain for more than 4 days	0.78	0.54	1.70	0.41	n
	Palpable mass	0.40	0.76	1.67	0.79	n
	Vaginal discharge	0.60	0.61	1.54	0.66	n
	Irregular menses	0.43	0.70	1.43	0.81	n
Endometriosis (in infertile women)	Uterosacral nodularity	0.06	0.99	6.00	0.95	o
	Uterosacral pain	0.08	0.98	4.00	0.94	o
	Obstructed pouch of Douglas	0.06	0.98	3.00	0.96	o
	Retroverted uterus	0.19	0.88	1.58	0.92	o
	Cervical motion tenderness	0.07	0.94	1.17	0.99	o
	Dysmenorrhea	0.56	0.48	1.08	0.92	o

[a]Sensitivity and specificity are point estimates; values of 1.0 were changed to 0.99 to allow calculation of likelihood ratios.

REFERENCES

a. Bennett DH, Tambeur LJMT, Campbell WB. Use of coughing test to diagnose peritonitis. Br Med J 1994;308:1336.

b. Liddington MI, Thomson WHF. Rebound tenderness test. Br J Surg 1991;78:795–796.

c. Singer A, McCracken G, Henry M, Those HJ, Cabahug C. Correlation among clinical, laboratory, and hepatobiliary scanning findings in patients with suspected acute cholecystitis. Ann Emerg Med 1996;28:267–272.

d. Gruber P, Silverman R, Gottesfeld S, Flaster E. Presence of fever and leukocytosis in acute cholecystitis. Ann Emerg Med 1996; 28:273–277.

e. Adedeji OA, McAdam WA. Murphy's sign, acute cholecystitis, and elderly people. J R Coll Surg Edinb 1996;41:88–89.

f. Talley NJ, McNeil D, Piper DW. Discriminant value of dyspeptic symptoms: a study of the clinical presentation of 221 patients with dyspepsia of unknown cause, peptic ulceration, and cholelithiasis. Gut 1987;28:40–46.

g. Priebe WM, DaCosta LR, Beck IT. Is epigastric tenderness a sign of peptic ulcer disease? Gastroenterology 1982;82:16–19.

h. Eskelinen M, Ikonen J, Lipponen P. Contributions of history-taking, physical examination, and computer assistance to diagnosis of acute small-bowel obstruction. A prospective study of 1,333 patients with acute abdominal pain. Scand J Gastroenterol 1994;29:715–721.

i. Wagner JM, McKinney WP, Carpenter JL. Does this patient have appendicitis? JAMA 1996;276:1589–1594.

j. Wade DS, Marrow SE, Balsara ZN, Burkhard TK, Goff WB. Accuracy of ultrasound in the diagnosis of acute appendicitis compared with the surgeon's clinical impression. Arch Surg 1993;128:1039–1044; discussion 1044–1046.

k. Manning AP, Thompson WG, Heaton KW, Morris AF. Towards positive diagnosis of the irritable bowel. Br Med J 1978;2:653–654.

l. Kaplan BC, Dart RG, Moskos M, Kuligowska E, Chun B, Adel HM, et al. Ectopic pregnancy: prospective study with improved diagnostic accuracy. Ann Emerg Med 1996;28:10–17.

m. Barnhart K, Mennuti MT, Benjamin I, Jacobson S, Goodman D, Coutifaris C. Prompt diagnosis of ectopic pregnancy in an emergency department setting. Obstet Gynecol 1994;84:1010–1015.

n. Washington E, Berg AO. Preventing and managing pelvic inflammatory disease: key questions, practices, and evidence. J Fam Pract 1996;43:283–293.

o. Matorras R, Rodriguez F, Pijoan JI, Soto E, Perez C, Ramon O, et al. Are there any clinical signs and symptoms that are related to endometriosis in infertile women? Am J Obstet Gynecol 1996;174:620–623.

2% have gastric cancer (14), and up to 15% have esophagitis (15). These estimates are probably high, because patients referred for endoscopy tend to have more severe symptoms and a greater likelihood of organic disease. The remaining patients have "nonulcer dyspepsia," by far the most common cause of dyspepsia in the primary care setting. This is a heterogeneous diagnosis with a variety of possible etiologies, including gastric motor abnormalities, gastroesophageal reflux, gastric hypersensitivity, and psychologic distress.

Table 14.5.
Characteristics of Diagnostic Tests Useful in Patients with Abdominal Pain

Disease	Diagnostic Test	Reference	Sensitivity[a]	Specificity[a]	LR+	LR−
Cholelithiasis	CT scan	a	0.79	0.99	79.0	0.21
	Ultrasound	a	0.97	0.95	19.4	0.03
	Oral cholecystogram	a	0.9	0.95	18.0	0.11
Acute calculous	Cholescintigram	b	0.98	0.93	14.0	0.02
cholecystitis	Ultrasound	b				
	Gallstones plus either wall thickening or ultrasonographic Murphy's sign		0.78	0.93	11.1	0.24
	Gallstones only		0.93	0.73	3.44	0.10
	WBC > 11,000	c	0.69	0.68	2.16	0.46
Peptic ulcer	EGD		0.95	0.99	95.00	0.05
	UGI	d	0.85	0.95	17	0.16
Helicobacter pylori	Silver stain	e	0.93	0.99	93.1	0.07
infection	Urease (CLO) test	e	0.9	0.99	90.0	0.10
	Urea breath test	e	0.9	0.96	21.5	0.01
	Serum IgG	e	0.91	0.92	10.9	0.09
Gastric cancer	EGD	f	0.94	0.99	94.0	0.06
	UGI (if > 1 cm) (31)		0.95	0.99	95.0	0.05
	UGI (if < 1 cm) (31)		0.57	0.99	57.0	0.43
Acute pancreatitis	Contrast CT scan	g	0.92	0.99	92.0	0.08
	Ultrasound	g	0.8	0.97	26.7	0.21
	Serum lipase	h	0.94	0.96	24.0	0.06
	Serum amylase	h	0.82	0.91	9.1	0.2
Chronic pancreatitis	ERCP	i	0.9	0.99	90.0	0.10
	Plain x-ray	i	0.3	0.98	15.0	0.71
	CT scan	j	0.8	0.85	5.3	0.24
	Ultrasound	j	0.65	0.85	4.3	0.41
Pancreatic cancer	ERCP	k	0.95	0.97	32	0.05
	CT scan	k	0.85	0.9	8.5	0.17
	Ultrasound	k	0.7	0.85	4.7	0.35
Small bowel	Ultrasound	l	0.88	0.96	22.0	0.13
obstruction	CT	m	0.96	0.83	5.6	0.05
	Plain x-ray	l	0.96	0.65	2.7	0.06
Appendicitis	CT scan	n,o	0.91	0.93	13.0	0.10
	Sonogram	n,p,q	0.85	0.90	8.5	0.17
	Elevated CRP	r	0.79	0.64	2.2	0.33
	Elevated WBC	r	0.53	0.65	1.5	0.72
Ectopic pregnancy	Sonogram abnormal	s	0.67	0.99	67.0	0.33
	Sonogram abnormal or indeterminate	s	0.98	0.84	6.1	0.02
PID	Inflammation on endometrial biopsy	t	0.8	0.78	3.6	0.26
	Elevated CRP	t	0.86	0.72	3.1	0.19
	ESR > 15 to > 25	t	0.72	0.56	1.6	0.50

[a]The values for sensitivity and specificity listed are point estimates. In most conditions, these are from meta-analyses and other overviews. Point estimates are used to allow for calculation of likelihood ratios. Furthermore, many of the studies from which this data came were subject to verification bias; that is, the gold standard was only applied if the diagnostic test under investigation was positive. This leads to overestimation of sensitivity and underestimation of specificity (98). Values of 1.0 were changed to 0.99 to allow for calculation of likelihood ratios.

REFERENCES

a. Shea J, Berlin J, Escarce J, Clarke J, Kinosian B, Cabana M, et al. Revised estimates of diagnostic test sensitivity and specificity in suspected biliary tract disease. Br J Surg 1994;73:988–992.

b. Greene R, Griner P, Block E, Panzer R. Cholelithiasis and acute cholecystitis. In: Panzer RJ, ed. Diagnostic Strategies for Common Medical Problems. Philadelphia: American College of Physicians, 1991:120–130.

c. Grube P, Silverman R, Gottesfeld S, Flaster E. Presence of fever and leukocytosis in acute cholecystits. Ann Emerg Med 1996;28:273–277.

continued

Table 14.5. *(continued)*
Characteristics of Diagnostic Tests Useful in Patients with Abdominal Pain

d. Sox HJ, Blatt M, Higgins M, Marton K. Medical Decision Making, Newton: Reed Publishing, 1988:337–361.

e. Cutler AF, Havstad S, Ma CK. Accuracy of invasive and noninvasive tests to diagnose *Helicobacter pylori* infection. Gastroenterology 1995;109:136–141.

f. Tatsuta M, Iishi H, Okuda S, Oshima A, Taniguchi H. Prospective evaluation of diagnostic accuracy of gastrofiberscopic biopsy in diagnosis of gastric cancer. Cancer 1989;63:1415–1420.

g. Agarwal N, et al. Evaluating tests for acute pancreatitis. Am J Gastroenterol 1990;85:356–366.

h. Crosetti J, Arvan D. Acute pancreatitis. In: Panzer RMD, Black EMD, Griner PMD, eds. Diagnostic Strategies for Common Medical Problems. Philadelphia: American College of Physicians 1991:161–167.

i. Owyang C, Levitt MD. Chronic pancreatitis. In: Yamada T, Alpers DH, eds. Textbook of Gastroenterology, 2nd ed. Philadelphia: JB Lippincott, 1995;2091–2112.

j. Soll A. Medical treatment of peptic ulcer disease. JAMA 1996;275:622–629.

k. Boland CR, Scheiman JM. Tumors of the stomach. In: Yamada T, Alpers DH, eds. Textbook of Gastroenterology, 2nd ed. Philadelphia: JB Lippincott, 1995:1494–1522.

l. Ogata M, Mateer JR, Condon RE. Prospective evaluation of abdominal sonography for the diagnosis of bowel obstruction [see comments]. Ann Surg 1996;223:237–241. Comment in: Ann Surg 1996 Mar;223(3):235–236.

m. Frager D, Medwid SW, Baer JW, Mollinelli B, Friedman M. CT of small-bowel obstruction: value in establishing the diagnosis and determining the degree and cause [see comments]. Am J Roentgenol 1994;162:37–41. Comment in: Am J Roentgenol 1996;166(5):1227.

n. Balthazar EJ, Birnbaum BA, Yee J, Megibow AJ, Roshkow J, Gray C. Acute appendicitis: CT and US correlation in 100 patients. Radiology 1994;190:31–35.

o. Malone AJ Jr, Wolf CR, Malmed AS, Melliere BF. Diagnosis of acute appendicitis: value of unenhanced CT. AJR Am J Roentgenol 1993;160:763–766.

p. Wade DS, Marrow SE, Balsara ZN, Burkhard TK, Goff WB. Accuracy of ultrasound in the diagnosis of acute appendicitis compared with the surgeon's clinical impression. Arch Surg 1993;128:139–1044; discussion 1044–1046.

q. Crady SK, Jones JS, Wyn T, Luttenton CR. Clinical validity of ultrasound in children with suspected appendicitis. Ann Emerg Med 1993;22:1125–1129.

r. Chi CH, Shiesh SC, Chen KW, Wu MH, Lin XZ. C-reactive protein for the evaluation of acute abdominal pain. Am J Emerg Med 1996;14:254–256.

s. Kaplan BC, Dart RG, Moskos M, Kuligowska E, Chun B, Abel HM, et al. Ectopic pregnancy: prospective study with improved diagnostic accuracy. Ann Emerg Med 1996;28:10–17.

t. Washington E, Berg AP. Preventing and managing pelvic inflammatory disease: key questions, practices, and evidence. J Fam Pract 1996;43:283–293.

Peptic ulcer disease is most often caused by either *Helicobacter pylori* infection or nonsteroidal anti-inflammatory drug (NSAID) use; only very rarely is it caused by hypersecretion of stomach acid, as in Zollinger-Ellison syndrome. Among patients not using NSAIDs, nearly 100% with duodenal ulcers and 80% with gastric ulcers are infected with *H. pylori*; however, only 10 to 25% of individuals infected with this organism develop ulcers (16, 17).

The most common symptom of ulcer disease is abdominal pain. This is classically described as visceral epigastric pain that is provoked by fasting and relieved by eating or antacids. Other symptoms more likely in ulcer than nonulcer dyspepsia include pain at night and vomiting. However, the history alone has been shown to be less than 50% accurate in diagnosis (18). The physical examination is important to help you exclude serious disease, although it does not reliably distinguish ulcer from nonulcer dyspepsia, since epigastric tenderness is a nonspecific finding equally common in both groups of patients. "Red flags" from the history and physical examination that might indicate gastric cancer, complicated (obstructed, perforated, or bleed-

ing) ulcer, or complicated reflux include anorexia, early satiety, weight loss, dysphagia, severe pain, anemia, gross or occult gastrointestinal bleeding, a palpable abdominal mass, abdominal distention, peritoneal signs, or severe systemic illness (see Table 14.3).

Diagnosis of peptic ulcer disease can be made by upper gastrointestinal (UGI) series radiography or upper endoscopy (Table 14.5). The latter is more expensive and has a slight risk of complications (0.15%) (14), but in addition to increased accuracy, it can provide biopsies to test for malignancy. Patients who have gastric ulcers diagnosed by UGI should have endoscopic biopsies performed to exclude cancer. Infection with *H. pylori* can be accurately diagnosed either invasively (urease test or silver stain of an endoscopic biopsy specimen) or noninvasively (13-C labeled urea breath test or IgG serology; see Table 14.5).

Gastric cancer (adenocarcinoma) is twice as common in men as women and is rare before age 50. *H. pylori* infection and diet are the most significant risk factors; it is also more common among Asians. Symptoms consist of epigastric pain, early satiety, and abdominal bloating; these generally do not occur early in the disease. The diagnostic gold standard is endoscopy, although UGIs have similar accuracy for tumors greater than 1 cm in size (19). Because radiographically benign-appearing gastric ulcers may be malignant, all patients with this finding on UGI should undergo prompt endoscopy and biopsy.

Pancreatic Disease

Acute pancreatitis is a common disorder that may vary in severity from mild to fulminant. Most cases (80%) are caused by excessive alcohol use or gallstones. The remainder are caused by hypertriglyceridemia, trauma, a variety of drugs, and a host of uncommon causes; about 10% of cases are idiopathic. Approximately 25% of patients with an episode of acute pancreatitis develop severe complications; the overall mortality rate is 9% (20).

Most patients with acute pancreatitis have upper abdominal pain (90%), which often radiates to the back, anorexia (85%), nausea and vomiting (75%), and fever (60%). The pain is usually sudden in onset and increases in severity over several hours. Common signs include decreased bowel sounds (60%) and abdominal rigidity (50%). Less common presentations include shock (15%), jaundice (15%), and hematemesis (10%).

Lipase is the most accurate blood test for diagnosing acute pancreatitis (LR+ 24.0, LR− 0.06; see Table 14. 4). Abdominal and chest plain films may demonstrate suggestive findings (such as hemidiaphragmatic elevation, pleural effusion, sentinel loops of small bowel, or a colon cut-off sign) or pancreatic calcifications (which are diagnostic of chronic pancreatitis). The greatest use of plain films may be their ability to exclude pneumoperitoneum from a perforated viscus, as this can present similarly to acute pancreatitis. Ultrasound, when positive, is most helpful at ruling in acute pancreatitis (LR+ 26.7), but it does not rule out pancreatitis when normal (LR− 0.2). Ultrasound can also be useful in diagnosing cholelithiasis as a presumptive cause of pancreatitis. Abdominal computerized tomography (CT) scans, particularly if contrast-enhanced, are more accurate than ultrasound at diagnosing pancreatitis. They can also demonstrate the presence of complications, such as necrosis and pseudocysts, and can provide prognostic information. A CT scan is therefore recommended for patients with clinically severe disease, when the diagnosis is in question, or when patients do not improve within 48 to 72 hours.

Chronic pancreatitis is most often due to chronic, excessive alcohol consumption, and usually presents with recurrent upper abdominal pain (80 to 90%) and tenderness (21). Symptoms or signs of exocrine or endocrine insufficiency, such as steatorrhea, weight loss, or diabetes, may also be present after 90% of the gland is diseased (21). Serum amylase and lipase are often normal or only slightly elevated. Abdominal plain films are diagnostic if they demonstrate calcifications in symptomatic patients (LR+ 15.0), but cannot rule out disease if normal (LR− 0.71). Ultrasonography and CT scanning are somewhat more helpful at ruling out chronic pancreatitis if normal (LR− 0.4 and 0.24, respectively), and they are reasonably useful when positive (LR+ 4.3 and 5.3, respectively). The most accurate diagnostic test is ERCP (LR+ 90, LR− 0.1), but because of its invasiveness and cost, it is not recommended as a first-line test (22). Tests of exocrine function are rarely needed to make the diagnosis.

The incidence of pancreatic cancer is 11/100,000 and increasing. It is responsible for 5% of all cancer deaths and has the worst prognosis of all malignancies, with a 5-year survival rate of less than 5% (23).

Risk factors for pancreatic cancer include chronic pancreatitis, diabetes mellitus, and smoking (23). Most patients are 60 to 80 years old and present with weight loss (95%), abdominal pain (80%), or jaundice (50%). The visceral, epigastric pain radiates to the back in 50% of cases. Cancers in the head of the pancreas may cause jaundice and hepatomegaly (80%) and a palpable gallbladder, also called "Courvoisier's sign" (30%) (23). ERCP, the most accurate diagnostic procedure, is invasive, expensive, and can cause acute pancreatitis in 2 to 5% of patients (22). Of the commonly used noninvasive imaging tests, a CT scan (LR+ 8.5, LR− 0.17) is more accurate than a transabdominal ultrasound (LR+ 4.7, LR− 0.35; see Table 14.4). In particular, a normal ultrasound does not rule out cancer in a patient in whom you have a high clinical index of suspicion. Endoscopic ultrasonography and magnetic resonance imaging (MRI) are promising new diagnostic modalities, although their test characteristics have not been well described.

Bowel Obstruction

The most common cause of bowel obstruction is adhesions resulting from previous surgery (85%).

Other causes of bowel obstruction include neoplasms, gallstones, congenital bowel abnormalities, or even ingested materials. Pain is usually intermittent and either generalized or localized to the midabdominal area; it may be relieved by vomiting. The small bowel is the most common location. Large bowel obstructions have a less acute onset, with less frequent intervals of pain and less vomiting, but greater distention. Strangulation (vascular compromise by the obstruction) occurs early in patients with an obstructed hernia or volvulus and in up to one-third of patients with complete bowel obstruction. Strangulation becomes more likely as time progresses and requires immediate surgical intervention. Patients with strangulation may have more marked tenderness and signs of peritonitis. A tender, nonreducible inguinal mass is present if the strangulation is due to an inguinal hernia.

Plain radiographs may reveal air-fluid levels; their absence rules out obstruction (LR− 0.06) (24). Ultrasonography (LR+ 22, LR− 0.13) or CT (LR+ 5.7, LR− 0.05) may provide additional information regarding the cause of an obstruction, earlier detection of strangulation, or increased confidence in watchful waiting (25–27).

Appendicitis

Acute appendicitis is the most common condition leading to surgery among patients with abdominal pain. In considering this diagnosis, you must walk a fine line between overdiagnosis and underdiagnosis. Approximately 15 to 35% of appendectomies reveal a normal appendix, thus causing unnecessary morbidity. Conversely, mortality and significant morbidity are much more frequent if surgery is delayed until appendiceal perforation, which occurs in 17% to 40% of patients.

Distention of the appendix initially leads to poorly localized epigastric or periumbilical visceral pain, which may be accompanied by anorexia, nausea, or vomiting. Physical examination at this stage reveals no specific findings. With peritoneal involvement, the pain becomes localized to the right lower quadrant, often at McBurney's point (5 cm from the anterior superior iliac spine on a line running from the umbilicus). Physical examination at this point will frequently reveal guarding, rigidity, rebound tenderness, a positive cough test (pain with coughing), Rosving's sign (referred rebound tenderness on the right lower quadrant from palpa-

tion of the left lower quadrant), or a psoas sign (pain with resisted thigh flexion; see Table 14.4). With rupture of the appendix, the pain may decrease for a brief time, then become much more intense. The temperature rises, the patient shows increasing signs of toxicity, and the abdomen develops a board-like rigidity.

Not all patients experience this classic sequence. In some, the pain localizes immediately. Others, particularly those with a retrocecal, retroiliac, or pelvic appendix, may have poorly localizing or even left lower quadrant (LLQ) pain. For these patients, a rectal or pelvic examination may be helpful, with tenderness and fullness perceived on the right, but not the left, side. Diagnosis of appendicitis is more difficult in elderly patients, who often have more nonspecific presentations and a decreased febrile response. It is also more challenging in young women, who have a broader differential diagnosis including ovarian cysts, mittelschmerz, pelvic inflammatory disease, ectopic pregnancy, endometriosis, or other gynecologic conditions.

Almost half of patients with acute appendicitis will have a normal white blood cell count. Among patients who are operated on for suspected appendicitis, 97% who actually had appendicitis also had an abnormal C-reactive protein. However, this test has not been evaluated in the group of patients with suspected appendicitis, as not all of them go to surgery. Abdominal ultrasound or CT may be helpful, but neither is clearly superior to the clinical examination (see Table 14.5), and obtaining these tests may result in a delay in diagnosis and time to surgery. Laparoscopy may be useful at times in differentiating between appendicitis and other conditions, especially in young women.

Diverticulitis

Acute inflammation leading to symptoms of diverticulitis affects only a minority of patients with diverticulitis (annual incidence 14/100,000) (28). Over 90% of inflamed diverticula are located in the sigmoid colon and lead to left lower abdominal pain. Apart from location, the symptoms and signs of diverticulitis bear many similarities to those of appendicitis. Diverticular pain has a more gradual onset, and 50% of patients will have had some abdominal symptoms, low-grade fever, or altered bowel function for more than 1 month (29). Urinary frequency or urgency may be present if the inflamed bowel lies adjacent to the bladder. Tenderness is localized in 58% of patients, usually in the LLQ. Peritoneal signs (12%), fever (12%), or a mass (33%) may be present (30).

Laboratory investigations are often unhelpful. Only about 60% of patients with acute diverticulitis have an elevated white blood count, and plain radiographs are abnormal in only one-third of patients (31). CT and barium enemas have approximately equal sensitivity (60 to 80%) (31, 32). Mortality rates may be as high as 6 to 16%, especially in elderly or immunosuppressed patients. Diagnosis may be delayed in these groups because classic signs and symptoms are less likely to be present.

Irritable Bowel Syndrome

Irritable bowel syndrome (IBS), a functional gastrointestinal disorder characterized by chronic abdominal pain and altered bowel habits, affects 10 to 20% of adolescents and adults (2, 33). It may be due to altered gastrointestinal motility, visceral hypersensitivity, and/or luminal irritation. Psychiatric conditions are more common in patients who seek medical help for IBS than in controls, but are not more common in individuals who report IBS-compatible symptoms in population-based surveys. Thus, they appear to have more to do with the decision to seek care for IBS than with the etiology of the syndrome. Stress can exacerbate symptoms in individuals with IBS and in healthy people. Other functional conditions, such as nonulcer dyspepsia, fatigue, and urogenital dysfunction may coexist with IBS.

Formal diagnosis of IBS requires 3 months of symptoms including abdominal pain, diarrhea, constipation, or alternating diarrhea and constipation. The pain of IBS is variable, but commonly is in the lower abdomen and is cramp-like or aching. Manning's criteria are useful historical clues to the diagnosis, particularly in women and the nonelderly (see Table 14.4) (34). They are:

- pain relief with bowel action;
- more frequent stools with the onset of pain;
- looser stools with the onset of pain;
- passage of mucus;
- sensation of incomplete evacuation; and
- abdominal distention as evidenced by tight clothing or visible appearance.

Diagnosis involves consideration of Manning's criteria and exclusion of other potential causes of the patient's symptoms. Clues to other diagnoses include abdominal pain that is severe, localizing, or awakens the patient; weight loss; fever; diarrhea that awakens the patient; stools suggestive of malabsorptive or secretory diarrhea; or rectal bleeding (melena or hematochezia). The physical examination in patients with IBS is generally unremarkable; abdominal tenderness, when present, is unimpressive. Peritonitis, masses, organomegaly, heme-positive stools, and jaundice are not caused by IBS and should prompt an evaluation for other conditions. Flexible sigmoidoscopy with or without barium enema (or colonoscopy) should be strongly considered, especially in patients whose IBS first appears after age 40. If diarrhea is predominant, additional studies could include fecal studies for leukocytes, fat, and weight; ova and parasites; thyroid function studies; and sigmoidoscopic biopsies.

Ectopic Pregnancy

Ectopic pregnancy should be considered in the differential diagnosis of every woman of childbearing age who presents with lower abdominal or pelvic pain. Classic findings include pain in the lower abdomen, back, or pelvis; vaginal spotting or bleeding; and a missed menstrual period. Most women will have had pain for less than 4 days. Unfortunately, the diagnosis is initially missed in up to 40% of women because these symptoms are common with a spontaneous abortion or normal pregnancy (35). Conversely, it is important to note that 30% of women with an ectopic pregnancy will have either abdominal pain or vaginal bleeding but not both, and up to 15% will not have missed a period. Pelvic examination often reveals adnexal tenderness, a tender adnexal mass, or pain on movement of the cervix (see Table 14.4). Following rupture, patients have increased tenderness, rigidity, and other signs of generalized peritoneal irritation or shock.

Serum β-HCG and ultrasound (transabdominal or transvaginal) are the most helpful tests. A serum β-HCG that is negative or over 50,000 mIU/mL rules out an ectopic pregnancy because the patient is not pregnant or the conceptus is too large to fit in a fallopian tube. If the quantitative serum β-HCG is greater than 6500, a transabdominal ultrasound should be able to detect an intrauterine pregnancy if one is present; between 6500 and 1500, a transvaginal ultrasound is preferable because the conceptus is small enough to be missed with a transabdominal study (36). If the abdominal ultrasound shows clear evidence of an ectopic pregnancy, vaginal ultrasound may be omitted.

Pelvic Inflammatory Disease

Pelvic inflammatory disease (PID) is an infection of the female upper genital tract that affects over 1 million American women each year. Young women with multiple sexual partners who use nonbarrier contraceptive methods or intrauterine devices (IUDs) are particularly at risk. The clinical presentation of PID varies widely, ranging from mild lower abdominal or pelvic pain to acute illness with severe systemic symptoms. No single physical finding or diagnostic test can reliably establish the diagnosis. Laparoscopy is currently considered the gold standard test, but it is impractical for routine use with every suspected case of PID and may miss up to 20% of positive cases. Because of this uncertainty and the possibility that chronic pelvic pain, infertility, or ectopic pregnancy may result from delayed treatment, physicians should have a high index of suspicion for this condition. A woman who has lower abdominal tenderness, adnexal tenderness, cervical motion tenderness, and no other clear cause for these symptoms meets the Centers for Disease Control (CDC) "minimum criteria" for the diagnosis of PID. Fever (>38.3°C), cervical or vaginal discharge, elevated erythrocyte sedimentation rate, elevated C-reactive protein, or laboratory evidence of gonococcal or chlamydial infection may be present, but no single finding is sufficiently accurate to rule the diagnosis in or out (see Table 14.5).

Endometriosis

Endometriosis is characterized by the presence of endometrial glands and stroma outside the uterine cavity in a variety of locations, including the pelvic peritoneum, ovaries, and uterine ligaments. The cyclical growth and bleeding of these endometrial implants causes pain. Although the pathologic findings of endometriosis can be found in 5 to 15% of women by laparoscopy, many of these women have no symptoms, and not all women who have symptoms will seek medical care (37).

The classic presentation of endometriosis involves cyclical pelvic pain, dyspareunia, and infertility. Dysmenorrhea may also be present, but is not predictive of endometriosis. Pain associated with intercourse is described as deep pain, and may continue for several hours post coitus. Some women have abnormal menses or premenstrual spotting, whereas others may report pain on defecation or urination, hematuria, constipation, diarrhea, or urinary frequency. Abnormal physical findings are most likely to be present during menses. Painful nodules along the uterosacral ligaments (LR+ 6.0) or a fixed retroverted uterus (LR+ 4.0) are useful to rule-in the diagnosis when present (see Table 14.3). Laparoscopy is the gold standard for diagnosis of endometriosis; because of their low sensitivity, ultrasonography and MRI are not very useful.

MANAGEMENT

Principles of Management

Treatment of abdominal pain can either be directed specifically to the established diagnosis or used empirically if a determination of the exact diagnosis is not essential. In some cases, reassurance is the only treatment needed. Your treatment plan should always include appropriate follow-up for your patient; the most appropriate interval for follow-up depends on the seriousness of the problem. The evidence supporting outpatient treatment strategies for the most common causes of abdominal pain are summarized in Table 14.6. Drugs useful for specific conditions, along with appropriate dosages, are summarized in Table 14.7.

Management of Specific Common Conditions

Biliary Tract Disease

The treatment of choice for symptomatic cholelithiasis is cholecystectomy, usually performed laparoscopically (38). This operation successfully eliminates symptoms in over 90% of patients. Treatment options for patients who are too ill or unwilling to undergo surgery include dissolution therapy (either oral or contact) or lithotripsy. Nonoperative treatments are associated with gallstone clearance rates of 90 to 95%, but less than one-third of patients are appropriate candidates for these treatments, and stones recur in 50% (38).

Initial treatment of acute cholecystitis consists of bowel rest, intravenous hydration, broad-spectrum antibiotics, analgesics, and nasogastric

Table 14.6.
Therapeutic Options for the Outpatient Management of Various Causes of Abdominal Pain

Disease	Reference	Treatment Strategy	Level of Evidence for Effectiveness[a]	Comments
Duodenal or gastric ulcer	a	HP eradication	A	Triple therapy for at least 7 days (see Table 14.7). Also prevent recurrence
		Histamine-2 antagonists	A	Do not prevent recurrence unless used in maintenance dose
		Proton-pump inhibitors	A	Do not prevent recurrence unless used in maintenance dose
Nonulcer dyspepsia	b	Histamine-2 antagonists	A	Avoid long-term use if possible
		Lifestyle changes	B	
		Cisapride	A	
Irritable bowel syndrome	c	Pharmacotherapy	C	Psyllium for any IBS symptoms complex; dicyclomine or amitriptyline for pain-predominant IBS; loperamide, diphenoxylate, or cholestyramine for diarrhea-predominant IBS; cisapride for constipation-predominant IBS
Pelvic inflammatory disease	d	Inpatient antibiotics	A	
		Outpatient antibiotics	B	
Endometriosis	e,f	Oral contraceptives	A	
		Danazol	A	
		Metroxyprogesterone acetate	A	
		GnRH analogues	A	
		NSAIDs	B	
Diverticulitis	g,h	IV antibiotics, fluids for acute exacerbations	B	
		High-fiber diet	C	To prevent flare-ups

[a]Level of evidence for effectiveness: A, strong or moderate research-based evidence (consistent across several studies, including at least two randomized controlled trials); B, limited research-based evidence (less consistent or extensive evidence, but preponderance of evidence supports use of treatment); C, common practice with little or no research-based evidence; X, moderate or strong evidence suggesting that this treatment is not effective.

REFERENCES

a. Soll A. Medical treatment of peptic ulcer disease. JAMA 1996;275:622–629.
b. Scolapio JS, Camilleri M. Nonulcer dyspepsia. Gastroenterologist 1992;4:13–23.
c. Lynn RB, Friedman LS. Irritable bowel syndrome. Med Clin North Am 1995;79:373–390.
d. Washington E, Berg AO. Preventing and managing pelvic inflammatory disease: key questions, practices, and evidence. J Fam Pract 1996;43:283–293.
e. Lu PY, Ory SJ. Endometriosis: current management. Mayo Clin Proc 1995;70:453–463.
f. Olive DL, Schwartz LB. Endometriosis. N Engl J Med 1997;328:1759–1769.
g. Ambrosetti P, Robert JH, Witzig JA, Mirescu D, Mathey P, Borst F, et al. Acute left colonic diverticulitis: a prospective analysis of 226 cases. Surgery 1994;115(5):546–550.
h. Leahy AL, Ellis RM, Quill DS, Peel AL. High-fibre diet in symptomatic diverticular disease of the colon. Ann R Coll Surg Engl 1985; 67:173–174.

suction (if an ileus is present). Cholecystectomy is usually performed within 48 hours of admission. Acute cholangitis is treated similarly, although urgent endoscopic or percutaneous decompression is advocated for severe illness or when patients do not rapidly improve. A number of small studies have shown that most patients with biliary dyskinesia have resolution of symptoms following cholecystectomy (39, 40). Many clinicians also use antispasmodics.

Dyspepsia

The approach to the dyspeptic patient has evolved as the role of *H. pylori* in ulcer disease and gastric cancer has become clear. Because *H.*

Table 14.7.
Drug Therapy of Various Causes of Abdominal Pain

Indications	Drug	Trade Name	Dosage	Cautions/Adverse Effect
Duodenal or gastric ulcer	Bismuth subsalicylate and Metronidazole and Tetracycline and Omeprazole	Pepto-Bismol Flagyl Losec	2 tabs qid × 7 days 250 mg qid × 7 days 500 mg qid × 7 days 20 mg bid × 7 days	
	Metronidazole and Clarithromycin and Omeprazole	Biaxin	500 mg bid × 7 days 500 mg bid × 7 days 20 mg bid × 7 days	
	Amoxicillin and Clarithromycin and Omeprazole		1 gm bid × 7 days 500 mg bid × 7 days 20 mg bid × 7 days	
Nonulcer dyspepsia	Cimetidine	Tagamet	400 mg bid	Avoid long-term use, and
	Ranitidine	Zantac	150 mg bid	Remember non-pharmacologic
	Cisapride	Propulsid	5–10 mg qid	Therapy such as weight loss
Irritable bowel syndrome	Psyllium	Metamucil	1/2–1 tbsp qd-bid	For any IBS symptom complex
	Dicyclomine	Bentyl	10–20 mg tid-qid	For pain-predominant IBS
	Amitriptyline	Elavil	10–25 mg qhs	For pain predominant IBS
	Loperamide	Imodium	2 mg bid	For diarrhea-predominant IBS
	Diphenoxylate		2.5–5 mg qid	For diarrhea-predominant IBS
	Cholestyramine	Questran	1/2–1 pack qd–bid	For diarrhea-predominant IBS
	Cisapride		5–10 mg tid	For constipation-predominant IBS
Pelvic inflammatory disease	Cefoxitin Doxycycline Clindamycin and gentamycin		2 g IV q6h 100 mg IV or PO q6h 900 mg IV q6h 2 mg/kg loading dose, then 1.5 mg/kg q8h	Inpatient regimen Inpatient regimen
	Ceftriaxone and Doxycycline		IM once 100 mg PO bid	Outpatient 14 day regimen
	Ofloxacillin and Clindamycin or Metronidazole		400 mg PO bid 400 mg PO qid 500 mb PO bid	Outpatient 14 day regimen
Endometriosis	Oral contraceptives Danazol Medroxyprogesterone acetate GnRH analogues NSAIDs		1 tab po qd 400–800 mg/day 10–30 mg/day Varies	
Diverticulitis				

pylori infection is no more likely in patients with nonulcer dyspepsia than in the general population, the presence of infection can serve as a surrogate diagnostic test for the presence of ulcer or cancer (16). Dyspeptic patients without clinical "red flags" (see Table 14.3) who are negative for *H. pylori* based on noninvasive testing and who do not use nonsteroidal anti-inflammatory drugs (NSAIDs) have an extremely low likelihood (< 1% if younger than 45) of ulcer or malignancy (15, 41, 42). They can be managed presumptively for nonulcer dyspepsia, with endoscopy considered if symptoms do not resolve or if more serious symptoms develop.

Initial treatment for nonulcer dyspepsia should consist of reassurance and avoidance of precipitants (e.g., certain foods, alcohol, tobacco, NSAIDs). Although no pharmacologic agent has been approved by the U. S. Food and Drug Administration for the treatment of nonulcer dyspepsia, many clinicians offer a trial of antacids or H_2-receptor antagonists (H_2RAs). Antacids are not superior to placebo; both have success rates of up to 70% in this condition (43). H_2RAs, on the other hand, have been shown to be of modest benefit in many studies, and on meta-analysis were shown to be 18% more beneficial than placebo (44). Prokinetic agents such as cisapride have similar efficacy to H_2RAs and may be helpful for patients who do not respond to acid-suppression therapy (see Table 14.5 for information on dosing regimens) (43). Psychotherapy has also been shown to decrease pain and other complaints in patients with functional dyspepsia (45). The effectiveness of H. pylori eradication therapy in patients with nonulcer dyspepsia is still unclear.

Dyspeptic patients with H. pylori infection who do not use NSAIDs have a moderately high likelihood of ulcer (50 to 55%). Although randomized trials have not yet been done, cost-effectiveness analyses and well-designed case series studies suggest that the best approach is to eradicate H. pylori infection in this group, with endoscopy reserved for patients whose symptoms persist or worsen and those with signs of complication (hemorrhage, perforation, or obstruction, and those patients felt to be at risk for malignancy) (46–48).

Treatment of peptic ulcer disease consists of antibiotics and acid-suppressive therapy to eradicate H. pylori. This promotes healing, reduces or eliminates symptoms, and reduces the annual rate of symptomatic ulcer recurrence from over 50% to under 10% (49). Many different combination therapies are effective. One week of treatment with bismuth subsalicylate, metronidazole, tetracycline, and omeprazole has the highest cure rate (94 to 98%), but compliance is difficult. Simpler, but more expensive, 1-week regimens consisting of clarithromycin and either metronidazole or amoxicillin along with omeprazole have cure rates of 86 to 91% (see Table 14.6). Two-week regimens combining antibiotics and H_2-receptor antagonists (H_2RAs) are also effective. After eradication therapy is completed, patients generally continue taking acid-suppressive therapy for an additional 6 weeks, although this may be unnecessary if H. pylori is eradicated.

Dyspeptic patients taking NSAIDs should be told to stop these medications. If their symptoms do not resolve, management consists of eradication of H. pylori, if present, and prescription of H_2RAs or omeprazole (the latter for complicated, large, or refractory ulcers). Patients with persistent symptoms or signs of complicated disease should be considered for endoscopy.

The definitive treatment of gastric cancer is surgery. Early-stage cancers have a favorable prognosis (stage I: 80 to 90% 5-year survival rate; stage II: 65%). Unfortunately, by the time symptoms occur, many patients have late-stage disease, which has a much poorer prognosis (stage III: 30 to 50%; stage IV: 5%) (50).

Pancreatic Disease

Mild cases of acute pancreatitis respond to hydration, pancreatic rest, analgesia, and, if an ileus is present, nasogastric suctioning. In severe cases, broad-spectrum antibiotics, a 7-day peritoneal lavage, and endoscopic removal of impacted gallstones (if there is obstructive jaundice or sepsis) may be helpful. Severe cases can lead to multiorgan failure and generally require a critical care unit.

Treatment of chronic pancreatitis is directed at avoiding or controlling pain. Noninvasive options include abstinence from alcohol and other precipitating factors, analgesics, and nerve blocks. Patients who have chronic pain in spite of aggressive noninvasive therapy and evidence of ductal dilatation by ERCP may benefit from one of a variety of internal surgical-drainage procedures. Partial or total resection of the pancreas can be considered for patients with incapacitating pain. The exocrine insufficiency from chronic pancreatitis can be treated with low-fat diets, medium-chain triglycerides, and pancreatic enzyme replacements.

The only definitive treatment for pancreatic cancer is surgery. Unfortunately, only 10% of tumors are resectable once diagnosed, and even these cases have a dismal prognosis.

Bowel Obstruction

Patients whose obstruction is accompanied by vascular compromise of the bowel (strangulation) require immediate surgery. Some patients with a nonstrangulating bowel obstruction will respond to fluid replacement and bowel decompression, but surgery is indicated for any patient whose obstruction does not promptly resolve.

Appendicitis

Once appendicitis is diagnosed, early surgery provides the best opportunity to avoid the complications and increased risks of appendiceal rupture. If the diagnosis is unclear, a period of close observation with repeated examination by a skilled clinician can be helpful. Appendectomy is a relatively simple procedure and leads to few complications. Laparoscopic appendectomy is more expensive, and requires longer operating times, but may lead to less need for postoperative analgesics and a quicker return to work or usual activities (51–53).

Diverticulitis

Approximately 30% of patients with diverticulitis require immediate surgery. The remainder will respond to bowel rest, intravenous fluids, broad-spectrum antibiotics, and close clinical observation (see Table 14.6) (28). Although a low-fiber diet, or no feeding at all, is usually advocated during suspected episodes, a high-fiber diet may be helpful in preventing recurrences. It has also been traditional to counsel patients with diverticulitis to avoid seeds, nuts, and other foods that are presumed to occlude the diverticular orifices.

Irritable Bowel Syndrome

The most important component of managing irritable bowel syndrome (IBS) is a therapeutic physician-patient relationship. Treatment initially includes education, reassurance, and diet (to include a trial of additional fiber and/or lactose restriction). Pharmacotherapy has not been shown to benefit patients with IBS, but therapy directed at specific symptoms that impair functioning may be tried. Antispasmodics may help with pain, antimotility agents or bile resins with diarrhea, and prokinetic drugs with constipation. Antidepressants and other psychologic treatments may also be considered. See Table 14.6 for common drug regimens. Although some physicians may try empiric therapy with metronidazole to eradicate an undiagnosed *Giardia lamblia* infection, there is no evidence to support or refute this practice.

Ectopic Pregnancy

At one time, all ectopic pregnancies were treated with open salpingectomy. Laparoscopy is now used increasingly for both diagnosis and management. Alternatively, patients with a small unruptured ectopic pregnancy (<4-cm diameter) may be treated with systemic methotrexate and followed with weekly β-HCG determinations until no level is detectable.

Pelvic Inflammatory Disease

Antibiotics are the treatment of choice for PID. Because of the potentially serious complications from undertreatment, women who meet the CDC minimum criteria (lower abdominal tenderness, adnexal tenderness, cervical motion tenderness, and no other clear cause for these symptoms) should receive empiric antibiotic treatment. Outpatient treatment with antibiotics is effective for mild cases. Parenteral therapy should be used for patients who are severely ill or vomiting, have HIV infection or a suspected pelvic abscess, or do not respond to oral therapy. Hospital admission and parenteral therapy may also be needed for pregnant women, adolescents, and patients who may not comply with therapy or follow-up. See Table 14.7 for recommended antibiotic regimens.

Endometriosis

Management of endometriosis depends on the severity of symptoms and the woman's desire for future fertility. NSAIDs used perimenstrually usually control mild symptoms. Other drugs such as oral contraceptives, danazol, progesterones, and GnRH antagonists are also useful in controlling mild to moderate symptoms but do not improve fertility (see Table 14.6). For some patients, conservative surgery can remove endometrial implants and preserve fertility, but pain relief is often modest and short lived. Women with severe pain may require total abdominal hysterectomy with bilateral salpingo-oophorectomy.

SPECIAL CONSIDERATIONS

Although detailed discussion of abdominal pain in children is beyond the scope of this chapter, a few general comments are appropriate. Studies of acute abdominal pain in children show that approximately 30% of cases are due to appendicitis, 60% to nonspecific abdominal pain, and the remainder to a variety of causes that include urinary tract infection, intussusception, renal colic, incarcerated hernia, testicular torsion, peptic ulcer disease, Hirschsprung's disease, and

PID (54). Less than 10% of recurrent abdominal pain in children is due to clearly identifiable organic disease; anxiety is believed to be responsible for the majority of cases (55). Clinical presentations in children may also be different than in adults. For example, in appendicitis the pain is less likely to be steady and in the right lower quadrant (RLQ), and the examination is less likely to show rigidity and decreased bowel sounds. It is important to calm the child as much as possible prior to and during the examination. It may help to sit on the table next to the child, and you should begin palpation far away from the area of pain and be gentle throughout.

The differential diagnosis of abdominal pain in the elderly is likewise somewhat different than that of younger adults (see Table 14.2). The likelihood of malignancy, diverticulitis, and cholelithiasis all increase with age. Clinical presentations of severe disease may be more subtle in the elderly as well, with a less-prominent fever response and fewer peritoneal signs. Therefore, older patients with abdominal pain are often appropriately subjected to more aggressive evaluation and closer follow-up.

CASE STUDY 1

A previously healthy 35-year-old woman has severe RLQ abdominal pain that began yesterday and became worse today. She reports a low-grade fever and some nausea, but denies diarrhea, urinary complaints, respiratory or systemic symptoms, or use of any medications or illicit drugs. She has no history of prior abdominal or pelvic symptoms. Her last menses were 5 weeks ago, but she does not consider this unusual, because her cycles are irregular. On examination, she appears mildly uncomfortable. Vital signs are normal. She has RLQ tenderness, but no guarding or mass.

QUESTIONS

1. Which diagnoses should be considered in your differential diagnosis?
2. What steps would you take next to assist in arriving at the correct diagnosis?

DISCUSSION

Acute appendicitis, pelvic inflammatory disease, ectopic pregnancy, and renal colic are potentially serious diagnoses that must be considered. Diverticulitis is less likely because of the patient's age and the right-sided location of the pain. Gastroenteritis, ovarian cyst, or nonspecific abdominal pain are also in the differential diagnosis, but are less likely because of the severity of the pain. Urinary tract infection is also a possibility, but it is less likely because of the absence of urinary symptoms such as frequency or dysuria.

A serum β-HCG and a pelvic examination should be performed. A negative β-HCG would rule out ectopic pregnancy. Cervical motion tenderness and bilateral adnexal tenderness would suggest PID. Right adnexal tenderness or mass would be consistent with ectopic pregnancy, appendicitis, or PID with a tubo-ovarian abscess. If a mass is present, a sonogram may be helpful in differentiating between these conditions. An elevated white blood cell (WBC) count or C-reactive protein (CRP) would suggest an acute infectious process such as appendicitis or PID, but a normal WBC count would not rule out these diagnoses.

CASE STUDY 2

A 40-year-old man complains of recurrent, nonradiating, moderately severe epigastric pain for 2 months. It is usually relieved with over-the-counter H$_2$RAs. Food occasionally helps, but sometimes precipitates, the pain. Past medical history and review of systems are unremarkable. He does not use any other medications (including over-the-counter NSAIDs), tobacco, or alcohol. Physical examination reveals only some mild epigastric tenderness.

QUESTIONS

1. What are likely diagnoses?
2. What is a reasonable option for initial management?

DISCUSSION

The patient has dyspepsia, mostly likely nonulcer dyspepsia. Peptic ulcer disease is less likely (20%) and stomach cancer would be very unlikely at this age; biliary colic is also a possibility. Obtaining stool guaiac cards and possibly a hemoglobin to exclude gastrointestinal bleeding would be appropriate, as would checking a *H. pylori* IgG titer. If the titer is negative, the probability of ulcer or cancer is very low, and empiric treatment with acid-suppressive therapy, such as H$_2$RAs, is appropriate. If the *H. pylori* test is positive, eradication with antibiotics and acid-suppressive therapy is reasonable. If symptoms do not improve, further evaluation is indicated.

REFERENCES

1. Adelman A, Revicki D, Magaziner J, Hebel R. Abdominal pain in an HMO. Fam Med 1995;27:321–325.
2. Hyams JS, Burke G, Davis PM, Rzepski B, Andrulonis PA. Abdominal pain and irritable bowel syndrome in adolescents: a community-based study. J Pediatr 1996;129:220–226.
3. Adelman A. Abdominal pain in the primary care setting. J Fam Pract 1987;25:27–32.
4. Gorelik U, Ulish Y, Yagil Y. The use of standard imaging techniques and their diagnostic value in the workup of renal colic in the setting of intractable flank pain. Urology 1996;47:637–642.
5. Jess P, Bjerregarrd B, Sleen B. Prognosis of acute nonspecific abdominal pain—a prospective study. Am J Surg 1982;114:338–340.
6. Klinkman MS. Episodes of care for abdominal pain in a primary care practice. Arch Fam Med 1996;5:279–285.
7. Lukens TW, Emerman C, Effron D. The natural history and clinical findings in undifferentiated abdominal pain. Ann Emerg Med 1993;22:690–696.
8. Muris JW, Starmans R, Fijten GH. One-year prognosis of abdominal complaints in general practice: a prospective study of patients in whom no organic cause is found. Br J Gen Pract 1996;46:715–719.
9. Reilly BM. Abdominal pain. In: Practical Strategies in Outpatient Medicine, 2nd ed. Philadelphia: WB Saunders, 1991:700–787.
10. Greene R, Griner P, Block E, Panzer R. Cholelithiasis and acute cholecystitis. In: Panzer RJ, ed. Diagnostic Strategies for Common Medical Problems. Philadelphia: American College of Physicians, 1991:120–130.
11. Friedman G. Natural history of asymptomatic and symptomatic gallstones. Am J Surg 1993;165:399–404.
12. Watkins J, Blatt C, Layden T. Gallstones: choosing the right therapy despite vague clinical clues. Geriatrics 1993;48:48–54.
13. Kadakia LTCS. Biliary tract emergencies—acute cholecystitis, acute cholangitis, and acute pancreatitis. Med Clin North Am 1993;77:1015–1036.
14. Bhattacharya I. Evaluation and management of dyspepsia. Hosp Pract 1992:93–101.
15. Fraser AG, Ali MR, McCullough S, Yeates NJ, Haystead A. Diagnostic tests for *Helicobacter pylori*—can they help select patients for endoscopy? N Z Med J 1996;109:95–98.
16. NIH Consensus Conference. *Helicobacter pylori* in peptic ulcer disease. JAMA 1994;272:65–71.
17. Cohen JC. Evolving therapies for peptic ulcer disease: *Helicobacter pylori* treatment. Gastroenterologist 1995;3:289–300.
18. Katz J. The course of peptic ulcer disease. Med Clin North Am 1991;75:831–840.
19. Sox HJ, Blatt M, Higgins M, Marton K. Medical Decision Making. Newton: Reed Publishing, 1988:337–361.
20. Steinberg W, Tenner S. Acute pancreatitis. N Engl J Med 1994:1198–1209.
21. Steer M, Waxman I, Freedman ST. Chronic pancreatitis. N Engl J Med 1995;332:1482–1490.
22. Panzer RMD. Pancreatic cancer and chronic pancreatitis. In: Panzer RMD, Black EMD, Griner PMD, eds. Diagnostic Strategies for Common Medical Problems. Philadelphia: American College of Physicians, 1991:175–185.
23. DiMagno E. Pancreatic adenocarcinoma. In: Yamada T, Alpers D, eds. Textbook of Gastroenterology, 2nd ed. Philadelphia: JB Lippincott, 1995:2113–2130.
24. Harlow CL, Stears RL, Zeligman BE, Archer PG. Diagnosis of bowel obstruction on plain abdominal radiographs: significance of air-fluid levels at different heights in the same loop of bowel [see comments]. Am J Roentgenol 1993;161:291–295. Comment in: Am J Roentgenol 1994;163(1):223–224.
25. Frager D, Medwid SW, Baer JW, Mollinelli B, Friedman M. CT of small-bowel obstruction: value in establishing the diagnosis and determining the degree and cause [see comments]. Am J Roentgenol 1994;162:37–41. Comment in: Am J Roentgenol 1996;166(5):1227.
26. Ogata M, Imai S, Hosotani R, Aoyama H, Hayashi M, Ishikawa T. Abdominal ultrasonography for the diagnosis of strangulation in small-bowel obstruction [see comments]. Br J Surg 1994;81:421–424. Comment in: Br J Surg 1994;81(10):1545–1546.
27. Ogata M, Mateer JR, Condon RE. Prospective evaluation of abdominal sonography for the diagnosis of bowel obstruction [see comments]. Ann Surg 1996;223:237–241. Comment in: Ann Surg 1996;223(3):235–236.
28. Ambrosetti P, Robert JH, Witzig JA, Mirescu D, Mathey P, Borst F, et al. Acute left colonic diverticulitis: a prospective analysis of 226 cases. Surgery 1994;115(5):546–550.

29. Ozick LA, Salazar CO, Donelson SS. Pathogenesis, diagnosis, and treatment of diverticular disease of the colon. Gastroenterologist 1994;2(4):299–310.
30. Schoetz DJJ. Uncomplicated diverticulitis. Indications for surgery and surgical management. Surg Clin North Am 1993;73(5):965–974.
31. Morris J, Stellato TA, Haaga JR, Lieberman J. The utility of computed tomography in colonic diverticulitis. Ann Surg 1986;204:128–132.
32. Johnson DC, Baker ME, Rice RP, Silverman P, Thompson WM. Diagnosis of acute colonic diverticulitis: comparison of barium enema and CT. Am J Roentgenol 1987;148:541–546.
33. Lynn RB, Friedman LS. Irritable bowel syndrome [published erratum appears in N Engl J Med 1994;330(3):228] [see comments]. N Engl J Med 1993;329:1940–1945.
34. Talley NJ, Phillips SF, Melton LJ, Mulvihill C, Wiltgen C, Zinsmeister AR. Diagnostic value of the Manning criteria in irritable bowel syndrome. Gut 1990;31:77–81.
35. Kaplan BC, Dart RG, Moskos M, Kuligowska E, Chun B, Adel HM, et al. Ectopic pregnancy: prospective study with improved diagnostic accuracy. Ann Emerg Med 1996;28:10–17.
36. Barnhart K, Mennuti MT, Benjamin I, Jacobson S, Goodman D, Coutifaris C. Prompt diagnosis of ectopic pregnancy in an emergency department setting. Obstet Gynecol 1994;84:1010–1015.
37. Damewood MD. Pathophysiology and management of endometriosis [see comments]. J Fam Pract 1993;37:68–75.
38. NIH Planning Committee. National Institutes of Health Consensus Development Conference Statement on Gallstones and Laparoscopic Cholecystectomy. Am J Surg 1993;165:390–398.
39. Reed D, Fernandez M, Hicks R. Kinevac-assisted cholescintigraphy as an accurate predictor of chronic acalculus gallbladder disease and the likelihood of symptom relief with cholecystectomy. Am Surg 1993;59:273–277.
40. Sorenson M, Fancher S, Lang N, Eidt J, Broadwater JR. Abnormal gallbladder nuclear ejection fraction predicts success of cholecystectomy in patients with biliary dyskinesia. Am J Surg 1993;166:672–675.
41. Mendall MA, Jazrawi RP, Marrero JM. Serology for Helicobacter pylori compared with symptom questionnaires in screening before direct access endoscopy. Gut 1995;36:330–333.
42. Patel P, Khulusi S, Mendall MA, Lloyd R, Jazrawi R, Maxwell JD, et al. Prospective screening of dyspeptic patients by Helicobacter pylori serology. Lancet 1995;346:1315–1318.
43. Scolapio JS, Camilleri M. Nonulcer Dyspepsia. Gastroenterologist 1992;4:13–23.
44. Dobrilla G, Comberlato M, Steele A, Vallaperta P. Drug treatment of functional dyspepsia. A meta-analysis of randomized controlled clinical trails. J Clin Gastroenterol 1989;11:169–177.
45. Haug TT, Wilhelmsen I, Svebak S, Berstad A, Ursin H. Psychotherapy in functional dyspepsia. J Psychosom Res 1994;38:735–744.
46. Ebell MH, Warbasse L, Brenner C. Management of dyspepsia in the outpatient setting: a cost-utility analysis. J Fam Pract 1997;44(6):545–555.
47. Ofman JJ, Etchason J, Fullerton S, Kahn KL, Soll AH. Management strategies for Helicobacter pylori-seropositive patients with dyspepsia: clinical and economic consequences. Ann Intern Med 1997;126:280–291.
48. McColl KE, El-Nujumi A, Murray L, et al. The Helicobacter pylori breath test: a surrogate marker for peptic ulcer disease in dyspeptic patients. Gut 1997; 40: 302–306.
49. Soll A. Medical treatment of peptic ulcer disease. JAMA 1996;275:622–629.
50. Boland CR, Scheiman JM. Tumors of the stomach. In: Yamada T, Alpers DH, eds. Textbook of Gastroenterology, 2nd ed. Philadelphia: JB Lippincott, 1995: 1494–1522.
51. Cox MR, McCall JL, Toouli J, Padbury RTA, Wilson TG, Wattchow DA, et al. Prospective randomized comparison of open versus laparoscopic. World J Surg 1996;20:263–266.
52. Hansen JB, Smithers BM, Schache D, Wall DR, Miller BJ, Menzies BL. Laparoscopic versus open appendectomy: prospective randomized trial. World J Surg 1996;20:17–20; discussion 21.
53. Frazee RC, Roberts JW, Symmonds RE, Snyder SK, Hendricks JC, Smith RW, et al. A prospective randomized trial comparing open versus laparoscopic. Ann Surg 1994;219:725–728; discussion 728–731.
54. Dickson JAS, Jones A, Telfer S, de Dombal FT. Acute abdominal pain in children. Scand J Gastroenterol 1988;23(suppl 144):43–46.
55. Apley J. The Child with Abdominal Pain, 2nd ed. Oxford: Blackwell, 1975.

15. Addiction

ROBERT E. GWYTHER

Key Clinical Questions

1. Does the patient have a diagnosable drug and/or alcohol problem?
2. Are there significant, concomitant medical or psychiatric diagnoses?
3. Is immediate treatment indicated (e.g., thiamine, surgery, antibiotics, tranquilizers, etc.)?
4. Does the patient need drug substitution (e.g., methadone, benzodiazepines) or detoxification?
5. Is the patient a danger to self or others?
6. Is the patient willing and/or eligible to receive addiction treatment?
7. What is the best initial treatment plan for the patient?
8. How should this patient be treated in the future?
9. Are there legal and/or ethical considerations for the treating physician?

Substance abuse disorders are estimated to involve 15% of patients in outpatient settings, 25 to 40% of hospitalized patients and nearly 50% of patients in emergency rooms (1, 2). Indeed, substance abuse may be the presenting problem or an important underlying factor in the care of almost any patient.

Once you make a substance abuse diagnosis, future treatment of that patient is forever affected. Psychiatric diagnoses, such as depression, cannot be separated from the addiction problem. When treating addicts for medical problems, you must often modify your usual treatment regimen to avoid certain medications. For instance, patients who are in recovery from alcohol addiction may wish to avoid treatment with "mind altering" drugs because of the tenets of Alcoholics Anonymous to which they adhere; recovering patients with a history of opiate addiction may want reassurance that their pain will be treated appropriately, followed by a detoxification regimen should opiates be needed. Care of substance abusers is frequently accompanied by complicated social situations involving patients and their friends or family members; thus, disposition plans often include an evaluation of danger the substance abuser poses to himself or others.

If you find that a patient is addicted to a drug, addiction treatment should be considered. Important factors in deciding treatment(s) to recommend are the patients' willingness to undergo treatment, their social support networks, their personal financial resources, and programs available in their communities.

You will, in your professional lifetime, confront significant legal and ethical questions around substance abusers who are patients and/or professional colleagues. For instance, the diagnosis of opiate abuse made on a medical professional patient presents an ethical dilemma: breaking confidentiality on a colleague versus protecting the public from an impaired health professional. In addition, prescription of controlled substances is accompanied by a set of strict regulations and a professional reporting system. Pharmacists filling inappropriately large or frequent prescriptions for addicting substances are generally required to report the situation and the name of the prescribing physician to a governmental agency.

DEFINITIONS

Discussions of substance abuse and addiction are difficult because the terminology and meanings vary among health professionals, in the media, in the medical literature, and in society. The fourth edition of *Diagnostic and Statistical Manual of Mental Disorders (DSM-IV)* from the American Psychiatric Association contains nearly 100 pages of substance abuse diagnoses (3). Specific diagnostic terms (e.g., intoxication, withdrawal, dependence, etc.) are defined for each of 12 drug categories using a similar set of criteria. To make a diagnosis, the physician must determine the drug(s) involved, the duration of use of each, and the negative consequences on the patient's health and/or psychosocial well-being (e.g., emphysema, driver's license revocation, divorce, bankruptcy) that have been caused by using drugs.

While describing diagnoses, the DSM-IV does not define addiction, the title of this chapter and a word commonly used in medicine and in society in general. The American Society of Addiction Medicine defines addiction as "a disease process characterized by the continued use of a specific psychoactive substance despite physical, psychological, or social harm" (4).

This chapter focuses only on addiction to drugs, including ethyl alcohol (hereafter referred to simply as alcohol), nicotine (or its vehicle, tobacco), prescription and illicit drugs, and various other chemicals, such as aromatic solvents (glue sniffing). Nonpharmacologic behaviors to which people may become addicted (gambling, eating, or sexual practices) are not covered.

The following definitions are used in this chapter:

Use of a drug: intake by any route of administration.

Misuse of a drug: use other than as prescribed, such as in the wrong dosage or at improper time intervals.

Abuse of a drug: drug use that puts the user or others at risk; or, the use for a reason other than intended (e.g., using Percocet to get high, rather than for pain); or, use of an illicit drug, such as heroin.

Tolerance to a drug: this develops when the effect of a constant dose becomes diminished; or, an increasing dose is required to achieve the desired effect.

Cross-tolerance to a drug exists when the tolerance a patient has developed by using one drug confers tolerance to other drug(s) the patient has not used; or, withdrawal effects a dependent patient experiences after stopping the drug of abuse are relieved when the patient takes another drug (e.g., when benzodiazepines relieve alcohol withdrawal symptoms).

Dependence on a drug exists when a withdrawal syndrome (psychologic and/or physical symptoms) develops when the drug is discontinued.

Addiction is the continued practice of a *behavior* despite negative consequences.

Understanding the distinction between dependency and addiction is crucial. Many people become dependent on drugs they use frequently but are *not* addicted unless use of the drug leads to negative consequences. For instance, dependence on caffeine is illustrated by someone who omits drinking the usual morning coffee and gets a "withdrawal" headache by 2:00 PM; most consumers do not suffer negative consequences from using coffee and, thus, are not addicted. Another example of dependency is the Type I diabetic who would die without insulin, but who is not addicted because insulin has positive consequences (living), rather than negative ones.

ETIOLOGY

With the exception of alcohol, most drugs of abuse have been found to have specific binding sites in the brain. These sites are located in the "pleasure pathway" (median forebrain bundle, nucleus accumbens, ventral tegmental area, locus ceruleus, and the medial longitudinal fasciculus) and affect neurotransmitters, notably dopamine and serotonin. Use of addictive drugs provides "positive reinforcement" in the pleasure pathway by stimulation of neuroreceptors and the release of neurotransmitters. Thus, an addict receives positive reinforcement from use of a drug and continues using despite accompanying negative consequences.

Addiction does not involve higher cortical function; the pleasure pathway is located in lower brain centers, which explains why models of addiction are available in mice and rats as well as in primates. Most addicts state they do not "want" to be addicted; however, they are not able to stop using drugs even though they "know they should."

There seems to be at least a component of genetic predisposition to addiction. For instance, identical twins demonstrate a higher coincidence of alcohol addiction than fraternal twins, even when raised in separate households (5).

PREVALENCE

Figures 15.1 and 15.2 demonstrate the prevalence of use of several common drugs by twelfth graders over the past two decades. Experts believe the most important variable in drug use is the public's perception of the risk of using (6). The drop in cigarette use of the 1990s is thought to be due in large part to society's growing awareness of the dangers of smoking.

Studies consistently show that the incidence of alcohol use, tobacco use, and other drug abuse (ATODA) is greatest in the second decade of life. Highest consumption of drugs occurs in the third decade of life, then falls off steadily both because of discontinuation and because users die rela-

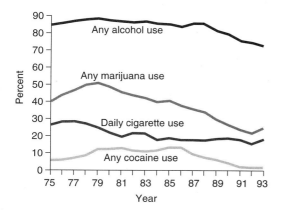

Figure 15.1. *Trends in selected measures of drug use for U.S. twelfth graders, 1975–1993.* (Reprinted with permission from Johnston LD, O'Malley PM, Bachman JG. National Survey Results on Drug Use from The Monitoring the Future Study, 1975–1993, Volume 1, Secondary School Students. Rockville, MD: National Institute on Drug Abuse, 1994.)

tively younger than nonusers. Clearly, the best time for prevention is during the grade school years, when children are most likely to start using drugs of abuse.

Physicians see a higher percentage of substance abusers than exists in the general population because of the negative physical and mental effects of abused drugs. The direct cost of medical treatment of ATODA in the United States is in excess of $136 billion annually (7). Adding such costs as law enforcement, interdiction programs, and decreased productivity in the work-

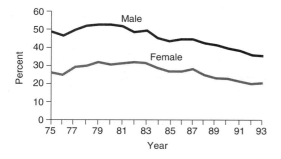

Figure 15.2. *Trends in use of alcohol for U.S. twelfth graders, 1975–1993 (by total and sex).* (Reprinted with permission from Johnston LD, O'Malley PM, Bachman JG. National Survey Results on Drug Use from The Monitoring the Future Study, 1975–1993, Volume 1, Secondary School Students. Rockville, MD: National Institute on Drug Abuse, 1994.)

force, the total cost of substance abuse is in excess of $240 billion/year (8).

DIFFERENTIAL DIAGNOSIS

Sometimes a drug-related diagnosis is obvious, with such conditions as emphysema in a long-time smoker or bleeding from esophageal varices in a patient who has Laënnec's cirrhosis. At other times, the diagnosis is more subtle, such as with decreasing school performance in an adolescent who is abusing marijuana. In some cases, one drug seems to be responsible (e.g., Laënnec's cirrhosis from alcohol), while in others, it is a synergism between more than one drug (e.g., oral cancer linked to both tobacco and alcohol consumption). At other times, it is the route of use that causes the problem (e.g., HIV from intravenous drug use), rather than an effect of the drug itself.

Addiction often goes undiagnosed. Physicians must be constantly vigilant, screen patients for substance abuse, and be aware of certain "red flag" diagnoses and laboratory results that correlate with substance abuse and should prompt investigation (Table 15.1). If you can diagnose drug abuse or addiction early, before irreversible organ damage or serious psychosocial consequences have occurred, you may be able to intervene successfully and prevent further deterioration.

PATHOPHYSIOLOGY

Although a thorough discussion of the effects of addictive drugs on the body is beyond the scope of this chapter, Table 15.2 reviews the most common causative mechanisms and associations.

CLINICAL EVALUATION

Screening

Screening for addiction begins with questioning patients about use of tobacco, alcohol, and licit and illicit drugs. Screening should be carried out with every new patient and updated at each "physical examination" for an existing patient; it should be done in any case of a "red flag" diagnosis or laboratory finding. Two screening tests for family physicians to use in the outpatient setting are the Cyr-Wartman questions and the CAGE questions (Table 15.3), which are demonstrated for alcohol but may be adapted for other drug abuse. The Cyr-Wartman screening test has

Table 15.1.
Red Flags for Addiction

HISTORY

Chief complaint: sleep disorder, pain, "nerves," trauma, rapid pulse, dizziness, shortness of breath, disorientation, tremor, palpitations, hematemesis, jaundice, melena, decreased libido, hallucinations

History of present illness: stopped drinking; "blackouts;" seizures

Past history: Recurrent pneumonia, recurrent peptic ulcers, variceal bleeding, recurrent trauma

Social history: family violence, family deterioration, financial deterioration, loss of job, frequent job changes, incarceration, deterioration of work or school performance

---

PHYSICAL FINDINGS

Vital signs: bradycardia, tachycardia; rapid, slow, shallow, or labored respirations; hypertension, hypotension

Skin: telangiectasias, "caput medusae," needle tracks, cellulitis, multiple ecchymoses and lacerations

Head and neck: caries, cheilosis, glossitis, leukoplakia, oropharyngeal mass, nasal ulcer, perforated nasal septum, myosis, mydriasis

Abdomen: enlarged or shrunken liver, ascites, splenomegaly

Genitorectal: testicular atrophy, hemorrhoids

Neurologic: agitation, delirium, obtundation, tremor, asterixis, seizures, ocular or radial nerve palsy

---

DIAGNOSES

Neurologic: encephalopathy, early stroke, new-onset seizures, overdose, syncope

Psychiatric: anxiety, panic disorder, depression, suicide attempt, acute psychosis, character disorder

Gastrointestinal: gastritis, ulcers, GI bleeding, cirrhosis, fatty liver, pancreatitis, oral or esophageal cancer

Cardiovascular: labile hypertension, supraventricular tachycardia, early myocardial infarction, esophageal varices, cardiomyopathy, bacterial endocarditis

Pulmonary: respiratory depression, aspiration pneumonia, gram-negative pneumonia, lung cancer, drowning

Genitourinary: erectile dysfunction

Infectious disease: HIV/AIDS, sepsis, endocarditis

Trauma: motor vehicle crashes (especially single vehicle), falls, gunshot, stabbing, beatings, on-the-job injury

Poisoning: methanol, ethylene glycol

Hematopoietic: macrocytic anemia

LABORATORY

CBC: macrocytic RBCs, thrombocytopenia

Chemistries: elevated transaminases (AST > ALT), GGT

Immunology: positive HIV, hepatitis B, hepatitis C

---

a sensitivity of 91.5% and a specificity of 89.7% (9). The CAGE screening test has a sensitivity of 85 to 94% and a specificity between 79 and 88% (10).

Neither the Cyr-Wartman questions nor the CAGE questions are diagnostic of alcohol addiction. Positive screens must be followed with questions to collect sufficient data to yield a DSM-IV diagnosis.

In the family medicine setting, positive responses to the mnemonic "UCR" (use, negative consequences, and repetition) should raise suspicion. When a patient has been using a drug and experiencing negative consequences as the result, yet continues to use the drug, the physician should strongly suspect addiction.

"Red Flag" Diagnoses

Certain diagnoses and clinical situations are associated with a high incidence of substance abuse and addiction. Table 15.1 lists some of the most common of these. The gastrointestinal system is especially hard hit by alcohol, and patients with esophagitis, gastritis, hepatitis, and pancreatitis should be queried for their drinking behaviors. Trauma, especially single car crashes and injuries sustained on the job, are highly correlated

Table 15.2.
Adverse Effects of Common Recreational Drugs

Drug	Is Strongly Associated with or Directly Causes
Tobacco	• Emphysema and chronic bronchitis • Coronary artery disease • Cancer of the lung, mouth, esophagus, and bladder • Decreased fetal weight
Alcohol	• Intoxication, leading to loss of judgment and inhibition (e.g., automobile crashes, drowning, suicide) and patients' putting themselves and others at risk from dangerous behaviors • GI tract diseases, especially gastritis, hepatitis, fatty infiltration of the liver, Laënnec's cirrhosis, esophageal varices, and pancreatitis • Hypertension and dilated cardiomyopathy • Central nervous system diseases, secondary to vitamin deficiencies (e.g., Wernicke's encephalopathy, Korsakoff syndrome) • Cancers, especially when used with tobacco (e.g., oral and esophageal carcinoma) • Fetal alcohol syndrome
Cocaine	• Seizures, acute psychoses • Vasospasm of cerebral and coronary arteries, leading to ischemia, stroke, myocardial infarction, cardiac arrhythmias, and sudden death • (In combination with alcohol, forming cocaethylene): necrotizing vasculitis, leading to stroke and myocardial infarction • Loss of appetite, loss of weight • Depression • Financial deterioration • Family and community violence and crime
Marijuana	• Pulmonary diseases such as asthma and bronchitis • Chronic underachievement • Other drug use
Heroin	• Overdose and respiratory depression, which may be fatal • Intravenous drug use sequelae, such as skin infections, endocarditis, hepatitis B, HIV, and AIDS • Violence and crime

Table 15.3.
Screening Questions for Alcohol Abuse

I. The Cyr-Wartman Questions
   1. When was your last drink of alcohol?   (Positive = yesterday or today)
   2. Have you ever had a problem with alcohol?   (Positive = "yes")

Interpretation: A positive response to either question is a positive screen and should prompt further questions about quantities and duration of alcohol use and any accompanying negative consequences of use.[a]

II. The CAGE Questions
   1. Have you ever tried to Cut down your use of alcohol?
   2. Have you ever been Annoyed by others criticizing your drinking?
   3. Have you ever felt Guilty because of your use of alcohol?
   4. Have you ever needed an "Eye opener" in the morning to settle your nerves?

Interpretation: A "yes" answer to two or more of these questions is a positive response and should prompt further questions about quantities and duration of alcohol use and any accompanying negative consequences of use.[b]

[a]Cyr MG, Wartman SA. The effectiveness of routine screening questions in the detection of alcoholism. JAMA 1988;259:51–54.

[b]Ewing JA. Detecting alcoholism. JAMA 1984;252:(14)1905–1907.

with drugs of abuse. Anyone seen in the emergency room with a history of multiple-trauma events should be closely questioned.

Physical violence, especially domestic violence and child abuse, are frequently linked to substance abuse, as are family disruption, marital discord, deteriorating financial status, and loss of employment.

Physical Findings

Table 15.1 lists physical findings that are commonly associated with addicts. Patients with these abnormalities should be questioned about their use of drugs and alcohol.

Laboratory Testing

Addiction is a clinical, rather than a laboratory, diagnosis. All laboratory results on an addicted patient can be completely normal. However, certain laboratory findings are suggestive of drug and alcohol abuse and, like "red flag" diagnoses, should tip you off to the likelihood of drug abuse or addiction (see Table 15.1).

Notable laboratory test abnormalities for alcohol abuse are increased RBC indices and thrombocytopenia and elevated liver enzymes (GGT, AST, ALT) with AST higher than ALT.

Table 15.4 lists various drug levels you can order on different laboratory specimens. Assays may be used to confirm that a patient has taken a drug (e.g., cocaine use in a young stroke victim) and/or aid in the management of a disease process (e.g., blood alcohol level in a comatose patient).

When ordering drug testing, have you made the patient vulnerable to criminal prosecution if an illegal drug such as cocaine is found? The answer is no. A patient may not be prosecuted in a criminal trial because of a positive drug test unless two conditions are met: (a) a "chain of custody" is established on the sample at the time of collection and carried through until the results are introduced into evidence; and (b) the drug assay method is approved by the state. Physicians ordering tests for medical reasons typically do not establish chain of custody on specimens; hospital and commercial laboratories may not use assay methods acceptable for a criminal trial.

Drug test results become available from a patient's medical record if subpoenaed by a court or when a patient signs a medical release of information form, such as those the insurance companies use routinely. Negative consequences of discovery do occur, such as loss of jobs, denial of health or life insurance benefits, or custody of dependent children. You should be aware of these consequences when ordering such laboratory tests and when you send results out of your office or hospital. You must realize, too, that drug levels may be required to properly diagnose and

Table 15.4.
Laboratory Testing for Substance Abuse

Specimen	Tests Available	Advantages	Disadvantages
Blood	Most drugs	Accuracy Easy access	Short window of positivity Slightly invasive

Urine	Cocaine
	Marijuana
	Opiates
	Barbiturates
	Benzodiazepines
	Phencyclidine
		Longer duration of positivity,
		  ranging from days (cocaine)
		  to weeks (marijuana)
			Observed or documented
			  specimen collection necessary

Saliva	Alcohol	Immediate results	Qualitative use only
Breath	Alcohol	Immediate results	Blood levels needed for accurate medical management

Hair	Cocaine
	Marijuana
	Opiates
	Amphetamines
	Phencyclidine
		Noninvasive
		Longest duration of positivity
		  (at least 90 days)
			Not widely available; quantitative
			  analysis invalid because amounts
			  of drug deposited vary with hair
			  color

manage a patient. Therefore, it is frequently appropriate to run the risk of ordering these tests in the patient's behalf.

MANAGEMENT

Management depends on the severity of the patient's addiction, the severity of concomitant medical and/or psychiatric problems, the necessity for treatment with vitamins or minerals, the necessity for substitution of cross-tolerant drugs to prevent or treat drug withdrawal, a determination of the threat the patient poses to himself or others, an assessment of the patient's resources, and an effort to direct the patient toward addiction treatment. An algorithm for decision making is presented in Figure 15.3.

Initial Decisions

Medical Stability

Initial management of an unstable patient follows guidelines for acute care. For instance, the comatose heroin addict may require intubation and/or treatment with naloxone for a presumed overdose. An alcoholic known to have esophageal varices, who is in shock after a bloody emesis, should initially receive volume expanders, followed by blood transfusions.

Patients in an acute care setting who might be chronic alcohol abusers should routinely be given 100 mg of thiamine to prevent Wernicke's syndrome. Also consider giving intramuscular or intravenous magnesium sulfate to prevent alcohol withdrawal complications.

In the family physician's office, medical management remains atop the list of considerations. Patients with gastritis from alcohol abuse or skin infections from injecting opiates must be evaluated and treated for their medical problems. They must also be evaluated for intoxication and withdrawal potential and treated with vitamins, minerals, and withdrawal prophylaxis. Initial steps in addiction treatment, discussed below, may be taken during the encounter.

Withdrawal Syndromes and Detoxification

Substance abusers must be evaluated for signs of a withdrawal syndrome. Withdrawal is most commonly seen in patients dependent on opiates or sedative-hypnotic drugs (including alcohol). Withdrawal syndromes from either category are uncomfortable, although sedative-hypnotic withdrawal is medically more dangerous. To treat a withdrawal syndrome, you should substitute a cross-tolerant drug using doses sufficient to alleviate the signs and symptoms of withdrawal. Initial loading doses are given both to increase patient comfort and, in the case of alcohol and sedative-hypnotic drugs, to prevent seizures and progression to delirium tremens, a potentially fatal complication (Table 15.5).

A patient withdrawing from opiate may experience mydriasis, "goose flesh," abdominal cramps, myoclonic jerks, and rhinorrhea. Patients dependent on opiates are usually stabilized in the hospital by being administered a daily dose of methadone to replace the amount of opiate drugs they were using prior to admission. Typically, patients addicted to opiates are maintained on this dose during the admission and subsequently discharged to methadone treatment programs. Alternatively, methadone may be tapered over 10 days, although relapse rates are very high.

Patients withdrawing from alcohol (or any sedative hypnotic drug) may experience tremor, tachycardia, nausea, diaphoresis, and fever. Assess the severity of the withdrawal syndrome by using a scale such as the revised Clinical Institute Withdrawal Assessment for Alcohol (CIWA-Ar) Scale (Table 15.6) (11). Subsequent decisions about when to use drug prophylaxis are based on the patient's blood alcohol level and the CIWA-Ar score at the time of assessment (12). Loading doses of (preferably long acting) cross-tolerant medication are used when CIWA-Ar scores exceed 25. Detoxification is completed by tapering patients off cross-tolerant drugs over a time period that depends on the drug of abuse. In the case of alcohol, detoxification is generally accomplished in less than a week; benzodiazepine detoxification can take months.

Psychiatric Stability

In acute situations, a patient's psychiatric status must be evaluated. Intoxicated patients manifest a spectrum of acute psychiatric symptoms depending on the abused drug(s). Cocaine and phencyclidine intoxication may cause euphoria, severe agitation, aggressive behavior and acute psychosis, whereas sedative hypnotic intoxication can induce depression and suicidal behavior. Many patients ingest multiple drugs (e.g., cocaine with marijuana or heroin), so the presentation can be mixed. As drugs are metabolized,

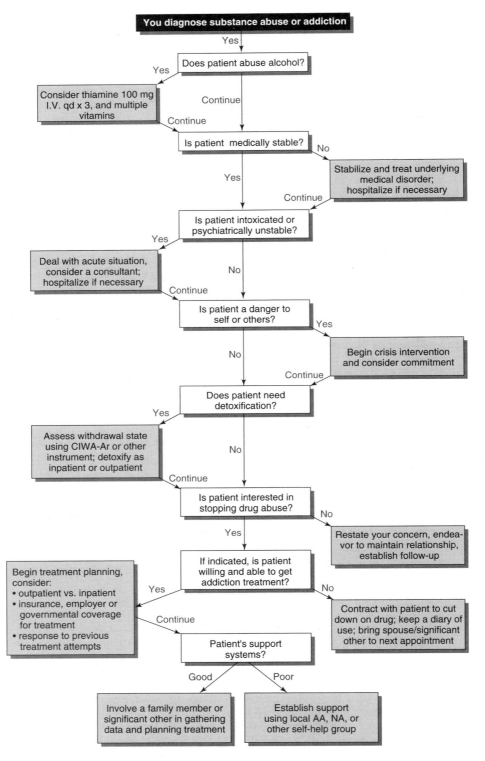

Figure 15.3. *An algorithmic approach for treating drug addicts.*

Table 15.5.

Example Regimens for Detoxification from Alcohol and Opiates

ALCOHOL
1. Thiamine: 100 mg IM on admission
2. Phenergan: 50 mg IM q6h prn nausea
3. Magnesium sulfate: 1 g IM q8h × 3 doses
4. Phenobarbital: 60 mg PO tid × 2 days
                   30 mg PO tid × 2 days
                   15 mg PO bid
5. Phenobarbital (injectable): 130–260 mg IM × 1 prn agitation (may need to repeat every 20 minutes until sedated after notifying physician)
6. Secobarbital: 100 mg PO or IM q HS prn sleep

OPIATES[a]
1. Methadone: 10 mg PO q2–4h, up to 3 doses in first 24 hr (titrate to relief of symptoms)
2. Methadone: total dose PO from day 1 every morning
3. Phenergan: 25–50 mg IM q6h, prn nausea
4. May discharge to methadone maintenance program on methadone, 30 mg PO qd, or
5. May taper methadone by 10% per day, starting on fourth day

---

[a] Adapted from Devenyi P, Saunders S. Physicians Handbook for Medical Management of Alcohol- and Drug-Related Problems. Toronto, Canada: Addiction Research Foundation and the Ontario Medical Association, 1986.

---

dependent patients may begin to exhibit psychiatric signs and symptoms of withdrawal, which are different and frequently opposite to those of the intoxicated state. Treatment with psychoactive drugs, such as haloperidol or benzodiazepines, may be necessary for intoxicated patients or those in withdrawal.

Some drug abusers are dangerous to themselves or others. In all cases, particularly in acute care settings, screening the patient for the potential to do harm must be made prior to finalizing treatment plans. Those admitted to hospitals may need suicide precautions or physical restraints, whereas others must be committed to protective custody to prevent harm to themselves or others. In no case should an intoxicated patient be discharged to drive home alone.

Addiction Treatment

Many times, addicted patients resolve their problems on their own. Over 80% of people who quit smoking cigarettes do so without consulting physicians (13). Even higher percentages of students who drank heavily in college have been shown to revert to low-risk drinking behavior when they leave college (14). Patients who present to the medical profession for help with addiction may have more severe problems than society in general.

Helping Patients Change

Family physicians confront addictive behaviors on a daily basis. Either the physician or the patient can address the subject initially, and then a search for a plan of action begins. The Readiness to Change Model, developed by Prochaska and DiClemente and discussed in detail in Chapter 6, Helping Your Patients Stay Healthy, is used for all types of behavior change, including addiction. The model suggests that behavior change occurs in stages. Current thinking is that patients rarely jump from the contemplation stage (realizing a problem exists) to permanently stopping the behavior during a single physician encounter. In terms of the Prochaska/DiClemente model, more realistic goals for success are helping the patient move along from stage to stage (15). Some drugs and some addiction problems may be addressed successfully within the context of a primary care practice; others are best referred to an addiction specialist or an addiction treatment program.

Initial Considerations in Addiction Treatment

Addicted patients have a history of continuing to use drugs despite negative consequences. Addicts are reluctant to stop using drugs even when their plights seem desperate. As physicians, we cannot

Table 15.6.
The Revised Clinical Institute Withdrawal Assessment Scale for Alcohol (CIWA-Ar)[a]

Clinical Dimension	Question and/or Observation	Score Range: 0–7
Nausea/vomiting	Ask, "Do you feel sick?" Observe for vomiting	0 = No nausea, no vomiting 1 = Mild nausea, no vomiting 4 = Intermittent nausea with dry heaves 7 = Constant nausea; frequent dry heaves and vomiting
Tremor	Arms extended and fingers spread apart	0 = No tremor 1 = Not visible, but can be felt fingertip to fingertip 4 = Moderate, with patient's arms extended 7 = Severe, even with arms not extended
Paroxysmal sweats	Observation	0 = No sweat visible 1 = Barely perceptible sweating; palms moist 4 = Beads of sweat obvious on forehead 7 = Drenching sweats
Anxiety	Ask, "Do you feel nervous?" Observation	0 = No anxiety; at ease 1 = Mildly anxious 3 = Moderately anxious, or guarded, so anxiety is inferred 7 = Equivalent to acute panic states, as seen in severe delirium or acute schizophrenic reactions
Agitation	Observation	0 = Normal activity 1 = Somewhat more than normal activity 4 = Moderately fidgety and restless 7 = Paces back and forth during most of the interview or constantly thrashes about
Tactile disturbances	Ask, "Have you any itching, pins and needles sensations, burning, or numbness, or do you feel bugs crawling on or under your skin?" Observation	0 = None 1 = Very mild itching, pins and needles, burning, or numbness 4 = Moderately severe hallucinations 7 = Continuous hallucinations
Auditory disturbances	Ask, "Are you more aware of sounds around you? Are they harsh? Do they frighten you? Are you hearing anything that is disturbing you? Are you hearing things you know are not there?" Observation	0 = Not present 1 = Very mild harshness or ability to frighten 4 = Moderately severe hallucinations 7 = Continuous hallucinations
Visual disturbances	Ask, "Does the light appear to be too bright? Is the color different? Does it hurt your eyes? Are you seeing anything that is disturbing you? Are you seeing things you know are not there? Observation	0 = Not present 1 = Very mild sensitivity 4 = Moderately severe hallucinations 7 = Continuous hallucinations
Headache, fullness in head	Ask, "Does your head feel different? Does it feel like there is a band around your head?" Do not rate dizziness or lightheadedness. Otherwise, rate severity.	0 = Not present 1 = Very mild 4 = Moderately severe 7 = Extremely severe
Orientation and clouding of sensorium	Ask, "What day is this? Where are you? Who am I?"	0 = Oriented and can do serial additions 1 = Cannot do serial additions or is uncertain about date 2 = Disoriented for date by no more than 2 calendar days 3 = Disoriented for date by more than 2 calendar days 4 = Disoriented for place and/or person

continued

Table 15.6. (*continued*)
The Revised Clinical Institute Withdrawal Assessment Scale for Alcohol (CIWA-Ar)[a]

Decision making[b]

Score	Category of Withdrawal	Treatment
< 20	Mild	No medication necessary
20–24	Moderate	Medication necessary
25–30	Severe	Medicate with loading doses
>30	Very severe	Consider hospital admission

[a] Adapted from Sullivan JT, Sukora K, Schneiderman J, Naranjo CA, Sellers EM. Assessment of alcohol withdrawal: the revised Clinical Institute Withdrawal Assessment for Alcohol (CIWA-Ar). Br J Addict 1989;84:1353–1357.

[b] Adapted from Patient Placement Criteria for the Treatment of Psychoactive Substance Use Disorders. Washington, DC: American Society of Addiction Medicine, 1991.

expect most patients to immediately change behavior because we say "quit." Although telling patients to stop using drugs may occasionally be successful, physicians can greatly improve a patient's chances for success in addiction treatment by learning "motivational techniques" such as those described by Miller and Rollnick (16). These strategies avoid polarization in the doctor-patient relationship through seeking common ground, rolling with resistance, and allowing patients to make decisions about their treatment.

When physicians refer patients to addiction treatment specialists, addicts are far more likely to show up for evaluation and treatment if the referring physician is actively involved in the process. Best results are obtained when the physician makes the initial contact with the referral source and, with the patient present, introduces the patient to the consultant by telephone or in person.

In recommending an addiction treatment program for a given patient, the following factors must be considered:

- Concomitant mental or medical illness. If significant medical or psychiatric complications exist, addicts are best treated in programs equipped to handle both the illness and the drug addiction.

- Previous addiction treatment history. Unlike many other diseases, an addict's chances for success in treatment improve with the number of previous treatment attempts, but addicts with prior treatment may benefit from a change of venue or program philosophy.

- Patient financial resources. Health insurance companies often limit addiction treatment, which dictates what many patients can afford. Some patients are eligible for employer or community-supported drug treatment, court-

ordered treatment, or programs sponsored by local or federal government.

- Family support. If an addict is fortunate enough to have a supportive family, programs that include a strong "family treatment component" increase the patient's chance of successful treatment (17).

- Living environment. Persons living in drug-infested environments should be placed in a drug-free location during treatment and after discharge.

Types of Addiction Treatment

Options for addiction treatment include office-based treatment, referral to self-help groups, or referral to formal addiction treatment programs. Addiction treatment programs can be inpatient or outpatient and use various strategies, such as pharmacotherapy, aversion therapy, cognitive-behavioral therapy, acupuncture, therapeutic communities and halfway houses, Outward Bound and "boot camp" techniques, or the "Minnesota Model." The following is a brief description of several common techniques used to treat addiction.

"SELF-HELP GROUPS"

In 1937, the modern "self-help" movement in alcohol treatment began in the United States with the creation of Alcoholics Anonymous (AA). Begun by a small group of alcohol addicts, including founders Bill Wilson and Dr. Bob Smith, AA conceived of "alcoholism" as a disease over which the sufferer (an "alcoholic") had no control. *Any* use of alcohol was thought to lead to uncontrolled use, which in turn led to further deterioration of the victim's life. The group developed 12 steps to recovery (Table 15.7), which, if followed, were a

Table 15.7.
The Original 12 Steps of Alcoholics Anonymous

1. We admitted we are powerless over alcohol—that our lives had become unmanageable.
2. We came to believe that a Power greater than ourselves could restore us to sanity.
3. We made a decision to turn our will and our lives over to the care of God.
4. We made a searching and fearless moral inventory of ourselves.
5. We admitted to God, to ourselves, and to another human being the exact nature of our wrongs.
6. We were entirely ready to have God remove all these defects of character.
7. We humbly asked Him to remove our shortcomings.
8. We made a list of all persons we had harmed, and became willing to make amends to them all.
9. We made direct amends to such people whenever possible, except when to do so would injure them or others.
10. We continued to take personal inventory and when we were wrong, promptly admitted it.
11. We sought through prayer and meditation to improve our conscious contact with God, praying only for knowledge of His will for us and the power to carry that out.
12. Having had a spiritual awakening as the result of these steps, we tried to carry this message to alcoholics, and to practice these principles in all our affairs.

Source: National Household Survey on Drug Abuse: Main Findings 1988. Rockville, MD: National Institute on Drug Abuse, 1990.

plan of action that could help the alcoholic stay sober. Members believe that lifelong attendance at AA meetings is necessary for the maintenance of sobriety and an improved way of living, including interactions with other people. Alcoholics Anonymous grew to become the largest and most widely available self-help movement in the world. Using similar precepts to AA, a number of other 12-step programs have grown as spin-offs of the organization, including Narcotics Anonymous (NA), Cocaine Anonymous, Overeaters Anonymous, and Gamblers Anonymous.

MINNESOTA MODEL

In 1948, a technique for treating alcoholic patients was developed at Willmar State Hospital in Minnesota. As the first program to have long-term success, it became the most common addiction-treatment technique in the United States. The "Minnesota Model" began with detoxified inpatients who were enrolled in a program lasting 4 weeks (hence the label "28-day program"). Treatment consisted of large-group activities in which patients were educated about the effects of alcohol, given the explanation for addiction as conceived by AA, and given a thorough indoctrination in the philosophy of AA. Each patient was assigned an individual counselor, frequently a recovering alcoholic, and, with the counselor's guidance, systematically worked through the first 5 steps of the AA program. Patients attended daily AA meetings, initially in the hospital and later in the community, so that, upon discharge, they could continue using ubiquitous AA meetings as support groups in their efforts to stay sober. Each patient was challenged to attend "90 meetings in 90 days" after leaving the program (18).

Variations on the Minnesota Model exist all over the United States. Some continue to be inpatient programs, but, because of expense, insurance companies have managed to force the creation of daytime or evening programs that eliminate the "hotel costs" and staff expenses of certified hospital treatment programs. Many "intensive outpatient programs" use Minnesota Model techniques, keep patients occupied 4 or 5 days of the week, train them to use self-help support groups, and refer program graduates to self-help groups.

COGNITIVE-BEHAVIORAL TECHNIQUES

Cognitive-behavioral therapy uses strategies to enable a patient's "higher cognitive function" to overcome the addiction. Patients are asked to "think" about their drug use, weigh the pros and cons of using, and change their behavior if they desire. Patients set individual drug-use goals (most commonly abstinence) and explore ways in which they can reduce or eliminate the use of drugs. As a part of the therapy, patients are taught "relapse prevention" techniques, such as changing their circle of friends, adjusting their daily work and personal lives, learning to drink soft drinks while others drink alcohol, and even practice at attending bars or restaurants without drinking.

AVERSION THERAPY

Aversion therapy involves using classic conditioning techniques to make patients averse to using drugs. Alcohol treatment is accomplished by giving patients emetine, which causes vomiting, and having them drink alcoholic beverages while they vomit frequently. For other drugs, the technique involves using their own drug paraphernalia and smoking or injecting simulated drugs, while electric shocks are administered to their body. Patients eventually become conditioned to avoid the drugs. Such programs have similar outcomes to Minnesota Model programs (19); their numbers peaked in the 1980s and then decreased as insurance company efforts reduced the availability of inpatient addiction treatment.

DRUG TREATMENT

Drugs used to treat addiction use different strategies such as adverse reaction, substitution, and blocking effects. Selection of a pharmacotherapy depends on the drug to which the patient is addicted.

Substitution Pharmacotherapy. Methadone is the classic example of a substitution pharmacotherapy. An opiate that causes relatively little euphoria, methadone is given to patients who are addicted to illicit opiates (e.g., heroin) or prescription opiates (e.g., morphine or oxycodone). Many patients succeed in methadone treatment programs and reverse the negative consequences of opiate use in their lives, regain employment, and become productive citizens. Unfortunately, some methadone programs have long waiting lists for admission, and because daily visits are required, many patients must drive long distances every day to obtain the drug. A cost-effective program, it is unfortunate that the federal government both restricts most physicians from prescribing methadone to opiate addicts and withholds funding for sufficient methadone treatment slots.

A second substitution strategy is nicotine replacement, which helps tobacco abusers discontinue smoking, chewing tobacco, or dipping snuff. Both transdermal patches and chewing gum are available to nicotine addicts whose goal is to discontinue nicotine by progressively lowering the concentration of nicotine in their patches or reducing the number of pieces of gum they use daily.

Adverse Reaction Pharmacotherapy. If taken in adequate dosage (125 to 500 mg/day) within 24 hours, disulfiram (Antabuse) causes patients to experience flushing, tachycardia, and nausea when they drink alcohol. It is used with some success by alcohol addicts who take disulfiram before they have an impulse to drink later in the day. It is also used by methadone treatment programs, mixed with methadone, in an effort to dissuade opiate addicts from drinking alcohol, because alcohol abuse is the most common cause of relapse in methadone patients. Disulfiram is easily defeated by the alcohol addict who simply avoids taking it if he or she decides to drink, and has fallen out of favor with many physicians.

Blocking Pharmacotherapy. Drugs that are competitive antagonists for binding sites are called blocking drugs. They bind to drug receptors in the brain, displacing the drug of abuse, but providing no stimulation of the receptor. Pharmacotherapies using blocking drugs have two uses in treating addicts. The first purpose is to immediately reverse the respiratory depressant effects of an overdose in an emergency situation. Naloxone (Narcan) is an opiate-receptor antagonist used to reverse opiate overdose, and flumazenil (Romazicon) is a benzodiazepine antagonist that reverses respiratory depression owing to benzodiazepine overdose. Both drugs may be lifesaving; both precipitate withdrawal symptoms in patients who are dependent on these drugs.

The second therapeutic use is to treat patients who agree to take the blocking agents regularly, thereby eliminating the pleasurable effects of drugs to which they are addicted. Patients are first detoxified, then begin taking the blocking drugs daily, knowing that if they take their drugs of abuse, they will not experience the desired effect. Like disulfiram in alcoholics, this strategy can be defeated by simply not taking the blocking drug before using the abused drug. However, certain groups of addicts seem to do well with blocking drugs, especially patients who have much to lose if they are found to relapse. The classic example of a successful blocking pharmacotherapy is the use of naltrexone (ReVia), an opiate antagonist, with addicted professionals such as physicians and lawyers. Such patients take 25 to 50 mg/day of naltrexone and are also subjected to a program of random urine testing. Relapse leads to loss of license to practice, which is a strong deterrent, and some success rates have been documented in excess of 95% (20).

Naltrexone has also been approved for treatment of alcohol addicts. It reduces the consumption of alcohol and is associated with more rapid reestablishment of sobriety following relapse in groups of patients who receive daily naltrexone therapy and simultaneous behavioral treatment (21). The mechanism of action of naltrexone is thought to be blockage of endogenous opioid-like neurotransmitters that positively reinforce alcohol use.

Brief Intervention

Many patients see a family physician early in their addiction, before serious medical or psychiatric sequelae have occurred. This is the ideal time to intervene in an attempt to get them to agree to treatment. Several "brief intervention" strategies have been tested and shown to be successful with some addicts. Essential elements include:

- Inform the patient of your concern about his or her drug use. Avoid parental or accusatory phrasing and, using the historical and laboratory data at hand, attempt to link drug use to negative physical, psychologic, or social consequences.

- Allow the patient to state his or her point of view.

- Assess the patient's readiness to change in terms of the Prochaska-DiClemente model (see Chapter 6), and use techniques to motivate the patient to reduce or stop using drugs.

- If the patient agrees with you, attempt to initiate planning toward discontinuation of drug use, such as setting a quit date for smoking or a visit to an open meeting of AA. This can be followed by a discussion of available addiction treatment methods.

- If the patient denies that a problem exists, but is willing to consider exploration, attempt to negotiate a commitment for cutting down or eliminating their drug(s). Suggest keeping a drug-use diary, noting urges to use, situations in which urges occur, responses, and both positive and negative consequences of use. Schedule a return appointment and attempt to include a spouse or significant other who can corroborate the diary and add to your understanding of the patient's problem.

- If the patient is unwilling to explore the problem, express your concern for his or her well-being and your willingness to reconsider the matter at a future date, and attempt to maintain a therapeutic relationship.

- Use follow-up visits to stay abreast of patient progress. Reinforce successes and be willing to change strategy if initial plans fail. Try to become a positive factor in the patient's attempts at recovery.

Success Rates of Addiction Treatment Programs

What do you tell your patients about their chances for success in addiction treatment? Most inpatient programs claim that 60 to 65% of their "graduates" are abstinent 1 year after completing treatment. Outpatient programs claim similar results, although their success may actually be 5 or 10% lower. One positive correlate with success in addiction treatment is the number of previous treatment attempts. That makes addiction treatment different from many other medical treatments, such as cancer chemotherapy.

Unfortunately the outcome statistics claimed by addiction treatment programs are not very accurate. Most programs determine success by interviewing their graduates on the telephone. When more sophisticated methods are used, such as interviewing friends, family, and coworkers or doing urine drug screens, success rates are far lower, sometimes in the range of 20 to 30%.

Abstinence-at-one-year has long been the standard of success for the addiction treatment field, largely based on the AA belief that any drinking leads to uncontrolled drinking ("one drink, one drunk"). Much research has shown that patients who stay sober for a year are more likely to regain employment and reestablish meaningful social networks. However, there are addiction treatment programs, notably in Great Britain, that claim success when their clients reduce intake and resume "social drinking." In the United States, the federal government has instituted new measures of success that are more objective and have more social significance than patient claims of abstinence, such as changes in crime statistics, rates of incarceration, and HIV conversion. In general, studies show that treatment has a positive effect on these outcome indicators.

Long-Term Treatment

All physicians treat patients who are addicted to drugs, whether or not the diagnosis has been made. Appropriate treatment of addicts differs from other patients, so physicians must endeavor to make the diagnosis in their own self defense as well as in behalf of the patient. The following are important considerations:

- Use nonpharmacotherapies whenever possible. Most addicts have long sought comfort from taking drugs; simply prescribing medication may be exactly the wrong tactic.

- Avoid prescribing "mind altering" substances to patients who are recovering addicts, because this practice has been associated with relapse. Drugs to avoid include elixirs containing alcohol, sedative hypnotic drugs, opiates, and antihistamines.

- Establish treatment contracts with patients involved in AA or NA. Be certain the recovering patient understands that you are committed to helping them while avoiding treatments that might trigger a relapse. Discuss how you will handle allergies, viral illnesses, anxiety, depression, insomnia, and pain—problems commonly treated by prescription of mind-altering substances.

- When treating opiate addicts in the hospital for painful conditions, use opiates only if necessary for adequate pain relief; then, use methadone to detoxify the patient once the painful episode has resolved.

- When admitting patients enrolled in methadone maintenance programs to the hospital, continue their current methadone dose to prevent a withdrawal syndrome. If needed, add opiate analgesics, starting with usual analgesic doses. Dose increases may be required because of tolerance induced by chronic methadone use.

- It is illegal to prescribe methadone to opiate-addicted outpatients. Although methadone may be prescribed to other outpatients for pain syndromes, methadone may be prescribed to outpatient addicts only in federally-monitored clinics.

PATIENT AND FAMILY EDUCATION

Family members and friends of drug addicts are invariably affected by the patients' drug use. Many times, these significant others are also abusing drugs. By virtue of their training and because they provide care for multiple family members, family physicians are in an excellent position to understand the dynamics between the people involved and to use close relationships on the behalf of their patients.

Problems among family members happen in many areas; notable among them are the following:

- Physical and emotional abuse, frequently perpetrated by male alcoholics against their spouses and/or children.

- Criminal behavior and subsequent legal troubles either from dealing drugs or stealing to acquire funds necessary to purchase them.

- Financial deterioration caused by the expense of illicit drugs, medical and legal bills, and/or the addict's failure to maintain a job.

- Infectious complications of intravenous drug use, including HIV and Hepatitis B or C, which are transmitted to the spouse and/or vertically to infants.

- Anxiety and depression in the spouse and/or children of the addict.

Following the creation of Alcoholics Anonymous, several offshoot organizations were developed to fulfill related needs. Prominent among these were 12-step organizations devoted to family members, including: Al-Anon, an organization for family members of alcoholics; Naranon, an organization for family members of drug addicts; and Alateen, an organization for teenagers with addicts in their families. These organizations subscribe to the precepts of AA and NA, and they focus on how family and friends "enable" addicts.

Enablers are people who live with addicts and, in many ways, make it possible for the addict to continue drinking or using drugs. For instance, enablers cook for and clean up after addicts, call the boss to report addicts ill when they are really intoxicated or hung over, or perform any number of supportive duties that spare addicts from having to deal with adverse situations of their own making.

Family physicians often refer family members of people with addiction problems to Al-Anon (Naranon, Alateen, etc.) so they can listen to family members of addicts in order to confirm suspicions about a family member; hear other viewpoints on users; understand that the drug use is not the "fault" of the family member; learn to stop enabling the addict; get tips on handling difficult situations at home; and learn how other families won or lost wars against addiction. The meetings are free, available almost everywhere, and have well-meaning members who are sympathetic and willing to help.

Treatment of the family's designated patient in an addiction treatment program is usually followed by a return to the addict's former living situation. Unless family members have developed insight into the problem of addiction and understand the patient's treatment, they may vent their resentment over past transgressions when the patient returns, increasing the chances of the patient's relapse. Treatment programs that include a significant "family component" have been shown to have increased effectiveness (23). Issues covered in the family component include:

- Teaching members about the disease concept of addiction. Patients are characterized as unable to change their propensity to use drugs, which is seen as intrinsic and probably genetic. Patients must be responsible for their actions but not considered "at fault," because they are unable to drink (or use drugs) without causing problems.

- An attempt is made to work on old relationship issues while the addict is still in the program and professional counselors are available.

- A plan for successful reimmersion into the family is developed before the patient returns home.

CASE STUDY 1

Rodney Clancy, a 43-year-old carpenter seen in the emergency room (ER) as an "unassigned patient," presented with abdominal pain and was worked up by the attending physician. You are asked to evaluate him for admission to your service. You elicit the following:

- History
  HPI: Increasing abdominal pain for the past 5 days, accompanied by nausea, then vomiting. Unable to hold anything down for the past 16 hours. Denies hematemesis or melena. Nobody at home or at work has been sick. Denies fever, cough, or chest pain.
  PMH: He has had hypertension for 10 years, poorly controlled. Denies diabetes, cancer, chronic obstructive pulmonary disease (COPD), ulcers. No

surgeries. Had a fractured ankle in an automobile crash when he was 28. Has used alcohol for 20 years, but denies seizures or reactions from alcohol withdrawal. Currently consumes a pint of liquor per day. "Gets shaky" if he goes without a drink in the morning.
  Medications: Atenolol, 50 mg qd for hypertension and Restoril 15 mg HS, prn for insomnia.
  Social history: Second marriage; two teenage sons reside with first wife; had a DWI 2 years ago and recently regained his license. First marriage broke up because of his drinking. Has worked as a carpenter his entire adult life; recently moved to town. Smokes a pack and a half of cigarettes per day since he was 15 years old; denies other drugs.

- Physical examination
  Vital signs: Pulse 108/min, regular; respirations 22/minute; BP 160/104; Temp. 37.9°C. Well-developed, well-nourished white male in some discomfort, lying on a gurney.
  Skin: No jaundice; heavy calluses on hands; superficial, pretibial ecchymoses.
  HEENT: Dental caries, tobacco stains on teeth, smells of tobacco; faint odor of alcohol.
  Heart: Regular rhythm; no murmurs or gallops.
  Lungs: Crisp rales at the bases that clear with coughing.
  Abdomen: Marked tenderness to direct palpation in the epigastric area, radiating to the left flank. No rebound. No masses. Liver about 3 cm. below the left costal margin with a 18 cm span.
  Genital/rectal: Testes slightly soft, prostate normal, no hemorrhoids; guaiac-negative stool.
  Neurologic: Oriented × 3. Cranial nerves intact. Strength 5/5 in all extremities. Full range of motion, reflexes brisk throughout, palpable tremor when extending fingers.

- Labs
  CBC: Hemoglobin 16 mg/dL, hematocrit 52%, WBC 14,500/HPF with increased

neutrophils, platelets 95,000/HPF;
MCV 104, MCH 33, MCHC, 28.
SMA7: Sodium 142 mEq/dL, potassium
4.3 mEq/dL, chloride 103 mEq/dL,
CO_2 28 mEq/dL, BUN 18 mg/dL, crea-
tinine 1.3 mg/dL, glucose 85 mg/dL.
Enzymes: SGOT (AST)—265 IU/dL;
SGPT (ALT)—182 IU/dL; Alk Phos—95
IU/dL; GGT—214 IU/dL; bilirubin 1.8
mg/dL; albumin 6.2 mg/dL.
Amylase: 435 IU/dL
Urinalysis: Normal
Blood alcohol level (BAL): 0.03 g/dL

QUESTIONS

1. How would you evaluate and treat Mr. Clancy's medical problems?
2. How would you evaluate and treat his psychiatric problems?
3. How would you evaluate him for addiction?
4. How would you involve his family?

DISCUSSION

The differential diagnosis of Mr. Clancy's abdominal pain includes pancreatitis, peptic ulcer disease, and perforated hollow viscus, as well as more obscure causes. He probably has nicotine dependency and alcohol dependency, based on his history of drinking a pint of liquor a day and shaking in the morning until he drinks alcohol. He has fever, early signs of asterixis, a slightly elevated WBC, low platelets, elevated liver enzymes with AST > ALT, and a blood alcohol of 0.03 g/dL after 16 hours of abstinence. All of this is consistent with alcohol abuse and dependence, but does not rule out a concomitant infectious process, gastrointestinal (GI) bleed, and/or disseminated intravascular coagulation (DIC). His enlarged liver and elevated liver enzymes indicate hepatitis, including several possible types; the transaminase ratio favors alcohol, but a hepatitis workup should probably include antigen and antibody tests for hepatitis B and C, because they can coexist with alcoholic hepatitis and/or fatty liver. Hepatitis B is more

common among drug abusers, and hepatitis C has an increased incidence in alcoholics.

Mr. Clancy should be given thiamine, 100 mg IV in the ER and daily for 3 days. He should be made NPO because of his pancreatitis, rehydrated, and continued on dextrose and isotonic IV fluids. Some physicians would use a nasogastric (NG) tube, depending on the amount of vomiting; if he developed a distended abdomen or his bowel sounds diminished, most would favor NG suction. While the patient is in the emergency room, flat-plate and upright radiographs of the abdomen should be ordered to rule out a perforation in his GI tract. If positive, he must go to surgery; if negative, he should be admitted to treat acute pancreatitis and follow his hematocrit and stool guaiacs carefully to watch for GI bleeding or DIC.

You should look for sources of infection in Mr. Clancy, because of the fever and the elevated WBC. Common sources include the lungs, abdomen, and urinary tract. A chest radiograph should be taken and blood and urine cultures ordered, and Mr. Clancy should be started on broad-spectrum antibiotics pending results of his cultures.

The tremor in Mr. Clancy's fingers is an early sign of alcohol withdrawal, occurring even in the presence of a 0.03 g/dL BAL. This is an indicator of significant dependency. He should receive withdrawal prophylaxis starting with a loading dose of a long-acting sedative hypnotic drug (phenobarbital or diazepam) sufficient to eliminate his tremor, yet not enough to suppress respirations. He also should be started on a regular dose of the same drug, given two to three times per day and tapered over about 5 days. Supplemental boluses of sedative hypnotics can be used if necessary to control the severity of the withdrawal syndrome. In addition, the patient may be more comfortable with a nicotine patch to diminish his craving for cigarettes. Mr. Clancy will need analgesia for his pancreatitis. You may need to use an opiate for severe pain, but be careful to monitor respirations because of the sedative hypnotics you are using simultaneously.

Initially, you will focus on urgent medical problems. However, you can collect more information from both Mr. Clancy and his wife about his use of alcohol, including past negative consequences. Many physicians would order a urine toxicology screen to determine whether he is using drugs other than alcohol and Restoril, which might influence his medical treatment. You may find out more from Mrs. Clancy concerning jobs, financial problems, relationships within the family, etc. You can assess Mr. Clancy's readiness for change. Using his diagnosis of pancreatitis as a new, negative consequence of drinking, it may be possible to begin to motivate Mr. Clancy to stop drinking. Other data you collect will direct the selection of motivational strategies you choose. Depending on Mrs. Clancy's perception of the problem and her propensity to seek help, she can be your ally in motivating him toward addiction treatment. She may be interested in attending an Al-Anon meeting.

During this admission, you should continue to work with Mr. Clancy to be certain he understands the negative influence of alcohol in life. You may want to elicit the help of a social worker, an addiction-oriented physician or counselor, or a member of AA. Mr. Clancy may be able to attend an in-house AA meeting if one is available.

Depending on Mr. Clancy's desires, his health insurance, and his financial situation, you may be able to enroll him in an addiction treatment program, once he is detoxified and medically stable. Even if he cannot afford to pay, most communities have some treatment available through local mental health centers. You can consider prescribing naltrexone as an adjunct to therapy if he chooses to enroll in an addiction treatment program.

CASE STUDY 2

Angela Hawkins is a 17-year-old patient. You have been her family doctor for the past 10 years, since starting your practice.

She has been healthy, seen only for physical examinations, viral illnesses, and mild acne. About 6 months ago, she approached you about birth control; you had a discussion about safe sex practices, recommended she have her partner use condoms regularly, and gave her a prescription for oral contraceptives. An above-average student, Angela saw her grades begin to slip last year, and Rita, her mother (also your patient), has been worried about it. Last week, Rita found some marijuana in a baggie while changing sheets in Angela's bedroom. Both of them are in the examination room; Rita is upset, and Angela looks embarrassed. Rita says she is afraid that Angela is on her way to becoming a drug addict and asks whether she "should be tested." Angela maintains that there is no problem and that "all of the kids smoke marijuana." Both look to you for the next move.

QUESTIONS

1. Who is/are the patient(s) in the case? What are her (their) expectations of you and what are her (their) rights?
2. Are there sufficient data to be concerned that Angela has more of a problem than just experimentation with marijuana?
3. How would you proceed from here?
4. Should you obtain samples for drug testing? If so, what would you order?
5. Would you use a consultant? Why or why not?

DISCUSSION

Both women are patients and each has specific needs. Although Angela may be the designated patient for this encounter, as family physician to both of them, you should try to address the needs of both. As a parent, Rita is appropriately concerned about her daughter's use of an illegal drug. She may be aware that marijuana is a "gateway drug," often the first illicit drug used by people who eventually develop addiction to one or more drugs. Rita wants to prevent her daughter from becoming a drug addict and is looking to you for help. Angela is correct that marijuana use by high school students is common (although the prevalence is about 35%, less than she states). Angela may want you to reassure her mother and get her out of an embarrassing situation.

Beyond marijuana use, there are two obvious "red flags" that are of concern: Angela's recent drop in school performance and her earlier request for birth control. Physicians should be aware that "amotivational syndrome" is one identifiable problem associated with using marijuana. As a former good student, Angela may be compromising future opportunities by her poor performance. Initiation of sexual activity should raise several concerns in your mind, including decreased impulse control secondary to marijuana intoxication and drug-related sexual activity.

The next step in this case is to gather more information. Interviewing adolescents is often more successful if the physician can interview them out of the presence of parents, siblings, or friends. In this case, you should listen initially as both patients express their concerns, then politely suggest that you talk to each one separately. The discussion with Angela should begin with a review of confidentiality of the doctor-patient relationship, which may even be accomplished before Rita leaves the room. Depending on state law, your discussions with an adolescent about drug use may be privileged, disallowing you to discuss matters with the parent. In any case, you should listen to Angela, establish rapport, and gather information about what drugs is she using and how does she use them, how long this has been going on, associated negative consequences, and her interest in stopping use. From Rita, you will want to learn about her fears, any information not yet confided, ideas she has about proceeding, and resources the family can put into the problem.

The question of drug testing often arises because parents want to know exactly what is going on with their child. The law usually allows parents to demand such testing, regardless of the wishes of a minor. However, a parental demand for testing is potentially divisive, depending on the adolescent's reaction. As their family physician, you will probably be able to influence the decision. In this case, Angela has admitted to marijuana use, which may be enough data for you to proceed. If you suspect other drugs, it might be worth getting a sample at your suggestion or on Rita's "demand" in order to gain perspective on the severity of the problem. If you find cocaine or opiates, you should have increased concern. A negative urine screen should not be too reassuring, because you may have missed the window of positivity.

Family physicians may choose to treat this case themselves or involve consultants, depending on their experience and comfort with adolescents and with drug abuse. If the family wants to obtain a referral, you should go along with the request, because potentially serious drug problems are involved and there is little to gain from refusing to refer Angela. In this case, you would pick a consultant who is knowledgeable about drug abuse and who has had experience and success working with adolescents.

REFERENCES

1. Fleming MF, Barry KL. Clinical overview of alcohol and drug disorders. In: Addictive Disorders. St. Louis: Mosby Year Book, 1992.
2. Moore RD, et al. Prevalence, detection, and treatment of alcoholism in hospitalized patients. JAMA 1989;261 (3):403–407.
3. American Psychiatric Association. Diagnostic and Statistical Manual of Mental Disorders, 4th ed. Washington, DC: American Psychiatric Association, 1994: 175–272.
4. Steindler MS. Addiction terminology. In: Principles of Addiction Medicine. Chevy Chase, MD: American Society of Addiction Medicine, 1994.
5. Knop J. Familial alcoholism: Family, twin adoption, and high-risk studies. EXS 1994;71:121–131.
6. Johnston LD, O'Malley PM, Bachman JG. National Survey Results on Drug Use from The Monitoring the Futures Study, 1975–1993. Rockville, MD: National Institute on Drug Abuse, 1994.
7. Kinney J. An overview of substance use and abuse. In: Clinical Manual of Substance Abuse. St. Louis: Mosby Year Book, 1991.

8. Substance abuse. In: Annual Report. Princeton, NJ: The Robert Wood Johnson Foundation Annual Report, 1992.

9. Cyr MG, Wartman SA. The effectiveness of routine screening questions in the detection of alcoholism. JAMA 1988;259:51–54.

10. Brown RL. Identification and office management of alcohol and drug disorders. In: Fleming MF, Barry KL, eds. Addictive Disorders. St. Louis: Mosby Year Book, 1992.

11. Sullivan JT, Sukora K, Schneiderman J, Naranjo CA, Sellers EM. Assessment of alcohol withdrawal: the revised Clinical Institute Withdrawal Assessment for Alcohol (CIWA-Ar). Br J Addict 1989;84: 1353–1357.

12. Hoffmann NG, Halikas JA, Mee-Lee D, Weedman RD. Patient Placement Criteria for the Treatment of Psychoactive Substance Use Disorders. Washington, DC: American Society of Addiction Medicine, 1991.

13. Marlatt GA, Curry S, Gordon JR. A longitudinal analysis of unaided smoking cessation. J Consult Clin Psychol 1988;56(5):715–720.

14. Fillmore KM, Bacon SD, Hyman K. Final Report: The 27-year Longitudinal Panel Study of Drinking by Students in College, 1949–1976. Rockville, MD: National Institute on Alcohol Abuse and Alcoholism, 1979.

15. Prochaska JO, DiClemente CC, Norcross JC. In search of how people change. Applications to addictive behaviors. Am Psychol 1992;47:1102–1114.

16. Miller WR, Rollnick S. Motivational Interviewing: Preparing People to Change Addictive Behavior. New York: Guilford Press, 1991.

17. Berenson D, Schrier EW. Current family treatment approaches. In: Principles of Addiction Medicine. Chevy Chase, MD: American Society of Addiction Medicine, 1994.

18. Institute of Medicine. Broadening the Base of Treatment for Alcohol Problems. Washington, DC: National Academy Press, 1990.

19. Smith JW. Treatment outcome of 600 chemically dependent patients treated in a multimodal inpatient program including aversion therapy and pentothal interviews. J Subst Abuse Treat 1993;10(4):359–368.

20. Reading EG. Nine years' experience with chemically dependent physicians: the New Jersey experience. Md Med J 1992;41(4):325–329.

21. O'Malley S, et al. Naltrexone and coping skills therapy for alcohol dependence. Arch Gen Psychiatry 1992;49: 881–887.

22. Berenson D, Schrier EW. Current family treatment approaches. In: Principles of Addiction Medicine. Chevy Chase, MD: American Society of Addiction Medicine, 1994.

23. Alcoholics Anonymous. New York: Alcoholics Anonymous World Services, 1976.

16. Ankle and Knee Pain

JAMES E. DUNLAP AND HENRY C. BARRY

Key Clinical Questions

1. Is the joint pain acute or chronic?
2. What is the likelihood of internal derangement or fracture?
3. Which patients need imaging studies?
4. Which patients need referral?

Ankle and knee pain are among the most common and important musculoskeletal complaints. Ankle sprains are the most common musculoskeletal injury seen in sports (1), and knee pain is the seventh most common complaint in ambulatory practice (2). In either joint, pain may be caused by acute injury, overuse injury, or other conditions such as arthritis.

Ankle and knee problems can be classified as traumatic and nontraumatic. Each of these, in turn, may be acute, chronic, or both. Among traumatic disorders are sprains, strains, dislocations, fractures, and overuse syndromes (such as tendonitis and stress fractures). Nontraumatic disorders include arthritis, osteomyelitis, and neoplasms. The differential diagnosis of ankle and knee pain is summarized in Table 16.1.

Ankle Pain

PATHOPHYSIOLOGY AND DIFFERENTIAL DIAGNOSIS

The ankle joint, depicted in Figure 16.1, includes the distal fibula, talus, and distal tibia. The mortise (combined joint structure) formed from these bones is stabilized on the lateral side by the anterior talofibular ligament, the calcaneal fibular ligament, the posterior talofibular ligament, and the peroneus longus and peroneus brevis. On the medial side, the deltoid ligament is composed of a superficial and deep layer of ligaments, which makes the ankle quite resistant to eversion stress. The mortise of the ankle joint allows dorsiflexion, plantar flexion, and internal and external rotation. The subtalar joint formed by the talus and calcaneus allows true inversion and eversion. The

distal tibia and fibula are stabilized by the syndesmosis, a thickened band of the interosseous membrane. Finally, the Achilles tendon attaches at the posterior portion of the calcaneus, assisting in plantar flexion.

Multiple factors influence the nature and degree of ankle injury: ankle flexibility; type of sport; shoe-surface interface; and prior injury. Acute injuries to the ankle can result in tears of the lateral or medial ligaments or the syndesmosis, tendonous injuries to the ankle or forefoot, or fractures of the ankle or midfoot. Approximately 90% of ankle injuries result from forced inversion with the ankle in plantar flexion. One common story is the basketball player who runs to make a basket and lands on another player's foot; in fact, the majority of individuals can accurately describe the trauma. The anterior talofibular ligament (ATFL) is the most vulnerable and most commonly injured ligament.

Achilles tendonitis is a common, often chronic, condition causing ankle pain. It is caused by repetitive eccentric microtrauma that stresses the peritendinous structures, resulting in inflammation and even partial tendon rupture. This may be the result of training errors, running in improper shoes, running on hills, and running on uneven or hard surfaces (3). Finally, Achilles tendon rupture has been reported as a complication of steroid injection (4, 5) and the use of fluoroquinolones (6, 7).

CLINICAL EVALUATION

You should perform a careful history and physical examination in all patients with ankle pain. The history should address the location, duration, character, and intensity of pain. It should also include a description of potential contributing mechanisms, ameliorating or exacerbating factors, previous injury, and current treatment. You also should address potential "red flags" (see Table 16.2). These conditions are serious and require early referral. Finally, you should ask all patients about their treatment and activity goals. For instance, an elderly patient with severe arthritis may wish only to be independent in transferring out of bed and in getting to the

Table 16.1.
Differential Diagnosis of Ankle and Knee Pain

Diagnosis	Frequency in Primary Care	Frequency in Emergency Departments
Ankle		
Inversion sprain	Frequent	Frequent
Avulsion fracture	Common	Frequent
Achilles tendonitis	Common	Common
Eversion sprain	Uncommon	Uncommon
Fibular fracture	Uncommon	Common
Syndesmosis sprain	Uncommon	Uncommon
Trimalleolar fracture	Rare	Uncommon
Knee		
Anterior knee pain[a]	Frequent	Frequent
Osteoarthritis	Common	Common
Patella tendonitis	Common	Common
MCL or LCL strain or tear	Common	Common
Meniscus tear	Common	Common
ACL strain or tear	Common	Common
Patella dislocation	Uncommon	Uncommon
Fracture	Uncommon	Uncommon

[a]Also known as patellofemoral dysfunction or chondromalacia patellae.

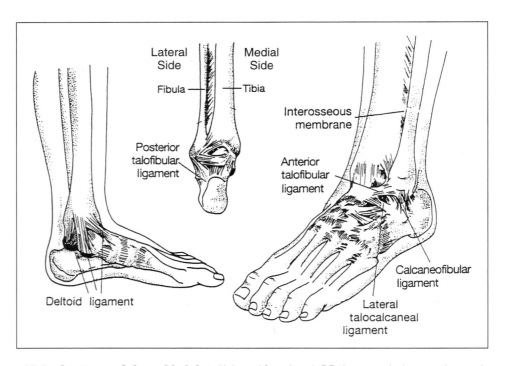

Figure 16.1. *Anatomy of the ankle joint.* (Adapted from Leach RE. A nonsurgical approach to early mobility: acute ankle sprain, treat vigorously for best results. J Musculoskel Med 1983;1(1):69.)

Table 16.2.
Red Flags Suggesting Progressive or Life-Threatening Disease in Patients with Ankle or Knee Pain

Red Flag	Diagnosis Suggested
Hemarthrosis	Internal Derangement
Knee pain and limp in child with normal knee examination	Hip disorder (e.g., Legg-Perthes, slipped capital femoral epiphysis)
Poor response to treatment	Internal derangement, malignancy (rare)
Bony swelling	Tumor
Fever	Osteomyelitis, septic arthritis
Rash, joint swelling	Collagen vascular disorders, gonococcal arthritis

bathroom. Others may desire return to full contact sports. In each circumstance, the management should be individualized and congruent with the patient's goals.

articulation where bones are united by ligaments.

History

The mechanism of injury is the single most important element of the history in the patient with a possible ankle sprain. You should also inquire about the chronicity of the symptoms and about changes in the level of activity (for instance, an increase in the number of miles or an increase in the intensity of work-outs). Further history should concentrate on previous injuries, whether a "snap" or "pop" was felt (suggesting ligament rupture), the time delay from injury to the onset of symptoms, and the initial treatment given. Symptoms such as an inability to bear weight immediately after the injury or a feeling that the ankle "gives way" are especially worrisome; the former is an important factor in distinguishing sprain from fracture (see Fig.16.2, Ottawa ankle rules). The Achilles tendon also can be a cause of ankle pain. Typically, the person will complain of pain in the posterior portion of the ankle.

Physical Examination

A solid knowledge of the functional anatomy of the ankle is imperative. Besides palpation, stress testing should be performed (Fig. 16.3). These stress tests include the talar tilt, anterior drawer, and the squeeze and Cotton tests. The talar tilt test

evaluates the calcaneofibular ligament (CFL) and is performed by stabilizing the distal lower leg in one hand while grasping each side of the foot at the talus with the thumb on one side and the forefingers on the other side. Varus stress is applied, and any qualitative difference between ankles suggests instability. The anterior drawer test is performed with the ankle slightly externally rotated and plantar flexed; a 3 mm difference between ankles suggests disruption of the ATFL.

To help distinguish ankle sprain from a fracture, you should palpate the posterior edge and the tip of each malleolus and the base of the fifth metatarsal. Tenderness in either location increases the likelihood of fracture. Finally, you should have the patient take four steps. The patient with a fracture is unlikely to be able to transfer weight twice onto each foot (see Fig. 16.2).

The squeeze test compresses the tibia and fibula above the midpoint of the calf. Pain indicates a syndesmosis sprain. The Cotton test for syndesmosis sprains is performed like the talar tilt test, except mediolateral force is applied, and any degree of motion over 3 mm is considered abnormal. Side-to-side comparisons should be performed in both of these tests. Injuries to the deltoid ligament result from dorsiflexion-eversion trauma, are relatively rare, and often are associated with fractures. Clinically, the components of the deltoid ligament are inseparable. Palpation of the tendon may reveal crepitus, tenderness, swelling, or a gap. The Thompson test (or midcalf compression test) assesses if the tendon is intact. This test is performed by compressing the gastrocnemius and soleus. If the foot plantar flexes, the test is negative (normal). If not, the test is positive, indicating complete or near complete rupture of the tendon.

Ankle sprains are classified by grade according to the degree of instability. Grade I injuries have minimal swelling and partial ligament tearing, but no clinical instability. Grade II injuries usually result from a complete tear of the ATFL and often have a positive anterior drawer test, ecchymosis, and swelling. This is also the most common type of injury diagnosed by physicians. Grade III injuries result from complete ligamentous disruption of the ATFL and CFL, with frank instability on stress testing. If a complete tear of the deltoid ligament is felt on eversion testing, radiographs should be ordered immediately to look for fracture.

Radiographic stress tests are radiographs obtained while placing the joint under manual

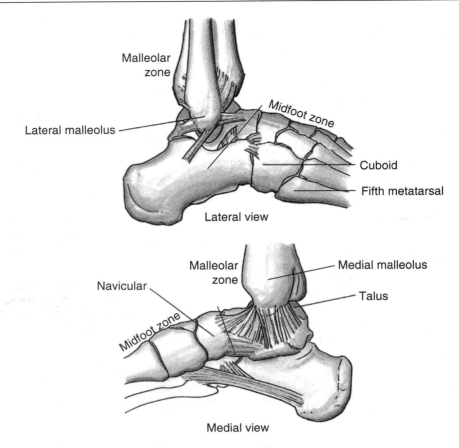

Malleolar zone

Lateral malleolus

Midfoot zone

Cuboid

Fifth metatarsal

Lateral view

Malleolar zone

Medial malleolus

Navicular

Talus

Midfoot zone

Medial view

Figure 16.2. *Ottawa ankle rules for radiographic series in acute injuries.*[a] You should perform a radiograph if the patient has pain in the malleolar or midfoot zone and *one* of the following:
- Bony tenderness at posterior edge or tip of either malleoli
- Bony tenderness over the navicular
- Bony tenderness at the base of the fifth metatarsal
- Inability to bear weight both immediately and in the emergency department (four steps), i.e., patient is unable to transfer weight twice onto each foot regardless of limping

[a]Text adapted from Stiell IG, McKnight RD, Greenberg GH, et al. Implementation of the Ottawa ankle rules. JAMA 1994; 271. Illustration reprinted with permission from Moore KL, Agur AMR. Essential Clinical Anatomy. Baltimore: Williams & Wilkins, 1995:276.)

stress (e.g., traction, eversion, or inversion). Although stress testing is generally recommended because it helps determine both the severity of injury and progress toward healing, several studies have shown that the interobserver agreement of these tests are poor. The nature of the studies do not allow for confident determination of test likelihood ratios. Although radiographic stress testing, arthrography, and arthroscopy have been used in some centers to assess injury severity, the results of such testing rarely change the conservative treatment given, and they are not recommended.

Radiologic Tests

The likelihood that a significant ankle fracture is present in a patient presenting with ankle injury (the pretest probability) is usually under 10%. To eliminate unnecessary use of radiographs and make the treatment of ankle injuries more cost effective, the Ottawa ankle rules (OAR; see Fig.

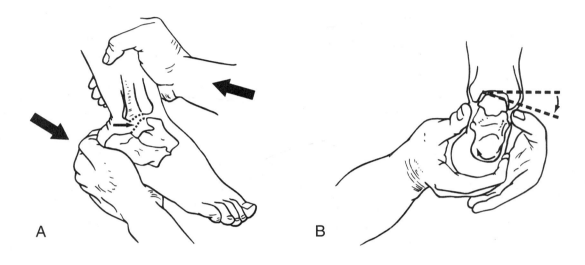

Figure 16.3. *Stress testing of the ankle.* A. Positive anterior draw sign (*small arrow*). The anterior draw sign test is used to evaluate the intactness of the anterior talofibular ligament. **B.** Test to evaluate the stability of the anterior talofibular and calcaneofibular ligaments. The ankle is unstable if the anterior talofibular and calcaneofibular ligaments are torn. (Reprinted with permission from American Osteopathic Association. Foundations for Osteopathic Medicine. Baltimore: Williams & Wilkins, 1997:638.)

16.2) have been developed and prospectively evaluated. Prospective multicenter evaluation of the OAR has yielded 93% to 100% sensitivities compared with 69% and 76% clinical examination sensitivities for ankle and midfoot fractures, respectively (Table 16.3) (8, 9). Additional validation of the OAR shows that the sensitivity of these rules for ankle fractures remains above 95%, but the sensitivity for midfoot fractures is slightly lower and more variable (10). In the emergency room setting, the percentage of patients with ankle injury for whom radiographs were ordered was reduced from 83 to 60%. In preliminary investigations, these rules also seem to be adequate for the pediatric population, but larger studies are needed (11).

Table 16.3.
Key Elements of the History and Physical Examination in Patients with Ankle Pain

Diagnosis	Test	Sensitivity	Specificity	LR+	LR−
Sprain vs. fracture	Ottawa ankle rule	1.00	0.39	1.64	0.0
	Clinical examination	0.69			

Keep in mind that the decision rule applies to an acutely injured ankle. You may wish to obtain radiographs when you find bone pain in the absence of injury, when the patient experiences night pain, or when symptoms do not fit conventional diagnoses or respond to treatment. These symptoms may indicate more serious conditions (see Table 16.2).

Ultrasound (12, 13) and magnetic resonance imaging (MRI) (14, 15) have been used to evaluate suspected Achilles tendonitis or Achilles tendon rupture. Although Kainberger (13) reports that ultrasound was fairly sensitive (72%) and specific (83%), there is no accepted gold standard, and the study did not include a wide spectrum of severity. Characteristics for MRI are not known. Most importantly, neither study is known to add significantly to the clinical examination.

MANAGEMENT

As with many other conditions, management of ankle pain begins with an assessment of goals. You should then proceed to address symptom relief (as that is usually the reason the patient seeks care), and then restoration of function. Table 16.4 summarizes some treatment options and the level of evidence for the interventions, and Table 16.5 summarizes commonly used drugs for ankle pain.

Ankle Sprains

Initial Management

Grade I and II lateral ankle sprains usually heal in an average of 8 and 15 days, respectively. Grade I sprains are treated symptomatically with ice, compression wraps, and elevation. You should recommend weight-bearing based upon the patient's tolerance. These sprains do not require immobilization. Grade II sprains should be treated with ice, compression, and elevation for 48 to 72 hours along with immobilization in a re-

movable splint (pneumatic or lace-up) for 2 to 7 days. Crutches will help the patient remain non-weight-bearing.

The management of grade III lateral ankle sprains is similar, although recovery is longer. The management of syndesmosis sprains follows that of third-degree sprains. Healing time is 6 to 8 weeks, and a longer period of immobilization is needed. Removable splints (i.e., posterior splint, pneumatic splint, or a Bledsoe brace) or casting facilitates progressive weight-bearing. Progressive weight-bearing as tolerated should be allowed and analgesics should be prescribed. Passive range-of-motion exercises (tracing the alphabet, drawing circles, etc.), especially dorsiflexion, should begin within a week of the injury. In all sprains, nonsteroidal anti-inflammatory drugs (NSAIDs) are commonly used for analgesia and to aid in reducing inflammation (see Table 16.5).

Long-Term Management

Further rehabilitation of the ankle joint is extremely important, and includes strengthening exercises, proprioception training, and func-

Table 16.4.
Management of Ankle Sprain

Treatment	Level of Evidence for Effectiveness[a]
NSAIDs	A
Splinting	A
Early mobilization	B
Physiotherapy	B
Ice	B
Compression	C

[a]Level of evidence for effectiveness: A, strong or moderate research-based evidence (consistent across several studies, including at least two randomized controlled trials); B, limited research-based evidence (less consistent or extensive evidence, but preponderance of evidence supports use of treatment); C, common practice with little or no research-based evidence.

Table 16.5.
Drug Therapy for Ankle or Knee Pain

Drug	Dosage	Cautions/Adverse Effects	Contraindications
Acetaminophen	325–650 mg every 4–6 hr	Liver dysfunction	
Aspirin	Up to 4 g/day (every 4–6 hr); maximum dose for alcoholics or those with liver disease = 2 g/day. (e.g., hepatitis)	Caution in pregnancy or lactation and in patients with asthma or ulcers. Gastrointestinal (GI) upset is common. Interferes with platelet aggregation. May cause tinnitus.	Allergy; third trimester of pregnancy; active ulcer; varicella or influenza infection in children or adolescents
NSAIDs		GI upset is common. Sodium retention; edema; may worsen congestive heart failure; renal or hepatic dysfunction; hypertension; bleeding. Many drug interactions: probenecid, oral anticoagulants, diuretics, methotrexate, lithium, and others. Caution in elderly.	Allergy to other NSAIDs; aspirin allergy; pregnancy; lactation; active ulcer
Ibuprofen (Motrin)	Up to 3200 mg/day (tid to qid)		
Naproxen	250–550 mg bid		
Tolmetin	600–1800 mg/day (tid)		
Diclofenac	50 mg tid		
Indomethacin	25–150 mg bid to qid, max 200 mg/day		History of proctitis, rectal bleeding (suppository)
Oxaprozin	1200 mg once daily	Special caution in the elderly	
Piroxicam	20 mg once daily	Depression, Parkinson's disease, epilepsy, sepsis	
Etodolac	600–1200 mg/day (bid to qid)		
Nabumetone	Up to 2 g/day (qd or bid)	Most useful for chronic pain	

tional exercises. The removable splints should be worn until the individual has been pain-free for at least 2 weeks. Sprains treated by cast immobilization alone take longer to return to full activity and have worse outcomes unless patients receive intensive rehabilitation and are closely monitored. To speed recovery and minimize time off work or sport, the use of physical therapy for this injury is strongly recommended. Recurrent ankle sprains and chronic pain after an ankle sprain usually are the result of inadequate rehabilitation. These individuals should receive more extensive supervised therapy. If pain persists after an injury despite adequate rehabilita-

tion, occult fracture should be suspected, especially talar dome fractures.

Ankle Fractures

Many fractures can be managed in the office without referral. Avulsion or chip fractures are the most common and can occur at the distal fibula below the level of the mortise, the distal portion of the tibial plafond, and the anterior surface of the talus. Regardless of size, these usually can be treated according to the degree of the associated ankle sprain. If the fragments are displaced more than 2 mm, immobilize the patient in a cast or posterior splint and refer to an orthopedic surgeon. Avulsion fractures of the peroneus brevis insertion from the fifth metatarsal head will heal without treatment but should be immobilized until weight-bearing can be tolerated. Nondisplaced navicular and cuboid fractures should be casted. Fractures of the talus within the mortise, the fibula at or above the joint or mortise surface, the tibial plafond near the joint line, and bimalleolar, trimalleolar, and any displaced fractures should be immobilized and referred. You should refer patients with fractures of the base of the fifth metatarsal (Jones' fracture) and of the growth plate (Salter-Harris fractures) to an orthopedic surgeon. Do not forget to provide analgesics for your patient (see Table 16.5).

Achilles Tendonitis

Management of Achilles tendonitis includes relative rest, rehabilitation of the gastrocnemius and soleus muscles, ice, heel lifts, and analgesics. Rehabilitation of the calf muscles begins with progressive stretching and range-of-motion exercises followed by strength training. NSAIDs may be helpful in reducing pain and inflammation (see Table 16.5). Steroid injection has been advocated by some, but is controversial (16). Attempts should be made to correct biomechanical abnormalities. Surgery is recommended only for those who fail conservative therapy and desire to continue running and those with Achilles tendon ruptures (17). The rate of rerupture is high among conservatively treated patients with Achilles tendon rupture, but casting may be reasonable in sedentary patients.

Knee Pain

PATHOPHYSIOLOGY AND DIFFERENTIAL DIAGNOSIS

The knee evolved to allow flexion and extension, movements that once were critical for walking and sprinting among hunter-gatherers. Today, the demands of sports and recreation have created additional stresses for a knee that is vulnerable to rotation, direct contact, and repetitive load. It should not be surprising that overuse and acute knee injuries are common. Although the history will provide major clues to the diagnosis, knowledge of the anatomy and examination of the knee are essential. Primary care physicians

can manage most knee injuries. Some acute knee injuries require surgery to restore function and allow return to work or play; this underscores the importance of an accurate diagnosis and knowledge of the appropriate criteria for referral.

The knee joint, depicted in Figure 16.4, consists of the patella, tibia, and femur. The patella is a sesamoid bone with a keel-shaped undersurface that fits between the medial and lateral femoral condyles. The primary stabilizers of the knee are the anterior and posterior cruciate ligaments (ACL and PCL, respectively), the medial and lateral collateral ligaments (MCL and LCL, respectively), the menisci, the joint capsule, and the medial and lateral retinaculum that attach to the patella. Secondary stabilizers of the knee include the iliotibial band (tensor fascia lata) and the quadriceps, hamstrings, and popliteus muscles.

The knee acts as a hinge that allows forward translation and internal rotation of the tibia during leg flexion and rearward translation and external rotation during extension. While the knee is flexed, the MCL and LCL provide stability to medially and laterally directed stress, respectively. The MCL and LCL also limit external and internal rotation during knee extension and flexion. The ACL is the only structure preventing anterior movement of the tibia on the femur. It also helps the MCL stabilize the knee during lateral stress when the knee is flexed. The PCL resists posterior movement of the tibia on the femur. The medial and lateral menisci act as shock absorbers but also stabilize the knee during movements such as pivoting. The popliteus muscle holds the lateral meniscus back during knee flexion, locks the knee in full extension, and unlocks the knee during the initiation of flexion.

Injuries to the knee ligaments and cartilage are common, although the exact frequency depends upon the population and activity. For example, skiers and football players have approximately 0.6 to 0.7 ACL injuries per 1000 days of sports participation (18), whereas in a 3-year period, one health maintenance organization (HMO) had an incidence of 0.4/1000 health plan members (19). Women are 2.5 to 4 times as likely as men to sustain ACL injuries in basketball and soccer (20). Isolated meniscus tears are the most frequent acute knee injury in an athletic population. Meniscus injuries are also discovered in 30 to 50% of patients with ACL tears. Nordic skiers have a high rate of knee injury (2.1 injuries per 1000 skier days), even though many people consider this activity to be "easy on the knees". Most

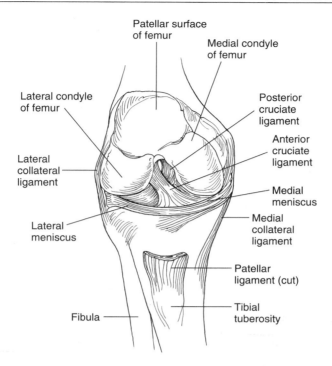

Figure 16.4. *Knee joint, anterior view.* (Reprinted with permission from Rucker LM. Essentials of Adult Ambulatory Care. Baltimore: Williams & Wilkins, 1997:556.)

(58%) of these injuries, however, are to the MCL (21). Anterior knee pain (a catch-all term that includes common conditions such as patellar tendonitis, patellofemoral dysfunction, chondromalacia patellae, etc.) and osteoarthritis of the knee are other common causes of knee pain and are seen in athletes and nonathletes alike.

Acute traumatic injuries to the knee include tears of the ACL, MCL, LCL, and menisci. Other examples of acute trauma include dislocation or subluxation of the patella and fractures of the patella, tibial plateau, femoral condyles, and fibular head. Common chronic traumatic injuries include patellar tendonitis and chondromalacia patellae. Anterior knee pain (AKP) is a heterogeneous group of disorders, but has become synonymous with chondromalacia patellae. Chondromalacia patellae is also called patellofemoral dysfunction (PFD), because the underlying cause of chondromalacia is thought to be poor tracking of the patella between the femoral condyles.

The mechanism of injury is an important clue to the specific diagnosis. Collateral ligament injuries result from medially or laterally directed stress to a planted knee, such as in football or skiing. Posterior cruciate injuries are rare and usually occur in a motor vehicle accident when a flexed knee hits a dashboard. The ACL can be injured by many mechanisms: an external force applied to a planted knee (e.g., during a football tackle); hyperextension and internal rotation (e.g., a basketball or volleyball player landing on somebody's foot); sudden deceleration with a flexed knee that pivots or rotates (e.g., a skiing fall); landing and pivoting or cutting (e.g., in soccer); or falling backward with a ski boot, displacing the tibia anteriorly. These mechanisms are not specific for ACL injuries, as sudden twisting or pivoting can also cause injuries to the menisci or cause patellar dislocation.

Chronic knee pain may be a long-term sequela of previous injury (especially if it was incompletely rehabilitated). Chronic knee pain is often associated with weak quadriceps muscles from disuse, resulting in PFD or AKP. The causes of osteoarthritis are multiple. The primary problem may, in fact, be genetic or trauma, rather than overactivity or exercise (22, 23).

CLINICAL EVALUATION

When evaluating a patient with knee pain, you should ask about the location, duration, character, and intensity of pain. You should also obtain a description of potential contributing mechanisms, ameliorating or exacerbating factors, previous injury, and current treatment. Potential "red flags," which are serious and may require early referral, are summarized in Table 16.2. Finally, you should determine the patient's treatment and activity goals, so management can be individualized.

History

The mechanism of injury and the presence of hemarthrosis are the two strongest determinants of internal derangement of the knee. Patients with hemarthrosis are likely to complain of sudden swelling (less than 24 hours after the injury) and bruising. Hearing or feeling a "pop" suggests an ACL tear, whereas locking of the knee typically is associated with meniscus injuries. Inability to bear weight and persistent giving way of the knee indicate internal derangement but are not specific for any one injury. Patients with anterior knee pain (AKP) often experience pain with specific actions: climbing up or down stairs, squatting, or prolonged sitting. They may also report snapping, popping, clicking, or catching sensations in the knee. Patients with osteoarthritis (OA) typically complain of stiffness with inactivity and pain with weight-bearing activity. In contrast to the stiffness associated with rheuma-

toid arthritis, that of osteoarthritis often improves after a few minutes of activity. Swelling of the knee is not common in OA except during an acute flare-up or in the presence of severe OA associated with bony changes.

Physical Examination

A skillful examination of the knee correctly identifies the diagnosis 90% of the time. Table 16.6 summarizes the characteristics of various components of the knee examination. The Lachman test for anterior cruciate ligament tears is sensitive and specific (LR+ 12, LR− 0.09) in experienced hands (24, 25). With the knee flexed to 20 to 30°, the top hand stabilizes the femur while the lower hand wraps around the inside of the proximal tibia with the thumb on top directing force anterior and slightly outward. When the leg is too large or the hands too small, place a knee or other firm support under the thigh, and with both hands placed near the tibial plateau, determine the amount of anterior translation and the firmness of the end point. A 3 mm side-to-side difference or the absence of a distinct stop (also called an end point) indicates an ACL tear. Before the Lachman test is performed, the knee should be flexed to 90° and the tibia pushed in a posterior direction (posterior drawer) to ensure PCL integrity. If the PCL is torn, the Lachman test is still accurate but must be done more carefully.

The presence of hemarthrosis suggests a significant knee injury that will require surgery 90% of the time. Patients with hemarthrosis usually have significant effusions and ecchymosis. Although

Table 16.6.
Key Elements of the History and Physical Examination in Patients with Knee Pain

Diagnosis	Test	Sensitivity	Specificity	LR+	LR−
Fracture	Ottawa knee rule (see Table 16.8)	1.00	0.49	1.98	0.00
ACL	Lachman test	0.92	0.92	12	0.09
"Internal derangement"	"Experienced" clinical examination	0.92	0.92	12	0.09
Acute meniscus injury	Joint line tenderness and positive McMurray test	0.92	0.93	13	0.04
	Joint line tenderness and negative McMurray test[a]	0.81	0.50	1.6	0.38
	No joint line tenderness and positive McMurray test	0.98	0.79	4.7	0.10
Chronic meniscus injury	Joint line tenderness	0.23	0.88	1.9	0.88
	Positive McMurray test	0.20	0.90	2.0	0.89

[a]Reported range of sensitivity 0.77 to 0.86; specificity 0.4 to 0.6.

McMurray — Fully flex, and apply lat or medial pressure.
Palpable click indicates a tear of meniscus.

distinguishing between effusion and hemarthrosis can be difficult, the presence of ecchymosis and rapid onset of swelling (less than 24 hours) will favor hemarthrosis. Approximately 70% of knee injuries with hemarthrosis represent ACL tears (26, 27). Osteochondral fractures are seen in about 10% of knee injuries with hemarthrosis. Although many studies report the prevalence of derangement in a series of subjects with hemarthrosis, one cannot calculate likelihood ratios without knowing about the other injured patients who did not have hemarthrosis. This is a common problem in the orthopedic literature.

Joint line tenderness (JLT) is present in 81% of meniscus tears; absence of this finding helps rule out meniscal tear (LR− 0.04) (28). Posterolateral or posteromedial pain that occurs at the extremes of flexion or extension also suggests meniscal injury. In a patient with anterior JLT, pain with squatting suggests chondromalacia rather than a meniscus tear. The McMurray test (see Fig. 16.5) is another physical examination maneuver for the detection of meniscal damage. To perform it, place the knee in full flexion. Using a combination of external rotation and valgus stress with the fingers along the lateral joint line and the lower hand cupping the heel, the knee is slowly brought into extension. A palpable click suggests a lateral meniscus tear. With the fingers along the medial joint line, the same maneuver is performed with internal rotation and varus stress to detect medial meniscus tears. If the range of motion of the knee is restricted, a McMurray test cannot be performed with any accuracy. The McMurray test has good specificity (approximately 90%), but is much less sensitive than JLT (approximately 30%) (28, 29). The results of joint line tenderness evaluation and the McMurray test are therefore complementary: a positive McMurray test is helpful in ruling in meniscal tear (LR+ 2.5 to 4), whereas the absence of joint line tenderness is more useful in ruling out meniscal tear (LR− 0.04).

When the history suggests a collateral ligament injury, the severity is determined by the examination. Side-to-side comparisons are essential. Individuals with a grade III or complete tear may actually walk into the office and not have any pain. Pathologic laxity is graded according to the amount of joint opening by a stress test with the knee in 30° of flexion, and is classified as 0 (normal), I (1 to 4 mm), II (5 to 9 mm), or III (10 to 15 mm). Grade I and grade II tears have definite end points, but grade III tears have soft or mushy end points (30). Allowing gravity to relax

the lower leg just off the table eliminates guarding for these tests.

If the diagnosis is uncertain (e.g., the patient is guarding too much or swelling prohibits adequate testing), application of ice, temporary immobilization, and the use of analgesics are common techniques for reducing the swelling and pain. The patient should return within a week for repeat evaluation.

Examination of the knee in patients with AKP often reveals atrophy of the quadriceps and crepitus with manipulation of the patella. Several clinical tests for AKP have been reported: patellar apprehension, patellar compression, and patellar laxity. These are qualitative tests. The patellar apprehension test is performed by applying inferiorly directed pressure at the superior portion of the patella. The patellar compression test is performed by having the patient contract the quadriceps muscle while the examiner firmly holds the patella in place. In either the patellar apprehension test or the patellar compression test, if the patient winces, grabs the knee, or otherwise voices displeasure, the test is considered positive. Patellar laxity is tested by manipulating the patella and determining the degree of movement, and the opposite knee is used for comparison.

Imaging of the Knee

Characteristics of imaging studies for the evaluation of the injured knee are shown in Table 16.7. Stiell (31, 32) developed the Ottawa knee rules (Table 16.8) to assist in the evaluation of acute knee injuries. They have been well validated and are 100% sensitive for fracture, with a specificity that approaches 50%. Further, clinicians correctly interpret the rule 96% of the time (33).

Multicenter prospective evaluation of these rules is needed, however, before they become a gold standard. In adolescents with open growth plates, a more conservative approach should be taken because no clinical prediction rules have been developed for this population. Also keep in mind that the decision rule applies only to an acutely injured knee. You may wish to obtain radiographs when you find bone pain in the absence of injury, when the patient experiences night pain, or when the patient's symptoms do not fit conventional diagnoses or respond to treatment. These symptoms may indicate the presence of more serious conditions (see Table 16.2).

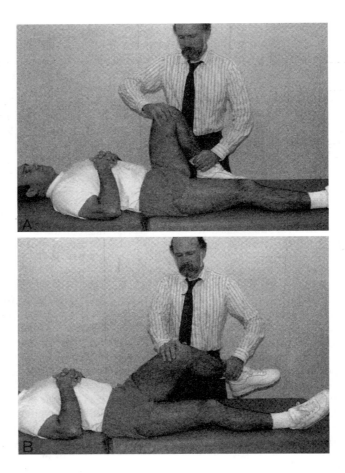

Figure 16.5. *McMurray test.* **A.** Starting position. **B.** Extension of the leg with valgus and internal rotation evaluates the medial meniscus, while extension of the leg with varus force and external rotation evaluates the lateral meniscus. (Reproduced with permission from Hyde TE, Gengenbach MS. Conservative Management of Sports Injuries. Baltimore: Williams & Wilkins, 1997:392.)

Table 16.7.

Characteristics of Diagnostic Tests in Patients with Knee Pain

Diagnosis	Test	Sensitivity	Specificity	LR+	LR−
"Internal derangement"	MRI	0.82	0.87	6.3	0.2
Acute meniscus tear	MRI[a]	0.89	0.92	11.0	0.1
Chondromalacia patellae	MRI[b]	0.29	0.97	9.6	0.7
	MR arthrogram	0.69	0.99	70	0.3
	CT arthrogram	0.65	0.99	65	0.3

[a]Reported range of sensitivity 0.82 to 0.95, specificity 0.87 to 0.95.

[b]Reported range of sensitivity 0.19 to 0.38.

In the absence of fracture, radiographs rarely alter the management of an acute knee injury. If internal derangement of the knee is suspected, the question of performing MRI arises. Although MRI is sensitive and specific for anterior cruciate ligament (ACL) tears, several studies have found it to be less accurate than the clinical examination (33 to 36). The literature on diagnostic testing suffers from many flaws, including the lack of an accepted gold standard, the absence of a wide spectrum on injury severity, and the role of examiner experience.

MRI should not be used to diagnose a suspected isolated ACL tear. If an examiner is not certain that there is an ACL tear, referral to a physician with more experience is usually more cost effective than ordering an MRI (36). The MRI has been used to look for associated meniscal lesions or bone contusions because the presence of these lesions is a relative indication for surgical ACL repair. This approach is being abandoned now because most ACL tears are repaired. An exception is the patient who initially elects not to have surgery for an ACL tear. If meniscal damage is seen on the MRI along with the ACL tear, surgical repair should be strongly encouraged.

Magnetic resonance imaging also will detect meniscal lesions. The sensitivity and specificity vary from 82 to 95% and 87 to 95%, respectively. This is not significantly different from the clinical examination in which a good history and the presence of a positive McMurray test or joint line tenderness yields a probability of meniscal tear of 75 to 99% (LR+ 10, LR− 0.1). An MRI can be helpful if a patient with a good history and persistent pain has a negative clinical examination and poor response to conservative therapy (several weeks of rest followed by physical therapy).

Although AKP is best diagnosed clinically, it should come as no surprise that several radi-

ographic procedures are also available: plain radiography, MRI, CT scan, sonography, and scintigraphy. None are needed in most patients with AKP. Imaging should be reserved for those who fail to respond to therapy or if the diagnosis is in doubt. The characteristics of these tests are summarized in Table 16.7. Although radiographs using Merchant's views (37) have been a standard among orthopedists for years, the findings rarely alter the initial conservative management. Merchant's views are performed with the knees flexed 45° and the x-ray beam declined 30°. More than 16° of subluxation is considered abnormal. Gagliardi (38) compared MRI, MR arthrography, and CT arthrography to surgical findings in patients with AKP ranging from mild to severe. MRI was relatively insensitive (19 to 38% depending upon severity) but very specific (97%). MR arthrography was more sensitive (69%) and was also specific (99%). CT arthrography was most sensitive (65%), and had 100% specificity. Thus, each procedure was very good at ruling in disease if positive (LR+ 7 to 14 for MRI, and 60 to 70 for CT or MR arthrography)

Table 16.8.

The Ottawa Knee Rules

Obtain a radiograph of the knee if the patient has *any* of the following characteristics:
- Age 55 years or older
- Tenderness at the head of the fibula
- Isolated patella tenderness
- Inability to flex to 90°
- Inability to bear weight both immediately and in the emergency department (four weight transfers onto each leg, regardless of limping)

Adapted from Stiell IG, Greenberg GH, Wells GA, et al. Derivation of a decision rule for the use of radiography in acute knee injuries. Ann Emerg Med 1995;26:405–413.

but was less helpful when normal (LR− 0.3 to 0.8).

All the following may be found on radiographs of patients with OA: normal; sclerotic joint margins; asymmetric joint space narrowing; subchondral cyst formation; osteophytes; bone destruction. None of these findings are specific, and they may be found in many other arthritides.

MANAGEMENT

You should begin by assessing the patient's goals and current level of function. You should then address symptom relief (as that is usually the reason the patient seeks care), followed by return to function. Table 16.9 summarizes the available treatment options and the level of evidence to support them; medications commonly used for management of knee pain are listed in Table 16.5.

Indications for Knee Surgery Referral

There are five major reasons to refer a patient for knee surgery:

- Hemarthrosis or rapid fluid accumulation;
- ACL or meniscus tears;
- Third-degree collateral ligament injuries;
- Uncertainty about the diagnosis; or
- Poor response to conservative treatment.

Appropriate surgical referral thus depends on the ability of the primary care physician to perform an accurate and complete history and physical examination of the patient with knee pain.

Initial Management of Knee Injuries

The initial management of an acute knee injury depends upon the type and severity of the injury. Fractures should be immobilized in a long leg splint, patients referred immediately to an orthopedist, and appropriate analgesia given (see Table 16.9). Collateral ligament tears, whether grade I or grade II, should be treated with a knee immobilizer and crutches until the pain has subsided enough to permit weight-bearing. Ice, compression, and elevation also help reduce pain and swelling. Keep in mind that when you are unable to adequately examine an acutely injured knee, you should begin symptomatic therapy and reexamine within a week. To prevent weakness of the quadriceps and secondary AKP, isometrics and leg raises (one leg at a time) should be begun while wearing the immobilizer. As the pain dissipates, range-of-motion exercises should be started followed by a progression of bike riding and resistance exercises before returning to sports-specific training. Grade I sprains usually heal in a week or less, whereas grade II injuries may take 2 to 3 weeks to heal.

Table 16.9.
Management of the Most Common Causes of Knee Pain

Diagnosis	Treatment	Level of Evidence for Effectiveness[a]	Recommendations or Comments
ACL	Surgery	B	
	Physical therapy	C	
Meniscus tear	Surgery	B	
	Physical therapy	C	
Osteoarthritis	NSAIDs	C	Reserve for acute flare-ups or when other analgesics are no longer effective
	Physical therapy	C	
Severe osteoarthritis	Surgery	B	For severe disease requiring knee replacement
Anterior knee pain	Patellar taping	A	
	Physical therapy	B	
	NSAIDs	C	
	Surgery	C	

[a] Level of evidence for effectiveness: A, strong or moderate research-based evidence (consistent across several studies, including at least 2 randomized controlled trials); B, limited research-based evidence (less consistent or extensive evidence, but preponderance of evidence supports use of treatment); C, common practice with little or no research-based evidence.

Grade III injuries should generally be referred to an orthopedist. These injuries are usually treated with a brace that allows 30° of flexion for 2 weeks. The brace is then unlocked to allow 30 to 90° of flexion. Return to full activity may take up to 9 weeks.

The initial management of an ACL tear is immobilization and referral to an orthopedic surgeon. Factors associated with a greater likelihood of success with surgical reconstruction of the ACL include isolated injury (versus multiple derangements); younger patient age; type of activity (cutting or jumping); greater degree of displacement of the tibia on the femur; physically demanding work activity; and likely compliance with a rehabilitation program. Surgery is also indicated in an individual who elects not to have surgery but then goes on to have repeated episodes of the knee "giving out" or is unable to perform daily activities.

The initial management of meniscus tears is controversial. In most instances, rest and protected weight-bearing combined with a short course of physical therapy comprise the initial treatment. If locking, pain, or inability to return to sports or work activity persists beyond 3 to 4 weeks, the patient should be referred.

Patellar dislocations are treated both surgically and conservatively. They may be associated with a tear of the medial retinaculum or of the insertion of the vastus medialis. Although the redislocation rate may be as high as 25 to 35% with conservative treatment, conservative therapy consists of a brief period of immobilization, ice, and compression, followed by bracing the patella with a lateral buttress knee sleeve and starting a functional rehabilitation program. Patients usually are able to return to full activity after recovery.

Long-Term Management of Knee Disorders

Overall, unless a patient is older than 50 and sedentary, the outcome of surgery for ACL tears is better than conservative treatment (38–41). Physical therapy is usually indicated for individuals undergoing casting or surgical procedures. Although physical therapy to strengthen quadriceps and hamstrings in the ACL-deficient knee can allow the individual to return to sports or full activity, several prospective longitudinal studies have shown that the incidence of meniscal tears, degenerative arthritis, pain, and disability are significantly greater in those who elect conservative treatment. This is particularly true for those who have meniscus tears associated with the initial ACL tear. Prophylactic bracing has not been shown to stabilize the anterior cruciate deficient knee or prevent these detrimental effects (40, 41).

Anterior knee pain is generally managed conservatively: analgesics (see Table 16.5), quadriceps-strengthening exercises, patellar taping, and ice. Particularly useful are eccentric exercises that strengthen the quadriceps near the patellar insertion (42). These are performed by having the patient stand on one leg and then squat partially. Surgical intervention is usually not needed, and is reserved for those who fail conservative therapy or for those with anatomic defects (such as patella alta or severe genu varum) (43).

Osteoarthritis (OA), is a chronic, degenerative condition. NSAIDs are commonly prescribed, but no studies have evaluated their impact on functional outcomes or disease progression. As OA is not an inflammatory condition, NSAIDs may be no better than acetaminophen for long-term management of OA. A short NSAID course (1 to 2 weeks) may be beneficial during an acute flare-up. Corticosteroid injections are rarely indicated; although intra-articular steroids may provide pain relief, the effect is brief and does not alter the course of the disease, and recurrent steroid use can damage articular cartilage. Physical therapy, flexibility, and strength training may help to maintain function. Patients with refractory pain, impaired mobility, and severe OA on radiograph should be referred to an orthopedic surgeon for possible joint replacement.

CASE STUDY 1

A 23-year-old athlete limps into your office complaining of ankle pain. The ankle was injured while playing basketball. The athlete went up for a rebound and came down on another athletes' foot. There was no pop, but the ankle was painful over the lateral portion and began to swell. The athlete was able to limp off the court. On examination you observe swelling and ecchymosis over the lateral malleolus, but find no bony tenderness. Anterior draw test shows the same amount of movement as the opposite ankle. The squeeze test is negative.

QUESTIONS

1. Would you x-ray the ankle?
2. What do you tell the athlete who wants a radiograph?
3. What initial course of treatment would you recommend?

DISCUSSION

This athlete's history is a classic inversion stress injury. The history and examination suggest a grade I ankle sprain. The ability to bear weight and the absence of bony tenderness yields a "negative" Ottawa ankle rule, indicating a negligible likelihood of fracture. Many athletes expect a radiograph, but when given explanation about the nature of injury, the findings, and those findings' lack of association with fracture, will often be satisfied. In fact, the more time you spend going over the rehabilitation, the greater their satisfaction! The initial treatment should consist of ice application, a removable splint, and pain medication. The athlete should be instructed in weight-bearing within tolerance and on early mobilization. Instruct the athlete in range-of-motion exercise and offer to call in a day or two to monitor progress.

CASE STUDY 2

A 43-year-old limps into your office complaining of pain and swelling of the right knee. The knee was injured yesterday while skiing. The skier was not sure of the order of events as the injury occurred quickly, but the skier thinks the knee was twisted while planting for a turn. The knee swelled immediately, and the skier was initially unable to bear weight, but is walking now. The knee is still swollen and is bruised. On examination, you observe a puffy knee, and the patella appears to be "floating." There is moderate ecchymosis. The range of motion appears normal, but there is a lot of spasm and guarding. You find no tenderness of the patella nor at the head of the fibula. You find no joint line tenderness, but on Lachman testing, the knee slides forward 1 cm and feels like it would keep sliding. The degree of guarding is such that you are unable to do a McMurray test.

QUESTIONS

1. Would you x-ray the knee?
2. What initial course of treatment would you recommend?
3. What is the most important course of action to take?

DISCUSSION

This unfortunate person has an acute injury with what appears to be a hemarthrosis and marked laxity of the anterior cruciate ligament. This person has a high probability of having an acute rupture of the anterior cruciate ligament. The degree of guarding prevents you from being able to tell if there are other derangements (such as meniscal tears). The spasm and guarding is normal, but should not divert your attention from a serious injury. The Ottawa knee rule is negative, so a radiograph is not necessary. This person needs to have the knee immobilized and should be on crutches. Give the patient something for pain, and arrange for orthopedic evaluation.

REFERENCES

1. Holmer P, Sondergaard L, Konradsen L, Nielsen PT, Jorgensen LN. Epidemiology of sprains in the lateral ankle and foot. Foot Ankle Int 1994;15:72–74.
2. National Ambulatory Medical Care Survey. Hyattsville, MD: National Center for Health Statistics, 1993.
3. Nichols AW. Achilles tendinitis in running athletes. J Am Board Fam Pract 1989;2:196–203.
4. Gibson T. Is there a place for corticosteroid injection in

the management of Achilles tendon lesions? Br J Rheumatol 1991;30:436.

5. Murtagh J. Injection for Achilles tendinitis. Aust Fam Physician 1992;21:798.

6. Huston KA. Achilles tendinitis and tendon rupture due to fluoroquinolone antibiotics. N Engl J Med 1994; 331:748.

7. Pierfitte C, Gillet P, Royer RJ. More on fluoroquinolone antibiotics and tendon rupture. N Engl J Med 1995; 332:193.

8. Stiell IG, Greenberg GH, McKnight RD, et al. Decision rules for the use of radiography in acute ankle injuries. Refinement and prospective validation. JAMA 1993; 269:1127–1132.

9. Stiell IG, McKnight RD, Greenberg GH, et al. Implementation of the Ottawa ankle rules. JAMA 1994;271: 827–832.

10. Pigman EC, Klug RK, Sanford S, Jolly BT. Evaluation of the Ottawa clinical decision rules for the use of radiography in acute ankle and midfoot injuries in the emergency department: an independent site assessment. Ann Emerg Med 1994;24:41–45.

11. Chande VT. Decision rules for roentgenography of children with acute ankle injuries. Arch Pediatr Adolesc Med 1995;149:255–258.

12. Fornage BD. Achilles tendon: U.S. examination. Radiology 1986;159:759–764.

13. Kainberger FM, Engel A, Barton P, Huebsch P, Neuhold A, Salomonowitz E. Injury of the Achilles tendon: diagnosis with sonography. AJR Am J Roentgenol 1990; 155:1031–1036.

14. Keene JS, Lash EG, Fisher DR, De Smet AA. Magnetic resonance imaging of Achilles tendon ruptures. Am J Sports Med 1989;17:333–337.

15. Berthoty D, Sartoris DJ, Resnick D. Fast scan magnetic resonance of Achilles tendonitis. J Foot Surg 1989;28: 171–173.

16. DaCruz DJ, Geeson M, Allen MJ, Phair I. Achilles paratendonitis: an evaluation of steroid injection. Br J Sports Med 1988;22:64–65.

17. Galloway MT, Jokl P, Dayton OW. Achilles tendon overuse injuries. Clin Sports Med 1992;11:771–782.

18. DeLee J, DeLee D. Orthopedic Principles and Practice. Philadelphia: WB Saunders; 1994.

19. Hirschman H, Daniel D, Miyasaka A. The fate of unoperated knee ligament injuries. In: Daniel D, Akezon W, O'Connor J, eds. Knee Ligaments: Structure, Function, Injury, and Repair. New York: Raven Press, 1990:481–503.

20. Arendt E, Dick R. Knee injury patterns among men and women in collegiate basketball and soccer. NCAA data and review of literature. Am J Sports Med 1995; 23:694–701.

21. Pigman EC, Karakla DW. Skiing injuries during initial military nordic ski training of a U.S. Marine Corps Battalion Landing Team. Mil Med 1990;155: 303–305.

22. Panush RS, Schmidt C, Caldwell JR, et al. Is running associated with degenerative joint disease? JAMA 1986;255:1152–1154.

23. Lane NE, Bloch DA, Hubert HB, Jones H, Simpson U, Fries JF. Running, osteoarthritis, and bone density: initial 2-year longitudinal study. Am J Med 1990;88: 452–459.

24. Hardaker WT Jr, Garrett WE Jr, Bassett FHd. Evalua-

25. Noyes FR, Bassett RW, Grood ES, Butler DL. Arthroscopy in acute traumatic hemarthrosis of the knee. Incidence of anterior cruciate tears and other injuries. J Bone Joint Surg Am 1980;62:687–695, 757.

26. DeHaven KE. Diagnosis of acute knee injuries with hemarthrosis. Am J Sports Med 1980;8:9–14.

27. Stanitski CL, Harvell JC, Fu F. Observations on acute knee hemarthrosis in children and adolescents. J Pediatr Orthop 1993;13:506–510.

28. Anderson AF, Lipscomb AB. Clinical diagnosis of meniscal tears. Description of a new manipulative test. Am J Sports Med 1986;14:291–293.

29. Stratford PW. Prospective evaluation of the McMurray test. Am J Sports Med 1994;22:567–568.

30. Hughston JC, Andrews JR, Cross MJ, Moschi A. Classification of knee ligament instabilities. Part I. The medial compartment and cruciate ligaments. J Bone Joint Surg Am 1976;58:159–172.

31. Stiell IG, Wells GA, McDowell I, et al. Use of radiography in acute knee injuries: need for clinical decision rules. Acad Emerg Med 1995;2:966–973.

32. Stiell IG, Greenberg GH, Wells GA, et al. Derivation of a decision rule for the use of radiography in acute knee injuries. Ann Emerg Med 1995;26:405–413.

33. Stiell IG, Greenberg GH, Wells GA, et al. Prospective validation of a decision rule for the use of radiography in acute knee injuries. JAMA 1996;275:611–615.

34. Terry GC, Tagert BE, Young MJ. Reliability of the clinical assessment in predicting the cause of internal derangements of the knee. Arthroscopy 1995;11:568–576.

35. Liu SH, Osti L, Henry M, Bocchi L. The diagnosis of acute complete tears of the anterior cruciate ligament. Comparison of MRI, arthrometry, and clinical examination. J Bone Joint Surg Br 1995;77:586–588.

36. Gelb HJ, Glasgow SG, Sapega AA, Torg JS. Magnetic resonance imaging of knee disorders. Clinical value and cost-effectiveness in a sports medicine practice. Am J Sports Med 1996;24:99–103.

37. Merchant AC, Mercer RL, Jacobsen RH, Cool CR. Roentgenographic analysis of patellofemoral congruence. J Bone Joint Surg Am 1974;56:1391–1396.

38. Gagliardi JA, Chung EM, Chandnani VP, et al. Detection and staging of chondromalacia patellae: relative efficacies of conventional MR imaging, MR arthrography, and CT arthrography. AJR Am J Roentgenol 1994;163:629–636.

39. Andersson C, Odensten M, Good L, Gillquist J. Surgical or nonsurgical treatment of acute rupture of the anterior cruciate ligament. A randomized study with long-term follow-up. J Bone Joint Surg Am 1989;71: 965–974.

40. Hawkins RJ, Misamore GW, Merritt TR. Follow-up of the acute nonoperated isolated anterior cruciate ligament tear. Am J Sports Med 1986;14:205–210.

41. Sommerlath K, Lysholm J, Gillquist J. The long-term course after treatment of acute anterior cruciate ligament ruptures. A 9- to 16-year follow-up. Am J Sports Med 1991;19:156–162.

42. Fyfe I, Stanish WD. The use of eccentric training and stretching in the treatment and prevention of tendon injuries. Clin Sports Med 1992;11:601–624.

43. Dehaven KE, Dolan WA, Mayer PJ. Chondromalacia patellae and the painful knee. Am Fam Physician 1980;21:117–124.

tion of acute traumatic hemarthrosis of the knee joint. South Med J 1990;83:640–644.

17. Anxiety and Depression

THOMAS L. SCHWENK

Key Clinical Questions

1. Could anxiety or depression be the primary cause of vague symptoms?
2. Could anxiety or depression be a factor affecting recovery and response to treatment in a patient who has a major medical diagnosis?
3. When do the symptoms of anxiety or depression cause enough functional impairment to warrant treatment?
4. When does a patient who has anxiety or depression warrant referral to specialized psychiatric services?

Anxiety and depression can be considered together because they are closely related biologically, epidemiologically, diagnostically, and therapeutically. Depressed patients often present with anxiety, and anxious patients may have depressed mood. The effects of both anxiety and depression on the treatment and rehabilitation of concomitant biomedical disease are similar. The neurotransmitter abnormalities in both diagnoses are similar or overlapping, and the primary pharmacologic approach to most anxiety and depressive disorders is an antidepressant. Occasionally, a patient may receive a discrete anxiety or depression diagnosis, but usually he or she can be placed along a continuum rather than into a discrete diagnostic "box." These diagnoses are common and important, cause significant dysfunction, and are eminently treatable, so they are worthy of diagnostic and therapeutic attention.

The majority of primary care patients have some elements of psychologic upset and dysfunction. This psychosocial component of medical care ranges from worry about a potential medical problem, to a coexistent psychiatric diagnosis such as major depressive disorder (MDD), to a primary psychiatric problem requiring referral such as bipolar disorder (1). One third of all primary care patients have a diagnosable anxiety disorder, and one quarter have a di-

agnosable depressive disorder (1). In neither of these groups, however, does a diagnosis have to be made in order to provide general, supportive treatment, nor does a specific diagnosis necessarily require specific treatment.

Primary care physicians underdiagnose psychiatric disorders, but the importance of this underdiagnosis with regard to the patient's functional outcome is unclear. Those patients whose diagnoses are missed usually have mild or self-limited disease and will respond to supportive care and watchful waiting (2). Within the highly prevalent group of primary care patients who have worry and mild psychiatric disease are a subset of patients requiring specific diagnosis and treatment—perhaps 5 to 8% for major depressive disorder, and 4 to 6% for generalized anxiety disorder or panic disorder. A much larger proportion, perhaps 15 to 20%, have more minor or subsyndromal diagnoses that do not quite meet usual diagnostic criteria; however, they may cause significant functional impairment in the patient's life, as well as in the patient's response to chronic disease treatment and rehabilitation, work responsibilities, and family roles (3). These symptoms can be addressed through the supportive counseling and patient education that occur as a part of almost every primary care office visit.

PATHOPHYSIOLOGY

Both depression and anxiety can range in severity from minor symptoms that result from external events or circumstances, to severe diseases caused by neurotransmitter dysregulation, particularly that of serotonin, dopamine, and norepinephrine. Depression is more likely to be precipitated by external stressors when it occurs earlier in one's life, with such stressors being identifiable in 60% or more of first episodes, but in only 25% of third or subsequent episodes. Anxiety symptoms are a natural reaction to real or potential threats in one's surroundings, but they can take on a life of their own and become more destructive and distressing than the original threat. Although synaptic serotonin, dopamine, and norepinephrine changes can be measured in patients who have depressive and anxiety disorders, and early work with positron emission tomography suggests that biochemical processes in the brain can be drastically altered by these diagnoses, the symptoms, onset, impairment, and recovery from the disease should not be considered separately from the patient's stresses, support, history, and genetic susceptibility.

Many patients (as well as physicians) ask whether these problems are physical or psychologic, for which a simple answer is rarely appropriate. The best response is probably, "Everyone feel anxious (or depressed) at times. Sometimes your susceptibility to anxiety (or depression), which is due to your genetic makeup or past experiences, interacts with stresses, losses, and changes in your life and can lead to a separate disease. This disease can cause severe physical and psychologic symptoms and impairment, and requires specific treatment." Unlike many biomedical diseases, for which a clear understanding of pathophysiology is necessary for treatment, the critical issue in depression and anxiety is to assess the severity of the symptoms and the resulting functional impairment, and to treat primarily on that basis.

DIFFERENTIAL DIAGNOSIS

There is not a standardized system for diagnosing depressive and anxiety disorders. Patients who have dysphoria (a general term for feeling "off," uncomfortable, lacking in energy, and disturbed in mood) or anxious symptoms can be assessed using a series of questions to determine if a primary anxiety or depressive disorder is present and whether specific treatment is required.

Many studies show that primary care physicians begin to develop a fairly specific differential diagnosis within 20 to 30 seconds of walking into an examination room and hearing the patient's concerns (4). Given the high prevalence of anxiety and depressive disorders in primary care practice, these conditions should be included in the differential diagnosis of nearly all patients, perhaps excluding those whose problems seem self-evident (e.g., lacerations, sore throats), although even those situations may have hidden elements that become more evident as the encounter evolves.

Having a high level of suspicion for depression and anxiety is the most critical step in the diagnostic process. If anxiety or depression is not considered early in the diagnostic process, it will likely not come up again until much later, at which point the patient will feel that the diagnosis is one purely of exclusion and therefore less important or legitimate. Recent large studies have confirmed the impression of experienced physicians that many patients view psychiatric diagnoses as less worthy or important, do not believe these diagnoses cause significant symptoms or dysfunction, and do not have faith that much can be done for these problems (5). Therefore, the outcome is likely to be better if you consider a psychiatric diagnosis and begin patient education as early as possible.

The relative likelihood of various anxiety and depressive disorders is shown in Table 17.1. Panic disorder, depression secondary to a medical condition, major depressive disorder, dysthymia (or minor depression), seasonal affective disorder, and bereavement (or grieving) are most commonly seen in primary care practice. In total, these common diagnoses may be present in 40% or more of primary care patients, although they often occur concomitantly with medical disorders (1). Brief descriptions of the most common diagnoses appear next.

Major Depressive Disorder (MDD)

MDD is a severe form of depression with strong biologic origins that occurs in a setting of significant psychosocial loss but can become recurrent irrespective of psychosocial loss or stress. The functional impairment from MDD varies widely but can be significant, leading to extensive and expensive medical care utilization, days in the

Table 17.1.
Prevalence of Depressive and Anxiety Disorders in Primary Care Practice

Common (5–10%)
  Mood disorder due to a general medical condition
  Major depressive disorder
  Mood disorder secondary to alcohol abuse

Less common (2–5%)
  Panic disorder
  Seasonal affective disorder
  Bereavement
  Dysthymia
  Mood disorder secondary to medications or other substances besides alcohol
  Adjustment disorder with mixed anxiety and depressed mood

Least common (1–2%)
  Bipolar disorder
  Generalized anxiety disorder
  Obsessive-compulsive disorder

hospital, and days not fulfilling usual family and work roles. Both psychotherapy and pharmacotherapy have been shown to be effective treatments, and both together are often needed.

Seasonal Affective Disorder (SAD)

SAD is a seasonal form of major depression with features similar to MDD but occuring on a cyclical basis related to ambient light deprivation during winter months. Both phototherapy and pharmacotherapy are frequently used.

Dysthymia

This condition is a chronic, "smoldering" form of minor depression with symptoms less severe than MDD but functional impairment that can equal MDD. Treatment regimens are less well established, and fewer dysthymia patients than MDD patients respond to antidepressants. Patients often move back and forth between dysthymia and MDD.

Mood Disorder Secondary to a General Medical Condition

This disorder is similar to MDD but is related to the onset of a major medical condition such as cancer, stroke, myocardial infarction, major trauma, multiple sclerosis, or certain medications such as oral contraceptives, antihypertensives, and alcohol. Distinguishing depression that occurs with a medical comorbidity from depression that occurs secondary to a comorbidity is difficult, and both often require specific treatment separate from that for the medical condition.

Panic Disorder Without Agoraphobia

This condition is characterized by panic attacks, at least some of which occur spontaneously. The patient has persistent concern about having future attacks or worry about the implication of the attacks, losing control, or "going crazy." The panic disorder patient usually has anxiety about a potentially serious medical disorder, such as cardiac, pulmonary, gastrointestinal, or neurologic disease, and is often seen by many physicians and consultants before the diagnosis is finally made.

Generalized Anxiety Disorder (GAD)

GAD is an anxiety disorder characterized by 6 or more months of chronic, fluctuating but generally excessive anxiety and worry about many aspects of life. The anxiety felt is out of proportion to the apparent threat, and this disorder is associated with many of the physical or psychologic symptoms of anxiety, such as chest pain, breathlessness, sweating, palpitations, nausea, or dizziness.

CLINICAL EVALUATION

Patients who have anxiety or depression may deny mood or psychiatric symptoms because of the stigma described previously, or because they truly do not feel the mood disturbance or psychiatric distress that physicians expect to find. To help identify anxiety or depression, you should assess patients for the following clues.

- Symptoms from multiple organ systems (particularly neurologic, gastrointestinal, and cardiac) that are difficult if not impossible to ascribe to a single medical condition

- Patients who are emotionally flat and verbally unproductive or who have worry and upset out of proportion to the apparent severity of the problem

- Sleep disturbance

- Frequent patient-initiated visits for reasons unclear to the physician

- Frequent emergency room or unscheduled office visits

- Patients labeled by the physician as "difficult" or a "problem"

- Patients who have cognitive or emotional dysfunction, such as forgetfulness, irritability, and loss of motivation or energy

- History of similar episodes or unspecified "breakdowns"

- Family history of psychiatric disease, suicide, or abuse of any kind (sexual, physical, substance)

Laboratory tests have no value in the diagnosis of depression or anxiety, beyond their judicious use to rule out medical conditions that might cause the same symptoms.

Determine if a Primary Medical Condition Should Be Considered Before Making a Primary or Concomitant Psychiatric Diagnosis

Depression commonly coexists with certain medical conditions, including myocardial infarction, stroke (particularly left frontal lobe), cancer, major trauma, multiple sclerosis, or any major new diagnosis, particularly if hospitalization is involved. Many physicians explain the depression on the basis of the psychologic trauma of such medical situations, but if the depression is severe and untreated, it becomes a significant condition in itself. Furthermore, depression can interfere with effective treatment of the primary medical condition, delaying recovery and significantly increasing morbidity. Depression is a more powerful predictor of mortality from myocardial infarction than physiologic measures such as cardiac ejection fraction, although it is not yet known whether treatment of the depression changes this risk (6). Medications are a common cause of depression as well, and you should always consider the medications listed in Table 17.2 as possibly causing depression.

Anxiety is less frequently associated with medical conditions than is depression, although you should consider hyperthyroidism, hypoglycemia, asthma, menopause, caffeinism, angina, gastroesophageal reflux, pulmonary embolism, and various neurologic diseases. Patients with chest pain who are not found to have ischemic disease often have panic disorder, but patients with ischemic heart disease also often have panic or anxiety symptoms. You should look for affective content out of proportion to the apparent severity of the symptoms, phobic behavior associated with the symptoms, and symptoms described in peculiar or inconsistent ways (intermittent stocking and glove paresthesias, or chest pain "like a rat nibbling at my heart") as clues to a possible primary anxiety disorder. Epidemiology is also critical: A 30-year-old woman who has chest pain is overwhelmingly more likely to have panic disorder than ischemic heart disease.

Overall, symptom-sign mismatch, in which the patient has many, seemingly severe, symptoms, negative findings on physical examination, and an increasingly long list of normal laboratory tests should alert you to a high likelihood of depression or anxiety, while you maintain the usual vigilance for undiagnosed medical disease.

Determine if the Anxiety or Depressive Symptoms Are Due to Another Psychiatric Condition

Substance abuse is the most common and most important psychiatric diagnosis that must be ruled out before a diagnosis of depression or anxiety is made (see Chapter 15, Addiction). There is some controversy regarding the use of antidepressants in alcoholic patients who cannot stay sober, on the assumption that their alcohol use is a form of self-medication for an untreated depression. Traditional teaching suggests that primary treatment for depression should not occur until the patient has successfully completed detoxification, but recent studies suggest that concomitant or even primary treatment for depression should take precedence (7). Other diagnoses that also should be considered include eating disorders, bipolar disorder, and schizophrenia.

Make a Primary Diagnosis of Depression or Anxiety, Determining the Type as Specifically as Possible

After making a primary or significant secondary diagnosis, you need to develop a more complete picture of the symptoms, precipitating events, psychosocial context and resulting illness behaviors such as phobias or work and home dysfunction. With depression, the most critical issue is to consider the possibility of bipolar disorder before initiating antidepressant medication that could unmask a serious mania and result in significant illness or suicide.

Table 17.2.
Common Medications That Can Cause or Worsen Depression

Drugs of abuse	Alcohol
	Amphetamines
	Cocaine
	Marijuana
Steroid hormones	Prednisone (or any glucocorticoids)
	Oral contraceptives
Psychoactive drugs	Opiate analgesics (e.g., codeine)
	Sedative-hypnotics (e.g., triazolam)
	Barbiturates
	Anxiolytics (e.g., diazepam)
Antihypertensives	β-Adrenergic blockers (especially those with lipophilic properties [e.g., propranolol])
Antihistamines	Chlorpheniramine
	Diphenhydramine
Cancer chemotherapy	

A specific depression diagnosis is based on the severity, duration, and nature of the symptoms, time course, and seasonal cycle. Diagnostic criteria for major depressive disorder are shown in Table 17.3. Many depressed patients in primary care will not fit any diagnostic pattern exactly, but will have severity of symptoms that mandates treatment targeted at improving function and quality of life.

For anxiety disorders, you should also try to make a specific diagnosis according to *Diagnostic and Statistical Manual of Mental Disorders* (DSM-IV) criteria (Tables 17.4 and 17.5). Because there is significant overlap and comorbidity among the anxiety diagnoses, and similar treatments (cognitive behavior therapy and antidepressants) are used for most entities, precision is not always necessary, and you may decide to treat based on the severity of the symptoms and the degree of functional impairment.

The recent clinical guidelines for depression developed by the Agency for Health Care Policy and Research recommend that the diagnosis and treatment of depression take precedence over that of anxiety, particularly because the use of antidepressants is effective for both conditions (8).

Table 17.3.
Diagnostic Criteria for Major Depressive Disorder

I. At least five of the following nine symptoms have been present nearly every day during the prior 2 weeks and have caused a significant deterioration in functioning. One of the symptoms must be *a* or *b*.
  a. Depressed mood
  b. Markedly diminished interest or pleasure in all, or almost all, activities
  c. Significant undesired weight change (±5%)
  d. Sleep disturbance (either loss of or excessive sleep)
  e. Psychomotor agitation or retardation
  f. Fatigue or loss of energy
  g. Feelings of worthlessness or guilt
  h. Cognitive dysfunction
  i. Strong suicidal ideation, plan, or attempt
II. Symptoms are not accounted for by mood disorder due to a general medical condition, substance abuse, or bereavement.
III. Symptoms are not better accounted for by a psychotic condition.

Adapted from American Psychiatric Association. Diagnostic and Statistical Manual of Mental Disorders (DSM-IV), 4th ed. Washington, DC: American Psychiatric Association, 1994.

Table 17.4.
Diagnostic Criteria for Generalized Anxiety Disorder

I. Excessive anxiety and worry occurring more days than not for the past 6 months about several different activities or events
II. Difficulty in controlling anxiety
III. At least three of the following six symptoms associated with anxiety
  a. Restlessness or feeling edgy
  b. Fatigue
  c. Difficulty concentrating
  d. Irritability
  e. Muscle tension
  f. Sleep disturbance
IV. Anxiety not part of another psychiatric disorder, such as panic disorder or posttraumatic stress disorder
V. Anxiety that causes significant functional impairment
VI. Anxiety not due to substance use or abuse, or a general medical condition

Adapted from American Psychiatric Association. Diagnostic and Statistical Manual of Mental Disorders (DSM-IV), 4th ed. Washington, DC: American Psychiatric Association, 1994.

MANAGEMENT

Management of these patients requires consideration of five major therapeutic actions: (a) general supportive counseling and education, (b) symptom control, (c) specific pharmacologic regimens, (d) targeted psychotherapy, and (e) referral to a mental health specialist.

Table 17.5.
Diagnostic Criteria for Panic Disorder

I. Recurrent panic attacks[a] with associated worry about having another attack or losing control that lasts for more than 1 month
II. Panic attacks not due to substance use or abuse or a general medical condition
III. Anxiety or panic attacks not better accounted for by another psychiatric disorder, such as obsessive-compulsive disorder or posttraumatic stress disorder

Adapted from American Psychiatric Association. Diagnostic and Statistical Manual of Mental Disorders (DSM-IV), 4th ed. Washington, DC: American Psychiatric Association, 1994.

[a]Panic attacks characterized by four or more of the following symptoms occurring over 10 minutes: palpitations, sweating, shaking, sensations of shortness of breath, feelings of choking, chest pain, nausea or abdominal distress, dizziness, depersonalization, fear of losing control, fear of dying, paresthesias, chills, or hot flushes.

Supportive Counseling and Education

Many studies of the treatment of psychiatric illness in primary care have shown that specific psychotherapy and full therapeutic use of medication are often difficult to document from chart review (9). However, physician interviews and office visit videotapes show that most physicians provide substantial informal counseling, support and education. The specific value of supportive counseling is difficult to prove with regard to treatment success or patient improvement, yet it seems to be an inherently valuable and important part of the overall compassionate care of these patients. You should devote a few minutes of each office visit with these patients to a discussion of interval stresses, new demands or upsets in the patient's life, and efforts to develop support from family members and friends. In addition, you can make nonspecific suggestions for ways to solve work and family problems, as well as recommendations for stress reduction such as exercise, relaxation therapy, meditation, or yoga. You can also make recommendations for reading as a way of helping patients understand their disease. *Feeling Good: The New Mood Therapy* (10) by David Burns and *How to Heal Depression* (11) by Harold Bloomfield and Peter McWilliams are excellent references that are widely available to patients. Finally, you can encourage the patient by explaining that these diseases are usually highly responsive to treatment, and express your commitment to keep working on effective treatment.

An absolutely critical interviewing skill is assessing the depressed patient for suicidal risk at each visit, at least until a treatment response is achieved. You do not need to be fearful of raising this issue with the patient, because literally every patient who has a mood disturbance has thought of suicide in at least a general way, if only to wish that their misery would just end by some unspecified means. Risk factors for suicide in depressed patients are shown in Table 17.6. You should consider referral for a patient who has several of these factors or whose presentation raises doubts in your mind of their stability and safety.

Symptom Control

Patients who have depression may not be sufficiently ill to need specific pharmacologic treatment, yet may have annoying or disruptive symptoms that need to be alleviated. Sleep disturbance, chronic pain such as myofascial pain

Table 17.6.
Factors Increasing the Risk of Suicide in Depressed Patients[a]

1. Increased age (over age 70 in men, age 60 in women)
2. Gender (women make more attempts; men are more often successful)
3. Poor social support
4. Lack of marital support or absence of children
5. Chronic physical illness or chronic pain
6. Alcoholism or substance abuse
7. History of prior attempts
8. Specific plan or explicit communication about intent
9. Family history of successful suicide

[a]Several risk factors together are particularly significant, e.g., a recently widowed, 70-year-old man who drinks excessively is an extremely high suicide risk and requires specific assessment.

(as in fibromyalgia), headache, and low back pain are particularly common. Many physicians use a variety of pain control medications, such as nonsteroidal anti-inflammatory drugs, or sedatives to control these symptoms. Although this may be appropriate at times, you should consider using tricyclic antidepressants (TCAs) in smaller than usual doses (e.g., imipramine 25 to 50 mg at bedtime) for both sleep and chronic pain control. The same approach applies to patients with anxiety, particularly those who have disturbance of sleep initiation. The regular use of TCAs may be equally effective and less hazardous than potentially addictive drugs like benzodiazepines. In addition, the patient may be found to be more profoundly depressed as the investigation proceeds, and the TCA can be increased to full dosage, or a different antidepressant added to the regimen in a simple fashion.

Specific Pharmacologic Treatment

Patients with severe depressive or anxiety symptoms and/or functional impairment for at least 1 month should receive full-dose antidepressant therapy. The treatment regimens for major depressive disorder, dysthymia, generalized anxiety disorder, and panic disorder are essentially the same (although the response rate for dysthymia is less than that for MDD, perhaps 30 to 40% compared with 80%). A TCA, selective serotonin reuptake inhibitor (SSRI), or one of the newer antidepressants such as venlafaxine or nefazodone may be used. These medications are equally effective on a population basis, but individual patients have varying responses. In addition, the likelihood that a particular patient will experience certain adverse effects is difficult to predict, so an empiric approach is often necessary. A selective list of antidepressants is shown in Table 17.7, with associated common effects, advantages, and disadvantages (12).

For depressed patients, the following features or information may help to select a first medication:

- History of a prior response to a specific drug

- Success of a drug in a first-degree biologic relative (that may predict a response on a genetic basis or at least enhance compliance)

- Presence of comorbid psychiatric disease (e.g., chronic pain patients may respond well to a TCA such as imipramine)

- Coexisting medical conditions (e.g., cardiac patients may have significant conduction disturbances exacerbated by TCAs)

- Using side effects to treat specific symptoms (e.g., the anorectic effect of fluoxetine in a patient who needs to lose weight)

- Presence of atypical features, such as hyperphagia or hypersomnia (for which an SSRI is indicated)

- Potential for drug-drug interactions (e.g., for a patient taking warfarin, the use of an antidepressant with low protein binding, such as venlafaxine, should be considered)

- Cost

Note: Although the direct cost of TCAs is much lower than that of SSRIs, some studies have shown overall costs to be lower with SSRIs when effectiveness, number of follow-up visits and dosage adjustments, complications, hospitalizations, and risk of suicide are taken into account (13).

When a patient does not respond to an adequate dose of an antidepressant in 6 weeks, you should consider either a switch to a different medication or a referral, depending on your comfort and expertise (see Indications for Referral, which is presented later). If the patient has had a partial response, a further dosage increase may be helpful, as well as an assessment of compliance. For the patient who responds fully and reaches a satisfactory level of function, treatment should be continued for at least 9 to 12 months. The risk of recurrence after one episode is approximately 25%, but rises to 75% or higher with three prior episodes of MDD (14). For patients with a first episode, medication may be stopped until, and if, a second episode occurs. After a second episode, many patients and physicians will

Table 17.7.
A Selection of Commonly Used Antidepressants

Generic Name	Brand Name	Common Dosage Range	Common Adverse Effects
Tricyclic antidepressants			
Imipramine	Tofranil	150–250 mg qhs	Sedation, dry mouth, orthostatic hypotension, prolonged QT interval
Desipramine	Norpramin	50–300 mg qhs	Similar to imipramine
Nortriptyline	Pamelor, Aventyl	l75–125 mg qhs	Fewer side effects compared to imipramine, commonly used in elderly
Selective serotonin reuptake inhibitors			
Fluoxetine	Prozac	10–40 mg qam	Tremulousness, GI upset, difficulty sleeping, sexual dysfunction
Paroxetine	Paxil	10–30 mg qam	Same as fluoxetine, usually more sedating
Serotonin-norepinephrine reuptake inhibitors			
Nefazodone	Serzone	150–300 mg bid	None consistently
Venlafaxine	Effexor	25–75 mg tid	Sedation, hypertension
Other			
Trazodone	Desyrel	300–500 mg qhs or in divided doses	Sedation (often used in low doses for sleep), orthostatic hypotension
Bupropion	Wellbutrin	50–150 mg tid	Agitation, lowered seizure threshold

choose to consider long-term maintenance therapy at full therapeutic doses. Some patients will choose to do this after one or two episodes because they do not wish to experience a recurrence for even a short time before treatment is restarted.

Antidepressants are also the most appropriate pharmacologic treatment of anxiety and panic disorders. Tricyclic antidepressants have been studied the most and are still prescribed frequently. They often have intolerable adverse effects, however (e.g., sedation, dry mouth). The use of desipramine can sometimes lessen these adverse effects, but at the cost of significant stimulation in many patients, causing the very symptoms—such as palpitations, tachycardia, and agitation—for which these patients sought help. For these reasons, most panic disorder patients are best treated with an SSRI. Benzodiazepines are often recommended for treating panic disorder and generalized anxiety disorder (GAD), particularly alprazolam (Xanax), but the potential for tolerance characteristic of the chronic use of all of the benzodiazepines makes them useful only for limited, short-term symptom control while primary treatment with an antidepressant is being started. β-Adrenergic blockers can be used in limited circumstances, such as in the patient who has infrequent attacks or one who requires symptom control while primary antidepressant treatment is being started, but these agents do not constitute adequate treatment for the underlying neurotransmitter dysregulation thought to cause panic disorder.

The same strategy for drug treatment of patients with panic disorder applies to those with GAD, although the number of patients with GAD and no evidence of concomitant MDD or other psychiatric disease requiring primary treatment (particularly substance abuse) is extremely small. For this reason, a primary, isolated diagnosis of GAD should always be questioned.

Benzodiazepines may be more appropriate for the rare patient who has primary GAD, as opposed to their secondary role in panic disorder. Buspirone may be a helpful alternative, but patients who have already taken benzodiazepines rarely make an effective switch to buspirone.

Specific Psychotherapy

Although much of the supportive counseling and education described previously can be useful, two specific forms of problem-focused, time-limited, outpatient psychotherapy have been studied, with good results. Whether you choose to seek training in one or both of these therapies is dependent on your interests, but these skills are attainable and practical in primary care practice.

The first type of specific psychotherapy is interpersonal therapy (IPT), which focuses on practical resolutions of problematic interpersonal relationships or other stressful events. The therapist seeks to:

- Identify specific events or relationships that stimulate abnormal amounts of stress or grief
- Encourage specific discussions about the nature and origin of the stress reaction
- Move through mutual problem resolution strategies to actively resolve the stressful situation or relationship.

For example, a common source of interpersonal stress is social isolation. Practical suggestions for such a situation might include calling a friend with whom the patient has lost contact, joining a social club specific to an interest the patient may have but has neglected recently, volunteering for a community or religious group, or enrolling in adult education classes. Another common problem to which IPT is often directed is marital stress, which may be somewhat more complicated, but still benefits from an outside person (e.g., the primary care physician) engaging in mutual problem solving. IPT may seem simplistic at times, but patients can be very appreciative of this problem-solving approach when they have lost the motivation or cognitive function to identify and resolve the source of their distress.

The second type of short-term therapy is cognitive-behavioral therapy (CBT), which is based on the observation that depressed patients suffer from an unrelenting and unjustifiably negative view of the world around them. CBT has been tested in both MDD and panic disorder patients and found to be as effective as antidepressant medication in mild to moderate disease (15). The main function of the therapist is to provide "homework" assignments to the patient that require him or her to gather and process information about his or her situation and relationships in a way that leads to new cognitive views of their surroundings, new relationships, or new social skills. This may require basic information provided in a didactic way by the therapist, such as knowledge about the origin of symptoms in panic disorder as a way of allaying fears about "going crazy" and losing control of one's body or mind. Therapists also teach patients new ways of self-talk—positive self-statements made before, during, and after stressful events that would normally provoke significant symptoms. Sometimes the therapist actually encourages the patient to seek stressful events, after much practice and preparation, as a way of testing new skills and achieving new levels of comfort in daily responsibilities. CBT is most successful if it is framed as exercises or assignments, if the therapist is very specific about the assignments and sees the patient frequently to provide appropriate feedback, and if the patient is deeply engaged in negotiations about the way the problems are addressed.

Indications for Referral

Eighty to ninety percent of patients who have depressive or anxiety disorders can be successfully treated and/or cared for by primary care physicians. This is similar to the success rate of primary care physicians in caring for most common problems. The remainder of patients will require referral, usually for one or more of the following reasons:

- Severe symptoms with a history of chronic disease unresponsive to prior treatments, especially with a high suicide risk

- Lack of response to initial treatments, even when different medications have been pushed to therapeutic doses

- Psychiatric comorbidity, such as substance abuse and eating disorders, that complicate treatment plans and lower the likelihood of a response

- Medical comorbidity that complicates treatment, such as severe heart disease

- Preference by the patient for a referral to specialized mental health providers

- Need for complex behavioral or psychiatric therapy, such as for severe phobias, obsessive-compulsive disorder, or posttraumatic stress disorder

- Severe symptoms that suggest hospitalization and/or electroconvulsive therapy is necessary, such as psychotic features or inability to care for oneself

If a referral is necessary, try to make it early in the process of care, so the patient does not feel abandoned or that the need for a consultant repre-

sents yet another failure in life. Arrangements are similar to other specialty consultations, with extra attention to the patient's need for a consultant with a specific style, approach, or gender. The possibility of a consultation should be presented to the patient in a matter-of-fact fashion, recognizing the inevitable stigma that many patients attach to psychiatric disease. Statements about the difficulty of the problem, the need for specialized help, and the value of a second opinion can be helpful.

CASE STUDY

M.S. is a 40-year-old woman who is married to a physician and is the mother of three children ranging in age from 8 to 14. Her chief complaint is sleep disturbance and lack of energy. The lack of energy shows up primarily in having no energy for activities related to her children or to the family's building a new house. She does not work outside the home, but has extensive volunteer responsibilities and now feels no motivation to pursue them. She reports a lack of sexual interest, which is very disturbing to her and her husband, although he has tried to be supportive of her situation. She has lost her appetite and approximately 10 lbs over the past 3 to 4 months. She feels quite hopeless and discouraged about the situation although not overtly suicidal.

M.S. believes that her problems began during extensive rehabilitation from a knee reconstruction to repair an anterior cruciate ligament torn while she was playing in an adult soccer league. During the early rehabilitation period she was unable to run and exercise as she had done before the injury. Her history reveals that she has a lifelong problem with a chronic low level of depression, dating back to high school, with some periods of psychotherapy related to relationships with her mother, whom she believes to be hypercritical. She tries consciously not to emulate her mother's behavior with her children but feels that she is beginning to do so. She requests an antidepressant.

DISCUSSION

The four considerations described earlier must be answered in order to make the correct response to this patient's request. The patient's symptoms clearly fit the criteria for major depressive disorder, as described in Table 17.3, including the number and type of symptoms, as well as their duration. We need to know about her medical history and medications (both negative), and other medical symptoms (none) in order to focus on MDD as the primary diagnosis. Her symptoms and functional impairment are clearly of sufficient duration and severity to warrant treatment of some type, and they do not suggest other psychiatric diagnoses as being likely or possible. The patient appears to have a history of dysthymia that has increased in severity and breadth so as to meet criteria for MDD, or she may be experiencing what is sometimes called double depression, meaning dysthymia and MDD concomitantly.

At this point the working diagnosis is MDD, which requires both psychotherapy (because of the issues raised by the patient concerning her relationship with her mother) and an antidepressant (because of the patient's significant physical symptoms and profound functional impairment). A good choice would be one of the mixed serotonin-norepinephrine agents such as nefazodone or venlafaxine, because they do not produce sexual dysfunction as a side effect (and the patient reports satisfactory sexual function as an important aspect of her marriage).

FOLLOW-UP

The patient was started on nefazodone at 100 mg bid, and the dose was increased over a few weeks to 250 mg bid, during which time her symptoms resolved quickly and dramatically. Her energy increased, as did her functional status with home and volunteer responsibilities and her sexual interest. Her husband and children continued to be supportive, and, as the patient began to feel better, she asked for a referral to a therapist to deal with some old issues with her mother. During this time her parenting behavior improved considerably, to her satisfaction and that of her children.

REFERENCES

1. Kessler RC, McGonagle KA, Zhao, et al. Lifetime and 12-month prevalence of DSM-III-R psychiatric disorders in the United States: results from the National Comorbidity Survey. Arch Gen Psychiatry 1994;51:8–19.
2. Schwenk TL, Coyne JC, Fechner-Bates S. Differences between detected and undetected patients in primary care and depressed psychiatric patients. Gen Hosp Psychiatry 1996;18:407–415.
3. Coyne JC, Fechner-Bates S, Schwenk TL. Prevalence, nature and comorbidity of depressive disorders in primary care. Gen Hosp Psychiatry 1994;16:267–276.
4. Feightner JW, Barrows HS, Neufeld VR, Norman GR. Solving problems: how does the family physician do it? Can Fam Physician 1977;23:67–71.
5. Endicott J, Blumenthal R. Barriers to seeking treatment for major depression. Depression Anxiety 1996–1997; 4:273–278.
6. Pratt LA, Ford DE, Crum RM, et al. Depression, psychotropic medication, and risk of myocardial infarction. Circulation 1996;94:3123–3129.
7. Mason BJ, Kocsis JH, Ritvo EC, Cutler RB. A double-blind, placebo-controlled trial of desipramine for primary alcohol dependence stratified on the presence or absence of major depression. JAMA 1996;275:761–767.
8. Depression Guideline Panel. Depression in Primary Care, Vol. 1. Diagnosis of Major Depression. Clinical Practice Guideline no. 5, Agency for Health Care Policy and Research publication no. 93–0551. Rockville, MD: Department of Health and Human Services, Public Health Service, Agency for Health Care Policy and Research, 1993.
9. Rost K, Smith GR, Mathews DB, Guise B. The deliberate misdiagnosis of major depression in primary care. Arch Fam Med 1994;3:333–337.
10. Burns DD. Feeling Good: The New Mood Therapy, 2nd ed. New York: William Morrow, 1992.
11. Bloomfield HH, McWilliams P. How to Heal Depression. Los Angeles: Prelude Press, 1994.
12. Depression Guideline Panel. Depression in Primary Care, Vol. 2. Treatment of Major Depression. Clinical Practice Guideline no. 5, Agency for Health Care Policy and Research Publication no. 93–0552. Rockville, MD: Department of Health and Human Services, Public Health Service, Agency for Health Care Policy and Research, 1993.
13. McFarland BH. Cost-effectiveness considerations for managed care systems: treating depression in primary care. Am J Med 1994;97(S6A):47S–58S.
14. Kupfer DJ, Frank E, Perel JM, et al. Five year outcome for maintenance therapies in recurrent depression. Arch Gen Psychiatry 1992;49:769–773.
15. Robinson LA, Berman JS, Neimeyer RA. Psychotherapy for the treatment of depression: a comprehensive review of controlled outcome research. Psychol Bull 1990;108:30–49.

18. Arthritis and Rheumatism

PETER CURTIS

Key Clinical Questions

1. What are the major differences in clinical findings between osteoarthritis and rheumatoid arthritis?
2. Which laboratory tests are most useful in the diagnosis of arthritic disorders?
3. What can the clinician do to reduce pain and minimize disability in arthritis patients?

CLINICAL EVALUATION

Most rheumatic complaints are first seen in primary care practice. Connective tissue diseases are encountered only rarely. The most common problems include degenerative osteoarthritis, soft tissue syndromes such as bursitis and myofascial trigger points, gout, and rheumatoid arthritis. Many disorders, however, often cannot be clearly categorized or distinguished from each other (1) (Table 18.1). Often the diagnosis becomes apparent only after symptoms have been present for some time.

In general, women suffer more frequently from rheumatic complaints than men, and the incidence for all patients rises rapidly above the age of 50.

This chapter describes a general approach to the diagnosis and treatment of arthritis and rheumatism and then reviews management of each of the problems seen most frequently in the office.

History

In evaluating a patient with rheumatic complaints or arthritis, pay particular attention to specific symptoms and findings. The onset, location, duration, migration, and quality of pain should be clarified. Stiffness unrelated to pain occurs particularly after inactivity of the joints ("morning stiffness") in conditions such as rheumatoid arthritis, generalized osteoarthritis, ankylosing spondylitis, and polymyalgia rheumatica. Fatigue is a common symptom associated with rheumatic problems, especially in the morning, whereas weakness may be a direct result of the disease process affecting muscle, or it may be wasting secondary to joint pathology and disuse.

Other important aspects of the history to check include any family history of arthritis (gout and rheumatoid arthritis are often familial), performance of activities of daily living, type of employment and work capacity, sexual function, and the patient's emotional state.

Physical Examination

Arthritic joints are usually characterized by swelling, which can be further exaggerated by adjacent muscle wasting. The swelling may also be close to the joint (periarticular), caused by diffuse and usually symmetric enlargement of the synovial membrane. It can occur as irregular discrete nodules or enlargements on tendon sheaths or in bursae. Synovial swelling has a jelly-like feel and is often tender and warm to the touch, but may not be painful when the joint is moved passively.

Effusions are intra-articular collections of fluid, sometimes associated with synovial thickening. The joint capsule is distended and the fluid can be milked to different parts of the joint. Effusions in large joints occur when more than 20 mL of synovial fluid is present and are caused by inflammatory disease or trauma to the joint. Irregular bony enlargement can coexist with synovial swelling and occurs most frequently in osteoarthritis of the knees and interphalangeal joints of the hand.

Depending on the patient's pain tolerance, local areas of soreness over the joint or soft tissue usually indicate inflammation. In acute inflammatory arthritis, the skin overlying the joint may be reddened or edematous.

It is important to analyze the motion of affected joints because this has major implications for rehabilitation, function, and prognosis. Motion restriction can be caused by intra-articular factors such as damage to cartilage, loose fragments, excess synovial membrane, or substantial effusions. Extra-articular causes of limited motion include contractures of the joint capsule, shortened ten-

Table 18.1.

Incidence of Rheumatic Disorders Per 1000 Population

Soft Tissue Rheumatism	Per 1000 Population
Nonarticular	13.2
Bursitis, tendonitis, synovitis	10.9
Shoulder syndromes	6.6
Humeral epicondylitis (tennis elbow)	4.0
Arthritis	
Osteoarthritis Knee	2.0 (>65 years: 95)
Hip	0.7 (>65 years: 55)
Hand	0.9
Gout	9.4
Rheumatoid arthritis	1.0
Ankylosing spondylitis	0.9
Reiter's syndrome	0.35
Connective Tissue Disease	
Systemic lupus erythematosus	0.04
Polymyalgia rheumatica	0.2–0.7[a]
Giant cell arteritis	0.05–0.1[a]
Polymyositis/dermatomyositis	0.001

[a]For people over 50 years old.

dons, and muscle spasm secondary to pain. Passive motion testing is the best indicator of joint damage, because this maneuver excludes the part played in the disorder by muscle and periarticular problems. Some joints may be hypermobile because of instability caused by (a) dislocation or subluxation, (b) weakening or damage to ligaments, or (c) muscle wasting. This often leads to the permanent deformities characteristically seen in rheumatoid arthritis (RA) (wrists, fingers, and feet) and osteoarthritis (hands, knees, and feet).

Finally, crepitus, a grating sensation, can sometimes be felt when palpating a joint. The feel of the crepitus depends on the disease process within the joint—for instance, a "grinding" sensation is caused by the motion of eroded cartilage and adjacent bone surfaces in osteoarthritis. Crepitus can also be felt in inflamed tendon sheaths.

An algorithm to distinguish different rheumatic disorders by history and examination is shown in Figure 18.1. In this evaluation process, there may be clues that suggest the presence of a connective tissue disorder, such as Raynaud's phenomenon (blanching of the fingers) associated with scleroderma or nail pitting associated with psoriatic arthropathy. Arthritis may be only one small component of these systemic disorders, which are quite rare in primary care practice. Typical nonarticular features of rheumatic disorders are shown in Table 18.2.

Laboratory Tests

In rheumatic disorders, the history and clinical examination are the keys to effective diagnosis, whereas laboratory tests and radiographs are used mainly to clarify and confirm a diagnosis. Specific historical, clinical, and laboratory criteria have been developed by the American College of Rheumatology for a wide range of connective tissue and joint disorders (1, 2). These criteria (Table 18.3) are considerably more sensitive than either laboratory testing or imaging in establishing a diagnosis, with high sensitivity (90%) and specificity (75 to 98%) (1, 2).

Many laboratory tests used in rheumatologic diagnosis lack sensitivity and specificity for the general population of patients seen in the office. Much clinically obvious arthritis is associated with normal laboratory profiles, and radiographic evidence appears late in the disease process.

The erythrocyte sedimentation rate (ESR) and C-reactive protein tests are based on the action of proteins produced by the liver in response to inflammation. These are sensitive screening tests for inflammation but have poor specificity for disease; they are often used to monitor progression and therapy of an established disease rather than to support a diagnosis. The normal ESR is 20 mm/hour, but the normal value rises by 5 mm/hr every decade in patients over the age of 40 years.

Although immunologic testing has become increasingly sophisticated and useful for studying certain unusual connective tissue disorders, results are difficult to untangle and are not helpful for the common rheumatologic problems seen in primary care. Rheumatoid factor (RF) and antinuclear antibody (ANA) are characteristic of certain inflammatory and connective tissue diseases, although they represent more of a general autoimmune reaction rather than being a specific indicator. A number of subsets of ANA subclassified by nuclear pattern and type are used to distinguish rare connective tissue disorders (3).

Rheumatoid factor only becomes positive some time after the onset of RA, occasionally sev-

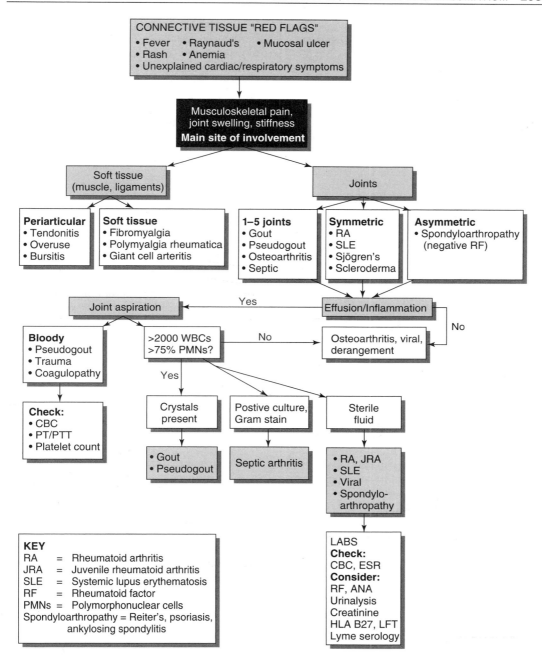

Figure 18.1. *Initial approach to joint problems.* (Adapted from American College of Rheumatology, Ad Hoc Committee on Clinical Guidelines. Guidelines for the initial evaluation of the adult patient with acute musculoskeletal symptoms. Arthritis Rheum 1996;39:1–8.)

eral years later. In fact, 25% of patients with RA never have a positive RF. The titer is only moderately significant at 1:160 and more diagnostic at 1:320. Raised levels are found in the healthy elderly population and in 3% of people with no joint disease. Thus, RF has a sensitivity of 28% and a specificity of 87% (LR+ 2.1; LR− 0.8) for RA and other rheumatic disorders. Its positive

Table 18.2.
Nonarticular Features of Rheumatic Disorders

Feature	Possible Diagnosis
Skin and nail changes	Psoriasis, scleroderma, SLE, Reiter's syndrome
Cutaneous/subcutaneous nodules	Gout, RA
Conjunctivitis/uveitis/ dry eyes	RA, Sjögren's/Reiter's syndromes
Chest pain, cough, dyspnea	RA, SLE
Diarrhea/abdominal pain	Scleroderma, RA, Reiter's syndrome
Dysuria/urethral discharge	Reiter's syndrome

predictive value (PPV) in unselected patients is only 24% (negative PPV 89%). ANA shows a sensitivity of 100% and specificity of 86% for systemic lupus erythematosus (SLE). In other rheumatic disorders, these figures are 45% and 85% respectively (4, 5).

When used in combination as a "rheumatic panel," often offered as a package test by commercial laboratories, RF, ANA, and uric acid (for gout) tests will have a positive predictive value of only 34.6% in identifying gout, rheumatoid arthritis, or SLE in a population presenting with joint pain and an estimated total prevalence of 10%. Thus, 65.4% of the population with a positive test result would not have even one of these diseases. Another point to remember is that serial testing (rather than ordering several tests at the same time) reduces false positive tests by about 9% and halves errors of classification. Consequently, these tests should only be ordered if there already is a strong suspicion of the diagnosis (6).

Table 18.3.
Diagnostic Criteria for Rheumatoid Arthritis

- Morning stiffness of at least 1 hour
- At least three joints involved in soft tissue swelling or effusion (joints: PIP, MCP, wrist, elbow, knee, MTP)
- At least one joint affected in wrist/MCP/PIP distribution
- Symmetric involvement of the same joint; both sides of body
- Nodules found subcutaneously or over bony points
- Rheumatoid factor positive
- Bone changes (erosions/decalcification) in hand/wrist radiographs

In testing for gout, serum uric acid levels are notoriously variable from week to week in the same individual, and high levels are found in renal disease, blood disorders, lymphoma, diabetes, and hypertension in the absence of gout. This test has a poor correlation with diagnosing acute gout.

Other tests, such as HLA-B27, Lyme or parvovirus serology, and antiphospholipid antibodies are only indicated if there is a high suspicion for the disease based on the history and physical examination (2, 3, 7).

Joint Fluid

Other than the history and clinical findings, analysis of fresh (within 2 hours) synovial fluid is the single most important diagnostic procedure in the assessment of joint problems. Sterile precautions during the aspiration procedure are essential. Access is easiest at sites showing capsular distention. If no fluid can be aspirated (often the case in acute gout), irrigating the joint with 2 mL of sterile saline will help obtain material for crystal analysis, white cell counts, and bacterial culture. Several arthritic disorders can be differentiated by synovial fluid analysis (Table 18.4).

Radiology

Radiographs can demonstrate a number of findings in rheumatic disorders. In soft tissues, fluid, subcutaneous nodules, calcifications, and synovial thickening can be identified. Affected joints will show increased or decreased articular space. Subchondral bone cysts caused by hypertrophic synovium are seen in RA. In gout, punched-out erosions may be identified on the bony margins of small joints.

Radionuclide scanning of bones and joints can be helpful in revealing inflammation, even when subclinical. Test sensitivity for joint problems is only moderate, because positive scans can be produced by other forms of osteoblastic activity (fracture, joint trauma, and osteoarthritis). Bone scans are useful for excluding osteomyelitis, metastases, infarcts, or necrosis, although in general specificity is poor.

GENERAL MANAGEMENT

Management depends on the number of joints involved and the frequency and severity of at-

Table 18.4.
Findings in Synovial Fluid

Diagnosis	White Cell Count	% PMN	Glucose Level	Other Findings
Normal	0–200	0–25	Normal	None
Trauma	>5,000	50	Normal	Red blood cells
Osteoarthritis	500–2,000	25	Normal	Cartilage debris
Acute rheumatic fever	2,000–15,000	50	Usually normal	None
Gout	2,000–50,000	75	Low	Urate crystals
Pseudogout pyrophosphate	2,000–50,000	75	Normal	Ca^{++} crystals
Septic arthritis	20,000–50,000	90	Low	+ culture in 80% +Gram's stain in 70%
Rheumatoid arthritis	1,000–5,000	50	Normal	Mucin clot, often xanthochromic; increased protein

tacks. Most patients in a medium-sized primary care practice will have transient or limited episodes involving one to three joints, and not more than 10 patients will have disabling disease. Broad goals of management include the following:

- Symptom relief—medication, rest, splinting
- Restoration/maintenance of function—physical/occupational therapy
- Prevention/correction of deformities—physical therapy, surgery
- Suppression of symptoms—medication
- Emotional health—education, social work, physical conditioning, counseling on employment, and sexuality

A great deal of information is available on self care, and the Arthritis Foundation publishes valuable educational materials as well as a regular newsletter. Physicians can also obtain useful information and catalogues of assistive devices for their patients (Arthritis Foundation (800)283-7800; Website—http://www.arthritis.org).

In practice, the family physician should be able to identify the major rheumatic disorders, arrange a program of pain relief (physical modalities, injections, and analgesics), advise on appropriate rest and disease-specific therapy, and provide patient education. Referral to a rheumatologist is important (a) when the diagnosis is unclear, (b) when the disease is severe or progressive, (c) if dangerous and complex therapy is needed, and (d) to undertake special studies or procedures.

Medication

Medications can help relieve the symptoms of arthritis in three ways: pain relief, anti-inflammatory effects, or attacking hypertrophic synovial tissues.

In most cases, simple analgesia can be used in combination with rest and local heat. Aspirin, acetaminophen, or nonsteroidal anti-inflammatory drugs (NSAIDs) can be quite effective for analgesia, whereas higher doses produce an anti-inflammatory effect. Aspirin is still widely prescribed, although some NSAIDs are better tolerated. Gastrointestinal side effects can be countered by prescribing misoprostol, an analogue of prostaglandin E, 200 μg given four times daily. Commonly used NSAIDs, doses, and relative costs are shown in Table 18.5.

Systemic corticosteroids reduce inflammation by inhibiting migration of neutrophils and monocytes and inhibiting prostaglandin synthesis. These drugs are used predominately in RA, connective tissue disease, and inflammatory muscle disorders (polymyalgia rheumatica, polymyositis) (2, 8). There are a variety of regimens, most designed to avoid or reduce the adverse effect of adrenal suppression (see Table 18.5). Steroids can also be used in joint injections, as adjunctive management when one or two joints are not responding to systemic therapy, or

Table 18.5.
Selected Nonsteroidal Anti-inflammatory Drugs (NSAIDs) Used to Treat Rheumatoid Arthritis

NSAID	Dosages (mg)	Schedule	Cost of Average Monthly Dose[a] ($)	GI[b]	Renal[c]
Naproxen sodium	275, 550	275–550 bid	23.99	++	++
(Anaprox, Naprosyn)	250, 375, 500	250–500 bid	10.22		
Ibuprofen (Motrin)	200, 400, 600, 800	200–800 q4–6h	26.99	++	++
Flurbiprofen (Ansaid)	50, 100	50–100 q4–8h	81.99	++	++
Diclofenac potassium	50	50 q6–8h	72.99	+++	++
(Cataflam)					
Diclofenac sodium	25, 50, 75	50 q6–8h	25.39		
(Voltaren)		75 bid			
Nabumetone (Relafen)	500, 750	1000 qd	72.99	+−++	+−++
Ketoprofen					
(Orudis)	25, 50, 75	50–75 q6–8h	95.99	+++	++
(Oruvail)	100, 150, 200 (extended release)	200 mg qd			

[a]Cost based on lowest possible price of average monthly therapy (generic, if available).

[b]Gastrointestinal adverse effects: reflux, diarrhea, ulceration.

[c]Renal effects: proteinuria, renal failure, fluid retention (most prevalent).

for the local treatment of myofascial and periarticular syndromes (9). Again, sterile techniques are important.

ALTERNATIVE THERAPIES

Because of the chronic, debilitating nature of arthritis and the lack of a permanent "cure," many patients seek alternatives to help function and reduce their suffering. Forty to 84% of patients with musculoskeletal complaints use alternative/complementary therapies (10, 11). Unorthodox therapies abound, including:

- Dimethyl sulfoxide
- Vitamins
- Honey/vinegar protocol
- Acupuncture
- Copper bracelets
- Insect venoms
- Herbal remedies
- Zinc
- Avoidance of food antigens
- Shark cartilage

It is known that certain minerals (zinc and copper) affect the immune system, whereas certain foods (wheat, milk, beef, alfalfa) cause inflammatory tissue responses. Except for acupuncture, the few randomized controlled studies that

have been done show no significant advantages to these therapies, although individual case series report that some patients respond dramatically after orthodox treatment has failed. However, there is increasing evidence that there is toxicity associated with a number of herbal and dietary regimens (12).

SOFT TISSUE SYNDROMES

These consist of a collection of discernible patterns of local musculoskeletal pain, stiffness, and tenderness separate from joints. Although the epidemiology is not well known for individual syndromes, these problems are frequently seen in primary care (see Table 18.1). There may be an association with a systemic disease, rheumatic disorder, repetitive trauma, or stress, but most frequently, the etiology is unclear. The tissues involved are muscle (usually tender "trigger" or myofascial points) in the neck, shoulder, and low back region, ligaments or tendons that become inflamed, and bursae that cause pain and swelling close to the joints (9, 13). The distribution of the most common syndromes is shown in Figure 18.2.

Clinical Evaluation

Myofascial Trigger Points

The patient will describe the onset of pain and aching in muscles, sometimes following trauma,

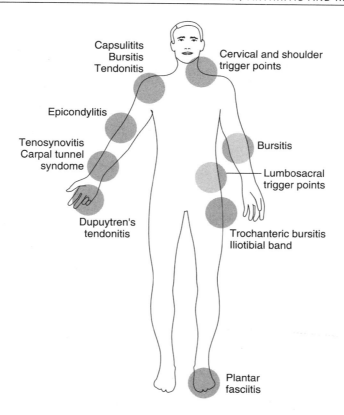

Figure 18.2. *Distribution of soft tissue syndromes.*

but most often arising spontaneously. The areas most affected are the neck and shoulder region, interscapular muscle, and the lower back and buttocks. A trigger point is an area of very localized muscle spasm, often involving only a few fibers. Palpation (approximately 4 kg of pressure) of the muscle usually elicits point tenderness, and the clinician may feel a "trigger or flick" against the examining finger (9). Deep pressure on a trigger point will cause pain of reproducible distribution and quality. Many clinicians believe that these problems are secondary to poor posture and deconditioning, often associated with stress or psychosomatic disorders.

The syndrome of fibromyalgia is characterized by widespread pain with at least 11 painful trigger points in the following muscle areas: suboccipital, paraspinal (C4–C7), trapezius, supraspinatus, lateral epicondyle, gluteal, greater trochanter, and knee (2). There is often an associated sleep disturbance with early morning waking.

Bursitis, Epicondylitis, Tendonitis

These conditions cause pain and reduced motion because of injury or inflammation of the structures close to joints. Motion testing and palpation reveal pain on active movement and local tenderness (13). The most common sites and symptoms are as follows:

- Capsulitis/bursitis of the shoulder—secondary to trauma or inflammation, producing pain and limited motion, often involving the biceps or supraspinatus tendons.

- Epicondylitis—pain over the wrist extensor insertions on the lateral epicondyle of the humerus ("tennis elbow").

- Tenosynovitis—usually involves the extensor or abductor tendon sheaths in the wrist area; caused by inflammatory disease (rheumatoid arthritis) or repetitive trauma.

- Carpal tunnel syndrome—compression of the median nerve in the wrist; may be caused by fluid retention, overuse, hypothyroidism, and diabetes. This produces pain (often nocturnal) in the wrist and hand, often with numbness and weakness of the thumb and index finger.

- Dupuytren's tendonitis or contracture produces fibrosis and shortening of one or more of the flexor tendons of the hand, leading to deformity.
- Iliotibial band is a fascial strain over the external aspect of the hip. It produces pain down the side of the leg. In the same area, trochanteric bursitis causes local pain directly over the greater trochanter and difficulty in walking.
- Plantar fasciitis is an inflammatory process occurring spontaneously, after trauma, or as a symptom of seronegative spondyloarthropathy (i.e., ankylosing spondylitis, Reiter's syndrome). The patient will have severe pain on walking and local tenderness to palpation.

Management

Trigger points will often respond to a graded exercise and conditioning program with local acupressure and deep massage. Acetaminophen, aspirin, or NSAIDs may give relief, although no strong evidence supports this approach. Muscle relaxants are not effective. Local injections of lidocaine, crystalline steroid, or just plain needling can produce immediate relief, but the trigger points often return. In the case of fibromyalgia with definite clinical sleep disturbance, antidepressant medication will help the patient return to a rapid eye movement (REM) sleep pattern, often with relief of the pain.

Bursitis and tendonitis usually respond well to initial rest, splinting, and NSAIDs. If there is no improvement after 2 weeks of therapy, a local lidocaine/steroid injection will often give relief. There should be a graded return to full activities with a gentle exercise program directed by a physical therapist.

OSTEOARTHRITIS (DEGENERATIVE JOINT DISEASE)

Osteoarthritis (OA) is the most common arthritic disorder. Although there are specific contributing factors, most healthy asymptomatic people will have developed some evidence of this degenerative process by the age of 50.

Pathophysiology

The exact cause is still unknown, but biomechanical and immune damage to the articular cartilage, bone, and synovium is thought to be the mechanism. Bone and cartilage are worn away in conjunction with synovial thickening. Bony spurs form at the articular edges, with local inflammation involving the joint capsule and adjacent ligaments.

Clinical Evaluation

Diagnosis depends on a careful history and examination. The distribution of joints affected in the hands and feet in osteoarthritis (distal interphalangeal [DIP] and proximal interphalangeal [PIP] joints) is different from rheumatoid arthritis, and the enlargement is hard and cool to the touch. It also more likely than other arthritides to affect large joints such as the knee or hip.

History

Osteoarthritis usually presents in a middle-aged person with mild, dull, aching pain in one or a limited number of joints. Pain worsens with activity, improves with rest, and can be aggravated by damp, cold weather. There are no systemic symptoms or signs. Stiffness comes from inactivity but improves after about 15 minutes of exercise, in contrast to inflammatory arthritis, in which stiffness is prolonged (>30 minutes). The patient complains of pain and reduced function and, in the case of knee and hip disease, difficulty walking. Usually the symptoms will wax and wane with increasing involvement of more joints. However, the patterns and trajectory of the disease are highly variable and often cannot be predicted. Risk factors include obesity, competitive contact sports, genetic inheritance, and diabetes. Osteoarthritis can be either primary (arising without obvious reason), or secondary to trauma or inflammation. Categories of primary OA are: peripheral joints, spine, generalized, and erosive. Categories of secondary OA are posttraumatic (injured joints only); rheumatic disorders; crystal deposition (gout, pseudogout); neuroarthropathy (strokes, proprioceptive loss); metabolic/endocrine disorders affecting bone (hemachromatosis, acromegaly, diabetes).

Physical Examination

Findings will be limited only to joints and musculoskeletal structures. The joint will be swollen and cool, and motion may be limited. Crepitus is a common and sensitive criterion for the disease. There may be effusions in large joints. Clinical signs include:

- Hands—enlargement of the DIP and/or PIP joints; carpometacarpal joint of the thumb often with some deviation of the phalanges; pain on motion (Fig. 18.3)

- Feet—Swelling (bunion) of the big toe and DIP joints

- Knees and Hips—pain and crepitus on passive motion; tenderness to palpation at the joint line; muscle atrophy. Hard swelling is caused by bone spurs, whereas soft swelling comes from effusions. There is significant limitation of range of motion on active and passive testing.

- Spine—degenerative change is common, leading to limited motion and stiffness of the neck or lower back. Osteophytes (bony spurs) at the facet joints can produce local pain as well as compression of spinal nerve roots, causing neuropathy (weakness and sensory loss). When disc degeneration and osteophyte formation are severe, spinal canal stenosis can cause direct injury to the spinal cord in the neck or lumbar spine areas (see Chapter 33, Neck Pain).

- Osteoarthritis of the wrists, ankles, and shoulders is usually the result of trauma or other secondary causes.

If internal derangement of the joint is suspected (i.e., torn meniscus), referral for arthroscopy is indicated.

Laboratory Tests

Synovial fluid analysis is useful in ruling out inflammatory arthritis (see Table 18.4). The fluid has good viscosity and a low white-cell count. The ESR is normal except in the rare case of erosive osteoarthritis or primary generalized osteoarthritis, which may have an inflammatory presentation much like rheumatoid disease. However, the ANA and rheumatoid factor tests will be negative. A "screening" arthritis test panel is not appropriate because of the high rate of false positives. Other tests are of little value. Their results are usually normal unless there is underlying metabolic or systemic disease, which will be suggested by history and physical examination. Early changes do not appear on radiograph, but as the disease progresses, radiographs will show narrowing of the joint space, increased density of articular surfaces, and spur formation at the joint margins. Radiology is useful to confirm diagnosis but is also positive for arthritic changes in elderly asymptomatic patients. CT scan and magnetic resonance imaging should be used only to evaluate symptoms and possible spinal stenosis.

Management

Randomized controlled studies have shown improved outcomes (increased strength and pain reduction) with exercise programs, the use of braces and taping, and low-impact aerobic conditioning (2, 14, 15). Exercise should be done twice daily over a period of several months. Activity that causes pain for longer than 2 hours should be avoided. Attention to supportive shoes and orthotics can relieve pain from asymmetric walking patterns. Obese patients should lose weight, especially when needing orthopedic surgery (criterion < 200 lbs.).

Pharmacotherapy is directed toward pain relief; using acetaminophen 4000 mg/day is as effective as NSAIDs. If there is a poor response,

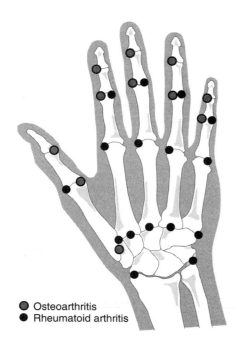

● Osteoarthritis
● Rheumatoid arthritis

Figure 18.3. *Distribution of joint involvement in rheumatoid arthritis and osteoarthritis.*

NSAIDs can be used, basing the dose for each patient on response (see Table 18.5). For OA of the knee, topical analgesics have been shown to be effective (salicylate or capsaicin cream applied four times daily) (15). Intra-articular steroid injections can be used for joints with effusion and inflammation. Another option is to use intra-articular lavage with sterile saline, which has been shown to be more effective, although more costly, than standard medical therapy (16).

Patients with severe OA not responding to medication, or those with serious functional impairment, should be referred to an orthopedic surgeon for osteotomy or arthroplasty.

GOUT

Gout is another common problem, affecting about 2.2 million people in the United States. This includes 5% of all males over 65 years old. The disease is more prevalent in males and African-Americans and is increasing in conjunction with a population rise in uric acid levels (2). Gout is often a familial disorder (40% of cases).

Pathophysiology

Symptoms are caused by the deposition of urate crystals in connective tissues, which induces local inflammation, necrosis, fibrosis, and subchondral bone destruction. Gout is associated with abnormal amounts of urates in the body resulting from defective metabolism of uric acid. It can also occur as a result of acquired causes of hyperuricemia-cancer (multiple myeloma, blood disorders), chronic renal disease, psoriasis, alcoholism, and certain medications (diuretics and antimetabolites such as cyclosporine). Uric acid is excreted mainly through the kidneys.

Differential Diagnosis

Criteria for diagnosis of acute gouty arthritis are:

- More than one attack of acute arthritis
- Maximum inflammation within 24 hours
- Monoarthritis
- Redness over joints
- First metatarsophalangeal (MTP) joint involved
- Unilateral first MTP joint attack
- Unilateral tarsal joint attack
- Tophus identified
- Hyperuricemia
- Asymmetric swelling in joint on radiograph
- Subcortical cysts on radiograph
- Urate crystals in joint fluid
- Joint fluid culture negative

Excluding the first two criteria, the presence of six of 11 of the above criteria confirm gout with a sensitivity of 98% and specificity of 95% (LR+ 19.6; LR− 0.02) (2).

Clinical Evaluation

History

Gout often starts as an acute attack developing over several hours. Sometimes there is a prodromal phase with arthralgias, fever, and chills. An affected joint is swollen, red, hot, and cannot be touched without pain. The attack will subside in a few days with desquamation of the skin. It usually affects one to three joints of the fingers and/or toes. Other joints in the feet, ankle, elbows, wrists, and, rarely, the sacroiliac joints, can be affected. The great toe is involved in 75% and the knee and ankle in 50% of attacks. The disease usually starts after age 30 in men and age 50 in women. For many patients, the natural course of the disease is of increasingly frequent and severe episodes (60% recur in the first, and 25% in the second years). For other patients, there may be no clear pattern. Patients who develop polyarticular gout usually have other complex medical problems such as hypertension, cardiac disease, obesity, and renal disease, which modify and complicate uric acid metabolism.

Physical Examination

This should be focused on the acutely tender, red, swollen joint(s). The patient may have fever, chills, and a flushed face. Chronic gout may be associated with swollen, intermittently painful joints in the hands and feet as well as "tophi." The latter are urate deposits in the soft and cartilaginous tissues that cause local nodular swelling and may discharge white material. The prevalence of tophi is closely linked to increasing levels of plasma urate. They are usually found at the first MTP joint, the elbow, the tendons of the hands, and on the ears. About 70% of patients have no tophi for 5 years after the onset of gout, although the rate of progression is increased by renal disease.

Uric acid stones form in the kidney in 25% of gouty subjects and may precede the first joint attack in 30% of these individuals as an episode of renal colic. Production of stones is closely related to high uric acid levels. About 20% of gouty subjects also have some renal damage leading to proteinuria and eventually renal insufficiency. The differential diagnosis of gout is shown in Table 18.6.

Laboratory Tests

An elevated uric acid level is suggestive of gout. Normal plasma uric acid levels should not exceed 6 mg/dL for women and 7 mg/dL for men, and a raised level (up to 18 mg/dL) is due to overproduction or underexcretion. Serum uric acid testing lacks sensitivity as a diagnostic test for gout; it will be normal in 25% of acute attacks. The ESR and white blood cell count are usually raised but are nonspecific in supporting the diagnosis. The definitive diagnosis is made by identifying the needle-like monosodium urate crystals from synovial fluid or a tophus, which, on microscopy, are negatively birefringent in polarized light (yellow against red background). However, crystals cannot be identified in 15% of patients with acute gout.

Imaging early in the disease is often normal. Later, periarticular swelling is seen with punched-out areas on the surface of articular bone (most frequently on the first metatarsal). Pure urate renal stones are radiolucent unless coated with calcium oxalate. Retrograde pyelography or CT scan

may be needed to evaluate the stones' distribution and size.

Management

Acute Gout

Acute gout can be treated with NSAIDs (usually indomethacin 25 to 50 mg every 6 to 8 hours) or colchicine 1 mg and then 0.5 mg every 2 hours, given until there is relief or gastrointestinal symptoms occur. The usual total dose of colchicine is 6 mg and should not exceed 8 mg. After the attack has subsided, colchicine 0.5 mg is continued twice daily. Dosages must be reduced by 50% in the presence of renal disease. Opioids may be needed if the pain is excruciating. Corticosteroids can be used as an intra-articular injection or as a 7-day taper if the patient cannot tolerate NSAIDs or colchicine (16). Bed rest is needed for an extra day after subsidence of the attack to prevent relapse.

Chronic Gout

The cornerstone of treatment in chronic gout is to prevent attacks. Review medications that may affect uric acid levels; recommend that the patient reduce high-purine foods (which contribute only 1 mg/dL to uric acid level) and lower alcohol intake (which contains purines and blocks renal excretion of uric acid); advise a high fluid intake; and stop aspirin (which can provoke acute attacks). This may be enough to control symptoms in patients who have reasonable uric acid levels and have suffered only one or two attacks of gout.

Table 18.6.
Differential Diagnosis of Gout

Problem	Characteristics
Cellulitis	Usually if no joint involved; motion not very painful; culture negative; a typical hot, red appearance of skin and soft tissues
Septic arthritis	Very painful joint motion; positive culture and high white blood cell count in joint fluid; blood culture may be positive
Rheumatoid arthritis	Often prior history of mild arthritis; typical joint distribution involving hands; slow onset of symptoms; RF usually positive
Pseudogout	Often clinically similar to gout; crystal refraction (blue on red background) in joint fluid shows short rods; crystals opaque on radiograph; there is a poor response to colchicine
Acute rheumatic fever	Fever; skin rash; polyarticular distribution; responds rapidly to salicylate therapy

Colchicine can be used to prevent recurrences. For patients with mild hyperuricemia and occasional attacks, the dose is 0.6 mg twice daily. It is also used initially to suppress attacks when starting other types of medications for gout.

The choice of drugs to lower the serum uric acid depends on the result of a 24-hour urinary uric acid study. A level higher than 600 mg/24 hr indicates that there is an overproduction of uric acid, requiring allopurinol, whereas a level lower than 600 mg/24 hr indicates the need for uricosuric drugs (see below) to block tubular reabsorption of filtered urate in the kidney.

- Uricosuric drugs (probenecid, 0.5 g daily, increasing to 2 g; or sulfinpyrazone, 50 to 100 mg twice daily, increasing to 200 to 400 mg twice daily) will lower the uric acid level as well as reduce tophi. These drugs can be used in combination with colchicine to reduce the frequency and severity of attacks. High fluid intake (2000 mL/day) and potassium citrate are also needed with these drugs to prevent crystal precipitation in the kidney. Adverse effects include rash (5%) and gastrointestinal problems (10%).

- Allopurinol—this drug quickly lowers plasma and urinary urates, facilitating mobilization of tophi and renal stones. The initial dose is 100 mg/day for 1 week, increasing to 300 mg/day depending on serum uric acid level. In combination with uricosuric drugs, allopurinol will "dissolve" tophi. Allopurinol in combination with ampicillin will produce skin rash in 20% of patients. The most common adverse effect is an acute gouty attack soon after the medication is begun, so colchicine or indomethacin should be administered in prophylactic doses during the first 3 months of allopurinol.

PSEUDOGOUT (CHONDROCALCINOSIS)

The presence of calcium deposits in cartilage is associated with a familial incidence and a variety of metabolic problems (diabetes, hyperparathyroidism, true gout). It occurs in older people (>60 years) involving large joints, especially shoulders and knees. It can be precipitated by stress or trauma and presents as acute and recurrent attacks of joint pain and effusion. Diagnosis is based on identifying calcification of cartilage and osteoarthritis in the joints on radiograph and finding characteristic crystals in synovial fluid

(see Table 18.4). Preferred treatment is with NSAIDs or colchicine 0.6 mg twice daily. Aspiration of the joint and intra-articular steroids can relieve local symptoms effectively.

RHEUMATOID ARTHRITIS

Although RA is a systemic disease, it mostly affects the synovial membrane of joints. It is three times more frequent in women than in men, and commonly (70% of cases) begins between 25 and 50 years of age.

Pathophysiology

In the affected joint, the synovial membrane becomes inflamed, forming a pannus of granulomatous tissue that erodes cartilage, ligaments, tendons, and eventually bone. These granulomas can also develop as subcutaneous nodules and lesions in other organs such as lungs, heart, and bowel. Effusions are present in the joints, and surrounding muscles atrophy from disuse. Severe musculoskeletal deformities can eventually occur, ending in fibrous fusion (ankylosis) of joint surfaces. In the hands, these are characterized by ulnar deviation, hammer fingers, and boutonnière and swan-neck deformities of the fingers (Fig. 18.4). The disease causes flexion deformities of the toes, valgus deviation of the foot, and fixation of the ankle joint. Vasculitis caused

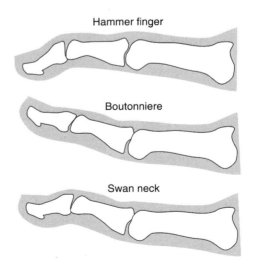

Hammer finger

Boutonniere

Swan neck

Figure 18.4. *Finger deformities in rheumatoid arthritis.*

by granulomas can lead to skin ulcers, scleritis in the eye, pleuritis, pericarditis, osteoporosis, and splenomegaly.

Differential Diagnosis

This is extensive because of the varied nature of the disease and the large number of other arthropathies and connective tissue diseases that have similarities with RA (see Fig. 18.1). The various causes of joint pain and swelling, myalgia, fatigue, fever, and weight loss must all be considered. The American College of Rheumatology has produced a set of criteria to promote diagnostic accuracy. When all are present, there is a sensitivity of 90% and specificity of 89% in making the diagnosis (LR+ 8.9; LR− 0.11) (2,18). These criteria are shown in Table 18.3.

Clinical Evaluation

RA
Early morning stiffness
Pannus?
Effusions

History

The onset is usually unremarkable, with aches and pains in the muscles and joints, low-grade fever, early morning stiffness, and weight loss in 70% of patients. It may be triggered by a stressful incident or viral infection. Subsequently, there will be symmetric joint swelling, usually involving the proximal interphalangeal (PIP) and metacarpophalangeal (MCP) or metatarsophalangeal (MTP) joints of the hands and feet (see Fig. 18.3). Wrists, knees, and ankles may also be affected. Rarely is only one joint involved. The patient typically complains of pain in the joints, fatigue, and a reduction in activities of daily living. The patterns of progression and joint involvement are quite variable:

- Episodic—lasting a few months, then resolving only to return at shorter intervals

- One or two joints remain inflamed for several months before others are affected

- Morning stiffness and fatigue for many months, but with no pain

- Malaise, fever, weight loss for several months preceding joint involvement

- Progressive subtle swelling of the joints

- Severe onset, getting progressively worse without relief

Some patients suffer from rheumatoid arthritis for some years, and then the disease becomes inactive or "burned out." Patients may develop

signs and symptoms of extra-articular involvement that lead to pulmonary, cardiac, and bowel symptoms.

Physical Examination

Findings include joint swelling, tenderness to palpation, loss of motion, effusions, muscle atrophy, inflammation of the tendons and tendon sheaths, and deformities in 20% of cases. Rheumatoid nodules can be found on the forearm and elbow area in 25% of patients with RA. An enlarged spleen may be felt in the abdomen, and vasculitis can cause peripheral neuropathy (sensory and motor loss) in the legs or arms. Cardiac arrhythmias, pericarditis, and pleurisy are other results of vasculitis.

Laboratory Tests

Apart from the variable results of RF, ANA, ESR, and C-reactive protein tests described earlier, there is usually a hypochromic anemia with a normal white blood cell count, unless splenomegaly is present (causing leukopenia). Joint fluid will show typical inflammatory changes (see Table 18.4). Radiograph changes are specific but not sensitive. Over half of patients have no detectable erosions in the first 6 months, with the most rapid progression occurring over the first 2 years (19). Early findings involve the hands or feet and show demineralization and swelling close to the joints. Joint spaces become narrowed, and erosions develop close to articular surfaces.

Management

Medication

Until recently, medication was traditionally given in a stepwise fashion, first to suppress symptoms and subsequently to use second-line drugs only if radiograph changes appeared. It is now known that the first-line drugs (aspirin, NSAID therapy, or even low-dose steroids) do not reduce progression of bone erosion or alter the natural history of the disease, so current opinion supports the early use of second-line drugs to reduce morbidity. The first-line agents are aspirin and NSAIDs. Second-line agents are antimalarials, sulfasalazine, methotrexate, gold salts, D-penicillamine, and azathioprine. Steroids options are low-dose, pulsed IV/IM, or intermittent high-dose steroids. Initially, the patient is started on aspirin or NSAIDs, and then the dosage is maximized.

There may be significant individual variability of response to different NSAIDs (see Table 18.5). If the patient has not improved in 2 to 3 weeks, second-line drugs are started, usually sulfasalazine or chloroquine. If these fail to control the symptoms and disease progression, methotrexate is required. Second-line drugs all have significant adverse effects, and the patient must be monitored carefully (Table 18.7).

Low-dose corticosteroids are generally used to bridge the time period in which the peak response is developing to the second-line drugs. If second-line drugs are ineffective, steroids are needed. Regimens are shown in Table 18.8. Local joint flares can be treated with intra-articular injection. Glucocorticoids (steroids) are effective and widely used in rheumatology, but 30 to 50% of patients on oral medication will develop osteoporosis (20). The most rapid bone mineral loss occurs in the first 6 to 12 months of therapy. The mechanism of this effect is suppression of osteoblastic proliferation and reduced intestinal calcium resorption. However, intra-articular injections will also temporarily suppress osteoblastic activity in the affected joint. When the oral dose is over 30 mg/day, there is a 20 to 50% reduction in bone mineral density (BMD) (20). When the dose is less than 10 mg/day, there is only a 10% reduction in BMD. Risk factors for steroid-induced osteoporosis include:

- Prolonged therapy
- Postmenopausal status
- High daily dose
- Young age of disease onset
- Low calcium intake
- High caffeine intake
- Smoking
- Alcohol abuse

Recommendations for preventing and treating steroid-induced osteoporosis are:

- Use the lowest dose of steroids for the shortest period of time
- Minimize the risk factors (see above)
- Ensure positive calcium balance (1500 mg elemental calcium) and vitamin D (400 to 800 IU)/day)
- Provide hormone replacement therapy to postmenopausal women
- Perform annual bone densitometry to monitor bone mass
- Consider using calcitonin (200 IU intranasally daily) or bisphosphonate (alendronate 10 mg daily)

Although randomized controlled studies show that second-line drugs are 30 to 40% more effective than placebo in improving symptoms and controlling progression of the disease, effectiveness is not as well proven for low-dose steroids (8).

Monitoring the progress of the disease and response to therapy requires repeated measures of joint involvement (inflammation, motion limitation, stiffness, deformity), pain level, results of

Table 18.7.
Treatment Regimens for Rheumatoid Arthritis

Drug	Peak Response	Dose	Laboratory Checks
Antimalarials	2–3 months	200–400 mg daily hydroxychloroquine (chloroquine)	Ophthalmic check, LFT, creatinine every 6 months
Sulfasalazine	4–5 months	500 mg/day with weekly increase to 2–3 g/day	LFT, CBC, creatinine every 3 months
Methotrexate	3–6 weeks	7.5 mg/week building to 20 mg every 2 weeks; IV for severe arthritis	LFT, CBC, creatinine every 4–8 weeks
Gold salts	5–8 months	IV/IM 50 mg/week, then monthly sodium thiomalate, aurothioglucose	Urine, CBC, LFT every 4 months
Azathioprine	4–6 months	1–2.5 mg/day to 5 mg/kg/day	CBC, differential every 2 months
Cyclosporin A	4–6 months	2.5 mg/day to 5 mg/kg/day	CBC, differential every 2 months

Table 18.8.
Regimens for Corticosteroid Therapy[a]

Preparation	Schedule	Usual Dosage	Indication
Prednisone	Daily low dose	<7.5 mg	Maintenance therapy
Prednisone	Short term	20–30 mg (1–2 weeks) with taper over 7–10 days	Short flare
Prednisone	Alternating	5–10 mg every other day	Maintenance therapy
Prednisone	High dose	>60 mg daily	Severe, acute illness
Methylprednisolone sodium succinate (Solu-Medrol, others)	IV pulse	500–1,000 mg/day for 3 days	Severe flare
Triamcinolone	IM pulse	80 mg alternate days two times	Severe flare
Medrol[b]	Intra-articular injection	40–80 mg/mL	Soft tissue articular injection

[a]Adverse effects: skin—thinning, striae, acne, hirsutism, bruising; cardiovascular—hypertension, edema; musculoskeletal—osteopenia, myopathy; personality—mood disorder, insomnia, euphoria; gastrointestinal—ulcer, bleeding; ophthalmic—glaucoma, cataract; endocrine—adrenal suppression, perforation, pancreatitis; metabolic—diabetes, obesity, menstrual disorders, hyperlipidemia.

[b]A variety of articular steroid preparations with different half-lives and costs are available.

acute-phase reactant tests (ESR, C-reactive protein) and radiographic evidence of damage.

Orthopedic Measures

Although levels of inflammation vary over the course of the disease, structural damage is permanent. Orthopedic intervention involves synovectomy to reduce further damage to the joint, resection arthroplasty, joint fusion, and joint replacement (21). Synovectomy is mostly palliative for only 1 to 3 years. Tenosynovectomy involves débriding tendon sheaths to improve motion. Resection arthroplasty removes the damaged part of a non–weight-bearing joint, and arthrodesis relieves pain by fusing the joint. Joint replacement using silastic prostheses has been the major innovation in arthritis care in recent years, leading to significant pain relief and improved function. However, long-term outcomes are not known.

Supportive Management

Physical and occupational health specialists play an important role in helping patients with rheumatoid disease function at home and at work. The following classification has been developed for assessing functional status describing the overall consequences of the disease (22):

Class 1—Completely able to perform usual activities of daily living, including work and recreational activities

Class 2—Able to perform usual self-care and work activities, but limited recreational activity

Class 3—Able to perform usual self care, but limited work and recreational activities

Class 4—Limited ability to perform usual self-care, work, and recreational activities

Supportive care includes splinting to preserve joint function (especially of the wrists) and protect and rest inflamed joints. There is no evidence that this ultimately reduces deformities, however. Assistive devices are useful for enabling the patient to undertake cooking, eating, house or yard work, and a number of other motion and fine-hand activities. There may be a need for modification of the home (bathroom, kitchen, and doorways, as well as a ramp for a wheelchair) and the controls of the patient's automobile.

Patients suffering from chronic arthritis often have significant psychosocial problems involving their own body image, depression, social interactions, and sexuality. Individual and group therapy may be very useful, antidepressant medication may be needed, and it is essential that the personal physician maintain an open and caring approach to these patients and their families.

Prognosis

About 5% of patients will be in remission within 2 years of the first attack, 15 to 25% will have progressive disease despite maximal therapy, and the remainder will follow a varying course. A poor prognosis is indicated by a high-titer RF, extra-articular involvement, persisting acute phase reactants, more than 20 joints involved, and significant functional disability within 1 year of onset.

CASE STUDY 1

Mr. M., aged 50 years, comes to the office for a routine physical examination. He is an executive and maintains a healthy lifestyle, playing a variety of sports regularly. However, he has noticed increasing pain in the right groin, buttock, and knee for about 18 months. He wonders if he has sciatica.

Mr. M. gives no history of previous significant trauma that might explain his pain. There is no family history of medical problems or cancer, but his father (age 72) has just had bilateral hip and knee replacement surgery for arthritis. When Mr. M. gets up in the morning, he experiences some stiffness that quickly wears off, but his pain worsens during the day. He has found that occasional ibuprofen 400 mg is effective in controlling the pain. Examination reveals normal straight leg raises in both legs and no weakness or neurologic deficits. He has marked limitation of internal and external rotation of the right hip, producing hip and knee pain. The knee is normal. There is tenderness to palpation in the groin over the joint capsule. All other joints are normal except for some prominent nontender bony swellings at the distal interphalangeal joints. The rest of his physical examination is normal.

QUESTIONS

1. What areas of history and physical examination should you focus on to assess his pain?
2. What tests and initial management would be appropriate and cost effective?

DISCUSSION

The physical findings of limited motion and local tenderness at the right hip with referred pain to the knee strongly suggest osteoarthritis. This diagnosis is supported by the bony "nodes" at the PIP joints and the family history of severe joint disease (in his father).

Radiographs of both hips should be done to reveal the extent of the degeneration and provide a baseline for monitoring progress. A CBC and urinalysis are low-cost baseline tests that may be useful reference points when on future medication. However, they add nothing to the diagnosis. Referral to physical therapy to design a remedial and exercise program, together with a more regular regimen of NSAIDs, will help control the pain. If there is no change in his condition over several months, referral to an orthopedic surgeon is indicated. An important issue here is the patient's understanding of his diagnosis and his perceptions and beliefs about his new "disability" and its effects on his athleticism. Because he may envision suffering the same fate as his father, Mr. M. must be helped to adjust and adapt to this chronic problem.

CASE STUDY 2

Mrs. G. is an overweight 35-year-old factory worker. She complains of increasing pain and stiffness in her shoulders, wrists, hands, knees, and ankles for 5 months, especially on getting up in the morning. It takes her about 2 hours to "get going." She also feels tired all of the time. Clinical examination is normal except for fusiform swelling of her fingers (PIP joints), an effusion in the right knee, and puffiness of the ankles. There is some pain and limitation of motion in her wrists and knees. There is no family history of arthritis. Analgesics and NSAIDs have not relieved her pain and dysfunction.

QUESTIONS

1. What is the likely diagnosis and how should it be evaluated?
2. What treatment options are there for this patient?

DISCUSSION

The distribution of joint symptoms, early-morning persistent stiffness, and fatigue strongly suggest an inflammatory arthritis. A radiographic survey of her joints shows adjacent tissue swelling, little evidence of osteoarthritis, but no erosions or radiolucencies. Her chest radiograph is normal, and there are no other systemic signs of rheumatism. Laboratory tests reveal a mild anemia, an ESR of 36 mm/hr, and a negative RF and ANA. Analysis of joint fluid from tapping the effusion reveals some increased protein, with 1000 leukocytes, a nonspecific, mildly abnormal result. These findings do not meet the criteria of rheumatoid arthritis, so she has a seronegative polyarthropathy; the diagnosis is unclear at this stage.

Treatment should be supportive, including an exercise program and referral to an occupational therapist to help the patient adjust her daily activities. Steroids or second-line drugs (i.e., gold salts) should not be considered at this stage because of the lack of a diagnosis and the drugs' adverse effects. Opioid medication is a reasonable option, as is maximizing anti-inflammatory therapy with NSAIDs. Regular follow-up may subsequently reveal systemic evidence of a rheumatic disorder or a change in her serology.

Referral to a rheumatologist will be useful in recommending more esoteric testing. It is important to discuss the implications and prognosis of this problem on work and home life with the patient. Such a forecast will not be easy, given the uncertainty of the diagnosis at this stage.

REFERENCES

1. Silman AJ, Hochberg MC. Epidemiology of the Rheumatic Diseases. New York: Oxford University Press, 1993.
2. Koopman WJ, ed. Arthritis and Allied Conditions. Baltimore: Williams & Wilkins, 1996.
3. Noe DA, Rock RC, eds. Laboratory Medicine. The Selection and Interpretation of Clinical Laboratory Studies. Baltimore: Williams & Wilkins, 1994.
4. Shmerling RH, Delbanco TL. How useful is the rheumatoid factor? Arch Intern Med 1992;152: 2417–2420.
5. Slater CA, Davis RB, Shmerling RH. Antinuclear antibody testing. A study of clinical utility. Arch Intern Med 1996;156:1421–1425.
6. Lichtenstein MJ, Pincus T. How useful are combinations of laboratory tests in "rheumatic panels" in the diagnosis of rheumatic disease? J Gen Intern Med 1988;3;435–442.
7. Weinblatt ME. Treatment of rheumatoid arthritis. In: Koopman WJ, ed. Arthritis and Allied Disorders, 13th ed. Baltimore: Williams & Wilkins, 1996.
8. Saag KG, Criswell LA, Sems KM, Nettleman MD, Kolluri S. Low-dose corticosteroids in rheumatoid arthritis. Arthritis Rheum 1996;39:1818–1825.
9. Travell JG, Simons DG. Myofascial Pain and Dysfunction. The Trigger Point Manual. Baltimore: Williams & Wilkins, 1983.
10. Eisenberg D. Alternative medical therapies for rheumatological disorders. Arthritis Care Res 1996; 9:1–4.
11. Marti JE. Alternative Health and Medicine Encyclopedia. Detroit: Visible Ink Press, 1995.
12. Panush RS, Endo LP. Diet and other controversial remedies. In: Katz WA, ed. Diagnosis and Management of Rheumatic Diseases. Philadelphia: JB Lippincott, 1988.
13. Cailliet R. Soft Tissue Pain and Disability, 3rd ed. Philadelphia: FA Davis Co, 1995.
14. Hochberg MC, Altman RD, Brandt KD, et al. Guidelines for the medical management of osteoarthritis, part 1: osteoarthritis of the hip. Arthritis Rheum 1995;38:1535–1540.
15. Hochberg MC, Altman RD, Brandt KD, et al. Guidelines for the medical management of osteoarthritis, part 2: osteoarthritis of the knee. Arthritis Rheum 1995;38:1541–1546.
16. Ike RW, Arnold WJ, Rothschild EW, et al. Tidal irrigation versus conservative medical management in patients with osteoarthritis of the knee: a prospective randomized study. J Rheumatol 1992;19:772–779.
17. Fam AG. Current therapy of acute microcrystalline arthritis and the role of corticosteroids. J Clin Rheum 1997;3:35–40.
18. American College of Rheumatology, Ad Hoc Committee on Clinical Guidelines. Guidelines for the initial evaluation of the adult patient with acute musculoskeletal symptoms. Arthritis Rheum 1996;39:1–8.
19. Fex E, Jonsson K, Johnson U, Eberhardt K. Development of radiographic damage during the first 5–6 years of rheumatoid arthritis. A prospective follow-up study of a Swedish cohort. Br J Rheum 1996;35:1106–1111.
20. Werth VP. Glucocorticoid-induced osteoporosis. Evaluation, prevention and treatment. J Clin Rheumatol 1997;3;S69–S73.
21. Anderson RJ. The orthopedic management of rheumatoid arthritis. Arthritis Care Res 1996;9:223–228.
22. Hochberg MC, Chane RW, Dwosh I, et al. The American College of Rheumatology 1991 revised criteria for the classification of global functional status in rheumatoid arthritis. Arthritis Rheum 1992;25:498–502.

19. Asthma and Chronic Obstructive Pulmonary Disease (COPD)

DOROTHY E. VURA-WEIS

Key Clinical Questions

1. What conditions can cause wheezing, shortness of breath, or frequent cough?
2. What trigger factors can be identified and modified to prevent future episodes and progression of asthma and COPD?
3. How can the patient or family monitor the disease in order to initiate early intervention for exacerbations?

Asthma is reversible obstructive lung disease that worsens in response to a number of stimuli (such as infection, allergies, and irritants), and improves spontaneously, by withdrawal of the offending stimulus, or with treatment. It is also sometimes called "reactive airway disease" and "bronchospastic disease." The prevalence of asthma increased 42% from 1982 to 1992 in the United States, with corresponding increases in mortality. Approximately 5% of the American population, or 15 million people, have asthma. Prevalence is higher in African-Americans (6.1%) than in Caucasians (5.0%) and higher in those under 18 (7.2%) (1). Prevalence rates for Hispanics are variable but generally higher than for Caucasians. Hospitalization and mortality rates for African-Americans are double those for Caucasians. These differences are especially pronounced among those living in inner cities and with limited access to health care.

Chronic obstructive pulmonary disease (COPD), which includes emphysema and chronic bronchitis, is characterized by obstruction to airflow that is chronic and not easily reversible with treatment. Although asthma of longer duration and greater severity may have a chronic component, the presence of significant reversibility is the defining characteristic. In addition, some people have both asthma and COPD.

COPD affects approximately 14 million Americans (2). About 100,000 deaths per year are attributed directly to COPD, and it is a contributing factor in at least that many more. Eighty to 90% of COPD is associated with tobacco smoke, although only about 15% of smokers are affected. Because men have smoked more in the past than women, more men are currently affected by COPD; this difference is decreasing due to changes in smoking habits. Prevalence and death rates from COPD have increased significantly in the last 20 years.

In 1991, the National Institutes of Health convened an expert panel to make recommendations on the diagnosis and management of asthma (3). In 1997, the second Expert Panel Report, "Guidelines for the Diagnosis and Management of Asthma," was published, based on new research findings and an evaluation of the effects of the earlier recommendations (4). The American Thoracic Society updated its recommendations for diagnosis and care of COPD in 1995 (2). Relevant information from those documents are referenced in this chapter.

Asthma

PATHOPHYSIOLOGY

Asthma is defined as "a lung disease with the following characteristics: (a) airway obstruction that is reversible (but not completely in some patients) either spontaneously or with treatment; (b) airway inflammation; and (c) increased airway responsiveness to a variety of stimuli" (3).

The role of inflammation in the etiology of asthma is important. A variety of triggers, mainly allergic but also sometimes infectious, irritant, or emotional, can initiate the events that result in obstruction to airflow. These effects together result in wheezing and shortness of breath. Once the inflammatory cycle has been activated, the lungs react more easily and dramatically to further stimuli. Small airways under 2 mm in diameter do not have cartilage for support and are affected earliest and most severely. Young children have a higher proportion of airways in this size range, which partly explains their greater susceptibility to asthma. Asthma symptoms are often worse at night. Even people without asthma have a diurnal pattern with airway resistance highest at night and lowest in early afternoon; this effect is much more pronounced in people with asthma.

Some patients experience only an immediate reaction to an allergen or irritant, or "early asthmatic response," which resolves with removal of the stimulus. Others have a later increase in obstruction, termed the "late asthmatic response" or "late-phase reaction," which occurs 4 to 8 hours after the initial stimulus. If the triggering exposure is continuous, the inflammatory response is perpetuated. Permanent changes in lung histology and physiology can develop, and after a number of years, the obstruction may not be completely reversible.

The role of infection in the development of asthma is complex and not completely understood. The first episode of wheezing in children is often associated with bronchiolitis, usually a result of a respiratory syncytial virus infection. A prospective study of infants tested at 1, 6, and 12 months of age showed that respiratory function was decreased even before the episode of bronchiolitis (5). In another study, antibodies to egg proteins and dust mites were more likely to be found in children after they had a respiratory syncytial virus infection, even in those without a family history of allergy, than in children without a history of respiratory syncytial virus (RSV) infection. This suggests that the infection increased the risk of sensitization (6).

The two primary risk factors for wheezing in children under 3 years of age are a positive family history of asthma and exposure to tobacco smoke. More than half of affected children will cease wheezing by age 6, and those that continue wheezing are likely to be the ones with symptoms of atopy (eczema, allergic rhinitis, or allergic conjunctivitis) and with a family history of allergy (7, 8). In children over 6 with asthma, up to 85% have other evidence of atopy (9). Boys are affected more commonly than girls. Longitudinal studies of children with asthma show that many improve in adolescence or early adulthood but may have recurrences in middle age, often triggered by an infection. Among asthmatic adults, approximately 50% have coexisting allergic disease.

CLINICAL EVALUATION

Asthma is diagnosed by a combination of history, physical findings, and pulmonary function test results (Table 19.1). As with most conditions, the history is most important.

History

The usual symptoms of asthma are difficulty breathing, wheezing, and cough, either in combination or alone, especially with exertion. A chronic cough lasting several months and occurring mainly at night may be the only symptom. Parents may report that their infants and young children have "chest congestion" and rapid or labored breathing, often with wheezing. In children and adolescents, chest pain with exercise may be the presenting symptom. When adults with asthma describe their breathing, they often express difficulty in getting enough air, feeling the breath does not go out all the way, or having to work harder or concentrate more in order to breathe (10).

If asthma is suspected, the initial history should include the following areas:

- Nature of symptoms, including shortness of breath, wheezing, cough, and chest pain
- Time (day vs. night) and location (home, work, school) when symptoms are noted
- Precipitating factors or "triggers" (Table 19.2)
- Recent infections, including sinusitis and bronchitis
- Symptoms attributed to chronic infections
- Symptoms of allergic diseases, including history of milk allergy or seasonal symptoms
- Measures or medications that have been helpful
- Previous diagnosis of asthma
- Family history of allergies and/or asthma
- Tobacco use or exposure

Exposure to workplace irritants or allergens may cause symptoms either on the job or several hours later as a late-phase reaction, which may make it difficult to identify the connection between the trigger and the symptoms. Exercise irritates the airways through the loss of heat and moisture during increased ventilation and can also cause both early and late asthmatic responses.

Most asthma patients have a limited perception of the degree of airway obstruction. They recognize a rapid worsening of obstruction more accurately than either a slow deterioration or the

Table 19.1.

Key Elements in the History and Physical Examination for Asthma or COPD

Question/Maneuver	Purpose
Detailed history of wheezing, shortness of breath, frequent cough, and character of sputum	To identify patterns relating time of day, activity, or exposure to allergens, irritants, or infection, and to identify frequent mucus production
Personal or family history of atopy (allergic conjunctivitis or rhinitis, eczema) or family history of asthma	To identify increased risk for asthma
Family history of COPD—at what age?	To determine likelihood of AAT (α_1-antitrypsin) deficiency or of familial tendency for less-severe COPD
Previous diagnosis of asthma or use of inhalers	To elucidate the time course and to help differentiate between transient wheezing and true hyperresponsive airways
Smoking history—either by patient or by household members	To identify a trigger for asthma, which should be avoided; to identify risk for COPD; and to begin the process for helping the patient stop smoking
In older adults, history regarding cardiac symptoms (chest pain, palpitations, ankle swelling, etc.).	To differentiate asthma/COPD from coronary artery disease or congestive heart failure
Assessment of heart rate, respiratory rate, cyanosis, and use of accessory muscles of breathing	To identify patients needing prompt intervention
HEENT and skin examination	To identify sinusitis, allergic rhinitis or conjunctivitis, and eczema
Lung examination for wheezing, prolonged expiration, increased resonance to percussion, and low diaphragm	These findings support a diagnosis of obstructive airways disease
Lung examination for basilar or other localized rales, decreased resonance	These findings would suggest CHF or infection.

absolute degree of obstruction. As an attack is resolving, they may believe they are back to normal despite the presence of significant obstruction. Nevertheless, it is important to ask the patient about the time course of symptoms and whatever exacerbating and alleviating factors they have noticed (11, 12).

Physical Examination

Few data are available on the sensitivity and specificity of physical findings pertinent to initial diagnosis. Physical examination may be remarkably normal even in patients with definite disease: up to one quarter of asthma and COPD patients have a normal examination even when obstruction can be demonstrated on pulmonary functions tests (13, 14).

During an acute episode, the patient may look anxious, with rapid or labored breathing, sitting upright or standing holding on to a chair or table

to maximize the efficiency of the thoracic muscles. Use of accessory muscles, with intercostal and supraclavicular retractions and tightening of the sternocleidomastoid muscle, often accompanies moderate-to-severe disease, especially in children with asthma. Vital signs are important: respiratory rate and heart rate may be increased, and a fever may be present if infection is the trigger. Pulsus paradoxus, the difference between systolic pressure in inspiration and in expiration, may be increased over 10 mm Hg with significant airway obstruction. Cyanosis is rare, but if present indicates a very sick patient.

Auscultation is the most useful technique for evaluating obstructive airway disease. Decreased intensity of breath sounds is the most common finding in asthma and COPD, present in 33 to 65% of patients (13, 14). Wheezes during expiration are characteristic of obstructive airway disease, especially if they take up a large part of the expiratory phase or if they are present

Table 19.2.
Asthma Triggers

Allergens
  Pollens
  Animal dander
  Dust mites
  Cockroaches
  Molds
Irritants
  Tobacco smoke
  Wood stove smoke
  Air pollution
  Perfumes
  Chemical vapors
Physical factors
  Cold air
  Exercise
Infections
  Viruses
  Possibly chlamydia and mycoplasma
Emotions
  Fear
  Anxiety/stress
  Anger
  Hard laughing or crying
Drugs
  Aspirin and NSAIDs (e.g., ibuprofen)
  β Blockers (e.g., propranolol)
  Sulfite additives in foods and beverages

in both inspiration and expiration. (Inspiratory wheezes not accompanied by expiratory wheezes are more likely to indicate upper airway obstruction caused by mucus or laryngeal obstruction). Wheezing is heard in 21 to 70% of COPD and asthma patients and is more often present with greater severity of illness. During a severe exacerbation, however, there may be so little air moving in and out of the lungs that no wheezing is heard. Wheezing on forced expiration suggests asthma or COPD, but this may be a normal finding if the wheezing is short, monophonic, and present only at the end of a maximal forced expiration (15).

Test forced expiratory time by having the patient exhale as hard and long as possible, while listening with a stethoscope placed over the trachea in the suprasternal notch until the last moment that sounds are audible. Forced expiratory time prolonged over 6 seconds has a sensitivity of 74 to 92% in patients detecting asthma or COPD, but a specificity of only 43 to 75%. Sensitivity can be raised to 98% by using a cutoff value of 4 seconds, making this a useful screening maneuver, but only half of the patients identified will actually have obstructive airway disease (the shorter cutoff value results in lower specificity) (16).

Rhonchi are often present during an exacerbation of either asthma or COPD. Inspiratory crackles may indicate either localized infection or atelectasis owing to airways being closed by secretions and bronchospasm. Some COPD patients have chronic coarse crackles in early-to-mid inspiration. A prolonged expiratory phase compared to the duration of the entire respiratory cycle is significant, but needs to be interpreted carefully because children normally have a longer expiratory phase than adults.

Chest percussion discloses hyperresonance owing to increased lung inflation in about a third of patients (34% sensitivity, 94% specificity) (14). This is likely to be accompanied by a low diaphragm (owing to increased residual volume) and decreased diaphragmatic excursion during respiration (owing to a smaller inspiratory reserve volume) in about a sixth of patients with COPD and one quarter of patients with asthma (13).

The point of maximal impulse (PMI) of the heart found in the subxiphoid area correlates with obstructive disease and is specific but not sensitive. Signs of severe disease include a heart rate over 100, a respiratory rate over 20, cyanosis, and pulsus paradoxus. Nasal examination may disclose pale boggy mucosa or nasal polyps, suggesting atopy in asthmatic patients. Skin examination may show eczema.

Patients with COPD often have evidence of smoking-related cardiovascular disease, such as carotid bruits, abdominal bruits, and decreased peripheral pulses. Although no single finding on physical examination is reliable for diagnosing obstructive airways disease, the more findings that are present—especially in conjunction with typical history—the more likely the patient is to have asthma or COPD.

Laboratory Evaluation

Pulmonary Function Tests

Studies to assess air flow are used to make the diagnosis of asthma and COPD and then to monitor severity and effects of medication. The standard test is spirometry, which can be performed by the clinician or a trained nurse in an office setting using low-cost equipment. The patient breathes in and out through tubing connected to sensors that measure air flow over time. The test is repeated after administering two puffs of a short-acting bronchodilator such as albuterol. Results are compared with normal predicted values for persons of the same age, height, gender, and race. They are also presented in graph format, either as volume/time graphs (Fig. 19.1), or as flow/volume loops.

The most important values in the study are forced expiratory volume in the first second (FEV_1), the forced vital capacity (FVC), the ratio FEV_1/FVC, and the peak expiratory flow rate (PEFR or peak flow). In obstructive disease, the FVC is usually normal, but the FEV_1 is decreased. Normal persons can exhale 65 to 75% or more of their breath in the first second of a forced expiration (that is, FEV_1/FVC is 65% or more). This ratio is decreased in both asthma and COPD patients. If the FEV_1 returns back to the normal range with bronchodilator therapy, the patient has asthma. If it increases by more than 12% but does not reach normal, the patient has either COPD with a prominent reversible component or asthma with some permanent airway obstruction (differentiation is complex and involves other historical and clinical factors). In pure COPD, there will be less than a 12% improve-

ment after a bronchodilator. The FEV_1 is the measurement used to define severity and response to treatment.

The PEFR is closely related to the FEV_1, with correlation coefficients of approximately 0.8 in a study comparing percent-predicted peak flow with percent-predicted FEV_1 before, during, and after treatment of asthma exacerbations (17). Peak air flow (or velocity) occurs at the time of the steepest slope of the spirogram curve, near the beginning of the forced expiration. Like the FEV_1, peak flow is reduced significantly by bronchospasm. Measurements can be made both in the office and by the patient at home to aid in diagnosis and to monitor the course of the disease. Peak flow meters are portable and relatively inexpensive.

If asthma is still suspected in spite of normal office spirometry, patients can record peak flow measurements twice a day for 2 weeks at home (in the morning before medications and in the early afternoon or evening after two puffs of albuterol) and also during episodes of breathing difficulty. Three measurements are made each time, and the highest is recorded. A peak flow variation of 20% indicates hyperresponsiveness consistent with asthma. If these results are not diagnostic, the patient may be referred to a pulmonologist for

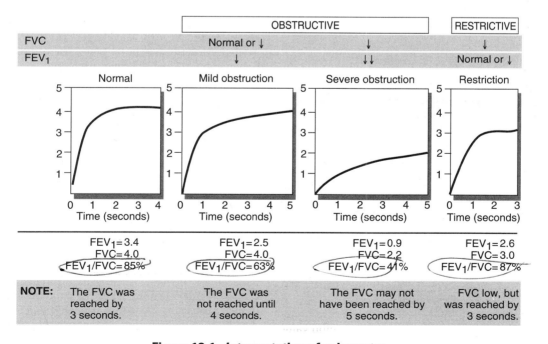

Figure 19.1. *Interpretation of spirometry.*

provocative tests to determine if the airways have an increased degree of reactivity or bronchospasm. The provocative test uses methacholine, which stimulates cholinergic receptors in the bronchioles and causes bronchospasm. The concentration of methacholine that causes a 20% reduction in FEV_1 is noted; a concentration less than 10 mg/mL is usually considered diagnostic of asthma.

Children under 5 are not usually able to perform pulmonary functions tests. In these young children, diagnosis is based primarily on history and physical examination.

Other Tests for Asthma

Further laboratory evaluation is needed only for specific indications. Pulse oximetry is useful to assess patients with rapid respiratory rate, cyanosis, or any respiratory distress. A complete blood count and differential is sometimes useful to differentiate infectious versus atopic etiology; eosinophilia may be seen with allergies and increased neutrophils with infection. Occasionally a total IgE level is obtained to evaluate the allergic component of disease and to add data in questionable cases. Chest radiographs show hyperinflation in about 45% of patients with asthma and are needed only when pneumonia or other processes are suspected or as a baseline in patients with severe asthma.

DIFFERENTIAL DIAGNOSIS

Other causes of wheezing and shortness of breath include congestive heart failure, airway obstruction (due to foreign body, tumor, epiglottitis, or laryngeal muscle spasm), and pulmonary embolus. Chronic cough may be due to postnasal drip, sinusitis, gastroesophageal reflux, or angiotensin-converting enzyme (ACE) inhibitors. These should be considered in the initial evaluation or if the patient doesn't respond to asthma treatment. In addition, some patients wheeze during a single acute infection and for several weeks afterward, but do not have persistent symptoms or any evidence of obstruction on spirometry if provocation tests are done. They may eventually develop criteria for asthma, but unless that happens, they should not be labeled as asthmatics.

MANAGEMENT

The NIH Expert Panel suggests four components of management:

- Controlling factors that contribute to asthma severity (such as allergens and irritants) to improve baseline respiratory status and decrease the frequency of exacerbations

- Monitoring respiratory status with objective measures of lung function for diagnosis, for classification of severity, and to assess response to treatment

- Using pharmacologic therapy in a way that reflects an understanding of the inflammatory nature of asthma

- Providing education for a partnership in asthma care, so that the patient and family understand the disease well enough to be motivated to make changes, use medications wisely, and work collaboratively with the physician

Several clinical trials to determine the effectiveness of the recommendations are promising: asthmatics with frequent emergency room (ER) visits in Memphis who received a 1-hour education session on the use of peak-flow meters, anti-inflammatory medication, use of inhalers, and treatment of exacerbations had fewer ER visits and hospital admissions in the following year than a control group (18). A few studies of comprehensive asthma management using the four principles show decreased symptoms and improved pulmonary function, with accompanying lower costs (19, 20), but larger studies are needed. Most studies of the daily use of peak-flow meters suggest that they are helpful in improving outcomes of moderate and severe asthma. Daily symptom monitoring has been shown to be helpful for some patients (21, 22).

Controlling Factors That Affect Asthma Severity

The best way to prevent allergen or irritant-induced asthma is to avoid exposure. Pets should be kept outdoors (or at least out of bedrooms) or given away. Patients should stop smoking and get the agreement of family members to stop smoking in the house. Dust mites and cockroaches and their excretions are common asthma triggers. Exposure can be limited by careful, regular cleaning when the patient is not in the house using a vacuum cleaner with a fine dust filter, using nonallergenic pillows and nonpermeable covers on mattresses and pillows (or washing the pillow itself every week), avoiding lying on overstuffed furniture, and removing carpeting and replacing it with washable throw rugs, especially in the bedroom.

Skin testing for indoor allergens is recommended for patients with moderate and severe asthma to identify which housekeeping measures are most important and to guide consideration of immunotherapy or "allergy shots." Skin testing is done by injecting a small amount of purified antigen intradermally and noting the size of any reaction (consisting of erythema and a wheal) at each site. If a decision is made to use immunotherapy, the patient is given subcutaneous injections of a dilute solution of the offending allergen, usually twice a week, with a very slow increase in the dose. When the maximum dose is reached, injections are gradually spaced to every 2 to 4 weeks. Treatment is continued for at least 3 years. Effectiveness of immunotherapy has been shown only for treatment with single allergens identified by history and skin testing together (23).

If occupational exposures are triggering asthma, the patient should be given a letter recommending a change in work assignment. Once a patient is sensitized to airborne particulate irritants or allergens, improved work-site ventilation is unlikely to provide adequate relief. Latex, in the form of gloves and other protective equipment, has become a frequent allergen. Because some patients have only a late-phase reaction to occupational stimuli, it can be difficult to connect symptoms that do not occur until the patient is at home; improvement on weekends and vacations provides the clue.

Other conditions associated with asthma exacerbations should be controlled or treated. These include gastroesophageal reflux, allergic rhinitis, nasal polyps, and sinusitis. If attacks are frequently triggered by emotional reactions, individual or family counseling can be very useful. Patients with asthma should receive annual influenza vaccine, because influenza can trigger an exacerbation.

Monitoring Asthma Status with Objective Measures of Lung Function

Determining baseline asthma severity is based on a combination of the patient's FEV_1 and FVC or peak flow measured in the office and the variability in peak flows measured by the patient at home, as described above. This information is combined with patient history to assess the pretreatment severity of asthma according to the criteria indicated in Table 19.3. The pretreatment severity is used to define the condition as mild, intermittent, mild persistent, moderate, or severe. Long-term management can then be initiated.

To determine the severity of an *exacerbation*, the patient checks peak flow values during a symptomatic episode and compares them with his or her personal "target" value (either the patient's best performance or the predicted level of function). A "zone" system, patterned after the red-yellow-green lights of a traffic signal, can be used to determine what intervention, if any, is needed according to whether the result is >80% (green zone), 50 to 80% (yellow zone), or < 50% (red zone) of the target. The zone system is used to guide management of acute exacerbations (Fig. 19.2). Even patients with mild intermittent asthma can have severe exacerbations that may require intubation.

Pharmacotherapy

Medications should be categorized by use, either for long-term control or for quick relief of exacerbations. Medications used for long-term control and for acute treatment with efficacy ratings are shown in Table 19.4, and specific medication dosages are listed in Table 19.5.

Whenever possible, medications are given by inhalation to increase delivery to the lungs and decrease systemic adverse effects. Metered-dose inhalers, or MDIs, are small and very portable, but are difficult for some patients to use effectively. Adding a large-volume spacer (e.g., Aerochamber, others) is helpful: the MDI is inserted in one end of the spacer, and the patient puts the other end in his or her mouth, presses down on the MDI to release the medication into the spacer, and then breathes in deeply and holds the breath in the lungs until the count of 10. After a few normal breaths, the process is repeated. Most patients, even young children, can use this successfully with either a standard mouthpiece or a mask (Fig. 19.3). Some inhalers are "breath-activated" and do not release medication until the patient inhales with the inhaler in the mouth. They may use a powder form of medication, in which case they are called "dry-powder inhalers," or DPIs.

Inhaled medications can also be delivered using a nebulizer machine; this is most appropriate for children under 5 and for patients who become very anxious during asthma attacks and have trouble coordinating the MDI with inspiration. Several studies have shown that an MDI with a spacer is equally or more effective than a nebulizer in most situations.

Table 19.3.
Classification and Long-Term Control Strategies for Asthma

Category	Pretreatment Symptoms	Pretreatment Lung Function	Long-Term Control Medications
STEP 1: Mild intermittent	Symptoms ≤ 2 times a week Asymptomatic and normal PEF between exacerbations Exacerbations brief (from a few hours to a few days); intensity may vary Nighttime symptoms ≤ 2 times a month	FEV_1 or PEF ≥ 80% predicted PEF variability < 20%	(NO LONG-TERM CONTROL MEDICATIONS INDICATED) Use β_2 agonists as needed for symptoms If needed more than twice a week, the patient may need to be reclassified as Step 2: mild persistent
STEP 2: Mild persistent	Symptoms > 2 times a week but < 1 time a day Exacerbations may affect activity Nighttime symptoms > 2 times a month	FEV_1 or PEF ≥ 80% of predicted PEF variability 20–30%	Anti-inflammatory: either low-dose inhaled corticosteroid (beclomethasone) or cromolyn or nedocromil (children usually begin with a trial of cromolyn or nedocromil) Or may consider zafirlukast or zileuton for patients ≥ 12 years old, or sustained-release theophylline
STEP 3: Moderate persistent	Daily symptoms Daily use of inhaled β_2 agonists Exacerbations affect activity and occur two or more times a week, may last days Nighttime symptoms > 1 time a week	FEV_1 or PEF 60–80% predicted PEF variability > 30%	Anti-inflammatory: medium dose inhaled corticosteroid Consider long-acting inhaled β_2 agonist, sustained-release theophylline, or long-acting β_2 agonist tablets (especially for nighttime symptoms).
STEP 4: Severe persistent	Continual symptoms Limited physical activity Frequent exacerbations Nighttime symptoms frequent	FEV_1 or PEF < 60% predicted PEF variability > 30%	Anti-inflammatory: high-dose inhaled corticosteroid AND long-acting bronchodilator (either long-acting inhaled β_2 agonist, sustained-release theophylline, or long-acting oral β_2 agonist tablets). If still uncontrolled, consider oral corticosteroid (e.g., prednisone).

Adapted from National Asthma Education and Prevention Program. Expert Panel Report II: Guidelines for the Diagnosis and Management of Asthma. Washington, DC: US Department of Health and Human Services, 1997.

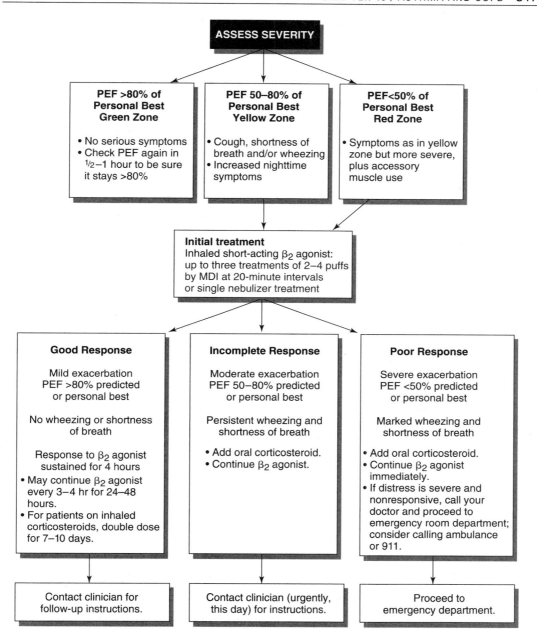

Figure 19.2. *Management of asthma exacerbations: home treatment.* (Adapted from National Asthma Education and Prevention Program. Expert Panel Report II: Guidelines for the Diagnosis and Management of Asthma. Washington, DC: US Department of Health and Human Services, 1997.)

Long-Term Control Medications

ANTI-INFLAMMATORY MEDICATIONS: CORTICOSTEROIDS

Inhaled corticosteroids block many steps in the inflammatory process. Initially they prevent only the late asthmatic response. After regular use, they also prevent the immediate response (24). Adverse effects of inhaled corticosteroids include hoarseness and candidiasis of the posterior pharynx, which can be decreased by using a spacer and by rinsing the mouth with water after

Table 19.4.
Management of Asthma

Treatment Strategy	Level of Evidence for Effectiveness[a]	Recommendations and Comments
Long-term control		
Cromolyn and nedocromil	A	Cromolyn more effective in children than adults
Inhaled corticosteroids	A	Effective in children and adults (also appear to prevent structural changes in airways that would lead to chronic obstruction)
Inhaled long-acting β_2 agonist (salmeterol)	A	Useful for control of nocturnal symptoms, prevention of exercise-induced symptoms, and to decrease dosage requirements of corticosteroids. No definite clinical evidence of tolerance with prolonged use.
Oral corticosteroids	A	Effective, but serious adverse effects with chronic use, so lowest effective dose should be used on an every-other-day schedule if possible.
Leukotriene modifiers (zafirlukast and zileuton)	B	Studies indicate decreased β_2-agonist use may reduce need for inhaled or oral corticosteroids.
Methylxanthines (theophylline)	B	Effective, especially for nocturnal asthma, but with more side effects than β_2 agonists. Less expensive than most alternatives.
Quick-relief medications		
Inhaled β_2 agonists	A	Effectiveness established. Long-term use may result in some degree of tolerance.
Systemic corticosteroids (e.g., IV methylprednisolone)	A	Effectiveness established. Usually 3–10 days of treatment is adequate, and it can be stopped without tapering.
Ipratropium bromide	B	May be useful in conjunction with β_2 agonists, especially in severe exacerbations
Methylxanthines (e.g., theophylline)	C	Not as effective as above medications. Toxicity is common and often outweighs benefits. Monitoring blood levels is essential.
Monitoring		
Peak expiratory flow (PEF) monitoring to guide therapy	B	Effectiveness of daily PEF monitoring difficult to isolate from other measures studied in clinical trials; several studies support effectiveness in moderate-to-severe asthma.
Symptom monitoring	B	Useful for indicating need to check PEF more frequently; not adequate to determine severity of obstruction. Variable reliability in different patients

[a]Level of evidence for effectiveness: A, strong or moderate research-based evidence (consistent across several studies, including at least two randomized controlled trials); B, limited research-based evidence (less consistent or extensive evidence, but preponderance of evidence supports use of treatment); C, common practice with little or no research-based evidence; X, moderate or strong evidence suggesting that this treatment is not effective.

Table 19.5.
Medications Used for Asthma

Medication	Adult Dose	Children's Dose
Cromolyn and nedocromil		
Cromolyn (Intal) MDI 1 mg/puff Nebulizer solution 20 mg/ampule	2–4 puffs tid-qid 1 ampule tid-qid	1–2 puffs tid-qid 1 ampule tid-qid
Nedocromil (Tilade) MDI 1.75 mg/puff	2–4 puffs bid-qid	1–2 puffs bid-qid
Inhaled corticosteroids[a]	(Low-dose regimens)[b]	
Beclomethasone dipropionate (Vanceril, Beclovent) 42 μg/puff or 84 μg/puff	4–12 puffs/day of 42 μg 2–6 puffs/day of 84 μg	2–8 puffs/day of 42 μg 1–4 puffs/day of 84 μg
Budesonide turbuhaler 200 μg/dose	1–2 inhalations/day	1 inhalation/day
Flunisolide (Aerobid)	2–4 puffs/day	2–3 puffs/day
Fluticasone propionate (Flovent) MDI: 44, 110, 220 μg/puff DPI: 50, 100, 250 μg/dose	2–6 puffs/day of 44 μg 2 puffs/day of 110 μg 2–6 inhalations of 50 μg	2–4 puffs/day of 44 μg 2–4 inhalations of 50 μg
Triamcinolone acetonide (Azmacort), 100 μg/puff	4–10 puffs/day	4–8 puffs/day
Long-acting β_2 agonists		
Salmeterol (Serevent) MDI 21 μg/puff DPI 50 μg/blister	2 puffs every 12 hours 1 blister every 12 hours	1–2 puffs every 12 hours 1 blister every 12 hours
Sustained-release albuterol 4 mg tablet	4 mg every 12 hours	0.3–0.6 mg/kg/day, not to exceed 8 mg/day
Leukotriene modifiers		
Zafirlukast (Accolate) 20 mg tablet	20 mg bid	(not approved for children)
Zileuton (Zyflo) 600 mg tablet	600 mg qid	(not approved for children)
Methylxanthines		
Theophylline 50–300 mg; sustained-release capsules or tablets	100–300 mg qhs or bid (follow serum levels [trough] if bid)	10 mg/kg/day and adjust per serum levels; can open capsules onto food
Systemic corticosteroids		
Prednisone, prednisolone, or methylprednisolone tablets or liquid	Short course for quick relief: 40–60 mg/day once daily (60 mg can be split bid)	Short course for quick relief: 1–2 mg/kg/day once daily or split bid
	Long-term control: 7.5–60 mg qd or qod	Long-term control: 0.25–2 mg/kg/day or qod
Short-acting inhaled β_2 agonists		
Albuterol (Proventil, Ventolin) MDI: 90 μg/puff DPI: 200 μg/capsule (Rotahaler)	Prior to exercise: 2 puffs or 1–2 capsules	Prior to exercise: 1–2 puffs or 1 capsule
	For exacerbation: 2 puffs or 1–2 capsules tid-qid	For exacerbation: 2 puffs or 1 capsule tid-qid

continued

Table 19.5. *(continued)*
Medications Used for Asthma

Medication	Adult Dose	Children's Dose
Nebulizer solution: 5 mg/mL (0.5%)	1.25–5 mg in 2–3 mL saline every 4–6 hours	1.25–2.5 mg (.05 mg/kg) in 2–3 mL saline every 4–6 hours
Bitolterol (Tornalate)	2 puffs every 6–8 hours	—
Pirbuterol (Maxair MDI or DPI)	2 puffs every 4–6 hours	—
Terbutaline (Brethaire)	2 puffs every 4–6 hours	—

[a]Most regimens are split bid.

[b]For medium dose, you generally can increase the low dose by 50%. For high dose, increase up to approximately double the low dose.

How to position the inhaler:

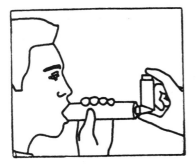

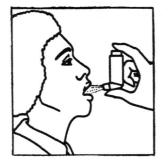

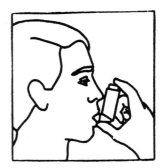

A. Use spacer. This is especially recommended for young children, for others who have difficulty coordinating inhaler use, and for all corticosteroid inhalers.

B. Open mouth with inhaler 1–2 inches away.

C. In the mouth. Do not use with inhaled corticosteroids. Use this position for breath-activated inhalers.

Figure 19.3. *Steps for using a metered-dose inhaler (MDI).* (Adapted from National Asthma Education and Prevention Program. Expert Panel Reports I & II: Guidelines for the Diagnosis and Management of Asthma. Washington, DC: US Department of Health and Human Services, 1991 and 1997.)

1. Remove the cap, hold the inhaler upright, and shake it.
2. Tilt the head back and breathe out.
3. Position inhaler according to one of the above pictures. A or B is best for MDIs.
4. Press down on the inhaler to release medication as you start to breathe in slowly. Continue breathing in for 3 to 5 seconds. (Note: If you are using a spacer, as illustrated in part A, you can press down on the inhaler just before you breathe in. If your MDI is 1 to 2 inches from your mouth, as in part B, you can press down on the inhaler just after you start to breathe in.)
5. Hold your breath for 10 seconds to allow the medicine to reach deeply into your lungs.
6. Repeat puff as directed. Waiting 1 minute between puffs may permit the second puff to penetrate your lungs better. NOTE: If your inhaler is a breath-activated dry-powder inhaler (DPI), exhale normally, then place the inhaler in your mouth as in part C, with your lips closed around it. Inhale rapidly and steadily, then hold the breath in your lungs for 10 seconds. Repeat after 1 minute if needed.

each dose. Even with proper technique, a small amount of steroid is absorbed through the respiratory tract, the mouth, and the pharynx, so concerns over systemic effects have been raised. Doses of beclomethasone of 800 µg/day in adults and 400 µg/day in children have been found to be safe in most studies of adrenal function. Higher doses may cause suppression of the hypothalamic-pituitary-adrenal axis. Children with moderate-to-severe asthma have a slower growth velocity during early-to-middle adolescence, but height by age 20 is unchanged compared to controls. Use of inhaled corticosteroids does not change this pattern at usual doses (24).

Severe chronic asthma may require oral steroids to deliver a higher total dose and to reach small airways inaccessible to inhaled medications in the presence of obstruction. In view of the serious adverse effects of long-term systemic steroids, they should be replaced by inhaled forms as soon as possible. If that is not possible, the lowest effective dose (e.g., 5 to 10 mg prednisone) should be given, preferably on an alternate-day schedule or as a single daily dose in the morning or early afternoon to decrease adrenal suppression (25).

Other Anti-inflammatory Medications

Alternative anti-inflammatory medications are cromolyn sodium, nedocromil, zafirlukast, and zileuton. Cromolyn (Intal) stabilizes mast cells and decreases the release of inflammatory mediators, resulting in inhibition of both the early and late-phase reactions. It can be inhaled 5 to 15 minutes before activity as prophylaxis for exercise-induced asthma. For chronic asthma, it is usually taken three to four times a day, which makes compliance a challenge. The full effect is not seen for 4 to 6 weeks, but because it has no serious adverse effects and is effective for many patients, it is a useful medication. It is most effective in children.

Nedocromil (Tilade) is similar to cromolyn, but also blocks the neurally mediated component of cough-variant asthma. As with cromolyn, adverse effects are rare. After the first month of use four times a day, the beneficial effects can often be maintained with two doses per day.

Leukotriene inhibitors and antagonists are a new group of anti-inflammatory medications that block part of the inflammatory cascade in both the early and late asthmatic response. Zafirlukast (Accolate) is a leukotriene D_4 antagonist prescribed as one 20 mg tablet twice a day; it has

minor adverse effects (i.e., headache, nausea, diarrhea) but does have several drug interactions (e.g., aspirin and warfarin). Zileuton (Zyflo) inhibits the synthesis of leukotrienes and is prescribed as 600 mg orally four times a day. Monitor liver enzymes before treatment begins, monthly for just 3 months of therapy, and then every 2 to 3 months for the remainder of the first year. Zileuton is effective at preventing aspirin and NSAID-related bronchospasm. In early trials, use of both leukotriene modifiers decreased the need for quick-relief medications, and zileuton decreased the need for oral corticosteroids.

Bronchodilators

Inhaled short-acting β_2 agonists like albuterol are no longer recommended as part of a scheduled chronic maintenance program because of decreasing effectiveness when used in this way. The new long-acting inhaled β_2 agonist salmeterol (Serevent) taken at bedtime decreases nocturnal symptoms during its 12-hour action. Some patients benefit from twice daily dosing for better daytime control, including prevention of exercise-induced asthma. Tolerance to its effectiveness has not been seen. Because salmeterol has a slow onset of action, it is not effective for acute exacerbations. In these cases, a short-acting β_2 agonist such as albuterol would be preferred. Albuterol is also available as a sustained-release tablet for use orally to control nighttime symptoms.

The methylxanthines include oral theophylline and parenteral aminophylline. They were once the mainstay of asthma management, but because of frequent adverse effects such as tremors, palpitations, nausea, and, rarely, seizures, they are now used only occasionally to control persistent nocturnal symptoms in asthma and to increase diaphragmatic muscle effectiveness in COPD patients.

Quick-Relief Medications

Short-acting β_2 agonists are used for control of acute symptoms. They act directly at the smooth muscle of the bronchioles to oppose the bronchoconstriction caused by the inflammatory mediators. Quick-onset, short-acting inhaled preparations such as albuterol (Proventil or Ventolin, known generically as salbutamol outside the United States) are used to treat acute episodes and to pretreat patients with exercise-induced asthma 5 to 15 minutes before activity.

Ipratropium bromide (Atrovent) is an inhaled anticholinergic medication that blocks the bronchoconstriction caused by cholinergic stimulation of the more proximal bronchioles. It is a first-line medication in COPD, and it is useful in some patients with severe asthma exacerbations (older patients may benefit more, as the receptors for β_2 agonists decrease with age but the cholinergic receptors continue to be active). It is also used for exacerbations caused by the use of β blockers.

Systemic corticosteroids are used to treat exacerbations that do not respond to short-acting bronchodilators. Depending on the situation, either oral steroids (usually prednisone) or intravenous corticosteroids (usually methylprednisolone) are used. A typical adult dose is 40 to 60 mg of prednisone per day until the peak flow has returned to over 80% of the patient's personal best. The dose can be stopped abruptly without danger of adrenal suppression if it has been used for less that 2 weeks. Tapering the dose to avoid rebound bronchospasm has been common practice, but this approach is not supported by clinical trials.

Long-Term Treatment Regimens

The most important part of asthma management is to develop a chronic treatment regimen that allows the patient to maintain a normal activity level and prevent exacerbations. Avoiding asthma triggers is essential. Except for those with mild intermittent asthma, all patients should be on a medication that decreases the inflammatory response of the airways to various stimuli. In addition, patients with moderate-to-severe asthma should maintain a record of their peak flow readings for early detection of deterioration.

β_2 Agonists can be used initially three to four times a day until the anti-inflammatory medication takes effect (3 to 4 weeks), and then should be withdrawn and saved for use during exacerbations. Several studies have shown gradual improvement of "personal best" peak flows or FEV_1 with continuing use of inhaled corticosteroids up to 9 months, followed by a plateau in pulmonary function (26).

The patient should be reminded to bring the peak-flow meter and diary to each visit for review of technique and results. Patients should measure and record peak flow twice a day when medications are changed. If asthma remains well-controlled for several months, try reducing medications, documenting the patient's status

with peak flow or spirometry measurements before and after the change is made.

Consultation with a pulmonary or allergy specialist is indicated if a patient's diagnosis is in doubt, the history suggests immunotherapy may be beneficial, the asthma does not come under control within 3 to 6 months of appropriate treatment, or the patient has severe asthma.

Managing Acute Exacerbations

A written "asthma control plan" for use when the patient has an exacerbation is an excellent mechanism for providing the patient reassurance and involving him or her in the treatment. In order to use the plan, the patient needs a peak-flow meter and a short-acting β_2 agonist inhaler (e.g., albuterol) accessible at all times. If severe exacerbations have occurred in the past, the patient should also have a supply of oral prednisone available to be used according to the plan. When a patient has respiratory symptoms, he or she should check a peak flow value, compare it with the target value, and follow the appropriate plan as outlined in Figure 19.2. If the peak flow drops into the yellow zone frequently, an increase in long-term control medications or improvement in avoiding triggers is needed.

Clear-cut instructions for how and when to contact the primary doctor or emergency room need to be included in the action plan. If a patient has limited resources to purchase the medications and equipment, is in a chaotic home environment, or has any psychiatric problems, extra efforts should be made to help him or her understand and prepare for treating the exacerbations.

When patients come to the office or emergency room with an acute exacerbation, higher doses of β_2 agonists are given by inhalation using a nebulizer machine and either a mouthpiece or a mask to reverse the bronchoconstriction. If the patient will be going home, a short course of prednisone is usually prescribed to break the cycle of inflammation and hyperresponsiveness of the airways. Frequent asthma exacerbations are a sign that the long-term management plan is not adequate. The physician should review the environmental measures to decrease asthma triggers, and add or increase the dosages of long-term control medications. If the patient has any of the "red flags" that indicate increased risk of death (Table 19.6), management should be coordinated with appropriate specialists, health educators, and home health or school nursing clinicians.

Table 19.6.
"Red Flags" for Increased Risk of Death from Asthma

1. History of previous life-threatening exacerbation with
   - sudden onset,
   - intensive care unit admission, or
   - intubation
2. Frequent unscheduled care manifest as
   - two or more hospitalizations in past year
   - three or more emergency visits in past year
   - emergency visit or hospitalization within month
3. High medication need, seen as
   - use of two or more MDIs of β_2 agonists per month
   - current use or recent withdrawal from systemic corticosteroids
4. Behavioral issues
   - serious psychiatric disease (including depression and psychosis)
   - illicit drug use
5. Social factors
   - low socioeconomic status
   - urban residence
   - limited access to ongoing medical care
6. Cognitive problems
   - difficulty perceiving changes in airflow obstruction
   - inability of patient or caretaker to understand instructions

Adapted from National Asthma Education and Prevention Program. Expert Panel Report II: Guidelines for the Diagnosis and Management of Asthma. Washington, DC: US Department of Health and Human Services, 1997.

Patient Education

As with any chronic condition, the patient (or parents) do the major work of controlling the disease. Asthma differs from most other chronic diseases in that the exacerbations may be dramatic and even terrifying, thus posing a true challenge to the patient to respond calmly and appropriately. Several points deserve special mention:

- The difference between dosage schedules for chronic versus acute management is confusing to patients, especially because β_2 agonists and corticosteroids are used in both situations. Written instructions should be provided, with prominent headings such as "LONG-TERM CONTROL PLAN: Use these medications every day" on one section and "QUICK-RELIEF PLAN: Follow this plan when you have breathing problems" on the other. Make photocopies for the patient to keep in several locations.

- Few asthma patients use their MDIs correctly on a regular basis. Have patients bring their inhalers to every visit to review their use, preferably with a spacer.

- Similarly, patients need reinforcement for how to use the peak-flow meter and why it is important to keep a diary if they have moderate or severe asthma. If they realize that a decrease in peak-flow value or an increase in symptoms can predict an asthma attack, they may be motivated to check their peak flow and use medication more appropriately.

- Parents become understandably frantic when their child does not respond to quick-relief medications in his or her usual manner. It is important to let them know ahead of time that each attack is likely to be a little different, that the written instructions will indicate the proper response, and that a phone consultation with the physician is encouraged whenever they are unsure how to proceed.

- Asthma has a major impact on family relationships, especially when the patient is a child. Parents often need to be encouraged to be consistent in their expectations and their response to any unacceptable behavior, to provide frequent positive feedback to the child separate from dealing with the asthma, and to avoid being manipulated by the child. Providing education and clear-cut guidelines for the asthma management can help to reduce their anxiety level. They should be reassured that most children with asthma can maintain normal activity levels and keep up with their peers.

- Environmental measures to decrease exposure to allergens and irritants should be reviewed every 6 to 12 months to reinforce their importance.

- Health educators can reinforce and expand on the education done in physicians' offices, both in classes and in individual sessions, in an office setting or in the patient's home.

SPECIAL CONSIDERATIONS

Pregnant women with asthma can be treated with the same protocols as other patients. All of the inhaled asthma medications can be used in pregnancy. Very little oral prednisone crosses the placenta, so it is also considered safe in pregnancy. Conversely, poorly controlled asthma is a known risk factor for intrauterine growth retardation and premature delivery.

Chronic Obstructive Pulmonary Disease

The American Thoracic Society defines COPD as "a disease state characterized by the presence of airflow obstruction due to chronic bronchitis or emphysema; the airflow obstruction is generally progressive, may be accompanied by airway hyperreactivity, and may be partially reversible." This definition acknowledges the overlap between asthma and COPD but emphasizes the progressive nature of the disease (whereas well-controlled asthma is not believed to result in permanent or progressive injury). Chronic bronchitis is defined by its clinical presentation as involving "a productive cough for 3 months in each of 2 successive years in a patient in whom other causes of chronic cough have been excluded." Emphysema is defined by its histopathology as "abnormal permanent enlargement of the airspaces distal to the terminal bronchioles, accompanied by destruction of their walls, and without obvious fibrosis" (2).

PATHOPHYSIOLOGY

The airways in patients with COPD have a number of characteristics that are similar to those in asthma: hypertrophy and overactivity of the mucus glands, increased numbers of goblet cells, smooth muscle hypertrophy, small airways clogged with mucus, and sloughing of the ciliated epithelium. During COPD exacerbations, the mucus contains primarily neutrophils rather than the eosinophils seen in asthma. Chemical substances elaborated in the inflammatory cells (such as neutrophil elastase) destroy the supporting attachments of the alveoli, resulting in decreased elastic recoil; they may also destroy the alveolar cells themselves, resulting in less surface area for gas exchange. Airflow obstruction is due partly to the increased secretions and bronchoconstriction as in asthma. In addition, with lack of external support, the small bronchioles collapse even with the normal increase in intrathoracic pressure that occurs during expiration. As obstruction increases and intrathoracic pressure during expiration rises, this effect is even more pronounced.

As indicated earlier, tobacco smoke is responsible for 80 to 90% of cases of COPD. The incidence and severity of COPD increase with longer duration of smoking and higher number of packs smoked.

Approximately 1% of people with COPD have a severe deficiency of α_1-antitrypsin (AAT), which is a protease inhibitor. AAT is a glycoprotein which inhibits neutrophil elastase; without adequate amounts of AAT, the elastase destroys alveolar tissue. The disease tends to occur earlier than in other COPD patients, often without smoking exposure, and it progresses more rapidly. Screening by testing AAT serum levels is indicated if a patient has unusually severe disease compared to age and smoking history (before age 50 in smokers and in any nonsmoker) or has a positive family history of AAT deficiency. Only severe deficiency, consistent with homozygous disease, is improved by treatment with replacement therapy.

Other cases of COPD may be related to occupational exposure, high concentration of indoor pollutants like wood-burning stove smoke, or bronchial hyperresponsiveness (suggesting some overlap with asthma). The contribution of passive smoking or outdoor environmental pollution in initiating COPD is unclear.

CLINICAL EVALUATION

History

The possibility of COPD is most often entertained in patients over age 50 who have dyspnea on exertion and a history of significant smoking (>30 pack-years). The breathing difficulty is often described as an inability to get enough air or as "air hunger," along with a sensation that breathing requires more work or effort than normal. Many also describe wheezing or tightness in the chest (10). A history of cough with mucus production for more than 3 months per year for 2 years places the patient into the category of chronic bronchitis by definition (assuming that no other etiology for the cough has been found). A family history of severe emphysema raises the possibility of α_1-antitrypsin deficiency.

Smokers over age 50 are also at risk for coronary artery disease and lung cancer, which can cause similar symptoms, so it is important to question the patient about chest pain, palpitations, or dyspnea on exertion, which would point to these conditions.

Physical Examination

The majority of the physical examination for COPD was discussed in the corresponding section on asthma. Because of the association with cigarette smoking, the patient suspected of COPD should also be evaluated for vascular diseases by evaluating the carotid, femoral, and pedal pulses and listening for an abdominal bruit. The oropharynx should be examined for tobacco-induced cancers.

Laboratory Evaluation

Spirometry is used to establish a baseline and classify severity of disease. If the FEV_1 is 50 to 90% of expected, the patient is considered to have mild disease; 35 to 50% is moderate, and less than 35% is considered severe. Other tests of lung function are not used routinely, but if a spirogram suggests restrictive or mixed disease, full pulmonary function tests with total lung capacity and inspiratory and expiratory reserve are needed.

Chest radiograph is used largely to rule out other diagnoses, such as lung tumor, congestive heart failure, evidence of restrictive disease, or infection. It is nonspecific in most cases of COPD, but in AAT deficiency, it may show hyperinflation with increased radiolucency in the bases. In other cases it may demonstrate bullae or blebs that predispose the patient to pneumothorax.

Arterial blood gases are used in patients with $FEV_1 < 50\%$, predicted to determine the baseline status and to identify "CO_2 retainers." (These are people with long-standing, severe COPD whose respiratory drive is stimulated only by low blood oxygen levels and not by elevated carbon dioxide levels. If they are given enough supplemental oxygen to achieve normal blood oxygen levels, they have no stimulus to breathe and therefore retain carbon dioxide and become acidotic and stuporous.) Arterial blood gases are also used to determine the need for continuous oxygen therapy.

Sputum Gram's stain is sometimes used to guide antibiotic therapy during exacerbations, although most often antibiotics are chosen empirically. Sputum culture and sensitivity are indicated only in patients who are severely ill and require hospitalization, especially if pneumonia is suspected.

MANAGEMENT

The most important step in managing patients with COPD is smoking cessation, both to improve current function and to slow the deterioration of FEV_1. Physician advocacy and referral to stop-smoking programs are valuable. Summaries of the management strategies, their effectiveness ratings, and medication dosages are shown in Tables 19.7 and 19.8.

Long-Term Management

As with asthma, treatment depends on both severity and frequency of symptoms. Patients who have only intermittent symptoms may be managed with inhaled β_2 agonists, such as albuterol, on an as-needed basis up to eight puffs in 24 hours. Often, these patients are just learning that they have COPD and are still smoking, so major emphasis should be placed on education about smoking cessation.

Patients with continual or frequent symptoms are treated with ipratropium bromide by MDI, two to six puffs four times a day on a scheduled basis, with β_2 agonists added up to 16 puffs a day for additional symptom control. If this regimen is not effective, a long-acting oral medication such as theophylline or sustained-release albuterol is added. The serum theophylline level (trough) should be less than 12 µg/dL to minimize adverse effects including nausea, tremor, palpitations, and insomnia.

Ten to 25% of patients with COPD have a significant improvement when treated with corticosteroids (27, 28). In some studies, the responders have been identified by giving patients an inhaled β_2 agonist and looking for a response of >20% improvement in FEV_1. Alternatively, the patients can be tried on prednisone 40 mg/day for 10 to 14 days, with objective monitoring of FEV_1 or PEFR before and after treatment to determine effectiveness (as noted previously, the patient's symptoms report is not a reliable means of assessing response). In view of the serious adverse effects of chronic steroid use, only those patients with a documented response should be continued on it after the 2-week trial. The prednisone should be tapered as much as possible, aiming for a low dose such as 7.5 mg every other day or a substitution of inhaled corticosteroids. Another approach is to use the 20% response to β_2 agonists as an indication to go directly to inhaled steroids, again monitoring response by FEV_1.

In cases of severe α_1-antitrypsin deficiency, intravenous replacement therapy with α_1-protease inhibitor (Prolastin) is given once a week.

Table 19.7.
Management Regimens for COPD

A. ✔ For all patients	Stop smoking; avoid second-hand smoke
B. Chronic management	
Mild COPD: intermittent symptoms (less than daily), FEV$_1$ usually > 50% predicted	Inhaled β$_2$ agonist as needed for symptoms, 1–2 puffs qid, not to exceed 8 puffs per day
Mild-to-moderate COPD: symptoms most days, FEV$_1$ usually 35–50% predicted	Ipratropium 2–6 puffs tid-qid, not to exceed 18 puffs per day
	Add β$_2$ agonist as needed or scheduled 1–2 puffs tid-qid
Moderate COPD: symptoms persist despite inhaled medications, FEV$_1$ usually 35–50% predicted qhs or bid	Consider long-acting oral medication: sustained release theophylline qhs or bid or sustained release albuterol
Severe COPD: continuing symptoms while on above medications, with diagnosis confirmed by obstructive pattern on spirometry with FEV$_1$ < 35% predicted	Consider trial of oral steroid for chronic management (see text)
	Evaluate need for oxygen therapy
C. Management of exacerbations	
Moderate	Add β$_2$ agonist if not already in use
	Oral antibiotics if sputum increased or changed color
	Consider short course of oral corticosteroids
	Consider mucokinetic agent if sputum very viscous
Severe	Increased bronchodilator doses: β$_2$ agonist (except salmeterol) 6–8 puffs every ½–2 hr and/or ipratropium 6–8 puffs every 3–4 hr (both agents with spacer, or by nebulizer). Albuterol and ipratropium available together in a metered-dose inhaler (Combivent). Hospitalization for intravenous corticosteroids, intensive bronchodilator management, antibiotics, mucokinetic agent and oxygen as indicated, intubation if necessary and per patient wishes

The disease usually stabilizes if the patient has stopped smoking.

Patients with severe disease may require continuous oxygen therapy, which has several beneficial effects: improved symptoms, increased exercise tolerance, and decreased pulmonary artery pressures (to decrease the development or severity of cor pulmonale). The general criteria for home oxygen are a pO$_2$ ≤ 55 mm Hg or SaO$_2$ ≤ 88%. If the pO$_2$ is 55 to 59% and the patient has evidence of tissue hypoxia (such as mental status changes, right heart failure from cor pulmonale or other causes, or polycythemia), continuous oxygen is also indicated. The patient uses the oxygen continuously, day and night, usually at 1 to 2 L/min, to keep the SaO$_2$ > 90% (corresponding to pO$_2$ > 60 mm Hg). The flow is often increased by 1 L/min during sleep and exercise to prevent hypoxia at those times. If the patient is a CO$_2$ retainer, caution must be with oxygen therapy. Patients on home oxygen are usually co-managed with a pulmonologist.

Treating Exacerbations

Moderate exacerbations of COPD are treated by increasing the frequency of inhaled anticholinergic (up to every 3 to 4 hours) and β$_2$ agonists (up to every 4 hours) to decrease bronchospasm, while initiating a course of oral corticosteroids at 40 mg of prednisone per day. The inhaled medications should be decreased to four times a day as soon as possible, and the prednisone can be stopped abruptly, without tapering, if given for less than 2 weeks. A number of clinicians prefer to taper prednisone after the patient's disease has stabilized in order to decrease the likelihood of recurrence, but this approach has not yet been supported by clinical studies.

Infections can cause COPD exacerbations by

Table 19.8.
Management of COPD

Treatment Strategy	Level of Evidence for Effectiveness[a]	Dosage	Recommendations and Comments
Smoking cessation (nicotine patches, nasal spray, gum)	A	Dosage dependent upon cigarette use and formulation	Initial improvement, then slowing of future deterioration
Ipratropium bromide for maintenance	A	2-4 puffs three to four times a day, up to 6 puffs tid (maximum 18 puffs per day)	Improves current symptoms and reduces obstruction, but no evidence that it changes long-term outcome
β₂ agonists:			
Albuterol inhaler	A	1-2 puffs three to four times a day, up to 4 puffs four times a day for exacerbation	Use for acute symptoms; no evidence that it improves or worsens long-term outcome
Oral albuterol, sustained-release preparation	—	4-8 mg qhs or bid	
Broad-spectrum antibiotics (amoxicillin, doxycycline, trimethoprim-sulfamethoxazole, cephalexin, and others) for exacerbations with sputum changes	B	Standard oral doses for 7 days for exacerbations if sputum increased or changed color	Meta-analysis shows statistically significant improved outcome.
Corticosteroids			
Oral (e.g., prednisone)	A	40 mg/day, then taper quickly for acute exacerbation (or for 14 days to test for steroid responsiveness, then taper to lowest effective dose)	
Inhaled corticosteroids (e.g., beclomethasone)	B	2-6 puffs bid if response to oral prednisone is documented by spirometry	
Intravenous (e.g., methylprednisolone)	A	60-120 mg IV every 6-12 hr for severe acute exacerbations; taper as soon as tolerated	
Continuous oxygen therapy	A	1-2 L per minute for continuous home use, or according to oxygen saturation monitoring. As needed in ER or hospital for exacerbations	Prolongs life, prevents development of pulmonary hypertension
Pulmonary rehabilitation programs	B		
Theophylline—sustained release preparation	C	200-450 mg qhs or bid, monitor serum levels and keep at 10-12 μg/mL	Small improvement in obstruction and in respiratory muscle function
Other agents:			
Guaifenesin (Robitussin, other formulations)	—	200-400 mg every 4 hr	
Acetylcysteine (Mucomyst)		3-5 mL of 20% solution every 6-8 hr for 24 hr, administered by aerosol with bronchodilator (caution: may cause bronchospasm)	

[a]Level of evidence for effectiveness: A, strong or moderate research-based evidence (consistent across several studies, including at least two randomized controlled trials); B, limited research-based evidence (less consistent or extensive evidence, but preponderance of evidence supports use of treatment); C, common practice with little or no research-based evidence; X, moderate or strong evidence suggesting that this treatment is not effective.

increasing mucus production and causing bronchoconstriction. Although many of the infections are viral, it is common practice to prescribe antibiotics for patients to keep at home so they can initiate treatment when mucus production increases and changes to a yellow or green color without having to wait for a doctor's appointment. A meta-analysis of well-designed clinical trials showed a small but statistically significant improvement in outcome with antibiotic use as compared to placebo, lending support to this practice (29).

If the above measures are not effective or the patient's condition deteriorates rapidly, hospitalization may be necessary to give more intensive bronchodilator therapy, intravenous antibiotics, steroids, and oxygen therapy. Intubation and mechanical ventilation may be necessary, but should be avoided because of the difficulty in weaning a COPD patient off the ventilator.

Patient Education

The most important intervention is education about smoking cessation. In addition, in order to participate in a collaborative partnership with the physician, the patient needs to understand the proper use of inhalers, home management of medications, avoidance of respiratory irritants, and how and when to contact the physician. Pulmonary rehabilitation programs that include these educational components along with exercise programs tailored to the severity of disease can improve the patient's functional status, exercise tolerance, and symptoms of breathlessness (30). Patients should receive influenza vaccine every year and polyvalent pneumococcal vaccine once. Patients with moderate-to-severe COPD deserve a discussion (when they still feel well, if at all possible) of their desires regarding intubation and resuscitation should they develop respiratory failure.

CASE STUDY

D.S. is a 35-year-old single postal worker who has had asthma for at least 20 years. She enters your practice on a number of asthma medications: an albuterol inhaler eight to sixteen puffs a day, long-acting theophylline at bedtime, and an antihistamine/decongestant. Wheezing occurs most days, and she is sometimes short of breath with moderate activity. She has been seen in urgent care clinics about three to four times a year and in the emergency room about once a year for the past several years for asthma exacerbations and sinus infections. She is interested in a more effective management regimen. On examination, she is comfortable; HEENT shows pale and swollen nasal mucosa, and there is no tenderness on percussion of the paranasal sinuses. Lung examination shows mildly decreased breath sounds, moderate air movement, wheezes during the last two-thirds of forced expiration, and increased resonance to percussion. Her peak flow readings in the office are 320, 300, and 330 L/min, which are about 70% of the value predicted for her age and height.

She reports that she sometimes has more trouble breathing when she sorts dusty batches of mail at the post office. She also has more problems when air pollution levels are higher. She has two dogs that do not sleep in her bedroom; she has never noticed increased wheezing when she is around them.

QUESTIONS

1. Into what category of asthma does D.S. fit?
2. What contributing causes can be identified and modified?
3. What treatment should be initiated at this visit?

DISCUSSION

In view of the frequency of her symptoms, D.S. has persistent asthma. The peak flow readings place her in the moderate persistent category. (This is not a true pretreatment evaluation, but will be adequate to guide initial changes in therapy.) The apparent contributing factors are dust exposure at work, allergic rhinitis, possible sinus infection, and air pollution. Her dogs may also be an unrecognized allergic problem.

Treating allergic rhinitis can have beneficial effects on asthma both directly and also through decreasing the frequency of sinus infections. The antihistamine-decongestant that she is taking is probably helping (theoretic concerns about antihistamines causing problems with dried secretions and worsening asthma are seldom confirmed in practice, so this can be continued), but the pale boggy nasal mucosa are an indication for additional therapy. An anti-inflammatory nasal spray, either a corticosteroid or cromolyn, should be prescribed for daily use.

Workplace interventions can be tension-provoking because of concern that they will lead to jobs with lower pay or less opportunity for advancement, especially in small companies that do not have alternative jobs available. In this case, however, a letter to her employer was effective in obtaining some accommodation for D.S. by assigning her to a different area when dust levels were high.

D.S. agrees to check peak flow readings before and after spending time with her dogs and record the information for review at the next visit. Unfortunately, other than documenting changes in peak flow levels when air pollution levels are high and staying in air-conditioned areas at those times, there is very little that can be done about pollution on a short-term basis.

Because D.S. has persistent asthma, she will benefit from using a corticosteroid inhaler on a daily basis. Her technique for using the inhaler is reviewed.

In order to have baseline information for future visits, spirometry is done before D.S. leaves the clinic. She is given a prescription for her own peak flow meter and taught how to use it. A personalized plan for both long-term control medications and management of exacerbations is written out and reviewed with her.

REFERENCES

1. Data Fact Sheet. Bethesda, MD: National Heart, Lung, and Blood Institute, October, 1995.

2. American Thoracic Society. Standards for the diagnosis and care of patients with chronic obstructive pulmonary disease. Am J Respir Crit Care Med 1995;152 (5):S80.

3. National Asthma Education and Prevention Program. Expert Panel Report: Guidelines for the Diagnosis and Management of Asthma. Washington, DC: US Department of Health and Human Services, 1991.

4. National Asthma Education and Prevention Program. Expert Panel Report II: Guidelines for the Diagnosis and Management of Asthma. Washington, DC: US Department of Health and Human Services, 1997.

5. Young S, O'Keeffe PT, Arnott J, Landau LI. Lung function, airway responsiveness, and respiratory symptoms before and after bronchiolitis. Arch Dis Child 1995;72:16–24.

6. Noma T, Mori A, Yoshizawa I. Induction of allergen-specific IL-2 responsiveness of lymphocytes after respiratory syncytial virus infection and prediction of onset of recurrent wheezing and bronchial asthma. J Allergy Clin Immunol 1996;98(4):816–826.

7. Martinez FD, Wright AL, Taussig LM, et al. Asthma and wheezing in the first six years of life. N Engl J Med 1995;332:133–138.

8. Soyseth V, Kongerud J, Boe J. Postnatal maternal smoking increases the prevalence of asthma but not of bronchial hyperresponsiveness or atopy in their children. Chest 1995;107:389–394.

9. Brooke AM, Lambert PC, Burton PR, Clarke C, Luyt DK, Simpson H. The natural history of respiratory symptoms in preschool children. Am J Respir Crit Care Med 1995;152:1872–1878.

10. Simon PM, Schwartzstien RM, Weiss JW, Fencl V, Teghtsoonian M, Weinberger S. Distinguishable types of dyspnea in patients with shortness of breath. Am Rev Respir Dis 1990;142:1009–1014.

11. Li JT, O'Connell E. Clinical evaluation of asthma. Ann Allergy Asthma Immunol 1996;76:1–14. Turcotte H, Boulet L. Perception of breathlessness during early and late asthmatic responses. Am Rev Respir Dis 1993; 148:514–518.

12. van Schayck CP, van Weel C, Harbers HJM, van Herwaarden CLA. Do physical signs reflect the degree of airflow obstruction in patients with asthma or chronic obstructive pulmonary disease? Scand J Prim Health Care 1991;9:232–238.

13. Badgett RG, Tanaka DJ, Hunt DK, et al. Can moderate chronic obstructive pulmonary disease be diagnosed by historical and physical findings alone? Am J Med 1993;94:188–196.

14. King DK, Thompson BT, Johnson DC. Wheezing on maximal forced exhalation in the diagnosis of atypical asthma. Ann Intern Med 1989;110;451–455.

15. Schapira RM, Schapira MM, Funahashi A, McAuliffe T, Barkey B. The value of the forced expiratory time in the physical diagnosis of obstructive airways disease. JAMA 1993;270:731–736.

16. Nowak RM, Pensler MI, Sarkar, DD, et al. Comparison of peak expiratory flow and FEV_1 admission criteria for acute bronchial asthma. Ann Emerg Med 1982;11: 64–69.

17. Kelso TM, Self TH, Rumbak MJ, Stephens MA, Garrett W, Arheart K. Educational and long-term therapeutic

intervention in the ER: Effect on outcomes in adult indigent minority asthmatics. Am J Emerg Med 1995; 13:632–637.

18. Lahdensuo T, Haahtela T, Herrala J, et al. Randomized comparison of guided self management and traditional treatment of asthma over one year. BMJ 1996; 312:748–752.

19. Gillies J, Barry D, Crane J, et al. A community trial of a written self-management plan for children with asthma. Asthma Foundation of New Zealand Children's Action. N Z Med J 1996;109:30–33.

20. Charlton I, Charlton G, Broomfield J, Mullee MA. Evaluation of peak flow and symptoms-only self-management plans for control of asthma in general practice. BMJ 1990;301:1355–1359.

21. Grampian Asthma Study of Integrated Care. Effectiveness of routine self-monitoring of peak flow in patients with asthma. BMJ 1994;308:564–567.

22. Abramson MJ, Pay RM, Weiner JM. Is allergen immunotherapy effective in asthma? A meta-analysis of randomized clinical trials. Am J Respir Crit Care Med 1995;151:969–974.

23. Barnes PJ, Pedersen S. Efficacy and safety of inhaled corticosteroids in asthma. Am Rev Respir Dis 1993; 148:S1–S26.

24. Beam WR, Weiner DE, Martin RJ. Timing of prednisone and alteration of airways inflammation in nocturnal asthma. Am Rev Respir Dis 1992;146(6):1524–1530.

25. Dompeling E, van Schayck CP, van Grunsven PM, et al. Slowing the deterioration of asthma and chronic obstructive pulmonary disease observed during bronchodilator therapy by adding inhaled corticosteroids. Ann Intern Med 1993;118:770–778.

26. Weiner P, Weiner M, Azgad Y, Zamir D. Inhaled budesonide therapy for patients with stable COPD. Chest 1995;108:1568–1571.

27. Callaghan CM, Dittus RS, Katz BP. Oral corticosteroid therapy for patients with stable chronic obstructive pulmonary disease. Ann Intern Med 1991;114:216–223.

28. Saint S, Bent S, Vittinghoff E, Grady D. Antibiotics in chronic obstructive pulmonary disease exacerbations. JAMA 1995;273:957–960.

29. Ries AL, Kaplan RM, Limberg TM, Prewitt LM. Effects of pulmonary rehabilitation on physiologic and psychosocial outcomes in patients with chronic obstructive pulmonary disease. Ann Intern Med 1995;122: 823–832.

KENDRA L. SCHWARTZ

Key Clinical Questions

1. Is the primary symptom pain, discharge, or a mass?
2. Is the symptom cyclic or noncyclic?
3. Is the symptom unilateral or bilateral?
4. Could the symptom(s) be due to cancer?
5. Does a palpable mass need excisional biopsy?

The three most common presenting problems related to the female breast are breast pain, nipple discharge, and a palpable mass (1). Nonpalpable breast abnormalities are becoming more common as increasing numbers of women obtain mammograms, but their management will not be discussed here. An important concern for women with a breast symptom is whether this represents a malignancy. This concern may be openly stated, but is often left unspoken, and an important part of the management involves acknowledging and appropriately addressing these fears.

BREAST PAIN

Mastalgia is a symptom complex of breast pain and tenderness, with or without nodularity. It is the most common breast problem in primary care practice (1, 2). Many women are concerned about cancer; in breast cancer patients, however, it is rare for pain to be the only presenting symptom (3). Mastalgia is either cyclic or noncyclic, and the management is related to this categorization. Reassurance, after appropriate evaluation, that the pain is not due to cancer will be sufficient for most women; roughly 15% will require further treatment (4).

Pathophysiology and Differential Diagnosis

Approximately two-thirds of women presenting with breast pain have cyclic mastalgia, which is bilateral pain that varies in intensity throughout the menstrual cycle and is thought to be hormonally mediated. Fibrocystic changes may also play a causative role, but histopathologic studies have shown no association. Numerous studies of levels of circulating progesterone, estrogen, prolactin, or quantity of hormone receptors have yielded conflicting results (5, 6), although altered hormone receptor sensitivity remains a possibility. A hormonal etiology is biologically plausible, because regularly ovulating women are most often affected, with the premenstrual time of their cycle the most painful. The usual age at presentation is 33 to 35 years, although the condition has been reported in postmenopausal women on hormone replacement therapy.

Noncyclic mastalgia occurs less often than the cyclic form and is usually unilateral. It typically occurs in women over the age of 40 years, and is not temporally related to the menstrual cycle. Several causes have been described; their relative frequency is summarized in Table 20.1. Postsurgical breast pain may occur at the site of an incision, particularly if the lines of Langer have been crossed. Mondor's disease (a phlebitis of the thoracoepigastric vein) may be related to a history of breast surgery, trauma, or radiation (7). Subclinical operable cancer may present with noncyclic breast pain of recent onset. It is rare, however, that pain is the only presenting symptom in malignancy; just 7% of women with breast cancer presented with pain as their only symptom in a study of 240 women over a 4-year period (3) Costochondritis (Tietze's syndrome) reportedly accounts for approximately 7% of noncyclic mastalgia patients (8). Note: If pain accompanies nipple discharge or a palpable mass, the management should be as outlined in those sections of this chapter.

Clinical Evaluation

A thorough history will help you classify the mastalgia as cyclic or noncyclic. The physical examination is also important in determining the appropriate management strategy for your patient. Several causes of noncyclic breast pain can be differentiated by physical examination. Although no single history or examination component will determine if cancer is present, a finding

331

Table 20.1.
Differential Diagnoses in Patients with Breast Pain

Diagnosis	Frequency	Specific Features
Cyclic	Common (67%)	Age < 40, bilateral, related to menstrual cycle
Noncyclic	Somewhat common (33%)	Age > 40, unilateral, unrelated to menstrual cycle
Cancer	Rare	Constant position, persistent
Costochondritis	Rare	Costochondral junction tenderness
Other musculoskeletal	Uncommon	Reproduction of pain with palpation
Trauma	Rare	History of trauma or previous surgery
Duct ectasia	Rare	Subareolar pain; discharge may be present
Cervical radiculopathy	Rare	Arm and neck pain present

of noncyclic pain that is recent in onset in a postmenopausal women should raise concern. Of course, if a dominant mass accompanies the mastalgia, cancer must be strongly considered. Key elements of the history and physical examination are summarized in Table 20.2.

History

Cyclic mastalgia is typically most severe premenstrually and subsides during the menses. It is usually described as bilateral, in the upper outer breast quadrants, and is often associated with nodularity. Women often characterize the pain as dull, aching, heavy, or sore. The range of severity can be from mild to severe enough to limit clothing selections, sleep positions, or hugging. Patients should therefore be questioned regarding the affect on their lives. Obtain a history of current hormone replacement or oral contraceptive therapy, and previous history of breast problems or surgery. You should also ask about a family history of breast problems, including cancer.

Women with noncyclic mastalgia are more likely to describe their pain as unilateral, with no temporal relationship to their menstrual cycle. It may be constant or remitting, but the periods without pain are not related to the menses. The pain is often described as sharp, burning, or drawing and is more commonly located in the subareolar or medial portion of the breast. Non-breast causes may result in symptoms such as radiation to the arm or axilla or pain with deep inspiration. As with cyclic mastalgia, patients should be questioned regarding previous breast problems or surgery and any family history of breast problems or cancer.

Physical Examination

The clinical breast examination (CBE) should include both inspection and palpation. Inspection of the breasts should be directed at searching for evidence of trauma or old surgical scar; both are related to noncyclic mastalgia. Whether the history is consistent with cyclic or noncyclic mastalgia, you should thoroughly palpate the breasts. Nodularity is common with both complaints, but if a dominant mass is found, the appropriate management protocol should be followed to rule out malignancy. Pain reproduced by palpation of the costochondral junction or the lateral chest wall suggests a musculoskeletal etiology such as

Table 20.2.
Key Elements of the History and Physical Examination for Breast Pain

Question/Maneuver	Purpose
Age, position of pain, laterality, character of pain, relation of pain to menstrual cycle	Differentiate between cyclic and noncyclic mastalgia
Evidence of trauma or previous surgery	Indicates noncyclic mastalgia
Reproducible chest wall pain	Indicates costochondritis
Reproduction of pain with neck movements	Indicates cervical radiculopathy
Thorough palpation of breasts	Screen for dominant mass

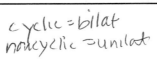

costochondritis. If you suspect that the pain is due to cervical radiculopathy, examine the range of motion of the patient's neck to determine if the pain is exacerbated by specific neck movements.

Laboratory Tests

Laboratory and imaging tests are not necessary unless a dominant mass is found. (See the section on Palpable Mass.)

Management

For the majority (85%) of women with breast pain, whether cyclic or noncyclic, reassurance from the physician that the pain is not due to cancer is sufficient treatment (4). For the remaining women, additional treatment will be needed. Management depends on whether the pain is cyclic or noncyclic. Keeping a pain calendar or diary for several months is often recommended to establish whether the pain is cyclic. The diary should include a rating of the pain (mild, moderate, and severe) along with the patient's menstrual calendar.

Cyclic Pain

NONPHARMACOTHERAPY

Very few clinical trials have been performed in patients with cyclic mastalgia, so objective evidence is lacking regarding the efficacy of most therapies. Therefore, before pharmacologic therapy is initiated, you should consider the following nonpharmacologic interventions. First, the patient should keep a diary of her pain, preferably with a severity scale. A record of the amount of pain on a daily basis for a minimum of a 2-month period may convince the woman that her pain is cyclic in nature and not severe enough to

warrant pharmacologic treatment, especially if that treatment has adverse effects. A second intervention at the initial evaluation is a proper-fitting brassiere. In an English study of 100 patients with breast pain, 75 found relief after being professionally fitted, regardless of their age, cup size, or underlying breast disease (9).

A third intervention that may be helpful, although not of proven benefit, is diet modification. The suggested dietary changes are based on studies of women with breast pain, although many studies were not randomized or placebo controlled. However, the diet modifications recommended have no known adverse side effects and may be prudent changes as a preventive measure for other diseases. The two most common recommendations are to remove methylxanthines (caffeine has been studied the most) and to adopt a very low-fat diet. Vitamin E and B supplements have also been advocated, but there is no evidence of effectiveness in several controlled trials, and high doses of these vitamins may have adverse effects.

PHARMACOTHERAPY

Many medications have been tried in the treatment of cyclic breast pain including oral contraceptives, progesterone, danazol, bromocriptine, thyroid hormones, tamoxifen, evening primrose oil, diuretics, and analgesics. Five medications (see Table 20.3) are known to be beneficial in controlled studies, two of which (bromocriptine and tamoxifen) are not generally recommended because of their adverse effects. The remaining three are oral contraceptives, danazol, and evening primrose oil. It should be kept in mind that some studies have noted a significant placebo effect (up to 20%) (10). There is no evidence to support the use of thyroid hormones, progesterone, diuretics, or analgesics in the treatment of cyclic mastalgia.

Table 20.3.
Medications Used in the Treatment of Cyclic Mastalgia

Medication	Common Dose	Possible Adverse Effects
Evening primrose oil	1 g q 8 hr	Nausea, bloating
Danazol	50–100 mg q 12 hr	Weight gain, menstrual irregularity
Oral contraceptive	1 q day	If weight gain and/or breast pain, shift to a lower estrogen and lower estrogenic progesterones
Bromocriptine	1.25–2.5 mg q hs	Nausea, vomiting, headache
Tamoxifen	10 mg q day	Long-term use associated with endometrial cancer and osteoporosis

Evening primrose oil is thought to exert its effect by normalizing lipid metabolism. In several controlled trials, it has been found to be effective (6). It is also well tolerated, has few adverse effects (nausea and bloating being the most common) (11), and is available over the counter. The usual dose is 3 g/day in three divided doses.

Danazol, a synthetic androgen, is the only drug approved by the U.S. Food and Drug Administration for mastalgia. It is thought to act by inhibiting the midcycle luteinizing hormone (LH) surge and by competitively binding estrogen and progesterone receptors in the breast. Its overall improvement rate is estimated at 70% (5). The starting dosage is 50 mg twice a day, with titration upward as tolerated. The usual maintenance dose is 100 mg twice daily; if there is no improvement in 1 month, the dose can be increased to 200 mg twice daily. If there still is no improvement at 2 months, stop the medication. If there is symptom improvement at 200 mg/day, the dose may be gradually lowered to 100 mg/day. The most common adverse effects are weight gain and menstrual irregularity.

Oral contraceptives have been used effectively, and birth control users, in general, have a decreased incidence of fibrocystic changes and fewer breast biopsies. However, oral contraceptives can also be a cause of breast pain in some patients. Because of their fairly safe side-effect profile, oral contraceptives may be tried as treatment for breast pain and are especially appropriate for patients wanting contraception. They may be used in combination with evening primrose oil.

Bromocriptine, the prolactin inhibitor, has been successfully used in treating cyclic breast pain. The relatively high incidence (20 to 33%) of adverse effects, such as nausea, vomiting, headache, and postural hypotension, has limited its use. In addition, bromocriptine is no longer indicated for use in lactation cessation due to its association with seizures, strokes, and fatalities. Starting doses are 1.25 mg with food at night for the first week, then 2.5 mg at night for 2 months.

Tamoxifen is an estrogen agonist/antagonist that inhibits the effect of estradiol on the breast. In one well-designed crossover study of 60 women, approximately twice as many women taking tamoxifen (71%) had relief of their mastalgia compared to those taking a placebo (38%) (12). However, because of concerns regarding its effect on bone density and possible association with endometrial cancer, it is not recommended for more than short-term use in the treatment of severe mastalgia and is recommended only if all other therapies have failed.

Noncyclic Breast Pain

Noncyclic breast pain is managed by treating the underlying cause. If the pain is found to be musculoskeletal (estimated as up to 90% of unilateral noncyclic cases), analgesics and/or anti-inflammatory drugs are recommended. Local injections of combination steroid and anesthetic have proven beneficial in prospective studies (13). Although evidence is lacking from randomized trials, both evening primrose oil and danazol have helped women with pain that is localized to the breast; danazol may be slightly more effective (5). Figure 20.1 is an algorithm for the diagnosis and treatment of mastalgia.

In general, surgical intervention is not recommended for treatment of mastalgia, except in the case of a dominant mass or mammary duct ectasia (both are addressed later in this chapter). In the past, procedures such as a subcutaneous mastectomy have been attempted as pain treatment, often with the result of a painful scar. Table 20.4. summarizes the treatment options for mastalgia.

NIPPLE DISCHARGE

Nipple discharges, secretions from the breast(s) of a woman who is not lactating, are often categorized as either physiologic or nonphysiologic/pathologic. Physiologic discharges are characterized as nonspontaneous, often bilateral, and arising from multiple ducts, whereas pathologic nipple discharges are typically spontaneous, unilateral, and usually from a single duct.

The majority of nipple discharges are due to benign conditions, but discharge is understandably a cause of concern. The discharge is often discovered upon manipulation of the breast. Once it is discovered, the anxious patient may manipulate the breast and nipple frequently to test if the discharge is still present, which may provoke more discharge. It is difficult to determine how common breast discharge is among women because many may not seek medical advice when they experience it. The prevalence also depends on the examination technique; discharge will be obtained more frequently if the breasts are expressed. In one study of 2,685 women undergoing a routine health examination that included breast compression toward the nipple, nipple discharge was present in 10% (14). Breast secretion may be present in as many as 50 to 70% of

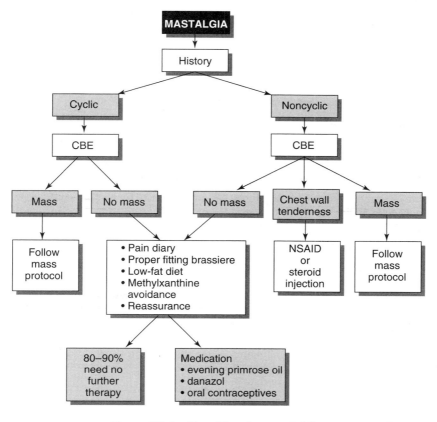

Figure 20.1. *Algorithm for mastalgia.*

Table 20.4.
Treatment Options for Breast Pain

Symptom	Treatment	Level of Evidence for Effectiveness[a]	Comments/Adverse Effects
Cyclic pain	Evening primrose oil	A	Minimal adverse effects of nausea, bloating
	Danazol	A	Significant adverse effects of menstrual irregularities, water retention, acne
	Proper-fitting brassiere	B	No adverse effects
	Bromocriptine	B	Significant adverse effects of nausea, headache, dizziness
	Oral contraceptives	C	Minimal adverse effects
	Methylxanthine withdrawal	C	Minimal adverse effects
	Vitamin supplements	X	Controlled studies indicate not effective
Noncyclic pain localized to breast		B	Trial of above medications starting with danazol, but difficult to treat
Noncyclic pain due to other underlying cause		B	Treat underlying problem

[a]Level of evidence for effectiveness: A, strong or moderate research-based evidence (consistent across several studies, including at least two randomized controlled trials); B, limited research-based evidence (less consistent or extensive evidence, but preponderance of evidence supports use of treatment); C, common practice with little or no research-based evidence; X, moderate or strong evidence suggesting that this treatment is not effective.

women if nipple aspiration by pump expression is performed (5). The significance of the finding of nipple discharge depends on the age, gravidity, parity, and menopausal status of the woman, as well as the characteristics of the discharge itself. Older postmenopausal women (over 60 years) who present with a discharge are approximately three times more likely to have breast cancer than women who are younger (15).

Pathophysiology and Differential Diagnosis

Physiologic breast secretions are typically bilateral, involve multiple ducts, and are not spontaneous. The discharge must be expressed by either gentle massage or by a device such as a breast pump. Galactorrhea, a milky discharge, is the most common physiologic discharge and requires investigation for an endocrine abnormality or a pharmacologic cause. A physiologic discharge more serous in character can result from frequent breast manipulation or medication.

Physiologic discharges are related to hormonal influences on breast tissue; hyperprolactinemia is usually the cause. Even a transient hyperprolactinemia may result in nipple discharge. Increased prolactin levels may be due to a physiologic, pathologic, or pharmaceutical event. Physiologic causes include nipple stimulation, sexual orgasm, sleep, exercise, and food ingestion. Pathologic events associated with increases in prolactin include hypothalamic lesions, pituitary tumors, chest wall trauma, hypothyroidism, renal failure (decreased prolactin clearance), and anovulatory syndromes such as polycystic ovaries. Many medications are associated with hyperprolactinemia, including dopamine-blocking drugs (e.g., phenothiazines, metoclopramide), dopamine-depleting drugs (e.g., reserpine, methyldopa), and drugs that increase prolactin secretion (e.g., opiates, amphetamines, verapamil). Other physiologic peptides that have prolactin-releasing activity include thyroid-releasing hormone (TRH), serotonin, vasoactive intestinal peptide (VIP), and vasopressin.

Pathologic discharges can originate either from the nipple and areola region or from a breast duct. These discharges are typically unilateral; evolve from a single duct; are bloody, serosanguinous, or watery; are either spontaneous or intermittent; and are often associated with a mass. Eczema, nipple adenoma, and Paget's disease can cause erythema and ulcera-

tion of the nipple skin, with an associated bloody discharge. Ductal diseases associated with nipple discharge are duct ectasia, sometimes called periductal mastitis, duct papilloma, and early ductal carcinoma. Duct papilloma and early ductal carcinoma usually involve only a single duct and cause a serosanguinous or sanguinous discharge (5). Duct papilloma is a benign condition of epithelial hyperplasia within the ducts. Papillomas that occur more centrally are usually solitary, benign, and not associated with the development of cancer. Papillomas that occur more peripherally are usually multifocal and have an increased risk for breast cancer. In situ ductal carcinoma is responsible for between 5 and 10% of unilateral nipple discharges (5). Studies of single-duct discharges (16) and pathologic discharges (17) have found similar rates of cancer (9% and 10%, respectively).

Infection and abscess can also lead to a purulent discharge. Mastitis is more common in the puerperium, but can occur after weaning. Finally, fibrocystic changes have also been associated with a nipple discharge (18). Table 20.5 includes the differential diagnosis of nipple discharge.

Clinical Evaluation

History

As Table 20.6 illustrates, important points to cover in the history of a woman presenting with nipple discharge include her age, whether both breasts have secretions, the characteristics of the secretion, recent pregnancy, current medications, menstrual cycle, menopausal status, exercise and sleep habits, sexual activity, and recent surgery or trauma.

Galactorrhea is more common in women of childbearing age and may occur for 1 to 2 years or longer following childbirth. Although both breasts are usually involved, the discharge may be unilateral. Amenorrhea, headaches, visual disturbances, and changes in appetite or temperature regulation should increase suspicion for a pituitary or hypothalamic problems. You should ask about the use of the following medications that can increase prolactin levels:

- Phenothiazines
- Haloperidol
- Metoclopramide
- Reserpine
- α-Methyldopa

Table 20.5.

Differential Diagnosis of Nipple Discharge

Diagnosis	Frequency in Office Primary Care (% Within Physiologic or Pathologic Category)	Typical Presentation
Physiologic		
Idiopathic	Common (40–45%)	Bilateral, milky or watery
Galactorrhea (prolonged lactation)	Somewhat common (25–30%)	Bilateral, milky
Medication	Uncommon (10–15%)	Bilateral, milky or watery
Anovulatory syndromes	Rare (1–2%)	Bilateral, milky or watery, irregular menses
Sella turcica lesions	Rare (1–2%)	Bilateral, milky or watery, irregular menses
Pathologic		
Duct papilloma	Common (40–45%)	Unilateral, serous or bloody
Fibrocyst	Uncommon (15–25%)	Usually unilateral, greenish or serous
Duct ectasia	Uncommon (15–20%)	Usually bilateral, multicolored, sticky
Eczema	Rare	Usually unilateral, bloody, crusting
Paget's disease	Rare	Usually unilateral, bloody, crusting
Early ductal carcinoma	Rare (5–10%)	Unilateral, serous or bloody
Infection/inflammation	Rare (5–10%)	Usually unilateral, purulent

Adapted from Newman HF, Klein M, Northrup JD, Ray BF, Drucker M. Nipple discharge: frequency and pathogenesis in an ambulatory population. NY State J Med 1983;83:928–933; Seltzer MH, Perloff LJ, Kelley RI, Fitts WT. The significance of age in patients with nipple discharge. Surg Gynecol Obstet 1970;131:519–522; Fung A, Rayter Z, Fisher C, King DM, Trott P. Preoperative cytology and mammography in patients with single-duct nipple discharge treated by surgery. Br J Surg 1990;77:1211–1212.

- Verapamil
- H$_2$-receptor antagonists
- Opiates
- Amphetamines
- Cocaine
- Hallucinogens
- Tricyclic antidepressants
- Oral contraceptives

Increased exercise, sleep, feeding (especially high-protein), sexual orgasm, nipple stimulation, and ovulation can affect prolactin secretion, so you should ask about recent changes in these functions or a temporal association between them and the discharge.

Complaints of breast skin changes along with nipple discharge should raise your suspicion for nipple adenoma, Paget's disease, or eczema. A colored (green, yellow, or brown), sticky, non-bloody secretion from both breasts is often due to mammary duct ectasia, a benign disease caused by inflammation and dilatation of a terminal duct that usually occurs in postmenopausal women. A unilateral, serous, watery, bloody, or serosanguinous discharge from one breast, espe-

Table 20.6.

Key Elements of the History and Physical Examination for Nipple Discharge

Question/Maneuver	Purpose
Spontaneous or expressed	Spontaneous is more suspicious of cancer
Bilateral or unilateral	Unilateral is more suspicious of cancer
Characteristics of discharge	Milky suggests galactorrhea
	Serous, bloody, watery increases suspicion for cancer
	Multicolored suggests duct ectasia
Irregular menses in premenopausal woman	Suggests hyperprolactinemia
Medications	May be cause of discharge
Skin changes	May suggest adenoma, eczema, Paget's disease
Recent pregnancy or weaning	Suggests galactorrhea or mastitis
Palpable mass	Increases suspicion for cancer

cially in a postmenopausal woman, is the most concerning presenting complaint.

Physical Examination

A complete clinical breast examination (CBE) is important to determine if there is a palpable mass present, especially in the case of a unilateral discharge. Inspection of the breasts to determine any skin changes, including retraction, should be performed. Each quadrant should be carefully palpated to ascertain if the discharge appears to be confined to a single duct, as in ductal papilloma or carcinoma. Special attention should be paid to the subareolar region to identify the area at which pressure produces the discharge and to palpate for masses.

Laboratory Tests

If the history and physical examination are consistent with galactorrhea, and all physiologic and pharmacologic causes have been excluded, use a prolactin level to rule out hyperprolactinemia. For women who are experiencing amenorrhea or other symptoms indicating pituitary or hypothalamic dysfunction, the prolactin and thyroid-stimulating hormone (TSH) levels should be checked to rule out hyperprolactinemia and hypothyroidism, respectively. Both tests are done by radioimmunoassay (RIA) and are very accurate. The prolactin specimen should be drawn fasting and 2 hours after awakening because both feeding and sleep can increase the level. If both the prolactin and TSH are normal and the patient is having regular cycles, a diagnosis of idiopathic galactorrhea can be made, and no further testing is indicated. If the patient has irregular menses and an elevated prolactin level, either a CT or an MRI of the brain is warranted to look for pituitary tumor. The higher the prolactin level, the greater the chance of pituitary adenoma; levels over 200 ng/mL are highly predictive of a positive finding. In several series, however, normal prolactin levels were found in patients with prolactinomas (19).

Discharges that are more suspicious for cancer (i.e., unilateral, spontaneous, bloody, serosanguinous, or watery) can first be tested with a guaiac card for the presence of blood, although reports are inconsistent as to the predictive value of this test. The percent of cancers whose discharges tested positive for hemoglobin ranges from 53% to 100% in the literature (16, 18, 20). Fluid cytology can also be obtained, although its clinical utility is debatable. Although the sensitivity of cytology is low (false-negative rate up to 35% in patients with carcinoma), the specificity is high (96 to 97%) (16, 21). Thus, it is more useful when positive and does not rule out malignancy when negative (LR+ 6.3, LR− 0.7). If cytology is negative and a bloody nipple discharge persists, an excisional biopsy should be performed. Additionally, cytology cannot differentiate between in situ and invasive cancer.

Surgical duct excision, which is the most specific diagnostic test, has traditionally been the method of choice to evaluate pathologic discharges. Both galactography and mammography have been advocated as noninvasive techniques to evaluate the patient with a suspicious discharge prior to surgery in an effort to decrease the number of surgeries for benign lesions. Galactography, a radiographic procedure that involves injection of a radiopaque into a suspicious duct, is not always helpful in differentiating between a benign and malignant neoplasm. Additionally, the procedure is not always available. The advantage of galactography is better localization of the lesion, which allows a more conservative surgical excision.

Mammography, which is often more readily available than galactography, should be ordered in women whose history and CBE raise suspicion of cancer. However, the sensitivity of mammography for detecting cancer in patients with a nipple discharge varies considerably in the literature, from 13% (16) to 90% (22), whereas the specificity is over 95%. Given the potentially high false-negative rate, perhaps the best use of mammography is to determine if there are other nonpalpable abnormalities present, increasing the suspicion for cancer.

Management

Management is dependent on the type of discharge. If the history, CBE, and discharge indicate galactorrhea, a cause for hyperprolactinemia should be sought, and if found, the necessary steps taken to remedy the hyperprolactinemic state. Such steps may include change of medication or lifestyle or evaluation and referral for pituitary tumor. When all laboratory tests and the menstrual cycle are normal, a diagnosis of idiopathic galactorrhea can be made and reassurance given. If, from the laboratory tests administered, including the imaging study of the brain, the only abnormal result is an elevated prolactin level in a normally menstruating woman, a diagnosis of idiopathic hyperprolactinemia can be made. However, the patient should be followed closely for further increases in the prolactin level and signs or symptoms of pituitary tumor.

In the case of clear or blood-related (serous, serosanguinous, or sanguinous) spontaneous discharges, especially unilateral, a mammogram and/or galactogram (if available) should be ordered. If either is suspicious, surgical excision of the abnormal area is necessary for definitive diagnosis. Cytology can also be ordered, but given the high false-negative rate, prolonged observation should not be based on the results. This is also true of the other noninvasive tests, mammography and galactography. If the discharge persists, the patient should be referred for a surgical evaluation. If a mass is palpable in a woman with a pathologic discharge, she should be managed as below. Figure 20.2 is an algorithm for nipple discharge.

PALPABLE BREAST MASS

Breast cancer is the most common malignancy in women and the second leading cause of cancer death. The majority of cases present as a palpable mass, usually found by the patient. For this reason, most women are frightened upon discovering a breast mass. Among the common presenting breast complaints, breast mass ranks second to breast pain (1). A complaint or finding of breast mass must always be taken seriously. The literature and lay press contain numerous reports of missed diagnoses of breast cancer. Delay in the diagnosis of breast cancer is one of the most common reasons for medical malpractice claims in the United States, and the majority of claimants are premenopausal women (23).

Pathophysiology and Differential Diagnosis

Because breast cancer is the most common cancer in women, palpable abnormalities found on the clinical breast examination should always raise the concern of malignancy. The risk of breast cancer varies considerably with age, and postmenopausal women presenting with a mass are much more likely to have cancer than are premenopausal women. A mass in a woman less than 30 years of age rarely (<2%) represents cancer, whereas a woman of 70 years or older with a mass will have cancer more than 85% of the time (24). Other causes of a breast mass include breast

cyst, fibroadenoma, fibrocystic mass, and duct papilloma. Duct papillomas typically occur in the late menstrual years and are one of the most frequent causes of nipple discharge (see section on Nipple Discharge). Breast cysts and carcinoma tend to occur later in life, whereas fibroadenomas and fibrocystic masses are more common in younger women. In fact, fibroadenoma and fibrocystic masses are the most common causes of a breast mass in women younger than age 25 (25). Table 20.7 shows the differential diagnosis of a breast mass by age groups.

Clinical Evaluation

History

You should obtain a breast cancer risk factor assessment in every woman with a breast mass. The incidence of breast cancer increases with age, with the majority of breast cancer occurring in women over age 50. Family history of breast cancer in a first-degree relative increases the risk about two to three times; if two first-degree relatives have been affected, the risk increases up to sixfold. A diagnosis of breast, ovarian, or endometrial cancer has been associated with an increased risk of subsequent breast cancer. History of pregnancy before age 30 is protective, as is a fewer number of years menstruating (26, 27).

In addition, the patient should be questioned regarding nipple discharge and pain in the affected breast. Nipple discharge may accompany duct papilloma or cancer. If pain is present, you should ask if it coincides with the patient's menstrual cycle, because masses associated with fibrocystic changes are often painful in the premenstrual period.

Physical Examination

The clinical breast examination should include inspection and palpation of both breasts as well as palpation of the axillary and supraclavicular lymph node regions. Skin retraction, dimpling, edema (*peau d'orange*), and bloody nipple discharge should make you suspicious for malignancy. If a mass is found, carefully palpate the opposite breast to determine if a symmetric mass is present. If a mirror-image mass or thickening is found, the risk of cancer is very low.

The typical malignant mass is immobile and rock hard with irregular borders. With this finding on CBE, especially in the presence of enlarged ax-

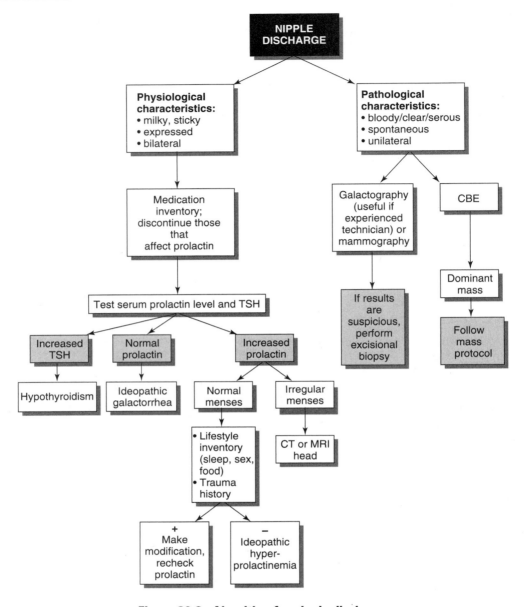

Figure 20.2. *Algorithm for nipple discharge.*

illary nodes, an immediate referral to a surgeon for biopsy would be the most prudent course. However, physical characteristics alone should not dictate the workup of a breast mass. Malignant masses can resemble breast cysts (soft and well-defined) or fibrocystic masses (soft and irregular) on physical examination. Breast cancer is least likely to imitate fibroadenomas in their physical characteristics (smooth and mobile), although any

breast mass deserves further investigation. Table 20.8 lists key elements of the history and physical examination for palpable mass. Table 20.9 outlines "red flags" suggestive of breast cancer.

The test characteristics of palpation for identification of malignant masses have been published based on examinations primarily by surgeons and gynecologists. Overall, the results of physical examination are accurate [(true positive

Table 20.7.
Differential Diagnosis of Breast Mass

Diagnosis	Age Group (years)	Likelihood of Diagnosis (%)	Usual Characteristics of the Mass
Breast cancer	(Common in older women)		Unilateral, hard, and immobile
	<25	<1	
	26–40	5–10	
	41–50	10–20	
	51–70	50–80	
	>70	>80	
Breast cyst	(Somewhat common in perimenopausal women)		Unilateral, soft, and well-defined
	<25	1–4	
	26–40	2–5	
	41–50	10–20	
	51–70	7–12	
	>70	<10	
Fibroadenoma	(Common in young women)		Unilateral, smooth, and mobile
	<25	50–75	
	26–40	15–30	
	41–50	10–20	
	51–70	<5	
	>70	<1	
Fibrocystic changes	(Common in young women)		Bilateral, soft, and irregular; change with cycle
	<25	10–25	
	26–40	30–40	
	41–50	Uncommon	
	51–70	Uncommon[a]	
	>70	Rare	
Duct papilloma		Uncommon for all ages, but most frequent at ages 30–50	Unilateral subareolar mass with discharge

Adapted from Byrne C. Breast. In: Cancer Rates and Risk. Harras A, Edwards BK, Blot WJ, Ries LAG, eds. National Cancer Institute. NIH publication no. 96–691, May, 1996:120–123; Devitt JE. Benign breast disease in the postmenopausal woman. World J Surg 1989;13:731–735; Hindle WH. Other benign breast problems. Clin Obstet Gynecol 1994;37:916–924; Ligon RE, Stevenson DR, Diner W, Westbrook KC, Lang NP. Breast masses in young women. Am J Surg 1980;140:779–782; Ferguson CM, Powell RW. Breast masses in young women. Arch Surg 1989;124:1338–1341.

[a]More frequent in women on hormone replacement therapy

+ true negative)/total patients] in only 60 to 80% of cases (28, 29) (Table 20.10). Additionally, there is often poor agreement among experienced examiners. In one study of four surgeons, there was agreement on the need for biopsy in only 11 of 15

masses that were subsequently found to be malignant (30). If the woman is premenopausal and the mass does not have the typical characteristics of malignancy, a reexamination of the breasts is recommended within the next month, during the

Table 20.8.
Key Elements of the History and Physical Examination for Palpable Mass

Question/Maneuver	Purpose
Age; previous or family history of breast, endometrial, or ovarian cancer; menstrual history	Determine if increased risk of breast cancer
Pain or tenderness	Suggests fibrocystic mass or fibroadenoma
Nipple discharge	Suggests duct papilloma or carcinoma
Mirror image mass in opposite breast	Suggests fibrocystic changes

Table 20.9.
"Red Flags" Suggestive of Breast Cancer

Symptom	Characteristics
Pain	Unilateral, noncyclic
Nipple discharge	Unilateral
	Watery, serous, serosanguinous, bloody
	Single duct
Breast mass	Unilateral
	Hard, immobile
	Noncystic
History	Postmenopausal
	Previous patient history of breast cancer
	Family history of breast cancer

time of least hormonal influence (3 to 10 days after the onset of menses) (25).

Laboratory Tests

The first step in the evaluation of a breast mass, especially in a perimenopausal or older woman, is to determine whether the mass is cystic or solid. Breast cyst aspiration can be performed in the office using a 22-gauge needle and syringe. The location of the mass should be carefully documented in case of a bloody aspirate. In order to rule out intracystic carcinoma (which is rare), you should send all bloody aspirates and any aspirate obtained from a postmenopausal woman not on hormone replacement therapy for cytology.

Alternatively, an ultrasound can also be obtained to determine if the mass is cystic. Aspiration has the advantage of therapeutically draining the cyst and providing a more expedient diagnosis. If the ultrasound demonstrates a cyst, the cyst should still be aspirated and cytology performed as indicated previously. In fact, the role of ultrasound in the diagnosis of breast cancer is primarily to characterize nonpalpable masses found on screening mammography (31). It has much less of a role in cases of palpable masses.

Mammography is obtained to evaluate for clinically occult malignancies, not to characterize the mass. It is not recommended in women less than 25 to 30 years of age or in pregnant women unless malignancy is strongly suspected, because the increased density of the breast tissue in these women renders the mammogram difficult to interpret. In addition, the breast is more radiosensitive in younger women, with a resulting theoretically increased risk of cancer from mammograms. A negative mammogram should not be interpreted as reassuring in the presence of a breast mass. An interval of 2 weeks between a mammogram following cyst aspiration is recommended, as aspiration can sometimes result in hematoma formation, which could confuse mammographic interpretation. The test characteristics for mam-

Table 20.10.
Characteristics of Diagnostic Tests Used to Identify Malignancy in a Woman with a Breast Mass

Test	Sensitivity	Specificity	LR+	LR−
Clinical breast examination (CBE)	0.92	0.65	2.6	0.12
Mammography	0.89	0.65[a]	2.5	0.17
Fine-needle aspiration (FNA)	0.83[b]	0.90[c]	27	0.17
Ultrasound	0.78	0.89	7.1	0.25
CBE + FNA + mammography (one or more individual tests positive is a positive "triple test;" all tests negative is a negative "triple test")	>0.99	0.98	50	0.02

Adapted from van Dam PA, Van Goethem MLA, Kersschot E, Vervliet J, Van den Veyver IBM, De Schepper A, Buytaert P. Palpable solid breast masses: retrospective single- and multimodality evaluation of 201 lesions. Radiology 1988;166:435–439; Wolberg WH, Tanner MA, Loh WY. Fine-needle aspiration for breast mass diagnosis. Arch Surg 1989;124:814–818; Kaufman Z, Shpitz B, Shapiro M, Rona R, Lew S, Dinbar A. Triple approach in the diagnosis of dominant breast masses: combined physical examination, mammography, and fine-needle aspiration. J Surg Oncol 1994;56(4):254–257; Hammond S, Keyhani-Rofagha S, O'Toole RV. Statistical analysis of fine-needle aspiration cytology of the breast. A review of 678 cases plus 4,265 cases from the literature. Acta Cytol 1987;31:276–280; Butler JA, Vargas HI, Worthen N, Wilson SE. Accuracy of combined clinical-mammographic-cytologic diagnosis of dominant breast masses. Arch Surg 1990;125:893–895.

[a]Range 0.55–0.74.

[b]Range 0.65–0.99.

[c]Range 0.55–0.97, but more recent work suggests a higher specificity.

mography in women with a palpable mass are shown in Table 20.10. Mammography is more likely to err toward a false positive result rather than a missed cancer (false negative).

Fine-needle aspiration (FNA) is recommended as the third component of the triple approach (along with CBE and mammography) in the workup of a breast mass. FNA should be performed by a clinician comfortable with and experienced in the procedure, usually a surgeon. One review (32) found that the sensitivity and specificity of FNA range from 77% to 99% and from 55% to 99%, respectively, although recent publications show improved specificity (see Table 20.10). The ranges are dependent on the experience of the person performing the aspiration and the cytopathologist interpreting the sample. The most common reason for a false-negative reading is an inadequate sample. If the cytopathologist indicates inadequate sample, the procedure must be repeated or an open biopsy performed. Additionally, well-differentiated tumors may lead to false-negative FNA results. If there is any question of atypia, excisional biopsy should be performed. If the results of the FNA show malignancy, treatment options can be discussed with the patient and definitive surgery planned.

Excisional biopsy is the gold standard for diagnosis of a breast mass. However, it has been estimated that if all "lumps" were biopsied, only 20 to 25% would be malignant (33). Because of this fact, the triple approach to a breast mass (as outlined in the following section) has advanced in recent years.

Management

The management recommendations for the evaluation of a breast mass are consistent. A triple approach is recommended that includes CBE, mammography, and fine-needle aspiration (FNA) to minimize both the number of excisional biopsies done for benign disease and the number of missed cancers. In a series of 234 patients who underwent an excisional biopsy in addition to this triple approach, a sensitivity of 100% was demonstrated: all patients who had breast cancer had at least one positive test. Although the specificity for the triad of tests was only 57%, the negative predictive value was 100%: all patients who had negative findings for malignancy in the three tests were found to have benign lesions (34). Figure 20.3 is an algorithm for the management of palpable breast mass.

Prior to the triple approach, if the mass feels cystic, you may perform a needle aspiration in the office. If the needle aspiration reveals clear fluid and the mass disappears after aspiration, the patient can be reassured. You may also want to obtain a mammogram approximately 2 to 4 weeks after aspiration in women over 30 years of age. In all cases, the patient should be rechecked 4 to 6 weeks following the initial aspiration. If the cyst has recurred, mammography and excisional biopsy should be recommended. Intracystic or partially cystic cancers should be suspected if the aspirate is bloody or a residual mass persists directly following aspiration. In those cases, you should recommend mammography and excisional biopsy.

The appropriate number of women who should be referred for biopsy is unknown. In addition to the components of the diagnostic triad, the breast cancer risk factors of the women must also be considered. If any of the components of the diagnostic triad of CBE, mammography, and FNA are suspicious or consistent with malignancy, the mass should be biopsied. If all three are negative, the mass can be closely followed with CBE by the same examiner every 3 months for two visits, then again in 6 months to determine if it is stable. Benign breast masses may spontaneously resolve over time.

SPECIAL CONSIDERATION: THE LACTATING BREAST

One of the most common problems a breast-feeding woman can encounter is mastitis. Mastitis is a cellulitis of the interlobular connective tissue within the mammary gland. The clinical spectrum can range from focal inflammation to systemic flu-like symptoms of fever, chills, and muscle aches. The affected breast will usually exhibit a tender, erythematous, wedge-shaped swelling. Estimates of the incidence of mastitis range from 2.5% to 33% of breast-feeding women; the actual value is probably closer to 10% (35, 36). Most cases occur within the first 2 months postpartum. The infection is bacterial, usually staphylococci; the breast skin and the infant's mouth have been proposed as the source. The key to the management of mastitis is complete emptying of the breast, warm compresses, early antibiotics, and bedrest. The patient should be advised to continue breast-feeding (37, 38); stopping breast-feeding would put her at increased risk of abscess formation. In fact, some experts recommend increased feedings on the af-

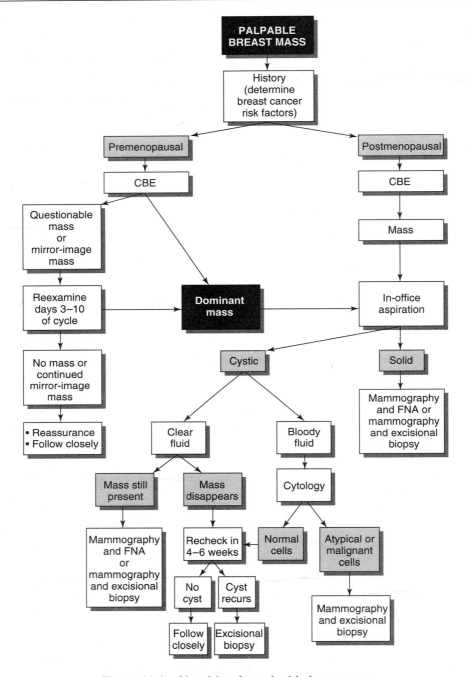

Figure 20.3. *Algorithm for palpable breast mass.*

fected side to minimize stasis. Others recommend starting feedings with the unaffected breast in order to allow the affected breast to "let down," thereby diminishing any pain accompanying feeding. Antibiotic coverage of gram-positive organisms with an agent such as dicloxacillin or erythromycin will usually control the infection and be safe for the infant. The antibiotic should be given for at least 10 days to minimize the chance of relapse.

CASE STUDY 1

Ms. S. is a 39-year-old mother of two who presents to your office complaining of a lump in her right breast, which she first noticed about 1 month ago. She has been checking it almost daily during that time and has not noticed a change in the shape or consistency. She notes that it was not painful when she first discovered it, but more recently it is minimally tender when she palpates her breast. She denies any discharge.

She does not have a family history of any cancer and has herself been very healthy all her life. A previous doctor has told her that she had evidence of fibrocystic changes on her breast examination, and she feels that this mass is most likely related to that previous diagnosis. Ms. S. has never had a mammogram. On examination, a 1-cm mass is palpated in the upper outer quadrant of the right breast. It is firm but somewhat mobile. No enlarged axillary nodes are present. An aspiration is attempted, but no fluid is returned.

QUESTIONS

1. What should you tell Ms. S. regarding the possibility of cancer?
2. What tests should you order next?

DISCUSSION

The incidence of breast cancer in this age group is quite low, and Ms. S does not have any risk factors for breast cancer. The characteristics of the mass are not typical for a malignant mass, but cancer can occur in a mass with these characteristics. In her age group, the diagnoses with the greatest pretest probability are fibrocystic disease and fibroadenoma (Table 20.7). Because you were unable to obtain fluid from the mass, it is probably not cystic, and your examination is more consistent with fibroadenoma. The next step is to order a mammogram and refer the patient to a surgeon who is experienced in fine-needle aspiration (FNA). Mammograms are recommended in this age group; the breast

tissue is not as dense as in women under 30. Ms. S. should be informed that if either FNA or the mammogram is abnormal, she will need an open biopsy.

Both the mammogram and FNA results are reported as benign and consistent with fibroadenoma. Ms. S. should be followed regularly with monthly self-examination and annual CBE and mammography. You should tell her that if she develops pain or the mass increases in size (fibroadenomas can grow so large they distort the appearance of the breast), she may have it surgically removed. The typical natural history of a fibroadenoma is to decrease in size as the woman ages and to calcify after menopause.

CASE STUDY 2

Ms. J. is a 50-year-old woman who presents to your office with a complaint of nipple discharge from her left breast for the past 2 to 3 weeks. She describes the discharge as thin and dark green in color. She first noticed it as a stain in her brassiere, but is able to elicit the discharge by squeezing her breast toward the nipple. She denies any pain and has not felt a mass.

QUESTIONS

1. What should you tell Ms. J. about the possible causes of her discharge?
2. How much of the workup can be done in the office, and what testing should be referred out?

DISCUSSION

Given the patient's description of the discharge, it is most likely a nonphysiologic discharge. You obtain more history from her and find that she is widowed for 2 years, is not sexually active, and has two adult children. Her menstrual cycles are regular, and she is not experiencing menopausal symptoms. On examination, her breasts appear normal with no skin changes. No masses are palpated. By milking the left breast, you are able to elicit a sticky, dark greenish discharge that appears to originate from multiple ducts. Similar maneuvers on the right breast do not elicit any fluid. The discharge tests negative for occult blood.

At this point, you can reassure the patient that her history and the discharge are most consistent with a diagnosis of mammary duct ectasia (periductal mastitis), an inflammatory process within the mammary ducts. You prescribe ibuprofen 600 mg every 4 hours for up to 7 days and advise the patient to use an ice pack for 15 minutes every hour, to avoid nipple manipulation, and to contact you if she is no better in 3 days or if she develops a fever above 101°F. She is sent for a mammogram, which is normal. If her symptoms persist after several weeks, she may need referral for surgical excision of the involved ducts. At that time, a galactogram may be obtained to better identify the inflamed mammary ducts.

REFERENCES

1. Roberts MM, Elton RA, Robinson SE, French K. Consultations for breast disease in general practice and hospital referral patterns. Br J Surg 1987;74:1020–1022.
2. Nichols S, Waters WE, Wheeler MJ. Management of female breast disease by Southampton general practitioners. BMJ 1980;281:1450–1453.
3. Preece PE, Baum M, Mansel RE, Webster DJT, Fortt RW, Gravelle IH, Hughes LE. Importance of mastalgia in operable breast cancer. BMJ 1982;284:1299–1300.
4. BeLieu RM. Mastodynia. Obstet Gynecol Clin North Am 1994;21:261–477.
5. DeVane GW. Breast dysfunction: galactorrhea and mastalgia. In: Blackwell RE, Grotting JC, eds. Diagnosis and Management of Breast Disease. Cambridge, MA: Blackwell Science, 1996:19–76.
6. Klimberg VS. Etiology and management of breast pain. In: Harris JR, Lippman ME, Morrow M, Hellman S, eds. Diseases of the Breast. Philadelphia: Lippincott-Raven, 1996:99–106.
7. Fiorica JV. Special problems: Mondor's disease, macrocysts, trauma, squamous metaplasis, miscellaneous disorders of the nipple. Obstet Gynecol Clin North Am 1994;21:479–485.
8. Wisbey JR, Kumar S, Mansel RE, Peece PE, Pye JK, Hughes LE. Natural history of breast pain. Lancet 1983;2:672–674.
9. Wilson MC, Sillwood RA. Therapeutic value of a supporting brassiere in mastodynia. BMJ 1976;2:90.
10. Pye JK, Mansel RE, Hughes LE. Clinical experience of drug treatments for mastalgia. Lancet 1985;2:373–377.
11. Gately CA, Miers M, Mansel RE, Hughes LE. Drug treatments for mastalgia: 17 years experience in the Cardiff mastalgia clinic. J R Soc Med 1992;85:12–15.
12. Fentiman IS, Caleffi M, Brame K, Chaudary MA, Hayward JL. Double-blind controlled trial of tamoxifen therapy for mastalgia. Lancet 1986;1:287–288.
13. Maddox PR, Harrison BJ, Mansel RE, Hughes LE. Noncyclical mastalgia: an improved classification and treatment. Br J Surg 1989;76:901–904.
14. Newman HF, Klein M, Northrup JD, Ray BF, Drucker M. Nipple discharge: frequency and pathogenesis in an ambulatory population. NY State J Med 1983;83: 928–933.
15. Seltzer MH, Perloff LJ, Kelley RI, Fitts WT. The significance of age in patients with nipple discharge. Surg Gynecol Obstet 1970;131:519–522.
16. Fung A, Rayter Z, Fisher C, King DM, Trott P. Preoperative cytology and mammography in patients with single-duct nipple discharge treated by surgery. Br J Surg 1990;77:1211–1212.
17. Paterok EM, Rosenthal H, Sabel M. Nipple discharge and abnormal galactogram. Results of a long-term study (1964–1990). J Obstet Gynecol Reprod Biol 1993; 50:227–234.
18. Gupta RK, Pant CS, Tandon US, Singh B. Diagnostic value of galactography in patients with nipple discharge. Indian J Cancer 1987;24:22–29.
19. Blackwell RE. Diagnosis and management of prolactinomas. Fertil Steril 1985;43:5–16.
20. Chaudary MA, Millis RR, Davies GC, Hayward JL. Nipple discharge: the diagnostic value of testing for occult blood. Ann Surg 1982;196:651–655.
21. Winchester DP. Nipple discharge. In: Harris JR, Lippman ME, Morrow M, Hellman S, eds. Diseases of the Breast. Philadelphia: Lippincott-Raven, 1996:106–110.
22. Leis HP. Management of nipple discharge. World J Surg 1989;13:736–742.
23. Osuch JR, Bonham VL. The timely diagnosis of breast cancer. Principles of risk management for primary care providers and surgeons. Cancer 1994;74:271–278.
24. Donegan WL. Diagnosis. In: Donegan WL, Spratt JS Jr, eds. Cancer of the Breast, 3rd ed. Philadelphia: WB Saunders, 1988:125–166.
25. Osuch JR. Abnormalities on physical examination. In: Harris JR, Lippman ME, Morrow M, Hellman S, eds. Diseases of the Breast. Philadelphia: Lippincott-Raven, 1996:110–114.
26. Byrne C. Breast. In: Harras A, Edwards BK, Blot WJ, Ries LAG, eds. Cancer Rates and Risk. National Cancer Institute. NIH publication no. 96–691, May, 1996:120–123.
27. Bradley AL, Sharp KW. Office gynecology: breast disease. Med Clin North Am 1995;79:1443–1455.
28. van Dam PA, Van Goethem MLA, Kersschot E, Vervliet J, Van den Veyver IBM, De Schepper A, Buytaert P. Palpable solid breast masses: retrospective single- and multimodality evaluation of 201 lesions. Radiology 1988;166:435–439.

29. Donegan WL. Evaluation of a palpable breast mass. N Engl J Med 1992;327–942.

30. Boyd NF, Sutherland HJ, Fish EB, Hiraki GY, Lickley HLA, Maurer VE. Prospective evaluation of physical examination of the breast. Am J Surg 1981;142:331–334.

31. Sickles EA. Imaging techniques other than mammography for the detection and diagnosis of breast cancer. Recent Results Cancer Res 1990;119:127–135.

32. Wolberg WH, Tanner MA, Loh WY. Fine-needle aspiration for breast mass diagnosis. Arch Surg 1989;124: 814–818.

33. Muskowitz M. Predictive value, sensitivity, and specificity in breast cancer screening. Radiology 1988;167: 576–578.

34. Kaufman Z, Shpitz B, Shapiro M, Rona R, Lew S, Dinbar A. Triple approach in the diagnosis of dominant breast masses: combined physical examination, mammography, and fine-needle aspiration. J Surg Oncol 1994;56(4):254–257.

35. Foxman B, Schwartz K. Looman SJ. Breastfeeding practices and lactation mastitis. Soc Sci Med 1994;38:755–761.

36. Fulton AA. Incidence of puerperal and lactational mastitis in an industrial town of some 43,000 inhabitants. BMJ 1945;1:693–696.

37. Lawrence R. Mastitis. In: Breastfeeding: A Guide for the Medical Profession, 4th ed. St. Louis: CV Mosby, 1994;260–265.

38. Marshall BR, Hepper JK, Zirbel CC. Sporadic puerperal mastitis: an infection that need not interrupt lactation. JAMA 1975;233:1377–1379.

21. Chest Pain

LEE A. GREEN

Key Clinical Questions

1. Is it acute cardiac ischemia?
2. Is it panic disorder?
3. Is it gastroesophageal reflux?
4. Is it a life-threatening disease?

Chest pain is one of the most common problems with which patients present to their family physician. It is also one of the most challenging; the differential diagnosis covers the entire spectrum of family medicine, from acute life-threatening conditions to somatoform sensations and worries.

The possibility of acute cardiac ischemia (ACI), a term that encompasses myocardial infarction (MI) and unstable angina, overshadows the evaluation of chest pain. Patient worries, as well as most clinical writing and research work related to chest pain, focus on ACI and coronary artery disease (CAD) because of their life-threatening nature. However, much in the chest besides the heart can hurt, and the origin of chest pain is by no means limited to structures in the chest. Heart disease is actually one of the less common causes of chest pain in the primary care setting.

In particular, both panic attack and gastroesophageal reflux can closely mimic ischemic heart disease, and both are more common than ACI. Untreated reflux can progress to Barrett's esophagus and ultimately malignancy or perforation in rare cases. Untreated panic disorder can be exceptionally disabling. Any noncardiac cause of chest pain not correctly diagnosed can cause iatrogenic harm by subjecting the patient to ill-advised, and often repeated, invasive cardiac workups.

The general approach to the patient with chest pain is rapid assessment of the likelihood of ACI, with immediate treatment if that likelihood is significant, or careful and judicious evaluation for other causes if it is not. In the case of noncardiac chest pain, thorough evaluation using the biopsychosocial model will allow most patients to be diagnosed and helped. However, the designation "noncardiac chest pain" is not an adequate stopping point for the family physician's evaluation.

PATHOPHYSIOLOGY

Pain in the chest may emanate from the heart, great vessels, lungs, pleura, ribs, shoulders, muscles, esophagus, or proximal stomach. Some patients will perceive pain in almost any of the upper abdominal structures (particularly the spleen) as chest pain. Pain may also be perceived in the chest as part of systemic processes such as panic attacks. In addition, "chest pain" might also be applied to an inflamed cyst in the skin of the thorax, breast pain, or contusions from trauma. However, these causes of pain are clinically quite distinct and not what the doctor or patient typically mean by the term chest pain; we will not consider them here.

Acute Cardiac Ischemia

The pain of ACI reflects hypoperfusion and consequent lack of oxygenation of the myocardium. Most often this results from acute occlusion of a coronary artery. The currently dominant theoretic model involves the rupture of an atherosclerotic plaque. Thrombus forms on the ruptured surface, occluding the artery and producing ischemia in the area of myocardium supplied by the artery (if collateral circulation is not adequate). Alternatively, thrombus may form on the rough surface of an unrupted plaque.

The afflicted myocardium progresses through a well-defined series of ischemic changes. If perfusion is not restored within 3 to 6 hours, loss of cell integrity as evidenced by leaking of cardiac troponins, myoglobin, and later creatine kinase occurs. Cell death in the affected area is the final stage, at which point ACI becomes infarction.

The term "unstable angina" does not correspond directly to a pathophysiologic process. It includes rest pain for 20 minutes or more which is likely to be thrombotic in origin and represent ACI. However, unstable angina also includes new onset, effort-dependent angina,

349

and a recent (within 2 months) clinically significant increase of chronic angina (1). Such "accelerations" of angina may represent rupture or other acute changes in plaques or formation of thrombus not fully occluding an artery; alternatively, they may represent simple progression of atheroma. Although it is generally not possible to differentiate between these mechanisms, they have very different prognostic implications for the patient.

The mortality of unstable angina in the form of rest pain or ACI is substantial and not greatly less than that of infarction (2, 3). The distinction between the two major forms of ACI, unstable angina and myocardial infarction, can often be made only in retrospect. Clinically, the distinction is not immediately important; appropriate and swiftly initiated treatment for ACI is. Variant angina, also known as vasospastic or Prinzmetal's angina, is the diagnosis commonly considered when chest pain is evaluated and coronary arteries are found to be without stenosis. In the case of variant angina, ischemic pain is produced by smooth muscle spasm narrowing the artery acutely, rather than by thrombotic occlusion. Despite the frequency with which it is considered, careful study demonstrates that very few chest pain patients without coronary occlusions actually have coronary vasospasm (4).

Stable Angina

Stable angina, also known as chronic effort-dependent angina, is a supply-demand imbalance between myocardial oxygen needs and delivery. Coronary arteries narrowed by atheroma, or capillaries compromised by left ventricular hypertrophy, allow sufficient blood flow for normal function of the myocardium at low levels of activity. This condition is often called coronary artery disease, or CAD. When the myocardium demands additional oxygen during physical activity, perfusion cannot increase commensurately, and the afflicted region becomes ischemic. Energy metabolism in the cardiac muscle cell becomes impaired, producing the characteristic electrical changes on electrocardiogram (ECG) (ischemic muscle conducts electricity differently) and wall motion abnormalities on echocardiography (ischemic muscle does not contract normally). Provocation of these changes using exercise or medications such as dipyridamole is the basis for noninvasive exercise testing for coronary artery disease.

Panic Disorder

The cause of the chest pain experienced in a panic attack is not known. The causes of panic attacks also are unknown and remain a subject of active controversy and research (5). The debate is between the theory of a primary psychologic cause with secondary physical response and a primary physiologic or autonomic cause with secondary psychologic interpretation as fear. Panic attacks may occur in isolation, as part of panic disorder, or as part of other anxiety disorders. Even in referral-biased populations, panic disorder is present in more than 30% of chest pain patients and may coexist with CAD (6).

Gastroesophageal Reflux Disease and Esophageal Spasm

Reflux of gastric acid contents into the distal esophagus is a commonplace phenomenon. The acid is a direct irritant to the mucosa, causing inflammatory infiltrates and sloughing of epithelium. Additional pain can be produced by smooth muscle spasm in reaction to this irritation. When a patient has reflux occurring severely and frequently enough, it becomes designated gastroesophageal reflux disease (GERD). Perhaps 10% of the adult population experiences this degree of symptoms, although less than 1% seek medical attention for it (7, 8). Reflux can be exacerbated by agents that relax the lower esophageal sphincter, most notably caffeine. Adrenergic agonists such as decongestants may also worsen reflux, as may theophylline. *Helicobacter pylori* infection, a cause of peptic ulcer disease, is not involved in GERD.

Musculoskeletal Pain

Although often attributed to inflammation of the costal cartilage or costochondral joints or to the intercostal muscles, the actual mechanism of musculoskeletal chest pain remains unknown. Musculoskeletal chest pains are prevalent in the community, and most people who have them do not present for medical evaluation.

Mitral Valve Prolapse

Mitral valve prolapse (MVP) is often given as a cause of chest pain among young people (especially young women) on the basis of retrospective findings of MVP in patients with noncardiac pain. MVP, however, is common in the general population, too. Prospective studies fail to demonstrate MVP to be more common among chest pain patients, and there is evidence that reflux may be the actual cause of most pain attributed to MVP (9).

Pleural and Pulmonary Pain

Pulmonary embolism may produce pain, usually pleuritic in nature. The clinical manifestations of pulmonary embolism are notoriously variable and entirely absent in at least half of cases. Shortness of breath and tachypnea are the most frequent manifestations. Pleuritic pain can also be produced by inflammation from an infectious process or by neoplasm. Spontaneous pneumothorax is uncommon and is associated with vigorous exercise, primarily (by a ratio of 5:1) in males in their twenties.

Rare Causes

Chest pain can also result from dissection of the thoracic aorta (almost exclusively found among hypertensive patients; Marfan's syndrome and syphilis are very rare causes); vertebral or rib metastases from any of several different malignancies; enlarged mediastinal nodes owing to lymphoma; sarcoidosis; and collagen-vascular diseases.

DIFFERENTIAL DIAGNOSIS

The clinical epidemiology of chest pain in family practice involves four entities: ischemic heart disease, panic, reflux, and musculoskeletal pain. Musculoskeletal pain is the most common, followed by reflux and panic. Heart disease is the most life-threatening, although panic causes substantial morbidity, which is often inadequately recognized.

Perhaps nowhere in medicine is the clinical epidemiology of a problem as varied, or as important in diagnosis, as in the case of chest pain. The prior probabilities of the various causes differ sharply across the clinical settings in which chest pain is commonly encountered. Research and teaching regarding chest pain have traditionally centered on emergency departments (ED) and referral centers, where the prevalence of serious pathology is high. For example, acute chest pain in emergency departments represents acute cardiac ischemia in one-quarter to one-third of cases (10). However, the prior probability of

acute ischemia in the primary care office setting is only 1.5% (11), and decisions appropriate in the ED may not be valid in the office.

Table 21.1 presents the final diagnoses of cases of chest pain from a network of family physicians' offices (11). Gastroesophageal reflux alone accounts for at least 13% of all patients. Most of the psychosocial category, and likely many of the nonspecific cases as well, represent panic attacks, either isolated or in the setting of panic disorder. Pulmonary causes were pleuritic for the most part. Causes such as aortic dissection and pneumothorax are very rare in family practice, not being observed at all in the 399 cases used to construct Table 21.1. By contrast, typically about 30% of patients seen in the emergency department with chest pain will have heart disease, and 15% or more will actually suffer MI (10).

Acute chest pain that is present while the patient is being seen or occurring just prior to being seen, and chronic or recurrent pain, in which the patient comes for a scheduled appointment to be evaluated, are very different clinical problems and must be approached with a different diagnostic mindset. Unfortunately, although good diagnostic research has been done on the detection of ACI, few objective data are available regarding the predictive values or key differentiating cues for nonacute pain.

In the case of acute chest pain, although GERD is a more common cause than either ACI or panic, the latter two threaten more adverse outcomes. The rapid detection of ACI is the first overriding

Table 21.1.
***Differential Diagnosis in Patients
with Chest Pain***

Diagnostic Category	% of Episodes in Family Practice Settings
Musculoskeletal	36
Gastrointestinal	19
Nonspecific chest pain	16
Stable angina	11
Psychosocial	7
Pulmonary	5
Nonischemic cardiac	4
Acute cardiac ischemia	2

Reprinted with permission from Klinkman MS, Stevens D, Gorenflo DW. Episodes of care for chest pain. J Fam Pract 1994;38: 344–352.

concern. Hence, the evaluation of acute chest pain is divided into two phases: rapid assessment for ACI, and complete evaluation. Initiation of treatment may follow the rapid assessment but precede complete evaluation. In the acute setting the physician must also bear in mind uncommon but dangerous causes such as aortic dissection and potential red herrings such as pericarditis.

In the nonacute situation, CAD (without the threat of immediate MI) must be detected if present, but GERD, panic, and musculoskeletal causes are more prominent. The evaluation of nonacute chest pain is not divided into rapid assessment and complete evaluation phases; thorough evaluation typically precedes initiation of therapy. For both acute and nonacute cases of chest pain, intelligent evaluation of chest pain is dependent upon a sound understanding of prior probabilities and how findings on history and examination modify them.

CLINICAL EVALUATION

Because the causes of chest pain are varied, evaluation involves a complete medical history and physical examination, which are time-consuming. Thrombolysis or acute revascularization can improve outcomes for properly selected patients, but only if those patients are identified quickly. Hence, the evaluation of the chest pain patient proceeds in two steps: (a) rapid evaluation using a few key predictors of ACI, followed by immediate initiation of treatment if indicated (ideally within 10 to 20 minutes of initial presentation); and (b) a complete evaluation once ACI has either been excluded or treated. Starting treatment for ACI should never be delayed while the complete evaluation phase is being done, unless serious doubt of the presence of ACI exists and information from the complete evaluation is crucial to resolving it.

Traditionally, physicians have relied on many history, examination, and laboratory clues in assessing patients for ACI; however, decision-making tools have identified a small set of factors that are of genuine predictive utility for ACI in a primary care setting (10, 12). Although published data do not include individual likelihood ratios for these findings, their weights in regression models do allow estimates for which findings are the most important. Table 21.2 presents these validated diagnostic cues in approximate order of importance for both rapid and detailed evaluation. Table 21.3 shows the acute cardiac ischemia, time-insensitive predictive instrument (ACI-TIPI),

Table 21.2.

Key Elements of the History and Physical Examination of the Patient with Chest Pain

Rapid evaluation for potential acute cardiac ischemia
History
  Character of pain
  Prior history of coronary artery disease
ECG findings (in descending order of importance)
  ST segment elevation or depression of ≥1 mm in at least two leads
  Q waves in at least two leads, not including aV$_R$, not known to be old
  T wave hyperacuity or inversion in at least two leads, not including aV$_R$
  New bundle-branch block

Complete evaluation
History
  Anxiety symptoms (choking feeling, fear, lightheadedness, paresthesias)
  Nighttime symptoms
  Previous episodes; age at onset
  Tachycardia
  Acid regurgitation, heartburn
  Relationship to activity
  Relationship to respiration
  Cardiac risk factors (hypertension, diabetes, smoking, family history, hyperlipidemia)
  Claudication
  Use of cocaine
Physical examination
  Blood pressure
  Heart murmurs
  Third, fourth heart sounds
  Stigmata of vascular disease (bruits, diminished pulses, arterial changes or A-V nicking on retinal examination, skin changes or ulceration of lower extremities)
  Earlobe creases
  Xanthelasma
  Edema
  Obesity

a well-validated clinical prediction rule for estimating the likelihood of ACI in patients with chest pain in the emergency department. The ACI-TIPI can be used in primary care settings, although its positive predictive value is lower owing to the lower incidence of MI.

History

Rapid Evaluation

ACI pain is dull, aching, pressing, squeezing, or heavy and steady. It is rarely burning. Pain or pressure may be located in the chest with radia-

Table 21.3.
The Acute Cardiac Ischemia Time-Insensitive Predictive Instrument (ACI-TIPI)[a]

The ACI-TIPI can be used to estimate the probability of ACI for the patients in the emergency department. The probability of ACI (%) is equal to

$$\text{Factor} = \exp(-3.933 + b_1x_1 + b_2x_2 + b_3x_3 + \ldots)$$
$$\text{Risk of ACI (\%)} = 100 \times [1 - 1/(1 + \text{Factor})]$$

This formula is more readily managed by programming into a handheld calculator or spreadsheet. The factors x_i with their weights b_i are shown below (ECG findings must be present in at least two leads; not due to block, LVH, or pacer; and T inversion in aV_R is excluded):

Variable	Weight (b_i)	Value (x_i)
Chest or left arm pressure or pain present	1.231	1
Not present		0
Chest or left arm pain is chief complaint	0.882	1
Not chief complaint		0
Male	0.712	1
Female		0
Age < 40 yr	−1.441	1
Age > 40 yr		0
Age > 50 yr	0.667	1
Age < 50 yr		0
Male patient, age > 50 yr	−0.426	1
Otherwise		0
ECG Q waves > 1 mm	0.616	1
Otherwise		0
ST segment elevated 2 mm or more	1.314	2
Elevated 1–2 mm		1
Otherwise		0
ST segment depressed 2 mm or more	0.993	2
Depressed 1–2 mm		1
Depressed 0.5–1 mm		0.5
Otherwise		0
T waves hyperacute (>50% QRS deviation)	1.095	1
Otherwise		0
T waves inverted 5 mm or more	1.127	2
Inverted 1–5 mm		1
T waves flat		0.5
Otherwise		0
Both STDEP and TWINV, not 0	−0.314	1
Otherwise		0

[a]Adapted from Braunwald E, Mark DB, Jones RH, et al. Unstable Angina: Clinical Practice Guideline no. 10. Washington, DC: Agency for Health Care Policy and Research, 1994.

tion elsewhere, or it may be located entirely outside the chest in the upper epigastrium, shoulder, upper arm, or neck. Pain is usually severe, but some patients present their discomfort as pressure or heaviness rather than pain. Asking only about "pain" will fail to identify many of these patients. The pain is often accompanied by palpitations, diaphoresis, pallor, dyspnea, and a feeling of impending doom ("angor animi"). Less severe and less persistent pain of the same type, triggered by activity and relieved by rest, is characteristic of chronic stable angina.

Compared to men, women are more likely to report their ischemic cardiac pain in the neck or back (13). Diabetic patients may have little or no pain, and elderly patients often present with shortness of breath rather than chest pain (14). Atypical chest pain (anginal-type pain appearing in patterns other than exertional angina) suggests a lower probability of ACI, but does not rule it out. Such atypical pain may be right-sided or midepigastric. Inferior MI may present with only a profound sense of unease, accompanied by nausea and vomiting. Well-localized sharp or pleuritic pain suggests noncardiac causes. Similarly, very brief pains lasting a few seconds each or pain present continuously for days are unlikely to represent ACI.

Not all heart pain is ischemic: pericarditis should be considered as well. A pattern of diffuse ST changes across the precordium, pain that is worse when recumbent and decreases with sitting or leaning forward, and low-grade fever is typical. Diagnosis may be difficult at first, only confirmed once enzymes have excluded MI while extensive ECG changes persist. A tearing or cutting pain, perhaps felt posteriorly in the chest, is felt to be associated with aortic dissection.

A history of established coronary artery disease is influential in decision making, but not always easily elicited. Ask the patient about a history of prior MI, abnormal noninvasive tests, and the results of previous catheterizations. Some patients may present only a history of nitroglycerin use for pain relief. The likelihood of ACI increases with age for both men and women, although it is not a powerful predictor. Premenopausal women can be regarded as having roughly the same risk as a man with the same history and examination findings but 10 years younger. Postmenopausally, women's risks converge over time to become similar to men's among the elderly.

In the acute setting, epidemiologic risk factors such as smoking, family history, hyperlipidemias, diabetes, and hypertension are good predictors of long-term risk of developing CAD; however they are minimally (for men) to not at all (for women) useful in discriminating between ACI and non-cardiac chest pain (15, 16). These traditional risk factors are important to assess when counseling patients both in primary prevention and after the diagnosis of CAD is established, but they should not color the evaluation of a patient who has chest pain acutely.

The chest pain of a panic attack mimics ACI. This mimicry is heightened by the other typical symptoms of panic attack, which include fear of imminent death, a choking feeling, shortness of breath, palpitations, sweating, and lightheadedness. The patient may also tremble and feel nauseated, symptoms often found in ACI as well. Paresthesias are sometimes part of panic attacks, but are uncommon with ACI. Fear of going crazy, derealization (feelings of unreality) and depersonalization (feelings of being outside of or detached from oneself) are not found in ACI in general, but may occur with panic attack. Sometimes panic attacks occur without subjective feelings of fear at all, and patients may not identify them as panic. Panic attacks may occur at any age; they usually begin in the patient's teens or twenties. Age of onset of symptoms makes a useful differential point; ACI is rare before age 35 in men or 45 in women, and uncommon until 10 years later than that.

Chest pain is also a common feature of somatization disorders. Onset at a young age, associated depression, and a medical record revealing multiple somatoform complaints across organ systems (and often multiple abdominal or pelvic surgeries) should prompt investigation for somatization.

The pain of GERD is classic "heartburn," a midepigastric to lower-thoracic burning pain that can be quite severe. It tends to occur after meals or when supine rather than with exertion, and it may be accompanied by acid regurgitation (17). When accompanied by severe, prolonged spasm of the esophageal smooth muscle ("nutcracker esophagus"), it can cause diaphoresis, pallor, and a sensation of squeezing or tightness, producing a clinical picture closely resembling angina pectoris. Esophageal spasm can be partially relieved by nitroglycerin, furthering its mimicry of ACI. Relief with antacids also suggests GERD, although its absence does not exclude the diagnosis.

Musculoskeletal pain can be sharp or dull, whereas ACI is not sharp. Musculoskeletal pain can often be localized with one finger; if this is true, ACI is thought to be very unlikely, although specific test characteristics have not been defined. Movement of the thorax or upper extremities (including breathing movements) can provoke musculoskeletal pain. Pulmonary causes of pain may behave like musculoskeletal pain, but are more often pleuritic (sharp pain worsened by breathing). Tachycardia and tachypnea are "red flags" for pulmonary embolism or pneumonitis. See Table 21.4 for other "red flags."

Complete Evaluation

The history of chest pain is structured around the differentiating points discussed above. The most important is the nature and character of the pain. For example, typical exertional anginal pain has a positive likelihood ratio of over 100 for the presence of coronary stenosis, whereas atypical pain has a positive likelihood ratio of 14 to 15 (18).

The best-studied element of history is that of typical angina as a predictor of coronary artery disease. Figure 21.1 presents the likelihood of CAD for men and women of varying ages and symptom descriptions (18). The positive likelihood ratio for typical anginal symptoms is 115 for men and 120 for women; for atypical angina, the ratios are 14 and 15, respectively. The practical importance of these symptom distinctions is readily apparent in Figure 21.1. "Typical anginal symptoms" (substernal dull, heavy, or squeezing chest pain/pressure appearing with exertion and relieved by rest) are highly predictive of CAD; "atypical angina" (anginal-type pain that occurs without exertion) is

Table 21.4.
"Red Flags" Suggesting Life-Threatening Disease in Patients with Chest Pain

Finding	Diagnosis Suggested
Hypotension, poor tissue perfusion, pulmonary, edema, or oliguria	Decreased cardiac output, possible large anterior myocardial infarction
Tachycardia, tachypnea, hypoxia	Pulmonary embolism
ECG changes, especially ST segment elevation or new LBBB	Myocardial infarction
New systolic mitral murmur	Ruptured papillary muscle
Arrhythmia and/or chest pain in younger patient	Cocaine abuse

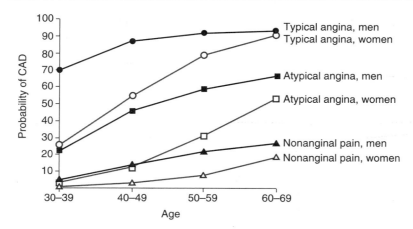

Figure 21.1. *Likelihood of coronary artery disease by patient and symptom characteristics.* Definitions: *typical angina,* substernal dull, heavy, or squeezing chest pain or pressure appearing with exertion and relieved by rest; *atypical angina,* anginal-type pain appearing in patterns other than on exertion; *nonanginal pain (atypical chest pain),* pain whose character is not that of typical angina (e.g., chest wall pain or epigastric burning).

moderately predictive; pain that is nonanginal in character is rarely caused by CAD.

The temporal pattern—whether the pain is constant or intermittent, brief or long-lasting, or associated with particular times of day—may help differentiate causes. Fleeting pains or pain continuously present for days are unlikely to be due to coronary disease, although the latter may be seen in patients with pericarditis. Fleeting pains are common and are thought to be musculoskeletal, although this has not been definitively established. Nighttime pain or pain in the supine position suggests reflux, as does postprandial pain (although this can occur with angina as well).

You should ask the patient about the frequency of recurrence and any changes in frequency (such as acceleration of angina or increasingly frequent panic attacks). If the pain is exertional in nature, you should ask how much exertion is required to bring it on and how much rest is needed to relieve it. Angina that occurs after less-strenuous exertion than before suggests progression of the disease and compels further investigation.

Exacerbating and relieving factors also help differentiate causes. Pain occurring with specific movements suggests musculoskeletal causes, and pain with respiration suggests pulmonary etiologies. Reflux is commonly worse after fatty or large meals and while bending at the waist; it usually is improved with antacids.

Associated symptoms such as paresthesias and palpitations (panic), leg swelling or pain (pulmonary emboli—PE), cough (pulmonary em-

boli), shortness of breath (PE, pneumothorax) and so forth should also be noted. Absence of subjective fear does not exclude panic, as up to a third of patients have the subtype of "nonfear panic disorder" (4). Diminution (though not disappearance) of the pain with sitting up and leaning forward is typical of pericarditis. Regurgitation of acid and even food into the pharynx is highly specific for GERD.

The patient's medical history also includes clues to the differentiation of chest pain. You should ask the patient about hypertension, diabetes, claudication, cerebrovascular disease, and other history suggesting vascular disease. Prior deep venous thrombosis or pulmonary embolism, recent surgery or childbirth, prolonged immobility, or a history of hypercoagulable states (e.g., malignancy, lupus anticoagulant, antithrombin III deficiency, protein C or S deficiency) all suggest pulmonary embolism. A recent viral illness or prodrome suggests either pleuritis or pericarditis. A history of multiple complaints across organ systems should prompt inquiry for primary somatization disorder or somatization as a manifestation of depression.

Coronary risk factor assessment is useful when addressing your patient's long-term risk of developing CAD. These include family history, hyperlipidemia, and smoking in addition to the medical history described above. Cocaine abuse should also be noted, because it can cause cardiac death in young patients. Caffeine intake predisposes to GERD, but does not increase the risk of CAD.

Physical Examination

Rapid Evaluation

The most important part of the physical examination is the patient's overall appearance. If the pain is present at the time of examination, is the patient simply describing a pain which is annoying, or is he or she pale and sweaty? Patients with ACI may press at their precordium, although this may be observed in panic and reflux as well.

The examination of the rapid evaluation phase should be brief, directed specifically toward the "red flags" of immediate danger (see Table 21.4). Test characteristics for these findings are generally not defined. However, the findings of sudden or "flash" pulmonary edema, a new mitral regurgitant murmur, hypoxia, bradycardia, hypotension, or a new S3 are ominous.

Complete Evaluation

The patient's vital signs, especially any changes in them during observation, should be noted. Sinus tachycardia in particular is characteristic of panic and pulmonary embolism (the latter especially when accompanied by tachypnea). Hypertension can occur as a result of acute pain, but stigmata of chronic hypertensive target organ damage (e.g., in the retinal vessels) should be noted. Such patients are at risk for aortic dissection.

Palpate pulses in all four extremities, and listen for bruits over the carotids, abdominal aorta, and renal vessels. Reduction or absence of pedal pulses or an audible bruit suggests vascular disease. The sensitivity and specificity of these findings is unknown, but sensitivity is probably poor and specificity is probably good, making the finding more useful when present (absence in no way rules out disease). An exception is young patients with scaphoid abdomens, many of whom have bruits on auscultation, although essentially all have normal vessels. Reduction or disappearance (perhaps intermittent) of the brachial and carotid pulses is associated with aortic dissection, as is inequality of blood pressure in the two arms in patients with chest pain.

Cardiac auscultation is ordinarily normal or nonspecific in the chest pain patient. Although a mitral click might be found, it is probably not causally associated with chest pain (9). A new murmur, while uncommon, is a "red flag" for adverse outcome, and a rub may aid in the diagnosis of pericarditis. Pulmonary auscultation is typically normal as well, but rubs, rales, and consoli-

dation should be sought. Percussion of the chest can reveal the rare spontaneous pneumothorax.

Earlobes should be examined for creases in the patient suspected of CAD. Although not a sensitive finding, and of unknown mechanism, they are very specific (70 to 90%) (19, 20) for coronary artery disease. Even in low-prevalence primary care populations, up to 50% of chest pain patients with such a crease will have CAD.

Laboratory Testing

Rapid Evaluation

The sole laboratory investigation in the rapid evaluation phase is a twelve-lead electrocardiogram (ECG). If there is no reason to doubt an ACI diagnosis, initiation of therapy should not be delayed while awaiting radiographs or other testing. An ECG should be performed on any patient in whom ACI is suspected, and should be completed and read within minutes of the patient's arrival.

Three features of the ECG are established predictors of ACI (Table 21.5). Of these, ST segment changes (or new left bundle-branch block [LBBB]), either ≥ 0.5-mm elevation or ≥ 1-mm depression in at least two leads is the most important. T wave hyperacuity (at least 50% of QRS amplitude) or inversion, again in at least two leads (excluding aV_R, in which the T wave is normally inverted) is second. Q waves of ≥ 1 mm in at least two leads is third. ST segment elevation during chest pain is 91% specific for acute MI (LR+ 5.1, LR− 0.59) (21). ST segment depression is associated with ischemia but less specifically with infarction.

Complete Evaluation

Chest radiographs will reveal widening of the mediastinum in half of the patients with aortic dissection (22). Other useful findings include consolidation in patients with pneumonia; the boot-shaped shadow of a fluid-filled pericardium; a tumor producing pleural irritation; a pneumothorax; or rarely the wedge-shaped shadows of pulmonary infarcts from emboli. Although unnecessary in pain that is clearly panic or reflux on clinical evaluation, a chest film is probably useful in most other situations. The actual frequency with which it is useful is undefined except in the ICU setting.

The standard laboratory test for confirming MI is the level of creatine kinase (CK) and the percent of CK present as the cardiac-muscle-

Table 21.5.
Characteristics of Diagnostic Tests Useful in Patients with Chest Pain

Test	Sensitivity	Specificity	LR+	LR−
Stress testing for angiographically significant coronary artery obstruction				
Nonsloping ECG ST segment depression[a]				
>2.5 mm	0.20	0.99	39	<0.81
2–2.5 mm	0.33	0.99	11	0.68
1.5–1.99 mm	0.42	0.98	4.2	0.59
1–1.49 mm	0.65	0.89	2.1	0.39
0.05–0.99 mm	0.86	0.77	0.9	0.18
Reversible perfusion defect on thallium scintigraphy[a]	0.71	0.94	11.8	0.31
Reversible wall motion abnormality on stress echocardiography[b]	0.81	0.89	7.4	0.21
Serum markers				
Myoglobin in normal range and not doubling over 2 hr within 6 hr of presentation[c]	0.86	0.95	17	0.147
Rapid (2 hr from symptom onset) bedside cardiac troponin T assay[d]	0.33	0.95	6.3	0.8
CK-MB single test in ED[e]	0.34	0.88	2.8	0.75
Simple CK serial determinations in CCU[e]	0.98	0.67	3.0	0.03

[a]Diamond G, Forrester J. Analysis of probability as an aid in the clinical diagnosis of coronary artery disease. N Engl J Med 1979; 300:1350–1358.

[b]O'Keefe JH. Comparison of stress echocardiography and stress myocardial perfusion scintigraphy for diagnosing coronary artery disease and assessing its severity. Am J Cardiol 1995;75:25D–34D.

[c]Tucker JF, Collins RA, Anderson AJ, et al. Value of serial myoglobin levels in the early diagnosis of patients admitted for acute myocardial infarction. Ann Emerg Med 1994;24:704–708.

[d]Antman EM. Evaluation of a rapid bedside assay for detection of serum cardiac troponin T. JAMA 1995;273:1279–1282.

[e]Sox HC. Common diagnostic tests: use and interpretation. Philadelphia: American College of Physicians, 1990.

specific MB isoenzyme. Cardiac-specific troponin T and troponin I assays are beginning to become available. These assays become positive sooner in the course of MI and persist longer than CK-MB. Normal CK levels without elevation of MB fraction at 24 hours from onset of symptoms essentially excludes MI. However, patients with ST segment elevation who do not elevate their CK-MB may elevate their troponins; these patients have a prognosis for adverse outcome approximately equal to that of those who suffer MI (23).

In the emergency department, elevated myoglobin levels 4 to 6 hours after presentation or levels doubling within 2 hours (and not accounted for by muscle trauma) even if still within the normal range offer a positive predictive value of 60 to 80%. Only 3% of patients in this setting without such findings will have an MI (24). In the primary care office where the prevalence of MI is much lower, positive predictive value may be poor, but the negative predictive value (the likelihood that patients with a normal CK do not have MI) is

virtually 100%. Rapid myoglobin determination, presuming normal CK levels, will "rule out" most patients not suffering MI within 6 hours of presentation, while capturing virtually all patients who will suffer MI. Although there is enthusiasm in some centers for echocardiography or other noninvasive imaging modalities in the acute setting, the value of such studies is not yet established, and they cannot be recommended for general clinical use at this time (25).

Testing for CAD may be done by exercise ECG, exercise echocardiography, or gated blood pool scanning; by any of these, substituting pharmacologic stress for exercise; or with the addition of thallium or 99m-technetium imaging. Graded exercise ECG using the Bruce or equivalent graduated protocols is the test of choice (1). Pharmacologic stress should be reserved for patients whose orthopedic or other conditions preclude adequate levels of exertion. Thallium scintigraphy can reveal areas of ischemic myocardium, and offers some increased specificity. Although widely used, in most cases it adds little to ECG testing for most patients. It is most useful for those whose bundle blocks, paced rhythm, or other artifacts render ECG interpretation problematic. Stress echocardiography reveals areas of wall motion abnormality induced by ischemia and may play a more prominent role in the future. At present, however, its utility is still being defined, and stress ECG remains the primary choice. The likelihood ratios for findings on stress ECG and echocardiogram are presented in Table 21.5.

Five-year mortality prognosis can also be estimated for outpatients from exercise ECG data (26). Angina is scored 0 for none, 1 for angina induced by but not limiting the treadmill test, and 2 for angina that limits the test. The score is (exercise in minutes) − (5 × maximal ST deviation) − (4 × angina score). Patients with scores greater than +5 have a 5-year survival of 99%; those with scores of −10 to +4 have a 95% 5-year survival; and those with scores of −10 or lower confer only a 79% 5-year survival.

Arterial blood gas testing or transcutaneous oxygen saturation measurement may be helpful in the outpatient setting if pulmonary embolism is considered, although test characteristics are not well defined. Suspected dissection of the aorta can be evaluated with angiography, transesophageal echocardiography, helical-scan computerized tomography (CT), or magnetic resonance imaging (MRI). Although all perform well in high-risk groups and effectively rule out the diagnosis when normal (1), angiography performs surprisingly poorly as the likelihood of disease drops. Only MRI appears to offer better than a 50% positive predictive value when the risk of aortic dissection is low (< 1%) (27).

Most GERD does not require laboratory testing; diagnosis based on symptoms is sufficient to initiate treatment, and if symptoms are controlled, further study is probably not warranted. There is no real "gold standard" diagnostic test for GERD. In fact, patients with demonstrable reflux of acid on 24-hour ambulatory pH monitoring are often free of mucosal injury and symptoms, whereas approximately a quarter of patients with demonstrable esophagitis have "normal" levels of acid reflux (28). The significance of reflux of barium is unknown (28); it is present in as many as 20% of normal controls, whereas only 30% of patients with mild esophagitis have an abnormal study (29). Radiographically demonstrable hiatus hernia is common, and

is found in up to 40% of normal controls. Although it is not very predictive of disease when positive (low positive predictive value), only 5% of patients without hiatus hernia have esophagitis (29). The Bernstein test (provocation of symptoms with infusion of dilute HCl) can establish that symptoms are related to reflux (LR+ 5.5, LR− 0.26) (30), but it is inconvenient and does not distinguish degrees of reflux or severity of esophagitis. Esophageal manometry is of low sensitivity and specificity and is not recommended (28).

MANAGEMENT

Management of the patient with chest pain is very different for each of the many causes previously discussed. Key elements in managing chest pain are listed in Table 21.6. Figure 21.2 illustrates the approach to the patient. The basic principles of therapy for the few most important causes of chest pain in primary care are summarized here.

ACI

All patients with suspected ACI should receive aspirin, 325 mg swallowed or chewed, immediately and then continued daily indefinitely. Aspirin therapy offers an absolute risk reduction (the difference in the event rate between control and treatment groups), depending on patient population, of three to 10 deaths or MIs prevented per 100 ACI patients, making it the most effective medical intervention available (31–35). It should only be withheld for true absolute contraindications, such as anaphylaxis, other major allergic reaction, or current active gastrointestinal bleed (not positive occult blood or history of bleed).

The patient with ST segment elevation or new LBBB, and perhaps with ST depression in anterior V leads suggesting posterior MI, should be considered for thrombolytic therapy at once. These indications are very narrow, and for patients outside them, thrombolysis is contraindicated (1, 25). Other contraindications include active gastrointestinal and genitourinary bleeding (not menses), abdominal or thoracic surgery within 1 month, head trauma, recent stroke, hypertensive crisis, aortic dissection, and pancreatitis. Age is not an absolute contraindication. Thrombolytic therapy reduces in-hospital and 1-year mortality (although probably not at

Table 21.6.
Key Elements in Management of Chest Pain, by Cause

Target Disorder	Intervention	Level of Evidence for Effectiveness[a]	Comments
ACI, CAD	Aspirin	A	Withhold only for absolute contraindication
ACI, CAD	β Blockers	A	Withhold only for absolute contraindication
ACI, CAD	Nitroglycerin	B	Pain relief and improvement of hemodynamic indices; unclear if improves survival
CAD	Coronary revascularization (bypass or angioplasty)	A	For patients meeting very specific selection criteria
CAD	Lipid lowering	A	Reduce LDL cholesterol to < 100 mg/dL if baseline > 130
CAD	Smoking cessation	A-	Largest absolute risk reduction of any treatment if patient successfully quits
ACI	Heparin	A	Unclear if adds benefit if aspirin already in use
ACI	Morphine	C	Clearly effective for pain and anxiety relief, although not formally studied; inadequate dosing common and inexcusable
ACI	Thrombolytics for patients not definitely meeting protocol criteria	X	Close is not close enough
MI	ACE inhibitors	A	Improve survival post-MI in anterior infarcts with ejection fraction <40%
MI	Thrombolysis for patients with ST segment elevation meeting protocol criteria	A	Most effective if initiated within 4 hrs of onset; weak effect 6–12 hr after onset
GERD	H$_2$-receptor antagonists	A	
GERD	Proton pump inhibitors	A	
GERD	Elevation of head of bed	B	
GERD	Decreased fat intake	B	
GERD	Avoidance of chocolate, onions, peppermint, and garlic	B	
Panic	Benzodiazepines	A	High rate of placebo response, and much
Panic	Tricyclic antidepressants	A	better short-term than long-term
Panic	Cognitive therapy	A	success for all modalities; combined
Panic	Combined drug and cognitive therapy	A	most successful
Musculoskeletal pain	NSAIDs	C	

[a]Level of evidence for effectiveness: A, strong or moderate research-based evidence (consistent across several studies, including at least two randomized controlled trials); A-, nonrandomized; B, limited research-based evidence (less consistent or extensive evidence, but preponderance of evidence supports use of treatment); C, common practice with little or no research-based evidence; X, moderate or strong evidence suggesting that this treatment is not effective.

3-year follow-up) by approximately six per 100 patients treated (36). Hospitals typically administer thrombolysis (usually with streptokinase or r-tPA) under specific protocols; see your institution's policy for details. Emergent balloon angioplasty is an alternative with potential advantages in the relatively few centers suitably staffed, equipped, and experienced.

β Blockade should be initiated within 12 hours of the onset of ACI in the absence of contraindications. β Blockers are also of proven benefit, reducing mortality among patients with documented MI by approximately six deaths per 1000 patients in the first week (37, 38), as well as reducing progression to MI among patients with unstable angina (39). Patients with severe bradycardia,

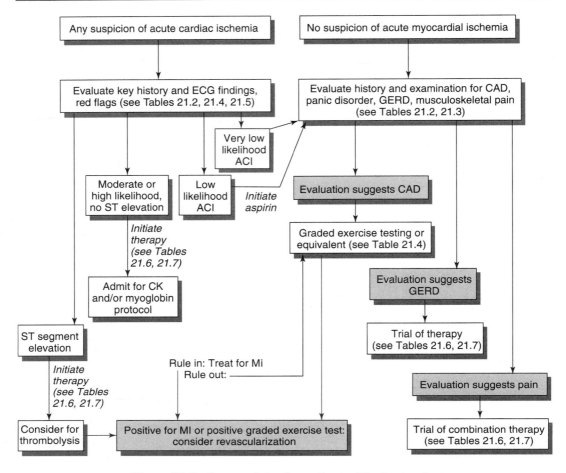

Figure 21.2. *Approach to the patient with chest pain.*

second- or third-degree AV block, first degree with a PR interval > 0.24 seconds, shock, or severe congestive heart failure (CHF) should probably not receive β blockers until these conditions have been resolved. CHF per se is not a contraindication, and may in fact benefit, but both CHF and chronic obstructive pulmonary disease (COPD) patients should have β blockers introduced cautiously, perhaps with the ultrashort-acting agent esmolol given intravenously. The usual choices for intravenous initiation and oral continuation therapy are atenolol and metoprolol (owing to their generally favorable adverse effect profiles), but all β blockers (i.e., now ISA β blockers) probably have similar beneficial effects.

Nitroglycerin provides some favorable hemodynamic effects (preload and afterload reduction) and significant relief of chest pain for ACI. MI patients commonly receive it intravenously, but

most chest pain patients initially receive up to three sublingual tablets over 15 minutes. It should not be given to hypotensive (SBP < 90 mmHg), bradycardic, or tachycardic patients, and it is dangerous in right ventricular infarction.

Heparin is similar to aspirin in its risk reduction for mortality among ACI patients, but it appears to add little benefit to patients already receiving aspirin (40, 41). If used, full-dose heparinization administered either intravenously or subcutaneously is required. ACE inhibitors are indicated within 24 hours of onset for patients who sustain MI, but not for ACI in general. For patients with large anterior infarcts, ejection fractions below 40%, or transient LV dysfunction, they provide an approximately 0.5% absolute risk reduction for mortality (42, 43). Benefit for other MI patients is unclear, and ACE inhibitors are contraindicated in hypotensive patients.

Oxygen (usually 2 L/min by nasal prongs) and bed rest are traditionally prescribed for ACI patients. These are not of proven benefit, although some physiologic rationale supports oxygen. Morphine has an important role in the control of pain and anxiety and is commonly underused both in dose and frequency because of an exaggerated fear of respiratory depression. Doses of 2 to 4 mg IV repeated every 20 to 30 minutes as needed are appropriate.

Calcium channel blockers do not generally improve outcomes and may increase mortality among patients with LV dysfunction or pulmonary edema (1). They should generally not be used in ACI, except for specific indications such as atrial arrhythmias and genuine variant angina (which is rare). Prophylactic administration of lidocaine is contraindicated because it increases mortality (44). Antiarrhythmic therapy should be reserved for sustained, symptomatic ventricular arrhythmias (25).

Coronary Artery Disease

Therapy for coronary artery disease (CAD) is aimed at controlling symptoms that interfere with the patient's function and reducing the risk of death or infarction. Aspirin, 80 to 325 mg taken orally daily, is a mainstay and should be given to all patients who do not have absolute contraindications (see those listed previously) (45). β Blockers, because of their proven mortality-reducing effect, are the first-choice antianginal drugs.

Smoking cessation, although challenging to accomplish, is essential. Smokers with CAD who quit reduce their absolute risk of death over the ensuing decade by more than 11% and perhaps as much as 16%, making smoking cessation the single most important intervention in this group (46, 47). The effect of smoking cessation is even greater for nonfatal morbidity such as disability and hospitalizations.

In patients with known CAD and baseline levels on diet alone ≤ 130 mg/dL, reduction in LDL cholesterol to below 100 mg/dL can prevent four deaths in 100 patients treated for 5 years (48). HMG-CoA reductase inhibitors ("statins") used in combination with diet are the preferred agents, as they are the only agents demonstrated to achieve this level of benefit.

Nitrates are used for additional symptomatic relief. Sublingual or spray forms are used for acute symptoms, and long-acting oral agents or transdermal patches are used for daily prevention. If patches are used, they should be removed at night to prevent disappearance of effect due to tachyphylaxis. Calcium channel antagonists are also useful for symptomatic relief, and long-acting agents appear to be safe, but the short-acting agents should be avoided because case-control studies suggest a nearly fourfold increase in odds ratio for cardiovascular mortality among hypertensive patients (49).

Revascularization offers mortality reduction for patients with 50% or greater left main coronary artery stenosis, three-vessel disease and diminished LV function, or two-vessel disease involving the left anterior descending artery (1, 25). Symptom improvement may be achieved for patients with any degree of CAD who suffer lifestyle-limiting anginal symptoms not adequately controlled by medical therapy. In general, the debate between coronary artery bypass graft (CABG) and angioplasty is beyond our scope here, but it should be noted that diabetic patients requiring insulin or oral agents appear to have a lower mortality with CABG (50).

Panic

The two primary approaches to treatment of panic disorder are cognitive therapy and pharmacologic therapy. The best results are obtained by combining the two modalities, as they have been shown to be mutually potentiating in the few trials in which they were combined (51).

Cognitive therapy is specifically aimed at teaching the patient to interpret the somatic sensations that accompany an attack as something other than evidence of serious illness. Panic patients have been demonstrated to interpret such sensations in much more alarming ways than nonpanic patients do. Cognitive therapy has been shown both to successfully change those interpretations and to provide improvement similar to pharmacologic therapy (52).

Pharmacologic management employs either antidepressants or anxiolytics, and is often necessary for more than 6 months. Treatment with either class of agent is more effective than placebo among patients in blinded trials willing to maintain treatment; however, dropout rates for placebo are over 80%, whereas active treatment dropouts are roughly 65% (53).

Tricyclic antidepressants are the best-studied antidepressants for panic disorder. Therapy should be initiated at low doses, and you should be careful to explain the expected adverse effects as normal so that panic patients do not interpret them as serious. Benzodiazepines are the primary anxiolytic class; buspirone may be useful but is not well studied yet. Alprazolam is often used for panic disorder, but it is likely that all members of the class are effective. Although tolerance is common with long-term use and tapering may be necessary to prevent withdrawal, addiction (increasing dose requirements, behavioral "drug-seeking," concealment of multiple sources, etc.) is uncommon. Benzodiazepines should be used on a fixed schedule, never prn, for panic disorder treatment.

Relaxation therapy has been shown to improve patients' ability to tolerate anxiety, but not to reduce the frequency or severity of panic attacks. It is therefore not a primary treatment recommendation for panic disorder, although it may be for other anxiety disorders.

Gastroesophageal Reflux Disease (GERD)

The first line of treatment for patients with GERD is modification of factors that exacerbate it. Elevation of the head of the patient's bed by 25 to 30 cm (54, 55), decreased fat intake (56), and smoking cessation (57) are known to reduce acid reflux. Avoiding caffeine is often advocated based on physiologic studies of lower esophageal tone (58, 59), but this has not been demonstrated to reduce clinical symptoms in adults. Antacids and alginic acid also provide symptomatic relief superior to placebo (60), and are sufficient in approximately 20% of patients.

Acid suppression with H_2-receptor antagonists, given either in divided doses or at bedtime, is effective for both symptom control and healing of esophagitis in 60% and 50% of patients, respectively (vs. 24 to 27% placebo response). Proton-pump inhibitors (e.g., omeprazole and lansoprazole) are even more effective: 83% and 78% for symptom control and healing, respectively (28). Because of their longer clinical track record of safety and lower expense, H_2 blockers are the first choice.

Promotility agents have not yet established a place in GERD treatment. Neither bethanechol (61) nor metoclopramide (62) is superior to placebo in symptom control, and both have significant adverse effects. Cisapride and domperidone are better tolerated and provide symptom relief superior to placebo in patients with nonulcer dyspepsia and GERD (28).

Musculoskeletal Pain

Musculoskeletal chest pain is traditionally treated with nonsteroidal anti-inflammatory drugs or acetaminophen. It is unclear what fraction of patients derive symptomatic improvement from this therapy. Considerable attention to the patient's worry about heart disease, with appropriate reassurance, is an important part of management. Table 21.7 summarizes drug therapy for chest pain.

CASE STUDY

Mr. S. is a 58-year-old man who presents to your office late on a Friday afternoon complaining of chest pain. His pain was dull and aching in character, midsternal, without radiation. It came on at rest while at work, and was of moderate severity. It lasted about fifteen minutes. For several years he has had very brief episodes of similar pain, lasting perhaps less than a minute, but they have been infrequent. He did not sweat or feel nauseated with the episode, but did notice his heart seeming to beat fast. He feels fine now. He does not have any pains when climbing stairs, but does get out of breath easily.

His history as recorded in his chart reveals a normal number of visits for musculoskeletal aches and pains, viral respiratory illnesses, and health maintenance examinations. His father had a heart attack in his late sixties. Mr. S. himself does not smoke, drinks little, does not exercise (despite your encouragement at each of his health maintenance examinations), and has a recent cholesterol of 210 mg/dL with an HDL of 40.

On examination, he is normotensive and 20 kg overweight. His pulse is 82 bpm, respirations 18/min, and he is in no distress. His fundi are benign, he has no bruits, and cardiac examination reveals only a regular rhythm with no murmurs or third (S3) or fourth (S4) heart sounds. Pulmonary auscultation reveals normal vesicular breath sounds in all fields.

You perform an ECG at once, while he chews four baby aspirin (80 mg each). The

Table 21.7.
Drug Therapy of Chest Pain, by Cause

Drug	Dose Range	Comments
ACI		
β Blockers		
Atenolol	Acute: initiate with 5 mg IV over 10 min, repeat over 5 min; then 50 mg PO stat, and 25–50 bid thereafter	Monitor for hypotension, bradycardia, and rales during IV loading
	Chronic: 50–100 mg PO qd	
Metoprolol	Acute: 5 mg IV every 2 min for three doses, then 50 mg PO bid starting 15–60 min after last IV dose	Monitor as for atenolol
	Chronic: 50–100 mg PO qd	
Esmolol	0.1 mg/kg/min, titrate up by 0.05 mg/kg/min every 10–15 min until HR < 60 or 0.2 mg/kg/min reached	Monitor as for atenolol Very short-acting, IV only
Aspirin	160–325 mg daily	Effect disappears at doses >325 mg/day
Nitroglycerin	IV: 5–10 μg/min, titrate up by 10 μg/min every 10 min until relief is achieved or headache or hypotension occur	Monitor for SBP < 90, or 30% below baseline in hypertensive patients
	Oral: 0.4 mg sublingual stat	Three doses usual maximum
ACE inhibitors		
Enalapril	5 mg PO qd, titrate to max 30 mg/d	
Lisinopril	5 mg PO qd, titrate to max 20 mg/d	
Enalapril	2.5–5 mg daily, to max of 40 mg/d in single or divided dose	
Morphine sulfate	2–4 mg IV every 10–20 min as needed	Underdosing common 10–30 mg may be required
GERD		
H₂ antagonists		
Famotidine	20 mg bid	20 mg hs may be effective for maintenance
Ranitidine, nizatidine	150 mg bid (or 300 hs)	150 hs may be effective for maintenance
Cimetidine	400–800 mg bid	800 hs may be effective for maintenance
Proton pump inhibitor		
Omeprazole	20 mg qd	
Lansoprazole	30 mg qd	
Panic disorder		
Tricyclics		
Imipramine	100–200 mg/day (hs or divided); initiate at 50 and titrate up by 25 every few days	Rather sedating
Desipramine	Same as imipramine	Less sedating; not as well investigated for panic
Benzodiazepines		
Diazepam	2.5–5 mg tid	Many other benzodiazepines are available and probably equally effective
Alprazolam	0.25 mg tid, titrated to max of 4 mg/d	Some antidepressant effect; may require careful dose adjustment for panic
Clonazepam	0.5 mg tid, titrated to maximum of 20 mg/d	
Anxiolytics		
Buspirone	15–30 mg/d divided bid–tid	See text

ECG reveals normal sinus rhythm, without ischemic changes.

QUESTIONS

1. Should you admit Mr. S. to hospital to rule out infarction?
2. How should you advise Mr. S. today?
3. What diagnostic workup should you pursue?

DISCUSSION

Mr. S.'s pain is consistent with myocardial ischemia, and it occurred at rest. Unstable angina is definitely a possibility, but MI is very unlikely given his short duration of pain and normal ECG. Because he has no high-risk features (remember that long-term risk factors contribute little here; it is MI in male relatives before age 55 or in female relatives before age 65 that confers increased risk in any case), outpatient management is appropriate. However, outpatient management is dependent upon his adherence to advice and follow-up; if these are in doubt, he should be admitted until CAD has been detected or excluded. A 6-hour myoglobin rule-out protocol is not appropriate because if admission is required, it would be for evaluation for CAD rather than to rule out infarction.

Mr. S. should know that you are concerned about possible coronary artery disease, and that there are other possibilities that require evaluation as well. He should remain on daily aspirin until the matter is settled. You will have to emphasize to him that aspirin could be very important to his survival (he believes it to be "just aspirin," after all!), that the protective effect of aspirin against heart attack is only present at low doses, that more is not better, and that he should take acetaminophen instead of more aspirin if he requires a pain reliever for headache or other minor condition. Mr. S. should also be instructed to go directly to the emergency room, without calling for advice first, if he has pain lasting 20 minutes or more (63).

Mr. S. has no indications for imaging nor contraindications to exercise testing. Hence, you schedule him for exercise treadmill testing on Monday and a follow-up in your office Tuesday morning.

OUTCOME

Mr. S. reappears in your office on Tuesday, having had no more pains. He does bring with him a copy of the treadmill report. He reached 11 mets and had 1 mm of ST segment depression. This is reported as an "equivocal" result, and the cardiologist reading it recommends cardiac catheterization. Mr. S. is very worried about the report, so you proceed with the referral.

His catheterization shows an isolated 40% occlusion of his left anterior descending coronary artery with a smooth surface. Unconvinced that this explains his pain, you schedule him for a longer visit and take a very detailed history. He describes several episodes from his early twenties to the present wherein he would have spells of "feeling unreal," accompanied by palpitations and shortness of breath with brief aching chest pains, once or twice a week. These episodes lasted a few weeks to 2 months each, and resolved spontaneously. You schedule him to meet with your practice's psychologist partner, and in the meantime start him on 50 mg of desipramine at bedtime. ⇒ anxiety!

REFERENCES

1. Braunwald E, Mark DB, Jones RH, et al. Unstable Angina: Clinical Practice Guideline no. 10. Washington, DC: Agency for Health Care Policy and Research, 1994.
2. White L, Lee T, Cook E, et al. Comparison of the natural history of new onset and exacerbated chronic ischemic heart disease. The Chest Pain Study Group. J Am Coll Cardiol 1990;16:304–310.
3. Karlson B, Herlitz J, Pettersson P, et al. A one-year prognosis in patients hospitalized with a history of unstable angina pectoris. Clin Cardiol 1993;16:397–402.
4. Beitman BD, Mukerji V, Russell JL, Grafting M. Panic disorder in cardiology patients: a review of the Missouri Panic/Cardiology Project. J Psychiatr Res 1993; 27(suppl)1:35–46.
5. Ballenger JC. Overview of panic disorder. Trans Am Clin Climatol Assoc 1993;105:36–51.

6. Fleet RP, Dupuis G, Marchand A, Burelle D, Beitman BD. Panic disorder, chest pain, and coronary artery disease: literature review. Can J Cardiol 1994;10:827–834.

7. Isolauri J, Laippala P. Prevalence of symptoms suggestive of gastro-oesophageal reflux disease in an adult population. Ann Med 1995;27:67–70.

8. Petersen H. The prevalence of gastro-oesophageal reflux disease. Scand J Gastroenterol Suppl 1995;211:5–6.

9. Woolf PK, Gewitz MH, Berezin S, et al. Noncardiac chest pain in adolescents and children with mitral valve prolapse. J Adolesc Health 1991;12:247–250.

10. Selker H, Griffith J, D'Agostino R. A tool for judging coronary care unit admission appropriateness, valid for both real-time and retrospective use. Med Care 1991;29:610–627.

11. Klinkman MS. Episodes of care for chest pain. J Fam Pract 1994;38:345.

12. Goldman L, Weinberg M, Weisberg M. A computer-derived protocol to aid in the diagnosis of emergency room patients with acute chest pain. N Engl J Med 1982;307:588–596.

13. Everts B, Karlson BW, Wahrborg P, Hedner T, Herlitz J. Localization of pain in suspected acute myocardial infarction in relation to final diagnosis, age and sex, and site and type of infarction. Heart Lung 1996; 25:430–437.

14. Weaver WD, Litwin PE, Martin JS, et al. Effect of age on use of thrombolytic therapy and mortality in acute myocardial infarction: the MITI Project Group. J Am Coll Cardiol 1991;18:657–662.

15. Green LA, Yates JF. Influence of pseudodiagnostic information on the evaluation of ischemic coronary disease. Ann Emerg Med 1995;25:451–457.

16. Jayes RLJ, Beshansky JR, D'Agostino RB, Selker HP. Do patients' coronary risk factor reports predict acute cardiac ischemia in the emergency department? A multicenter study. J Clin Epidemiol 1992;45:621–626.

17. Klauser AG, Schindlbeck NE, Muller-Lissner SA. Symptoms in gastro-oesophageal reflux disease. Lancet 1990; 335:205–208.

18. Diamond G, Forrester J. Analysis of probability as an aid in the clinical diagnosis of coronary-artery disease. N Engl J Med 1979;300:1350–1358.

19. Moraes D, McCormack P, Tyrrell J, Feely J. Earlobe crease and coronary heart disease. Ir Med J 1992;85: 131–132.

20. Tranchesi B Jr, Barbosa V, de Albuquerque CP, et al. Diagonal earlobe crease as a marker of the presence and extent of coronary atherosclerosis. Am J Cardiol 1992;70:1417–1420.

21. Rude RE, Poole WK, Muller JE, et al. Electrocardiographic and clinical criteria for recognition of acute myocardial infarction based on analysis of 3,697 patients. Am J Cardiol 1983;52:936–942.

22. Luker GD, Glazer HS, Eagar G, Gutierrez FR, Sagel SS. Aortic dissection: effect of prospective chest radiographic diagnosis on delay to definitive diagnosis. Radiology 1994;193:813–819.

23. Ravkilde J, Nissen H, Horder M, Thygesen K. Independent prognostic value of serum creatine kinase isoenzyme MB mass, cardiac troponin T, and myosin light chain levels in suspected acute myocardial infarction. Analysis of 28 months of follow-up in 196 patients. J Am Coll Cardiol 1995;25:574–581.

24. Tucker JF, Collins RA, Anderson AJ, et al. Value of serial myoglobin levels in the early diagnosis of patients admitted for acute myocardial infarction. Ann Emerg Med 1994;24:704–708.

25. Ryan TJ, Anderson JL, Antman EM, et al. ACC/AHA guidelines for the management of patients with acute myocardial infarction: a report of the American College of Cardiology/American Heart Association Task Force on Practice Guidelines (Committee on Management of Acute Myocardial Infarction). J Am Coll Cardiol 1996;28:1328–1428.

26. Mark DB, Shaw L, Harrell FE Jr, et al. Prognostic value of a treadmill exercise score in outpatients with suspected coronary artery disease [see comments]. N Engl J Med 1991;325:849–853.

27. Barbant SD, Eisenberg MJ, Schiller NB. The diagnostic value of imaging techniques for aortic dissection. Am Heart J 1992;124:541–543.

28. DeVault KR, Castell DO. Guidelines for the diagnosis and treatment of gastroesophageal reflux disease. Practice Parameters Committee of the American College of Gastroenterology. Arch Intern Med 1995;155: 2165–2173.

29. Ott DJ, Wu WC, Gelfand DW. Reflux esophagitis revisited: prospective analysis of radiologic accuracy. Gastrointest Radiol 1981;6:1–7.

30. Richter JE. Acid perfusion (Bernstein) test. In: Castell DO, Wu WC, Ott DJ, eds. Gastroesophageal Reflux Disease: Pathogenesis, Diagnosis, and Therapy. London: Futura Publishing, 1985:139–148.

31. ISIS-2 (Second International Study of Infarct Survival) Collaborative Group. Randomised trial of intravenous streptokinase, oral aspirin, both, or neither among 17,187 cases of suspected acute myocardial infarction: ISIS-2. Lancet 1988;2:349–360.

32. Lewis HD Jr, Davis JW, Archibald DG, et al. Protective effects of aspirin against acute myocardial infarction and death in men with unstable angina. Results of a Veterans Administration Cooperative Study. N Engl J Med 1983;309:396–403.

33. Wallentin LC. Aspirin (75 mg/day) after an episode of unstable coronary artery disease: long-term effects on the risk for myocardial infarction, occurrence of severe angina, and the need for revascularization. Research Group on Instability in Coronary Artery Disease in Southeast Sweden [comments]. J Am Coll Cardiol 1991;18:1587–1593.

34. Cairns JA, Gent M, Singer J, et al. Aspirin, sulfinpyrazone, or both in unstable angina. Results of a Canadian multicenter trial. N Engl J Med 1985;313:1369–1375.

35. Theroux P, Ouimet H, McCans J, et al. Aspirin, heparin, or both to treat acute unstable angina. N Engl J Med 1988;319:1105–1111.

36. Cerqueira MD, Maynard C, Ritchie JL, Davis KB, Kennedy JW. Long-term survival in 618 patients from the Western Washington Streptokinase in Myocardial Infarction trials. J Am Coll Cardiol 1992;20:1452–1459.

37. First International Study of Infarct Survival Collaborative Group. Randomised trial of intravenous atenolol among 16,027 cases of suspected acute myocardial infarction: ISIS-1. Lancet 1986;2:57–66.

38. The TIMI Study Group. Comparison of invasive and conservative strategies after treatment with intravenous tissue plasminogen activator in acute myocardial

infarction. Results of the thrombolysis in myocardial infarction (TIMI) phase II trial. N Engl J Med 1989;320: 618–627.

39. Yusuf S, Wittes J, Friedman L. Overview of results of randomized clinical trials in heart disease. II. Unstable angina, heart failure, primary prevention with aspirin, and risk factor modification. JAMA 1988;260:2259–2263.

40. Gurfinkel EP, Manos EJ, Mejail RI, et al. Low-molecular-weight heparin versus regular heparin or aspirin in the treatment of unstable angina and silent ischemia. J Am Coll Cardiol 1995;26:313–318.

41. O'Donnell CJ, Ridker PM, Hebert PR, Hennekens CH. Antithrombotic therapy for acute myocardial infarction. J Am Coll Cardiol 1995;25:23S–29S.

42. Ball SG, Hall AS, Murray GD. Angiotensin-converting enzyme inhibitors after myocardial infarction: indications and timing. J Am Coll Cardiol 1995;25:42S–46S.

43. LeJemtel TH, Hochman JS, Sonnenblick EH. Indications for immediate angiotensin-converting enzyme inhibition in patients with acute myocardial infarction. J Am Coll Cardiol 1995;25:47S–51S.

44. Hine LK, Laird N, Hewitt P, Chalmers TC. Meta-analytic evidence against prophylactic use of lidocaine in acute myocardial infarction. Arch Intern Med 1989; 149:2694–2698.

45. Antiplatelet Trialists' Collaboration. Collaborative overview of randomised trials of antiplatelet therapy—I: Prevention of death, myocardial infarction, and stroke by prolonged antiplatelet therapy in various categories of patients. BMJ 1994;308:81–106.

46. Cavender JB, Rogers WJ, Fisher LD, Gersh BJ, Coggin CJ, Myers WO. Effects of smoking on survival and morbidity in patients randomized to medical or surgical therapy in the Coronary Artery Surgery Study (CASS): 10-year follow-up. CASS Investigators. J Am Coll Cardiol 1992;20:287–294.

47. Daly LE, Mulcahy R, Graham IM, Hickey N. Long-term effect on mortality of stopping smoking after unstable angina and myocardial infarction. BMJ (Clin Res Ed) 1983;287:324–326.

48. Scandinavian Simvastatin Survival Study Investigators. Randomised trial of cholesterol lowering in 4444 patients with coronary heart disease: the Scandinavian Simvastatin Survival Study (4S). Lancet 1994; 344:1383–1389.

49. Alderman MH, Cohen H, Roque R, Madhavan S. Effect of long-acting and short-acting calcium antagonists on cardiovascular outcomes in hypertensive patients. Lancet 1997;349:594–598.

50. National Heart, Lung, and Blood Institute, Clinical Alert, September 21, 1995.

51. Mavissakalian M. Combined behavioral therapy and pharmacotherapy of agoraphobia. J Psychiatr Res 1993; 27(suppl)1:179–191.

52. Gelder MG, Clark DM, Salkovskis P. Cognitive treatment for panic disorder. J Psychiatr Res 1993;27 (suppl) 1:171–178.

53. Curtis GC, Massana J, Udina C, Ayuso JL, Cassano GB, Perugi G. Maintenance drug therapy of panic disorder. J Psychiatr Res 1993;27(suppl)1:127–142.

54. Stanciu C, Bennett JR. Effects of posture on gastro-oesophageal reflux. Digestion 1977;15:104–109.

55. Johnson LF, DeMeester TR. Evaluation of elevation of the head of the bed, bethanechol, and antacid form tablets on gastroesophageal reflux. Dig Dis Sci 1981; 26:673–680.

56. Becker DJ, Sinclair J, Castell DO, Wu WC. A comparison of high- and low-fat meals on postprandial esophageal acid exposure. Am J Gastroenterol 1989;84: 782–786.

57. Waring JP, Eastwood TF, Austin JM, Sanowski RA. The immediate effects of cessation of cigarette smoking on gastroesophageal reflux. Am J Gastroenterol 1989;84:1076–1078.

58. Thomas FB, Steinbaugh JT, Fromkes JJ, Mekhjian HS, Caldwell JH. Inhibitory effect of coffee on lower esophageal sphincter pressure. Gastroenterology 1980; 79:1262–1266.

59. Cohen S. Pathogenesis of coffee-induced gastrointestinal symptoms. N Engl J Med 1980;303:122–124.

60. Kitchin LI, Castell DO. Rationale and efficacy of conservative therapy for gastroesophageal reflux disease. Arch Intern Med 1991;151:448–454.

61. Farrell RL, Roling GT, Castell DO. Cholinergic therapy of chronic heartburn. A controlled trial. Ann Intern Med 1974;80:573–576.

62. Bright-Asare P, El-Bassoussi M. Cimetidine, metoclopramide, or placebo in the treatment of symptomatic gastroesophageal reflux. J Clin Gastroenterol 1980;2: 149–156.

63. Dracup K, Alonzo AA, Atkins JM, et al. The physician's role in minimizing prehospital delay in patients at high risk for acute myocardial infarction: recommendations from the National Heart Attack Alert Program. Ann Intern Med 1997;126:645–651.

22. Chronic Cardiac Disease

RICHARD W. PRETORIUS AND MICHAEL J. FRANKLIN, JR.

Key Clinical Questions

1. What are the four common syndromes of heart disease?
2. What are the most effective treatment strategies for heart failure?
3. How are arrhythmias best managed?

The management of both acute and chronic cardiac disease is usually done by primary care physicians (family physicians and internists). Although some interventions require the assistance of subspecialists (e.g., invasive monitoring, catheterization, angioplasty, balloon pumps, open heart surgery), the primary care physician, who regularly sees the patient, can best handle the comorbid conditions, medications, lifestyle issues, values, and ethical concerns that affect the heart's function. The accomplished family physician understands the dynamic relationship among heart and other organ systems and understands the evolution of the disease process over time. The family physician uses this knowledge to frequently make incremental changes in medications in the outpatient setting—particularly in the elderly—and then monitors the patient closely over time for the expected physiologic and functional changes.

Cardiac disease remains the leading cause of morbidity and mortality in the United States and accounts for nearly half of all deaths per year (about 500,000). As we are not able to defeat death, the thoughtful physician must recognize the limits of the human heart and the limitations of medical science. The patient, rather than the diagnosis, should always be the focus of the management of cardiac ailments. Knowledge of a patient's spiritual beliefs, personal goals, and psychosocial support systems is a prerequisite to giving good medical care.

PATHOPHYSIOLOGY AND DIFFERENTIAL DIAGNOSIS: THE FOUR COMMON SYNDROMES OF HEART DISEASE

To manage patients with heart problems, conceptualize four separate (but interrelated) systems: (*a*) a muscular *pump* to push fluid (blood) around the body; (*b*) a *network of electrical wiring* to coordinate the muscles; (*c*) a *plumbing system of vascular pipes* to supply the muscles with oxygen and nutrients; and (*d*) a *series of gates or valves* to regulate the flow of fluid (1). Derangements of each system cause distinct syndromes, but as with any complex machine, failure in one system often leads to problems with another. In managing your patients, you should attempt mentally to separate the heart's function into each of these four systems. As you develop a diagnostic and therapeutic plan, keep in mind the relationship of these four systems with each other as well as with other organ systems in the body (especially the lung, kidneys, brain, and liver), seeking to integrate their function back into a whole interconnected unit (Fig. 22.1).

Pump problems result from either damaged heart muscle (e.g., from myocardial infarction or cardiomyopathy) or weakened heart muscle (e.g., from hypertension, tight heart valves, leaky heart valves). The location of the pump problem has traditionally been used to classify heart failure (HF) as right-sided, left-sided, or biventricular, and they produce different symptom complexes:

- When the blood backs up behind the left ventricle (left-sided heart failure), increased hydrostatic pressure in the pulmonary veins causes fluid to collect in the alveoli and/or the pleural spaces. Clinically, this increased fluid presents as dyspnea on exertion, paroxysmal nocturnal dyspnea, orthopnea, rales, and/or pleural effusions.

- When blood backs up behind the right ventricle (right-sided heart failure), fluid collects in the venous system, and passive congestion develops in the liver, abdomen, and legs. Clinically, this increased fluid presents as peripheral edema, ascites, hepatic enlargement, and/or engorged neck veins.

- When blood backs up behind both the right and left ventricle (biventricular failure), then both of the above symptom complexes develop. Although right-sided failure will occasionally occur in isolation because of damage

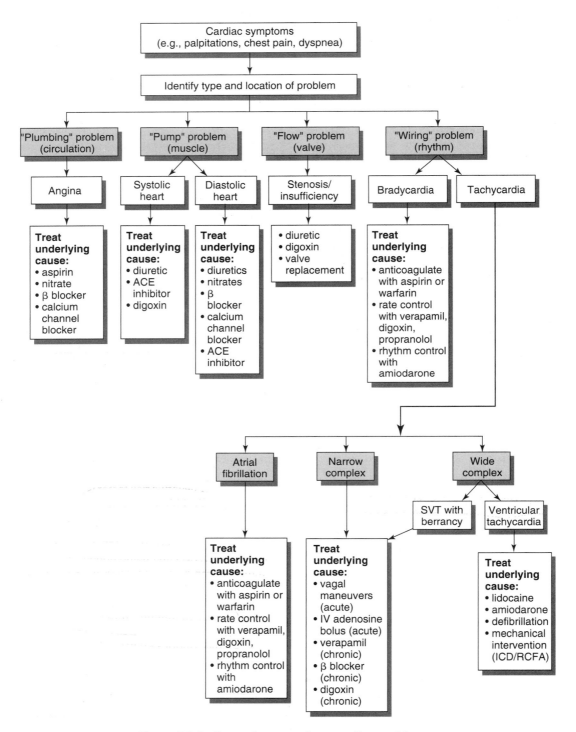

Figure 22.1. *General approach to cardiac problems.*

to the right ventricle (e.g., right-sided my-ocardial infarction or cor pulmonale), damage to the powerful left ventricle will typically cause back-up of fluid into both the lungs and the venous system.

Problems with the initiation of the electrical impulse or the conduction of the impulse through the heart's "wiring" result in arrhythmias of various types, usually with a fairly good correlation between the anatomic location of the insult and the type of arrhythmia produced. Arrhythmias interfere with the normal rhythm of the pump and produce clinically important syndromes, primarily because of the decreased amount of fluid pushed out of the heart. Main symptoms of rhythm disturbances include:

- A sensation of fluttering or thumping in the chest owing to awareness of the heart's irregular or rapid beating;

- Lightheadedness or syncope owing to temporarily inadequate perfusion of the brain; and

- Symptoms of left-sided congestive heart failure (see previously described symptom complexes).

If the heart's demand for blood exceeds the ability of the coronary circulation to deliver the blood, it suffers either pain (angina) or cell death (myocardial infarction). The most common alteration in this balance occurs when atherosclerotic plaque in the coronary arteries diminishes the available blood supply to the myocardium. Any stress on the heart will increase the myocardial workload and can unmask the inadequacy of the coronary arteries to carry an adequate supply of oxygen to the heart. Increased stress on the heart can result from intrinsic damage to the heart muscle (prior myocardial infarction, heart failure, cardiomyopathy), extrinsic oxygen demand (infection, hyperthyroidism, physical exertion), diminished oxygen supply (pneumonia, pulmonary edema, anemia), or excessive work demand of the heart muscle (chronic uncontrolled hypertension, valvular heart disease, emotional stress). Angina reflects hypoxia of heart muscle regardless of whether the patient experiences chest discomfort (70% of cases) or not (30% of cases, particularly patients with diabetes) (2).

The heart valves maintain a unilateral direction of flow and separate the pumping chambers when the muscle is contracting. Any damage to the heart valve will affect the direction of flow as well as the functional integrity of the individual chambers. The increased cardiac workload from a defective valve will usually cause congestive heart failure, angina, or both. The therapeutic interventions discussed in this chapter are used to treat HF and angina in patients with and without valvular disease, with one or two exceptions.

ANGINA PECTORIS

The evaluation of chest pain is discussed in Chapter 21. This chapter addresses the management of angina pectoris. General goals of patient management in angina pectoris, after the diagnosis has been made, include:

- Aggressively reducing risk factors for atherosclerosis

- Minimizing the frequency and intensity of anginal pain

- Maximizing the patient's functional ability

- Preventing premature death

Identifying and modifying cardiac risk factors are two major preventive functions performed by the family physician. Five major positive risk factors have independent correlation with coronary artery disease: advanced age (male over 45 years of age or female over 55 years of age); family history (first-degree relative with coronary artery disease); cigarette smoking; hypertension; and hyperlipidemia (particularly a high-density lipoprotein [HDL] level less than 35 mg/dL) (2). The one major negative risk factor is HDL greater than 60 mg/dL. Although age and family history cannot be altered, the other risk factors can. Smoking cessation strategies can be implemented; blood pressures of less than 135/85 can be pursued; and glycosylated hemoglobins of less than 6.0 mg/dL can be sought. High lipid levels can be lowered by a low-fat diet (less than 30% fat in the diet—read the labels on food!), consistent exercise (at least 30 minutes, three times a week), and weight reduction (decrease the total caloric intake by 1000 calories a day until a target weight is achieved).

Management

According to the guidelines established by the National Cholesterol Education Committee, patients with one or no cardiac risk factors should reduce their low-density lipoproteins (LDL) to below 160 mg/dL (2). If a patient has two or more risk factors, his or her goal should be less than 130 mg/dL. Lastly, if a patient has known ischemic coronary disease or a previous myocardial infarction, the goal should be 100 mg/dL. If the patient's LDL remains greater than 30 mg/dL above his or her respective LDL goal, lipid-lowering medications should be considered. In postmenopausal women, hormone replacement therapy should be strongly considered, as estrogens can reduce the risk of atherosclerosis by at least 30%. Niacin (in doses of 2 to 3 g a day) can be an excellent choice in patients with increased triglycerides or decreased HDL; it is inexpensive and over-the-counter. HMG CoA reductase inhibitors (the so-called "statin" class of lipid-lowering agents) block the synthesis of cholesterol in the liver and are a good choice if the LDL is elevated. These agents are more expensive (a minimum of $30 a month) and require monitoring of liver enzymes, although they can reduce the LDL by 30% or more depending on the agent and the dose used.

Nitrates, β-adrenergic antagonists, and calcium channel antagonists are the primary antianginal medications used to control symptoms, decrease recurrence, and increase longevity. When prescribing these medications and monitoring their effects, you should be alert for possible adverse effects and drug interactions. Among the important issues to keep in mind are the following:

- Tolerance has been described in patients on long-acting dinitrates. To prevent this, patients on these medications should have a period of at least 6 to 8 hours a day without the medication. This is less of a problem with mononitrates if they are used once a day.

- β-Adrenergic blocking drugs reduce myocardial oxygen consumption by limiting the heart's rate and contractility. Therefore, they must be used with caution in patients who also have heart failure. Propranolol is a good choice because it is considerably less expensive, although it requires twice-a-day dosing and has a slightly increased rate of side effects. Metoprolol and atenolol offer some advantages in dosing and adverse-effects.

- Among the calcium channel blockers, diltiazem is often the best choice because it causes less hypotension and less reduction in cardiac contractility than other agents and has the greatest benefit on coronary vasodilatation.

- In patients who also have congestive heart failure, medications to improve contractility and reduce myocardial demands, such as digoxin, diuretics, and angiotensin-converting enzyme (ACE) inhibitors may have a salutary effect on angina as well.

Aspirin also contributes to an improved prognosis in persons with coronary artery disease. Patients with known coronary artery disease have a lower incidence of myocardial infarction (by 30%) and death (by 15%) when taking one aspirin per day compared to a placebo (3). In addition to being a good agent for secondary prevention of thrombosis formation (i.e., after coronary artery disease is diagnosed), aspirin appears to be a reasonable agent for primary prevention (i.e., in the asymptomatic patient without known coronary artery disease), particularly in men over the age of 50. It is also used as a therapeutic agent in patients with acute onset of chest pain: 160 mg of chewed aspirin at home (i.e., two baby [81 mg] aspirin tablets), before leaving to go to the emergency room, can decrease the risk of myocardial infarction by one fourth. Table 22.1 lists medications to use for angina.

Mechanical Interventions

An estimated 300,000 percutaneous transluminal coronary angioplasty (PTCA) and 300,000 coronary artery bypass operations are performed each year in the United States. PTCA is a technique of inflating a balloon inside a stenotic lesion to restore patency of the coronary artery. It is performed in the catheterization laboratory and is useful for selected patients with one- or two-vessel disease. PTCA offers a patient who does not wish to undergo a major operation an alternate successful treatment. In addition, the procedure is less expensive, decreases hospital stay, and significantly reduces recovery time. The most common problem with the procedure is the rapid restenosis rate, which reaches approximately 30% at 6 months (3). A newer procedure that involves inflating a wire mesh cage called a stent inside the coronary artery is gaining popularity, as its restenosis rate is slightly better than angioplasty: 25% at 6 months (3). Coronary artery bypass grafting (CABG) is useful in patients with three-vessel disease or in those with left main coronary disease. It provides excellent relief to patients with severe angina; its long-term benefits are less clear.

Table 22.1.

Medications Commonly Used to Treat Angina, Heart Failure, and Arrhythmias

Drug	Typical Dosage Range	Typical Number of Daily Doses	Approximate Monthly Cost Range ($)	Common Adverse Effects
Nitrates				
Nitroglycerin	0.4 mg sublingual	prn	7 per 100 tablets	Headache, transient hypotension
Isosorbide dinitrate (Isordil)	40–160 mg/day	2–4	2–8	Same
Isosorbide mononitrate (Isordil)	30–120 mg/day	1–2	15–44	Same
Transdermal nitroglycerin	0.2–0.8 mg/day	1	37–55	Headache, contact dermatitis
Beta blockers				
Propranolol (Inderal)	80–480 mg/day	2	4–26	Bronchospasm, fatigue
Metoprolol (Lopressor)	100–200 mg/day	2	20–40	Same
Atenolol (Tenormin)	25–100 mg/day	1	9–29	Same
Calcium channel blockers				
Diltiazem (Cardizem)	120–360 mg/day	1–4	16–90	Hypotension, headache
Verapamil (Calan)	120–240 mg/day	1–3	9–18	Conduction problems, bradycardia
ACE inhibitors				
Captopril (Capoten)	25–150 mg/day	2–3	20–74	Cough, hypotension, renal insufficiency
Enalapril (Vasotec)	2.5–20 mg/day	2	14–43	Same
Benazepril (Lotensin)	10–40 mg/day	1	20 all strengths	Hypotension, renal insufficiency
Moexepril (Univasc)	7.5–30 mg/day	1	7–30	Same
Diuretics				
Hydrochorothiazide	12.5–50 mg/day	1	0.25–0.60	Hypotension, hypokalemia, dehydration
Furosemide (Lasix)	20–600 mg/day	1–2	1–30	Same
Metolazone	2.5–20 mg/day	1–2	7–34	Same
Inotropes				
Digoxin (Lanoxin)	0.125–0.25 mg/day	1	3 both strengths	Confusion, yellow-green vision, GI upset, arrhythmias
Antiarrhythmic agents				
Adenosine	6–12 mg IV bolus		25–50 per dose	Transient chest pain, flushing
Amiodarone (Cordarone)	100–400 mg/day	1	46–184	Corneal microdeposits, hypothyroidism or hyperthyroidism or pulmonary fibrosis

The costs are based on average wholesale price to the pharmacist. The retail cost to the patient will be 20–100% higher. Generics are used when available. The lower price often reflects half of a tablet of a higher strength. Table prepared with the assistance of Michael Kelly, Pharm.D.

HEART FAILURE

As a pump with four chambers, the heart depends on having strong ventricular contractions, walls with just the right amount of compliance, appropriately proportioned chamber sizes, and valves that open fully and do not leak. When the pump fails to keep up with the demands of the body, heart failure results. Pump damage can occur suddenly from acute myocardial infarction; over weeks to months from alcoholic, viral, infiltrative, or inflammatory cardiomyopathy; or over decades from hypertension and valvular heart disease. Severity of heart failure is rated based on patient function (Table 22.2). The success of a treatment program depends on both preventing additional injury to the heart and shoring up the strength and function of the remaining healthy heart tissue.

Table 22.2.
Functional Criteria for Patients with Heart Disease: New York Heart Association Criteria

Class	Functional Limitation	Description
I	No limitation	Intensive physical activity (e.g., aerobic exercise, manual labor) may cause symptoms.
II	Slight activity limitation	Moderate activity (e.g., climbing stairs) causes symptoms.
III	Marked activity limitation	Very modest activity (e.g., walking across room, taking a bath) causes symptoms.
IV	Limitation at rest	Symptoms at rest in bed.

Adapted from Braunwald E, ed. Heart Disease, 3rd ed. Philadelphia: WB Saunders, 1988:12.

History and Physical Examination

In keeping with the underlying mechanism of injury, the onset of symptoms of HF can be sudden, gradual, slow, or even nonexistent. The classic findings of cough, shortness of breath, dyspnea on exertion, paroxysmal nocturnal dyspnea, and orthopnea are actually late findings and are relatively uncommon in the patient with chronic, progressive heart failure. The early findings—weakness and easy fatigability—are subtle and can easily be overlooked. An elderly patient who develops fatigue will often attribute it to aging, although an organic cause, including HF, is actually more likely.

Similarly, the classic physical findings of new-onset S3 or S4, diastolic regurgitation murmur, jugular venous distention, hepatojugular reflux, and hepatomegaly are also late findings. The more common early findings are subtle and include peripheral edema, increased intensity of heart sounds, lateral displacement of the point of maximal impulse (PMI), and an unexplained increase in weight. Although gravity and mild venous insufficiency are the most common causes of peripheral edema, a careful evaluation of heart function must be considered, for example, in a laconic farmer who complains of his boots being too tight.

Laboratory and Ancillary Tests

Helpful tests usually include an ECG (looking for rhythm disturbances, old or new myocardial infarctions, left ventricular hypertrophy), chest radiograph (looking for venous congestion, intestinal edema, pleural effusion, and cardiomegaly), cardiac enzymes (looking for muscle damage from a recent myocardial infarction), electrolytes (looking for altered sodium and potassium levels), blood urea nitrogen (BUN) and creatinine (assessing the degree of renal impairment), complete blood count (CBC—looking for physiologic or dilutional anemia), thyroid function (looking for hypo- or hyperthyroidism), liver enzymes (looking for passive hepatic congestion), digoxin level (looking for a therapeutic level, if the patient is on digoxin), echocardiogram (looking for valvular abnormalities, ventricular wall motion, and estimated left ventricular ejection fraction), and exercise stress test (looking for myocardial ischemia). Although these tests can usually be done on an outpatient basis, patients with new HF are commonly admitted to the hospital overnight under a rule-out-MI protocol, since myocardial infarction and myocardial ischemia are often associated with new-onset HF (4).

If the initial workup is unrevealing and the patient does not show evidence of underlying coronary artery disease but is hypertensive, you should consider a diagnosis of hypertensive cardiomyopathy, as this is the second most common cause of HF (5). Because hypertension can cause systolic dysfunction, diastolic dysfunction, or both (and the treatment differs depending on the cause), a patient with a hypertensive cardiomyopathy must be further classified into one of these categories, which is not always an easy task. As a general rule, however, a patient with a systolic dysfunction will usually have a low ejection fraction (less than 40%) and an enlarged cardiac silhouette on chest radiograph, whereas a patient with diastolic dysfunction will usually have a normal or elevated ejection fraction (greater than 60%) and a normal cardiac silhouette on chest radiograph (6). The echocardiogram is by far the most commonly used test to determine an ejection fraction because a radionuclide scan is more expensive (although it is a little more sensitive) and a cardiac catheterization is an invasive procedure. Although the echocardiogram is a helpful test, the ejection fraction by this method is only an approximation (up to one third are probably uninterpretable), so you must remember to treat the patient and not the test (7).

Management of Heart Failure Due to Systolic Dysfunction

Systolic dysfunction, the most common and the best studied form of HF, is treated with one, two, or three agents: diuretics, ACE inhibitors, and digoxin. Diuretics are the usual first-line agent, as most patients present with some degree of fluid overload (5). Hydrochlorothiazide is occasionally used with mild HF, but it is not very potent and may also lower the blood pressure (which already may be low from decreased cardiac output). Furosemide is the preferred diuretic for moderate or severe HF. It is normally begun at a dose of 20 to 40 mg per day, although elderly patients may be started at 10 mg per day. There is no standard target dose, and the goal is to use as much (or as little) as needed to remove the excess fluid. Doses of up to 600 mg per day or higher may occasionally be needed, particularly in patients with concomitant renal insufficiency. If the total daily dose exceeds 80 mg, divided doses given at breakfast and lunch should be used. If the total daily dose exceeds 160 mg, an additional agent, such as metolazone given 1 hour before the furosemide, is helpful. Potassium supplements will be required in almost all patients to maintain a serum potassium greater than 4.0 mEq/L, and potassium levels should be checked frequently (every 3 to 5 days initially, then every 3 months) (5).

Careful monitoring and frequent dosage adjustments of diuretics are often required to straddle the fine line between fluid overload and fluid depletion. Just as the key diagnostic endpoint in diabetes is the blood glucose and in asthma it is the peak flow, so the most critical piece of information in HF is establishing an appropriate "dry weight" and in monitoring the level of control. Daily home weights coupled with careful attention in the office to skin turgor (by pinching the skin on the forearm), ankle edema (by pushing on the skin of the ankle with one's thumb), and orthostatic blood pressures will provide important clues as to whether more or less diuretic is needed. Carefully watching the serum BUN and creatinine is also useful, although you must remember that both will rise in the fluid-overloaded patient as well as the fluid-depleted patient: in the first case because of decreased

cardiac output and in the second, from decreased intravascular volume.

ACE inhibitors are commonly used as either first- or second-line agents. All symptomatic patients as well as asymptomatic patients with systolic dysfunction who have an ejection fraction less than 40% should be treated with an ACE inhibitor to reduce the chance of additional deterioration in heart function (strength of evidence = A) (8). Although it is usually used with a diuretic, an ACE inhibitor may be used as sole therapy in the subset of patients who present with fatigue or mild dyspnea on exertion, yet do not have any other signs or symptoms of volume overload (strength of evidence = C) (8). Large-scale clinical trials used captopril and enalapril (in doses of 50 mg three times a day and 10 mg twice a day, respectively), but all ACE inhibitors are likely to be effective in treating systolic heart failure, and no particular agent is recommended over another (5). ACE inhibitors are contraindicated in severe renal insufficiency, symptomatic hypotension, and hyperkalemia greater than 5.5 mEq/L; so carefully monitoring of BUN, creatinine, potassium, body weight, and hydration status (similar to using diuretic therapy) can allow titration up to an optimal dose. Once again, patience and careful monitoring are required, as the full effect of ACE inhibitors on functional status may not be seen for several months.

Digoxin is a useful third-line agent. Although there is no evidence that digoxin decreases mortality in patients with systolic dysfunction, it can improve symptoms and prevent clinical deterioration (strength of evidence = A) (9). Thus, it should be added to the medical regimen of patients with mild or moderate heart failure who remain symptomatic after they are treated with optimum doses of ACE inhibitors and diuretics, and it should be used routinely in patients with severe heart failure. Drug levels and potassium levels should be monitored carefully because of digoxin's low toxic-to-therapeutic ratio and the increased toxicity in the setting of hypokalemia. Renal function (BUN and creatinine) should be monitored as well, since a decline in renal function from worsening HF can increase the digoxin level. In addition, drug interactions are common and must be watched for. Table 22.1 lists drug therapies.

In addition to medication interventions, addressing lifestyle issues may be of some benefit, although the evidence is less certain. In general, patients with HF should be discouraged from using more than 2 g of sodium a day, consuming more than one alcoholic drink a day, and drinking excessive fluids (strength of evidence = C) (10). Regular exercise should be encouraged in all patients, except those with dyspnea at rest (strength of evidence = B), although there is insufficient evidence at this time to recommend the routine use of formal rehabilitation programs (10).

Management of Heart Failure (HF) Due to Diastolic Dysfunction

Diastolic dysfunction is the second major class of HF, affecting up to 40% of patients, particularly elderly patients with long-standing hypertension (11). It occurs in the setting of a stiff, noncompliant ventricle with decreased end-diastolic volume and increased end-diastolic pressure. A number of common processes have detrimental effects on ventricular diastolic function, and the differential diagnosis is the same as in systolic dysfunction: coronary artery disease, hypertension, valvular disease, hypertrophic cardiomyopathy, infiltrative cardiomyopathy, and restrictive cardiomyopathy.

The diagnosis is difficult, and a high index of clinical suspicion is necessary. Unless the diastolic dysfunction occurs simultaneously with systolic dysfunction, the echocardiogram will show a normal ejection fraction, the chest radiograph will show a normal-sized heart, and the ECG will not show signs of hypertrophy. Thus, the diagnosis is suggested when the signs and symptoms of heart failure are present in the setting of a normal radiologic evaluation, and it is confirmed when the signs and symptoms of heart failure improve after a therapeutic trial of appropriately selected medications for diastolic dysfunction.

The optimum treatment of diastolic dysfunction is not well defined and currently remains largely trial and error. Although diuretics are still used in the setting of fluid overload, additional agents commonly considered include β blockers, calcium channel blockers, long-acting nitrates, and ACE inhibitors (strength of evidence = C) (6, 12). β Blockers (e.g., propranolol) and calcium channel blockers may enable the stiff left ventricle to fill adequately by delaying the conduction of the electrical impulse across the atrioventricular node; long-acting nitrates may allow the stiff left ventricle to relax in patients who have compromised myocardial function due to chronic small vessel ischemia; and ACE inhibitors may improve left ventricular function, paradoxically, by de-

creasing afterload. Although both β blockers and calcium channel blockers can have negative inotropic effects (and therefore are contraindicated in pure systolic heart failure), they appear to benefit diastolic heart failure.

ARRHYTHMIAS

Arrhythmias typically present as fluttering or palpitations in the chest, although they can present as lightheadedness or syncope if cerebral perfusion is compromised and occasionally as angina if coronary artery perfusion is compromised. Many arrhythmias are asymptomatic; however, because cardiac output and heart rate are only minimally affected; examples include premature heart beats, some forms of heart block, and runs of ventricular tachycardia that are too short (6 to 10 beats) to produce symptoms. Although arrhythmias can arise from extrinsic causes (e.g., certain medications, particularly antiarrhythmic agents themselves, or hyperthyroidism), they usually result from conduction system disease, which can be caused by any of the other three heart syndromes discussed in this chapter. They can be caused by ischemia (because myocardial cells starved for oxygen have difficulty generating a normal electrical impulse), by infarction (because dead myocardial cells cannot generate any electrical impulse), and by heart failure or valve problems that alter the anatomy of the normal conduction pathways.

The arrhythmias are typically classified by two physical findings—rate (fast, slow, or normal) and regularity (or irregularity) of the heart beat—and by two electrocardiographic findings—location (supraventricular or ventricular) and morphology (wide complex or narrow complex) of the electrical impulse. The physical findings are determined by carefully auscultating the heart; the ECG findings are determined by looking for the presence or absence of P waves and measuring the width of the QRS complex .

Premature Heart Beats

Premature atrial contractions (PACs) and premature ventricular contractions (PVCs) are fairly common. They are typically asymptomatic and incidental, with little or no clinical significance. Because they can be provoked by caffeine, nicotine, and emotional stress, lifestyle issues typically need to be addressed. Persistent PACs and PVCs are a little more worrisome and may necessitate an exercise stress test to investigate the possibility of coronary artery disease. This is particularly true if the PVCs are multifocal or occur more than six times a minute.

Bradycardia

Bradycardia (ventricular rate less than 60 beats per minute) is commonly due to medication, ischemia, sinus node dysfunction, and atrial-ventricular (A-V) block. Medication-induced bradycardia is treated by making the appropriate medication adjustment. Ischemia is treated by addressing the underlying cause, although atropine may need to be used temporarily. Sinus node dysfunction and high-grade A-V block are treated with a permanent pacemaker (if the bradycardia is symptomatic).

Regular Narrow Complex Tachycardia: Supraventricular Tachycardia

Narrow complex tachycardias are almost exclusively supraventricular in origin. With the exception of atrial fibrillation, these tachycardias are regular, with a rate that varies depending on the etiology. If the rate is under 180 beats per minute and there is a P wave in front of each QRS complex, it is a sinus tachycardia and is controlled by treating the underlying cause; if there is no P wave, it is a reentry tachycardia and is treated by using medications to slow down the conduction; if the rate is between 150 and 250 beats per minute, there is no P wave, and there is a sawtooth pattern in between the QRS complex, it is atrial flutter and is treated by electrocardioversion (because medications do not work, unlike with atrial fibrillation).

In a reentry tachycardia, various techniques are used to break the fast heart rhythm. Vagal maneuvers are commonly used in the office. The old standby is to vigorously massage the carotid sinuses (although there is a slight risk of dislodging an atherosclerotic plaque using this technique). A more effective vagal maneuver is having the patient lie supine and bear down with the Valsalva maneuver, which has a 55% success rate (13). If these maneuvers are unsuccessful, then either an intravenous (IV) adenosine bolus or an IV diltiazem drip can be used to block the A-V node and slow the heart rate. Once the heart rate is slowed to normal, it can be maintained by blocking the A-V node with digoxin, a β blocker, or a calcium channel blocker, with verapamil being the most effective in preventing recurrence.

Irregular Narrow Complex Tachycardia: Atrial Fibrillation

Atrial fibrillation, which usually presents as a tachycardia, is the most common arrhythmia requiring treatment, affecting approximately 2.2 million persons in the United States (almost 1% of the entire population). Because it is primarily a manifestation of an aging heart (except when it is caused by hyperthyroidism), it is found in the second half of life and occurs with increasing prevalence in each successive decade of life beginning at age 40. It occurs in 5% of patients in their seventies, 10% of patients in their eighties, and 15% of patients in their nineties (14).

Like other arrhythmias, the primary therapeutic objective is to treat the underlying injury to the heart. Other than hyperthyroidism and the occasional reentrant tachyarrhythmia, the disruption of the normal electrical pathway of the left atrium is due to weakening of the atrial muscle from chamber enlargement (atrial size > 4.0 cm), to coronary artery disease, or to both. Chamber enlargement occurs from congestive heart failure, hypertensive heart disease, and/or valvular heart disease.

The workup for new-onset atrial fibrillation simply involves an investigation for the above mechanisms of injury. Typical studies to consider include electrolytes (looking for alteration in sodium, potassium, calcium, and magnesium), glucose (looking for diabetes), thyroid function (looking for hyperthyroidism), ECG (confirming the rhythm and looking for chamber enlargement, myocardial infarction, and left ventricle [LV] strain), echocardiogram (looking for the size of the left atrium and for valvular disease), and exercise stress test (looking for coronary artery disease).

After the underlying injury has been addressed and treated, the management of persistent atrial fibrillation involves three strategies: control of the heart rate if the patient has a rapid ventricular rate (which most patients do), appropriate anticoagulation, and possible cardioversion using chemical or electrical interventions. The first of these, control of the heart rate to less than 90 at rest, is achieved fairly easily by using a loading dose of a rate-controlling agent (e.g., digoxin 0.5 mg initially and then 0.25 mg every 4 hours times two), followed by a maintenance dose of digoxin (0.125 to 0.5 mg/day), verapamil (120 to 240 mg/day), or propranolol (80 to 320 mg/day). Digoxin has the advantage of not adversely affecting blood pressure but has the disadvantage of being less effective than a calcium channel blocker or β blocker in regulating paroxysmal (i.e., intermittent) atrial fibrillation or controlling heart rate during exercise. Table 22.1 lists drug therapies for arrhythmias.

Anticoagulation is usually necessary because of the risk of stroke from embolism of a left atrial thrombus. The risk of stroke averages 4.5% per year for untreated patients with atrial fibrillation (14). Although aspirin or no medication can be used in the patient less than 65 years old who has no other risk factors (i.e., an otherwise healthy heart and no known atherosclerosis), patients with comorbid heart disease or over age 65 should be treated with warfarin, thinning the blood to a target international normalized ratio (INR) between 2.0 and 3.0 (strength of evidence = A). Although warfarin is not a benign medication (average rate of intracranial hemorrhage = 0.3% per year), it can decrease the annual risk of stroke by two thirds (15). The use of warfarin is also expensive and labor intensive, as it requires monthly phlebotomies for INR levels to prevent either overcoagulation or undercoagulation. It may not be a good idea in the frail elderly patient who falls frequently.

Because the presence of atrial fibrillation will increase the risk of stroke and decrease the cardiac output by 10%, many patients are considered for chemical or electrical cardioversion if they do not spontaneously convert after decreasing the stress on the left atrium by controlling the heart rate, improving oxygenation, and diuresing excessive fluid. Anticoagulation with warfarin is typically initiated as the first step in preparation for cardioversion. Therapeutic INR levels (in the 2.0 to 3.0 range) are desirable for 3 weeks before cardioversion and should be continued for 4 weeks after successful cardioversion. Although older agents such as quinidine and flecainide were once commonly selected for chemical cardioversion, they have been associated with a 1 to 6% yearly proarrhythmia risk (and a 0.8% increased annual mortality rate), and more recent approaches have favored amiodarone (strength of evidence = C), which does not appear to have a proarrhythmic effect even in the setting of congestive heart failure (14). If amiodarone is unsuccessful after a typical dose of 400 mg/day for 4 weeks, then direct current electrocardioversion is a good option, with a 90% success rate. Bear in mind that an elderly patient with an increased atrial diameter of more than

4.0 cm is likely to reconvert to atrial fibrillation and so may not be a good candidate for cardioversion. In even the best of situations, cardioversion is associated with about a 50%-per-year risk of reconverting to atrial fibrillation. Preliminary studies suggest that a maintenance dose of amiodarone (100 to 200 mg/day) may maintain sinus rhythm in as many as 80% of patients at 1 year (strength of evidence = C) (15).

Wide Complex Tachycardia

A wide complex tachycardia, which is frequently fatal, occurs when the ventricular heart rate is over 100 beats per minute and the duration of the QRS complex is greater than 120 msec (i.e., greater than three small boxes on a standard ECG). An irregular wide complex tachycardia is due to ventricular fibrillation, is hemodynamically unstable (i.e., causes hypotension), and must be treated immediately with electrical cardioversion. A regular wide complex tachycardia is due to ventricular tachycardia in 80% of the cases, particularly when there is preexisting coronary artery disease. The other 20% of regular wide complex tachycardias are caused by supraventricular tachycardia (SVT) owing to a preexisting electrical short circuit, from either a bundle branch block or a preexcitation syndrome such as Wolff-Parkinson-White (WPW) syndrome. Reviewing an old ECG should indicate whether there is prior coronary artery disease, bundle branch block, or preexcitation syndrome.

If the wide complex tachycardia is hemodynamically unstable (e.g., the cardiac output is insufficient to deliver adequate blood flow to vital organs, particularly the brain, heart, and kidney), then defibrillation with 200 to 360 Joules is indicated regardless of its cause. Regular ventricular tachycardias that are hemodynamically stable do not require immediate defibrillation and should be treated with intravenous lidocaine, intravenous amiodarone, and—if necessary—synchronized defibrillation at 50 Joules. Wide complex tachycardia due to SVT associated with a bundle branch block is treated with the usual protocols for narrow complex SVT. Wide complex tachycardia due to a preexcitation syndrome is treated with an intravenous β blocker such as esmolol or metoprolol.

Although there is no harm in treating a wide complex tachycardia of supraventricular origin with protocols for one of ventricular origin, the converse, treating a wide complex tachycardia of ventricular origin with protocols for one of supraventricular origin, is not benign because medications that block the A-V node (e.g., β blockers and calcium channel blockers) have negative inotropic effects that can cause deterioration of the fragile ventricular function in a ventricular tachycardia. Adenosine, which has an extremely short half-life of 9 seconds, can be used sometimes with reasonable safety to briefly block the A-V node and take a "quick look" at whether the heart rate slows, indicating a true SVT. As a rule of thumb, however, all new-onset wide complex tachycardia, especially if symptomatic, should be considered ventricular in origin until proven otherwise.

The traditional three treatment options of observation, medication, and electrical cardioversion for wide complex tachycardia are now augmented with a fourth option: direct mechanical intervention through the use of radiofrequency catheter ablation (RFCA) or an implantable cardioverter-defibrillator (ICD). RFCA is primarily useful in the subset of patients with recurrent tachyarrhythmias who have an accessory pathway (less than 5% patients with tachyarrhythmias). An ICD, although expensive (nearly $50,000 per implantation), has been useful in preventing fatal arrhythmias in survivors of cardiac arrest as well as in patients who have an inducible (i.e., reproducible) ventricular tachycardia in the laboratory. The Food and Drug Administration has recently approved the ICD for nonsustained, asymptomatic ventricular tachycardia in the postmyocardial patient, as a preliminary research study has shown a 50% decreased death rate in this population (16).

VALVULAR HEART DISEASE

With the advent of widespread treatment of streptococcal pharyngitis in the modern era, the incidence of rheumatic heart disease has dropped dramatically. Although valvular heart disease can still occur from congenital causes (A-V cushion defect in Down's syndrome), other infectious causes (endocarditis), and papillary muscle injury (myocardial infarction), the current most common cause is aortic stenosis due to the calcification associated with the aging process. Similar to other chronic cardiac diseases, the diagnosis of aortic stenosis is often subtle and dependent upon observing the gradual development of HF in the setting of a patient with a harsh systolic murmur in the aortic region of the precordium. Treatment is

directed toward controlling the resultant heart failure, which includes the judicious use of diuretics and digoxin. ACE inhibitors should be avoided because they only increase the pressure drop across the aortic valve and do not decrease the workload on the myocardial muscles. Serial echocardiograms (once a year or so) are useful to monitor the aortic valve area. Uncontrolled symptoms or an aortic valve area of less than 0.75 cm^2 is considered an indication for valve replacement unless age and comorbid conditions contraindicate surgery.

CASE STUDY

Mr. Smith is a 60-year-old, mildly obese diabetic patient with no previous cardiac history who presents to your office with a 2-week history of progressive shortness of breath on exertion, associated ankle swelling, and a 12-pound weight gain. He has not had chest pain but does recall an episode of acute diaphoresis and nausea that occurred while shoveling snow 2 weeks ago. He felt quite anxious at the time, but his symptoms resolved within 3 hours at home with rest. Over the past 2 days, he has become short of breath after walking more than a few steps, and he has noticed a fluttering in his chest. He slept in a chair last night so that he could breathe easier.

On physical examination, his blood pressure is 100/60, his heart rate 110, his respirations 28, and his temperature 37.2°C. He appears mildly breathless but otherwise is cooperative and does not appear in acute distress. His neck is supple, but he has jugular venous distention to the angle of his jaw. Lung examination shows bilateral rales two-thirds the way up his posterior hemithorax, dullness to percussion at the left lung base when compared to the right, and slight wheezing on expiration. Palpation of his anterior chest shows his PMI to be displaced to the left axillary line at the 6th intercostal space. Percussion confirms an enlarged cardiac silhouette, and auscultation reveals an irregularly irregular heart rhythm that is slightly fast, an early diastolic murmur at the apex that is new, and a faint S3. Abdominal examination shows mild hepatomegaly and slight dullness at the flanks, but no fluid wave. The extremity examination is remarkable for 2+ edema to the midthighs bilaterally and slightly diminished peripheral pulses, but no cyanosis.

QUESTIONS

1. What heart syndromes are involved?
2. What was the probable sequence of events?
3. How will you treat each of the heart syndromes?

DISCUSSION

Based on the history and physical alone, you should be able to determine that Mr. Smith is suffering from all four heart syndromes. In regard to coronary circulation, Mr. Smith describes a 3-hour history of angina which sounds as if, as subsequent events showed, he had a myocardial infarction. Because he is diabetic, you are not surprised that he did not have chest pain. In regard to his cardiac pump, you deduce that he has had a pump failure with diminished cardiac output resulting in hypotension, pulmonary edema, hepatomegaly, ascites, and peripheral edema. You diagnose class III heart failure, most likely systolic in origin. In regard to his heart rhythm, you diagnose an atrial fibrillation with a rapid ventricular rate. In regard to his heart valves, you diagnose a mitral insufficiency.

The sequence of events appears to have been initiated by the silent myocardial infarction. You suspect that a moderately large portion of the myocardium has been involved, since Mr. Smith has gradually slipped into heart failure, but not a massive amount, because he did not develop acute pulmonary edema. Because a large portion of the heart has been affected, you expect the ECG to show an anterior wall myocardial infarction with either a septal or lateral wall extension to have damaged

the mitral valve leaflets, resulting in the mitral insufficiency. The atrial fibrillation may have resulted from the circulation problems but appears to be a more recent development, likely resulting from atrial distention form the increasing fluid overload.

Treatment of the heart failure will involve using diuretics to remove the excess fluid, and the patient will likely need an ACE inhibitor and possibly digoxin (depending on the degree of heart failure still present once the patient has been stabilized). Treatment of the angina that has developed into a myocardial infarction will require aspirin, a β blocker, and possibly a nitrate (if there is a suspicion of ongoing ischemia). Treatment of the atrial arrhythmia will require warfarin because the mitral insufficiency represents comorbid heart disease. A rate-controlling agent will not be indicated initially because the mild tachycardia is likely a compensatory increase in heart rate to maintain a more-adequate cardiac output in the setting of decreased blood pressure. Likewise, medical or electrical cardioversion should be postponed because diuresis of the excess fluid will decrease the distention of the left atrium and may very well cause spontaneous conversion to a normal sinus rhythm. Treatment of the mitral insufficiency will be directed to treating the heart failure with diuretics and ACE inhibitors, although the degree of dysfunction will need to be carefully monitored, and valve replacement could conceivably be needed in the future.

You admit the patient to your local hospital to complete the workup, to stabilize the patient, and to confirm your suspicions.

Acknowledgments

We wish to acknowledge Dr. Donald O. Kollisch for the conceptual framework used in this chapter.

REFERENCES

1. Kollisch D, Sloane PD. Chronic cardiac disease. In: Sloane PD, Slatt LM, Curtis P, eds. Essentials of Family Medicine, 2nd ed. Baltimore: Williams & Wilkins, 1993.

2. Braunwald E, et al. Unstable Angina: Diagnosis and Management. Clinical Practice Guideline, no. 10. ACHPR publication no. 94–0602. Rockville, MD: US Department of Health and Human Services, Public Health Service, Agency for Health Care Policy and Research, March 1994:1–154.
3. Ryan TJ, et al. ACC/AHA guidelines for the management of patients with acute myocardial infarction. J Am Coll Cardiol 1996;28(5):1328–1428.
4. Parmley WW. Pathophysiology of congestive heart failure. Clin Cardiol 1992;15(suppl I):I-5-I-12.
5. Kelly RA, Smith TW. Digoxin in heart failure: implications of recent trials. J Am Coll Cardiol 1993; 22(suppl A):107A–112A.
6. Stevenson LW. Modern management of heart failure. Hosp Pract 1996;31(3):103–119.
7. Karon BL. Diagnosis and outpatient management of congestive heart failure. Mayo Clin Proc 1995;70: 1080–1085.
8. Lange RA, Hillis LD. Management of dilated cardiomyopathy. Hosp Pract 1993;28(5A):45–53.
9. Garg R, Gorlin R. The effect of digoxin mortality and morbidity in patients with heart failure. N Engl J Med 1997;336(8):525–533.
10. Baker DW, et al. Management of heart failure. I. Pharmacologic treatment. JAMA 1994;272(17):1361–1366.
11. Udelson JE, Bonow RO. Diastolic dysfunction as a cause of heart failure. Hosp Pract 1993;28(10A):49–56.
12. Mair FS. Management of heart failure. Am Fam Physician 1996;54(1):245–254.
13. Delbridge TR, Yealy DM. Wide complex tachycardia. Emerg Med Clin North Am 1995;13(4):903–923.
14. Pieper SJ, Stanton JS. Narrow QRS complex tachycardias. Mayo Clin Proc 1995;70:371–375.
15. Ukani ZA. Contemporary management of atrial fibrillation. Med Clin North Am 1995;79(5):1135–1152.
16. Biblio LA, et al. Treating ventricular arrhythmias in primary care. Patient Care 1996:10–30.

23. Diabetes Mellitus

SAMUEL S. WEIR AND TIMOTHY J. IVES

Key Clinical Questions

1. Which type of diabetes does this patient have?
2. How is this patient coping with diabetes?
3. For this patient, what is the hardest thing about living with diabetes?
4. How can I (we) support this patient's attempts to care for his or her condition?
5. How can I (we) help this patient to reduce the risks of complications from diabetes?
6. How can I (we) help this patient to maintain acceptable levels of blood lipids, blood glucose, and blood pressure?

BACKGROUND

Diabetes mellitus is a common, chronic, and incurable medical condition that often is accompanied by severe complications. It includes three separate conditions: type I, or insulin-dependent diabetes (IDDM); type II, or non-insulin-dependent diabetes mellitus (NIDDM); and gestational diabetes. Management of diabetes includes both lifestyle adjustment and medications. Nearly all patients with diabetes benefit from a low-fat, high-fiber diet with reduced intake of simple carbohydrates. Increasing physical activity reduces the insulin resistance of NIDDM and gestational diabetes and reduces the need for exogenous insulin among those with IDDM. The most successful clinicians work to support and encourage each patient's coping strategies and help their patients problem solve the day-to-day issues involved in living with diabetes.

Management focuses on metabolic control, on supporting self care, and on preventing complications. A team approach is essential in caring for diabetic patients. The goal of this chapter is to provide a general approach to the primary care of patients with diabetes.

EPIDEMIOLOGY AND PATHOPHYSIOLOGY

In 1995, about 16 million persons in the United States had diabetes mellitus. Ninety-five percent of these cases were type II, or NIDDM (1). Type II diabetes is a disease of adults (usually over age 40) that presents insidiously and occurs more commonly in obese persons, sedentary persons, and those with a high-fat diet. African Americans, Hispanics, and Native Americans are all at increased risk, as are those with a family history of type II diabetes. As the population in the United States ages and fattens, the prevalence of type II diabetes is increasing and has been recently estimated at 7% (2).

In contrast, 5% of cases are type I, or IDDM. Type I diabetes occurs more commonly in those under age 40, presents acutely as weight loss, polyuria, polydipsia, and polyphagia, and can present as an emergency in the form of diabetic ketoacidosis.

Diabetes is both a disease and a risk factor for other diseases. Both type II and type I diabetes accelerate atherosclerosis in major blood vessels, making diabetes an important risk factor for ischemic heart disease, peripheral vascular disease, and stroke. These macrovascular complications are the major cause of death among persons with diabetes (1). As many as 75% of persons with diabetes die as a result of these cardiovascular complications (3). Premenopausal women with diabetes lose their gender advantage over men relative to cardiovascular disease rates by virtue of their disease, and they have nearly the same cardiovascular disease rates as similarly aged men without diabetes (4). Diabetes is the leading cause of lower extremity amputations in the United States, with diabetic patients being at 15 times' greater risk than nondiabetic patients (1).

Besides these macrovascular complications, diabetes mellitus affects small blood vessels, leading to blindness, nephropathy, and neuropathy. Renal failure is the second most common cause of death and disability, occurring in about 10% of persons with diabetes. African-American women are at greatest risk of this complication. In 1992, 56,059 people with diabetes were treated with dialysis or transplantation for end-stage renal disease: 36% of all cases of end-stage renal disease in this country (1). Annual mortality for patients with diabetes and end-stage renal failure (ESRF) in the United States is 25% (5). Diabetic retinopathy is the most frequent cause of new blindness in American adults (aged 20 to 74), with approximately 20,000 new cases per year (1).

In addition to these complications, diabetes often clusters with other risk factors for vascular disease. Sixty-five percent of persons with diabetes also have high blood pressure—increasing the risk of cardiovascular disease, stroke, peripheral vascular disease, end-stage renal failure, and blindness (1). Close to 55% of patients with diabetes have significantly raised blood lipid levels (Weir S, LaForge B, Hafer K. Diabetes Registry from Kaiser Foundation Health Plan of North Carolina. Unpublished data, 1997). This clustering of cardiovascular risk factors among patients with type II diabetes has been referred to as "syndrome X" (6).

The central feature of all types of diabetes is hyperglycemia. Many variables, ranging from biologic to psychosocial, affect blood glucose levels among patients with diabetes. Commonly encountered biologic factors include level of physical activity, physiologic stress (e.g., infection, surgery, trauma), hormonal changes (e.g., the menstrual cycle), other medications, and meal timing, composition, and amount. Psychosocial factors include depression, acute stress, and anxiety.

Type I or Juvenile-Onset Diabetes Mellitus (IDDM)

Type I diabetes occurs primarily in children and young adults. Sophisticated twin studies indicate a very strong genetic component to the etiology to type I diabetes (6). It is more common in those with certain HLA types and is the result of autoimmune destruction of the beta cells of the pancreas. Currently, this genetic susceptibility is thought to be activated by viral infections (e.g., Coxsackie virus) that trigger an autoimmune destructive process. The usual abrupt clinical onset of IDDM as diabetic ketoacidosis (DKA) is usually preceded by a more gradual loss of beta cell function over several months to years. As a result of this beta cell damage, patients are totally insulin deficient and require multiple insulin injections (at least twice a day) to survive.

Type II or Non-Insulin-Dependent Diabetes Mellitus (NIDDM)

Type II diabetes (NIDDM) has both genetic and environmental causes. Twin studies demonstrate a greater than 30% concordance among monozygotic twin pairs in the expression of type II diabetes (7). Type II diabetes is rare in persons less than age 30, and if it does present in this age group, it is termed maturity-onset diabetes of youth (MODY). Incidence of type II diabetes increases with increasing age and with increasing body mass index (2). Certain racial groups, as previously mentioned, are at increased risk for type II diabetes. Both a sedentary lifestyle and a high-fat diet increase the risk of type II diabetes (6, 7). Finally, both impaired glucose tolerance and glucose intolerance of pregnancy are risk factors for subsequent type II diabetes (6–8).

The inherited trait(s) causing type II diabetes are forms of insulin resistance. This insulin resistance occurs at different sites within the body, including the muscle (decreased uptake and storage of glucose) and the liver (inappropriate increased glucose production) (9). It is unclear whether this insulin resistance is primary or secondary to high circulating levels of free fatty acids (10). The trait of insulin resistance (the so-called "thrifty gene") may have conferred a survival advantage in an environment of frequent feast-famine cycles in past centuries (11). Unfortunately, in the current environment of all feast with no famine, it may lead to central obesity and type II diabetes in those with less pancreatic reserve.

CLINICAL EVALUATION

History

Type II diabetes has mild, nonspecific symptoms of gradual onset; the disease often goes undetected for years. The average case of type II diabetes in the United States has been present for more than 5 years prior to detection (2). Therefore, clinicians should foster a high index of suspicion for the disease among patients with one or more risk factors. The following signs and symptoms should alert the clinician to possible type II diabetes:

- *General:* weight loss, fatigue, chronic malaise, gradually increasing thirst
- *Dermatologic:* recurrent fungal infections (vaginal, dermatophytic, intertrigo, etc.), slow healing of skin injuries

- *Ophthalmologic:* recent visual changes (often requiring a change in refractive correction), blurred vision (caused by osmotic and fluid changes in the lens due to hyperglycemia)
- *Dental:* periodontal disease
- *Urinary:* nocturia and polyuria
- *Neurologic:* burning, tingling, numbness in feet and/or hands

Less commonly, and most often in geriatric populations, type II diabetes may present acutely as nonketotic, hyperosmolar, hyperglycemic syndrome, with confusion, lethargy, prostration, malaise, and occasionally coma. Such patients have profound dehydration and weight loss. Hyperglycemia is marked (as high as 2000 mg/dL), with hyperosmolality and little or no ketosis.

In contrast, IDDM typically presents acutely as diabetic ketoacidosis (DKA). Patients with IDDM, usually children or adolescents, describe a rapid onset of some or all of the classic symptoms of diabetes: polyuria (frequent urination), polydipsia (frequent drinking due to chronic excessive thirst), polyphagia (frequent eating), weight loss, and fatigue. The seasonal incidence of type I diabetes parallels that of viral infections, with more cases presenting in winter and early spring.

In newly diagnosed patients, take a careful history of prior symptoms of diabetes. Patients with newly discovered NIDDM can often recall months or even years of previous nocturia, visual difficulties, or recurrent candidal vaginitis before the discovery of their disease. Ask patients about their family history of diabetes and its complications. This underscores the complications for which they are at risk and brings out their previous experience with diabetes.

Evaluation of risk factors for vascular complications should include careful questioning of smoking habits, previous blood pressures, previous lipid measurements, and family history of cardiovascular disease. Assessment of current complications can begin with history items aimed at discovering visual difficulties, problems with periodontal disease, cardiovascular history, sexual dysfunction, and problems with peripheral neuropathy. Prior ophthalmologic, dental, or podiatric care should be noted. A recent population-based epidemiology study found that the simple question, "Thinking now of *both* legs or *both* feet, have you had pain or discomfort such as numbness, burning, or tingling when you are not walking in the past 6 months?" is a valuable predictor of the presence of peripheral neuropathy. This history question had a 97% sensitivity when compared with the gold standard of a formal neurologic examination by a neurologist (13).

Physical Examination

Pay particular attention to the patient's blood pressure, weight, and height. (Body mass index is calculated as weight (kg)/[height (m)]^2; those with values less than 27 are not considered to be obese, those with a body mass index (BMI) of 27 or greater are obese.)

Examination of the eyes (dilated), dentition, heart and peripheral pulses, feet and legs, and the peripheral neurologic system should be meticulously documented at the initial evaluation because these organs are the targets of microvascular disease.

The monofilament foot examination identifies patients at high risk of subsequent foot ulcer and provides an opportunity for teaching foot care to patients (12). A nylon monofilament is held perpendicular to the skin surface and pressed against the skin of the foot until it buckles. The inability of a patient to feel the end of the monofilament while buckled predicts a higher risk of subsequent foot ulcer (13). Compared with the measurement of pedal pulses and vibration perception threshold, the monofilament examination had over 85% reproducibility between different examiners and different times and was the only test judged to be satisfactory (14, 15).

All type II patients should have a retinal screening examination as part of the initial evaluation and annually thereafter. Either a dilated retinal physical examination or the examination of retinal photographs may be used for this screening (16). Examination of retinal photos has a sensitivity of 100% and a specificity of 82% for serious retinopathy requiring intervention compared with the gold standard of a dilated examination by an ophthalmologist. In many health care systems, retinal photography is more convenient and accessible than an ophthalmologist, and is also less expensive (17).

Although the history and physical examination may raise strong suspicions for diagnosis of diabetes, it can only be confirmed by laboratory testing (Fig. 23.1).

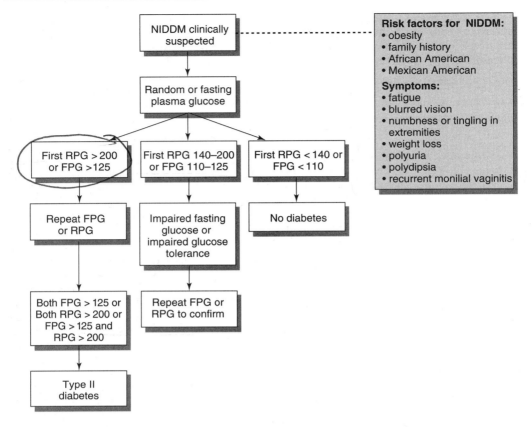

Figure 23.1. *Diagnosis of diabetes by laboratory testing.*

Laboratory Tests

The criteria for diagnosis of diabetes mellitus or impaired glucose tolerance in the nonpregnant adult are at least two occasions on separate days in which one of the following is observed:

- A random plasma glucose measurement greater than or equal to 200 mg/dL plus the classic symptoms (polyuria, polydipsia, and unexplained weight loss) of diabetes, or

- A fasting plasma glucose measurement greater than or equal to 126 mg/dL (fasting is defined as no caloric intake for at least 8 hours), or

- A 2-hour postglucose load measurement greater than or equal to 200 mg/dL. The test is performed using a glucose load containing the equivalent of 75 g of anhydrous glucose dissolved in water (18).

The oral glucose tolerance test (OGTT) is not recommended for routine use because of its poor reproducibility (18). Despite the fact that a HbA_{1C} level greater than or equal to 7.0% is a very sensitive and specific measure of diabetes, it has not been chosen as a criterion for making the diagnosis of diabetes because of lack of standardization of the test (18).

However, an oral glucose tolerance test may be helpful if the initial plasma glucose results are equivocal. The OGTT consists of drinking a 75-g oral glucose load after an 8-hour fast, with plasma glucose measured beforehand (fasting) and 2 hours afterward. For a diagnosis of diabetes, the 2-hour measurement must equal or exceed 200 mg/dL on at least two occasions.

Laboratory Monitoring

The HbA_{1C} test documents the average blood glucose levels in the 3 months immediately prior to testing. Similar tests include the total glycosylated hemoglobin test and the fructosamine test, which measure the percentage of serum proteins that are glycosylated (19). The reported value is directly proportional to the average blood glucose concentration over the life span of the patient's circulating red cells (120 days).

The HbA$_{1C}$ assay (or the related assays mentioned above) does not give any information about the range of blood glucose levels over the same period. A mean glucose level of 150 mg/dL might occur with a range between 100 and 200; the same mean concentration could occur with a range that varied between 50 and 250. These two vastly different situations call for different therapeutic responses, but they both result in the same HbA$_{1C}$ result. Despite these limitations, the HbA$_{1C}$ test is an important tool in managing diabetic patients. Regular use of this test results in improved glucose control in patients with IDDM (20).

A random urine albumin/creatinine ratio can document the presence or absence of microalbuminuria and thus monitor renal damage (5). In one study of Pima Indians, this test had a sensitivity of 82% and a specificity of 76% for subsequent nephropathy at 4.2 years of follow-up (21). This test represents a significant improvement over the 24-hour collection and is now considered the screening test of choice (2). Figure 23.2 summarizes the use of the albumin/ creatinine ratio to screen for microalbumin.

Differential Diagnosis

Diabetic ketoacidosis needs to be distinguished from other forms of ketosis, especially alcoholic ketosis and poisoning with methanol. Hyperosmolar nonketotic hyperglycemic syndrome should to be suspected in any elderly patient with delirium or unexplained recent changes in behavior.

Acute hyperglycemia in a patient presenting in stress due to trauma or pain may not represent previously undiagnosed diabetes. A HbA$_{1C}$ test can be useful in assessing whether the hyperglycemia is due to an acute stress or diabetes. In the hospital, acute hyperglycemia occurs most commonly on the cardiac care unit. Unfortunately, many of these patients will discover that they have not only heart disease but also previously undetected NIDDM.

Diabetes mellitus is usually unrelated to other disease processes but occasionally may be secondary to steroid therapy and to other conditions such as hypothyroidism or hemochromatosis. Other signs and symptoms of hypothyroidism include being cold natured, having noted dry-

ness of the skin and hair, and experiencing constipation, fatigue, and delayed relaxation of the deep tendon reflexes, especially at the ankle. Hemochromatosis, a disease of iron overload, often presents with liver disease, joint complaints, and occasionally diabetes mellitus (22).

The physician is responsible for communicating the diagnosis in a way that the patient can understand. The diagnosis of diabetes mellitus should not be made prematurely, as it labels a patient, from employment and insurance perspectives, as being at high risk for cardiovascular and other diseases. On the other hand, diabetes is a serious condition, and it is inappropriate to tell patients that they have "just a touch of sugar."

Most people with diabetes experience the discovery of their disease as a loss and can be expected to have reactions that will likely include anger, depression, and denial. A perceptive physician will be aware of these emotions and help the patient cope with these natural emotional responses. In addition to assessing the emotional response of the patient, it is appropriate for the health care team to express understanding and empathy regarding the patient's situation. Many patients with newly discovered diabetes have family members who have experienced complications of the disease, and their diagnosis will bring these memories to the forefront.

MANAGEMENT

The diagnosis of diabetes mellitus prompts a comprehensive initial management plan. With type II diabetes, the most appropriate strategy is to briefly discuss the diagnosis and initial therapy with the patient and to schedule a return visit as soon as possible for a full evaluation (Fig. 23.3). This initial medical evaluation has three goals:

- Assessing the patient's psychologic reactions to the diagnosis of diabetes
- Assessing associated risk factors for macrovascular and microvascular disease
- Assessing any current complications

In addition, *and when they are receptive to learning more about their disease,* newly diagnosed patients deserve thorough education about the disease, its behavioral treatment, and the signs and symptoms of hypoglycemia, hyperglycemia, and common complications. Most often, this education

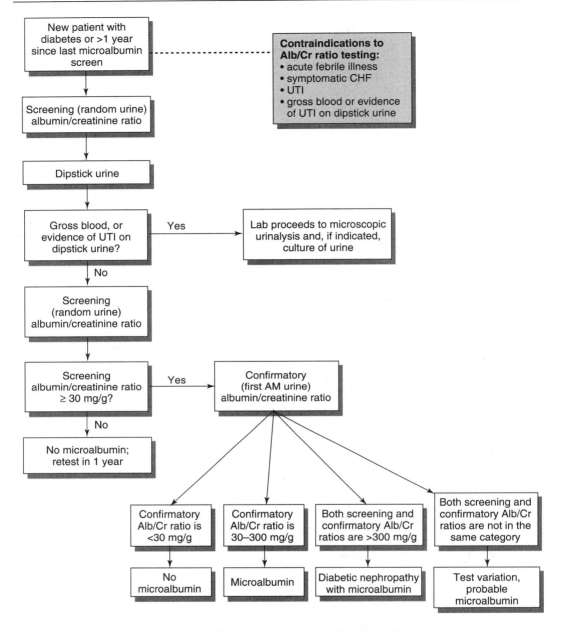

Figure 23.2. *Monitoring renal function in diabetes.*

is done by a member of the physician's staff, preferably one who is a certified diabetes educator. A team approach is appropriate in educating and caring for patients with diabetes, but the patient **must receive** two consistent messages from everyone: (a) diabetes is a serious medical condition, and (b) lifestyle modification (eating habits,

activity level) plays a crucial part of the management of diabetes (23).

Therapeutic Considerations

As the primary care physician of a patient with diabetes, you should work with the patient to

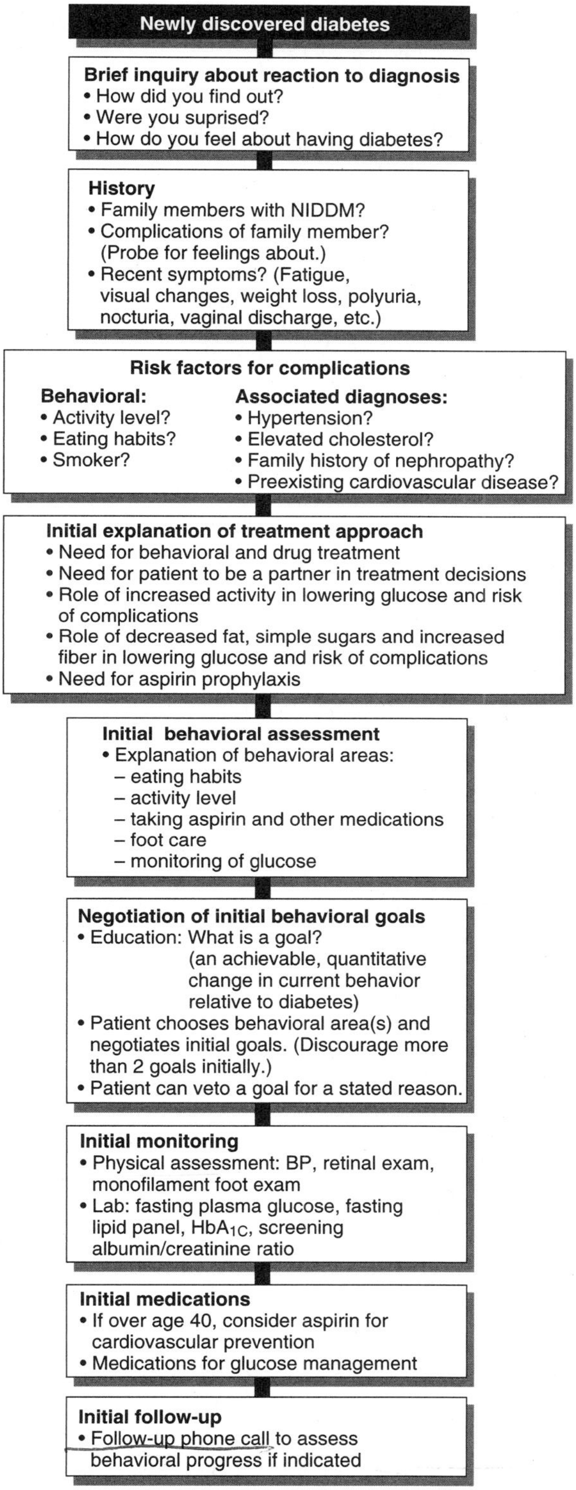

Newly discovered diabetes

Brief inquiry about reaction to diagnosis
• How did you find out?
• Were you suprised?
• How do you feel about having diabetes?

History
• Family members with NIDDM?
• Complications of family member?
  (Probe for feelings about.)
• Recent symptoms? (Fatigue,
  visual changes, weight loss, polyuria,
  nocturia, vaginal discharge, etc.)

Risk factors for complications

Behavioral:
• Activity level?
• Eating habits?
• Smoker?

Associated diagnoses:
• Hypertension?
• Elevated cholesterol?
• Family history of nephropathy?
• Preexisting cardiovascular disease?

Initial explanation of treatment approach
• Need for behavioral and drug treatment
• Need for patient to be a partner in treatment decisions
• Role of increased activity in lowering glucose and risk
  of complications
• Role of decreased fat, simple sugars and increased
  fiber in lowering glucose and risk of complications
• Need for aspirin prophylaxis

Initial behavioral assessment
• Explanation of behavioral areas:
  – eating habits
  – activity level
  – taking aspirin and other medications
  – foot care
  – monitoring of glucose

Negotiation of initial behavioral goals
• Education: What is a goal?
            (an achievable, quantitative
            change in current behavior
            relative to diabetes)
• Patient chooses behavioral area(s) and
  negotiates initial goals. (Discourage more
  than 2 goals initially.)
• Patient can veto a goal for a stated reason.

Initial monitoring
• Physical assessment: BP, retinal exam,
  monofilament foot exam
• Lab: fasting plasma glucose, fasting
  lipid panel, HbA_{1C}, screening
  albumin/creatinine ratio

Initial medications
• If over age 40, consider aspirin for
  cardiovascular prevention
• Medications for glucose management

Initial follow-up
• Follow-up phone call to assess
  behavioral progress if indicated

Figure 23.3. *Management of the newly discovered diabetic patient.*

achieve a level of blood glucose that is normal as much of the time as possible, while avoiding severe hypoglycemic episodes. There are two reasons for this overall goal.

First, the patient will feel better. Explain to patients that they can look forward to sleep uninterrupted by nocturia, vision that is clear, and enough energy to complete their daily activities. Normalizing blood glucose concentrations improves quality of life for these patients.

Second, patients will reduce their risk of microvascular complications. The Diabetes Care and Complications Trial proved that sustained levels of values of HbA_{1C} below 8% are associated with a decreased incidence and progression of retinopathy, nephropathy, and neuropathy in patients with IDDM (24, 25).

The major unresolved controversy is how to apply the results of this significant research to the much larger population of patients with NIDDM. Although most diabetologists agree that intensive insulin therapy and improved glucose levels will reduce the risk of microvascular complications in patients with type II diabetes, there is much debate about the value of intensive insulin therapy in cardiovascular complications (26).

Data from both cross-sectional and prospective observational studies suggest an association between glycemic control and cardiovascular mortality (27). Unfortunately, because glucose concentrations increase with increasing duration of NIDDM, it is unclear whether these observations indicate a direct relationship between blood sugar concentrations and the risk of cardiovascular disease or a relationship between duration of NIDDM (and its associated clustering of other known vascular risk factors) and cardiovascular disease.

The ongoing United Kingdom Prospective Diabetes Study should help answer the important question of whether NIDDM should be managed with "tight" glycemic control (28).

Behavioral Management

The cornerstone of diabetes management in all patients is the modification of behavior. The crucial nature of managing and monitoring their own behavior must be repetitively stressed to patients. Increasing physical activity and eating foods that are low in fat, low in concentrated sugars, and high in fiber are central features of virtually all diabetes care plans.

Exercise

Increased physical activity reduces insulin resistance by depleting muscle glycogen and inducing the enzymes associated with glucose storage. Its practical value can be demonstrated to patients with a treadmill session in the office or, more commonly, a 15- to 20-minute walk. Capillary glucose is measured before and after 20 minutes of activity and almost always documents a significant decrease in the patient's blood glucose. For patients with type II diabetes, additional benefits to exercise include reductions in blood pressure and body weight and an increase in the HDL cholesterol.

Walking, stretching, calisthenics, and swimming are excellent activities. For older patients or those not in good physical condition, exercise should begin slowly and only after an evaluation of their cardiovascular status. Patients at significant risk for ischemic heart disease (over age 40 with other risk factors or over age 50) should be evaluated with a formal exercise stress test prior to strenuous exercise.

Two possible complications of exercise are unique to diabetes. First, patients taking insulin or oral hypoglycemic agents should be warned about hypoglycemia during or after exercise. They should be instructed to have a form of glucose or sucrose available (e.g., Life-Saver candies or fruit). Second, in IDDM patients who have little or no insulin in their systems (i.e., no injection within 12 hours), preexercise glucose values greater than 250 mg/dL combined with exercise can result in hyperglycemia and ketosis.

Diet

Dietary management of patients with NIDDM should focus on four general principles:

- Increasing the proportion of calories from complex carbohydrates (e.g., pasta, whole-grain bread, grains) and avoiding simple sugars (e.g., cakes, cookies, pies, pastries, regular sodas, candy).

- Avoiding fat, especially saturated (meat and dairy) fats

- Managing weight

- When on insulin, synchronizing meals with the peak action of insulin

Dietary guidelines for patients with diabetes are provided in Table 23.1. Avoiding simple carbohydrates and encouraging the eating of com-

Table 23.1.
American Diabetes Association Dietary Guidelines

Nutrient	Recommended Distribution of Calories (%)
Carbohydrates	55–60
Protein	15–20
Fat (total)	<30
Saturated fat	<10
Polyunsaturated	<10
Monounsaturated	10–15

Nutrient	Recommended Daily Intake
Protein	0.8 g/kg of ideal body weight
Fiber	35–40 g/day, with 50% coming from soluble fibers such as dried beans, lentils, oats, guar gum
Cholesterol	<300 mg/day
Sodium	<3000 mg/day

plex carbohydrates and high-fiber foods will reduce insulin resistance and, calorie for calorie, will improve serum glucose levels. Low fat consumption, favoring polyunsaturated and monounsaturated fats (e.g., canola oil or olive oil), will reduce insulin resistance and help normalize plasma lipid values. For patients who are obese (BMI > 27), weight loss improves insulin sensitivity. The dietary guidelines published by the American Diabetes Association (see Table 23.1) should be reviewed with patients.

The final principle applies to patients maintained on insulin therapy, especially IDDM patients. The number of calories consumed should remain fairly constant from day to day, and the timing of meals (or snacks) should correspond to the times when the action of insulin, either regular or long-acting, is at its peak. Individuals taking multiple daily injections of regular insulin or those on an insulin infusion device have greater flexibility in the timing of meals.

These dietary principles can be highlighted and reinforced by the physician, but they also need to be supplemented by detailed suggestions for behavioral change by a diabetes educator who can tailor these nutritional principles to the patient's own situation. Dietary change rarely occurs quickly; gradual changes in eating habits are more common. Negotiating one to three goals at each office visit is reasonable.

Although type II patients are often overweight and weight loss is an appropriate therapeutic goal for clinicians, weight loss (or a particular target weight) is seldom a useful goal *for the patient*. The patient's progress toward achieving behavioral goals is of greater importance. Patients find it difficult to lose weight, and this is even more difficult after blood glucose values are normalized. The goal is to provide each patient with a success that he or she can savor. Define success in behavioral terms: starting a walking program or changing to a lower-fat milk.

Pharmacotherapy of Diabetes

For many patients, behavioral management alone will not be enough. Fasting plasma glucose levels will remain above 150 mg/dL, and symptoms such as nocturia or vulvar candidiasis will remain. For these patients or those with a HbA_{1C} level above 7.0%, drug therapy is recommended to supplement the behavioral methods outlined above. There are now four different classes of oral agents available in the outpatient setting: the sulfonylureas, a biguanide (metformin), a thiazolidinedione (troglitazone), and an α-glucosidase inhibitor (acarbose).

Sulfonylurea Drugs: The Original Oral Hypoglycemic Agents

Sulfonylureas lower blood glucose by stimulating insulin secretion by the pancreas and by increasing tissue sensitivity to insulin. Seven different sulfonylurea agents are available; they are divided into first-generation drugs (acetohexamide, chlorpropamide, tolazamide, and tolbutamide) and second-generation drugs (glipizide, glyburide, and glimepiride) primarily by virtue of their date of introduction.

Although sharing a common mechanism of action, these agents vary in their relative potency, duration of action, metabolism, route of excretion, and adverse effects. The family physician should become familiar with several of these agents (Table 23.2) to accurately monitor efficacy and select the best regimen for the individual patient.

Several general principles guide the use of these agents. First, choose an agent with a relatively short half-life (e.g., tolazamide, glipizide), especially in the elderly, as the most common adverse effect is hypoglycemia. With longer-acting agents (e.g., chlorpropamide), this unfortunate adverse effect can become prolonged and may re-

Table 23.2.
Oral Hypoglycemic Agents

Drug	Daily Dose (mg)	Half-life (hr)	Metabolism/Excretion	Duration of Action (hr)	Equivalent Dose (mg)	Cost (30-Day Supply, Generic if Available)
Acetohexamide	250–1500 in 1–2 doses	1.6 (1–2.5) Metabolite: 5.3 (2–12)	Active liver metabolites	12–18	500	$19.68
Chlorpropamide	100–750 in 1 daily dose	25–62 (av = 34)	70% hepatic metabolism, 30% excreted unchanged via renal elimination (tubular secretion)	24–72	250	$7.95
Tolazamide	100–1000 in 1–2 doses	7	Metabolized to active and inactive products; renal excretion (tubular secretion)	10–24	250	$9.31
Tolbutamide	500–2000 (3000) in 2–4 doses	7 (4–24)	Metabolized to inactive products	6–12	1000	$9.25
Glipizide	2.5–40 in 1–2 doses	6	Converted to inactive metabolites (90% liver/10% kidney)	8–12	5	$23.62
Glyburide	1.25–20 in 1–2 doses	10	Converted to inactive metabolites (50% liver/50% kidney)	10–22	5	$22.24
Glyburide (micronized)	0.75–12 in 1–2 doses	4	Same as with regular-release glyburide	24	3	$22.98
Glimepiride	1–4 in a single daily dose	9	Converted to inactive metabolites	2–3	2	$27.23
Metformin	500–2550 in 1–2 daily doses	4.5	Excreted unchanged in urine	8–12	—	$37.55
Troglitazone	200–600 in a single daily dose	16–34	85% hepatic metabolism	24	—	$116.19

[Handwritten margin notes:]

Sulfonylurea — stimulate insulin secretion from pancreas

Metformin — ↓ hepatic GNG, ↑ peripheral glucose utilization

Troglitazone — ↓ insulin resist in skeletal muscle & adipose

αGlucosidase — Delays digestion & absorption of complex carbs quire hospitalization. Second, several of these agents are now available generically and are much less expensive than their newer counterparts. For patients with limited finances, these agents are still the drugs of choice. Third, start with a low dose, administered 30 minutes prior to the morning meal, with dosage increases every 5 to 7 days. More rapid dosage adjustments are inappropriate and may lead to hypoglycemia after a "steady-state" has been reached. Fourth, when splitting these agents into a twice-daily regimen, give the second dose 30 minutes before the largest meal of the day, usually dinner. Finally, the dosage of these agents may be reduced or the agent discontinued in some patients who become more active and change their eating habits.

The newest agent in this class is glimepiride (Amaryl). It is thought to induce less insulin secretion, supposedly because of a different binding site on cells. Clinical practice, however, has not borne out a distinct advantage over glipizide or glyburide to date. The average daily dose is 4 mg, given in a once-daily regimen (t½ = approximately 9 hours).

A 30-day generic supply of the lowest daily dosage of tolbutamide costs the patient approximately $9.50. With the exception of glimepiride, all of these agents are available generically (29).

Biguanide Drugs: Metformin

Metformin (Glucophage, Bristol-Myers Squibb) is a biguanide agent similar to phenformin, an agent removed from the market in October 1977 due to numerous reports to the Food and Drug Administration (FDA) of fatal lactic acidosis. This agent's primary actions are decreasing hepatic gluconeogenesis and increasing peripheral glucose utilization. As monotherapy or when combined with an oral sulfonylurea, metformin initially reduces mean fasting plasma glucose levels by 60 to 90 mg/dL (a 2.0 to 3.0% reduction in HbA_{1C}) (30). Metformin decreases blood pressure and triglycerides and increases HDL cholesterol (31). Metformin also decreases tissue plasminogen activator, decreases platelet aggregation, and raises plasminogen activator inhibitor-1 (PAI-1), producing a decrease in abnormal clotting activity and an enhanced fibrinolysis. As metformin is renally eliminated, patients with renal insufficiency (i.e., serum creatinine > 1.5 for males or 1.4 for females) are not considered candidates for metformin therapy.

The most common adverse drug events seen with metformin include nausea (seen in 30 to 35% of patients, initially), vomiting, anorexia, diarrhea (30%), and a metallic taste. These effects tend to be transient over 2 to 4 weeks and are often dose-related. If gastrointestinal adverse effects persist, one can try reducing the dose or stopping the drug temporarily. Metformin does not induce hypoglycemia, nor does it prevent hypoglycemia from oral sulfonylurea agents or insulin. As this agent and all biguanides inhibit lactate metabolism, lactic acidosis is seen but is very rare with metformin (three cases per 100,000 patient years).

The following patient-related risk factors are associated with a higher incidence of lactic acidosis: patients with renal impairment, concurrent use of intravenous iodinated contrast media; hemodynamically unstable patients, use of diuretics, acute gastrointestinal distress, septicemia, impaired hepatic function, metformin overdose, hypoxemia, and alcohol abuse. In all of these cases, it may be preferable to consider an alternative therapy, such as troglitazone or a sulfonylurea agent. While taking metformin, regular (every 3 to 6 months) monitoring of liver function tests, creatinine, and HbA_{1C} is recommended. In addition, annual monitoring of CBC, fasting plasma lactate, and vitamin B_{12} is appropriate (32).

Metformin is indicated in type II diabetics not responding to a reasonable trial of a diabetic diet for at least 6 to 12 weeks. Metformin may be added to a sulfonylurea in patients who fail to meet treatment goals despite maximal doses of these agents.

The initial oral dose is 500 mg twice daily, with breakfast and dinner, or 850 mg once daily, with breakfast. Some patients may be started on only 500 mg at dinner to decrease the risk of adverse gastrointestinal events. With the 500 mg strength, make dosage increases on a weekly basis only to minimize gastrointestinal adverse drug events and to titrate to the minimum effective dose. With the 850 mg dose, after 2 weeks, increase to one tablet PO twice a day, one with breakfast and one with supper, if the patient is tolerating the drug and the fasting blood glucose > 140 mg/dL. The maximum total daily dose is 2,550 mg, given in divided doses with meals. The 30-day cost of the lowest daily dosage of metformin is $45.05—approximately 4 times the price of generic tolazamide (29).

Thiazolidinediones: Troglitazone

Troglitazone (Rezulin, Parke-Davis), a thiazolidinedione derivative, acts primarily by decreasing peripheral insulin resistance in skeletal muscle and adipose tissue, without augmenting insulin secretion (33). Secondarily, by enhancing insulin action in the liver, the exaggerated glucose production in the liver is lessened. As with metformin, serum triglycerides (20 to 25% reduction) and blood pressure may be lowered and HDL cholesterol may be increased (6 to 18% increases have been observed). Troglitazone therapy lowers blood glucose levels by about 40 mg/dL (1.3% of HbA_{1C}). Other agents in this class, including ciglitazone and piaglitazone, are in clinical trials.

Unlike metformin, troglitazone does not cause lactic acidosis. Because it is excreted by the liver, it is not contraindicated in patients with renal insufficiency. However, liver enzyme elevations (1%) and, rarely, jaundice (0.1%) have been reported with troglitazone. Serum cholesterol may increase while on this drug. As troglitazone is hepatically cleared, obtain a baseline liver panel before initiating therapy. Although troglitazone does not itself induce hypoglycemia, it may increase the effectiveness of insulin, and patients may need to have their insulin regimens adjusted downward to avoid hypoglycemic episodes.

Troglitazone is indicated for the treatment of type II diabetics with poor glycemic control (i.e., $HbA_{1C} > 8.5$) who have to use >30 units/day of insulin. It is not indicated for patients with IDDM. Troglitazone may be appropriate in patients with NIDDM with central adiposity, hypertension, and hypertriglyceridemia who have not met therapeutic goals despite multiple daily insulin injections. Unfortunately, the cost limits its usefulness role even in this population.

The initial dose is 200 mg once daily, with increases, if necessary, up to 600 mg/day. The average dose is 400 mg/day. There is little dose-related increase in effect, with 200 mg having as great a benefit as 400 or 800 mg/day. The bioavailability of this agent is increased when it is taken with food. The cost to the patient for a 30-day supply of the lowest daily dose of this drug is $118.00, more than 40 times the cost of a month supply of generic tolazamide (29). There are no studies showing that patients treated with metformin or troglitazone enjoy better clinical outcomes than patients treated with sulfonylureas.

α-Glucosidase Inhibitors: Acarbose for Miglitol

This class of drugs delays the digestion and absorption of complex carbohydrates (34). These orally administered agents, used primarily as an adjunct in type II patients, work only in the upper gastrointestinal tract, where they inhibit the breakdown of complex carbohydrates from food into simple sugars such as glucose by temporarily inhibiting intestinal α-glucosidase, the primary enzyme that breaks down carbohydrates in the small intestine. Both acarbose (Precose, Bayer) and a second α-glucosidase inhibitor, miglitol (Glyset, Bayer), which entered the market in June, 1997, are available in the United States. Acarbose prevents rapid postprandial blood glucose increases by slowing the rate of digestion and absorption of carbohydrates from the stomach. This mechanism of action is very similar to high (30 g/day) levels of dietary fiber, which also slow the rate of absorption of carbohydrates into the circulation. Use of acarbose lowers fasting blood glucose levels by 15 to 30 mg/dL and postprandial blood glucose by 40 to 54 mg/dL, an effect greater in patients with diets high in complex carbohydrates (equivalent to a reduction of HbA_{1C} of 0.5 to 1.5%). Other potential benefits include no risk of hypoglycemic episodes, no changes in weight, a decrease in nutrient-stimulated insulin secretion, decreased fasting serum triglycerides and cholesterol, and decreased fasting plasma glucose.

Many patients taking acarbose experience gastrointestinal adverse effects such as nausea, diarrhea, borborygmus (loud bowel sounds), bloating, and flatulence ("loud, not smelly"), which occur in over 75% of patients initially and may persist in up to 30% of patients after 6 months of therapy. Increases in liver transaminases (3.8%), and anemia (1%) are also seen; it is unknown if this effect is related to malabsorption of iron. When used in combination with a sulfonylurea or insulin, acarbose potentiates the risk of hypoglycemia from the other agent. Patients taking acarbose need to know that when they experience mild to moderate hypoglycemia, they cannot use table sugar (i.e., sucrose) to treat it. Acarbose inhibits the absorption of table sugar. Oral glucose is appropriate. Because of this, it is appropriate to encourage patients on combination therapy (sulfonylurea and acarbose or insulin and acarbose) to measure blood glucose levels prior to each meal.

Acarbose has been used as monotherapy for mild type II diabetes or added to sulfonylurea therapy. The older regimen starts with 25 mg (i.e., 1/2 tablet) PO three times a day, chewed with the first mouthful of food at a meal. The newer alternative dosing option starts at 25 mg PO every day at the largest meal of the day (usually dinner) for 1 week, with gradual upward titration each week by 25 mg, up to a maximum of 100 mg PO three times a day. Slow titration of the dose (i.e., over the course of 6 to 9 weeks) up to 100 mg three times a day is recommended to minimize the risk of the gastrointestinal complaints that increase the risk of nonadherence to the regimen. Monitor the effects and titrate the dose based upon the results of a 1-hour postprandial plasma glucose reading. These agents may be used in conjunction with oral hypoglycemic agents in moderate to severe type II diabetes, and might be used alone in patients with mild or early-onset cases with high postprandial glucose surges, but normal fasting levels (i.e., <200 mg/dL), such as in cases of gestational diabetes mellitus. A 1-month supply of the lowest daily dose of acarbose costs $47.82. Assuming that this low dose will reduce HbA_{1C} by 0.5%, this corresponds to a cost to the patient of $95.00/1.0% reduction in HbA_{1C} per month (29).

Insulin

All patients with type I diabetes (IDDM) and patients with type II (NIDDM) diabetes who fail behavioral management alone or in combination with oral hypoglycemic agents will require insulin. Many patients fear injecting themselves and face the prospect of using insulin with trepidation. Such patients deserve reassurance that being on insulin will almost certainly not be as bad as they fear, and that insulin will help them feel better and lower their risk of complications. In some cases, the need for insulin will need to be discussed at one or two clinic visits before beginning insulin therapy to allow the patient to get used to the idea.

Although insulin therapy is often thought of as the "last resort" in patients with NIDDM who fail other modalities (i.e., exercise, dietary management, and weight control), it may be appropriate to use a short course of insulin therapy during times of acute stress and when rapid normalization of blood glucose is appropriate (for example, with infections, surgery, or hospitalization). The development of human insulins via recombinant DNA technology has made this short-term, intermittent use of insulin practical by significantly reducing the risk of developing anti-insulin antibodies and subsequent insulin allergy.

Rational therapy with exogenous insulin requires some knowledge of the physiology of endogenous insulin secretion. Endogenous insulin secretion follows two patterns: (a) small amounts of basal insulin are secreted continuously during the fasting state, and (b) postprandial boluses of insulin are secreted in response to a meal. Patients with IDDM and some patients with 15 to 20 years of NIDDM need to have both of these physiologic patterns of insulin secretion replaced by exogenous insulin. Most patients with NIDDM who have recently failed sulfonylurea therapy need only to have basal insulin secretion replaced. For patients with NIDDM, replacing basal insulin allows the pancreas to "rest" so that it can handle postprandial insulin requirements with endogenous insulin secretion (although simplistic, this model of insulin therapy is logical and effective).

Replacing basal insulin is relatively simple with one evening (when used in combination with an oral agent) or two (when used alone) daily injections of an intermediate to long-acting insulin or of a fixed (70/30 neutral protamine Hagedorn [NPH]/regular) mixture insulin preparation. Initial basal insulin therapy might begin at about 0.3 to 0.4 units of insulin/kg of ideal body weight per day divided into two nearly equal doses. Basal insulin requirements are about the same at night as they are during the day; therefore, the total dose should be distributed in proportions of about 60 to 65% in the morning and 35 to 40% in the evening. Nocturnal hypoglycemia is rarely a problem if one starts with this dosing regimen.

Replacing total insulin is necessary in patients with IDDM or in those with long-standing NIDDM who are poorly controlled with basal insulin therapy alone. These patients will require at least two injections a day, often with mixtures of short- and long-acting insulin at each injection ("split-mixed" insulin therapy). This regimen provides the best control but is more difficult to administer. In this method, the total daily insulin requirement (initially this can be estimated at 0.5 to 0.6 units per kg of ideal body weight per day) is split into a morning (0.6 total dose) and evening (0.4 total dose) dose; each dose is a mixture of NPH (0.6 to 0.7 of the dose) and regular (0.3 to 0.4 of the dose) insulin (Table 23.3). Many patients with IDDM (and a few with NIDDM) will require three or four injections a day to achieve acceptable blood glucose control. The most common three-injection-a-day regimen is a

Table 23.3.
Insulin Pharmacokinetics

Insulin	Route/Onset (hr)	Peak (hr)	Duration (hr)
Rapid-acting	SQ/0.5	1–2	4–7
Regular (neutral)	IM/0.1–0.5	0.5–1	2–4
	IV/Immediate	<1	
Semilente (insulin zinc suspension prompt)	SQ/1–1.5	4–9	12–16
Intermediate-acting			
NPH (isophane insulin suspension)	SQ/1–1.5	4–14	18–24
Lente (insulin zinc suspension)	SQ/1–2.5	7–15	18–24
Long-acting			
Ultralente (insulin zinc suspension extended)	SQ/4–6	10–30	>36

lispro works VERYfast.

morning injection of NPH and regular insulin, an injection of regular insulin before supper, and a bedtime injection of NPH. The most common four-injection-a-day regimen is evening NPH (or in some cases Ultralente) with three premeal injections of regular insulin to cover postprandial insulin requirements.

A new "wrinkle" in insulin therapy emerged in late 1996 with the addition of lispro (pronounced "lice pro") insulin, an insulin analogue, which has a faster onset than regular insulin (15 minutes vs. 30 to 60 minutes), allowing administration other than before mealtimes. Lispro gets through subcutaneous tissue faster and clears the bloodstream faster with low immunogenicity and a lower incidence of postprandial hypoglycemia, which can be problematic with regular insulin (35). The clinical significance of this development is that lispro more closely emulates the pattern of insulin secretion seen in nondiabetic individuals after a glucose challenge.

Lispro insulin is most appropriately given 15 minutes before eating and should be injected subcutaneously into the abdomen for the best rate of absorption and onset of action (36). It is eliminated more rapidly than regular human insulin (i.e., Humulin R or Novolin R) and thereby reduces the risk of hypoglycemia 2 to 3 hours after meals. As lispro has not been well studied in children under age 12 or in pregnancy, its use in these populations cannot be recommended. Because of the risk of hypoglycemia, recommend that patients monitor their blood glucose postprandially (i.e., after 2 to 3 hours) when using lispro.

When switching from regular human insulin to lispro, a unit-for-unit switch is recommended.

The pharmacodynamic profile of lispro versus regular human insulin is outlined in Table 23.4.

Interestingly, when mixing lispro with NPH insulin, the stabilization of blood glucose is delayed. A recent study on this effect has produced a different dosing regimen when using this combination: 20 to 40% NPH and 60 to 80% lispro is injected before each meal (37). This regimen addresses the drawback of lispro's short duration of action (i.e., 4 hours) and allows it to be used in a twice-daily (i.e., "split and mixed") regimen with NPH or even when the evening NPH injection is moved to bedtime.

When mixing lispro with human NPH insulin or human Lente insulin, the injection should be given within 5 minutes after mixing and within 15 minutes before a meal. At present, the manu-

Table 23.4.
Pharmacodynamic Profile of Lispro vs. Regular Human Insulin

	Lispro	Regular Human Insulin
Onset	2–15 minutes	30–60 minutes
Peak	30–90 minutes	120–240 minutes
Duration	2–4 hours	6–8 hours

Blood Glucose (mg/dL)	Timing of Injection Before Eating	
	Lispro[a]	Regular Human Insulin
>200	20 minutes	About 1 hour
150–200	10 minutes	45 minutes
<150	5 minutes	30 minutes

[a]Based on the preprandial blood glucose level.

facturer does not recommend premixing lispro with intermediate-acting insulin (e.g., NPH) in prefilled syringes that will be stored in a refrigerator for several days before use, as it is unknown how the pharmacodynamics of the mixture will change over time.

With any of these more complex insulin regimens, self-monitoring of blood glucose levels with adjustment of insulin dosages based on glucose results is essential. A typical algorithm suggests the patient make daily adjustments in the regular insulin by decreasing the usual regular insulin dose by two units if the blood glucose level is less than 70, by making no change for blood glucose levels between 70 and 150, and by increasing the dose by one unit for blood glucose levels between 150 and 200, by two units for blood glucose levels between 150 and 200, by three units for blood glucose levels between 200 and 250, etc. These adjustments may also need to be tailored to the individual patient, based on individual sensitivity to insulin.

Adjustments in the NPH component of an insulin regimen are made every 5 to 7 days and only if there is a clear pattern (50% of the blood glucose results out of the target range). For example, for a patient using daytime sulfonylureas and bedtime insulin, the evening NPH dose would be increased by 10% if 50% of the fasting glucose readings are above 150 mg/dL for a given 5- to 7-day period.

Glucose Monitoring

Glucose monitoring is essential for both the patient and the physician. Three strategies exist for monitoring blood glucose levels in NIDDM: (a) periodic testing of glycosylated hemoglobin, (b) periodic office measurement of fasting blood glucose levels, and (c) self-blood glucose monitoring at home. The first two should be recommended for all patients; the home monitoring is optional unless required for particular situations (e.g., patients requiring total insulin therapy). Table 23.5 summarizes these tests and gives a range of values for "nondiabetic," "acceptable," and "poor" for each.

Whatever monitoring methods are used, each patient **must have** knowledge of his or her current blood glucose levels after every office visit. A patient education handout will communicate this important information. For home monitoring, a log book helps summarize the results of glucose monitoring over time.

Fasting Blood Glucose Levels

Periodic measurements of fasting glucose concentrations are useful in patients with NIDDM. During initiation of an oral agent or titration, the fasting glucose level is relatively stable and a general indication of the severity of disease. This is not the case for patients with IDDM, in whom fasting glucose concentrations are much more variable.

Home Blood Glucose Monitoring

Home blood glucose monitoring is essential for IDDM patients and useful for many patients with NIDDM. These hand-held monitors are now widely available and easy to use, and newer models (e.g., One Touch II) require no wiping or timing to produce very acceptable results (cost: around $50.00 with a manufacturer's coupon). Home monitoring educates patients about how various activities (e.g., cutting the grass, eating a piece of cheesecake) can affect blood glucose.

The patient must record the results in a log book (or store the results in the machine's memory) for review and documentation by the physician. The most appropriate use of results is to help develop individualized patient guidelines (e.g., "If your fasting glucose is less than 140 and

Table 23.5.
Indices of Metabolic Control in Diabetes

Test	Nondiabetic	Acceptable	Poor
Fasting plasma glucose (mg/dL)	115	140	>200
2-hr postprandial plasma glucose (mg/dL)	140	200	>235
Glycosylated hemoglobin (%)	6	7	>10
Fasting plasma cholesterol (mg/dL)	200	<240	>240
Fasting plasma triglyceride (mg/dL)	150	200	>250

if you plan to exercise between breakfast and lunch, take only one-half tablet instead of one whole tablet" or, "If your blood glucose reading before supper is greater than 250, take your medication and either eat less for supper or take a 30-minute brisk walk after supper").

Encourage patients to record not only their blood glucose values but also their insulin doses, mealtimes, and exercise sessions. Additionally, lipid values, blood pressure, weight, and smoking status should be checked regularly in these patients.

Preventing Complications

Several preventive strategies effectively lower the risk of diabetes complications. The annual influenza and regular (every 6 years) pneumococcal vaccines are appropriate for adults with diabetes. Screening tests of proven value in detecting early signs of microvascular complications include regular retinal examinations to identify patients who will benefit from laser therapy for retinopathy, urine testing for microalbuminuria to identify patients with early signs of nephropathy, and monofilament foot examinations to identify patients at high risk for amputation (effectiveness rating: A). Screening tests for cardiovascular risk factors include assessing smoking status, measuring fasting lipid levels, and regularly measuring blood pressure. Behavioral preventive strategies include smoking cessation, increase in low-fat, low-cholesterol foods, increase in physical activity, and daily foot care.

Because cigarette smoking is an important risk factor for both macrovascular and microvascular complications, smoking cessation is an important part of prevention. If the patient is physically addicted to nicotine, nicotine patches can help ease withdrawal during the initial weeks. Formal group smoking-cessation programs may help if the patient is unable to quit alone (see Chapter 6, Helping Your Patients Stay Healthy).

Aspirin (80 to 325 mg/day) is an effective chemoprophylactic agent to reduce the risk of coronary and cerebral vascular disease and is appropriate for patients with diabetes at higher risk of these complications (see Chapter 22, Chronic Cardiac Disease). In the largest study evaluating the use of aspirin in patients with diabetes, aspirin (325 mg twice a day) was associated with a 27% reduction in myocardial infarction risk and a 10% reduction in mortality. Enteric-coated as-

pirin is associated with a lower risk of gastrointestinal adverse effects. It should be recommended for most diabetic patients to reduce the incidence of macrovascular disease.

Hypertension should also be controlled aggressively, especially in patients with evidence of early nephropathy. In these patients, maintaining blood pressures of 130–135/80–85 mm Hg has been shown to slow the progression of nephropathy.

The most common lipid abnormality seen with NIDDM is a pattern of elevated triglycerides, decreased HDL cholesterol, and mild to moderately elevated LDL cholesterol (type IV hyperlipidemia). As activity increases and eating habits are modified, these risk factors will likely improve, but repeated monitoring and drug intervention may be necessary (38).

Amputation rates are reduced significantly when patients take regular care of their feet. Educational interventions that encourage and support foot care have been shown to reduce amputation rates among patients with diabetes (14). Any complex or chronic foot problem should be referred to a podiatrist or orthopaedist with an interest in diabetic foot care.

In addition to these important efforts at tertiary prevention, the family physician is in the unique position to practice primary prevention of NIDDM among two populations at especially high risk: family members of patients with NIDDM, women with a history of gestational diabetes, and obese patients with hypertension. Increased activity (e.g., aerobic exercise, walking, stretching, gardening) reduces the risk of subsequent NIDDM; it should be routinely recommended for all siblings and children of patients with NIDDM, especially those who are obese (4). An example of an initial exercise regimen would be walking for 30 minutes at least three or four times a week.

LONG-TERM MANAGEMENT

Physicians often expect a great deal from their patients with diabetes. These patients are expected to know all the signs and treatment of hypoglycemia. They must modify their eating habits in ways that are strikingly different from the patterns of their family and friends. They are encouraged to perform at higher levels of physical activity than those of their peers. Patients receiving insulin therapy are expected to inject themselves up to four times a day. Many are asked to draw their own capillary blood, test it for glucose, record the results, and adjust their activity, diet, or dosage of medication based on the results three or four times a day. Finally, these patients are asked to initiate and maintain these complex new behaviors, not for a period of several weeks or months, but indefinitely (see Fig. 23.3)!

Unfortunately, when patients have trouble with these difficult challenges, they are often labeled as "noncompliant" or "difficult." At a time when the patient is already keenly aware of his or her failure with a nearly impossible task, many physicians express their frustration, either explicitly or implicitly, adding to a patient's sense of failure and further lowering an already compromised self-esteem. It is no wonder that many patients with diabetes also struggle with depression and other forms of stress (23).

If patients and their family members are to make these difficult behavioral changes, they must have an understanding and empathic physician who will not abandon them when they fail. These changes in lifestyle require instruction, encouragement, and reinforcement. In the office setting, these crucial activities are often best accomplished by a health care team consisting of a health educator (this can be a nurse), a dietitian, and a physician.

Patients vary in their levels of intellectual functioning, social support, daily routines, and socioeconomic status. At the time of diagnosis and initial evaluation, many patients will require intensive, frequent office visits; others will require only one or two visits. All patients need periodic updates in their knowledge and their individual behavioral treatment plan.

To help patients adhere to behavioral changes, it is crucial to reassess diabetes-related behavior at each follow-up visit. One mechanism to do this is to use "behavioral vital signs." After assessing a patient's behavioral status, it is appropriate to let the patient choose a behavioral domain (i.e., diet, exercise, glucose monitoring) they may want to work on for the next period of time. Once a behavioral domain has been chosen, the patient can negotiate a specific behavioral goal with the health care professional and can discuss likely barriers or problems and their solutions. In many settings, a nurse or dietitian can provide this focused behavioral counseling.

PUTTING IT ALL TOGETHER: THE ROUTINE OFFICE VISIT

Goals of Ongoing Diabetes Care

Busy primary care physicians have to prioritize their time constantly. Given a 15-minute follow-up appointment with a diabetic patient, what is the most valuable way to spend that time? What interventions are most effective at improving either the quantity or quality of a diabetic person's life (39)? Let's look at a hypothetic patient, a man, aged 45, with diabetes:

- Smoking counseling with successful cessation results in a gain of 3.39 years of life expectancy.

- Counseling to take aspirin as chemoprophylaxis against coronary disease adds 1.19 years of life expectancy.

- Treatment to lower systolic blood pressures greater than 142 mm Hg results in about 9 months of increased life expectancy.

- Lowering HbA_{1C} by 2.0% points (if a newly discovered diabetic) will increase life expectancy by 6 months.

- Cholesterol reduction adds an additional 2 months of increased life expectancy.

Clearly, a consistent approach to counseling cigarette smokers and increasing the use of aspirin is the most useful preventive intervention.

Organizing the Office Visit

Diabetic patients should be seen at least every 4 months. Ideally, these visits are preceded by laboratory testing so that you can review the results with the patient (Table 23.6).

At the beginning of a visit, ask how the patient is doing and briefly check on family and home activities. Has there been any significant nocturia, polyuria, or other problems? Next, quickly ascertain the pattern of blood glucose levels since the last visit and get a sense of the average fasting concentration and the average blood glucose reading before dinner. Check on number and type of hypoglycemic episodes. Occasional (two to three times a month) mild reactions are nearly unavoidable if one is going to achieve acceptable or excellent ranges of glucose concentration. Discuss the results of previous tests if performed.

There will not be enough time for a complete physical examination at each visit. Try to alternate between the anatomic regions targeted by

Table 23.6.
Organizing the Office Visit

1. How are things going?	General perceptions Symptoms Complaints Problems Urinary symptoms

2. Review recent blood glucose readings.	Review log/printout
	Average
	   I. Fasting glucose
	   II. Before-dinner glucose
	Hypoglycemic episodes

3. Review recent laboratory results.	HbA$_{1C}$ Lipids Urine

4. Physical examination.	Check one per visit of
	   I. Eye/teeth
	   II. Cardiovascular system
	   III. Lower extremities

5. Review previous behavior goals.	Smoking Weight Exercise Stress
6. Review medications.	
7. Summarize findings and agree on clinical behavioral plans (<3 per visit).	
8. Schedule next visit with encouragement.	

diabetes or presenting symptoms. In this way, important areas gets documented at least once a year. During the examination, discuss the appropriate care of that area of the body. Patients should also be encouraged to keep regular visits with their ophthalmologist and dentist.

Next, review the patient's previous behavioral goals in a friendly, nonjudgmental way (e.g., "How are you doing with your smoking? I remember last time you said you wanted to cut back to one-half pack a day," or "How is your walking program going? Have you been able to do what you wanted to with that?"). This part of the visit should be friendly and nonconfrontational. Patients should feel comfortable enough to share with you their failures as well as their successes. When problems are uncovered, move into a collaborative, problem-solving mode. For example, say "So it's just not working out for you to walk after work? You are probably too busy getting supper ready for the family. I can understand that. Perhaps you might consider some other time to walk." To be successful with this as-

pect of patient care, it is essential to work with patients to help solve their problems; do not try to solve their problems for them.

Review the use of insulin or oral medications, checking on adherence to the regimen and the need for changing dosage levels. Summarize your findings to the patient. Ideally, patients should be given visual, printed feedback about their range of blood glucose concentrations and how their level corresponds to what is desirable. The important behavioral domains that influence glucose concentrations should be reviewed: activity level, eating habits, and stress management techniques.

Goals should be negotiated and summarized. The patient may choose to reaffirm a previous goal that was difficult to meet or to set a new behavioral goal that moves beyond the current program. The physician's role at this point is to clarify the goal, to make it as specific as possible, and to write the goal down legibly for the patient to review later. Limit the number of goals to three per visit.

CONCLUSIONS

All physicians will care for patients with diabetes. Although the diagnosis of diabetes is straightforward, the evaluation of these patients requires a comprehensive, systematic approach. Treatment is complex and requires continuity in a relationship with a primary care physician. A friendly, nonthreatening doctor-patient relationship is important to maximize adherence to complex behavioral and medical treatment plans. As in many areas of primary care, a preventive, self-care approach involving both patient and family members is critical to successful management. By remembering the principles of family medicine, the care of these patients can be a rewarding and enjoyable experience, providing the satisfaction that comes from preventing tragic complications.

CASE STUDY

A 48-year-old, slightly overweight office manager comes to the office complaining of blurred vision. On questioning, she admits to increased fluid intake, urinary frequency, and a vaginal discharge. A urine dipstick test reveals significant glycosuria.

STUDY QUESTIONS

1. How will you make the diagnosis in this patient?
2. What type of diabetes does she have?
3. What are your plans for clinical evaluation?
4. What will you discuss with the patient?

DISCUSSION

This is a typical presentation of type II diabetes (NIDDM). Although the glycosuria is strong evidence for diabetes, you should arrange one or more fasting plasma glucose levels. A random plasma glucose might immediately provide the answer if it is greater than 200.

Clinical evaluation should include a comprehensive physical examination, an initial urinalysis, HbA$_{1C}$, and lipid panel. However, there will be little time to imple-

ment all these activities at this visit; a longer return visit within the next 2 or 3 days should be scheduled. The most immediate talk is to reassure the patient that there is no acute danger, and help her process the diagnosis. She may have a lot questions and concerns. It is a good opportunity to take a family history and check her knowledge of the disease.

Some physicians would start immediate treatment with a low-dose oral hypoglycemic, so that the patient is reassured that active management is underway. This should be accompanied by education about hypoglycemia, another time-consuming activity.

Finally, you should discuss the diagnosis, with implications, and then clarify the strategy for future visits, tests, referral to an ophthalmologist, and broad-management issues of diet, exercise, and medication. Finally, give the patient some well-designed educational material aimed at her literacy level that she can review at home with her family in preparation for the next visit.

REFERENCES

1. National Diabetes Information Clearinghouse. Diabetes Statistics. NIH publication no. 96-3926. Washington, DC: US Department of Health and Human Services, Public Health Service, National Institutes of Health, 1995.
2. Harris MI. Undiagnosed NIDDM: clinical and public health issues. Diabetes Care 1993;16:642–652.
3. Harris MI, Entmacher PS. Mortality from diabetes. In: Harris MI, Hamman RF, eds. Diabetes in America. NIH publication no. 85–1468. Washington, DC: US Government Printing Office, 1985:1–48.
4. Barrett-Connor EL, Cohn BA, Wingard DL, Edelstein SL: Why is diabetes mellitus a stronger risk factor for fatal ischemic heart disease in women than in men? The Rancho Bernardo Study. JAMA 1991;265:627–631.
5. Bennett PH, Haffner S, Kasiske BL, Keane WF, Mogensen CE, et al. Screening and management of microalbuminuria in patients with diabetes mellitus: recommendations to the Scientific Advisory Board of the National Kidney Foundation from an ad hoc committee of the Council on Diabetes Mellitus of the National Kidney Foundation. Am J Kidney Dis 1995;25:107–112.
6. Hawkes CH. Twin studies in diabetes mellitus. Diabetic Med 1997:347–352.
7. Reaven GM. Role of insulin resistance in human disease. Diabetes 1988;37:1595–1607.

8. Helmrich SP, Ragland DR, Leung RW, Paffenbarger RS Jr. Physical activity and reduced occurrence of non-insulin-dependent diabetes mellitus. N Engl J Med 1991;325:147–152.

9. Marshall JA, Hamman RF, Baxter J. High-fat, low-carbohydrate diet and the etiology of non-insulin-dependent diabetes mellitus: the San Luis Valley Diabetes Study. Am J Epidemiol 1991;134:590–603.

10. Henry RH. Glucose control and insulin resistance in non-insulin-dependent diabetes mellitus. Ann Intern Med 1996;124:97–103.

11. Unger RH. Lipotoxicity in the pathogenesis of obesity-dependent NIDDM. Diabetes 1995;44:863–870.

12. Franklin GM, Kahn LB, Baxter J, Marshall JA, Hamman RJ. Sensory neuropathy in non-insulin-dependent diabetes mellitus: the San Luis Valley Diabetes Study. Am J Epidemiol 1990;131:633–643.

13. Caputo GM, Cavanagh PR, Ulbrecht JS, Gibbons GW, Karchmer AW. Assessment and management of foot disease in patients with diabetes. N Engl J Med 1994;331:854–860.

14. Duffy JC, Patout CA. Management of the insensitive foot in diabetes: lessons learned from Hansen's disease. Milit Med 1990;155:575–580.

15. Klenerman L, McCabe C, Cogley D, Crerand S, Laing P, White M. Screening for patients at risk of diabetic foot ulceration in a general diabetic outpatient clinic. Diabetic Med 1996:561–563.

16. Peters AL, Davidson MB, Ziel FH. Cost-effective screening for diabetic retinopathy using a nonmydriatic retinal camera in a prepaid health-care setting. Diabetes Care 1993;16:1193–1195.

17. Singer D, Nathan J, Fogel H, Schachat A. Screening for diabetic retinopathy. Ann Intern Med 1992;116:660–671.

18. Expert Committee on the Diagnosis and Classification of Diabetes Mellitus. Report of the Expert Committee on the Diagnosis and Classification of Diabetes Mellitus. Diabetes Care 1997;20:1183–1194.

19. Peters A, Davidson M, Schringer D, et al. A clinical approach for the diagnosis of DM: an analysis using glycosylated hemoglobin levels. JAMA 1996;276:1246–1252.

20. Larsen ML, Horder M, Mogensen EF. Effect of long-term monitoring of glycosylated hemoglobin levels in insulin-dependent diabetes mellitus. N Engl J Med 1990;323:1021–1025.

21. Nelson RG, Knowler WC, Pettitt DJ, Saad MF, Charles M, Bennett PH. Assessment of risk of overt nephropathy in diabetic patients from albumin excretion in untimed urine specimens. Arch Intern Med 1991;151:1761–1765.

22. Case Records of the Massachusetts General Hospital. Weekly clinicopathological exercises. Case 31–1994. A 25-year-old man with the recent onset of diabetes mellitus and congestive heart failure. N Engl J Med 1994;331:460–466.

23. Jacobson AM. The psychological care of patients with insulin-dependent diabetes mellitus. N Engl J Med 1996;334:1249–1253.

24. Diabetes Control and Complications Trial Research Group. The effect of intensive treatment of diabetes on the development and progression of long-term complications in insulin-dependent diabetes mellitus. N Engl J Med 1993;329:977–986.

25. Kroleweski AS, Laffel LMB, et al. Glycosylated hemoglobin and the risk of microalbuminuria in patients with IDDM. N Engl J Med 1995;332:1251–1255.

26. Genuth S. Exogenous insulin administration and cardiovascular risk in non-insulin-dependent diabetes mellitus and insulin-dependent diabetes mellitus. Ann Intern Med 1996;124:104–109.

27. Laakso M. Glycemic control and the risk for coronary heart disease in patients with non-insulin-dependent diabetes mellitus: the Finnish studies. Ann Intern Med 1996;124:127–130.

28. Turner R, Cull C, Holman R. United Kingdom prospective diabetes study 17: a 9-year update of a randomized, controlled trial on the effect of improved metabolic control on complications in non-insulin-dependent diabetes mellitus. Ann Intern Med 1996;124:136–145.

29. Troglitazone for non-insulin-dependent diabetes mellitus. Med Lett Drugs Ther 1997;39:49–51.

30. DeFronzo, RA, Goodman AM, et al. Efficacy of metformin in patients with non-insulin-dependent diabetes mellitus. N Engl J Med 1995;333:541–549.

31. Turner RC, et al. UK prospective study of therapies of maturity-onset diabetes 1: effect of diet, sulfonylurea, insulin or biguanide therapy on fasting plasma glucose and body weight over one year. Diabetologia 1983;24:404–411.

32. Dunn CJ, Peters DH. Metformin: a review of its pharmacological properties and therapeutic use in non-insulin-dependent diabetes mellitus. Drugs 1995;5:722–749.

33. Saltiel AR, Olefsky JM. Thiazolidinediones in the treatment of insulin resistance and type II diabetes. Diabetes 1996;45:1661–1669.

34. Balfour JA, McTavish D. Acarbose: an update on its pharmacology and therapeutic use in diabetes mellitus. Drugs 1993;46:1026–1054.

35. Fineberg NS, Fineberg SE, Anderson JH, Kirkett MA, Gibson RG, Hufferd S. (1996). Immunologic effects of insulin lispro [Lys (B28), Pro (B29) human insulin] in IDDM and NIDDM patients previously treated with insulin. Diabetes 1996;45:1750–1754.

36. Ter Braak E, Woodwroth JR, Bianchi R, Cerimele B, Erkelens DW, Thissjssen JHH, et al. Injection sites on the pharmacokinetics and glucodynamics of insulin lispro and regular insulin. Diabetes Care1996;19:1437–1440.

37. Torlone E, Pampanelli S, Lalli C, Del Sindaco P, Di Vincenzo A, Rambotti AM, et al. Effects of the short-acting insulin analog [Lys (B28), Pro (B29)] on postprandial blood glucose control in IDDM. Diabetes Care 1996;19:945–952.

38. American Diabetes Association: nutritional recommendations and principles for individuals with diabetes mellitus: 1986. Diabetes Care 1987;10:126–132.

39. Yudkins JS. How can we best prolong life? Benefits of coronary risk factor reduction in non-diabetic and diabetic subjects. BMJ 1993;306:1313–1318.

24. Dizziness

ALEXANDER W. CHESSMAN AND PHILIP D. SLOANE

Key Clinical Questions

1. Can your patient's dizziness be classified as vertigo, presyncope, or disequilibrium? If so, does its classification assist you in creating a differential diagnosis?
2. How can you effectively and efficiently rule out serious causes of dizziness in this patient?
3. When is medication useful in the treatment of nonspecific dizziness? Which medications should you prescribe?

Dizziness is a difficult condition to diagnose properly because of

- the confusing words patients use to describe the symptoms
- a lack of consistent definitions of the symptom
- an incomplete understanding of many of the common diagnoses
- the inability of laboratory testing to contribute meaningfully in many difficult cases, and
- cultural differences in interpretation of the term "dizziness"

Yet dizziness is one of the most common presentations in ambulatory care, accounting for 1% of all office visits (1). It is largely managed at the primary care level: of those patients with dizziness who present for medical care, approximately 70% see family practitioners or general internists, and only 4% are referred to a consultant (2). Therefore, it is important for primary care physicians and those studying this discipline to develop a systematic approach to this complex problem.

A useful first step in evaluating patients with dizziness is to categorize the symptom as either vertigo, presyncope, disequilibrium, and other. Distinguishing among these dizziness subtypes will often define a pathophysiologic mechanism, help narrow the differential diagnosis, and/or suggest appropriate laboratory tests and treatments. For this reason, this chapter is organized based on these dizziness subtypes.

Occasionally, dizziness represents a warning sign of a serious problem, such as an impending stroke (3). Clinicians should be alert for these "red flag" diagnoses, but they should also be aware that such instances are rare, and so should work to avoid overtesting. Even when dizziness does not signify a dangerous underlying cause, the dizziness itself can interfere greatly with daily activities, causing significant patient concern, and often can respond to appropriate treatment.

Very little objective data exist on the evaluation and management of dizziness. Little is known about the sensitivity and specificity of historical and physical examination maneuvers or of how and when to select laboratory tests. This lack of knowledge is largely because dizziness presents so many diagnostic possibilities, the most serious of which are uncommon, and because dizziness is only one way that these diseases can present. Thus, dizziness remains a problem that challenges the art more than the science of medicine.

PATHOPHYSIOLOGY AND DIFFERENTIAL DIAGNOSIS

The first step in evaluating dizziness is to clarify exactly what the patient means by dizziness. The patient's words provide a clue to pathophysiology and differential diagnosis. There are four general types of dizziness: vertigo, presyncope, disequilibrium, and other (4).

Vertigo

Vertigo is a feeling that the body or environment is moving; the most typical description is of the room spinning. Vertigo usually implies disease of the inner ear, the brainstem, or the nerve connections between them. Common causes of vertigo include ear disorders, such as neurolabyrinthitis, benign positional vertigo, and otitis media (when it affects the adjacent inner-ear structures), and diseases affecting the brainstem, such as migraine and transient ischemic attacks. Vertigo has also been described in persons with neck problems and panic disorder.

Texts written by otolaryngologists and other subspecialists often differentiate between central and peripheral vertigo. Central vertigo is described as less intense, more often continuous, and associated with vertical nystagmus. Peripheral vertigo is described as more intense, more often episodic, and associated with horizontal or rotatory nystagmus. Unfortunately, trying to differentiate clinically between peripheral and central vertigo in primary care is not useful. Most primary care vertigos are peripheral; so clinical measures to distinguish central vertigo would have to be quite sensitive and specific to be helpful, and they are not. Indeed, central vertigo presents in a wide variety of ways, ranging from catastrophically severe (e.g., cerebellar infarction) to minimal (e.g., lightheadedness noted months after a stroke) and may or may not be accompanied by nystagmus.

The one value of differentiating between "central" and "peripheral" vertigo is that the distinction may help you think anatomically when creating a differential diagnosis:

- Central causes of vertigo (in approximate order of frequency in primary care) include anxiety/panic disorder, transient ischemic attacks, migraine (including atypical migraine not accompanied by headache), medications (e.g., phenytoin), alcoholism, stroke, and tumors (e.g., acoustic neuroma, which generally presents as unilateral hearing loss with tinnitus and not as dizziness).

- Peripheral causes of vertigo (in approximate order of frequency in primary care) include neurolabyrinthitis (injury to the semicircular canals due to either a virus or infarction of a tiny arteriole), benign paroxysmal positional vertigo (a unique syndrome characterized by short episodes of vertigo brought on by certain head movements), serous otitis media/sinusitis (for unclear mechanisms), recurrent vestibulopathy (a poorly understood syndrome of episodes of vertigo lasting about a day and occurring up to several times a year), Ménière's disease, and medications (e.g., gentamicin).

Presyncope

Presyncope is the feeling of being about to pass out or of almost passing out. The description is of a kind of lightheadedness. Often the sensation occurs when the patient is on his or her feet; in such situations, it is accompanied by a desire to sit or lie down. It implies a temporary restriction of circulation to the cerebral cortex.

Presyncope is the precursor to syncope and shares the same pathophysiology. Syncope is the transient loss of consciousness with loss of postural tone, and its major mechanism is cerebral hypoxia. It can arise as a result of the decreased overall capacity of the blood to carry oxygen, decreased cardiac output, reduced cerebral blood pressure, or carotid artery narrowing. Presyncope also can occur in anxiety disorders.

The most common causes of presyncope in primary care are, in approximate descending order by frequency:

- Postural hypotension associated with acute viral illness or a medication

- Vasovagal reactions (sudden lowering of blood pressure due to a stimulus such as abdominal pain, sudden emotional upset, having blood drawn, or just having urinated or had a bowel movement)

- Impaired cardiac output because of dehydration, anemia, acute myocardial infarction, infection, or congestive heart failure

- Cardiac arrhythmias

Disequilibrium

Disequilibrium is a feeling of imbalance. It is described by the patient as more of a problem below the neck than above the neck. This sensation is almost always improved by sitting down and worsened by standing upright. It implies one or more lesions in the balance system, which means that a whole variety of structures can be affected: the cerebellum (e.g., by multiple sclerosis, alcoholism, stroke, or certain drugs such as phenytoin), proprioceptive fibers in the facet joints of the neck (e.g., by arthritis or muscle spasm), muscle weakness (e.g., physical deconditioning), proprioceptive problems in the lower extremities (e.g., diabetes or other peripheral neuropathies), or lesions that typically cause vertigo because they affect the brainstem or inner ear (e.g., after the acute vertigo from a neurolabyrinthitis or stroke has faded, imbalance often remains).

Disequilibrium is relatively rare as an isolated type of dizziness in primary care, so it is difficult to estimate what the most common causes are. Much more common than isolated disequilibrium is a feeling of imbalance that accompanies other types of dizziness such as severe vertigo. In the elderly, nearly all dizziness syndromes include a component of imbalance. Pure disequilibrium in younger persons is usually due to neurologic disease, especially if it is associated with objective physical findings such as ataxia, a positive Romberg test, or dysdiadochokinesis.

Other/Vague Dizziness

Other forms of dizziness tend to be vague and difficult to describe. The most common descriptive terms used are "floating" or a vague lightheadedness. Such forms of dizziness may reflect the fact that the patient is inarticulate and medically unsophisticated. However, vague forms of dizziness are most commonly associated with emotional disorders such as anxiety and depression.

Dizziness That Has Multiple Components

The above classification of dizziness types is based on the patient history and can help guide your evaluation. This delineation is especially

useful in persons who are young or middle aged. Unfortunately, in older persons, dizziness tends to be more difficult to categorize and often involves multiple symptoms; in one series of older persons with dizziness, 42% could not be classified as exclusively vertigo, presyncope, disequilibrium, or other (5). Thus, in older patients and others with complex dizziness syndromes, the history must often be more extensive and the physical examination more important.

CLINICAL EVALUATION

The differential diagnosis of dizziness is immense. Table 24.1 lists the most common causes of dizziness and their approximate prevalence among three subgroups of primary care patients: all patients seen in office practice, those whose dizziness is chronic, and those who present to emergency departments.

Dizziness rarely represents a life-threatening condition. In one study of 144 patients with

Table 24.1.
Estimated Frequency of Various Causes of Dizziness in Three Settings Based on Published Epidemiologic Studies (Estimated Percent of Patients, by Diagnosis and Setting)

	Estimated % of Patients with the Diagnosis		
	In Primary Care Office Settings		In Emergency Departments[d,e]
Diagnosis	All Patients[a,b]	Chronic Dizziness[c]	
Labyrinthitis/vestibular neuronitis	23	3	9
Benign paroxysmal positional vertigo	7	16	6
Recurrent peripheral vertigo (includes Ménière's disease)	2	14	4
Psychiatric	13	17	11
Cerebrovascular disease (includes migraine)	8	10	4
Viral syndrome	4	—	10
Otitis media/sinusitis	10	—	4
Other acute infections	1	—	4
Medication side effects	6	—	8
Multicausal	—	13	—
Vasovagal	5	6	3
Hypertension	3	—	2
Cardiac ischemia/congestive heart failure	2	—	3
Anemia	2	—	5
Diabetes/hypoglycemia	—	—	2
Other	8	3	2
No diagnosis made	6	18	23
Hospitalized for evaluation	1.5	—	15.5

[a]Sloane PD. Dizziness in primary care: results from the National Ambulatory Medical Care Survey. J Fam Pract 1989;29:33–38.

[b]Sloane PD, Dallara J, Roach C, et al. Management of dizziness in primary care. J Am Board Fam Pract 1994;7:1–8.

[c]Kroenke K, Lucas CA, Rosenberg ML, Sherokman B, Herbers JE, Wehrle PA, Boggi JO. Causes of persistent dizziness: A prospective study of 100 patients in ambulatory care. Ann Int Med 1992;117:898–904.

[d]Madlon-Kay DJ. Evaluation and outcome of the dizzy patient. J Fam Pract 1985;21:109–113.

[e]Skiendzielewski JJ. The weak and dizzy patient. Ann Emerg Med 1980;9:353–356.

dizziness (mean age 58.6 years) from primary care offices, only one death occurred in 6 months of follow-up. Still, you must be on the lookout for rare, life-threatening conditions as you conduct a dizziness evaluation. Table 24.2 identifies some of these rare but serious diagnoses and the "red flag" items from the history and examination that suggest the presence of each.

To help narrow your differential diagnosis, an important diagnostic first step is to characterize the dizziness based on the patient history. Important elements include:

- The dizziness subtype (vertigo, presyncope, disequilibrium, or other)

- Whether the dizziness is acute or chronic and, if it is chronic, what the previous evaluation has been

- Knowledge of the common causes of dizziness in the primary care population to which your patient belongs

Figure 24.1 provides a general approach to the patient with dizziness, based on characterization of the dizziness and key elements from the history and physical examination. Because dizziness does not fit well into algorithmic thinking, Figure 24.1 should be thought of only as a general guide. Sometimes the patient will present with a classic symptom pattern that suggests a specific diagnosis, and an algorithmic approach will be unnecessary. At other times, typing of the dizziness is not possible, and your history may need to be more extensive.

History

Initial questions in the history should include:

- Characteristics of the dizziness—ask in the most open-ended fashion possible for the patient to describe the dizziness. While the patient is talking, listen for words describing a sensation of spinning, fainting, or falling. Encourage the patient to continue describing the symptoms until you hear no new information, then offer specific prompts.

- Other characteristics—onset, severity, duration, precipitating factors, alleviating factors, and associated symptoms

- General health—cardiac or neurologic history. Risk factors for atherosclerosis (cholesterol, hypertension, obesity, diabetes mellitus, age, gender), previous history of myocardial infarction, transient ischemic attack, or cerebrovascular accident

- Medications—aspirin and quinine (tinnitus); antihistamines, tricyclic antidepressants, and antihypertensives (presyncope); aspirin, nonsteroidal anti-inflammatory drugs, and warfarin (gastrointestinal bleeding)

You should also be on the alert for "red flags" that suggest a potentially life-threatening disease (see Table 24.2). In addition, you should ask about the effect of the symptoms on the patient's life. Ask if the dizziness has kept the patient from work or other activities such as driving or socializing.

Table 24.2.
"Red Flags" Suggesting Progressive or Life-Threatening Illness in Patients with Dizziness

Diagnosis	"Red Flag" Symptoms/Signs
Central vertigo syndromes such as stroke or cerebellar degeneration	Cranial nerve and/or cerebellar symptoms or signs such as diplopia, ataxia, dysarthria, abnormal gait, dysdiadochokinesis, facial weakness, vertical nystagmus
Vertebrobasilar insufficiency	Episodes of vertigo lasting 10–120 minutes in older persons with risk factors for atherosclerosis, especially if accompanied by symptoms such as ataxia, visual loss, or dysarthria
Acoustic neuroma	Gradual onset of unilateral hearing loss and tinnitus; loss of corneal reflex
Cardiac arrhythmia	Palpitations; history of heart disease
Acute event with secondary hypotension (e.g., myocardial infarction, pneumonia, acute gastrointestinal bleed)	Fever, symptoms or signs of systemic infection; chest pressure, diaphoresis, nausea, shortness of breath; melena or blood in bowel movements

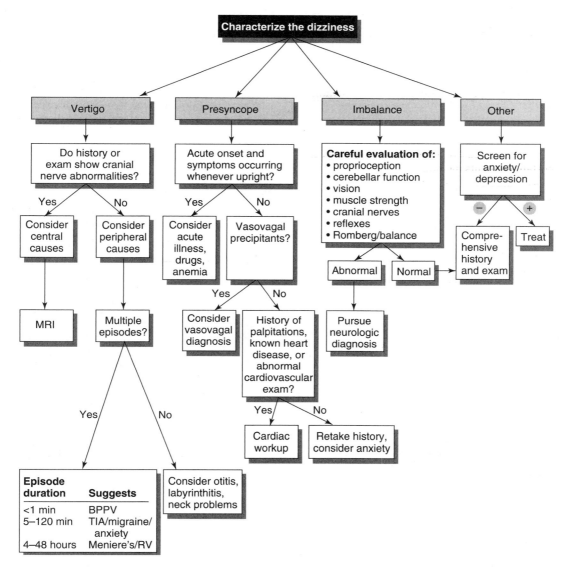

Figure 24.1. *General approach to diagnosis in patients with dizziness.*

Vertigo

In patients with vertigo, find out if the vertigo occurs in recurrent episodes. If so, ask about the duration and characteristics of the episodes. Often, the pattern of episodes will point to a specific diagnosis.

• *Benign paroxysmal positional vertigo* (BPPV) is a syndrome characterized by brief (less than 1 minute) episodes of vertigo brought on by head movement, especially by rolling over in bed or by bending over and straightening up.

Typically, the patient has severe symptoms for a few days, then gradually improves over a few weeks. Recurrences are common.

• *Transient ischemic attacks or migraine* (sometimes without headache) generally produce vertigo lasting between 5 and 120 minutes. Sometimes the vertigo is accompanied by other neurologic symptoms.

• *Episodes of vertigo without any other symptoms* that last between 6 and 48 hours and recur infrequently (typically around once a year) characterize a benign syndrome called recurrent vestibulopathy (RV). If episodes of similar duration are accompanied by tinnitus and a gradual hearing loss (often unilateral, and nearly always more profoundly affecting the lower pitches), then the diagnosis is Ménière's disease. =tinnitis, hearing loss, vertigo

A single episode of vertigo could be the first episode of one of the above conditions. If the vertigo is severe and accompanied by nausea and horizontal nystagmus, the diagnosis is usually acute neurolabyrinthitis.

Presyncope

Additional areas about which to question the patient with presyncope include:

- Anemia—heavy menstrual bleeding, gastrointestinal bleeding, jaundice

- Risk factors for postural hypotension—medications, viral symptoms

- Possible factors that would precipitate a vasovagal reaction—micturition, defecation, pain, or acute anxiety

- Cardiac symptoms—palpitations, a history of rheumatic heart disease or valvular problems, orthopnea, paroxysmal nocturnal dyspnea

- Risk factors for atherosclerosis

Be on the alert for anxiety or depression as well, because these common causes of dizziness can occasionally present as presyncope.

Disequilibrium

Because proper balance involves a smooth interaction between the visual, vestibular, and neuromuscular systems, your history should include an inquiry about each of these areas:

- Visual problems—cataracts, macular degeneration, or a new prescription for glasses

- Proprioceptive system problems—numbness in the feet or conditions that cause peripheral neuropathy, such as diabetes mellitus and alcoholism

- Vestibular system problems—look especially for one or more episodes of vertigo in the past, which could suggest labyrinthine damage or an old stroke

- Physical deconditioning—lack of exercise is the most treatable cause and/or contributing factor to disequilibrium in older persons; be sure to look for it.

Keep in mind that disequilibrium frequently results in older persons because problems exist in more than one part of the balance system. For example, someone with vestibular damage from neurolabyrinthitis decades ago may develop a balance problem when, in old age, vision declines.

Mixed/Other/Vague

In this case you will want to look for symptoms of anxiety and depression:

- Depressive symptoms—anhedonia, dysphoria, guilt, helplessness/hopelessness, concentration difficulty, appetite change, sleep change

- Symptoms of anxiety—jitteriness, excessive worry, headache, stomachaches, difficulty falling asleep, and tingling of the hands and mouth (due to hyperventilation)

If the patient does not express symptoms of anxiety or depression, you should take a comprehensive history, looking for clues to some other diagnosis such as a metabolic problem or a systemic illness.

Physical Examination

The physical examination in persons with dizziness should be focused and based on their symptoms. In patients in whom you do not have a good history or narrow differential diagnosis, a more comprehensive examination should be conducted that focuses on the cardiovascular, neurologic, visual, and otologic areas.

Vertigo

Concentrate on the cranial nerves, ears, and neck. If BPPV is suspected, do the Hallpike maneuver: Move the patient rapidly from a sitting position to a recumbent position, with the head turned at a 30° angle, first to the one side and then to the other. There are five elements to a positive Hallpike maneuver (not all will necessarily be present in every patient): precipitation of vertigo by the maneuver (often only with the head turned to one side), latency of vertigo onset of a few seconds, vertigo accompanied by rotatory nystagmus, resolution of the dizziness within less than a minute, and less acute dizziness with repeating the maneuver.

Presyncope

The physical examination for presyncope includes listening to the heart and checking for carotid bruits, assessing for relative or absolute volume depletion, particularly by checking orthostatic vital signs. Controversy exists about the standard method for checking for orthostatic hypotension and the accuracy of the test, because some patients have true orthostatic presyncope without meeting the criteria for orthostatic hypotension (a systolic blood pressure fall of at least 20 mm Hg or a diastolic drop of at least 10 mm Hg).

Disequilibrium

Conduct a careful neurologic examination, focusing on:

- Cerebellar signs and balance
- Proprioception and other peripheral nerve function
- Vision
- Cranial nerves (remember to check for nystagmus)
- Muscle strength and deep tendon reflexes

If the examination is abnormal, a neurologic diagnosis should be pursued. If it is normal, conduct a more comprehensive examination, and consider revising the history.

Laboratory or Other Diagnostic Tests

Practicing primary care physicians order relatively few laboratory tests on dizzy patients (3). This limited laboratory testing is probably because the history and physical examination often rule out life-threatening disease and lead to a presumptive diagnosis. A few tips about ordering tests follow.

- If a metabolic problem or an acute infection is suspected, order electrolytes, a serum glucose, and a CBC.
- If a cardiac arrhythmia is suspected, order an ECG and ambulatory rhythm (Holter) monitoring. Do not be surprised if you fail to find an arrhythmia; most suspected arrhythmias are not confirmed.
- If you want to rule out posterior fossa disease (e.g., an acoustic neuroma), order a magnetic resonance imaging (MRI) and not a CT scan, because the resolution is better.

MANAGEMENT

The key to appropriate management of persons with dizziness is making the correct diagnosis. We cannot discuss all the causes of dizziness here; however, we will comment on a few of the more common diagnoses.

Acute neurolabyrinthitis is a common dizziness problem. It involves permanent destruction of some or all of the balance mechanism of one inner ear. Although the lesion does not repair itself, the opposite inner ear and associated compensatory vestibular structures gradually learn to compensate for the deficit. Therefore, most patients gradually lose their vertigo, nystagmus, and imbalance. Young persons typically feel back to normal in a couple of weeks; older persons take longer and may remain with a persistent, mild imbalance. Treatment is symptomatic; the most common is to prescribe 25 to 50 mg of meclizine every 6 hours, tapering the dose as the patient improves. Activity should be as tolerated.

Benign paroxysmal positional vertigo (BPPV) is another self-limited problem. Because these patients are often elderly, fear of falling is often present. Speed of recovery from BPPV is accelerated by physical activity; so you should encourage your patients to move in spite of the dizziness. Exercises can be helpful: instruct your patient to sit on the bed and fall over repeatedly to whichever side provokes the most dizziness, falling several times a day and three to five times per session. This will desensitize the brain, allowing the patient to do daily activities with less dizziness. Meclizine is not indicated in patients with BPPV, because it only makes the patient drowsy and lightheaded without significantly reducing the vertigo episodes.

[handwritten margin note: Bnef periods of vertigo brought about by head movement]

Serous otitis media and sinusitis are also common causes of dizziness in primary care (3). Treatment of these conditions is outlined in Chapter 35. Anxiety (including panic disorder) and depression are among the most treatable causes of dizziness. Treatment of these conditions is outlined in Chapter 17.

Undiagnosed Dizziness

In primary care, it is not uncommon for a patient to be undiagnosed at the end of an office visit. We as physicians then face a dilemma. Because most dizziness gets better without treatment and is not life threatening, we do not want to order unnecessary tests; however, we want to do something.

Often, the patient is given a low dose (25 mg) of meclizine, told to take this "dizziness medication," and instructed to return if not better in a week or so. This practice is reasonable if the patient has peripheral vertigo. However, patients with presyncope and disequilibrium will get worse with meclizine, as will persons with anxiety or depression.

Bewar [margin annotation]

Some patients with undiagnosed dizziness have postural dizziness of the presyncopal type. These patients tend to be older and to have negative cardiac workups. They often act as though they have postural hypotension but do not meet diagnostic criteria for this disorder. In many cases, this postural lightheadedness is actually a type of imbalance, and its causes are the same as those of disequilibrium. In other cases, however, enough blood pools in the lower extremity to reduce cerebral blood flow without affecting the brachial artery blood pressure; such individuals respond to interventions such as support stockings, hydration, frequent contraction of leg muscles, cardioselective β-adrenergic blocking agents, and volume expansion with fludrocortisone acetate (6).

Chronic Dizziness

Patients with chronic dizziness are often both miserable and frustrating. Management of this problem is challenging, and a comprehensive approach is beyond the scope of this chapter. Here are a few general principles:

- A family physician is often the best physician for such a patient. Be thorough in your evaluation, but order tests and consultations judiciously. Subspecialists rarely have the breadth of approach that is necessary to sort out the multiple problems and possible diagnoses in a patient with complex dizziness or to understand when management is more important than diagnosis.

- Be sympathetic. Just because you cannot measure a patient's dizziness does not mean the patient is not suffering.

- Remember that the body uses the visual and proprioceptive systems to combat dizziness, so do what you can to maximize these areas. Correct refraction problems, recommend cataract surgery when appropriate, prescribe a cane or other proprioceptive aid, and be sure the patient has a night light.

- Over a third of patients will have a secondary psychologic disorder, usually depression or anxiety. Treating these disorders helps reduce the dizziness.

- Most patients will be physically deconditioned because they limit their activities too much. This physical deconditioning worsens postural lightheadedness and causes imbalance. A vigorous exercise program is often the most effective management available for persons with chronic dizziness.

CASE STUDY 1

Ms. S. is a 39-year-old woman who noted severe dizziness upon awakening yesterday. She felt so dizzy that she stayed in the house. Today she remains dizzy but feels improved enough to come to the office. The dizziness is made worse by sudden movements, and she reports that as long as she remains still she has relatively little dizziness. What concerned her is that her last episode occurred while driving and necessitated her pulling over to the side of the road.

In the office, she describes in her own words a sensation of spinning that lasts a few seconds but leaves her with a lightheaded feeling. She has been generally healthy, without history of ear problems (including hearing loss), recent upper respiratory infection, fever, or trauma. The only medication that she takes is an oral contraceptive. She denies symptoms of depression or anxiety.

General observation reveals a woman who appears to be uncomfortable. Although she moves slowly and carefully, her gait is normal. Examination of the ears and cranial nerves is normal. No nystagmus is noted.

QUESTIONS

1. What is your differential diagnosis? What serious causes can you already rule out on the basis of her history and physical examination findings?
2. What additional evaluation would you perform?

3. What should you tell Ms. S about the cause of her dizziness?
4. What should you recommend for treatment?

DISCUSSION

Ms. S describes definite vertigo. The history of acute onset and brief episodes brought on by movement suggests benign paroxysmal positional vertigo (BPPV). However, many vertiginous disorders are worsened by head movement; so your differential diagnosis at this point should include labyrinthitis and the first episode of recurrent vestibulopathy or Ménière's disease. Serious problems that appear unlikely based on the history and examination include cerebrovascular and cardiac disease, an acoustic neuroma, and central causes of vertigo.

The next step is to perform the Hallpike maneuver. This test elicits five beats of rotatory nystagmus and severe dizziness and nausea with her head turned to the left and hanging down, confirming a diagnosis of BPPV. At this point you can tell the patient that the problem is in the posterior semicircular canal on the left, that it will gradually resolve over days to weeks, and that remaining active will help her get better faster. You can show her vestibular training exercises. As there is no evidence to support its use, meclizine should not be prescribed. You ask her to telephone your office in follow-up after 5 to 7 days.

CASE STUDY 2

Ms. J. is a 77-year-old woman with an episode of dizziness early this morning. She went to the bathroom immediately upon awakening and felt so dizzy that she had to hold on to the sink to keep from falling.

In the office, Ms. J. describes a lightheadedness that felt as if she were about to "black out." She denies any palpita-

tions. During the previous 2 days, she had watery, frequent bowel movements. She has chronic two-pillow orthopnea, but has noticed no increase in dyspnea on exertion or paroxysmal nocturnal dyspnea. She has no melena or blood per rectum. She also has no history of transient ischemic attack or stroke.

Her past history is remarkable for chronic obstructive lung disease and hypertension. Her medications include a diuretic and a β-adrenergic agonist inhaler.

Her pulse and blood pressure are 90 and 150/90 (seated) and 105 and 135/80 (standing after 5 minutes), respectively. She has a right carotid artery bruit. Lung sounds are normal. There is a III/VI systolic murmur heard loudest at the right upper sternal border. The heart rate is regular. There is no increase in jugular venous distension, no hepatojugular reflux, and no peripheral edema.

QUESTIONS

1. What is the most likely cause of her dizziness?
2. What do you do next?

DISCUSSION

As is often the case with older patients, the diagnosis is not obvious from the history and examination. She describes presyncope that is present when on her feet, and she approaches but does not meet criteria for postural hypotension. Diarrhea, possibly due to a virus, appears a likely explanation. However, her age places her at higher risk for cardiovascular disease, so you obtain an electrocardiogram. It shows nonspecific S-T abnormalities, so she is admitted overnight for observation and to rule out myocardial infarction. At the same time, she is gently hydrated. By morning she is asymptomatic, her cardiac enzymes are normal, and you obtain a modified treadmill test, which is normal. You send her home with a presumptive diagnosis of gastroenteritis, encourage her to drink plenty of fluids, and ask her to return in a few days for a follow-up visit.

REFERENCES

1. Sloane PD. Dizziness in primary care: results from the National Ambulatory Medical Care Survey. J Fam Pract 1989;29:33–38.
2. McGee SR. Dizzy patients. Diagnosis and treatment. West J Med 1995;162:37–42.
3. Sloane PD, Dallara J, Roach C, et al. Management of dizziness in primary care. J Am Board Fam Pract 1994; 7:1–8.
4. Drachman DA, Hart CW. An approach to the dizzy patient. Neurology 1972;22:323–334.
5. Sloane PD, Baloh RW. Persistent dizziness in geriatric patients. J Am Geriatr Soc 1989;37:1031–1038.
6. Sloane PD. Evaluation and management of dizziness in the older patient. Clin Geriatr Med 1996;12:785–801.

25. Dysuria

GEORGE R. BERGUS

Key Clinical Questions

1. Is the dysuria related to the urinary system?
2. If the symptom arises from the urinary system, is it due to infection?
3. If the dysuria is from a urinary tract infection (UTI), does the infection involve the upper or lower urinary tract?
4. Is the UTI an isolated or recurrent episode?
5. Are there special concerns related to a UTI in the specific patient?

Dysuria is pain or discomfort associated with urination that is typically localized to the bladder or urethra. This is a common chief complaint in the primary care office setting (1). Approximately 3% of all office visits are in response to this symptom, with associated medical care costs in excess of $1 billion each year (2, 3). The task of the health care provider is to determine the source of the dysuria, the appropriate treatment, and the required follow-up.

The main focus of this chapter is on urinary tract infections (UTIs). These infections can be divided into four very broad categories: (a) acute uncomplicated lower tract infection in women, (b) recurrent uncomplicated lower tract infection in women, (c) acute upper tract infection (pyelonephritis) in women, and (d) UTIs in children, men and geriatric patients. Each of these large groups should be further divided into simple and complex infections, as there are important differences in their evaluation and treatment. Other causes of dysuria are discussed in the following chapters: vaginitis (Chapter 42), prostate infection (Chapter 34), and sexually transmitted diseases (Chapter 36).

PATHOPHYSIOLOGY AND DIFFERENTIAL DIAGNOSIS

Dysuria is caused by inflammation within the genitourinary (GU) system. Acute dysuria is often the result of an infection of the urinary tract.

It can also be due to other causes of inflammation in the vagina, perineal area, urethra, or prostate. The most common vaginal infections are bacterial vaginosis, vaginal candidiasis, and vaginal trichomoniasis. Other causes of dysuria include perineal trauma, senile vaginal atrophy, and the poorly understood "urethral syndrome." The latter syndrome has been ascribed to trauma, chemical irritation, low levels of urinary pathogens, or infection of periurethral tissue by unknown microorganisms (4). The sexually transmitted diseases herpes simplex, chlamydia, gonorrhea, and trichomoniasis can cause dysuria in either sex. Prostate infections can be associated with urinary symptoms including decreased urine flow, urgency, and hesitancy. Both acute prostatitis and upper tract UTI may present as fever and dysuria.

Pathophysiology

Most UTIs are caused by bacteria that normally inhabit the colon. Nearly 80 to 90% of community-acquired UTIs in adults and children are due to *Escherichia coli* (5, 6). The predominance of a single species of bacterium is important because it makes urine culture unnecessary for many patients. Other gram-negative organisms, including *Proteus* species, *Klebsiella pneumoniae,* and *Pseudomonas aeruginosa,* cause infections but are much less common except in hospitalized patients, immunocompromised patients, or patients who have undergone recent GU catheterization or instrumentation. Gram-positive organisms including *Staphylococcus saprophyticus, Staphylococcus aureus,* group B streptococcus, and *Enterococcus faecium* are also uropathogens, but are much less common causes of UTI than gram-negative organisms. Anaerobic bacteria predominate in the gut but almost never cause UTI.

The usual route of infection is one in which bacteria ascend from the perineum, pass through the urethra and invade the bladder. Only a small number of *E. coli* strains have glycolipid adherence factors that enhance their ability to bind to urinary epithelium; these strains cause most UTIs. Infections usually remain within the lower urinary tract, but can sometimes ascend through the ureters to invade the upper urinary tract. When the renal parenchyma becomes infected, the infection is called pyelonephritis. Infections within the urinary tract are rarely from a blood-borne source.

Differential Diagnosis

The differential diagnosis of dysuria is summarized in Table 25.1 for patients in the family practice office and emergency department. Approximately 70% of otherwise healthy younger women who present with a complaint of dysuria and no vaginal symptoms have a UTI. Females have a much higher risk for UTI than males at all ages except during the neonatal period. During the third and fourth decades of life this gender difference is at its maximum, with women at 40 to 50 times greater risk. Young adult women have the highest incidence of UTI of any group, and those who are afflicted by it average one infection every other year (7). Although not all women develop UTI, 20 to 30% of women will have at least one infection.

Individuals with certain physiologic risk factor are more prone to develop UTI. For example, 10 to 20% of women have an epithelium to which uropathogenic *E. coli* more easily adhere. A history of at least two prior UTIs is a marker for this type of epithelium and is a strong predictor of subsequent infections. Colonization of the vagina by uropathogens increases the risk of UTI. Other risk factors operate by way of perineal contamination of the urinary tract, e.g., sexual intercourse and fecal incontinence (7). Finally, stasis of urine in the bladder adds to risk by facilitating bacterial multiplication. Infrequent voiding or incomplete bladder emptying are two common causes of stasis. It should not be surprising that women who use a diaphragm and spermicide for contraception are at increased risk for UTI. The diaphragm can cause urinary stasis (particularly if it is too large); a spermicide promotes colonization of the vagina with uropathogens; and sexual activity increases the chance that uropathogens enter the urinary tract.

CLINICAL EVALUATION

History

Clinical evaluation of urinary symptoms is variable and depends largely on the clinical setting of the patient. UTI in healthy adults is typically accompanied by urinary frequency, nocturia, pain on urination, and suprapubic discomfort. The clinician can use the history to determine the probability of UTI and to exclude other causes for the symptoms. When an adult woman complains of dysuria and has no vaginal symptoms, little further clinical evaluation is needed if there are no risk factors for a complicated infection. In the absence of vaginal discharge or other vaginal symptoms, there is a 65 to 75% probability that acute dysuria is from a UTI (8, 9). If vaginal complaints are also present or the dysuria is described as external, a more thorough evaluation is needed to exclude sexually transmitted diseases (STDs) and vaginitis. When the patient complains of both dysuria and vaginal discharge, the probability of UTI drops to below 20%.

Elements of the history that suggest infection of the upper urinary tract (pyelonephritis) include fever, chills, abdominal pain, flank pain, and vomiting. However, over 30% of women with symptoms suggestive of lower tract infection have some degree of upper tract involvement, whereas conversely, in some studies, up to a third of patients with lower tract infections had fever and flank pain. Key elements of the history and physical examination of the patient with dysuria, including test characteristics when known, are shown in Table 25.2.

The seriousness of UTIs thought to be localized to the lower urinary tract can also be determined by the clinical evaluation. Markers of a serious infection include prepubertal or geriatric age, symptoms for more than 7 days, an immunosuppressing condition, an episode of acute pyelonephritis within the past year, known anatomic abnormality, pregnancy, a history of recurrent infections, and diabetes mellitus (3). "Red flags" for serious or complicated infection are summarized in Table 25.3.

Table 25.1.

Differential Diagnosis of Dysuria in Otherwise Healthy Women of Reproductive Age

Diagnosis	Frequency in Office or Emergency Department
Lower tract UTI	Very common
Vaginitis	Common
Upper tract UTI	Less common
Urethritis	Less common

Table 25.2.
Key Elements of the History and Physical Examination for Dysuria

Diagnosis	Question or Maneuver	Sensitivity	Specificity	LR+	LR−
UTI[a]	Nocturia	0.67	0.62	1.8	0.53
	Dysuria	0.80	0.50	1.6	0.40
	Urgency	0.39	0.71	1.3	0.86
	Frequency	0.87	0.32	1.3	0.41
	Offensive odor of urine	0.20	0.85	1.3	0.94
	Combination of dysuria, frequency, urgency	0.84	0.40	1.4	0.40
Pyelonephritis	Chills and rigors	0.32	0.87	2.5	0.78
	Fever	0.44	0.80	2.2	0.70
	Nausea and vomiting	0.24	0.84	1.5	0.90
	Flank pain	0.48	0.67	1.5	0.78
Urethritis	Mild symptoms	—	—	—	—
	Urethral discharge				
	Vaginal or urethral discharge	—	—	—	—
	New sexual partner	—	—	—	—
Vaginitis	Vaginal discharge	—	—	—	—
	Vaginal pruritus	—	—	—	—
	No associated urinary symptoms	—	—	—	—
Prostatitis	Associated with other urinary symptoms:				
	Nocturia, frequency, urgency	—	—	—	—
	Rectal pain	—	—	—	—
	Tender prostate	—	—	—	—

[a]Sources: Dobbs FF, Fleming DM. A simple scoring system for evaluating symptoms, history and urine dipstick testing in the diagnosis of urinary tract infection. J R Coll Gen Pract 1987;37:100–104; Österberg E, Aspevall O, Grillner L, Persson E. Young women with symptoms of urinary infection. Prevalence and diagnosis of chlamydial infection and evaluation of rapid screening of bacteriuria. Scand J Prim Health Care 1996;14:43–49; Bailey BL. Urinalysis predictive of urine culture results. J Fam Pract 1995;40:45–50.

Physical Examination

The physical examination in adult women with dysuria should be focused. You will need to obtain the patient's vital signs, palpate the midabdomen, and percuss the flanks of the patient. Tenderness at these last two sites suggests upper tract disease; however, suprapubic tenderness with an uncomplicated lower tract infection is common. You will need to perform a vaginal examination on women who also complain of vaginal discharge or irritation.

Laboratory Tests

Collecting a Specimen

Urine collection is the first step in the laboratory evaluation of a patient with dysuria or suspect UTI. Adults can provide noncontaminated specimens by catching a midstream specimen of urine in a sterile container (the first few seconds of urine is not collected, as it can contain bacteria from the distal urethra). Giving the

Table 25.3.
"Red Flags" for a Complicated Infection

- Male gender
- Prepubertal or geriatric age
- Symptoms for more than 7 days
- An immunosuppressing condition
- An episode of acute pyelonephritis within the past year
- Known anatomic abnormality
- Pregnancy
- Diabetes mellitus
- Fever
- Flank pain or tenderness

Adapted from Johnson JR, Stamm WE. Diagnosis and treatment of acute urinary tract infections. Infect Dis Clin North Am 1987; 1(4):773–791.

patient adequate instructions about cleansing the urethra and genitalia has been stressed in many textbooks, but controlled studies have not demonstrated a clear advantage to this practice (10).

Urinalysis

The urinalysis includes a dry reagent test strip (the dipstick) and microscopy of a centrifuged urine sample. The dipstick, which detects blood, nitrite, and leukocyte esterase in the urine, is simple to perform and takes less than 5 minutes from sample collection to test result. The sensitivity, specificity, and likelihood ratios for dipstick and microscopic urinalysis are summarized in Table 25.4.

The leukocyte esterase (LE) test detects the presence of an esterase found in white blood cells and has a reported sensitivity for detecting UTI in the range of 70 to 90% (11, 12). The LE is less sensitive in patients with only mild symptoms and more sensitive in patients with severe symptoms (13). It is likely that there is a relationship between the severity of symptoms and leukocyte counts in the urine, as both are related to urinary tract inflammation. False-positive results can occur because of contamination by vaginal leukocytes, leukocytes from chlamydial urethritis, and by a high urine pH, high levels of urine glucose, or from tetracycline, cephalexin, gentamicin, imipenem, or clavulanic acid in the urine (14).

Nitrite is found in the urine when dietary nitrates are excreted into the urine and converted by gram-negative bacteria. This conversion usually requires that the urine and gram-negative organisms have several hours of contact; therefore, the first voided specimen in the morning is most likely to be positive in a patient with UTI. The nitrite test has a sensitivity of only 30 to 40% (11, 15); gram-positive and *Pseudomonas* species will not be detected with this test, because these bacteria do not convert nitrates to nitrites. However, the specificity of this test is above 95%, so a positive nitrite test is highly suggestive of UTI (LR+ 8.8). Using the leukocyte esterase and nitrate in combination (the dipstick is considered positive if either test is positive) is a better predictor of UTI than either test individually (16).

Blood is detected by a dipstick using the peroxidase-like activity of hemoglobin in the urine. False-positive reactions can occur from the peroxidase-like activity of myoglobin or the presence of bacteria that produce peroxidase. The presence of blood is not very sensitive for UTI but, in the presence of dysuria, it is a fairly specific indicator of infection.

Direct microscopy of the urinary sediment is used to look for white cells (pyuria), red cells (hematuria), bacteria (bacteriuria) and white cell casts. The sediment is prepared by centrifuging a test tube of freshly voided urine, decanting the urine, and then resuspending the sediment with the urine, which adheres to the sides of the test tube. The microscopy results are influenced by how long the urine is allowed to sit after collection, the duration and speed of centrifugation, the technique used to decant the urine and resuspend the sediment, and the technique of the individual performing the microscopy.

Although the number of leukocytes per high-power field (400× magnification) in the resuspended urine sediment is commonly used to diagnose UTI, there is disagreement about how many leukocytes define the presence of infection.

Table 25.4.
Characteristics of Diagnostic Test Useful for Patients with UTI

Test	Sensitivity	Specificity	LR+	LR−
Dipstick[a]				
Leukocyte esterase	0.87	0.68	2.7	0.19
Nitrite	0.53	0.94	8.8	0.50
Sediment microscopy				
1 bacterium/HPF[b]	0.95	0.85	6.3	0.06
10 bacteria/HPF[b]	0.85	0.99	85	0.15
5 WBC/HPF[c]	0.91	0.48	1.7	0.19
10 WBC/HPF[b]	0.82	0.65	2.3	0.28
5 RBC/HPF[a]	0.44	0.88	3.7	0.60

[a]Source: Pfaller MA, Koontz FP. Laboratory evaluation of leukocyte esterase and nitrite tests for the detection of bacteriuria. J Clin Microbiol 1985;21(5):840–842.

[b]Source: Barry HC, Ebell MH, Hickner J. Evaluation of suspected urinary tract infection in ambulatory women: a cost-utility analysis of office-based strategies. J Fam Pract 1997;44(1):49–60.

[c]Source: Bailey BL. Urinalysis predictive of urine culture results. J Fam Pract 1995;40:45–50.

Some authors have suggested that as few as 2 white blood cells per high-power field (WBC/HPF) can be used to identify infected urine, whereas others feel that 5, 10, or 15 WBC/HPF are more appropriate cutpoints (17, 18). Instead of one rigid criterion, it is more appropriate to use the number of WBC/HPF to revise the probability of UTI (19). For example, in a woman with typical symptoms of UTI, 2 WBC/HPF might be considered positive because of the high pretest probability of UTI. On the other hand, in men and children with dysuria, a more stringent cutpoint of 5 WBC/HPF is appropriate to define a positive test and will reduce the number of false-positive results. Finally, in a patient without any symptoms, you might use 10 to 15 WBC/HPF to define pyuria.

The presence of bacteria at high power (400×) is also suggestive of UTI. Finding at least one bacterium under these conditions has a sensitivity of approximately 95% and a specificity of approximately 85%. Increasing the definition of bacteriuria to at least 10 bacteria/HPF improves specificity (99%) but is associated with a lower sensitivity (85%) (20). Therefore, if no bacteria are found in the sediment, a UTI is ruled out (LR− 0.06), and if 10 or more bacteria are seen per high-power field, the infection is ruled in (LR+ 85).

White cell casts can also be found in the urine sediment and are identified by their tube-like granular appearance. Their presence suggests inflammation within the kidney such that white blood cells are collecting within the renal tubules. Infection is the primary cause of these casts, although interstitial nephritis can also produce these casts.

Urine Culture

The gold standard for UTI is a "positive" urine culture, that is, a urine culture that grows at least 10,000 colony-forming units (cfu) of a pathogenic bacteria per milliliter (21). The way that a "positive" culture is defined has changed over time. Previously, growth of 100,000 cfu/mL was required before the culture was thought to indicate infection, but this higher colony count was based on studies of patients with pyelonephritis. More recent studies demonstrated that a cutoff of 100,000 cfu/mL will miss about one third of women with uncomplicated lower tract infections.

Urine cultures are useful if you have to confirm the infection, identify the organism and its antibiotic susceptibilities, or confirm successful treatment. A culture is not typically part of the evaluation of a premenopausal woman with acute dysuria from what appears to be an uncomplicated lower tract infection. First, culture results are not available at the time you prescribe antibiotic therapy and frequently are not even available by the end of the treatment. In addition, cultures have not been found to be highly predictive of the *clinical* outcome of antibiotic treatment in this group of patients (22). Because of these problems, urine cultures are not cost-effective in the routine care of UTI in healthy women (23). Cultures are necessary when evaluating dysuria in children, men, and older women and in younger women who have either a significant probability of an upper tract infection or infections with bacteria not likely to respond to the routine antibiotics.

MANAGEMENT

In managing a patient with UTI, you should consider the characteristics of both the patient and the infection, but customize the treatment plan for your patient and their infection. Treatment recommendations with their level of evidence are summarized in Table 25.5. An algorithm for management appears in Figure 25.1.

Much of the required clinical data about women with dysuria can be collected over the telephone, raising the possibility of diagnosing and treating a UTI without an office visit. The high pretest probability of infection in young, healthy women has led many health providers and some health care organizations to manage suspected UTI in selected female patients without an office visit. Although no controlled trials

Table 25.5.
Management of Urinary Tract Infection

Treatment Strategy	Level of Evidence for Effectiveness[a]
Oral antibiotics	A
Cranberry juice	B
Increased fluid intake	B

[a]Level of evidence for effectiveness: A, strong or moderate research-based evidence (consistent across several studies, including at least two randomized controlled trials); B, limited research-based evidence (less consistent or extensive evidence, but preponderance of evidence supports use of treatment); C, common practice with little or no research-based evidence; X, moderate or strong evidence suggesting that this treatment is not effective.

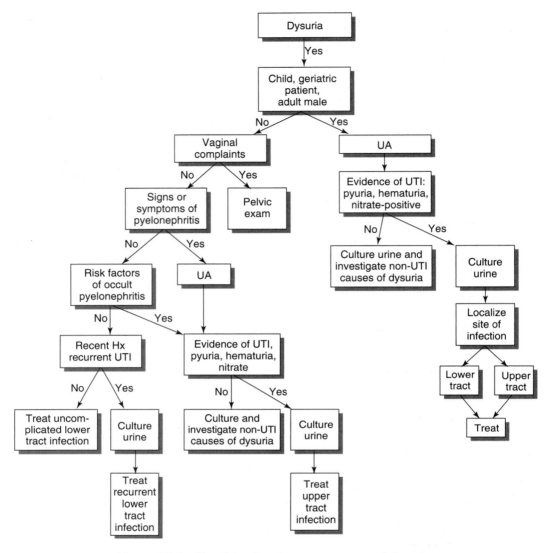

Figure 25.1. *Algorithm for the management of dysuria.*

have compared this treatment strategy to an office-based strategy, cost-effectiveness analyses support the empiric approach when it is physician monitored, but not when patients can access antibiotics directly (24, 25).

Acute Uncomplicated Lower Tract Infection in Otherwise Healthy Younger Women

Many uncomplicated lower tract UTIs in women are self limited or respond to home remedies. In fact, nearly 40% of lower tract infections will clear within 2 weeks without antibiotic treatment (26). Drinking cranberry juice (300 mL daily for 4 to 8 weeks) is a widely used home remedy, and research shows that this beverage is more likely to clear bacteriuria than water alone (27). Despite the utility of nondrug treatment, antibiotic therapy of UTI is the standard of care and is supported by the best evidence.

The specific antibiotic should be selected after considering antibacterial spectrum, safety, and cost. Trimethoprim/sulfamethoxazole (TMP/

SMX), trimethoprim alone, nitrofurantoin, or an oral cephalosporin (e.g., cephalexin) are frequently used for initial treatment of a lower tract UTI. Amoxicillin is not a good choice, since as many as 20 to 30% of the gram-negative organisms that cause UTI are resistant in some areas. A urinary analgesic, phenazopyridine, is useful for patients with significant dysuria to quickly provide symptomatic relief. Antibiotics for urinary tract infection are summarized in Table 25.6.

Three days of antibiotic treatment appears to be optimal for most acute uncomplicated cases of UTI. Three-day therapy results in a cure rate close to that achieved with 7 to 10 days of treatment but with many fewer antibiotic complications (28). TMP/SMX is preferred by most clinicians because of its low cost, high cure rate, and only moderate level of adverse effects (29). Generally, a follow-up visit is not required if the urinary symptoms resolve with the short course of antibiotics. Single-dose therapy has been widely used, but has a lower cure rate and a higher recurrence rate than multiple-day therapy.

The use of the fluoroquinolones for initial treatment of uncomplicated lower tract UTIs is effective and well tolerated, but this class of antibiotic is significantly more expensive than TMP/SMX. The increased drug expense of a fluoroquinolone is somewhat moderated by lower rates of treatment failure and adverse effects. As a result, 3 days of a fluoroquinolone and TMP/SMX have been reported to have similar average cost per patient (30). As bacterial resistance to TMP/SMX increases, the empiric use of the fluoroquinolones as therapy is likely to become more common. But resistance development is also an issue with fluoroquinolones.

Women with occult pyelonephritis form an important subgroup of women with symptoms typical of uncomplicated lower tract infections. Occult pyelonephritis is present in up to 30% of women with UTI seen in the office setting and 50% of women with UTI seen in emergency rooms (31). Women with risk factors for occult pyelonephritis (see Table 25.3) should receive 7 to 10 days of antibiotic treatment. Single-dose therapy has a high failure rate in these patients and should not be used (32). TMP/SMX is a reasonable first choice in this group, and the fluoroquinolones are a reasonable second choice. Nitrofurantoin should not be used for treating women at risk for occult pyelonephritis because it does not provide therapeutic drug levels within the upper urinary tract.

Recurrent Infections

Although repeated lower tract UTIs may be due to inadequately treated infections (and are therefore actually relapses), most repeat infections are

Table 25.6.
Oral Drug Therapy for UTI[a]

Drug	Indications	Dosage
Trimethoprim/sulfamethoxazole (TMP/SMX) (Septra, Bactrim, others)	Lower or upper tract infections	Adult: double-strength formulation bid Child: 8 mg TMP/40 mg SMX/kg/day; give bid
Trimethoprim (Trimpex, Proloprim, others)	Lower tract infections	Adult: 100 mg bid
Nitrofurantoin (Macrodantin, Macrobid, others)	Lower tract infections	Adult: 50–100 mg qid or 100 mg bid with Macrobid Child: 5–7 mg/kg/day; give qid
Cephalexin (Keflex, others)	Lower or upper tract infections	Adult: 250–500 mg qid Child: 25–50 mg/kg/day given qid
Ciprofloxacin (Cipro)	Lower tract Upper tract	Adult: 250 mg bid Adult: 500 mg bid
Amoxicillin/clavulanate (Augmentin)	Lower or upper tract infections	Adult: 875 bid Child: 45 mg of amoxicillin component in two divided doses

[a]Note: Length of treatment of outpatient with lower tract infection (oral antibiotics): female adult—3 days; male adult—10 days; geriatric patient or child—7–14 days. For outpatient with upper tract infection (oral antibiotics): adult—14 days; geriatric patient or child—14–21 days. For hospitalized patient with upper tract infection and initial IV antibiotics (switch to oral antibiotics when stable): female adult—14 days; male adult, geriatric patient, or child—21 days.

recurrences due to a new infection. Recurrent infections typically occur in women with the genetic or behavioral factors discussed earlier that place them at an increased risk for UTI. Only rarely do these women have anatomic abnormalities. As a result, extensive radiographic imaging and urologic evaluation have a low yield in women with recurrent lower tract infections and typically are not indicated.

Laboratory evaluation of women with recurrent infections is similar to the approach recommended for the isolated lower tract infection. At some point, however, you should obtain a urine culture to both clearly document the infection and identify the organism and its antibiotic susceptibility. This approach will prevent women with recurrent episodes of dysuria from causes other than UTIs from being inappropriately treated with antibiotics.

Recurrent infections can be treated with the same short courses of antibiotics recommended for isolated lower tract infections. Additionally, physicians can prescribe a short course of antibiotics that the patient keeps on hand to use once she develops her typical symptoms. This "patient-initiated treatment" is convenient for the patient, and studies have shown it to be safe and effective (33). If the patient has three or more UTIs in a year that are related to sexual intercourse, you can prescribe a single dose of antibiotics to be used routinely after intercourse. When a woman has recurrent infections that are not related to intercourse, daily antibiotic prophylaxis has been shown to be useful. The dosage in both of these treatment regimens is the same used for treatment of UTI, but is given only once postcoitally or once per day.

Acute Pyelonephritis in Younger Women

Acute pyelonephritis is a systemic disease and requires different management than a lower tract infection. Women with pyelonephritis should be placed into one of three groups:

1. Women who are febrile but medically stable and tolerating liquids by mouth
2. Women who, because of severity of infection or underlying disability, are not medically stable or are unable to take oral fluids or medications
3. Women who have infection complicated by abscess or obstruction, regardless of ability to take fluids by mouth

Medically stable women who maintain hydration on oral fluids can be treated as outpatients. Using oral antibiotics at home, these women do as well as if they were admitted to the hospital and treated with parenteral antibiotics (34). The choice of the oral antibiotic, the duration of treatment, and the patient's ability to return for frequent follow-up are all important for successful outpatient management of pyelonephritis. Fourteen days of TMP/SMX or a fluoroquinolone (e.g., Liprofloxacin) is generally effective, although resistance to TMP/SMX is becoming a problem in many communities. Amoxicillin alone has a high failure rate, but when combined with clavulanate, it can be used with good results. Parenteral ceftriaxone is widely used as a "loading" dose that is followed by oral antibiotics, but whether this combination has any advantage over oral therapy alone is not known. Regardless of the initial antibiotic selection, because pyelonephritis is a tissue infection, it is crucial to adjust antibiotic coverage with the aid of the urine culture and antibiotic sensitivity report.

Women with pyelonephritis need hospital care when they are not medically stable, are unable to remain hydrated on oral fluids, or have a complicated infection. The initial choice of antibiotic should be a fluoroquinolone, ampicillin and gentamicin, or a third-generation cephalosporin (all given parenterally). Fifteen percent of these patients will have bacteremia, so you should obtain blood cultures prior to starting parenteral antibiotics (30). Intravenous antibiotics should be continued until the patient has been afebrile for 24 hours; the patient can then be switched to an oral agent for an additional 14 days.

When patients do not improve after 72 hours of parenteral therapy, imaging is indicated to identify a perinephric abscess, an intrarenal abscess, an unrecognized anatomic abnormality, or ureteral obstruction. Either sonography or computed tomography (CT) can be used to identify these complications. Abscess or obstruction is an indication for urologic consultation. Complicated infections should be treated for at least 21 days.

To confirm cure after clinical resolution of pyelonephritis, a follow-up culture should be obtained 2 to 4 weeks after the end of antibiotic treatment. Imaging of the urinary tract after successful treatment is not recommended except in women with

- more than one episode of pyelonephritis
- a slow response to parenteral antibiotics

- abnormalities on their follow-up urinalysis
- a history of childhood urinary tract infection without previous imaging

SPECIAL CONSIDERATIONS

Adult Men with Urinary Tract Infections

A more extensive evaluation is warranted in men with dysuria because they are more likely to have a serious infection when they develop UTI. As with women, men should be identified as having either an upper tract or a lower tract infection. Other causes of dysuria, including prostatitis and urethritis, need to be excluded as causes of urinary symptoms.

An initial choice of antibiotic for a suspected lower tract infection is typically TMP/SMX or a fluoroquinolone. Pretreatment culture is recommended, and antibiotic treatment should be continued for 7 to 10 days; shorter-duration treatment is not well studied in men. Men with pyelonephritis can be treated as outpatients with a fluoroquinolone or in hospital with parenteral antibiotics if their symptoms are more severe. Those managed as outpatients should be treated for 10 to 14 days, whereas hospitalized patients should receive a total of 14 to 21 days of antibiotic therapy. After a second lower tract infection or a single episode of pyelonephritis, the adult male patient should undergo imaging to identify an anatomic abnormality or nephrolithiasis.

Urinary Tract Infections in Older Adults

In the geriatric population, UTI can present without urinary symptoms but as mental status changes, tachypnea, tachycardia, fever, gait instability, and falls. These symptoms can also be caused by many other conditions, including other infections, hypoxia, an adverse reaction to medications, or metabolic abnormalities. Diagnosis of UTI in this age group is challenging because the symptoms are nonspecific and asymptomatic bacteriuria is common, affecting 10% of elderly men and 20% of elderly women (35).

Lower tract UTI in older women (age > 50 years) should be treated for 7 to 10 days, whereas older men should be treated for 14 days. Shorter courses of treatment are not recommended in this age group. Urine culture should be obtained before treatment because the organism or its antibiotic sensitivity is not highly predictable.

Pending the culture results, these patients can be started on a fluoroquinolone, TMP/SMX, or amoxicillin/clavulanate. Older patients with upper tract infections should be treated using the same guidelines given for men in the preceding section.

Urinary Tract Infections in Children

Approximately 3 to 5% of girls and 1 to 2% of boys have at least one symptomatic UTI before puberty (36). Like adults, children can be at increased risk for UTI because of perineal colonization by uropathogens or urine stasis in the bladder. Young children are prone to perineal colonization because of stool incontinence, and several studies have also shown that noncircumcised male infants are at a higher risk for UTIs compared to their circumcised peers because they are more likely to harbor *E. coli* on their genitalia (37). Older children are prone to urine stasis because of infrequent voiding. Vesicoureteral reflux can also be responsible for incomplete bladder emptying and places children of all age groups at increased risk for UTI.

Clinical Evaluation

You should always perform a thorough history and physical in a child with suspected UTI to exclude other causes of the symptoms. In addition, children can have UTI without the dysuria and other urinary symptoms typically seen in adults. Neonates with UTI might present only with late-onset jaundice, fever, poor weight gain, irritability, or hypothermia. In infants, diarrhea, vomiting, fever, or failure to thrive might be observed (38). The classic urinary symptoms that typify UTI in adults are relatively uncommon in preschool children, with only 10% of UTIs presenting with these complaints. In school-age children, UTI can present with dysuria, but it can also present as abdominal pain or urinary incontinence. Urethral irritation from bubble bath irritation, vaginitis, pin worms, and trauma resulting from masturbation or sexual abuse are more common causes of dysuria in children than UTI.

Laboratory Tests

Urine samples from neonates and infants can be obtained by bladder catheterization. This method has a high success rate of obtaining a noncontaminated specimen and is safe (39). Suprapubic aspiration of the bladder is widely used, but is more invasive, requires more physician time, and is no more successful. A urine sample obtained by placing a plastic bag over a child's genitalia often provides confusing data, since contamination of the collected urine with bacteria from the skin is common.

Urinalysis is not a sensitive test for UTI in neonates and infants because 50% of the urinalyses of these young children with UTIs can be normal (40). Nor is this test specific for UTI; young children can develop pyuria after viral immunization or with nonurinary foci of infection. Therefore, urine culture is a routine part of the evaluation of ill children in these age groups regardless of the result of the urinalysis. In older children, the dipstick and microscopic urinalyses are useful tests for assessing infection and have similar test characteristics as those reported in adults (see Table 25.4).

Management

Noninfant children with lower tract UTI are treated along the same general guidelines as UTIs in men. When symptoms are mild and the urinalysis suggests an infection, 10 days of oral antibiotics should be prescribed after a urine sample is obtained for culture. TMP/SMX, amoxicillin/clavulanate, nitrofurantoin, or a cephalosporin are reasonable first choices for these infections. The fluoroquinolones should not be routinely used in children because of their toxicity to growing cartilage (see Table 25.6).

All neonates and infants with UTI need hospitalization and parenteral antibiotics. When a child is past infancy and has the manifestations of an upper tract infection, outpatient therapy is still possible as long as the child appears nontoxic and is tolerating oral fluids. Treatment duration is typically 14 to 21 days. If hospitalization is required owing to the age of the child (< 3 months old) or the severity of the infection, parenteral ampicillin and gentamicin or a third-generation cephalosporin should be used as initial coverage, with therapy later adjusted based on the culture and sensitivity results.

A urine culture should be obtained after completion of therapy in children to confirm successful treatment of the infection. Renal function should also be evaluated by measuring the serum creatinine. Imaging studies to detect anatomic or functional abnormalities such as vesicoureteral reflux are indicated for children with UTI with any of the following:

- Any UTI in a newborn or infant
- Recurrent lower tract infections in female children postinfancy
- Any lower tract infection in male children
- A single episode of pyelonephritis in any child

Although there are many different recommendations about imaging based on expert opinion, few randomized studies have been done (41). The many different recommendations are not totally consistent, and researchers have found that imaging is inconsistently used in children. The reasoning behind the recommendations for imaging is that early detection of urologic abnormalities will lead to interventions that improve long-term outcomes such as the prevention of chronic renal damage.

Renal sonography can be used to detect urinary tract obstruction. When significant abnormalities are visualized on the sonogram, additional information can be obtained using an intravenous pyelogram (IVP) or a nuclear renal scan. Voiding cystourethrography (VCUG) is used to define urethral and bladder anatomy. It needs to be delayed for 3 to 6 weeks after successful treatment of the infection to allow inflammation-related changes to abate.

Catheter-Associated UTI

Catheter-associated UTI is a common source of iatrogenic gram-negative bacteremia because catheters are frequently used in patients with diminished resistance to infection and the catheter provides an easy portal of entry for bacteria. You can prevent catheter-related infections by removing the urinary catheter as soon as possible or by not inserting it in the first place. Prophylactic antibiotics can reduce the risk of catheter-related infections in patients who have only a short-term need for a catheter, such as postoperative patients (42). Prophylaxis does not work with the long-term placement of a catheter; almost all catheterized patients will develop bacteriuria within 30 days. Intermittent catheterization will markedly reduce the risk of UTI and is preferable to a chronic, indwelling catheter.

Many catheter-associated infections occur in nursing homes. When the infection is mild, treatment with an oral fluoroquinolone is usually successful and hospitalization is not necessary. You should also replace the catheter if it has been in place for more than 2 weeks. Bacteria adhere to the surface of the urinary catheters and create a biofilm, which prevents antibiotics from reaching the embedded bacteria. Parenteral antibiotics are indicated for moderately severe infections; remember that most patients with catheters are elderly or medically compromised, and are usually less able to tolerate an infection than young adults.

Asymptomatic Bacteriuria

Asymptomatic bacteriuria can occur in all age groups. Screening for this condition is only recommended for several specific conditions. The U.S. Preventive Services Task Force recommends that all pregnant women be screened at 12 to 16 weeks' gestation with a urine culture. Screening in pregnancy is important because 6% of women will have asymptomatic bacteriuria, and over 20% of these women will develop acute pyelonephritis. Identifying and treating pregnant women with asymptomatic bacteriuria will significantly reduce the risk of pyelonephritis. In fact, only 6.5 women with asymptomatic bacteriuria need to be treated to prevent one case of pyelonephritis (43). Using the urinalysis alone for screening will miss 25 to 50% of women with asymptomatic bacteriuria (44).

An oral cephalosporin, nitrofurantoin, or TMP/SMX can be used for treatment, although the latter is avoided at term because of the concern that sulfonamides increase the risk of neonatal kernicterus. The duration of antibiotic therapy for asymptomatic bacteriuria is controversial, although 7 to 10 days of therapy are usually recommended. Treatment should be followed up by culture to confirm successful clearing of bacteriuria. Because women identified with asymptomatic bacteriuria at any point during pregnancy have an increased risk of redeveloping this condition after treatment, they should be repeatedly screened by urine culture. Antibiotic prophylaxis is an option for women who develop recurrent asymptomatic bacteriuria or pyelonephritis during pregnancy.

Screening for asymptomatic bacteriuria is also recommended in children with recurrent UTI (45). The child should bring a urine sample for culture at increasing intervals (e.g., 1 month, 3 months, 6 months, 12 months, and then yearly) because recurrent infection is common. Alternatively, home nitrite testing of first morning urine samples is an effective way to identify recurrent bacteriuria before the child becomes symptomatic.

Asymptomatic bacteriuria is also common in elderly patients, occurring in 10% of men and 20% of women. A higher prevalence of asymptomatic bacteriuria is found in nursing homes. Although this finding is a marker of poor health and a risk factor for death, there is good evidence that treatment of this condition with antibiotics does not improve health (46). Although the bacteriuria can be eradicated by the use of antibiotics, it tends to recur quickly. Screening is therefore not recommended in this group.

CASE STUDY 1

A 28-year-old woman presents with a 24-hour history of dysuria and urinary frequency. She has been forcing oral fluids without improvement. She denies fever, chills, or flank pain. She has been sexually active with one partner for 3 months and uses oral contraceptive pills for birth control.

QUESTIONS

1. What other data from the history and physical do you need to properly manage this patient?
2. What laboratory tests would you order?
3. If the patient is diagnosed with a UTI, how would you treat her?

DISCUSSION

The presence of these urinary symptoms in the absence of vaginal complaints makes UTI highly likely. You should identify whether she has risk factors that should warn you of a possible complicated UTI (see Table 25.3). For an uncomplicated UTI in a healthy woman, only limited laboratory investigation, if any, is warranted. Prior to obtaining any tests, the probability of UTI in this patient with dysuria and no vaginal symptoms is approximately 70%. If empiric therapy is not chosen, a reasonable strategy is to perform a dipstick evaluation of the urine. If this test is positive for blood, leukocyte esterase, or nitrite, you could presume the presence of

UTI. If all results are negative, you can perform a microscopic examination of the centrifuged sediment. If the patient has an uncomplicated lower tract infection, she should be treated with 3 days of TMP/SMX (one double-strength tablet, twice daily). No follow-up is needed unless symptoms do not resolve. If the patient is thought to be at risk for having a complicated UTI (despite having symptoms suggestive of only a lower tract infection), she should receive 7 days of treatment and be followed up to confirm cure.

the sediment for WBC casts, which would suggest pyelonephritis. A urine culture is necessary because pyelonephritis is a tissue infection, and you need to know about the antibiotic sensitivity of the infecting organism. If the patient is maintaining hydration and is not pregnant, she can be placed on 2 weeks of therapy with TMP/SMX or a fluoroquinolone pending sensitivities.

CASE STUDY 2

A 34-year-old woman who presents with 5 days of dysuria and malaise has some back pain today. She denies chills, nausea, and vomiting. On examination, she is not in distress and has the following vital signs: temperature 38°C, pulse rate 92 beats/minute, blood pressure 122/70, and respiratory rate 16. She has moderate right CVA tenderness to percussion and no abdominal tenderness.

QUESTIONS

1. What other data from the history and physical do you need to properly manage this patient?
2. How would you test her urine?
3. What antibiotic regimen does she need?

DISCUSSION

You should determine whether the patient is otherwise healthy, able to maintain oral hydration, and in a stable home situation with someone who is able to help care for her. You also need to know about her last menstrual period in order to assess her chances of being pregnant. A urinalysis is needed with both dipstick and microscopic examination of the sediment to look for evidence of infection. Also look at

REFERENCES

1. Stamm WE, Hooton TM. Management of urinary tract infections in adults. N Engl J Med 1993;329(18):1328–1334.
2. Patton JP, Nash DB, Abrutyn E. Urinary tract infection: economic considerations. Med Clin North Am 1991;75(2):495–513.
3. Johnson JR, Stamm WE. Diagnosis and treatment of acute urinary tract infections. Infect Dis Clin North Am 1987;1(4):773–791.
4. Gittes RF, Nakamura RM. Female urethral syndrome. A female prostatitis? West J Med 1996;164:435–438.
5. Wilkie ME, Almond MK, Marsh FP. Diagnosis and management of urinary tract infection in adults. BMJ 1992;305:1137–1141.
6. Todd JK. Management of urinary tract infections: Children are different. Pediatr Rev 1996;16(5):190–196.
7. Hooton TM, Scholes D, Hughes JP, et al. A prospective study of risk factors for symptomatic urinary tract infection in young women. N Engl J Med 1996;335:468–474.
8. Berg AO, Heidrich FE, Fihn SD, et al. Establishing the cause of genitourinary symptoms in women in a family practice. JAMA 1984;251(5):620–625.
9. Komaroff AL, Pass TM, McCue JD, Cohen AB, Hendricks TM, Friedland G. Management strategies for urinary and vaginal infections. Arch Intern Med 1978;138:1069–1073.
10. Bradbury SM. Collection of urine specimens in general practice: to clean or not to clean? J R Coll Gen Pract 1988;38(313)363–365.
11. Pfaller MA, Koontz FP. Laboratory evaluation of leukocyte esterase and nitrite tests for the detection of bacteriuria. J Clin Microbiol 1985;21(5):840–842.
12. Blum RN, Wright RA. Detection of pyuria and bacteriuria in symptomatic ambulatory women. Gen Intern Med 1992;7:140–144.
13. Lachs MS, Nachamkin I, Edelstein PH, Goldman J, Feinstein AR, Schwartz JS. Spectrum bias in the evaluation of diagnostic tests: lessons from the rapid dipstick test for urinary tract infection. Ann Intern Med 1992;117:135–140.
14. Beer JH, Vogt A, Neftel K, Cottagnoud P. False-positive results for leucocytes in urine dipstick test with common antibiotics. BMJ 1996;313:25.

15. Roy JB, Wilkerson RG. Fallibility of Griess (nitrite) test. Urology 1984;23:270–271.

16. Hurlbut TA, Littenberg B. The diagnostic accuracy of rapid dipstick tests to predict urinary tract infection 1991;96(5)582–588.

17. Alwall N. Pyuria: Deposit in high-power microscopic field—WBC/HPF versus WBC/mm^3 in counting chamber. Acta Med Scand 1973;194:537–540.

18. Wigton RS, Hoellerich VL, Ornato JP, Leu V, Mazzotta LA, Cheng IC. Use of clinical findings in the diagnosis of urinary tract infection in women. Arch Intern Med 1985;145:2222–2227.

19. Bergus GR. When is a test "positive"? The use of decision analysis to optimize test interpretation. Fam Med 1993;25:656–660.

20. Jenkins RD, Fenn JP, Matsen JM. Review of urine microscopy for bacteriuria. JAMA 1986;255(24):3397–3403.

21. Latham RH, Wong ES, Larson A, Coyle M, Stamm WE. Laboratory diagnosis of urinary tract infection in ambulatory women. JAMA 1985;254:3333–3336.

22. Schultz HJ, McCaffrey LA, Keys TF, Nobrega FT. Acute cystitis: a prospective study of laboratory tests and duration of therapy. Mayo Clin Proc 1984;59:391–397.

23. Carlson KJ, Mulley AG. Management of acute dysuria. Ann Intern Med 1985;102:244–249.

24. Rubin N, Foxman B. Pharmacoepidemiology reports: the cost-effectiveness of placing urinary tract infection treatment over the counter. J Clin Epidemiol 1996;49 (11):1315–1321.

25. Barry HC, Ebell MH, Hickner J. Evaluation of suspected urinary tract infection in ambulatory women: a cost-utility analysis of office-based strategies. J Fam Pract 1997;44(1):49–60.

26. Mabeck CM. Treatment of uncomplicated urinary tract infections in nonpregnant women. Postgrad Med J 1972;48:69–75.

27. Avorn J, Monane M, Gurwitz JH, Glynn RJ, Choodnovskiy I, Lipsitz LA. Reduction of bacteriuria and pyuria after ingestion of cranberry juice. JAMA 1994; 271(10):7514.

28. Norrby SR. Short-term treatment of uncomplicated lower urinary tract infections in women. Rev Infect Dis 1990;12(3):458–467.

29. Hooton TM, Winter C, Tiu F, Stamm WE. Randomized comparative trial and cost analysis of 3-day antimicrobial regimens for treatment of acute cystitis in women. JAMA 1995;273(1):41–45.

30. Johnson JR, Lyons MF, Pearce W, et al. Therapy for women hospitalized with acute pyelonephritis: a randomized trial of ampicillin versus trimethoprim-sulfamethoxazole for 14 days. J Infect Dis 1991;163:325–330.

31. Fihn SD, Johnson C, Roberts PL, Running K, Stamm WE. Trimethoprim-sulfamethoxazole for acute dysuria in women: a single-dose or 10-day course. Ann Intern Med 1988;108:350–357.

32. Ronald AR, Boutros P, Mourtada H. Bacteriuria localization and response to single-dose therapy in women. JAMA 1976;235:1854–1856.

33. Wong ES, McKevitt M, Running K, Counts GW, Tuck M, Stamm WE. Management of recurrent urinary infections with patient-administered single-dose therapy. Ann Intern Med 1985;102:302–307.

34. Pinson AG, Philbrick JT, Lindbeck GH, Schorling JB. Oral antibiotic therapy for acute pyelonephritis: a methodologic review of the literature. J Gen Intern Med 1992;7:544–553.

35. Boscia JA, Kobasa WD, Knight RA, Abrutyn E, Levison ME, Kaye D. Epidemiology of bacteriuria in an elderly ambulatory population. Am J Med 1986;80(2):208–214.

36. Jodal U, Winberg J. Management of children with unobstructed urinary tract infection. Pediatr Nephrol 1987;1(4):647–656.

37. Wiswell TE, Roscelli JD. Corroborative evidence for the decreased incidence of urinary tract infections in circumcised male infants. Pediatrics 1986;78(1):96–99.

38. Edelmann CM Jr, Ogwo JE, Fine BP, Martinez A. The prevalence of bacteriuria in full-term and premature newborn infants. J Pediatr 1973;82:125–132.

39. Pollack CV Jr., Pollack ES. Suprapubic bladder aspiration versus urethral catheterization in ill infants: success, efficiency and complication rates. Ann Emerg Med 1994;23:225–230.

40. Crain EF, Gershel JC. Urinary tract infections in febrile infants younger than 8 weeks of age. Pediatrics 1990;86 (3):363–367.

41. Dick PT, Feldman W. Routine diagnostic imaging for childhood urinary tract infections: a systematic overview. J Pediatr 1996;128:15–22.

42. Van Der Wal E, Verkooyen RP, Mintjes-De Groot J, Oostinga J, et al. Prophylactic ciprofloxacin for catheter-associated urinary-tract infection. Lancet 1992;339:946–951.

43. Smaill F. Antibiotic vs. no treatment for asymptomatic bacteriuria. In: Enkin MW, Keirse MJNC, Renfrew MJ, Neilson JP, eds. Pregnancy and Childbirth Module of the Cochrane Database of Systematic Reviews, 1995. London: BMJ Publishing Group, 1995.

44. Bachman JW, Heise RH, Naessens JM, Timmerman MG. A study of various tests to detect asymptomatic urinary tract infections in an obstetric population. JAMA 1993;270(16):1971–1974.

45. Kemper KJ, Avner ED. The case against screening urinalyses for asymptomatic bacteriuria in children. Am J Dis Child 1992;146:343–346.

46. Abrutyn E, Mossey J, Berlin JA, et al. Does asymptomatic bacteriuria predict mortality and does antimicrobial treatment reduce mortality in elderly ambulatory women? Ann Intern Med 1994;120:827–833.

26. Fatigue

DAVID N. LITTLE

Key Clinical Questions

1. What is the best initial approach to the workup of a patient with fatigue?
2. How do you distinguish psychologic causes of fatigue from physical and lifestyle causes in a cost-effective manner?
3. What is the best management strategy for a patient with fatigue whose workup does not reveal a specific underlying diagnosis?

The workup of fatigue demands a comprehensive approach on the part of the physician because there is a broad differential diagnosis that includes a spectrum of physical, psychologic, and lifestyle causes. While searching for and treating underlying diagnoses, you should incorporate a biopsychosocial approach and a cost-effective choice of laboratory studies. In some cases it will not be possible to identify a precise pathophysiologic mechanism for fatigue.

Fatigue (or tiredness or lassitude) is a common presenting complaint in family practices and other primary care settings. Community surveys have documented that 14 to 42% of persons report some degree of fatigue, but that only a small percentage bring their fatigue to the doctor for evaluation (1). Primary care studies show that 6.7 to 9.9% of adults coming to the office have fatigue as a chief complaint (2–5).

Studies of the outcome of fatigue demonstrate that 50 to 70% of patients fail to improve after 1 year of follow-up (6, 7). As a result, family physicians, with their longitudinal responsibility for patient care, will need to help many individuals cope with a disabling symptom. This includes using strategies such as chronic illness management, in which the doctor and patient share responsibility for symptom control and aim to enhance functional ability.

PATHOPHYSIOLOGY AND DIFFERENTIAL DIAGNOSIS

The underlying causes of fatigue can be divided into psychologic, physical, and lifestyle causes.

Table 26.1 illustrates the broad differential diagnosis you should consider when evaluating a patient with symptoms of fatigue. You should keep in mind that some patients will have contributing factors from both physical and psychologic diagnoses as well as lifestyles that add to the complexity of the diagnostic process.

Psychologic Causes

Community surveys have shown that patients with psychiatric disorders have a threefold to sixfold increased risk of feeling fatigued and that premorbid psychologic symptoms predispose patients to fatigue following infections (1). Patients with depressive disorders often complain of fatigue as part of a symptom complex that includes loss of energy, sleep problems, and poor appetite. Depression is the most common psychiatric illness in the outpatient setting, affecting at least 5% of outpatients in any 6-month period (8).

Anxiety disorders make up the second most common psychiatric illness in outpatients and may also be responsible for patients reporting tiredness as a primary symptom. You should also look for adjustment reactions to life changes (such as marital status change, birth or departure of children, death of a family member, job change), which can lead to psychologically dependent fatigue symptoms. You should investigate the role of substance abuse (caffeine, alcohol, illicit drugs), because overuse of these substances may produce symptoms of fatigue.

Physical Causes

Many different physical illnesses may cause symptoms of fatigue. Overall biomedical disorders account for 50% of primary care patients presenting with tiredness (2, 3, 5, 9, 10). The most common physical disorders causing fatigue are diabetes, acute infections, cardiovascular disease, and lung disease. In addition, physicians need to be alert for medications' side effects that are related to tiredness. Drugs commonly prescribed that may cause fatigue symptoms include analgesics, psychotropics, antihypertensives, and antihistamines.

Table 26.1.
Differential Diagnosis of Fatigue

Diagnosis	Frequency in Office Primary Care	% of Fatigued Primary Care Patients with this Diagnosis[a]
Depression	Very common	15.7
Diabetes	Very common	10.6
Acute infections	Very common	10.1
Adjustment reactions	Very common	9.6
Cardiovascular disease	Very common	7.9
Lifestyle causes	Very common	7.8
Anxiety	Common	6.1
Lung disease (COPD, asthma)	Common	4.9
Connective tissue disorders	Common	4.7
Malignancy	Somewhat common	3.2
Medication side effects	Somewhat common	2.8
Anemia	Somewhat common	2.8
Hypothyroidism	Somewhat common	2.6
Substance abuse	Somewhat common	2.2
Chronic infections (TB, HIV Disease)	Rare	1.8
Inflammatory disorders (inflammatory bowel disease, hepatitis)	Rare	1.6
Neurologic disorders	Rare	0.4
Psychosis	Rare	0.1
No diagnosis made	Very common	31.4

Adapted from Sugarman JR, Berg AD. Evaluation of fatigue in a family practice. J Fam Pract 1984;5:643–647; Morrison JD. Fatigue as a presenting complaint in family practice. J Fam Pract 1980;10:795–801; Bates DW, Schmitt W, Buchwald D, Ware NC, Lee J, Thoyer E, Kornish RJ, Komarof AL. Prevalence of fatigue and chronic fatigue syndrome in a primary care practice. Arch Intern Med 1993;153:2759–2765; Elnicki DM, Shockcor WT, Brick JE, Beynon D. Evaluating the complaint of fatigue in primary care: diagnoses and outcomes. Am J Med 1992;93:303–306.

COPD, chronic obstructive pulmonary disease; TB, tuberculosis.

[a]Percentages total more than 100% because some patients have more than one diagnosis.

Connective tissue disorders are an important cause of fatigue. You should consider the diagnoses of rheumatoid arthritis and systemic lupus erythematosus, both of which can lead to tiredness and may be accompanied by chronic anemia. Another disorder that contributes to fatigue is fibromyalgia, a chronic condition associated with a history of widespread pain and focal tenderness on digital palpation. Table 26.2 gives you the diagnostic criteria for fibromyalgia.

Less common disorders presenting as fatigue include inflammatory conditions such as rheumatic fever, chronic hepatitis, and inflammatory bowel disease. Neurologic disorders such as multiple sclerosis, Parkinsonism, and dementia may present as fatigue but usually have distinguishing signs and symptoms. Malignancy of various organ systems may cause tiredness, either as a manifestation of anorexia or in association with chronic occult blood loss (as with cancer of the colon). Hypothyroidism is a potential cause of fatigue, as are chronic infections such as tuberculosis and HIV disease. Obstructive sleep syndromes are manifested by morning tiredness, snoring, and headaches and should be considered, especially in obese patients presenting with fatigue. More subtle causes of physical fatigue include chemical and heavy metal toxicity such as carbon monoxide and lead poisoning.

Lifestyle Causes

Alterations in lifestyle may cause fatigue, although they less frequently lead to patients' seeking a medical consultation. Some of the causes to consider include an increase in physical exertion relative to the patient's established habits, inadequate rest, sleep pattern disruption, and effects of recent surgery or trauma. Studies show that fatigue may also be associated with environmental stresses such as excessive noise, heat, or cold (11). Ironically, people who have a sedentary lifestyle are more likely to report fatigue than those who are physically active. The probable explanations for this association include the antidepressant and anxiolytic effects

Table 26.2.
Criteria for the Diagnosis of Fibromyalgia

Both criteria must be present.
1. History of widespread pain.
   Definition. Pain is considered widespread when all of the following are present: pain in the left side of the body, pain in the right side of the body, pain above the waist, and pain below the waist. In addition, axial skeletal pain (cervical spine or anterior chest or thoracic spine or low back pain) must be present. In this definition, shoulder and buttock pain is considered as pain for each involved side. "Low back" pain is considered low segment pain.
2. Pain in 11 of 18 tender point sites on digital palpation.
   Definition. Pain, on digital palpation, must be present in at least 11 of the following 18 tender point sites:
   Occiput: bilateral, at the suboccipital muscle insertions.
   Low cervical: bilateral, at the anterior aspects of the intertransverse spaces at C5–C7.
   Trapezius: bilateral, at the midpoint of the upper border.
   Supraspinatus: bilateral, at origins, above the scapular spine near the medial border.
   Second rib: bilateral, at the second costochondral junctions, just lateral to the junctions on upper surfaces.
   Lateral epicondyle: bilateral, 2 cm distal to the epicondyles.
   Gluteal: bilateral, in upper outer quadrants of buttocks in anterior fold of muscle.
   Greater trochanter: bilateral, posterior to the trochanteric prominence.
   Knee: bilateral, at the medial fat pad proximal to the joint line.
   Digital palpation should be performed with an approximate force of 5 kg. For a tender point to be considered "positive," the subject must state that the palpation was painful. "Tender" is not to be considered "painful."

Adapted from Wolfe, et al. The American College of Rheumatology criteria for the classification of fibromyalgia: report of the Multicenter Criteria Committee. Arthritis Rheum 1990;33:160.

of regular exercise as well as the improved sleep habits of fit individuals.

Chronic Fatigue Syndrome (CFS)

In recent years, considerable attention has been focused on the chronic fatigue syndrome. You will find the official diagnostic criteria for this syndrome in Table 26.3. Patients must have unexplained persistent or relapsing fatigue that is not relieved by rest and is severe enough to reduce daily activity levels by at least 50%. In addition, they must demonstrate a total of eight associated minor symptoms and signs. Because there is no specific diagnostic test that clearly separates this group of patients from others with chronic fatigue who may lack all the criteria, you should think of this group as possibly representing more than one specific cause. Research studies to date have not identified a viral etiology but have suggested both qualitative and quantitative abnormalities of immunologic function (12). Although no specific treatment yet exists, making a diagnosis of CFS has several benefits: reducing unnecessary investigations, providing an explanation to the patient, in some cases providing support for disability, and identifying an approach to treatment.

CLINICAL EVALUATION

In most cases, the evaluation of fatigue will involve an extensive history and physical examination rather than the focused examination that is used for some other presenting complaints. When you perform this evaluation, you should keep in mind psychologic, physical, and lifestyle causes. The extent of your evaluation, as well as the focus of laboratory investigations, depends on the likely causes discovered by the history and physical.

History

You can use the key elements of the history listed in Table 26.4 to guide your approach to interviewing a patient with fatigue. Because of the prevalence of psychologic and lifestyle causes of fatigue, you should take a careful psychosocial history, focusing on symptoms of depression and probing for aspects of the patient's lifestyle, such as environmental stresses, impaired sleep, and inactivity, that can contribute to feeling fatigued. Unless you are already familiar with the patient's family and occupational history, you should cover these areas in your interview. You may want to ask your patient to keep a daily diary to

Table 26.3.
Criteria for Chronic Fatigue Syndrome[a]

Major Criteria (both criteria must be present)
- Persistent or relapsing fatigue or easy fatigability, not explained by other chronic conditions, lasting at least 6 months, that
  - Does not resolve with bed rest, and
  - Is severe enough to reduce average daily activity by at least 50%

Minor criteria (eight minor criteria without physical criteria *or* six minor criteria plus two physical criteria)
- Mild fever or chills
- Sore throat
- Lymph node pain anterior or posterior cervical or axillary chains
- Unexplained generalized muscle weakness
- Myalgia
- Prolonged (> 24 hours) generalized fatigue following previously tolerable levels of exercise
- New, generalized headaches
- Migratory, noninflammatory arthralgia
- One or more of the following neuropsychologic symptoms:
  Photophobia
  Tansient visual scotomata
  Forgetfulness
  Excessive irritability
  Confusion
  Difficulty thinking
  Inability to concentrate
  Depression
- Sleep disturbances (hypersomnia or insomnia)
- Patient describes initial onset as acute or subacute

Physical criteria
- Low grade fever
- Nonexudative pharyngitis
- Palpable or tender anterior or posterior cervical or axillary lymph nodes (<2 cm in diameter)

[a]Adapted from Epstein KR. The chronically fatigued patient. Med Clin North Am 1995;79:321.

help you determine precipitating factors and associations; such strategies have the added benefit of actively involving your patient in the diagnostic process.

You should be on the alert during your first visit with a fatigued patient for "red flags" that may indicate a need for urgent care. Table 26.5 gives warning signs and symptoms for major depressive episode, drug withdrawal syndromes, life-threatening infections, severe heart failure, and poorly controlled diabetes. Be sure to take a careful medication history, covering both prescription and over-the-counter drugs, in order to consider side effects explaining the patient's tiredness.

Use elements of the history to help differentiate psychologic from physical causes of fatigue. Table 26.6 lists key features of both major causal groupings. In the case of psychologic diagnoses:

- The complainant is more likely to be the patient.

- There is more likely to be a dysfunctional family setting and/or a previous history of functional health problems.

- The onset of the fatigue is more likely to be associated with stress and to be accompanied by multiple, nonspecific symptoms.

- The tiredness is more likely to have a recurrent pattern that is worse in the morning and fluctuates rather than progresses in intensity over time. Psychologically mediated fatigue is actually relieved by physical activity, whereas physical causes worsen with such activity and limit functional ability even in the face of strong desire on the part of the patient.

If your initial history suggests that the patient's fatigue is likely to be of psychologic origin, consider screening tests such as the Beck Depression Inventory. It is important to assess other expectations or concerns such as desire for refer-

Table 26.4.

Key Elements of the History and Physical Examination for Fatigue

Question/Maneuver	Purpose
Psychosocial history	Screen for psychologic and lifestyle-related causes
• Sadness or agitation	of fatigue
• Substance abuse	
• Life and environmental stresses	
• Activity/exercise level	
• Sleep habits, appetite	
• Anhedonia	
• Ability to concentrate	
• Feelings of worthlessness/hopelessness	
Look for "red flags" (see Table 26.5)	Screen for suicidality, withdrawal syndromes, life-threatening infections, poorly controlled heart failure or diabetes
Look for features differentiating physical from psychologic cases (see Table 26.6)	Assess likelihood of psychologic cause of fatigue
Medication use	Evaluate for medication side effects
Fever	Screen for acute infections
Weight loss	Screen for cancer, HIV disease
Pallor	Screen for anemia
Cough	Screen for TB, HIV disease, COPD
Joint pains/inflammation	Screen for connective disease disorder
Widespread pain, trigger points (see Table 26.2)	Screen for fibromyalgia
Exertional dyspnea	Screen for heart failure, COPD
Lymphadenopathy/hepatosplenomegaly	Screen for malignancy, infections
Thyromegaly, dry skin, delayed reflexes	Screen for hypothyroidism
Ear-nose-throat examination	Screen for otitis, pharyngitis, sinusitis
Cardiopulmonary examination	Screen for CHF, COPD, pneumonia

CHF, congestive heart failure; COPD, chronic obstructive pulmonary disease; TB, tuberculosis.

ral, work slip, symptom relief, and sexual or social problems. In some cases you may want to interview family members; in every case, you should discuss your plans with the patient to develop understanding and mutual agreement. You may refer your patient for a consultation in order to provide reassurance or to help make plans for counseling or lifestyle change.

Physical Examination

Because of the broad differential diagnosis of fatigue, you will need to examine several organ systems (see Table 26.4). Fever, weight loss, and cough may be seen in infections, malignancy, or chronic pulmonary disease. The musculoskeletal examination can be used to screen for signs of

Table 26.5.

"Red Flags" Suggesting Progressive or Life-Threatening Disease in Patients with Fatigue

Diagnosis	"Red Flags" Suggestive of the Disease
Major depressive episode	Suicidal ideation, social withdrawal
Withdrawal syndrome	History of alcohol, narcotic, or psychotropic drug abuse with recent discontinuation of use
Life-threatening infection	Fever > 39.5°C, meningitis, shock
Severe heart failure	Orthopnea, edema, cardiomegaly, auscultatory crackles
Poorly controlled diabetes	Polydipsia, polyuria

Table 26.6.
Features That May Help Differentiate Psychologic from Physical Causes of Fatigue

Features	Psychologic	Physical
Primary deficit	Desire	Ability
Onset associated with stress	Yes	No
Duration	Recurrent	Averages 2 months
Timing	Worst in morning	Worst in evening
Course	Fluctuating	Progressive
Physical activity	Relieves	Worsens
Associated symptoms	Nonspecific, multiple	Specific, few
Previous health problems	Often functional	Often organic
Family situation	Dysfunctional	Supportive
Physical appearance	Anxious, depressed	Ill, toxic

Adapted from Solberg LI. Lassitude. JAMA 1984;251:3274.

connective tissue disorder, whereas widespread pain and the presence of trigger points indicate a diagnosis of fibromyalgia (see Table 26.2). You should search for signs of hypothyroidism by palpation of the thyroid gland, examination for dry, coarse skin, and elicitation of delayed, deep-tendon reflexes. The lymphatic system should be checked for evidence of lymphadenopathy and an abdominal examination performed for signs of hepatic or splenic enlargement, both of which may indicate an underlying malignancy. The ear-nose-throat examination is used to screen for upper respiratory infection. You should perform a careful cardiopulmonary examination to screen for signs of heart failure, pneumonia, or chronic obstructive lung disease. You may need a second visit to allow sufficient time for performing these examinations.

Laboratory Tests

Due to the high incidence of psychologic causes and the broad differential diagnosis of physical causes, laboratory tests have a low yield in the workup of patients presenting with tiredness (2, 6). The only laboratory test that has been shown to have a greater yield in fatigued patients than in age/gender-matched controls is the monospot test for infectious mononucleosis. The yield, however, is no greater than 20%, and it is highly dependent on age and associated symptoms (13).

Despite the low predictive utility of laboratory tests, most physicians order a limited initial evaluation that includes a complete blood count, erythrocyte sedimentation rate, serum glucose (if the patient is obese), and thyroid-stimulating hormone (if the patient is over 40). This combination of tests will help you to confirm or rule out

the most common physical causes of fatigue discussed in Table 26.1. You may order other studies based on risk as defined during the initial history and physical examination. Examples of the latter include HIV serology, skin tests for tuberculosis, and Lyme Disease serology.

MANAGEMENT

An approach to management is shown in Figure 26.1, using a system of two office visits advocated by Ruffin and Cohen (11). In actual practice, you may have prior knowledge of the patient, and may therefore modify the approach to suit the circumstances as well as to reflect the likelihood of a particular etiology.

Initial Visit

The priorities for the initial visit are to establish a therapeutic relationship and to briefly assess elements of the history and physical examination that may indicate urgent problems. Once urgent issues are eliminated, you should plan a second visit by ordering laboratory studies and scheduling additional time to complete the history and physical examination. Patient education at this visit should emphasize the need for a comprehensive assessment, especially because some patients have limited willingness to accept the suggestion of a psychologic etiology.

Second Visit

During the second visit, you should complete your history and physical examination and review the laboratory studies. If needed, gather additional information regarding social profile, past

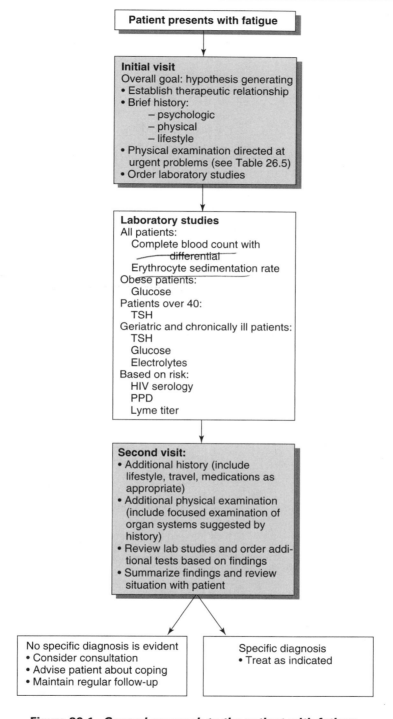

Figure 26.1. *General approach to the patient with fatigue.*

medical history, family history, review of systems, medication history, and lifestyle history.

It is important to meet with the patient toward the end of this visit to summarize the findings and make treatment suggestions based on the data. In some cases a specific diagnosis is evident and plans can proceed to begin appropriate therapy. At other times, either no specific diagnosis is found (in approximately ⅓ of patients—see Table 26.1) or the results of the evaluation suggest that there may be two or more contributing causes (in approximately ¼ of patients—see Table 26.1) . In these circumstances, you should discuss plans with the patient to develop understanding, enhance cooperation, and maintain a broad perspective on biomedical and psychosocial issues. Follow-up plans should be based on mutual agreement.

If the cause is physical, further investigation may be indicated. A consultation may be helpful to reassure you and your patient that no medical cause has been overlooked, although continuing to search for a "cure" may delay effective therapy and create unrealistic expectations.

For those patients in whom the pattern of the illness suggests a psychologic cause, other approaches have been previously discussed. In all cases, you should fully discuss plans and make a commitment to continuing care through follow-up visits.

Therapy for Chronic Fatigue

The medical literature contains no strong research studies to guide the treatment of chronically fatigued patients (Table 26.7). Cognitive behavior therapy has been shown to help individual patients. Tricyclic antidepressant medication has limited ability to relieve fatigue and some associated rheumatic symptoms such as myalgias, arthralgias, and headache (14, 15). The newer antidepressant medications that selectively block reuptake of serotonin have a more favorable adverse-effect profile, but good research-based evidence of effectiveness in treating chronic fatigue is lacking to date. Many physicians recommend an exercise program and supportive therapy, although randomized controlled trials of these approaches have not been performed.

In general, medical therapy is of extremely limited value in treating fatigue. You may wish to consider alternative therapies, with referral based on careful understanding of an individual's health beliefs and expectations.

Table 26.7.
Management of Chronic Fatigue

Treatment Strategy	Level of Evidence for Effectiveness[a]	Recommendations/Comments
Cognitive behavior	B	Patients are taught to gradually increase activity and to develop practical coping strategies
Antidepressant medication		
Tricyclics	B	Lower doses than used to treat depression
SSRIs	C	Favorable side-effect profile
MAO inhibitors	B	Difficult to utilize because of special diet
Exercise	C	Improves functional capacity, mood, and sleep habits
Supportive therapy	C	Emphasize improved function rather than care; discuss effects of fatigue on daily living
Immunotherapy (α-interferon, intravenous immunoglobulins)	X	Variable results, high toxicity and expense
Antiviral therapy	X	Not shown to be effective

Modified from Deale, A, et al. Cognitive behavior therapy for chronic fatigue syndrome. Am J Psychiatry 1997;154:408–414; Wilson A, Hickie I, Lloyd A, Wakefield D. The treatment of chronic fatigue syndrome. Am J Med 1994;544–550; Calabrese L, Danao T, Camara E, Wilke W. Chronic fatigue syndrome. Am Fam Physician 1992;45:1205–1213; Matthew DA, Manu P, Lane TJ. Evaluation and management of patients with chronic fatigue. Am J Med Sci 1991;302:269–277; Sharpe M, Hawton K, Sinkin S, Surawy C, et al. Cognitive behavior therapy for the chronic fatigue syndrome: a randomized controlled trial. BMJ 1996;312:22–26.

MAO, monoamine oxidase; SSRIs, selective serotonin reuptake inhibitors.

[a]Level of evidence for effectiveness: A, strong or moderate research-based evidence (consistent across several studies, including at least two randomized controlled trials); B, limited research-based evidence (less consistent or extensive evidence, but preponderance of evidence supports use of treatment); C, common practice with little or no research-based evidence; X, Moderate or strong evidence suggesting this treatment is *not* effective.

Coping Strategies for Chronic Fatigue

Because fatigue as a symptom has a high likelihood of persisting regardless of the specific etiology, patients benefit from learning coping strategies similar to those developed for patients with chronic pain syndromes. Such strategies involve active participation by the patient in developing habits, physical exercises, and mental techniques to improve quality of life and functional abilities. All such strategies have in common a focus on individual control and enhancement of self-esteem. In many cases, patients learn best through supportive counseling by professionals and by participation in support groups of individuals with similar chronic symptoms.

Patient Education

Physicians have an important role in educating and supporting their patients with complex chronic symptoms. In the case of the fatigued patient, the emphasis at the initial visit should be to assure the patient that a thorough evaluation will be performed and to explain the need to approach diagnoses with a comprehensive evaluation of biomedical and psychosocial factors. The emphasis in subsequent visits should be on continuity of the doctor-patient relationship, review of symptom diaries, advice for regular exercise, and assisting the patient to identify sources of support from family, friends, and support groups when appropriate.

CASE STUDY

Ms. K. is a 48-year-old woman who presents to the office with a 3-month history of tiredness. She works as a school administrator and typically maintains a 50- to 60-hour/week schedule, including several evening meetings. Recently she has felt that her ability to concentrate is diminished and she has been "too tired" to use her exercise bicycle when she gets home in the evening. Some days are better than others. She worries that she is losing interest in her professional work and her physical appearance.

Ms. K. is married without children. Her husband, employed as a bank manager, is supportive but sometimes distant. She recalls a 6-month "nervous breakdown" while she was in college but has otherwise been in good emotional health. She does not drink alcohol or use illicit drugs.

She had an upper respiratory illness 2 weeks ago and for the past year has had heavy, irregular menstrual periods. She typically gets 7 hours of sleep and occasionally experiences a problem with sleep onset. She takes acetaminophen for intermittent joint pains that mainly involve the large joints of upper and lower extremities.

On examination she is moderately overweight, afebrile, and normotensive. There are several 0.5 to 1.0 cm cervical lymph nodes. Her affect is somewhat flat, her thought content is normal, and she is without suicidal ideation. Otherwise her general health appears to be good.

QUESTIONS

1. What should you tell Ms. K. about her fatigue?
2. What is the best course of treatment?
3. What areas should be focused on at the time of a second visit?

DISCUSSION

The brief history and physical examination in this case do not yield a specific underlying cause for Ms. K.'s fatigue. A psychologic cause is suggested by her presenting herself for assistance, the fluctuating course, the vague history of psychologic disorder during college years, the nonspecific symptoms, and the possible work-related stress. Possible physical causes include cardiorespiratory illness (suggested by the loss of exercise capacity), postinfectious illness (suggested by the recent URI and lymphadenopathy), anemia (suggested by the history of menorrhagia), diabetes (suggested by obesity), menopause (suggested by her age), and connective tissue disorders (suggested by the history of joint pains). Lifestyle causes also need to be considered because of Ms. K's sedentary habits and sleep pattern disruption.

Statistically, she is most likely to be suffering from fatigue related to a psychologic disorder such as depression. However, further investigation by scheduling a complete history and examination is needed to exclude other disorders.

It is premature to prescribe treatment for Ms. K.'s fatigue, but you should reassure her that the initial visit does not indicate an urgent medical condition. In anticipation of a second visit, you should order laboratory studies, including complete blood count with differential, glucose, thyroid-stimulating hormone, erythrocyte sedimentation rate, monospot (because of the recent URI), and rheumatoid factor (because of the history of arthralgias). An additional goal for this initial visit is to establish a trusting relationship with Ms. K., because the prognosis of fatigue as a presenting complaint is uncertain and the condition may become chronic.

REFERENCES

1. Lewis G, Wessely S. The epidemiology of fatigue: more questions than answers. J Epidemiol Commun Health 1992;46:92–97.
2. Sugarman JR, Berg AD. Evaluation of fatigue in a family practice. J Fam Pract 1984;5:643–647.
3. Cathebras PJ, Robbins JM, Kirmayer L J, Hayton BG. Fatigue in primary care. J Gen Intern Med 1992;7:276–286.
4. Kroenke K, Mangelsdorff D. Common symptoms in ambulatory care. Am J Med 1989;86:262–266.
5. Morrison JD. Fatigue as a presenting complaint in family practice. J Fam Pract 1980;10:795–801.
6. Kroenke K, et al. Chronic fatigue in primary care. JAMA 1988;260:929–934.
7. Valdini AF, et al. A one-year follow-up of fatigued patients. J Fam Pract 1988;26:33–38.
8. Kamerow DB. Anxiety and depression in the medical setting. Med Clin North Am 1988;72:745–751.
9. Bates DW, Schmitt W, Buchwald D, Ware NC, Lee J, Thoyer E, Kornish RJ, Komarof AL. Prevalence of fatigue and chronic fatigue syndrome in a primary care practice. Arch Intern Med 1993;153:2759–2765.
10. Elnicki DM, Shockcor WT, Brick JE, Beynon D. Evaluating the complaint of fatigue in primary care: diagnoses and outcomes. Am J Med 1992;93:303–306.
11. Ruffin MT, Cohen M. Evaluation and management of fatigue. Am Fam Physician 1994;50:625–632.
12. Calabrese L, Danao T, Camara E, Wilke W. Chronic fatigue syndrome. Am Fam Physician 1992;45:1205–1213.
13. Lane TJ, Matthews DA, Manu P. The low yield of physical examinations and laboratory investigations of patients with chronic fatigue. Am J Med Sci 1990;299:313–318.
14. Goldenberg DL, Felson DT, Dimerman A. A randomized, controlled trial of amitriptyline and naproxen in the treatment of patients with fibromyalgia. Arthritis Rheum 1986;29:1371–1377.
15. Gracious B, Wisner KL. Nortriptyline in chronic fatigue syndrome: a double-blind, placebo-controlled single case study. Biol Psychiatry 1991;30:405–408.

27. Fever in Infants and Preschool Children

WILLIAM C. WADLAND

Key Clinical Questions

1. How can you differentiate between relatively benign viral illness and serious bacterial infection (SBI) in children with clinically significant fever?
2. When should inpatient care be considered?
3. What information should parents receive to help in the assessment, management, and follow-up care of their child?

Fever in infants and young children is the primary cause for unscheduled visits to family medicine, pediatrics, and emergency departments (1). Despite its frequency, the evaluation and management of fever in young children remains controversial. At least two-thirds of all children visit a physician for an acute illness with fever before they are 3 years of age, and for about 14% of these children, there is no obvious source of fever (1).

The clinical appearance of children with fairly benign viral infections may be quite similar to the appearance of those with serious bacterial infections (SBIs) (2). Febrile children younger than 3 months of age who appear "toxic" (severe lethargy, poor tone, and, inability to drink fluids) have a 17% probability of having an SBI (sepsis, bone or joint infections, urinary tract infection, pneumonia, or enteritis), and a 4% probability of having meningitis (1). Because physicians are fearful of missing potential serious infections, they often opt for more aggressive investigations and greater use of antibiotics than necessary (3).

This chapter describes several practice guidelines and observational scales that help clinicians take a rational and structured approach to the evaluation and management of the febrile child (4–8). The efficacy of these approaches, however, is limited when assessing nontoxic-appearing children (8). Primary care clinicians must, therefore, establish excellent rapport with parents and maintain close communication for follow-up to provide appropriate levels of care for diagnosis and treatment. Parents are reported to be very willing to accept approaches that inflict less discomfort and avoid unnecessary antibiotics (3, 9).

PATHOPHYSIOLOGY AND DIFFERENTIAL DIAGNOSIS

Definition and Measurement of Fever

Most clinicians define fever as $\geq$100.4°F (38.0°C) by rectal temperature; temperatures above 106°F (41.1°C) are called *hyperpyrexia*. Rectal temperatures are traditionally considered the most accurate means to detect fever but also the most inconvenient. Even though nonrectal thermometers are used frequently in the outpatient setting, their reliability, especially in children less than 36 months, is questionable. Several studies report poor correlations between oral, axillary, and rectal temperatures (10–12); the correlation coefficients were 0.74 for oral and axillary temperatures and 0.70 for rectal and axillary temperatures (10). The sensitivity to detect a fever (when defined as 37.4°C) by oral or axillary thermometers is less than 50%, resulting in a high false-negative rate and many undetected fevers (10). The tympanic thermometer is used frequently in outpatient, hospital, and emergency room settings. Several studies have found that the younger the child, the less accurate the aural thermometer, with reports of sensitivities ranging between 66 and 80% (11–14). The accuracy of aural thermometers varies greatly with the age of the child, the operator experience, and a special technique of "tugging the ear."

When talking to a patient by telephone, physicians often ask the parent to measure the child's temperature. However, only 10% of the mothers in one study were able to correctly read three preset thermometers, despite 67% stating they knew how to read them (15).

Differential Diagnosis

The risk of serious bacterial infection is greater in younger children, those who appear toxic, and those with rectal temperatures greater than 102.2°F (39°C). Febrile infants (100.4°F rectally)

435

less than 28 days of age, whether they appear toxic or not, have a high incidence of serious bacterial infections (4 to 20%) (4, 16). Febrile children less than 3 months old who appear toxic (lethargy, hypoventilation, or signs of poor circulation or cyanosis) have a 17% probability of serious bacterial infections, an 11% probability of bacteremia, and a 4% probability of meningitis (17). The risk of occult bacteremia in febrile children (102.2°F or 39°C) between 3 and 36 months of age who are nontoxic-appearing is approximately 7% (range 5 to 9%) (4). Table 27.1 summarizes the risks for SBI by age and clinical appearance of the febrile child.

The differential diagnosis of fever in children is summarized in Table 27.2. The frequency of specific diagnoses in infants and preschool children with fever varies with the age of the child. Serious bacterial causes such as meningitis, pneumonia, and urinary tract infections are more common in younger children.

Upper Respiratory Infections

Uncomplicated upper respiratory infections (URIs) are by far the most common cause of fever in preschool children. Over 300 types of viruses have been implicated, with rhinoviruses being the most common. Children have a higher incidence of URIs than adults because immunity occurs only after exposure. Preschool children commonly have 12 URIs per year, whereas adults may have only two to three per year. URIs (commonly called "colds") are spread by hand-to-face contact and not as previously thought by respiratory droplets.

Otitis Media

Otitis media (OM) usually occurs in children who have had a URI for several days. Retained secretions occur in one or both ears, causing full-ness, pressure sensations, mild fussiness, and low-grade fever. The fluid in the middle ear then becomes infected. Bacteria are implicated in two-thirds of cases, with *Haemophilus influenzae* and *Streptococcus pneumoniae* the most common isolates. It has also been reported that 40% of children with acute otitis media will have no apparent earache (18).

Acute Chest Infections: Bronchitis, Bronchiolitis, and Pneumonia

Chest infections can affect either the upper airways (bronchi and bronchioles), as with bronchitis and bronchiolitis, or the lung parenchyma, as with pneumonia. Bronchitis is characterized by rhonchi and bronchiolitis by wheezing, although the reliability of these symptoms is low. Children with upper airway infections usually are not seriously ill and can be managed as outpatients. Respiratory syncytial virus (RSV) causes relatively severe lower respiratory infections in infants. Pneumonia should be suspected in children with fever, retractions, cough, tachypnea, and general malaise. Pneumonia in children can be both viral and bacterial; bacterial pneumonia is often accompanied by bacteremia.

Other Serious Bacterial Infections

Typical symptoms of meningitis such as high fever, irritability, photophobia, vomiting, lethargy, and neck stiffness are often not present in infants. Meningitis can develop in children who present with only a mild respiratory infection and low-grade fever. You should carefully follow infants with fever and no clear etiology to ensure lack of progression to serious illness.

Bacteremia is more common in children under 2 years of age and those who appear toxic. Typi-

Table 27.1.
Risks for SBI by Age and Clinical Appearance of the Febrile (38°C or 100.4°F[R]) Child[a]

	Age < 3 Months		Age 3–36 Months	
	Toxic Appearance[a]	Nontoxic Appearance	Toxic Appearance	Nontoxic Appearance
SBI %	17.3 (8.0–30.0)	8.6 (3.7–15.6)	10% (5.0–90.0)	4.3 (3.0–11.0)[b]
Bacteremia %	10.7 (6.7–15.7)	2.0 (0.8–3.8)	—	—
Meningitis %	3.9 (1.7–7.1)	1.0 (0.2–2.4)	—	—

[a]Risk for SBI is less than 1.4% (0.4–2.7) if WBC is <15,000 WBC/mm^3, normal urine analysis, and stool screen (see References 1 and 4).

[b]Nontoxic-appearing children aged 3–36 months with a temperature of >102.2°F rectally have a slightly higher risk of bacteremia of 6.8% (4.6%–9.4%)

Table 27.2.
Most Frequent Diagnoses in Infants with Fever

Age ≤ 2 Months[a]		Age ≤ 1 Year[b]	
Diagnosis	% of Cases	Diagnosis	% of Cases
Nonspecific viral illness	36.7	Upper respiratory infection	38.6
Upper respiratory infection	24.8	Otitis media	32.9
Viral gastroenteritis	9.4	Nonspecific viral illness	15.9
Aseptic meningitis	8.5	Gastroenteritis	11.4
Otitis media	6.7	Pneumonia	1.6
Pneumonia	3.1	Bronchiolitis	1.2
Sepsis/meningitis	2.7	Croup	1.2
Bacterial gastroenteritis	2.7	Chickenpox	1.2
Other bacterial infections	2.7	Roseola	1.2
Urinary tract infection	1.7	Streptococcal pharyngitis	1.2

[a]Adapted from Kimmel SR, Gemmill DW. The young child with fever. Am Fam Physician 37(6):196–206, 1988.
[b]Data from Hoekelman RA. Infectious illness during the first year of life. Pediatrics 59:119–121, 1977.

cal organisms include *S. pneumoniae* (65 to 70%), *H. influenzae* (20 to 25%), *Neisseria meningitidis* (3 to 5%), and others (5 to 15%) (19). These patterns are changing with the increased use of the *H. influenzae* vaccine (20). Finally, urinary tract infections have been reported in up to 4% of children age 3 to 24 months with fever and no diagnosed source (19, 21) (see Chapter 25, Dysuria).

CLINICAL EVALUATION

The evaluation of fever in infants and preschool children requires a comprehensive history, complete physical examination, rational use of laboratory studies, and communication and follow-up with parents to assess any changes or progression in clinical status. Frequently, the complaint of fever in children originates from a telephone call by parents seeking advice. If the child has constitutional symptoms such as malaise, poor fluid intake, rapid respirations, or lethargy, then he or she must be seen by the physician for adequate evaluation.

History

Clinicians should inquire about the exact age of the child in months, the degree of temperature elevation, the route and reliability of reading the temperature, and the child's current health status, other concurrent illnesses, immunization status, birth history (such as prematurity), previous hospitalizations, focal signs of infections

(skin, bone, ears, etc.), feeding and drinking status, and general activity level. Because of the unreliability of history and increased risk of serious bacterial illness, infants less than 1 month of age who have fevers of 100.4°F or more rectally merit a full clinical evaluation, including laboratory studies and probable hospitalization (4).

Febrile children between the age of 28 and 90 days can be risk stratified (low-risk versus high-risk for SBI) based on historical and clinical appearance. Table 27.3 lists key elements of the history and physical examination that aid in classifying the level of risk for serious disease and identifying specific causes of fever.

There are conflicting reports in the literature on whether the height of fever is important (16, 17, 22, 23), with most authors agreeing that the incidence of SBI (reported range from 12 to 62%) increases considerably with hyperpyrexia (rectal temperature > 106°F or 41.1°C). Also, a positive response to antipyretics in patients with lower temperature does not necessarily rule out serious bacterial infection (24, 25).

Physical Examination

Age-specific vital signs should be evaluated and assessed. Symptoms suggestive of SBI include irregular respirations, stridor, retractions, cyanosis, altered consciousness, nasal flaring, poor muscle tone, and skin pallor (16, 17). The Yale Observation Scale (YOS) has been developed to identify febrile infants with SBI based on their clinical

Table 27.3.
Key Elements of the History and Physical Examination in Infants and Preschool Children with Fever

Question/Maneuver	Purpose
Age, degree of fever, or method of measurement	Risk of serious illness is greater if less than 28 days of age Rectal temperature of ≥100.4°F (38°C) defined as true fever Axillary and oral temperatures are unreliable in young children
Comorbidities such as concurrent illness, previous hospitalizations, prematurity, or recent immunization	These factors can contribute to an increased risk of serious illness.
Focal signs of infection such as skin lesions, joint swelling and redness, or pulling on ears	Indicates possible source of infection
Constitutional symptoms and feeding status (lethargy, irritability, inactivity)	May indicate dehydration and serious illness
Clinical observation for toxic findings such as rapid respirations, cyanosis, retractions of chest, altered consciousness, skin pallor, decreased activity, and responsiveness	Increased likelihood of serious illness
Inquiry about parents' capability to measure temperature, observe for changes, and return for follow-up	Ensures timely follow-up in case of progression and deterioration of clinical status

appearance. It includes factors such as quality of cry, reaction of parents, state variation, color, state of hydration, and response to social overtures. A score of 10 or above (out of a maximum of 30 points) is predictive of serious illness in toxic-appearing children.

However, the positive and negative likelihood ratios are only 3.0 and 0.41, respectively, for a YOS greater than 10. In nontoxic-appearing children, the sensitivity of the Yale scale is only 16.7%, and specificity improves to 91.9% (LR+ 2.06 > LR− .91). Therefore, the scale is of little use in ruling out serious illness in nontoxic-appearing children (26).

Table 27.4 lists criteria used at Rochester University to evaluate low-risk children for serious illness. These criteria should be applied to well-appearing children who are ≤ 60 days of age with rectal temperature ≥ 38°C. The Rochester criteria have a sensitivity of 92%, specificity of 54%, LR+ of 2, and LR− of 0.15 for the identification of children with SBI (7). The negative predictive value of the Rochester criteria is 98.9% (97.2 to 99.6%) for any SBI and 99.5% (98.2 to 99.9%) for bacteremia (7). Children who meet all of these low-risk criteria are unlikely to have SBIs. Therefore, the Rochester criteria are helpful for physicians who wish to exclude serious in-

Table 27.4.
The Rochester Criteria

1. Infant appears generally well
2. Infant has been previously healthy
   - Born at term (≥37 weeks' gestation)
   - Did not receive perinatal antimicrobial therapy
   - Was not treated for unexplained hyperbilirubinemia
   - Had not received and was not receiving antimicrobial agents
   - Had not been previously hospitalized
   - Had no chronic or underlying illness
   - Was not hospitalized longer than mother
3. No evidence of skin, soft tissue, bone, joint, or ear infection
4. Laboratory values
   - Peripheral WBC 5.0–15.0 × 10^9 cells/L (5000 to 15,000/mm³)
   - Absolute band form count ≤ 1.5 × 10^9 cells/L (≤1500/mm³)
   - ≤10 WBC/HPF (40×) on microscopic examination of a spun urine sediment
   - ≤5 WBC/HPF (40×) on microscopic examination of a stool smear (only for infants with diarrhea)

Adapted from Jaskiewicz JA, McCarthy CA, Richardson AC, White KC, Fisher DJ, Ragan R, et al. Febrile infants at low risk for serious bacterial infections—an appraisal of the Rochester criteria and implications for management. Pediatrics 1994;94:390–396.

fections during a period of continued observation and follow-up care.

Figure 27.1 provides an algorithm for management of the infant aged between 0 and 90 days, depending on toxic versus nontoxic appearance.

Laboratory Tests

Most infants and children with fever do not require laboratory investigations. Specific groups of children in whom laboratory investigation (CBC, blood cultures, and lumbar puncture) are warranted include:

- Temperature ≥ 100.4°F and under age 28 days
- Temperature > 100.4°F, age 28 to 90 days, and toxic-appearing

- Temperature > 102.2°F, age 91 days to 36 months, and toxic-appearing

Children aged 91 days to 36 months who are febrile but not toxic-appearing may require an intermediate level of workup, guided by the CBC and targeting evaluation of specific symptoms. Specific approaches to the management of fever in each age group are discussed later in this chapter.

The characteristics of diagnostic tests for the most important SBIs are presented in Table 27.5. The risk of SBI increases with a white blood count (WBC) > 15,000 cells/mm^3, although the prevalence of bacteremia may still be as low as 2 to 4%, with the majority of children with a WBC in this range free of serious illness. Extreme evaluations, WBC ≥ 35,000 to 50,000 cells/mm^3, are

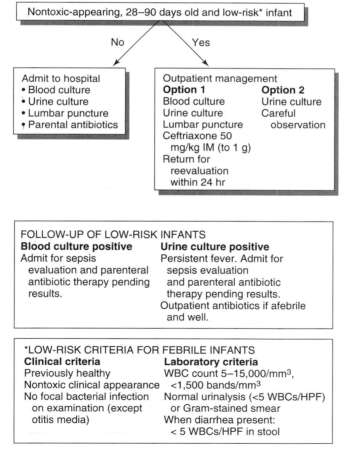

Figure 27.1. *Algorithm for the management of a previously healthy infant 0 to 90 days of age with fever without source ≥ 38.0°C.*

Table 27.5.

Characteristics of Diagnostic Tests Useful in Infants and Children with Fever Greater Than (100.4°F) 38°C[a]

Diagnostic Test	Sensitivity	Specificity	LR+	LR−
1. WBC > 15,000				
Viral infection	0.25	—	—	—
Pneumonia	0.64	—	—	—
UTI	0.62	—	—	—
Meningitis	0.50	—	—	—
Bacteremia	0.77	0.65	2.2	0.36
2. WBC > 25,000–35,000[a]	—	—	—	—
3. WBC > 35,000–50,000[a]	—	—	—	—
4. Temperature response to acetaminophen of 0.8°C	0.47	0.74	2.1	0.71
5. Blood cultures—in child Temp > 39.4°C, WBC > 10,500, and toxic appearance on Yale scale	—	—	—	—
6. UTI				
Standard U/A				
5 WBC/HPF in a spun urine	0.66	0.81	3.4	0.43
Enhanced U/A				
≥ 10 WBC/HPF and ≥ 10 bacteria on oil fluid/HPF in an unspun urine	0.84	0.93	12.1	0.17
7. Spinal fluid analysis	—	—	—	—
8. Chest radiograph				
Pneumonia	0.68	0.83	4.0	0.39

[a]Table is incomplete owing to lack of test characteristics reported in the literature. SBI risk increases 2.5 times if WBC ≥ 35,000/mm³ compared with WBC ≥ 15,000 < 25,000 (26).

associated with a 26% (reported range 19 to 50%) probability of SBI (27, 28).

As in Table 27.1, children between the ages of 3 months and 36 months who have a fever of 102.2°F (39°C) or greater and a toxic appearance should also be admitted for full sepsis workup. If there are no signs of toxicity, these children can be evaluated as outpatients with studies based on specific symptoms. One option is to obtain blood cultures on all children in this category, whereas another is to obtain blood cultures only on children with WBC ≥ 15,000. Children who appear nontoxic, have a temperature less than 102.2°F (39°C), and have no clear source of infection require no diagnostic tests. They can be given antipyretic medication alone and should be followed-up appropriately.

As Table 27.5 illustrates, many children with mild to moderate elevation of the white blood count are free of serious illness. The temperature response to antipyretics does not exclude serious illness (26). Even in toxic-appearing

children with a WBC > 15,000, only 57% of children with a positive blood culture are actually bacteremic (29). An "enhanced urine analysis" (unspun urine using oil immersion, with 10 bacteria and 10 white blood cells per high-power field (HPF), or spun urine ≥ 5 white blood cells/HPF) has better screening characteristics than the standard urinalysis (19). Spinal analysis will be positive for meningitis in only 8% of patients with indications for lumbar puncture, especially toxic-appearing infants less than 28 days of age. Many children with indications for lumbar puncture, even with negative meningitis, have associated higher risks for bacteremia (3.2%), bacteriuria (5.4%) and stool pathogen (14%) (30).

Chest radiograph (indicated for cough with retractions, tachypnea, rales, and marked rhonchi) is more accurate if read by a radiologist blinded to the diagnosis listed by the examining clinician (32). A positive chest radiograph is helpful at ruling in pneumonia (LR+ 4.0), although a negative chest radiograph does not rule out the diagnosis (LR− 0.4).

Fecal leukocytes and occult blood are not reliable predictors of enteric pathogens in children with diarrhea (32). Stool cultures and clinical evaluations are essential to make the correct diagnosis (32).

MANAGEMENT

There is no absolute standard of care for management of infants and children with fever. In fact, there is considerable variation in approaches and much latitude for clinical judgment reported in surveys of clinicians (33). The guidelines proposed in this section should be used as helpful suggestions for clinicians who must make judgments based on individual clinical findings and circumstances (4). According to at least one author, there may be little or no harm from a delay in antibiotic treatment in some meningitis patients, if they present initially with nonspecific symptoms and have close follow-up care for worsening symptoms (34).

Age < 28 Days

Children less than 28 days of age with fever (100.4°F or 38°C or greater) should be admitted to the hospital for a full sepsis evaluation (complete blood count, blood culture, and lumbar puncture), close observation, and initiation of parenteral antibiotics while awaiting culture results. An alternative in nontoxic-appearing infants is to withhold antibiotics pending laboratory results (4). One author proposes close observation alone without antibiotic interventions in "very low-risk" infants who have WBC < 15,000, normal urinalysis, and stool screen (35), because the likelihood of serious disease is low and intervention can be initiated with progression of clinical findings.

Age 28 to 90 days

All febrile, toxic-appearing infants aged 28 to 90 days should be admitted for full sepsis evaluation and initial parenteral antibiotics. Infants who are nontoxic-appearing with a WBC < 15,000 can be managed by either a full sepsis evaluation, parenteral therapy, and return to be reevaluated in 24 hours or by a urine culture, careful observation, and follow-up in 24 hours. Children with a higher WBC and temperature elevations increase the usefulness of sepsis evaluation, antibiotics, and possible hospitalization. This strategy is summarized in Figure 27.1.

Age 3 to 36 months

Figure 27.2 illustrates the approach for older children aged 91 days to 36 months. All toxic-appearing children in this age group merit hospitalization. Nontoxic-appearing children with a temperature ≤ 39°C (102.2°F) and no clear source of infection should receive antipyretics, no diagnostic tests, and close follow-up if fever persists in 48 hours. Nontoxic-appearing children with a temperature greater than 102.2°F (39°C) should have blood cultures, especially if the WBC is >15,000. Antibiotics (oral or parenteral) should be initiated pending changes in the patient's clinical appearance and positive cultures (see the next section for information on antibiotic selection). If empiric antibiotics are started and close follow-up is possible in a nontoxic-appearing child, blood cultures are usually not necessary.

Reducing Fever

Antipyretic therapy with either acetaminophen or ibuprofen effectively controls fever with little adverse effect (39.4%) (Tables 27.6 and 27.7). Parents frequently underdose antipyretics, using partial doses rather than full doses (36). You should therefore inquire about dosages and routes of administration (37, 38). Sponging by tepid water or alcohol is not recommended and has no efficacy (39); these practices should be abandoned.

Antibiotic Selection

Outpatient

For outpatients, antibiotic therapy can be initiated either orally with amoxicillin or intramuscularly with ceftriaxone, as illustrated in Figures 27.1 and 27.2. Amoxicillin has a greater likelihood of resistance to *H. influenzae*, especially in unimmunized children, and slightly higher rates of meningitis and bacteremia at follow-up reculturing (40). You should weigh the benefits of decreased resistance to newer-generation antibiotics versus the relatively low risks of missed treatments with amoxicillin. It is estimated that in febrile children (3 to 36 months) suspected of occult bacteremia, it would take 2,500 treatments

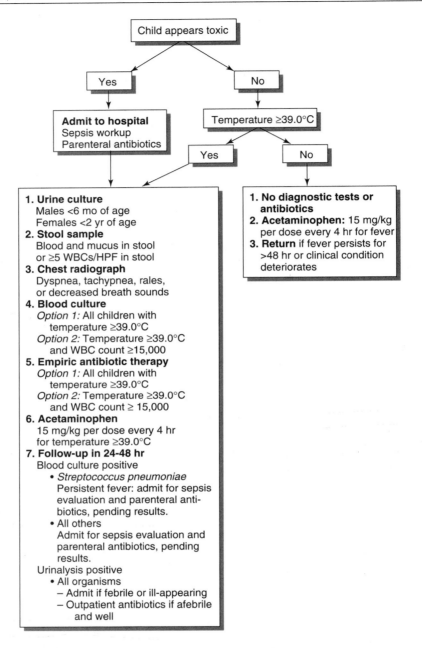

Figure 27.2. *Algorithm for the management of a previously healthy child 91 days to 36 months of age with fever without source.*

with empiric parenteral ceftriaxone versus no treatment to prevent four cases of meningitis (41).

All hospitalized infants and children who are toxic require intravenous antibiotics, as listed in Tables 27.6 and 27.7.

Follow-up

The clinician must ensure reliable follow-up of all patients managed expectantly as outpatients. Parents should be advised to check their child

Table 27.6.

Therapeutic Options Available for Management of Infants and Preschool Children with Fever

Treatment Strategy	Level of Evidence for Effectiveness[a]	Recommendation/Comments
Antipyretic medication (acetaminophen)	A	Advise giving adequate dose per kg and question dispenser size used. Aspirin not recommended due to Reye's syndrome risk.
Oral antibiotics	B	Some reports of failure to prevent *H. influenzae* bacteremia in unimmunized infants
Intramuscular antibiotics	A	Recommended as in Figures 27.1 and 27.2
Intravenous antibiotics	A	Recommended as an option for hospitalized patients, especially those with dehydration and documented bacterial meningitis
Oral hydration	A	Child must be "nontoxic" and tolerate oral fluids to prevent dehydration
Intravenous hydration	A	Hospitalization for dehydration
Sponging for fever control	X	Not recommended

[a]Level of evidence for effectiveness: A, strong or moderate research-based evidence (consistent across several studies, including at least two randomized controlled trials); B, limited research-based evidence (less consistent or extensive evidence, but preponderance of evidence supports use of treatment); C, common practice with little or no research-based evidence; X, moderate or strong evidence suggesting that this treatment is not effective.

every 4 hours for activity, rectal temperature, skin color changes, and adequate fluid intake. Parents should call if there are any concerns. Arrangements for timely follow-up in 24 to 48 hours should be made before leaving the office or emergency department. Children who are still febrile at follow-up visits and have worsening symptoms should have a complete sepsis evaluation and admission to the hospital.

CASE STUDY

Infant B. is a 10-month-old who was previously well and presents with a fever of 102.4°F (39.2°C) rectally. The mother reports poor fluid intake, and the child appears lethargic, has a weak cry, and is poorly responsive to stimulation. Additional clinical findings include very dry mucus membranes, diminished skin turgor, a bulging anterior fontanelle, and cyanotic skin with peripheral pallor. Vital signs include a pulse of 180 and a respiratory rate of 40, but no retractions or cough. There is no nuchal rigidity; in fact, the child seems flaccid with decreased tone of muscles. Chest examination is clear with no cardiac murmur. Otoscopy reveals otitis media bilaterally.

QUESTIONS

1. Is the presentation owing only to otitis media or to more serious bacterial illness?
2. What should be the clinical and diagnostic evaluation?
3. What is the appropriate level of care (outpatient versus inpatient) and follow-up?

DISCUSSION

Even though the patient is older than 90 days and there is a definite focus of infection (otitis media), the toxic appearance suggests serious illness. Therefore, the child should have a full sepsis evaluation, empiric antibiotics, and hospitalization. The relative dehydration merits intravenous fluids. This actual patient from my practice had meningitis due to *S. Pneumoniae* and responded well to intravenous antibiotics and hydration without residual sequelae.

Table 27.7.

Drugs Recommended for Use in the Management of Infants and Preschool Children with Fever

Drug (Common Trade Name)	Common Dosing Range[a]	Common Adverse Effects[a]	Cost (Generic Prices Unless Noted Otherwise)[b]
Nonnarcotic antipyretics			
Acetaminophen (Tylenol)	12.5 mg-15 mg/kg po q4–6h	Hepatotoxicity in overdose; contraindicated in G6PD deficiency	$3–$4/ 4-oz bottle
Ibuprofen(children's Advil or children's Motrin)	5 mg/kg if T° ≤ 39.2°C; if >39.2 °C, 10 mg/kg, 4–6 po every hr; maximum = 40 mg/kg/day	GI distress, ocular problems, granulocytopenia, anemia; inhibits platelet aggregation; use caution in ASA hypersensitivity or hepatic/ renal insufficiency	$5–$6/ 4-oz bottle
Initial antibiotic therapy			
Amoxicillin (Amoxil, Polymox)	20–40 mg/kg/day in a dosing regimen po q8h; given for 2 days, then reevaluate after laboratory results available	Similar to penicillin (with cross sensitivity), interstitial nephritis, diarrhea	Generic prices: 125 mg/5 mL susp. 150 mL = $3.56; 250 mg/5 mL susp. 150 mL = $6.10
Ceftriaxone (Rocephin)	50 mg–75 kg/kg (max. 2 g), intramuscular × 1 Await reevaluation as above	Use with caution in PCN-allergic patient or renal impairment; may cause reversible cholelithiasis, sludging in gallbladder, and jaundice. Use with caution in neonates at risk for hyperbilirubinemia. Painful on injection, especially in children.	1,000-mg vial for injection = $37.52 (trade brand)
Otitis media— ampicillin (Polycillin, Omnipen)	40 mg/kg/day po q6h	Same as amoxicillin	500-mg vial = $5.26
UTI—co-trimoxaxole = trimethoprim (TMP) and sulfamethoxazole (SMX) (Septra, Bactrim)	8 mg/kg TMP/40 mg/kg SMX per day, given in two divided doses, 12 hr apart (q12h)	Not recommended for infants < 2 mo. May cause kernicterus in newborns; may cause blood dyscrasias, crystalluria, glossitis, renal or hepatic injury, GI upset.	$4.07/120-mL bottle
Meningitis—cefotaxime (Claforan)	All given intravenously: 0–1 week: 50 mg/kg q12h 1–4 weeks: 50 mg/kg q8h 1 month to 12 years: 100–180 mg/kg/day in 4–6 divided doses	Similar to ceftriaxone. Use with caution in renal impairment or PCN allergy Toxicities similar to other cephalosporins; allergy, neutropenia, thrombocytopenia, eosinophilia, positive Coombs test, elevated BUN, creatinine, and liver enzymes.	$69.14/500-mg vial

[a]Dosages and cautions as listed in Johnson KB, ed. The Harriet Lane Handbook: A Manual for Pediatric House Officers. St. Louis: CV Mosby, 1993; Guide to Antimicrobial Therapy, 26th ed. 1996; Sanford JP, Gilbert DN, Moellering RC, Sandle MA. The Sanford Guide to Antimicrobial Therapy 1997. Dallas, TX: Therapy Antimicrobial, 1997.

[b]Prices quoted for prescription drugs are based on average wholesale price (AWP), which reflects the cost of the agent to the pharmacy. Most hospitals obtain these agents for considerably less.

REFERENCES

1. Baraff LJ. Management of infants and children 3 to 36 months of age with fever without source. Pediatr Ann 1993;22:497–498, 501–504.

2. Telle DW, Pelton SE, Grant MJ, Herskowitz J, Rosen DJ, Allen CE, et al. Bacteremia in febrile children under 2 years of age: results of cultures of blood of 600 consecutive febrile children seen in "walk-in" clinics. J Pediatr 1975;87:227–230.

3. Kramer MS, et al. Parents' versus physicians' values for clinical outcomes in young febrile children. Pediatrics 1994;93:697–702.

4. Baraff LJ, Bass JW, Fleisher GR, Klein JO, McCracken GF Jr., Powell Kr, et al. Practice guidelines for the management of infants and children 0–36 months of age with fever without source. Pediatrics 1993;92:1–12.

5. Baker MD, Bell LM, Avner JR. Outpatient management without antibiotics of fever in selected infants. N Engl J Med 1993;329:1437–1441.

6. Baskin MN, O'Rourke EJ, Fleisher GR. Outpatient intramuscular administration of ceftriaxone. J Pediatr 1992;120:22–27.

7. Jaskiewicz JA, McCarthy CA, Richardson AC, White KC, Fisher DJ, Ragan R, et al. Febrile infants at low risk for serious bacterial infections—an appraisal of the Rochester criteria and implications for management. Pediatrics 1994;94:390–396.

8. Teach SJ, et al. Efficacy of an observation scale in detecting bacteremia in febrile children three to thirty-six months of age, treated as outpatients. J Pediatr 1995; 126:877–888.

9. Oppenheim PI, et al. Incorporating patient preferences into practice guidelines: management of children with fever without source. Ann Emerg Med 1994;24:836–841.

10. Orgen JM. The inaccuracy of axillary temperatures measures with electronic thermometer. Am J Dis Child 1990;144:109–111.

11. Hooker EA, et al. Use of tympanic thermometers to screen for fever in patients in a pediatric emergency department. South Med J 1993;86:855–858.

12. Peterson-Smith A, et al. Comparison of aural infrared with traditional rectal temperatures in children from birth to age 3 years. J Pediatr 1994;125:83–85.

13. Terndrup TE, et al. The performance of two tympanic thermometers in pediatric emergency departments. Clin Pediatr 1991;30:18–23.

14. Terndrup TE, et al. Impact of operator technique and device on infrared emission detection tympanic thermometry. J Emerg Med 1992;10:683–687.

15. Baneo L, et al. The ability of mothers to read a thermometer. Clin Pediatr 1990;29:343–345.

16. Nocicka A. Evaluation of the febrile infant younger than 3 months of age with no source of infection. Am J Emerg Med 1995;13:215–218.

17. Baraff LJ, Oslund SA, Schreger DC, Stephen ML. Probability of bacterial infections in febrile infants less than three months of age: a meta-analysis. Pediatr Infect Dis J 1992;11:257–264.

18. Heikkinen T, et al. Signs and symptoms predicting acute otitis media. Arch Pediatr Adoles Med 1995;149:26–29.

19. Kramer MS, et al. Urine testing in young febrile children: a risk-benefit analysis. J Pediatr 1994;125:6–13.

20. Bacon MA, et al. Blood cultures in private pediatric practice: an eleven-year experience. Pediatr Infect Dis J 1989;8:2–7.

21. Marild S, et al. Fever, bacteriuria, and concomitant disease in children with urinary tract infection. Pediatr Infect Dis J 1989;8:36–41.

22. Alpert G, et al. Case-control study of hyperpyrexia in children. Pediatr Infect Dis J 1990;9:161–163.

23. Bonadio WA, et al. Systemic bacterial infections in children with fever greater than 41 degrees. Pediatr Infect Dis J 1989;8:120–122.

24. Baker MD, et al. Childhood fever: correlation of diagnosis with temperature response to acetaminophen. Pediatrics 1987;80:315–318.

25. Baker RC, et al. Severity of disease correlated with fever reduction in febrile infants. Pediatrics 1989;83: 1016–1019.

26. Mazur LJ, et al. Diagnostic tests for occult bacteremia: temperature response to acetaminophen versus WBC count. Am J Emerg Med 1994;12:403–406.

27. Kramer MS, et al. Role of the complete blood count in detecting occult focal bacterial infection in the young febrile child. J Clin Epidemiol 1993;46:349–395.

28. Jazur LJ, et al. Extreme leukocytosis in patients presenting to a pediatric emergency department. Pediatr Emerg Care 1991;7:215–218.

29. Baron MA, et al. Blood cultures in private pediatric practice: an eleven-year experience. Pediatr Infect Dis J 1989;8:2–7.

30. Barnett ED, et al. Serious bacterial infections in febrile infants and children selected for lumbar puncture. Pediatr Infect Dis J 1994;13:950–953.

31. Kramer MS, et al. Bias and "overcall" in interpreting chest radiographs in young febrile children. Pediatrics 1992;90:11–13.

32. Huicho L, et al. Occult blood and fecal leukocytes as screening tests in childhood infectious diarrhea: an old problem revisited. Pediatr Infect Dis J 1993;12:474–477.

33. Baraff LJ. Management of the febrile child: a survey of pediatric and emergency medicine residency directors. Pediatr Infect Dis J 1991;10:795–800.

34. Goodman JM. Commentary: legal aspects of bacterial meningitis. Pediatr Infect Dis J 1992;11:700–701.

35. McCarthy PL. The febrile infant. Pediatrics 1994;94: 397–399.

36. Hyam E, et al. What's in a teaspoon? Underdosing with acetaminophen in family practice. Fam Pract 1989;6:221–223.

37. Autret E, et al. Comparative efficacy and tolerance of ibuprofen syrup and acetaminophen syrup in children with pyrexia-associated infectious diseases and treated with antibiotics. Eur J Clin Pharmacol 1994;46: 197–201.

38. Lesko SM, et al. An assessment of the safety of pediatric ibuprofen: a practitioner-based randomized clinical trial. JAMA 1995;273:929–933.

39. Newman J. Evaluation of sponging to reduce body temperature. J Can Med Assoc 1985;132:641–642.

40. Fleischer GR, et al. Intramuscular versus nonantibiotic therapy for the prevention of meningitis and other bacterial sequelae in young febrile children at risk for occult bacteremia. J Pediatr 1994;124:504–512.

41. Ward ER, et al. Cautionary note on the use of empiric ceftriaxone for suspected bacteremia. Am J Dis Child 1991;145:1359–1361.

28. Headache

JOHN P. FOGARTY

Key Clinical Questions

1. Is there serious underlying pathology causing this patient's headache?
2. What tests, if any, should be considered in the evaluation of this patient to rule out serious causes of headache?
3. Are social and psychologic factors influencing this presentation?

Headaches afflict 75 to 90% of adults in the United States each year; about 50% of Americans have had severe or disabling headaches at some time in their lives. Most patients with headaches see their family physicians and not a specialist. Despite our preconception that headaches are usually a chronic problem, studies show that most people who consult a primary care physician for this symptom do so only once (1). Because headaches account for ten million visits to family doctors per year, they have an enormous financial affect on society, both directly in terms of office visits, medications, and medical testing, and indirectly in terms of days lost from usual activities and in chronic disability.

Knowing the presenting characteristics of the most common headache syndromes will help you make the correct diagnosis. Most patients presenting with headaches have no serious underlying medical problem. Although they are appropriate in selected patients, imaging and laboratory studies are not indicated for most patients with headache. The relationship between the patient and the physician is crucial in caring for patients with chronic or frequently recurring headaches. A trusting and open relationship will help you understand the progression of the headache, the response to treatment, the development and prevention of inappropriate coping strategies, the occurrence of new symptoms, and the potential need for referral.

In primary care settings, headaches can be classified as "primary" or "secondary" (Fig. 28.1). Primary headaches are generally benign, are not associated with underlying diseases, and account for over three-fourths of the headaches seen in primary care. Secondary headaches are symptoms of an underlying disease or physiologic disruption and account for the other one-fourth of presenting headaches.

PATHOPHYSIOLOGY

Primary Headaches

Migraine

Migraine headaches are no longer regarded as primarily of vascular origin. Patients with migraine have a genetic susceptibility and a lower threshold for responsiveness to the complicated neurochemical and neurocirculatory reactions that normally occur in the body, particularly those associated with the 5-hydroxytryptamine or serotonergic receptors in the central nervous system (2, 3).

Serotonergic receptor subtypes are found in both neuronal and vascular sites. They are associated with numerous precipitants or triggers of migraine headaches and include vascular, neuronal depolarization, and inflammatory components. Medications for acute or chronic symptoms may act either peripherally or centrally, whereas prophylactic medications are thought to act by "stabilizing" the serotonergic system.

Cluster

The mechanism of cluster headaches is unknown but is thought to be vascular, an unusual sensitivity to histamine, or abnormal activity of the sphenopalatine ganglion (4). Attacks may be precipitated by histamine, alcohol, nitroglycerin, smoking, or stress.

Tension

Tension or "muscle contraction" headaches have been attributed to contraction of scalp, facial, and/or posterior neck muscles. However, electromyography (EMG) studies and blinded studies that elicit scalp tenderness have shown equivocal results. Ischemia resulting from chronically

447

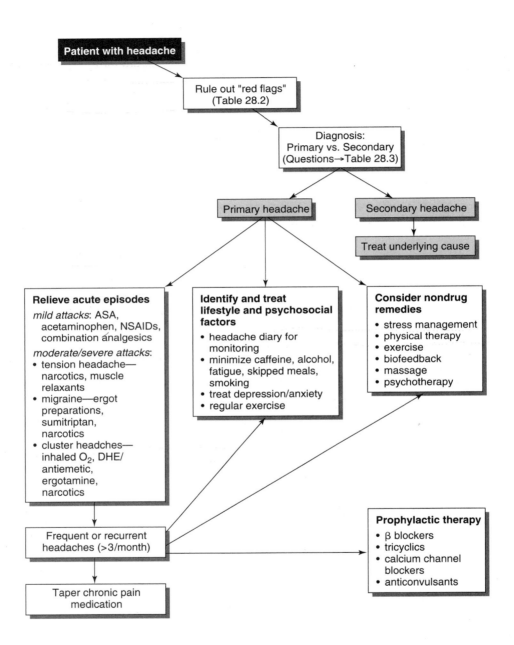

Figure 28.1. *General approach to the patient with headache.*

contracted muscles may play a role in patients with chronic tension headaches, and serotonin may be implicated in the etiology of tension headaches by its depletion in platelets and impaired binding to lymphocytes and monocytes in patients with this disorder. This "neuroreceptor/neurovascular" hypothesis may explain the symptom overlap frequently seen between migraine and tension headaches, and it also helps explain why medication that was previously believed to be specific for only one type of headache often alleviates both kinds (5).

Miscellaneous

Other, less common, benign headaches with no underlying pathology for which the causes and mechanisms are unknown include cough, exertional, coitus, and cold stimulus or "ice cream" headaches (6).

Secondary Headaches

Temporomandibular Joint (TMJ)

Headaches caused by TMJ disorders may be related to internal derangements of the TMJ itself or to myofascial pain dysfunction around the joint. Myofascial disorders are associated with an abnormal chewing motion, teeth grinding at night (bruxism), or locking on opening. With TMJ disease, actual joint pathology is present (7).

Temporal Arteritis (TA)

Temporal (giant cell) arteritis is a systemic panarteritis that selectively involves arterial walls with significant amounts of elastin. This painful inflammation of the temporal arteries occurs in about 3 to 5 persons per 100,000 over age 50 (8). About 50% of patients with TA have polymyalgia rheumatica, and about 15% of patients with polymyalgia rheumatica have TA. Both conditions occur almost exclusively in patients over 50 years old, with a mean age of onset of 70. The estimated prevalence of TA among patients over age 65 presenting with a "new" headache is 5 to 15% (9, 10).

Sinusitis

Acute infection of the bony sinuses of the face and head may cause localized headache. The headache may be caused by the inflammation associated with this infection, by pressure on contiguous structures in the enclosed bony sinuses, or indirectly by the fever and systemic symptoms of this infection.

Intracranial Masses

The greatest concern for many headache patients, including those who have had a comprehensive assessment, is that they may have a brain tumor. Although headache eventually occurs in 70% of brain tumor patients, it is the sole complaint in less than 20%. Only half of patients diagnosed with a malignancy have a headache at the time of diagnosis. The most frequent initial symptom of a brain tumor is seizure or neurologic dysfunction (11).

Subarachnoid Hemorrhage

Subarachnoid hemorrhage usually results from a ruptured berry aneurysm, arteriovenous malformation, or trauma. Acute headache may be preceded days to weeks earlier by a similar but less severe "sentinel" headache due to bleeding.

Trauma

Chronic headache develops in 30 to 50% of persons who sustain a head injury (12). Headaches may take on the characteristics of either migraine or tension. Patients may also describe dizziness, irritability, fatigue, insomnia, impaired concentration, or memory disturbance along with the headaches, and these symptoms may persist for months or years.

DIFFERENTIAL DIAGNOSIS

The four basic categories of primary headaches include migraine; tension/contraction; cluster; and miscellaneous headaches associated with environmental, physical, exertional, or psychologic precipitants. Tension headaches comprise the majority of headaches seen in a primary care office. Causes of secondary headaches include extracranial and intracranial structural abnormalities, infection, inflammatory diseases, trauma, tumors, intracranial bleeding, systemic diseases, drug abuse, environmental exposures, and psychosocial factors. Table 28.1 lists the differential diagnosis of primary and secondary headache with approximate percentages of presentation in the primary care office setting.

Table 28.1.

Differential Diagnosis in Patients with Headache

Headache Type	Primary or Secondary	Frequency in Primary Care (% of Headaches in Office)
Tension (muscle contraction) headache	Primary	45–50
Migraine, common (aura not present)	Primary	20–25
Sinusitis	Secondary	5–7
Withdrawal from caffeine, opiates, alcohol, marijuana	Secondary	5–8
Migraine, classic (aura present)	Primary	3–5
Arthritis/joint disease: Osteoarthritis of cervical spine, TMJ	Secondary	2–4
Posttraumatic headache	Secondary	2–5
Medications/chemicals: Vasodilators, nitrates/nitrites Monosodium glutamates	Secondary	2–5
Fever	Secondary	2–4
Cluster	Primary	2–3
Ophthalmologic (glaucoma, eye strain)	Secondary	1–2
Miscellaneous headaches: cough, exertion, "ice cream," sexual headache, hypothermia (common for patients, but rarely require an office visit)	Primary	<1
Meningitis/encephalitis	Secondary	<1
Migraine variants: ophthalmologic, hemiplegic, basilar	Primary	<1
Temporal arteritis	Secondary	<0.5
Subarachnoid/subdural bleeds	Secondary	0.5
Brain tumor	Secondary	0.46

Adapted from Becker LA, Iverson DC, Reed FM, Calonge N, Miller RS, Freeman WL. Patients with new headaches in primary care. J Fam Pract 1988;27:41–46; Dubose CD, Cutlip AC, Cutlip WD. Migraines and other headaches: approach to diagnosis and classification. Am Fam Physician 1995;51:1498–1504; Williams JW, Simel DL. Does this patient have sinusitis? Diagnosing acute sinusitis by history and physical examination. JAMA 1993;270:1242–1246.

Brain tumors, subarachnoid hemorrhage (SAH), and subdural hematoma (SDH) are rare. In a study of 2,800 patients presenting with "new" headaches to primary care offices, only 26 had one of these conditions (13). Sixteen of these patients had a normal neurologic examination. All 26 patients, however, had at least one of the following signs or symptoms: abnormal neurologic examination (10 patients), change in level of function (10 patients), loss of consciousness (six patients), papilledema (four patients), change in headache pattern only (three patients) or seizures (one patient). Patients without any of these symptoms therefore have very little risk of tumor, SAH, or SDH. "Red flags" to help you

consider more serious disease are summarized in Table 28.2.

CLINICAL EVALUATION

History

The history should include questions regarding onset, frequency, duration, quality, intensity, location, precipitating and ameliorating factors, and associated symptoms (14, 15). Additionally, inquire about the pattern of a usual or typical headache, any history of headache, specific neurologic symptoms, injuries, and allergies. Past and current medication use will guide therapy.

Table 28.2.
"Red Flags" Suggesting Serious Progressive or Life-Threatening Disease in Patients with Headache

Diagnosis	"Red Flags"
Intracranial hemorrhage	Headache that is abrupt, explosive, and extremely severe (i.e., "the worst headache of my life")
Sepsis, trauma	Headache in a drowsy or confused patient or associated with fever
Possible intracranial mass lesion	Headache, new in onset, that is constant, prevents sleep, and progressively worsens over several weeks. The "first" or "new" headache, especially over the age of 35. Focal neurologic signs, seizures, loss of consciousness, change in mental or functional status, and papilledema.
Temporal arteritis (TA), CVA	Headache in the elderly patient accompanied by focal neurologic symptoms (CVA), local tenderness, absence of temporal pulse, or jaw claudication (TA)
Meningitis, purulent sinusitis, otitis, dental abscess	Headache accompanied by fever or a stiff neck, altered mental status, targeted physical findings
Accelerated hypertension	Headache with abnormal physical signs (e.g., focal neurologic deficits, high blood pressure [>200 mm Hg systolic or >120 mm Hg diastolic])

In addition, medication overuse and misuse may worsen headaches.

Family history is useful, because migraine headaches tend to run in families. However, the relative roles of genetic and environmental factors are difficult to separate. Social and personal stresses may either precipitate or exacerbate the response to a typical headache. You should ask about job, family, and personal relationships along with sleep disturbances, dietary changes or patterns, and exercise habits. Use of alcohol, caffeinated beverages, tobacco products, and illicit drugs should be determined because use and/or withdrawal of these substances can cause headache. Finally, evaluate the patient's emotional state, psychologic status, and coping style.

Physical Examination

The physical examination confirms the clinical hypothesis and helps rule out a secondary cause. The content and extent of the physical examination is guided by the history, the setting (clinical office or emergency room), and your previous experience with the patient (long-standing or new patient).

Primary Headaches

There is little information in the literature that describes the value of specific signs and symptoms in the diagnosis of primary headache syn-

dromes. The following paragraphs describe patterns typical of migraine, cluster, and tension headaches.

Migraine

Migraine is characteristically unilateral, and the intensity of the acute attacks may be characterized as moderate, severe, or incapacitating. The typical attack lasts from 4 to 24 hours, although some patients experience prolonged attacks, lasting one or more days (status migraine). True migraine headaches can occur with an aura (classic migraine) or without an aura (common migraine). The aura, if present, consists of focal neurologic symptoms starting 5 to 30 minutes before the onset of the headache, lasting for 15 to 30 minutes, and usually resolving before the headache begins. The most common aura symptoms are visual (scotomata such as flashing lights, bars, or other patterns), but they may also include paresthesias, diplopia, syncope, or ataxia. Other symptoms include a pulsating quality, aggravation by activity, nausea, vomiting, and photophobia or phonophobia (3, 16).

Cluster

Cluster headache, also called Horton's headache and histamine cephalgia, is the most severe form of recurrent headache. Attacks consist of severe, strictly unilateral periorbital or temporal pain lasting 15 minutes to 3 hours. Cluster headaches occur in a range from once every other day to eight times daily, with a series lasting weeks or months, separated by remissions lasting months or years (hence the name). Attacks are associated with one or more of the following: conjunctival injection, lacrimation, nasal congestion, rhinorrhea, forehead and facial sweating, miosis, ptosis, or eyelid edema. The intensity of the pain may be excruciating and patients are typically unable to lie down, so they may pace the floor. Men are affected five to six times more frequently than women. Attacks may be precipitated by alcohol, histamine, nitroglycerin, smoking, or stress (4).

Tension

Tension headaches are either episodic or chronic. An episodic headache may last 30 minutes to 7 days. The pain is pressing or tightening in quality, mild to moderate in intensity, and usually not worsened by routine activity. The pain of episodic tension headache is usually bilateral and nausea is absent, but photophobia or phonophobia may be present. The patient usually has symptoms fewer than 15 days per month. The chronic, tension-type headache has the same clinical characteristics as the episodic form but it occurs more frequently (at least 15 days per month for at least 6 months per year). This has also been called chronic daily headache and is frequently associated with overuse of pain medications or ergot preparations. There is considerable overlap with migraine in these patients, and these headaches are frequently termed "mixed headaches" (5).

Secondary Headaches

Diagnosis of a primary headache assumes that a secondary cause has been excluded. A change in the severity, frequency, location, or quality of a patient's usual headache pattern with or without focal neurologic symptoms may portend a secondary cause. Table 28.3 provides the key elements of the history for discriminating between specific types of primary and secondary headache.

Sinusitis

Frontal and maxillary sinusitis may be accompanied by tenderness and/or headache over the frontal and maxillary areas. Pain may also radiate to the retro-orbital and vertex areas in frontal sinusitis, and the headache may be worsened by bending forward or jarring the head. Chronic sinus infection can cause dull headache or a feeling of pressure over the sinuses and may be mistaken for migraine.

Tumor

Headache is the sole initial complaint in fewer than 20% of patients with brain tumor. These patients most commonly present with either seizure or neurologic dysfunction (12). Traditional features of brain tumor (vomiting, papilledema, and headache that worsen with the Valsalva maneuver) are present in a minority of patients. Headaches caused by brain tumors are usually "new" or different from previous headaches, are

Table 28.3.

Key Elements in the History and Physical Examination for Headache	
Diagnosis	Question / Maneuver
1. Assist in narrowing differential, comparing previous presentations	1. Previous history of headache, types, frequency, treatment
2. Serious underlying pathology	2. Look for "red flags" (see Table 28.2)
3. Migraine	3. History of "throbbing," photophobia, associated nausea, unilateral pattern; positive family history for migraine
4. Analgesic rebound headache	4. History of medication use (types, frequency, quantity)
5. Assist in planning treatment and screen for depression, chronicity of headache, likelihood of compliance, and motivation for recovery.	5. Psychosocial history: previous history of anxiety/depression; substance abuse; current life stresses; activity/exercise level; patient's "worries" about the headache
6. Serious underlying pathology	6. Screening neurologic examination
7. TMJ, sinusitis, cervical arthritis, or temporal arteritis	7. Palpate head, neck, and scalp

usually subacute and progressive, and may be resistant to relief with the use of analgesics (11). Multiple studies reveal that very few patients presenting with headaches caused by brain tumors have normal neurologic examinations and no history of seizure, change in function, or loss of consciousness (13). Papilledema is found in 40% of brain tumor patients. Abnormal neurologic signs in a patient with a "new" headache that is severe and progressive should raise suspicion for a tumor (11).

Temporomandibular Joint Disorders

Temporomandibular joint (TMJ) disorders are common in the general population and include both joint and muscle disorders. There may be an opening or closing click or pop, pain with maximal opening, or pain with side-to-side motion of the jaw. Patients may often be anxious or depressed, and they frequently complain of tension-type headaches (7).

On physical examination, pain may be elicited by palpating over the lateral aspect of the TMJ or by palpating through the external auditory meatus. Tenderness of the muscles of mastication (masseter and pterygoid) may also be present. Because there is considerable overlap between TMJ and tension headaches, tenderness of the temporalis muscles is nonspecific and does not discriminate this type of headache (7).

The combination of reciprocal clicking of the TMJ, pain on jaw opening, and pain on palpation of the TMJ is 92% sensitive and 91% specific for internal derangement of the TMJ (LR+ 10.2, LR− 0.08). Similarly, the combination of pain on palpation of the TMJ, pain on jaw opening, and pain with lateral movement is 77% sensitive and 85% specific for myofascial dysfunction of the TMJ (LR+ 5.1, LR− 0.27) (7).

Hemorrhage

Headache associated with subarachnoid hemorrhage (SAH) is usually severe, unrelenting, and of abrupt onset. Accompanying symptoms may include nausea and vomiting, stiff neck, decrease in level of consciousness, and focal neurologic deficits. Approximately 50% of patients with subarachnoid hemorrhages have "sentinel bleeds" that may persist for hours or days, potentially providing warning signs to impending significant events (9, 11).

The classic headache following SAH is frequently associated with focal neurologic symptoms or loss of consciousness. Care must be taken to identify subtle neurologic signs, including brief loss of consciousness at the onset, nuchal rigidity, ocular motor palsy, or papilledema (12). One large series found that six of 17 patients with SAH did not present with a headache (13).

Laboratory Tests

The cause of most headaches can be determined by a careful history and supplemented by a general and symptom-focused neurologic examination. Inappropriate reasons for obtaining laboratory tests and imaging studies include anxiety of patients and family members and medicolegal concerns. When the diagnosis remains uncertain after the history and physical examination are completed, the optimal "test" is often a follow-up assessment within 1 to 2 weeks. Characteristics of the tests most useful in evaluating headache conditions are summarized in Table 28.4.

CT and MRI

Although CT and MRI are commonly performed for patients with headache, there are few recently published data either supporting or refuting this practice. Although the scans may relieve anxiety in some patients, the detection of "abnormal" clinically insignificant findings, the risk of adverse events with contrast, and the overall cost for society mandate careful use of these technologies (13). A series of over 3,000 scans in patients with headache as the only symptom (normal neurologic examination) demonstrated the following percentages of various pathologies: 0.8% tumor, 0.2% arteriovenous malformation, 0.3% hydrocephalus, 0.1% aneurysm, and 0.2% subdural hemorrhage (9). However, most patients with headache do not receive a CT scan (only 3% in one study), so the likelihood of these pathologies among all patients with headache is even lower (13).

Chronic headache patients with isolated headaches (those without neurologic symptoms, without an abnormal neurologic exam, persistent visual symptoms, personality change, recent head trauma, history of seizures, known history of cancer or HIV, history of subarachnoid bleed or previous neurosurgical procedure) have an extremely low yield of neuroimaging. Only 0.01% had an abnormality requiring neurosurgi-

Table 28.4.
Characteristics of Diagnostic Tests/Maneuvers Useful in Patients with Headache

Suspected Diagnosis	Test	Sensitivity	Specificity	LR+	LR−
Brain tumor	CT—best for bone abnormalities/SAH	0.75	0.60	1.88	0.42
	MRI—more sensitive for white matter abnormalities	0.95	0.80	4.8	0.06
Subarachnoid hemorrhage (SAH)	CT without contrast—within 72 hours[a]	0.90	0.80	4.5	0.13
	CT without contrast—after 72 hours	0.74			
	LP (specificity is for xanthochromia after 12 hours)[b]	1.0	1.0		
Mild head injury	Skull radiographs[c] CT[d]				

Adapted from Becker LA, Iverson DC, Reed FM, Calonge N, Miller RS, Freeman WL. Patients with new headaches in primary care. J Fam Pract 1988;27:41–46; Evans RW. Diagnostic testing for the evaluation of headaches. Neurol Clin 1996;14(1):1–26; Evans RW. Postconcussion syndrome and sequelae of minor head injury. Neurol Clin 1992;10:815–843; Schwartz RB. Neurobiology of brain tumors. Neurol Clin 1995;13:723–756; Miller J, Diringer M. Management of subarachnoid hemorrhage. Neurol Clin 1995;13:451–478.

[a]Indications: acute, "severe" worst headaches with or without neurologic symptoms; may have nausea, vomiting, or loss of consciousness. May have antecedent history of "sentinel headaches."

[b]Performed on all patients with new headache suspicious for SAH and a normal CT (CT performed first).

[c]Frequently performed, but probably not justified where CT is available. Moderate risks for abnormality include (a) history of loss of consciousness; (b) progressive headache; (c) alcohol or drug intoxication; (d) posttrauma seizure of amnesia; (e) serious facial injury; or (f) basilar skull fracture.

[d]Indications include history of loss of consciousness along with Glasgow coma scale < 15, focal neurologic signs, and abnormal mental status.

cal intervention (17). Studies in children with headaches without clinical evidence of a structural lesion also demonstrate the limited value of neuroimaging (18).

Neuroimaging is not warranted for patients with migraine who have a normal neurologic examination (19).

In the emergency situation, the most sensitive indications for the ordering of CT include positive neurologic findings coupled with unresponsiveness, intoxication, or amnesia (20).

Other Tests

An erythrocyte sedimentation rate (ESR) and temporal artery biopsy should be considered in patients over the age of 50 with new headaches, especially those with temporal tenderness or visual symptoms. The presence of at least three of five key criteria (age at least 50 years, new onset of localized headache, temporal artery tenderness or decreased pulse, ESR of at least 50 mm/hr, and positive histology) is 94% sensitive and 91% specific (LR+ 11.7, LR− 0.07) for the diagnosis of TA (21).

Electroencephalograms (EEGs) are not indicated in the routine evaluation of patients with headache. The contribution of EEG to diagnosis

and treatment in children with chronic headache is minimal and should not be routinely performed in these children (22, 23).

MANAGEMENT

Early follow-up is recommended in patients with new headaches to evaluate their response to therapy and to reconfirm the history and physical examination. Review of headache diaries, precipitating factors, and life events may help avoid the chronic headache. Patients with headache (especially primary headaches) should have a significant role in their own diagnosis and treatment plan. It may be important to reassure your patient that there is not a serious cause for the headaches such as cerebral neoplasm or aneurysm. However, patient education during an acute headache is not very effective. Subsequent visits to assess patient understanding, the response to therapy, and frequency of attacks can be therapeutic. The mutually cooperative, understanding relationship critical to long-term success can only be established with frequent visits at the onset of the headaches, followed by a gradually decreasing frequency of visits as the patient assumes more responsibility for headache management (Fig. 28.1) (24).

Nonpharmacotherapy

Patient education should include counseling to avoid specific precipitating factors such as alcohol, certain foods, fatigue, and particular life stressors. Encourage regular exercise and sleep routines, not skipping meals, smoking cessation, and limiting caffeine and alcohol intake. Biofeedback, stress management, and muscle relaxation techniques may also be useful adjuncts (25). The level of evidence to support different pharmacotherapy and nonpharmacotherapy approaches to the management of headache is summarized in Table 28.5.

Primary Headache

Migraine

Migraine has no "cure," so treatment goals should focus on control of pain and awareness of triggers.

Table 28.5.
Management of Headache

Treatment Strategy	Level of Evidence for Effectiveness[a]	Recommendations/Comments[b]
Pharmacotherapy		
Abortive therapy		
Simple analgesics	A	Mainstay of therapy for mild headaches
NSAIDs	A	Very effective, first-line therapy
Compound analgesics	A	Effective, but chronic use should be avoided
Ergot derivatives	A	Effective; limit daily and monthly usage
Sumatriptan	A	Effective both subcutaneously and orally. Use with caution in the face of possible coronary artery disease
Narcotic analgesics	A	May be the only effective medication for severe migraine, but limit long-term use
Prophylactic therapy		
β Blockers	A	Treatment of choice for migraine prophylaxis
Tricyclics	A	Useful with coexisting depression
SSRI antidepressant	B	May be particularly useful for mixed depression and tension type
Calcium channel blockers	B	Mixed results; nifedipine may cause headache
Nonpharmacotherapies		
Avoid "triggers"/diary (diet, alcohol, tobacco)	B	Allows patient to monitor and participate in treatment decisions and management
Patient education	B	Reassurance, support, alleviation of anxiety, improves compliance and outcome
Wellness program	B	Regular exercise, balanced meals, adequate sleep
Biofeedback	B	May reduce medication requirements
Transcutaneous electrical nerve stimulation (TENS)	B	Same as above
Relaxation, behavioral counseling	B	May be useful adjunct provided by primary physician
Acupuncture	C	Few studies to support, but frequently sought by chronic headache patients

[a]Level of evidence for effectiveness: A, Strong or moderate research based evidence (consistent across several studies, including at least two randomized controlled trials); B, Limited research based evidence (less consistent or extensive evidence, but preponderance of evidence supports use of treatment); C, Common practice with little or no research based evidence; X, Moderate or strong evidence that treatment is not effective

[b]Adapted from Capobianco DJ, Cheshire WP, Campbell JK. An overview of the diagnosis and pharmacologic treatment of migraine. Mayo Clin Proc 1996;71:1055–1066; Diamond S. Migraine headaches. Med Clin North Am 1991;75(3):545–563; McKenna JP. Cluster headaches. Am Fam Physician 1988;37:173–178; Saper JR. Chronic headache syndromes. Neurol Clin 1989;7:387–411; Silberstein SD. Overview in the diagnosis and treatment of migraine. Neurology 1994;44 (suppl 7):S6–S16; Williams JW, Simel DL. Does this patient have sinusitis? Diagnosing acute sinusitis by history and physical examination. JAMA 1993;270:1242–246; Silberstein SD. Office management of benign headache. Postgrad Med 1993;93:223–240; Gunderson CH. Management of the migraine patient. Am Fam Physician 1986;33:137–143.

Patient education about the condition, insight into family and life stresses, knowledge of environmental and emotional triggers, and counseling may help both decrease headache frequency and increase coping skills. Physicians should avoid the "quick fix" of focusing on medication first for the headache. Recent evidence suggests that analgesic overuse leads to rebound headaches, which are frequent, severe, and refractory and represent a major cause of chronic headache.

ACUTE THERAPY

The goal of acute (abortive) therapy in migraine is to terminate the attack or decrease its symptoms. The initial choice of medication depends on the presence or absence of nausea, prior treatments, comorbid conditions, and the severity of the current attack. Simple analgesics, acetaminophen, aspirin, and nonsteroidal anti-inflammatory drugs (NSAIDs) are considered first-line therapy. Ketorolac (Toradol), an NSAID available for parenteral administration, may be particularly effective for moderate migraine because it is rapidly absorbed, causes few adverse effects, and is not habituating. Combination analgesics, such as acetaminophen with isometheptene and dichloralphenazone (Midrin) or acetaminophen with butalbital and caffeine (Fioricet), are effective in the treatment of mild-to-moderate attacks, but both may cause a medication-induced or rebound headache if used frequently. Their use should therefore be limited to no more than 2 days per week (2, 26).

For moderate to severe migraine attacks that fail to respond to simple or combination analgesics, ergotamine tartrate, dihydroergotamine (DHE), and sumatriptan succinate (Imitrex) are effective agents. DHE may be given by intramuscular or intravenous means, whereas sumatriptan may be self-administered by auto-injector or given orally. Phenothiazines (e.g., chlorpromazine and prochlorperazine) given intravenously are also effective agents for acute attacks.

Effective symptomatic therapy must also consider the associated symptoms of migraine such as nausea and vomiting. Adjunctive measures include the use of antiemetic medications or caffeine; metoclopramide (Reglan) is effective in treating the gastrointestinal manifestations of migraine and potentiates the action of other agents by enhancing gastric motility and intestinal absorption. Medications and doses are found in Table 28.6.

PREVENTIVE THERAPY

Preventive therapy is indicated if the number of attacks exceeds three or four per month, it significantly impacts on quality of life or job attendance, or the headaches occur on a predictable schedule (e.g., with menses). Effective medications include β blockers, tricyclic antidepressants (TCA), calcium channel blockers, ergot derivatives, or corticosteroids. Cyproheptadine (Periactin) has proven useful in children. Calcium channel blockers are not as effective as β blockers for prophylaxis, but they are the agents of choice for those patients who are unable to take β blockers (e.g., patients with asthma, congestive heart failure, or insulin-dependent diabetes). Methysergide (Sansert) is very effective in refractory cases; this drug should not be used for longer than 6 months without a "drug holiday" because of adverse effects (3). See Table 28.6 for drug doses.

Cluster Headaches

Acute therapy for cluster headache is less well studied than therapy for migraine due to the relative rarity of this condition. Options include inhalation of 100% oxygen by mask at a rate of 7 to 10 L/min; DHE or ergotamine as used in migraine; and sublingual nifedipine, 10 mg (do not use together with ergotamine). Other medications used in treatment of acute migraine may also be helpful in cluster headache, although careful follow-up to evaluate effectiveness is important.

Prevention is the goal for any patient who has had a series of cluster headaches. Methysergide, lithium (monitor blood levels weekly to avoid toxicity), prednisone, and calcium channel blockers have been used, but supportive evidence largely comes from observational studies.

Tension Headaches

Acute drug therapy should begin with acetaminophen or adequate doses of NSAIDs. Some physicians use muscle relaxants for selected patients. Avoid propoxyphene because of its low potency and high abuse potential. Tension headaches often become chronic. Long-term use of narcotic analgesics may lead to dependence. Discontinuation of daily drug intake often results in headache improvement.

Medications used for migraine prophylaxis are also useful for patients with frequent, chro-

Table 28.6.
Drug Therapy for Headache

Indications/Contraindications	Drug (Common Trade Name)	Common Dosage	Cautions and Adverse Effects
Acute severe migraine	Sumatriptan (Imitrex) DHE	6 mg SC 25–50 mg PO 0.5–1.5 mg IM/IV 2–3 mg nasal spray	Not yet FDA approved
	Ergotamine tartrate (Wygraine)	Rectal: 1 suppository at onset; repeat 1 hour prn (max of 2/day, 12/mo) Sublingual: 1 tablet at onset; repeat once in 1 hour if needed (2- mg tablets)	Use minimum subnauseating dose
	Ketorolac (Toradol)	30–60 mg at onset; repeat 15–30 mg q6h	Abuse potential controversial
	Butorphanol (Stadol, Stadol NS)	1 spray (1 mg) in 1 nostril at onset; repeat in 1 hour (max 3 doses/day)	
Mild to moderate migraine	Chlorpromazine (Thorazine)	12.5 IV; repeat q30min to total dose of 37.5 mg	
	Prochlorperazine (Compazine)	10 mg IV by slow push	Antiemetic, potentiates other treatments
	Metoclopramide (Reglan)	10–20 mg IV/IM	
	Acetaminophen	650–1000 mg PO initially; repeat q6–8h	
	Acetaminophen, butalbital, and caffeine (Fioricet, Esgic)	2 tablets PO at onset; repeat 1q4–6h prn (max 5/day, 15/month)	
	Aspirin, butalbital, caffeine (Fiorinal)	2 tablets PO at onset; repeat 1q4–6h prn (max 5/day, 15/month)	
	Ibuprofen (Nuprin, Advil, Motrin)	600–800 mg at onset; repeat q6h	Combination analgesic vasoconstrictor
	Naproxen sodium (Anaprox, Aleve)	550–825 mg initially; repeat q8h	
	Acetaminophen, chloralphenazone, and isometheptene (Midrin, Isocom)	2 capsules at onset, followed by 1 every hour as needed, to a maximum of 5 capsules/day, 20/month	
Acute tension headache	Aspirin, NSAIDs, acetaminophen, combination analgesics	Dosages as above	
Prophylaxis	Propranolol (Inderal)	40–320 mg/day	
	Nadolol (Corgard)	40–240 mg/day	
	Atenolol (Tenormin)	25–200 mg/day	
	Metoprolol (Lopressor)	100–200 mg/day	
	Verapamil (Calan, Isoptin, Verelan)	240–480 mg/day	
	Amitriptyline (Elavil)	10–175 mg/day	
	Nortriptyline (Pamelor, Aventyl)	10–125 mg/day	
	Valproic acid (Depakene, Dephcote)	250–1500 mg/day	
	Cyproheptadine (Periactin)	2–16 mg/day	
	Methysergide (Sansert)	2–6 mg/day	
	Phenelzine (Nardil)	15–60 mg/day	MAO inhibitor

nic tension headaches. β Blockers and tricyclic antidepressants, alone or in combination, are especially beneficial. Physical therapy may be a useful adjunct in the management of chronic tension headaches along with biofeedback, relaxation, exercise, and other nonpharmacotherapy treatments.

Secondary Headaches

Once the diagnosis is established for secondary headaches, the best treatment approach is management of the underlying condition. Treatment of the multiple potential diagnoses is beyond the scope of this chapter and may involve primary therapy or specialty consultation.

Special Considerations

Headache in Children

Between 37 and 75% of children experience at least one headache before age 15. Recurrent headache occurs in 6 to 23% (27). Migraine in children is the most common diagnosis, comprising up to 70% of headaches in studies of patients presenting to a pediatric headache clinic (28). Key variables that distinguish migraine from other headaches in children include frequency, type of pain, neurologic deficits, nausea, and vomiting (28). Acute migraine attacks in children usually respond to simple analgesics. Acetaminophen is usually very effective, whereas NSAIDs may be needed for more severe headaches. Acute and preventive care programs must be clear; deal with medication management during school hours because of regulations concerning drug use in school. Cyproheptadine (Periactin) may be particularly effective for prophylactic therapy for migraine in children.

Headache in the Elderly

Headaches in the elderly are common and usually benign. Because the incidence of underlying organic disease increases with age, consider both organic and benign causes. Tension headache, the most common primary headache, may be aggravated by underlying cervical spine osteoarthritis and/or depression. Migraine variants can sometimes be confused with acute cerebrovascular events. Differentiating factors that favor migraine include a history of recurrent attacks; slow and progressive visual and other neurologic symptoms (versus an acute simultaneous onset); and a duration of more than 20 minutes with migraine accompaniments (versus less than 15 minutes for most transient ischemic attacks [TIAs]). Medications prescribed for migraine and tension headaches work well in the elderly, although sumatriptan is not recommended in patients with ischemic heart disease because of the risk of coronary vasospasm. Similarly, β blockers and calcium channel blockers for migraine prophylaxis must be used with caution in patients with a history of sinus bradycardia or left ventricular dysfunction (8).

CASE STUDY

Mrs. M. is a 27-year-old woman, married and the mother of two young children, who works full time as a junior executive at an advertising agency. She has noticed an increasing frequency of her headaches, which are becoming almost daily. She has a long history of migraine headaches and has tried multiple medications in the past, including a 6-month course of nortriptyline for prophylactic therapy, which worked well for her at that time. She is presently taking six to eight butalbital with acetaminophen (Fioricet) per day. She is under significant stress at work and is the main source of support for her children, taking them to preschool and after-school activities. Because of her schedule, she has discontinued her membership at the health club and has gained 20 pounds in the past year. She is sleeping poorly and frequently eats fast food.

When appearing for her appointment, she is harried in appearance and is quite impatient that she has had to wait an extra 15 minutes to see the doctor. She would just like a refill of her Fioricet and tried unsuccessfully to accomplish this through a telephone call. She describes her headaches as daily, occurring throughout the day, worse in the morning, and only partially relieved by the medication. She wants to know if there is anything stronger that she can take. She denies any aura, neurologic symptoms, nausea, or vomiting, and her pain is usually bilateral and radiates to her neck. She has had no fever, chills, or recent illnesses. Physical examination is limited to vital signs, head and neck, fundoscopy, and a brief neurologic examination. The results are normal.

QUESTIONS

1. What should you tell Mrs. M. about the cause for her headaches?
2. Would you order any laboratory or imaging studies?
3. What would be your treatment approach?

DISCUSSION

In spite of Mrs. M.'s long migraine history, her present headache pattern is not consistent with migraine. Stress from her job and family obligations, and sleep, nutrition, and exercise habits are probably all contributing to the development of this pattern. The first step in management will be to educate Mrs. M. to recognize the role of her behaviors and environment in her headache history. More history will be needed to explore her present relationship with her husband, his support of her career, and his willingness to help with home chores and child care duties. Exploration of their financial situation may allow consideration of other options for child care or part-time help at home. The role of the increasing use of compound analgesics must also be explored with the patient, with the suggestion that increasing her drugs may actually be making her headaches worse instead of better.

With the history and physical examination consistent with chronic tension or mixed headaches and no "red flags" present, no laboratory tests or imaging studies are indicated. A headache "diary" should be recommended to help sort out triggers for her headaches. Adjustments in sleeping, eating, and her work schedule may be

necessary to allow the patient to reestablish control over her life. Because chronic medications are a frequent factor in exacerbating headaches, her present medications must be strictly limited and gradually tapered over the next 2 to 4 weeks. An antidepressant may be added as an adjunct to help her taper the Fioricet, and NSAIDs could be prescribed as an alternative for pain relief when she has a more severe headache. Recommending that she resume her exercise program may also help this pattern. Close follow-up with the same physician to provide continuity in a supportive relationship will be critical to success.

REFERENCES

1. Becker LA, Iverson DC, Reed FM, Calonge N, Miller RS, Freeman WL. Patients with new headaches in primary care. J Fam Pract 1988;27:41–46.
2. Capobianco DJ, Cheshire WP, Campbell JK. An overview of the diagnosis and pharmacologic treatment of migraine. Mayo Clin Proc 1996;71:1055–1066.
3. Diamond S. Migraine headaches. Med Clin North Am 1991;75(3):545–563.
4. McKenna JP. Cluster headaches. Am Fam Physician 1988;37:173–178.
5. Saper JR. Chronic headache syndromes. Neurol Clin 1989; 7:387–411.
6. Pascual J, Iglesias F, Oterino A, Vazquez-Barquero A, Berciano J. Cough, exertional, and sexual headaches: an analysis of 72 benign and symptomatic cases. Neurology 1996;46:1520–1524.
7. Schiffman E, Haley D, Baker C, Lindgren B. Diagnostic criteria for screening headache patients for temporomandibular disorders. Headache 1995;35:121–124.
8. Ruoff GE. Headache in elderly patients. Postgrad Med 1993;94:109–121.
9. Evans RW. Diagnostic testing for the evaluation of headaches. Neurol Clin 1996;14(1):1–26.
10. Robb-Nicholson C, et al. Diagnostic value of the history and examination in giant cell arteritis: a clinical pathological study of 81 temporal artery biopsies. J Rheumatol 1988;15:1793–1796.
11. Dodick D. Headache as a symptom of ominous disease. Postgrad Med 1997;101:46–64.
12. Coutin IB, Glass SF. Recognizing uncommon headache syndromes. Am Fam Physician 1996;54:2247–2252.
13. Becker LA, Green LA, Beaufait D, Kirk J, Froom J, Freeman WL. Detection of intracranial tumors, subarachnoid hemorrhages, and subdural hematomas in primary care patients: a report from ASPN, part 2. J Fam Pract 1993;37:135–141.
14. Mondell BE. Evaluation of the patient presenting with headache. Med Clin North Am 1991;75(3):521–524.
15. Dubose CD, Cutlip AC, Cutlip WD. Migraines and

other headaches: approach to diagnosis and classification. Am Fam Physician 1995;51:1498–1504.

16. Silberstein SD. Overview in the diagnosis and treatment of migraine. Neurology 1994;44(suppl 7):S6–S16.

17. Weingarten S, Kleinman M, Elperin L, Larson EB. The effectiveness of cerebral imaging in the diagnosis of chronic headache. Arch Intern Med 1992;152:2457–2462.

18. Maytal J, Bienkowski RS, Patel M, Eviatar L. The value of brain imaging in children with headaches. Pediatrics 1995;96:413–416.

19. Quality Standards Committee of the American Academy of Neurology. Practice parameter: the utility of neuroimaging in the evaluation of headaches in patients with normal neurologic examinations (summary statement). Neurology 1994;44:1353.

20. Reinus WR, Erickson KK, Wippold FJ. Unenhanced emergency cranial CT: optimizing patient selection with univariate and multivariate analysis. Radiology 1993;186:763–768.

21. Hunder GG, Bloch DA, Michel BA, et al. The American College of Rheumatology 1990 criteria for the classification of giant cell arteritis. Arthritis Rheum 1990; 33:1122–1128.

22. Gronseth GS, Greenburg MK. The utility of the electroencephalogram in the evaluation of patients with headache. Neurology 1995;45:1263–1267.

23. Kramer U, Nevo Y, Neufeld MY, Harel S. The value of EEG in children with chronic headaches. Brain Dev 1994;16:304–308.

24. Silberstein SD. Office management of benign headache. Postgrad Med 1993;93:223–240.

25. Gunderson CH. Management of the migraine patient. Am Fam Physician 1986;33:137–143.

26. Diamond S, Diamond ML. Emergency treatment of migraine. Postgrad Med 1997;101:169–179.

27. Hanson RR. Headaches in childhood. Semin Neurol 1988;8:51–59.

28. Gladstein J, Holden EW, Peralta L, Raven M. Diagnoses and symptom pattern in children presenting to a pediatric headache clinic. Headache 1993;33:497–500.

29. HIV Disease

J. KEVIN CARMICHAEL

Key Clinical Questions

1. What signs and symptoms suggest HIV infection?
2. How should antiretroviral therapy be managed?
3. What opportunistic infections can be prevented, and how?
4. How may we optimize the quality of life for persons living with HIV infection?

The human immunodeficiency virus (HIV) is a retrovirus that is transmitted sexually or through the exchange of blood or other infectious body fluids. Transmission through unprotected sex with HIV-infected persons and injection drug use account for over 95% of HIV infections; vertical transmission from mother to child and accidental exposure to contaminated blood or blood products during health care delivery contributes the rest.

The World Health Organization estimates that 22 million people worldwide are infected with HIV. Of these, approximately 780,000 live in North America. In the United States, about 40,000 new HIV infections occur yearly, and AIDS is a leading cause of death for all persons between 25 and 44 years of age. Early in the epidemic in the United States, the risk group most affected was that of men who have sex with other men. This pattern is rapidly changing to reflect trends seen throughout the rest of the world, that is, heterosexual transmission and disproportionate representation of the poor and racial and ethnic minorities (1–3).

HIV infection is diagnosed by testing for the presence of antibodies to the virus. A screening test, the enzyme-linked immunosorbent assay (ELISA), is performed and a positive ELISA (false-negative rate .019, false-positive rate .0015) is confirmed by Western Blot testing (false-negative rate 0, false-positive rate 0.006). The period of time after infection and before detectable antibodies is about 6 weeks in most cases and rarely longer than 6 months.

Primary care physicians usually decide to test for HIV infection because of either risk factors or suspicious clinical signs or symptoms. Risk factors include injection drug use, unprotected sexual activity (particularly men who have sex with men, persons with multiple sexual partners, or prostitutes), and the receipt of unscreened blood or blood products (i.e., prior to 1985 in the United States). Suspicious clinical signs and symptoms include any sexually transmitted disease; pulmonary or extrapulmonary *Mycobacterium tuberculosis* infection; any young person with herpes zoster; severe seborrheic dermatitis of the face or scalp; bacterial pneumonia unless other risk factors exist; chronic unresponsive *Candida* infection of the skin, mouth, or vagina; thrombocytopenia; and unexplained fatigue, malaise, fevers, night sweats, diarrhea, or adenopathy. Inquiry about HIV risk factors and education about HIV transmission should be part of the health maintenance examination for all patients between ages 13 and 50.

CLINICAL EVALUATION

History

At the first visit with an HIV-infected patient, you should obtain a thorough medical history, including details of how HIV was contracted and any ongoing high-risk behaviors. Repeat HIV antibody testing is indicated in those instances in which clear documentation of HIV infection is unavailable. The occurrence of opportunistic infection or any other HIV-associated condition should be noted. Current medications should be listed, including vitamins or other substances taken for nutritional or medical purposes. You should pay particular attention to sexually transmitted diseases (hepatitis B and C, syphilis, genital warts, and herpes simplex) and fungal, parasitic, and mycobacterial diseases. The psychosocial history should include questions about living situation, support systems, and financial resources. The use of alcohol, tobacco, and other recreational drugs should be discussed. Table 29.1 lists key elements of the history and physical examination.

The review of systems must be comprehensive, as positive responses may provide clues to under-

Table 29.1.
Key Elements of the History and Physical Examination for HIV Infection

Question/Maneuver	Purpose
Date and place of HIV testing	The presence of HIV must be clearly documented. Cases of testing errors and of persons claiming HIV infection who are not infected have been reported.
History of or exposure to *Mycobacterium tuberculosis* and/or syphilis	Tuberculosis and syphilis are more difficult to treat in HIV-infected persons and require close observation.
History of unexplained fever for >2 weeks or oropharyngeal candidiasis	These symptoms indicate the need for PCP prophylaxis even if CD4 > 200.
History of opportunistic infection	Recurrence is common, and the possibility of recurrent disease must be considered when evaluating any new symptoms.
Careful examination of the fundi, mouth, lymphatic system, genitals, and rectum	Cytomegalovirus retinitis, oral candidiasis, infection or malignancy of the lymphatic system, and cervical and rectal cancer may be detected early by careful examination.

lying opportunistic infection, malignancy, or HIV-related central nervous system disease. Symptoms that should be specifically inquired about include fatigue, fever, night sweats, weight loss or gain, appetite, anxiety or depression, adenopathy, skin rash, bruises or bleeding from gums, oral sores or lesions, changes in the taste of food, visual changes, shortness of breath or cough, nausea and/or vomiting, diarrhea, genital or rectal sores, arthritis, discoordination, and changes in mental status such as forgetfulness or mental slowing.

Physical Examination

You should perform a complete physical examination at the initial visit (see Table 29.1). Vital signs, including weight and temperature, should be documented at each encounter. The key areas for examination in HIV-infected persons are the oral cavity, retina, chest, abdomen (liver and spleen), genital system, rectum, lymphatic system, skin, and the neurologic system, including mental status. In the mouth, you should look for candidiasis; the purple lesions of Kaposi's sarcoma; hairy leukoplakia on the lateral tongue; gingivitis; herpetic or aphthous ulcers; and occult lymphoma. Funduscopic examination commonly reveals cotton wool spots, but in patients with CD4 counts less than 50, you should look carefully for cytomegalovirus (CMV) retinitis. Hepatosplenomegaly is common in HIV-infected persons and warrants further evaluation for signs of systemic infection or malignancy.

Your genital system examination should look for ulcer disease or warts. Because women with HIV are at increased risk for cervical neoplasia, Papanicolaou (Pap) smears are indicated at least yearly and more frequently if any dysplasia is detected. The rectum may also have ulcerative disease or warts, and the incidence of rectal carcinoma is increased in men with HIV infection.

Although generalized lymphadenopathy is common in HIV-infected persons, single enlarged, painless lymph nodes should elicit your concern for lymphoma. Lymphadenopathy may also be found in other malignancies and in systemic infection. Focal neurologic findings suggest central nervous system (CNS) infection (e.g., toxoplasmosis or cryptococcus) or tumor. Peripheral neuropathy may be caused by the virus or as a consequence of antiretroviral therapy. Decreases in short-term memory, depression, dementia, and psychosis may be present and become more common in late-stage disease. Table 29.2 lists "red flags" suggesting life-threatening disease in patients with HIV infections.

Laboratory Testing

Initial laboratory testing of the HIV-positive patient should include repeat HIV-1 antibody testing if documentation is not available (to verify the diagnosis); HIV-1 RNA quantitation by either PCR, bDNA, or NASBA methodology; and CD4 enumeration (to help determine disease severity—see Table 29.3). In addition, the follow-

Table 29.2.
"Red Flags" Suggesting Progressive or Life-Threatening Disease in Patients with HIV Infection

"Red Flag"	Implication
Visual changes (particularly floaters and field deficits)	Suggests CMV retinitis—a sight-threatening complication (incidence increases at CD4 < 50).
Fever	Prolonged fever usually represents opportunistic infection.
Shortness of breath or dyspnea on exertion	Suggests pneumonitis (bacterial, mycobacterial, fungal, or protozoal)
Focal neurologic deficits	Possible CNS infection or tumor.
Odynophagia/dysphagia	Esophageal infection (most common with *Candida*, herpes simplex virus [HSV], or cytomegalovirus [CMV]).
Weight loss	Loss of >4 kg in <4 months suggests opportunistic infection.
Diarrhea	Bacterial, parasitic, or mycobacterial infection should be ruled out. Medication and diet-related diarrhea must also be considered.
Paresthesias of feet or hands	Medications (didanosine, stavudine, and zalcitabine) are a common cause of peripheral neuropathy, although HIV- related neuropathy may occur.

ing tests help screen for infection: CBC with platelets, chemistry panel and albumin to assess kidney and liver function and nutritional status, RPR, HBsAg and anti-HBc, toxoplasmosis IgG, a chest radiograph, and a tuberculin skin test (PPD), unless there is a reliable history of a previous positive test or of treatment for tuberculosis. Finally, as previously stated, women should have a Pap smear (4).

Prognosis

The prognosis for persons infected with HIV is changing. The development and widespread use of highly active antiretroviral therapy (HAART) has resulted in a decline of 23% in deaths during 1996 when compared with 1995 (the first decline since the epidemic began). The durability of this improved prognosis remains to be determined. Viral load and CD4 counts are both independent predictors of prognosis. Changes in viral load are indicative of an improved prognosis, with a 1 log decline in viral load decreasing the rate of progression to AIDS or death by 70%.

You should take the time to assess the patient's expectations about his or her illness, as many people still equate HIV infection with the immediate end of life. The data on survival with HAART should be explained to patients as essential information for the development of a treatment plan.

Table 29.3.
Diagnostic Tests Useful in Gauging the Severity of HIV Infection

Test	Explanation	Interpretation
CD4 enumeration	A measure of immune system status critical for the assessment of the risk of, and the need for prophylaxis of, opportunistic infection.	CD4 > 500 is associated with relatively good immune function. CD4 < 500 indicates the need for antiretroviral therapy. CD4 < 200 defines AIDS and indicates the need for opportunistic infection prophylaxis.
HIV-1 RNA viral quantitation by either PCR or bDNA	These tests measure the quantity of virus in 1 mL of blood. The amount of virus present and the degree to which it changes with treatment have clinical utility for prognosis and for evaluation of drug efficacy.	Viral loads of >10,000–30,000 indicate the need for therapy. The goal of therapy is to drive loads as low as possible for as long as possible.

MANAGEMENT

HIV infection presents a great challenge to health care providers. It is the most feared and stigmatized disease of our time. Although medical treatment is rapidly evolving, recent advances are expensive and of uncertain long-term value. Many emotions—including fear, disapproval, anger, pity, helplessness, and sorrow—may arise in you while caring for those with HIV infection. The principles of family practice—primacy of the patient, respect of autonomy, and an empathetic approach—all serve you well when caring for HIV-infected persons.

The five critical components of the care of HIV-infected persons include (a) prevention of transmission; (b) preservation of immune function; (c) prophylaxis against opportunistic infection; (d) early diagnosis and treatment of opportunistic infection; and (e) optimization of quality of life.

Prevention of Transmission

HIV is not yet curable, so prevention is the only method of decreasing the spread of the infection. Importantly, persons already infected are at risk for reinfection with strains of HIV that are resistant to some or all antiretroviral drugs. For this reason, patients should receive explicit instructions on the methods of HIV transmission and on how to minimize the risk of reinfection and of transmission to others. Physical barriers during sexual activity and clean, single-use needles for injecting drugs are mainstays for preventing HIV transmission. Because there are numerous public misconceptions about HIV, you should also discuss the many ways HIV is not transmitted (e.g., through casual social contact or via saliva, sweat, or tears).

Preservation of Immune Function

Preservation of immune function is primarily a function of antiretroviral therapy. There are data (strength of evidence = B) suggesting that adoption of a "healthy lifestyle"—including smoking cessation, moderation of alcohol intake, good nutrition, aerobic exercise, and stress reduction—helps maintain immune function and improves survival in HIV infection.

The goal of antiretroviral therapy is to maximally inhibit viral replication and minimize the development of resistant strains of HIV. There

are currently three classes of antiretroviral medications; nucleoside reverse transcriptase inhibitors (e.g., zidovudine), nonnucleoside reverse transcriptase inhibitors (e.g., nevirapine), and protease inhibitors (e.g., indinavir). Nucleoside reverse transcriptase inhibitors compete with nucleoside triphosphates, causing premature termination of viral-DNA chain synthesis. Nonnucleoside reverse transcriptase inhibitors are noncompetitive inhibitors of reverse transcriptase, inactivating a key catalytic site. Protease inhibitors block HIV protease from cleaving viral precursor proteins into the final viral elements. Because HIV-infected persons are often taking multiple medications, consideration of potential drug interactions is critical before adding or changing medications. Commonly used medications, with doses and adverse effects, are listed in Table 29.4.

The cost of antiretroviral therapy appears high ($9,000 to $12,000 yearly). New data reveal that, in part because of resultant declining hospitalization and opportunistic infection, antiretroviral treatment costs about $10,000 per year of life gained. This compares quite favorably with many other commonly accepted medical interventions, such as enalapril for congestive heart failure ($9,700 per year of life gained), lovastatin to prevent coronary disease ($21,000), screening mammography ($30,000), fecal occult blood testing combined with sigmoidoscopy ($43,000), renal hemodialysis ($50,000), prostate-specific antigen screening ($113,000), and coronary artery bypass surgery ($13,000).

Initiating Therapy

Current recommendations support the initiating therapy in patients with CD4 counts less than 350 (strength of evidence = A), patients with viral load in excess of 30,000 regardless of CD4 count (strength of evidence = A), and patients with symptomatic HIV disease (recurrent mucosal candidiasis, oral hairy leukoplakia, chronic unexplained fever, night sweats, or weight loss) regardless of CD4 count or viral load (strength of evidence = A). The recent trend has been toward earlier and more aggressive treatment. Many experts advise that all persons with HIV infection should be on antiretroviral therapy, although clinical data to support this recommendation are lacking (5). Figure 29.1 summarizes the approach to the patient.

Table 29.4.
Antiretroviral Therapy

Generic Name	Trade Name	Dose	Common Adverse Effects
Nucleoside reverse transcriptase inhibitors			
Didanosine (ddI)	Videx	200 mg bid[a]	Peripheral neuropathy, pancreatitis, diarrhea
Lamivudine (3TC)	Epivir	150 mg bid	Nausea
Stavudine (d4T)	Zerit	40 mg bid[a]	Peripheral neuropathy, nausea
Zalcitabine (ddC)	Hivid	0.75 mg tid	Peripheral neuropathy, mucositis, pancreatitis
Zidovudine	Retrovir	200 mg tid	Headache, anemia, nausea
(AZT, ZDV)		300 mg bid	Myopathy
Nonnucleoside reverse transcriptase inhibitors			
Nevirapine	Viramune	200 mg bid	Rash, elevated transaminases
Delavirdine	Rescriptor	400 mg tid	Rash
Protease inhibitors			
Indinavir	Crixivan	800 mg q8h	Elevated bilirubin, nephrolithiasis, nausea; owing to a high affinity for several of the cytochrome P450 isoenzymes, many hepatically metabolized drugs are contraindicated or require dose adjustments.
Nelfinavir	Viracept	750 mg tid	Nausea, diarrhea
Ritonavir	Norvir	600 mg bid	Circumoral paresthesia, hypertriglyceridemia, nausea, diarrhea; owing to a high affinity for several of the cytochrome P450 isoenzymes, many hepatically metabolized drugs are contraindicated or require dose adjustments.
Saquinavir	Invirase	600 mg tid	Nausea, diarrhea, elevated transaminases; due to a high affinity for several of the cytochrome P450 isoenzymes, many hepatically metabolized drugs are contraindicated or require dose adjustments.

[a]Reduce dose if patient weighs less than 60 kg.

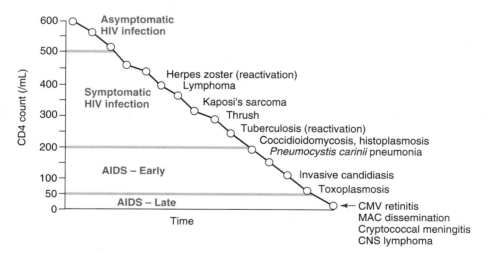

Figure 29.1. *Relationship between CD4 count and HIV-related conditions and opportunistic infections.*

Selecting and Monitoring Antiretroviral Therapy

The rapid rate of viral replication can quickly result in acquisition of antiretroviral resistance, especially in the face of suboptimal therapy. For this reason, combination therapy has emerged as the standard of care, but the optimal number of agents to use is not yet known. Current recommendations emphasize three-drug therapy (strength of evidence = A). Recommended combinations include two nucleoside analogues such as zidovudine/didanosine, zidovudine/zalcitabine, zidovudine/lamivudine, or stavudine/lamivudine, plus either a protease inhibitor or a nonnucleoside reverse transcriptase inhibitor. Treatment with two nucleoside analogues alone may be appropriate in some instances but is generally suboptimal (strength of evidence = A) (5).

Changes in plasma HIV RNA levels are the standard for determining the magnitude and duration of antiretroviral activity (strength of evidence = A). HIV RNA levels should be measured at baseline and 4 weeks after initiating or changing therapy. The biologic and intra-assay variability of this test require a 0.5 log or threefold change for significance. Therefore, the goal of antiretroviral therapy is a decline in HIV RNA of greater than 0.5 log and hopefully to undetectable levels. Although the majority of treatment-induced changes in HIV RNA occur in the first 4 weeks, it may take 3 to 6 months to see the maximal effects. In stable patients on antiretroviral therapy, HIV RNA levels and CD4 counts should be measured every 3 months. CD4 changes are now felt to be of less use in guiding antiretroviral therapy than HIV RNA levels, but they are still necessary to determine the need for prophylaxis and as a secondary measure of antiretroviral efficacy (6, 7).

Changing Therapy

Treatment failure, drug toxicity, intolerance, nonadherence, or current use of a suboptimal therapy all necessitate a regimen change. Treatment failure is defined as a rise in HIV RNA to within 0.5 log of pretreatment levels, a decrease in CD4 of >50%, or clinical deterioration as manifest by opportunistic infection or other HIV-related symptoms. When changing therapies, at least two new drugs should be added to any failing regimen (strength of evidence = C). Patients who have had experience with many drugs may

benefit from medications that they have not used for a prolonged period of time. Temporary interruption or cessation of effective antiretroviral therapy should be avoided, as viral resistance may be encouraged (strength of evidence = C). Although there are data demonstrating survival benefits from antiretroviral therapy even in advanced disease, cessation of antiretroviral therapy may be appropriate when toxicity or pill burden interfere with quality of life.

Prophylaxis Against Opportunistic Infection

The appropriate prophylaxis against opportunistic infection remains critically important when caring for people living with HIV infection. Currently prophylaxis against *Pneumocystis carinii* (PCP), *Mycobacterium tuberculosis*, and *Toxoplasma gondii* is standard of care (strength of evidence = A). Prophylaxis against *Streptococcus pneumoniae* and *Mycobacterium avium* complex should be considered in all patients (strength of evidence = B). Additionally, vaccination against hepatitis B and influenza virus is recommended for HIV-infected persons, even though these pathogens are not traditionally classified as opportunistic (strength of evidence = B). The specific indications and regimens are listed in Table 29.5. Prophylaxis against *Candida* species, *Cryptococcus neoformans*, *Histoplasmosis capsulatum*, *Coccidioides immitis*, cytomegalovirus, and herpesvirus is not recommended for most patients but may be considered in selected patients (e.g., persons with CD4 < 50 residing in endemic areas) (8).

Early Diagnosis and Treatment of Opportunistic Infection

Effective early diagnosis requires patient education, close patient follow-up, and a good patient-physician relationship. You should understand the relationship between CD4 count and various HIV-related conditions and opportunistic infections. Figure 29.2 illustrates these relationships. Patients should be educated about conditions they are at risk for and should be aware of symptoms that require immediate reporting to the physician. Persons living with HIV infection may at times seem overly concerned about symptoms. However, you must remember that people with HIV are at a much higher risk for real illness than noninfected persons, making careful evaluation of their complaints essential. Generally, patients

Table 29.5.
Opportunistic Infection Prophylaxis

Pneumocystis carinii
Indication:	CD4 < 200 or unexplained fever > 2 weeks or oropharyngeal candidiasis
First choice:	TMP/SMX DS (Bactrim DS, Septra DS, others) qd
Alternatives:	TMP/SMX DS 3 times a week, dapsone 100 qd, aerosolized pentamidine 300 mg every month via Respirgard II nebulizer

Mycobacterium tuberculosis
Indication:	Tuberculin skin test reaction of >5 mm; or prior positive skin test without treatment; or contact with case of active tuberculosis. If known drug-resistant strain, consult with public health authority.
First choice:	Isoniazid 300 mg plus pyridoxine 50 mg qd × 12 months or isoniazid 900 mg plus pyridoxine 50 mg twice weekly as directly observed therapy × 12 months
Alternatives:	Rifampin 600 mg qd × 12 months

Toxoplasma gondii
Indication:	IgG antibody to *Toxoplasma* and CD4 < 100
First choice:	TMP/SMX DS qd
Alternatives:	TMP/SMX DS 3 times a week, or dapsone 100 mg qd plus pyrimethamine 50 mg every week plus leucovorin 25 mg every week

Streptococcus pneumonia
Indication:	All patients
First choice:	Pneumococcal vaccine 0.5 mL IM × 1
Alternatives:	None

Mycobacterium avium complex
Indication:	CD4 < 50
First choice:	Azithromycin 600 mg every week or clarithromycin 500 bid
Alternatives:	Rifabutin 300 mg qd

Hepatitis B virus *(recommended although clinical efficacy has not been validated in this population.)*
Indication:	All anti-HBc-negative persons
First choice:	Energex-B 20 μg IM × 3, or Recombivax HB 10 μg IM × 3
Alternatives:	None

Influenza virus *(recommended although clinical efficacy has not been validated in this population.)*
Indication:	All patients annually before influenza season
First choice:	Whole or split virus 0.5 mL IM yearly
Alternatives:	None

TMP/SMX, trimethoprim/sulfamethoxazole.

should be seen every 1 to 3 months for routine follow-up and more frequently should problems arise. Staff must be aware of the increased risk of illness and facilitate communication of problems.

Optimizing the Quality of Life

HIV infection profoundly impacts on all areas of a person's life. Several studies have found an increased incidence of depression and suicide in HIV-infected persons. In addition, many persons living with HIV infection suffer significant declines in economic status with disease progression. Psychosocial issues, financial concerns, sexuality, and facing death must all be addressed. Psychologic support, nutritional support, social services, community-based organizations, home-nursing services, religious groups, and hospice care are all valuable resources for the support of persons living with HIV infection.

PATIENT EDUCATION

Patients and physicians both require continuing education as the care of HIV infection evolves. At a minimum, patients must understand how HIV is transmitted and how they can prevent transmission to others. They also should be taught the basic concepts of HIV management, including the central problem of viral resistance and the need for strict adherence to medication regimens to combat the development of resistance. You should work

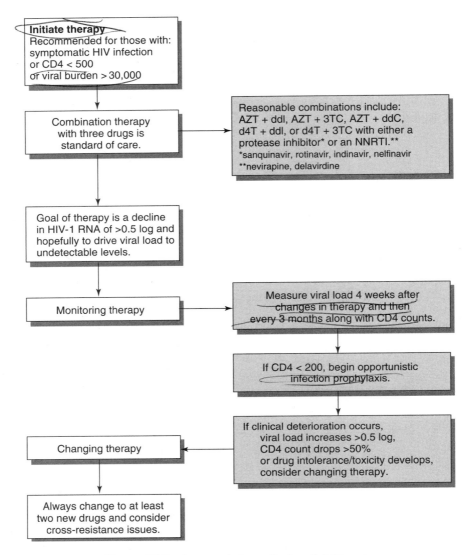

Figure 29.2. *Approach to antiretroviral therapy.*

to involve patients actively in their care, keeping them informed of results and implications of viral load testing and CD4 counts. Medication dosing, adverse effects, and interactions should be carefully explained and decisions about adjusting the treatment plan made jointly (Table 29.6).

SPECIAL CONSIDERATIONS

Pregnancy

According to the Centers for Disease Control and Prevention, approximately 7,000 infants are born

yearly to women with HIV infection. Without intervention, about 25% of these infants will become infected with HIV. High maternal viral load (>20,000 copies/mL), prolonged rupture of membranes, low maternal CD4 count, preterm delivery, and symptomatic maternal disease appear to increase the risk of transmission. In 1994, analysis of the AIDS Clinical Trial Group 076 study revealed that the administration of zidovudine to pregnant women and their newborns decreased transmission from 25% to 8% (4). Consequently, the U.S. Public Health Service (USPHS) has rec-

Table 29.6.
Counseling of Patients with HIV Infection

Prevention of HIV transmission	Use of barriers such as condoms during sexual activity. Use of clean needles during injection drug use. Methods by which HIV is *not* transmitted should also be covered.
Overview of HIV therapy	The care of persons living with HIV is rapidly evolving and the prognosis has improved markedly. All patients should be educated as to the therapeutic options available to them and the efficacy of these therapies.
Instruction on medication usage	Treatment often requires many medications with significant side effects and potential drug interactions. Instruct carefully on how to take medications and the need for adherence to the regimen.
Symptoms suggesting serious disease	"Red Flag" symptoms (Table 29.2) should be emphasized

ommended that all pregnant women be counseled and encouraged to be tested for HIV infection. If HIV infected, pregnant women should be offered a zidovudine protocol to reduce the risk of HIV transmission to their children.

The mechanism for the protection conferred by zidovudine is unclear. Some investigators feel that the primary factor is preemptive treatment of the infected neonate. There are concerns among many clinicians that zidovudine monotherapy may be suboptimal, and combination regimens are being evaluated in ongoing clinical trials. Owing to the rapid evolution of therapy, consultation with a knowledgeable specialist is clearly indicated for all pregnant women with HIV infection (9–11).

Occupational Exposure to Blood or Body Fluids

Accidental exposure to HIV during the provision of health care can infect physicians and other health care workers. The risk of acquiring HIV infection following a needle stick with a hollow-bore needle containing HIV-infected blood is about 1 in 250. This risk is increased by deep penetration, the presence of visible blood on the device causing injury, previous placement of the device in a blood vessel, and a source patient with a high viral titer and/or late-stage disease. Other types of exposures (e.g., solid-bore needles or splashes to the skin) have lower degrees of risk.

A case-controlled study recently concluded that the risk of transmission can be reduced by about 79% by postexposure prophylaxis. Based on these findings, the USPHS now recommends postexposure chemoprophylaxis with three anti-retroviral drugs (zidovudine, lamivudine, and indinavir or saquinavir) for the high-risk exposures (12, 13). Three-drug prophylaxis may be considered in less-risky exposures as well but is not recommended in very low-risk exposures. Postexposure prophylaxis should be initiated within 1 to 2 hours and continued for 4 weeks. Exposed workers should receive counseling and medical evaluation, including HIV antibody tests at baseline and at 6 weeks, 3 months, and 6 months after exposure. Clearly, however, it is best to avoid exposure to HIV through judicious use of universal precautions. Table 29.7 summarizes the USPHS recommendations.

CASE STUDY

A 22-year-old woman presents to your office with a history of a positive HIV test at the local health department. She is anxious but denies physical complaints. You elicit a history of recurrent vaginal candidiasis and an episode of herpes zoster about 1 year ago. Her CD4 count is 175 cells/mL and her HIV-1 RNA level is 150,000 copies/mL. She is currently not sexually active, lives with her mother and 4-year-old child, and works as a cashier in a local supermarket.

QUESTIONS

1. What additional tests would you recommend?

Table 29.7.
USPHS Recommendations for Chemoprophylaxis After Occupational Exposure to HIV

Type of Exposure	Source Material[a]	Antiretroviral Prophylaxis[b]
Percutaneous	Blood[c]	
	• Highest risk	Recommended ZDV + LMD + IDV
	• Increased risk	Recommended ZDV + LMD ± IDV
	• No increased risk	Offer ZDV + LAD
	• Fluid containing visible blood, other potentially infectious fluid[d], or tissue	Offer ZDV + LMD
	Other body fluid (e.g., urine)	Not offer
Mucous membrane	Blood	Offer ZDV + LMD ± IDV
	Fluid containing visible blood, other potentially infectious fluid or tissue	Offer ZDV ± 3TC
	Other body fluid (e.g., urine)	Not offer
Skin, increased risk[e]	Blood	Offer ZDV + LMD ± IDV
	Fluid containing visible blood, other potentially infectious fluid, or tissue	Offer ZDV ± 3TC
	Other body fluid (e.g., urine)	Not offer

[a]Any exposure to concentrated HIV (e.g., in a research laboratory or production facility) is treated as percutaneous exposure to blood with highest risk.

[b]Recommended—postexposure prophylaxis (PEP) should be recommended to the exposed worker with counseling.

Offer—PEP should be offered to the exposed worker with counseling.

Not offer—PEP should not be offered, as these are not occupational exposures to HIV.

Regimens—zidovudine (ZDV) 200 mg tid; lamivudine (LMV) 150 mg bid; indinavir (IND) 800 mg tid (If IND is not available, saquinavir may be used 600 mg tid); prophylaxis is given for 4 weeks. For full prescribing information, see package inserts.

[c]*Highest risk*—a significant volume of blood (e.g., deep injury with large-diameter hollow needle previously in source patient's vein or artery, AND containing high titer of HIV).

Increased risk—EITHER exposure to significant volume of blood OR blood with high titer of HIV.

No increased risk—NEITHER exposure to large volume of blood NOR blood with high titer of HIV (e.g., solid suture needle injury from source patient with asymptomatic HIV infection).

[d]Includes semen; vaginal secretions; cerebrospinal, synovial, pleural, peritoneal, pericardial, and amniotic fluids.

[e]For skin, risk is increased for exposures involving a high titer of HIV, prolonged contact, an extensive area, or an area in which skin integrity is visibly compromised. For skin exposures without increased risk, the risk for drug toxicity outweighs the benefit of PEP.

2. What medical therapies would you suggest?
3. In addition to medical therapy, what issues would you consider discussing?

DISCUSSION

Recommended additional testing would include CBC with platelets (if it was not reported with the CD4 count), chemistry panel including albumin, RPR, HBsAg, and anti-HBc, toxoplasmosis IgG, chest radiograph, tuberculin skin test (unless there is a reliable history of a previous positive test or of treatment for tuberculosis), and cervical Pap smear.

The patient's abnormal CD4 count and high viral load strongly support initiation of antiretroviral therapy. In this situation, a combination of two nucleoside analogs and a protease inhibitor would be reasonable. One such combination would be zidovudine 300 mg bid, lamivudine 150 mg bid, and indinavir 800 mg three times a day. This therapy might reasonably be expected to lower the viral load by 2 logs, possibly to undetectable levels. The resultant low viral load would result in much less viral replication and delay the development of viral resistance. Furthermore, a good response to this therapy may also include a rise in CD4 count. At her current CD4 count of 150, she also needs prophylaxis against PCP. Trimethoprim/sulfamethoxazole is the drug of choice; she should take one double-strength tablet daily, every Monday, Wednesday, and Friday. This PCP prophylaxis should be continued even if her CD4 count rises above 200. You should also recommend vaccination for *Streptococcus pneumoniae*, hepatitis B virus (if anti-HBc is negative), and influenza.

The diagnosis of HIV infection is devastating. You will need to allot time over several visits to answer questions and discuss important issues with this patient. She should understand the severity of the disease, the benefits of treatment, and her need for regular medical follow-up. She must be given careful instructions about the use of her medications and potential side effects. Also, you should encourage involvement with community organizations and support groups, and assess the need for individual supportive psychotherapy. Referral to a nutritionist is warranted as a complement to your discussion of healthy lifestyles. Before leaving the office, the patient should clearly understand how to prevent transmission and reinfection and the need to inform past, current, and future sexual partners. She should also be taught about contraception and the risk of perinatal transmission of HIV.

REFERENCES

1. Karon JM, Rosenberg PS, McQuillan G, Khare M, Gwinn M, and Petersen LR. Prevalence of HIV Infection in the United States, 1984–1992. JAMA 1996; 276:126–131.
2. UNAIDS Fact Sheet; the HIV/AIDS Situation in Mid 1996. Geneva, Switzerland: Joint United Nations Programme on HIV/AIDS, 1996.
3. Rosenberg PS. Scope of the AIDS epidemic in the United States. Science 1995;270:1372–1375.
4. Centers for Disease Control and Prevention. USPHS/IDSA guidelines for the prevention of opportunistic infections in persons infected with human immunodeficiency virus. MMWR 1997;46(RR-12):1–46.
5. Carpenter CJ, Fischl MA, Hammer SM, et al. Antiretroviral therapy for HIV infection in 1997. JAMA 1997;277:1962–1969.
6. Mellors JW, Kingsley LA, Rinaldo CR, Todd JA, Hoos BS, Kokka RP, et al. Quantitation of HIV-1 RNA in plasma predicts outcome after seroconversion. Ann Intern Med 1995;122:573–579.
7. Saag MS, Holodniy M, Kuritzkes DR, O'Brien WA, Coombs R, Poschner ME, et al. HIV viral load markers in clinical practice. Natl Med 1996;2:625–629.
8. Connor EM, Sperling RS, Gelber R, et al. Reduction of maternal-infant transmission of human immunodeficiency virus type 1 with zidovudine treatment. N Engl J Med 1994;331:1173–1180.
9. Centers for Disease Control and Prevention. Update: AIDS among women—United States, 1994. MMWR 1995;44:81–84.
10. Centers for Disease Control and Prevention. Recommendations of the US Public Health Service task force on the use of zidovudine to reduce perinatal transmission of human immunodeficiency virus. MMWR 1994; 43(RR-11):1–20.
11. Carmichael C. Preventing perinatal HIV transmission: zidovudine use during pregnancy. Am Fam Physician 1997;55:171–176.
12. Centers for Disease Control and Prevention. Case-control study of HIV seroconversion in health-care workers after percutaneous exposure to HIV-infected blood—France, United Kingdom, United States, January 1988–August 1994. MMWR 1995;44:929–933.
13. Centers for Disease Control and Prevention. Update: provisional Public Health Service recommendations for chemoprophylaxis after occupational exposure to HIV. MMWR 1996;45:468–472.

30. Hypertension

WARREN P. NEWTON AND TIMOTHY J. IVES

Key Clinical Questions

1. How should blood pressure be measured?
2. What should be included in the initial evaluation of a patient with hypertension?
3. What lifestyle modifications are effective for the treatment of hypertension, and what is their role in long-term management?
4. How should medications be chosen?
5. After blood pressure has been stabilized, how should the patient be monitored?

Approximately 50 million Americans have hypertension, defined as having a systolic pressure over 140 mm Hg and/or a diastolic pressure over 90 mm Hg and/or being on treatment (1). The prevalence increases greatly with age, changing from 15.2% of 18- to 24-year-old individuals to 60.2% for ages 65 to 74 years. About two-thirds of hypertensives have either mild hypertension (diastolic pressures from 90 to 100 mm Hg) or isolated systolic hypertension (systolic pressure above 140 mm Hg, diastolic below 90 mm Hg). As many as 35% of all people with hypertension are unaware of the problem, and only 21% are being treated adequately (1).

The importance of hypertension is that it is the first sign of a chronic progressive process that may end in stroke or renal failure and is a major risk factor for coronary artery disease (2). Moreover, treatment dramatically lowers end-organ complications. Nationally, the incidence of strokes has dropped by 57% in the last 20 years, and mortality from coronary heart disease has also declined significantly. Both changes are in part attributable to better detection and control of hypertension (1).

The major responsibility for detecting and treating hypertension does not rest with special hypertension clinics or programs, but rather with family physicians and other primary care clinicians who see patients in their own communities. This chapter focuses on what you should know about hypertension: making the diagnosis; the initial evaluation; recommending lifestyle modification and drug therapy; and planning long-term management.

MAKING THE DIAGNOSIS

The first step toward treating hypertension is finding it. Every family physician should have a strategy for detecting hypertension in his or her patient population. Most physicians screen for hypertension "opportunistically," in that patients presenting to the office for any reason have their blood pressure measured. This approach is similar to that used for rubella vaccination in women of childbearing years. It works well for those patients who come to the physician several times a year. Some groups, however, such as middle-aged men, underserved populations, and teenagers, do not see their physician regularly and may require special contacts with mailings, health fairs, or work-site screening. Identification of these patients is easier in practices in which the physicians have defined panels of patients such as health maintenance organizations or small communities.

The way that blood pressure is measured is crucial. Occasionally, a patient's blood pressure will be elevated by apprehension or previous activity, so make an effort to have your patient relaxed and at rest for 15 minutes when you make the measurement. Recent use of tobacco, caffeine, or decongestant therapy before measurement may give spuriously high blood pressure readings. The patient should be seated, with the arm bare and supported. The air bladder portion of the cuff should encircle 80% of the arm, and a wider cuff should be used for obese or thick arms. Too small a cuff will falsely elevate the readings by as much as 10 to 15 mm Hg. In contrast, a tight sleeve or other constriction of the upper arm may increase arterial blood turbulence and lower blood pressure readings. The cuff should be inflated to the pressure at which the radial pulse disappears so that the auscultatory gap does not confuse the systolic reading. Finally, the diastolic pressure should be noted at the disappearance of the sounds, not muffling, because disappearance is a more reliable criterion for diagnosis, and most studies of treatment have used it.

Once you have detected the patient with an elevated blood pressure, keep in mind that the final diagnosis of hypertension is a clinical one—a function of the actual blood pressure, risk factors, and the affect of the diagnosis on the patient (2, 3). Use caution in giving the label of hypertension, as this has been shown to increase absenteeism from work by 80% and may dramatically affect access to, or cost of, life insurance (3). A single, greatly elevated blood pressure reading (systolic greater than 200 mm Hg and/or diastolic greater than 120) is adequate to make the diagnosis of hypertension, but for most patients with somewhat elevated blood pressure (systolic greater than 140 mm Hg and/or diastolic greater than 90), an average of three readings over at least 6 weeks should be used. If the average systolic pressure is greater than 140 mm Hg and/or the average diastolic is greater than 90, the diagnosis is confirmed.

The term "isolated systolic hypertension" refers to a systolic blood pressure above 140 mm Hg when the diastolic blood pressure is less than 90. In practice, the weight of tradition has used the diastolic blood pressure to distinguish severity of hypertension, although longitudinal work shows systolic blood pressure may be a better predictor of future morbidity and mortality. The terms "mild" or stage I hypertension are used for diastolic pressures between 90 and 99 mm Hg, whereas "moderate" to "very severe" (stages II–IV) refer to diastolic pressures over 100 mm Hg.

INITIAL EVALUATION

Table 30.1 lists the key elements of history, physical examination, and laboratory tests that should be done on all patients with a new diagnosis of hypertension, together with a grade representing the strength of the evidence supporting the specific recommendation. Once you have diagnosed a patient as hypertensive, the initial evaluation should address the possibility of primary causes of hypertension, screen for end-organ damage and other cardiovascular risk factors, and begin the education of the patient and the family. As the table demonstrates, there is very little scientific evidence that addresses whether doing a particular component of the evaluation improves outcomes. The rationale for doing them is based on tradition

Table 30.1.
Key Features of Evaluation of Hypertension

History	Level of Evidence for Effectiveness[a]
Features suggesting of primary disease	C
Age < 25	
Malignant course	
Lack of response to therapy	
End-organ disease	C
Chest pain	
Orthopnea	
Paroxysmal nocturnal dyspnea	
Other cardiovascular risk factors	C
Diabetes	
Smoking	
Family history of early coronary artery disease	
History of elevated cholesterol	
Physical examination	C
Blood pressure	
Pulse	
Weight	
Height	
Cardiac: size, rhythm, S_3, JVD, edema	C
Vascular: carotids, peripheral pulses	C
Back: renal bruits	C
Fundus	C
Neurologic (strength, sensation, reflexes, gait, cranial nerves, speech, orientation)	C
Laboratory tests	
Urinalysis	C
BUN/creatinine	C
Potassium	C
Glucose	C
Total cholesterol/lipid panel	C
Electrocardiogram	C

[a]Level of evidence for effectiveness: A, strong or moderate research-based evidence (consistent across several studies, including at least two randomized controlled trials); B, limited research-based evidence (less consistent or extensive evidence, but preponderance of evidence supports use of treatment); C, common practice with little or no research-based evidence; X, moderate or strong evidence suggesting that this treatment is not effective.

and on an understanding of the natural history of cardiovascular disease.

Differential Diagnosis

First address the possibility of primary causes of hypertension. The most common primary causes are chronic renal disease, oral contraceptives with high levels of hormones, renovascular hypertension, hyperaldosteronism, and pheochromocytoma. Although not commonly considered in studies of primary causes of hypertension, heavy alcohol use may also cause hypertension. In primary care settings, however, the majority of newly diagnosed hypertensives will not have a primary disease, and workup is indicated only in the patient under 25, those in whom a primary disease is suspected on clinical grounds, such as lability or malignant course or lack of response to therapy, or those with physical findings of primary disease such as a renal bruit or a cushingoid appearance.

History

All patients should be asked about the use of alcohol, oral contraceptives, and response to previous therapy. Symptoms suggesting end-organ disease, such as chest pain, orthopnea, or paroxysmal nocturnal dyspnea, should be noted. Finally, other cardiac risk factors that interact with hypertension to promote atherosclerosis, such as smoking, diabetes, family history of early cardiac disease, and history of hyperlipidemia, should be identified.

Physical Examination

Physical features that suggest a primary cause of hypertension include cushingoid features, such as a moon facies and central adiposity, the diastolic abdominal bruit suggestive of renovascular hypertension, and the diminished femoral pulses with hypertension in the arms that suggest coarctation of the aorta. To assess end-organ damage, cardiovascular examination should include noting the cardiac size, the presence of an S_3 sound or other signs of cardiac failure, decreased pulses, and carotid bruits. Neurologic examination should address changes suggestive of a prior cerebrovascular accident (CVA) such as focal weakness or abnormal gait. Funduscopic examination may disclose hypertensive retinopathy.

Laboratory or Other Diagnostic Tests

Laboratory tests should include a urinalysis to identify proteinuria and hematuria, serum blood urea nitrogen (BUN), and creatinine to assess renal function and an ECG to check for left-ventricular hypertrophy and baseline ST changes. If clinical suspicion of left ventricular hypertrophy is high, an echocardiogram or chest radiograph may be appropriate. Obtain a fasting blood glucose

level and a screening cholesterol to detect silent diabetes mellitus and hyperlipidemia. There are no firm rules about additional tests. Most physicians screen for hyperaldosteronism and chronic renal disease with serum potassium and BUN/creatinine levels.

Patient Education

Hypertension is a difficult disease for patients to understand—it is without symptoms and, for most patients, the major issue is risk of stroke or heart attack in 15 to 20 years, far removed from their current experience. By taking time for a thorough history and physical examination, you underscore the importance of the hypertension and begin to teach the patient how lifestyle influences the problem. Over the long term, your effectiveness in managing the hypertensive patient depends on your ability to educate both your patient and the family. The first visits set the tone.

INITIAL TREATMENT
General Approach

After the initial evaluation, take time to develop an individualized treatment plan that contains elements of lifestyle modifications and, if appropriate, pharmacotherapy. Figure 30.1 provides a flow chart describing initial management. The overall goal of treatment is improving long-term survival and the quality of life rather than quickly lowering the blood pressure to a normal range. Indeed, if blood pressures are modestly elevated—e.g., diastolic less than 105 mm—a period of observation without therapy can be very valuable, as a substantial proportion of patients with mild hypertension will normalize without pharmacotherapy.

Almost all patients with moderate to severe hypertension benefit from pharmacotherapy. Using data from the Hypertension Detection and Follow-up Program (HDFP), for example, for patients with diastolic blood pressures between 115 and 129 mm Hg, the number (of patients) needed to treat (NNT) over 5 years to prevent one death, stroke, or infarction is 3 (4). For patients with mild or stage I hypertension, however, the benefit of treatment is less clear. The data from HDFP patients with diastolic pressures between 90 and 94 mm Hg show an NNT of 345, and those from other trials have yielded an NNT as high as 5,000 for mild hypertensives (5). What seems clear is that patients with mild hypertension have an

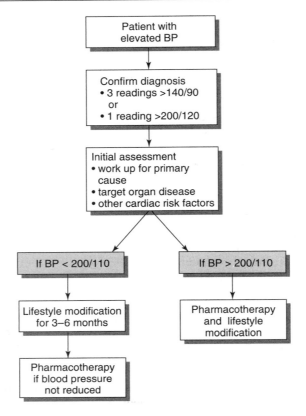

Figure 30.1. *General approach to a patient with elevated blood pressure.*

increased risk of stroke and the other sequelae of hypertension, but only patients with increased baseline risk—as with the presence of other cardiac risk factors such as smoking or end-organ disease—seem to benefit substantially from treatment with medication (6–10).

Treating isolated systolic hypertension in the elderly patient can reduce the incidence of strokes, although the adverse effects of some medications may be greater in this population (11). Lifestyle changes may be a reasonable place to start.

Lifestyle Modifications

Lifestyle modifications—especially exercise, weight loss, and potassium supplementation—should be considered for every patient with hypertension. Table 30.2 lists the strategies that have been tried along with a general assessment of the strength of the evidence supporting the effectiveness of each in improving long-term outcomes. In general, there is good evidence that specific strategies improve blood pressure over the short term—satisfying criteria for a "B" recommendation—but there is no evidence that any of these strategies change blood pressure over the long-term or that key long-term patient outcomes such as stroke or myocardial infarction are affected. In general, nonpharmacotherapies have fewer adverse effects and are cheaper; but they are not a panacea. In most cases, the proper use of lifestyle modifications, such as an exercise prescription or a weight loss program, requires a great deal of commitment by both physician and patient. Furthermore, some therapies, such as biofeedback, may be very expensive. More information is presented in Chapter 6, Helping Your Patients Stay Healthy, which discusses behavioral changes and lifestyle modification.

Exercise

A number of different trials have found that an exercise regimen lowers blood pressure in patients

Table 30.2.
Effectiveness of Nonpharmacotherapy

Therapy	Level of Evidence for Effectiveness[a]
Aerobic exercise	B
Potassium supplementation	B
Weight loss	B
Alcohol reduction (if > 6/day)	B
Calcium/magnesium supplementation	C
Stress reduction/biofeedback	X
Sodium restriction	X

[a]Level of evidence for effectiveness: A, strong or moderate research-based evidence (consistent across several studies, including at least two randomized controlled trials); B, limited research-based evidence (less consistent or extensive evidence, but preponderance of evidence supports use of treatment); C, common practice with little or no research-based evidence; X, moderate or strong evidence suggesting that this treatment is not effective.

with both normal and high initial blood pressures and may decrease the number of medications and the dosage necessary to achieve adequate blood pressure control (12). Other benefits of an exercise program include reducing life stress through improved psychologic health, helping weight loss, increasing serum HDL levels, and lowering overall mortality (13). Exercise is an appropriate first step for most hypertensive patients. An example of an initial, minimal exercise regimen would be walking briskly for 30 minutes three to five times a week (evidence rating = B).

Weight Loss

There is a strong correlation between obesity and hypertension, especially in people with centrally dependent body fat. Clinical trials of weight loss, often combined with exercise, have resulted in lowered blood pressure (14, 15). If a weight loss program is prescribed, a simple instruction like "you should try to lose some weight" is not sufficient. The physician should specify a target weight, coordinate a dietary intervention such as a 1,500-calorie diet, give an exercise prescription, and use frequent follow-up office visits (such as every 4 to 6 weeks) or local community groups such as Weight Watchers to help the patient lose weight (evidence rating = B).

Stress Reduction/Biofeedback

Some studies related to stress reduction have shown lowered blood pressure over several months, but longer-term studies have been disappointing (16). Techniques used include meditation, biofeedback, and patient education about stress and coping mechanisms (evidence rating = X).

Potassium Supplementation

Good evidence suggests that additional potassium in the diet, in the form of either additional potassium-rich foods or prescription supplementation, improves blood pressure on its own and in combination with medication (17, 18). Patients should therefore be counseled to eat foods rich in potassium, such as bananas, citrus juices, and leafy vegetables, and consideration should be given to a prescription of potassium (evidence rating = B).

Sodium Restriction

Population studies show a consistent correlation between salt intake and hypertension, but clinical trials of sodium reduction have shown a clinically insignificant long-term effect (19); the palatability of salt substitutes is poor, and long-term patient adherence to significant sodium restriction is very low. Although a few patients may be salt sensitive, emphasis should be placed on other lifestyle strategies for which better effectiveness has been demonstrated (evidence rating = X).

Calcium and Magnesium Supplementation

For calcium, evidence from trials is equivocal, but calcium supplementation may be attractive in situations in which there is another indication, as in the perimenopausal woman at risk for osteoporosis (20). For magnesium, similarly, early studies have raised the possibility of efficacy, but the relationship of magnesium to sodium or potassium, dosage, or other important aspects of treatment requires further clarification (evidence rating = C) (21, 22).

Alcohol Reduction

Alcohol acts as a vasopressor, and there is some good evidence that reduction of heavy alcohol use (six or more drinks a day) can improve high blood pressure (23–25). There is not yet evidence showing that reduction of mild-to-moderate alcohol intake lowers blood pressure (evidence rating = B).

Antihypertensive Medication

The most important principle in choosing a medication is to individualize the choice according to demographics, ability to pay, medical history, and lifestyle. Table 30.3 lists the key features of the major classes of medications. In general, only diuretics and β blockers have been proven to reduce adverse patient outcomes—stroke, myocardial infarction (MI), and death—over the long term and should, therefore, be considered first (26). Newer classes of agents are effective in re-

ducing blood pressure but have not been shown to have a long-term impact on outcomes. In short-term studies, moreover, different classes of agents have different effects with different populations and have greatly different costs and adverse drug-effect profiles (27, 28).

Patient Population

Thiazide diuretics and calcium channel blockers seem to be more effective for African-American populations. In contrast, β blockers and angio-

Blacks— thiazides, CCB
Whites — β blockers, ACE-I

Table 30.3.
Characteristics of Antihypertensive Medications

Drug	Major Disadvantages	Dosing Regimen	Generic Availability	Level of Evidence for Effectiveness[a]	Average Cost to the Patient[b]
Thiazide diuretics (e.g., hydrochlorothiazide [HCTZ])	Hypokalemia, hyperuricemia, hyperglycemia, elevation of low-density lipoprotein	qd	Yes	A	HCTZ[c] = $5.84
β Blockers (e.g., atenolol, metoprolol, propranolol)	Mood changes/depression, heart block, nightmares and sleep disturbances, increased bronchospasm, decreased cardiac output/ tolerance to exercise	qd to bid	Yes (for some agents)	A	Aronozol[c] = $9.23 Propranolol[c] = $7.05
Reserpine (Serpasil)	Mood changes/depression, sexual dysfunction (both male and female), nasal stuffiness, peptic ulceration	qd	Yes	A	Reserpine[c] = $6.92
ACE inhibitors (e.g., captopril, enalapril, fosinopril, lisinopril)	Rash, transient loss of taste, drug fever, proteinuria, cough	qd to tid	No	B	Captopril[c] = $10.05
Calcium channel blockers (e.g., diltiazem, nifedipine, verapamil)	Constipation, dizziness	qd to tid	Yes (for some agents)	B	Verapamil[c] = $26.60
α₁ Blockers (e.g., doxazosin, prazosin, terazosin)	Dizziness, headache, lethargy, syncope	bid to tid	Yes (for some agents)	B	Prazosin[c] = $7.97
Clonidine (available in both oral tablets and transdermal patches)	Mood changes/depression, sedation, hypertensive crisis with rapid withdrawal	qd to bid	Yes	B	Clonidine[c] (Tabnot) = $6.98 (Patch) = $31.40

[a]Level of evidence for effectiveness: A, strong or moderate research-based evidence (consistent across several studies, including at least two randomized controlled trials); B, limited research-based evidence (less consistent or extensive evidence, but preponderance of evidence supports use of treatment); C, common practice with little or no research-based evidence; X, moderate or strong evidence suggesting that this treatment is not effective.

[b]Prices for an average daily dose were obtained at a community pharmacy in Chapel Hill, NC on May 23, 1997, for one month of therapy.

[c]Generic drug product used in cost calculation.

tensin-converting enzyme (ACE) inhibitors may be more effective for Caucasian and younger patients. In older patients, the end point of therapy may be modified. For example, older persons with isolated systolic hypertension must be treated very cautiously to prevent postural syncope and falls. Also, some patients with multi-infarct dementia may benefit from diastolic blood pressures somewhat higher than usual (i.e., around 85 to 95 mm Hg).

Coexistent Medical Problems

β Blockers have been shown to reduce mortality in post-MI patients, and similarly, ACE inhibitors will benefit those with congestive heart failure with systolic dysfunction. In patients with diabetes mellitus, β blockers may mask hypoglycemic symptoms, and both thiazide diuretics and β blockers may mildly worsen glycemic control. An ACE inhibitor or dihydropteridine calcium channel blocker (e.g., nifedipine, felodipine, amlodipine) may be preferred in this population to reduce the rate of progression of nephropathy. In patients with asthma or chronic obstructive lung disease, β blockers may trigger bronchospasm. In patients with cardiac arrhythmias or those receiving digitalis, hypokalemia induced by thiazide diuretics and the hyperkalemia caused by ACE inhibitors may lead to serious arrhythmias. Cardiac conduction delay may be worsened by β blockers or calcium channel blockers, and in these cases, an ACE inhibitor may prove to be of benefit. Patients with depression or sleep disorders may be adversely affected by all adrenergic blocking agents, including clonidine, β blockers, methyldopa, and reserpine.

Effects on Normal Activities

Sexual dysfunction has been ascribed to all of the antihypertensive medications, particularly centrally acting agents such as clonidine, methyldopa, or β blockers and thiazide diuretics. You need to be able to talk openly to your patient about this adverse effect. Whether any of these adverse effects forces a change in the drug regimen depends upon the severity of symptoms and the importance to the patient. Sedation produced by clonidine or methyldopa may impair the manual coordination required at work by some patients; similarly, β blockers can make aerobic conditioning more difficult and so are less attractive for patients with occupations that require strenuous physical activity or those in athletic training. ACE inhibitors (e.g., captopril, enalapril) or α blockers (e.g., prazosin) may be preferred in these cases.

Dosing

Therapeutic regimens should be as simple as possible to enhance adherence. Dosing frequency is more important than the total number of medications used. If possible, prescribe a medication that is taken once daily (e.g., atenolol, metoprolol, enalapril, verapamil, nifedipine, prazosin, clonidine, thiazides, or reserpine.) Older antihypertensive agents have been reformulated into products that can be taken on a once-daily (or less) basis. These agents include diltiazem, verapamil, nifedipine, metoprolol, or propranolol (sustained-release tablets or capsule) or clonidine (transdermal patch applied weekly). Remember that improvements in formulation may also incur an added cost to the patient for these agents. Products consisting of a combination of antihypertensive agents, usually prescribed after titrating individual agents to achieve blood pressure control, may allow smaller doses of each drug to be used. This may decrease the overall drug cost.

Cost

Think in terms of monthly cost of the medication to the patient. Newer agents such as ACE inhibitors are effective but are currently much more expensive than older agents, primarily because of the lack of generic products available for substitution. Generic products, if available and of adequate quality, can save the patient up to 20-fold (e.g., $5.00 vs. $100.00/month).

After you have chosen a medication and started treatment, take care to bring the blood pressure down slowly. Lowering the blood pressure too rapidly can result in deleterious effects, such as postural hypotension, syncope, or other cardiac events, and is a common cause of nonadherence and failed therapy. Treatment is usually not urgent and the overall goal is to prevent long-term complications such as strokes. If control is not achieved after an adequate trial of a particular medication—i.e., 4 weeks—three options are available: increase the daily dosage, substitute another agent, or add a second agent. Usually, maximizing one agent should be tried first.

LONG-TERM MANAGEMENT

Initially, the patient should be seen every 1 to 2 weeks until the blood pressure is stabilized. Then, gradually decrease the frequency of visits to every 3 months for 1 year, and finally, to every 6 to 12 months. Ideally, patients should have their blood pressures checked occasionally between visits, either at work or at home. Reliable, home blood-pressure monitoring devices are readily available, and after you have determined that both the machine and the patient's measurement technique are acceptable, this will provide an excellent source of ongoing data. Patients should be told to always bring a record of their blood pressure readings and all of their medications with them to each visit.

In addition to a review of all medications and possible adverse effects, each visit should include a history of cardiac symptoms, blood pressure, heart rate, and cardiopulmonary examination, including rhythm, new murmurs, S_3, jugular venous distention (JVD), edema, and rales. A detailed examination should be performed annually to detect evidence of end-organ damage such as left-ventricular hypertrophy, stroke, or vascular disease. Urinalysis and BUN/creatinine levels should be screened annually, along with potassium if the patient is taking a diuretic or an ACE inhibitor. A flow sheet in the patient's chart will allow you to easily follow the patient's blood pressure, physical findings, laboratory studies, and prescribed treatments over time.

There are several ways to assess patient adherence with the treatment plan. Talking with family members about the actual usage of pills may be useful, as is counting the pills the patient brings to the office visit. Other tests of adherence include checking a serum uric acid level, which is almost always elevated in patients taking diuretics, or following the pulse rate of patients, which is often reduced in patients taking β blockers. Finally, if you are still concerned, calling the patient's pharmacy will reveal the frequency of refills.

Continuous 24-hour ambulatory monitoring of blood pressure is rapidly becoming available throughout the United States and may be helpful in managing hypertensive patients who are difficult to control. With a good monitor and use of the proper technique, ambulatory monitoring is accurate, but the prognostic significance of 24-hour blood-pressure readings remains unclear. Like many new technologies, the value of ambulatory monitoring in ongoing clinical practice is yet to be proved.

Over time, the key issues in the management of hypertension are patient education and patient involvement in his or her own care. As hypertension is a silent "disease," treatment does not usually make the patient feel better. The physician's task is to diagnose hypertension and then to educate the patient and family about its importance. Often the physician must persuade the patient to make major changes in lifestyle or to take medication that may be expensive or have long-term unpleasant adverse effects for the rest of his or her life. In this regard, it is important to encourage the patient's sense of responsibility for monitoring and treatment. Regular blood pressure measurements at home or work provide direct reinforcement for continuing a diet, exercise, or medication program. How well the physician educates and helps the patient maintain a normal blood pressure determines the success of the treatment plan at 5, 10, and 15 years.

CASE STUDY 1

L.J. is a 48-year-old African-American woman who works in an animal laboratory. She sustained a laceration at work; at the visits for the laceration repair and for suture removal, you note that her blood pressure has been elevated, 168/96 and 156/98, respectively. She has no history of hypertension and is not on any medications.

QUESTIONS

1. Would you diagnose hypertension now? If not, what would you do in order to establish the diagnosis?
2. Once the diagnosis has been established, what would your initial evaluation be?
3. Assuming that the initial evaluation does not turn up surprises, what should be your initial management of this patient?

DISCUSSION

Diagnosis requires three separate readings unless the level is markedly elevated, so the appropriate action is to have the patient return for follow-up. A third similar blood pressure would establish the diagnosis. The initial evaluation should consist of considering whether a workup should be done for a primary cause of hypertension, looking for signs and symptoms of end-organ disease, and exploring other cardiac risk factors. Initial management should be lifestyle modification, with emphasis placed on weight loss, exercise, and increased dietary potassium.

(atenolol 25 mg each day) are good first choices. They have been proven to reduce long-term outcomes such as stroke or myocardial infarction; they are inexpensive and need to be taken only once a day, and are generally well tolerated. For a patient with hypertension and angina, the β blockers become the best choice because they will treat both conditions. For patients with diabetes and hypertension, the ACE inhibitors are attractive because of their renal protective effects; in any case, the key issue is controlling blood pressure as tightly as possible.

CASE STUDY 2

R.T. is a 56-year-old construction worker whom you have diagnosed with hypertension, as his usual blood pressure is approximately 175/105. His serum potassium, blood urea nitrogen, creatinine, and glucose are normal; his total cholesterol is 243 mg/dL, and urinalysis does not show protein. He has no symptoms or signs of end-organ disease. A 6-month trial of exercise, weight loss, and increase of dietary potassium has been partially successful, with a reduction of blood pressure to approximately 165/100.

QUESTIONS

1. Should you start medication? If so, which one, at what dose, and why?
2. If R.T. had angina, what medication would you start and why?
3. If R.T. had diabetes, what medication would you consider?

DISCUSSION

Lifestyle modification has had a partial effect. The drop of blood pressure is clinically significant, but a further drop of blood pressure to below 140/90 would substantially reduce the risk of stroke and heart attack. Medication is therefore indicated. A diuretic (such as hydrochlorothiazide 25 mg each day) or a β blocker

REFERENCES

1. The Joint Committee on Detection, Evaluation, and Treatment of High Blood Pressure. The fifth report of the Joint National Committee on Detection, Evaluation, and Treatment of High Blood Pressure (JNC V). Arch Intern Med 1993;153:154–183.
2. Kannel WB. Blood pressure as a cardiovascular risk factor. JAMA 1996;275:1571–1576.
3. Haynes RB, Sackett DL, Taylor MA, et al. Increased absenteeism from work after detection and labeling of hypertensive patients. N Engl J Med 1978;299:(14): 741–744.
4. Laupacis A, Sackett DL, Roberts RS. An assessment of clinically useful measures of the consequences of treatment. N Engl J Med 1988;318:1728–1733.
5. Hoes AW, Grobbee DE, Lubsen J. Does drug treatment improve survival? Reconciling the trials in mild-to-moderate hypertension. J Hypertens 1995;13:805–811.
6. Veterans Administration Cooperative Study Group on Antihypertensive Agents. Effects of treatment on morbidity in hypertension. II. Results in patients with diastolic blood pressure averaging 90 through 114 mm Hg. JAMA 1970;213:1143–1152.
7. Langford HG, Stamler J, Wassertheil-Smoller S, Prineas RJ. All-cause mortality in the Hypertension Detection and Follow-up Program: findings for the whole cohort and for persons with less-severe hypertension, with and without other traits related to risk of mortality. Prog Cardiovasc Dis 1986;29(suppl 1):29–54.
8. Medical Research Council Working Party. MRC trial of treatment of mild hypertension: principal results. BMJ 1985;291:97–104.
9. Taguchi J, Freis ED. Partial reduction of blood pressure and prevention of complications in hypertension. N Engl J Med 1974;291:329–331.
10. Australian National Blood Pressure Management Committee. The Australian therapeutic trial in mild hypertension. Lancet 1980;1:1261–1267.
11. SHEP Cooperative Research Group. Prevention of stroke by antihypertensive drug treatment in older

persons with isolated systolic hypertension. Final results of the Systolic Hypertension in Elderly Program (SHEP). JAMA 1991;265:3255–3264.

12. Fagard RH. Prescription and results of physical activity. J Cardiovasc Pharmacol 1995;25(1):S20–S27.

13. Leon AS, Connett J, Jacobs DR Jr, Rauramaa R. Leisure-time physical activity levels and risk of coronary heart disease and death. JAMA 1987;258:2388–2395.

14. Reisen E, Abel R, Modan M, et al. Effect of weight loss without salt restriction on the reduction of blood pressure in overweight hypertensive patients. N Engl J Med 1978;298(1)1–6.

15. MacMahon S, Wilcken DEL, Macdonald GJ. The effect of weight reduction on left-ventricular mass. N Engl J Med 1986;314(6):334–339.

16. Van Montfrans GA, Karemaker JM, Wieling W, Dunning AJ. Relaxation therapy and continuous ambulatory blood pressure in mild hypertension: a controlled study. BMJ 1990;300:1368–1372.

17. Siani A, Strazzullo P, Giacco A, Pacioni D, Celentano E, Mancini M. Increasing the dietary potassium intake reduces the need for hypertensive medication. Ann Intern Med 1991;115(10):753–759.

18. Cappucio FP, MacGregor GA. Does potassium supplementation lower blood pressure? A meta-analysis of published trials. J Hypertens 1991;9:465–473.

19. Midgley JP, Matthew AG, Greenwood CMT, Logan AG. Effect of reduced dietary sodium on blood pressure. JAMA 1996;275:1590–1597.

20. NIH Consensus Development Panel. Optimal calcium intake. JAMA 1994;272:1942–1948.

21. Gilleran G, O'Leary M, Barlett WA, et al. Effects of dietary sodium substitution with potassium and magnesium in hypertensive type II diabetics: a randomised blind controlled parallel study. J Hum Hypertens 1996;10:517–521.

22. Geleijnse JM, Witteman JCM, Bak AAA, et al. Reduction in blood pressure with a low sodium, high potassium, high magnesium salt in older subjects with mild to moderate hypertension. BMJ 1994;309:436–440.

23. Potter JF, Beevers DG. Pressor effect of alcohol in hypertension. Lancet 1984;I:119–122.

24. Maheswaran R, Gill JS, Davies P, Beevers DG. High blood pressure due to alcohol: a rapidly reversible effect. Hypertension 1991;17:787–792.

25. Maherswaran R, Beevers M, Beevers DG. Effectiveness of advice to reduce alcohol consumption in hypertensive patients. Hypertension 1992;19:79–84.

26. Psaty BM, Smith NL, Siscovick DS, et al. Health outcomes associated with antihypertensive therapies used as first-line agents. A systematic review and meta-analysis. JAMA 1997;277:739–745.

27. Matterson BJ, Reda DJ, Cushman WC, et al. Single-drug therapy for hypertension in men. N Engl J Med 1993;328:914–921.

28. Edelson JT, Weinstein MC, Tosteson AN, et al. Long-term cost effectiveness of various initial monotherapies for mild to moderate hypertension. JAMA 1990;263:408–413.

31. Low Back Pain

PHILIP D. SLOANE

Key Clinical Questions

1. Is underlying visceral or systemic disease responsible for the pain?
2. Is there neurologic deficit involved? If so, is surgical evaluation necessary?
3. Are psychosocial factors contributing to or aggravating the pain?

Low back problems can be classified as acute, recurrent, or chronic. Most acute episodes improve regardless of the treatment used, and the patient resumes normal activity within 6 weeks. Recurrences of pain are quite common, however, making low back disorders a major cause of discomfort and disability. Chronic pain develops in only 10 to 15% of patients with low back pain, but it can cause significant distress and functional disability and requires aggressive treatment.

Making a specific anatomic diagnosis is often neither possible nor necessary in a patient with back pain. Nevertheless, you should carefully evaluate each new low back problem to rule out serious, life-threatening conditions, to assign the patient a working diagnosis, and to develop a management plan that is best suited for the individual patient.

Management of patients with acute back problems should provide pain relief and foster rapid return to normal activity. Recurrent problems are usually managed like new episodes, except that greater attention is given to long-term prevention. Management of patients with chronic back problems should focus on comfort, mobility, and prevention of disability, rather than on elimination of pain.

Low back pain is extremely common: 70% of the world's adults will experience at least one disabling episode in their lives. Back problems constitute the second most-frequent reason for physician visits in the United States (after upper respiratory infections) (1) and are the most common cause of disability in adults under the age of 45 (2). Because the majority of physician visits for low back pain are to generalists, the family physician must include among his or her skills a systematic and reasonable approach to the assessment and management of low back pain.

PATHOPHYSIOLOGY

It is helpful to think in terms of four general categories of back pain: uncomplicated back pain, complicated back pain, pain due to systemic disease, and referred pain. Most uncomplicated low back pain (98%) is due to some kind of structural problem (bone, muscle, joint, disc, nerves associated with lumbar vertebrae or pelvis, tendon, or ligament) (3). The term complicated back pain is used when structural back pain is associated with signs and symptoms of spinal nerve root compromise. Other kinds of low back pain may be due to systemic diseases affecting the spine or to referred pain from abdominal or pelvic pathology.

Uncomplicated Back Pain

Uncomplicated back pain (structural back pain without nerve root compromise) can arise by several mechanisms. Each adjacent pair of vertebrae articulates by way of three separate joints: the two facet joints posteriorly, and the intervertebral disc anteriorly. Firm, fibrous ligaments help support these joints, limiting range of motion. Around these structures are the paravertebral muscles, which provide further support and aid mobility (Fig. 31.1). Injury to any of these structures can cause similar symptoms. The most common are injury to muscles and ligaments, osteoarthritis, degenerative disc disease, and malalignment of spinal structures.

Injury to Muscles and Ligaments (Strain, Sprain, or Contusion)

Injury to muscles and ligaments can occur when performing day-to-day activities, such as bending or straining, or from direct trauma, such as a fall, and can result in a secondary muscle spasm and pain on movement. Injury to muscles and ligaments is the most common cause of acute low back pain, especially in young adults. Patients

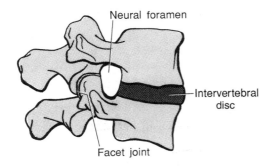

Figure 31.1. *The intervertebral motion segment: two vertebrae articulating via a disc and two facet joints.*

with muscle or ligament injuries usually develop pain after unusual physical activity.

Osteoarthritis (Degenerative Joint Disease)

Loss of articular cartilage, osteophyte formation, and articular surface irregularity impair joint function and at times can lead to inflammation and pain. Any of the intervertebral joints can be involved, but the facet joints of the lumbar spine are the most common location of degenerative joint disease. Radiographic evidence of arthritis is universal in persons over age 40 and therefore is of limited diagnostic value. Patients with osteoarthritis can experience pain in a variety of circumstances: chronically, after exertion, or after unusual positioning (such as sitting with the back unsupported, engaging in twisting, or even sleeping on a soft mattress). Degenerative joint disease is the most common cause of chronic low back pain in the elderly.

Degenerative Disc Disease

Weakening of the fibrous outer ring of an intervertebral disc (the annulus fibrosus) can cause the gelatinous center of the disc (the nucleus pulposus) to bulge abnormally or to herniate (extrude or rupture) into the spinal canal. The incidence of degenerative disc disease peaks in middle age (35 to 55); the discs most commonly involved are L3-L4, L4-L5, and L5-S1. The presence of disc disease does not necessarily imply that low back pain is present or that disc disease is the cause of back pain; magnetic resonance imaging (MRI) of asymptomatic adults indicates that 52% of normal subjects demonstrate bulging, 27% have a protrusion, and 1% have a

herniation (4). Disc disease can present chronically, after exertion, or after minor trauma. Often it is preceded by several years of recurrent attacks of acute back pain that last only a few days. The existence of significant nerve root compromise suggests disc disease, especially if the patient is under age 60.

Malalignment

Malalignment or motion restriction of spinal structures such as the facet joints, the sacroiliac joint, and/or the vertebral bodies themselves is not proven as a cause of low back pain. Chiropractic and osteopathic clinicians believe that the etiologic causes for low back pain are mainly due to reduced mobility or hypermobility of vertebrae; however, there is little objective evidence that this is a cause rather than an effect.

Other Causes

Other causes of uncomplicated low back pain include fracture (usually a compression fracture of the vertebral body, often due to minor trauma in older persons with osteoporosis) and myofascial syndrome (often called fibromyalgia, a chronic disorder characterized by muscle tenderness and painful "trigger points," which generally occurs in the upper rather than the lower back).

Certain patient characteristics increase the risk of uncomplicated back pain. Workers in occupations requiring lifting, such as nursing assistants and construction workers, have a high incidence of uncomplicated low back pain. Long-term heavy smokers are more likely to suffer from low back pain than nonsmokers, and smoking cessation may reduce risk. Likewise, obesity plays a role: increasing body mass index has been shown to correlate with increased prevalence of low back pain, and growing evidence exists that weight loss can reduce low back pain (5).

Complicated Back Pain

Complicated back pain (structural back pain with nerve root compromise, also called radiculopathy or sciatica) is a condition in which pain, numbness, paresthesia (commonly burning or tingling), and/or muscle weakness reflect injury to the spinal root of a peripheral nerve. Nerve root compromise is the most common physiologic complication of low back pain. It can be caused by any of the structural causes and by many of the systemic causes of low back pain; however, the most common causes are degenerative disc disease and arthritis. The 4th and 5th lumbar and the 1st sacral dermatome nerve roots are most commonly affected because the lower lumbar spine is subjected to the greatest physical stress during daily activities, such as sitting for long periods of time, and, consequently, is the most common site of both degenerative joint disease and degenerative disc disease. Nerve root compromise is thought to be significant if a neurologic (motor or sensory) deficit is present below the knee or if the knee or ankle jerk reflex is diminished.

Systemic Causes

Systemic causes of low back pain are rare (less than 1% of all cases) but important to detect, because they often need aggressive evaluation and management. They include cancer, which is less than 1% (6). Other rare causes are infection, inflammatory arthritis, and Paget's disease. Cancer associated with the lumbosacral spine is generally metastatic; in men, prostate cancer is most common; it women, it is breast cancer. Infectious causes of low back pain include osteomyelitis, paraspinous abscess, epidural abscess, and diskitis. The most common type of inflammatory arthritis is ankylosing spondylitis, a condition that begins in the lumbosacral spine and gradually progresses upward. Paget's disease is a poorly understood condition characterized by bony overgrowth; it is common in the elderly and generally runs a benign, asymptomatic course, but it can lead to significant pain in some individuals.

Referred Pain

Referred pain from abdominal or pelvic structures can arise from structures such as muscle, ligaments, or joint capsules. Acute conditions referring pain to the back, such as pancreatitis, pyelonephritis, nephrolithiasis, pelvic inflammatory disease, and dysmenorrhea, generally are associated with enough other symptoms to suggest the diagnosis. Subacute processes occasionally produce such prominent back symptoms, however, that the true diagnosis is initially overlooked. Such conditions include pancreatic cancer, posterior peptic ulcer disease, abdominal aortic aneurysm, prostatitis, and cholecystitis.

DIFFERENTIAL DIAGNOSIS

In recent years, the approach to low back pain has shifted away from making a specific diagnosis such as arthritis, muscle strain, or disc disease. This is because the structural causes of low back pain are often impossible to diagnose with precision, and because studies have indicated that, in the absence of "red flags," all patients with acute episodes of back pain can be managed similarly.

For this reason, the differential diagnosis of low back pain concentrates on:

- identifying or ruling out progressive or life-threatening disease
- identifying the small subgroup with significant neuromuscular injury due to complicated back pain (i.e., involving nerve root compromise)
- labeling all other patients as having uncomplicated back pain.

Uncomplicated back pain—i.e., that without evidence of life-threatening disease or significant nerve root compromise—is by far the most common diagnosis in primary care. It can be subdivided into acute (first episode, duration less than 12 weeks), recurrent (duration less than 12 weeks, but one or more prior episode), and chronic (duration of at least 12 weeks) (7). This approach to the differential diagnosis of low back pain is outlined in Table 31.1.

Acute low back pain only occasionally becomes chronic: of recent-onset back pain patients,

Table 31.1.
Differential Diagnosis of Low Back Pain

Diagnosis	Frequency in Office Primary Care
Acute uncomplicated backache	Very common
Chronic uncomplicated backache	Very common
Recurrent uncomplicated backache	Very common
Backache with nerve root compromise	Somewhat common
Referred pain from abdominal or pelvic disease	Somewhat common
Spinal fracture	Somewhat common
Paget's disease	Somewhat common
Inflammatory arthritis	Rare
Infection	Rare
Cancer	Rare
Cauda equina syndrome	Rare

14% have impaired function and 10% report high-intensity pain a year later (8). Chronic low back pain can be devastating, however; one third of patients whose low back pain is chronic consider themselves permanently disabled by the pain (9). The same structural factors that commonly cause acute pain are responsible for chronic pain; nearly all chronic back pain is due to uncomplicated backache. Risk factors for the development of chronic low back pain include psychologic factors (anxiety, fear of pain [10], a sense of being "always sick," [11], high scores on Minnesota Multiphasic Personality Inventory scales for hypochondriasis and hysteria) (12), manual labor (13), sedentary lifestyle before the injury (14), nerve root compromise, smoking, prior episodes of low back pain, and low education level (11).

CLINICAL EVALUATION

A careful history and physical examination are essential in the evaluation of all patients with low back pain. In the patient with acute or recurrent back pain, each new episode should be approached similarly. In the patient with chronic pain, it is important to review the diagnostic evaluation that has been done and to update yourself based on the patient's progress since previous visits. Key elements of the history and physical examination are presented in Table 31.2.

In many respects, your primary diagnostic goal of the initial evaluation of acute low back pain is triage. You must

- determine that the pain is intrinsic to the back and not refereed from a problem elsewhere

Table 31.2.
Key Elements of the History and Physical Examination for Low Back Pain

Question/Maneuver	Purpose
Information about age, duration and description of symptoms, history of back pain, response to treatment, medication/drug use, and general health	Assist in creating and narrowing differential diagnosis
Look for "red flags" (see Table 31.3)	Screen for cancer, infection, cauda equina syndrome, ankylosing spondylitis, and related arthritis, fracture, and referred pain due to abdominal, retroperitoneal, or pelvic structures
History of significant trauma prior to or at the onset of pain	Suggests musculoligamentous damage or fracture
History and distribution of numbness, tingling, and/or weakness below the knee	Screen for significant nerve root compromise (Sn-N-Out)
Psychosocial history • History of anxiety/depression • Substance abuse • Education level • Current life stresses • Work status; job tasks • Activity/exercise level • Worry about the pain • Pending litigation	Assist in planning treatment and in assessing for depression, noncompliance, and chronicity
Observe ambulation and mobility	Screen for unilateral leg weakness; estimate severity of pain
Temperature	Screen for infection
Limited neurologic examination • Straight-leg raising (Sn-N-Out) • Crossed straight-leg raising (Sp-P-In) • Strength testing of quadriceps, dorsiflexion of foot/great toe, and plantar flexion • Knee and ankle jerks	Abnormalities suggest significant nerve root compromise

Reprinted with permission from Sackett DL, Haynes RB, Guyatt GH, Tugwell P. Clinical Epidemiology: A Basic Science for Clinical Medicine, 2nd ed. Boston: Little, Brown & Co, 1991.

Sp-P-In, specific tests, when positive, rule disease in; Sn-N-Out, sensitive tests, when negative, rule disease out.

- rule out progressive and life-threatening disease
- determine whether nerve root compromise is present.

This diagnostic triage forms the basis for decisions to conduct further tests or refer to a specialist (Fig. 31.2). In addition, your evaluation visit must establish rapport with the patient; evaluate the onset, course, and severity of the problem; and identify psychosocial issues that may affect the prognosis and treatment plan.

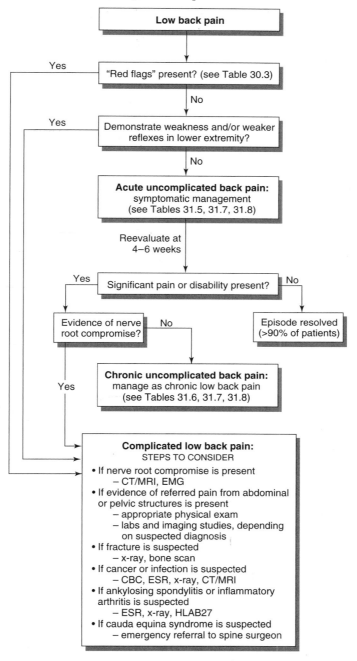

Figure 31.2. *General approach to the patient with low back pain.*

History

One useful strategy is to have a series of questions to ask yourself to be sure that your evaluation is sufficiently complete. These include:

- What is the most likely diagnosis, given the patient's age, presentation, and examination? What are the second and third most likely diagnoses?
- What serious disease should not be missed?
- What life stresses or psychosocial problems are present in this patient?
- What does this patient want and need from this visit?

To answer these questions, your history should inquire about the following areas:

- General health—age, weight, chronic illnesses and/or disabilities, appetite, malaise, fever, energy level
- Characteristics and history of the current problem—onset, pain pattern, severity, duration, radiation, impact on physical function (sleep, work, dressing, sex, recreation), factors improving or worsening the pain (e.g., relief on bending forward suggests facet joint arthritis; relief on bending backward suggests disc disease), beliefs about the pain
- History of back problems—episodes, tests, therapy, recovery, disability, pending litigation or workman's compensation
- "Red flags" (Table 31.3)—elements of the history that suggest a need for further evaluation to rule out progressive or serious disease
- Occupation/activity—work, job tasks, availability of sick time, job stresses, activity level off the job, exercise patterns
- Current psychosocial status—recent and past emotional problems, family function, current stresses, reaction to the illness, perception of the pain and its impact on life
- Medications/drugs—analgesics, steroids, nonsteroidal anti-inflammatory drugs (NSAIDs), recreational and over-the-counter drugs, alcohol.

The onset and characteristics of the pain itself are important in differentiating complicated from uncomplicated backache. Thus, your history should focus on the "red flag" conditions and also determine whether symptoms of nerve root irritation are present. Pain, numbness, and/or paresthesia radiating to the hip or upper leg are very common and nonspecific in low back pain patients; therefore, nerve root irritation is generally not considered to be significant unless these symptoms radiate below the knee and objective deficits can be found by the clinician.

Much is unproven about the value of specific questions in ruling in or out various diagnoses, so the recommendations in Tables 31.2 and 31.3 are largely empiric. However, the following data have been gathered from studies conducted in primary care settings:

- No single question can adequately screen for the possibility of cancer. Highly specific questions good at ruling in the possibility of cancer include: previous history of cancer (sensitivity 0.31, specificity 0.98, LR+ 15.5, LR− 0.70), and unexplained weight loss (sensitivity 0.15, specificity 0.94, LR+ 2.5, LR− 0.90) (15).
- No single question can adequately screen for ankylosing spondylitis and related inflammatory arthritis. More sensitive questions that help rule out the diagnosis include: age at onset <35 years (sensitivity 0.92, specificity 0.30, LR+ 1.3, LR− 0.27), no relief by lying down (sensitivity 0.80, specificity 0.49, LR+ 1.6, LR− 0.41), and duration of pain >3 months (sensitivity 0.71, specificity 0.54, LR+ 1.5, LR− 0.54) (15, 16). The combination of age over 35, relief when lying down, and 3 months' duration of pain effectively rules out the diagnosis (LR− 0.06)
- Sciatica (pain, tingling, numbness, or weakness) below the knee is the most reliable symptom of a herniated disc in patients with back pain, and the absence of this very sensitive symptom largely rules out this diagnosis. Deyo et al. report the sensitivity to be 0.95 and the specificity to be 0.88 (LR+ 7.9, LR− 0.06); however, these figures probably overestimate the true predictive power of this information in the primary care setting (15).

Physical Examination

A focused physical examination is adequate in patients with back pain whose history does not suggest referred pain or systemic disease (see Table 31.2). Elements of the physical examination should include a general assessment of (a) the location and severity of the pain (watch the patient walk, undress, and transfer on and off the exam-

Table 31.3.
"Red Flags" Suggesting Progressive or Life-Threatening Disease in Patients with Low Back Pain

Diagnosis	"Red Flags" Suggestive of the Disease
Referred pain from abdominal, retroperitoneal, or pelvic structures	Dysuria, fever, nausea/vomiting, chest pain, abdominal mass, localized tenderness on examination
Fracture	History of trauma, osteoporosis, long-term corticosteroid use, age >70
Spinal cancer (usually metastatic)	History of cancer, unexplained weight loss, pain unrelieved by bed rest or remaining motionless, age >50
Infection (diskitis, body, osteomyelitis, or abscess)	Fever, recent history of infection, pain unrelieved by bed rest or remaining motionless, immunosuppression, age >50
Ankylosing spondylitis or related inflammatory arthritis	Pain unrelieved by remaining motionless, night pain, morning stiffness, relief with exercise, especially in young men
Cauda equina syndrome	Acute onset of urinary retention or fecal incontinence; loss of anal sphincter tone; saddle anesthesia (numbness in the area of the anus, perineum, and genitals); global/progressive lower extremity weakness

ining table; palpate for muscle spasm); (b) temperature (to screen for infection); and (c) a neurologic examination focusing on the lower extremities (to screen for lumbar nerve root compromise).

Key elements of the neurologic examination include:

- The straight leg raising test (with the patient lying supine, flex the hip with the knee straight; the test is positive if <90° of flexion causes or aggravates sciatica below the knee or worsens back pain). Although studies of the characteristics of this test are largely limited to hospitalized patients, it appears to be the most sensitive screen for lumbar nerve root compromise, and its absence rules out the diagnosis (sensitivity 0.98, specificity 0.44, LR+ 1.8, LR− 0.04) (17, 18).

- The crossed, straight leg raising test (raising the opposite leg with the knee straight; the test is positive if this exacerbates the painful leg). The test has a high specificity and therefore confirms the existence of lumbar nerve root compromise and suggests acute disc herniation (sensitivity 0.43, specificity 0.94, LR+ 7.2, LR− 0.61) (17, 19).

- Strength and reflex testing in the distribution of the 4th and 5th lumbar and the 1st sacral nerve roots (Fig. 31.3).

In performing your examination, you should be aware that the interrater reliability of physical examination maneuvers is far from perfect. In general, weakness and straight leg raising have the best interobserver agreement (0.56 to 1.00); reflex testing and crossed straight leg raising have fair agreement (0.33 to 0.65); and muscle spasm, localized tenderness, and sensory deficits are the least-reproducible findings (18, 20).

Laboratory Tests

Most patients with low back pain do not need laboratory testing. The laboratory can be helpful in evaluating patients suspected of having nerve root compromise (to determine whether or not disc herniation is present) such as cancer, infection, or inflammatory arthritis (e.g., ankylosing spondylitis). Characteristics of the tests most useful in evaluating these conditions are summarized in Table 31.4. The following are general recommendations regarding laboratory tests:

- If an abdominal or pelvic cause of the pain is considered, testing should be appropriate for the differential diagnosis.

- The best primary care test for evaluating persons with suspected disk disease is the computed tomography (CT) scan, because its lower

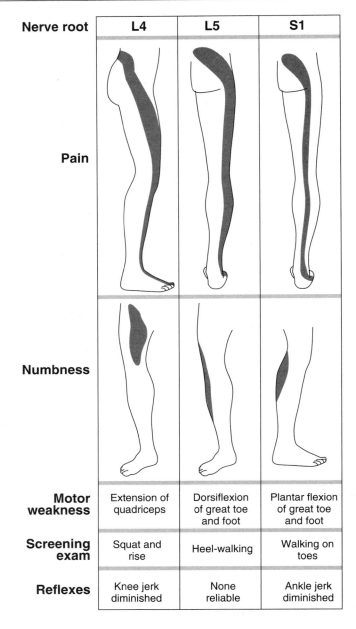

Nerve root	L4	L5	S1
Pain			
Numbness			
Motor weakness	Extension of quadriceps	Dorsiflexion of great toe and foot	Plantar flexion of great toe and foot
Screening exam	Squat and rise	Heel-walking	Walking on toes
Reflexes	Knee jerk diminished	None reliable	Ankle jerk diminished

Figure 31.3. *Testing for lumbar nerve root compromise.* (Adapted from Bigos S, Bowyer O, Braen G, et al. Acute Low Back Pain Problems in Adults. Clinical Practice Guideline, Quick Reference Guide no. 14, AHCPR publication no. 95–0643. Rockville, MD: US Department of Health and Human Services, Public Health Service, Agency for Health Care Policy and Research, December, 1994.)

cost and increased specificity outweigh the modest increase in sensitivity of the MRI scan. In general, patients should not be evaluated by CT unless they have either cauda equina syndrome, severe symptoms or significant signs of nerve root irritation in spite of 4 to 6 weeks of conservative management, or new onset of weakness in the affected extremity.

- If infection is suspected, a sedimentation rate should be obtained. Patients whose sedimen-

Table 31.4.
Characteristics of Diagnostic Tests Useful in Patients with Low Back Pain

Diagnosis the Test Is Trying to Detect (in Patients in Whom History and/or Physical Raises "Red Flags")	Test	Sensitivity[a]	Specificity[b]	LR+[c]	LR−[c]
Herniated disc	CT scan	0.80	0.71	2.76	0.20
	MRI scan	0.92	0.52	1.92	0.15
Spinal cancer	ESR ≥20	0.78	0.67	2.36	0.33
	ESR ≥50	0.56	0.97	18.7	0.45
	X-ray plain films (compression fracture or lytic/blastic lesion)	0.70	0.95	14.0	0.32
	Bone scan (if known cancer)	0.99	0.70	3.30	0.01
	CT scan	0.95	0.80	4.75	0.06
	MRI scan	0.95	0.95	19.6	0.05
Infection	MRI scan	1.00	—	—	0.00
	X-ray plain films	0.48	—	—	—
	Bone scan	0.86	0.49	1.68	0.31
Ankylosing spondylitis	HLA-B27 antigen	0.95	0.91	10.6	0.05

Data are from Thornbury JR, Fryback DG, Turski PA, et al. Disk-caused nerve compression in patients with acute low-back pain: diagnosis with MR, CT myelography, and plain CT. Radiology 1993;186:731–738; Schipper J, Kardaun JW, Braakman R, van Dongen KJ, Blaauw G. Lumbar disk herniation: diagnosis with CT or myelography. Radiology 1987;165:227–231; Deyo RA, Diehl AK. Cancer as a cause of back pain: frequency, clinical presentation, and diagnostic strategies. J Gen Intern Med 1988;3:230–238; Joines JD, McNutt RA, Carey TS, Deyo RA, Rouhani R. Finding cancer among ambulatory patients with low back pain: a comparison of diagnostic strategies. (unpublished article); Meyers SP, Wiener SN. Diagnosis of hematogenous pyogenic vertebral osteomyelitis by magnetic resonance imaging. Arch Intern Med 1991;151:683–687; Palestro CJ, Kim CK, Swyer AJ, Vallabhajosula S, Goldsmith SJ. Radionuclide diagnosis of vertebral osteomyelitis: indium-111-leukocyte and technetium-99m-methylene diphosphonate bone scintigraphy. J Nucl Med 1991;32:1861–1865. Torda AJ, Gottlieb T, Bradbury R. Pyogenic vertebral osteomyelitis: analysis of 20 cases and review. CID 1995;20:320–328; Gran JT, Husby G. HLA-B27 and spondyloarthropathy: value for early diagnosis? J Med Genetics 1995;32:497–501.

[a]Tests with high sensitivity are good for ruling out. A negative test effectively rules out the diagnosis (Sn-N-Out).

[b]Tests with high specificity are good for ruling in. A positive test makes the diagnosis very likely (Sp-P-In).

[c]The likelihood ratio enables you to modify your estimate of the probability that the patient has a specific diagnosis based on the test result. If the test result is positive, multiply your original (i.e., pretest) estimate of the probability of the disease by the LR+; if the test is negative, use the LR−.

tation rate is above 20 (30 if the patient's age is >65) should be considered for a bone scan, which has high sensitivity (but only modest specificity). A normal bone scan rules out all but the earliest infection.

- If tumor is suspected, plain film radiographs may be diagnostic; however, MRI provides the greatest specificity and sensitivity. One recommended strategy is to use the erythrocyte sedimentation rate (ESR) to risk-stratify patients suspected of having cancer; those with an ESR ≤20 can be screened with a radiograph; those with an ESR > 20 should have an MRI (6).

- Needle electromyelography (EMG) has a high specificity (true positive rates >90%) but low sensitivity (45 to 78%) in identifying nerve root compromise. It is indicated only in a few unusual situations: persons with multiple medical problems potentially causing reduced function (e.g., an older person with knee arthritis) and persons with subjective muscle weakness in whom you suspect lack of cooperation (21).

Plain films of the lumbosacral spine are of limited value. They can be used to screen patients for malignancy, but as noted in Table 31.4, sensitivity is low. They can identify the presence of osteoarthritis, but this finding is unlikely to alter the management of persons with low back pain. In a systematic review of 35 studies published between 1994 and 1996, van Tulder concluded that radiographic findings suggesting degenerative joint disease, such as subchondral sclerosis, joint space narrowing, and osteophyte formation consistently occur in higher prevalence in persons with low back pain than in controls. Evidence does not, however, support an association between spondylosis, spondylolisthesis, spina bifida, transitional vertebrae, or Scheuermann's disease and the incidence of low back pain; instead, these conditions occur in similar prevalences in normal populations (22).

MANAGEMENT

Low back pain varies in its severity and its effect on the patient's functional and psychologic status. Some patients are in excruciating pain with the smallest movement; others are able to go through their normal day with only mild or moderate pain. The prognosis is generally good, however; between 70 and 90% of acute problems resolve in a month, and nearly all chronic problems improve with appropriate treatment. In all cases, the goals of your management should be to relieve symptoms and to return the patient to normal function as early as possible.

Therapy must be individualized, taking into consideration the patient's symptoms, personal circumstances, and past history. When the pain is acute, the main issue is assisting the patient in recovering rapidly. When the pain is recurrent, your management should focus on both rapid resolution of the episode and the development of habits that will prevent future episodes. When the pain is chronic, your approach should involve understanding the biologic, psychologic, and social factors aggravating the pain and intervening in all these areas, with the goal of getting the patient to function optimally with as little pain as possible.

Acute Episodes

The management of acute low back pain involves a wide range of therapies. The existing literature on the effectiveness of these therapies was critically reviewed by a panel convened by the Agency for Health Care Policy and Research (AHCPR) as part of the development of clinical guidelines for the management of acute low back pain (2). The panel's conclusions on the effectiveness of various treatments are summarized in Table 31.5. In managing specific patients, you should individualize your therapeutic decisions based on the characteristics of the pain, the patient's history, and relevant occupational, psychologic, and social factors. Following are general recommendations:

- If the pain is mild or moderate (e.g., if the patient is able to carry out nonstrenuous daily tasks), a reasonable initial regimen would include (a) acetaminophen, aspirin, or another nonsteroidal anti-inflammatory drug (NSAID); (b) avoidance of strenuous activity until pain subsides (i.e., lift no more than 20 pounds); (c) limiting sitting to 20 minutes or less without getting up and moving around; (d) gentle stretching exercises (in moderate cases, start the exercises after a few days of rest); (e) education on avoidance of back strain (a written handout helps); and (f) a follow-up visit in a week. Spinal manipulation is a safe and effective alternative therapy method; it may be especially useful in persons with acute facet joint or sacroiliac joint symptoms (23).

- If the pain is severe (e.g., the patient is unable to change position without intense discomfort), a reasonable initial regimen might include (a) an opiate analgesic and/or muscle relaxant; (b) an NSAID; (c) bed rest for 2 to 4 days, followed by gradual increase in activity; (d) application of ice packs for 20 minutes at a time for 1 to 2 days; and (e) a return visit in 3 to 5 days. Generally the pain will be less intense by the return visit, and the patient can be managed as outlined in the previous recommendation for mild to moderate pain.

- The patient should be urgently referred to a specialist if signs of cauda equina syndrome (see Table 31.3) are present or if the patient has a rapidly progressing neurologic deficit.

- Patients with nerve root compromise who do not require urgent specialist referral should be managed no differently than those with uncomplicated backache; however, recovery is generally slower. Such patients should initially be reassessed weekly and their regimen modified based on change in symptoms. If the patient's function is not markedly improved, or if muscle weakness, reduced reflexes, and/or significant leg pain persist after 4 to 6 weeks, a CT or MRI scan or consultation with a back surgeon should be considered. Persons with severe radicular weakness and/or pain who are highly motivated to return quickly to a high level of physical

Table 31.5.

Therapeutic Options Available for the Management of Acute Low Back Pain

Treatment Strategy	Level of Evidence for Effectiveness[a]	Recommendations/Comments
Bed rest/activity recommendations	A	Gradual return to normal activities is superior to prolonged bed rest; bed rest should be used only for severe pain and limited to 2–4 days
Patient education about low back symptoms	A	Improves recovery and satisfaction; reduces MD visits; see Table 31.8
Spinal manipulation	A	Improves function and provides pain relief when used in first 2 weeks; not proven more effective than placebo beyond 2 weeks or if nerve root compromise present; risks low
Surgery for herniated disc	A	Referral recommended only if patient has (a) severe, disabling sciatica, with objective signs of nerve root compromise, and (b) failure to improve with at least 4 weeks' conservative treatment
Nonsteroidal anti-inflammatory drugs (NSAIDs)	B	Many choices; none superior to the others; may cause gastrointestinal irritation
Muscle relaxants	B	Probably of similar effectiveness to NSAIDs; may cause drowsiness
Opiate analgesics	B	Effectiveness probably similar to NSAIDs; significant abuse potential and adverse effects; use for short period and only for severe pain
Shoe insoles and lifts	B	Controversial; may be effective if (a) patient stands for prolonged periods of time, and (b) leg length discrepancy > 2 cm exists
Acetaminophen	C	Safe, inexpensive, nonnarcotic; effectiveness limited
Trigger point and/or facet joint injection with local anesthetic and/or steroid	C	Studies equivocal (trigger point) or absent (facet joint); use discouraged by AHCPR panel
Lumbar corsets and back belts	C	Unproven effectiveness; may weaken abdominal muscles; not recommended for acute low back pain
Physical therapy for pain relief (e.g., ice, heat, ultrasound)	X	Unproven benefit; significant cost
Traction	X	Studies indicate no better than placebo; adverse effects are those of prolonged bed rest
Transcutaneous electrical nerve stimulation (TENS)	X	Unproven benefit; significant cost
Oral corticosteroids	X	Not recommended
Antidepressant medication	X	Not recommended
Colchicine	X	Not recommended

[a]Level of evidence for effectiveness: A, strong or moderate research-based evidence (consistent across several studies, including at least two randomized controlled trials); B, limited research-based evidence (less consistent or extensive evidence, but preponderance of evidence supports use of treatment); C, common practice with little or no research-based evidence; and X, moderate or strong evidence suggesting that this treatment is not effective.

performance (e.g., professional athletes) may benefit from more rapid evaluation, because surgical removal of a herniated disc may reduce recovery time in such individuals. Most patients improve without surgery. The only valid randomized trial of surgery shows some benefit at 1 year, but no difference in outcome at 5 and 10 years (24).

- If the pain is recurrent (i.e., if the patient has had several other episodes of acute pain), the above principles apply, but your regimen should be tailored based on what has helped in the past, and your follow-up should be more intensive. Return office visits should emphasize physical comfort measures (e.g., lumbar support cushion, firm mattress, and getting up frequently when sitting for long periods), avoidance of mechanical back stress (e.g., proper lifting technique), and the development and maintenance of an exercise and prevention program (a physical therapist can be helpful here).

Table 31.6 lists some of the medications most commonly prescribed for patients with low back pain. In acute low back pain, opiates and muscle relaxants should be used only for short periods of time, when the pain is severe. If NSAIDs are prescribed, they should be tapered as soon as the patient regains mobility, and the patient should be warned about signs of gastritis (taking pills with meals may help).

In mild to moderate cases, reassure the patient that the pain will likely resolve over the next few weeks and encourage the patient to remain as active as possible without markedly worsening the pain. Bed rest causes deconditioning and can aggravate spasm, so it should be reserved for severe, debilitating back pain and should be limited to 2 to 4 days. Time off work depends on the nature of the job; persons who do manual labor

Table 31.6.
Drugs Recommended for Use in the Outpatient Management of Low Back Pain

Drug (common trade name)	Common Dosing Range (mg)	Type of Drug
For severe acute pain		
Oxycodone (Percodan/Percocet)	5–10 q 4–6 hrs	Opiate
Codeine (with acetaminophen Tylenol #3)	30–60 q 4–6 hrs	Opiate
Transdermal fentanyl (Duragesic)	25 µg/hr[a]	Opiate
Diazepam (Valium)	2.5–5 q 6–8 hrs	Muscle relaxant
For moderate acute pain		
Aspirin (various brands)	325–650 q 4 hrs	NSAID
Ibuprofen (Motrin)	400–600 q 4–6 hrs	NSAID
Naproxen (Naprosyn, Naprelan)	250–500 q 8–12 hrs	NSAID
Indomethacin (Indocin)	25–50 q 6–8 hrs	NSAID
Cyclobenzaprine (Flexeril)	10–20 q 8 hrs	Muscle relaxant
For mild acute pain		
Acetaminophen (Tylenol)	325–650 q 4–6 hrs	Nonopiate analgesic
Aspirin (various brands)	325–650 q 4–6 hrs	NSAID
Ibuprofen (Advil, Motrin IB, others)	200–400 q 4–6 hrs	NSAID
Naproxen sodium (Aleve, Anaprox)	200–400 q 8–12 hrs	NSAID
Chlorozoxazone (Parafon Forte)	250–500 q 6–8 hrs	Muscle relaxant
For severe chronic pain		
Oxycodone (Percodan/Percocet)	5–10 q 4–6 hrs	Opiate
Codeine (Tylenol #3)	30–60 q 4–6 hrs	Opiate
Methadone	2.5–10 q 6–24 hrs	Opiate
Transdermal fentanyl (Duragesic)	25 µg/hr[a]	Opitate
For mild/moderate chronic pain		
Diclofenac (Voltaren)	25–50 q 8 hrs	NSAID
Naproxen (Naprosyn, Naprelan)	250–500 q 8–12 hrs	NSAID
Acetaminophen (Tylenol)	325–650 q 4–6 hrs	Nonopiate analgesic
Aspirin (various brands)	325–650 q 4–6 hrs	NSAID
Ibuprofen (Advil, Motrin IB, others)	200–400 q 4–6 hrs	NSAID
Carbamazepine (Tegretol)	100–200 q 6 hrs	Anticonvulsant

[a]Transdermal patch. Initial dose should be 25 µg unless patient is already tolerant to opiate drugs; dose may be increased after a few days.

may require considerable release time, whereas persons who do not perform physical labor can often work while recovering. Sitting, however, is mechanically stressful for the back and can be a significant problem for persons with low back pain. Instructions should include using a chair with good lumbar support (and possibly using a lumbar support cushion), getting up and stretching frequently, and taking short walks (which often help limber the back). As symptoms decrease, activity should be gradually increased.

With extreme cases, avoidance of exercise should be recommended. As the pain begins to subside, however, muscle stiffness will benefit from gentle stretching. Other exercises, such as strengthening and aerobic activities, should be added once the pain is largely resolved. Athletes who do activities that are stressful for the back, such as soccer or football, should substitute a conditioning exercise like swimming or (if tolerated) cycling while the back episode is resolving. Persons with recurrent episodes of back pain should be encouraged, once the episode has improved, to develop an exercise and conditioning program that stretches and strengthens the back as an ongoing activity.

Chronic Pain

In 10 to 15% of persons with low back pain, the illness runs a chronic or relapsing course. Persons with chronic low back pain consume tremendous health care resources, often for unproven therapies. They often become permanently disabled (a patient who has been off work for 6 months for low back pain has a 50% chance of never returning to work). Yet with aggressive and appropriate management, most persons with chronic low back pain will be able to function normally (25).

Management of chronic low back pain has three cornerstones: exercise, education, and psychosocial support. Relatively few therapies have been demonstrated to be effective (Table 31.7), and medication is of limited value. Most effective is a coordinated, multidisciplinary effort. Such a program can be carried out by the family physician in consultation with a physical therapist and a behavioral scientist. In difficult cases, referral to a pain clinic may be helpful.

A critical component of effective management of chronic (and recurrent) low back pain is improvement of physical conditioning through an incrementally increased exercise program. If the patient is obese, a weight loss program should be instituted as well (see Chapter 43). Begin with low-stress aerobic activities, such as walking, swimming, or riding a bicycle, and increase the pace and duration as fitness improves. Next add exercises to condition the abdominal, pelvic, and paraspinous muscles. Finally, if necessary, add specific training undertaken by a physical or occupational therapist to assist the patient in safely carrying out strenuous work-related activities.

Attention to psychosocial issues is vital. Many persons with chronic low back pain have underlying stresses or psychologic problems or develop them after prolonged suffering. Many give a history of previous physical or mental abuse in childhood. Thus, regular office visits should include discussion of the patient's home, family, and work situation. Conducting a family conference can also be helpful in gaining insight into the patient's family relationships. In addition, a formal evaluation by a clinical psychologist or similarly trained behavioral scientist can sometimes help define psychologic issues and implement a formal therapeutic program. Behavioral treatment should assist the patient in learning to focus on function rather than pain, overcoming addiction to pain medication, learning nonpharmacologic strategies to combat pain (such as self-hypnosis and biofeedback), and managing underlying anxiety or depression.

Medications play an adjuvant role in the effective management of chronic low back pain. Many patients chronically use one or another pain medication. In severe pain, opiates sometimes are necessary; when used, they should be given regularly (never PRN) by the same clinician, with the dose gradually reduced over time. Rarely, a patient has to be maintained on a strict regimen of opiate medications. For mild and moderate pain, acetaminophen or an NSAID will usually suffice; however, long-term NSAID use often leads to gastritis or peptic ulcer disease. During an acute flare-up, pain medication and/or a muscle relaxant should be used. If the patient is clinically depressed, an antidepressant is indicated. If the patient is terminally ill, the chronic use of opiates is appropriate. Table 31.6 provides guidelines for selecting a medication for persons with chronic low back pain.

Similarly, the role of surgery is relatively minor. Although many persons with chronic pain have been operated on, most persons would have been functioning equally well 2 years later if they had avoided surgery. Therefore, a referral to a back surgeon should generally be limited to persons with intractable pain in spite of adherence to a comprehensive management program

Table 31.7.

Management of Chronic Uncomplicated Backache

Treatment Strategy	Level of Evidence for Effectiveness[a]	Recommendations/Comments
Exercise	A	Workers who exercise regularly have fewer days lost from work; little agreement on specific regimen; walking and swimming are the least mechanically stressful of aerobic exercises
Acetaminophen	A	Safest medication for long-term use
Nonsteroidal anti-inflammatory drugs	A	Significant risk of adverse effects such as gastritis and ulcer formation with long-term use
Behavioral therapy (relaxation training, imagery, coping skills)	B	
Lumbar support cushions and seating	B	Lumbar support cushions, footwear with impact-absorbent soles
Lumbar corsets and back belts	B	Effective primarily as a preventive when used on the job by persons who do frequent lifting
Biofeedback	B	Conflicting evidence from studies of effectiveness, but preponderance of evidence suggests some effect. Cost can be considerable.
Acupuncture	B	Studies indicate that needling improves pain, but that needling along appropriate Chinese meridians is not superior to misplaced needling
Muscle relaxant drugs	C	No evidence for effectiveness over placebo with chronic use
Opiate analgesics	C	No more effective when used chronically than acetaminophen; may be valuable for short periods of time during exacerbations
Manipulation	C	Randomized trials have only demonstrated effectiveness during first 2 weeks of an acute episode
Physical therapy modalities for pain relief	C	Cost outweighs potential benefits; patients should be taught application of cold and heat at home
Antidepressants	C	Most randomized trials show lack of effectiveness as treatment for pain; if clinical depression is present (frequency is increased in lower back pain), then they are indicated
Epidural steroid injections	C	Risks generally outweigh benefits
Back schools (structured education programs)	C	May be especially effective when integrated into the workplace
Transcutaneous electrical nerve stimulation	C	Randomized trials have failed to demonstrate effectiveness
Facet joint injections	X	Studies indicate no difference from placebo
Oral corticosteroids	X	Side effects are potentially severe, and effectiveness is unproven

Data are from Bigos S, Bowyer O, Braen G, et al. Acute Low Back Problems in Adults. Clinical Practice Guideline, Quick Reference Guide no. 14, AHCPR publication no. 95-0643. Rockville, MD: US Department of Health and Human Services, Public Health Service, Agency for Health Care Policy and Research, December, 1994; van Tulder MW, Koes BW, Bouter LM. On the accuracy of history, physical examination, and erythrocyte sedimentation rate in diagnosing low back pain in general practice. In: van Tulder, ed. Low Back Pain in Primary Care: Effectiveness of Diagnostic and Therapeutic Interventions. The Hague (Netherlands): EMGO Institute, 1996; Magni G. The use of antidepressants in the treatment of chronic pain. A review of the current evidence. Drugs 1991;42:730–748.

[a]Level of evidence for effectiveness: A, strong or moderate research-based evidence (consistent across several studies, including at least two randomized controlled trials); B, limited research-based evidence (less consistent or extensive evidence, but preponderance of evidence supports use of treatment); C, common practice with little or no research-based evidence; and X, moderate or strong evidence suggesting that this treatment is not effective.

or who show continued signs of nerve root compromise after 6 weeks of conservative therapy.

Patient Education

Education and emotional support are important components of effective patient management. Although you are unlikely to have a precise anatomic diagnosis, your patient needs an understandable explanation of what is happening, the prognosis, and what to do. If the initial diagnosis is uncomplicated backache, assure the patient that there is "no hint of a dangerous problem" and that "a rapid recovery can be expected." During follow-up visits, the pain may not resolve as quickly as the patient would like, and you may have to deal with frustration at continued disability. In such situations, it can be helpful to point out that pain and disability are less than they were before, and to reassure the patient that with time and adherence to a regimen, further improvement will occur. Another important element of education is to teach the patient to avoid mechanical factors that aggravate low back pain.

Table 31.8 outlines areas to emphasize in the education of patients with acute and chronic low back pain.

Table 31.8.

Instructing and Counseling the Patient with Low Back Pain

Condition	Key Points to Cover in Patient Education and Counseling
Acute low back pain	Reassure that the pain will improve—disability is not likely
	Provide a clear, confident explanation for the pain, using models or diagrams to explain the anatomy (if helpful to this patient)
	Explain the lack of need for special investigations unless "red flags" are present or symptoms do not resolve in 6 weeks
	Give clear instructions about prescribed activity level and therapy, including safe and effective methods of symptom control
	Activity instructions • Severe pain—bed rest for 2–4 days, then gradual increase in activity • Moderate pain—no strenuous activity; restricted activity and exercise initially, then gradual increase • Mild pain—continue daily routines, add stretching exercises
	Exercise instructions • Severe pain—none • Mild to moderate pain—stretching exercises (e.g., pelvic tilt, flattening lumbar curve, pulling one knee at a time to chest while lying on back, gentle rotation of hips); gradual increase in walking • Resolving pain (including residual stiffness)—stretching exercises plus gradual introduction of strengthening (e.g., half sit-ups) and increased aerobic (e.g., swimming, walking longer distances) activity
	Instruct about whether or not to take time off work; if so, offer to write a work excuse. Provide your best estimate as to how much time off is anticipated and whether activity restrictions will be recommended on returning to work
	"Red flags"—when to contact you prior to the next scheduled visit
	Date, time, and purpose of next visit
Chronic back pain	Emphasize that focusing on curing the pain is not helpful; instead try to focus on improving function
	Emphasize that function nearly always improves with time and with physical activity
	Discuss the effect of the back pain on work, household duties, transportation/driving, sleep, sex, socializing, leisure activity, and personal finances
	Activity instructions—encourage all activity that does not cause longstanding increase in pain or impairment of function (as opposed to merely temporarily increasing pain)
	Exercise instructions—gradual introduction of stretching, strengthening, and aerobic conditioning exercises by a physical therapist

CASE STUDY

Mr. S. was helping his daughter move into her dormitory room to begin college 1 week ago. While picking up a heavy box, he experienced a sudden, severe pain in his lower back. The next day the pain persisted and began to radiate into his buttocks and along the posterior and lateral aspects of his right thigh and lower leg. Over-the-counter ibuprofen helped, but he became concerned because of the persistence of the pain down his leg.

In the office Mr. S. states that he feels considerable relief when supine and motionless. He has no history of cancer, has no fever or known infection, has had no bowel or bladder dysfunction or weight loss, and has experienced no other neurologic symptoms other than those previously described. Besides the pain Mr. S. experiences from his lower back, his general health appears to be good.

General observation reveals a slight limp, as the patient does not completely extend his right leg when he walks. The straight leg raising test is positive in both legs, eliciting pain below the knee in the right leg at 40° extension on the right and 50° on the left. The patient complains of pain if his leg is extended while he sits. Mr. S. has difficulty going up on his tiptoes on the right leg, and his ankle reflex is diminished on that side.

QUESTIONS

1. What should you tell Mr. S. about the cause of his back pain?
2. What more serious etiologies are unlikely in light of the history and physical examination?
3. What laboratory tests should be ordered for Mr. S.?
4. What is the best course of treatment for Mr. S., and what is his prognosis?

DISCUSSION

The history of Mr. S.'s injury and the positive straight leg raising, as well as the pertinent negatives listed, confirm that this is a case of low back pain with significant nerve root compromise. Considering that cancer causes less than 1% of back pain, that Mr. S. was previously in good health, and that his pain was associated with a potentially injurious event (lifting the heavy box), malignant neoplasm is very unlikely. Likewise, spinal infection is improbable in light of Mr. S.'s lack of recent fever or known infection. Further evidence that systemic disease is not the cause here is his ability to find a comfortable stationary position (supine) that provides relief from pain. It is also of note that his general health, except for the back pain, appears good.

With the history and physical examination strongly suggestive of mechanical injury, and no "red flags" present, no laboratory tests are indicated at this point. The weakness and diminished reflexes in his right leg do suggest, however, that some type of imaging study and the consideration of surgery for disc disease must be considered. Exactly how to proceed in a case of this type is unclear; the majority of physicians would treat him conservatively for a short period of time (e.g., a week) and, if his neurologic findings did not resolve, would then obtain an MRI. The best initial course of treatment for Mr. S.'s lumbar disc herniation is a day or two of bed rest followed by a gradual increase in activities to the extent allowed by the pain. NSAIDs should be given to reduce inflammation and pain. This course of treatment should be followed and the patient reevaluated within a week.

Acknowledgment

Thanks to Marie Nash for assistance in reviewing the literature and in planning this chapter.

REFERENCES

1. Cypress BK. Characteristics of physician visits for back symptoms: a national perspective. Am J Public Health 1983;73:389–395.
2. Bigos S, Bowyer O, Braen G, et al. Acute Low Back Problems in Adults. Clinical Practice Guideline, Quick Reference Guide no. 14, AHCPR publication no.

95–0643. Rockville, MD: US Department of Health and Human Services, Public Health Service, Agency for Health Care Policy and Research, December, 1994.

3. Deyo RA. Back pain revisited: newer thinking on diagnosis and therapy. Consultant 1993;33:88–100.

4. Jensen MC, Brant-Zawadzki MN, Obuchowski N, Modic MT, Malkasian D, Ross JS. Magnetic resonance imaging of the lumbar spine in people without back pain. N Engl J Med 1994;331:69–73.

5. Deyo RA, Bass JE. Lifestyle and low-back pain. The influence of smoking and obesity. Spine 1989;14: 501–506.

6. Deyo RA, Diehl AK. Cancer as a cause of back pain: frequency, clinical presentation, and diagnostic strategies. J Gen Intern Med 1988;3:230–238.

7. Wheeler AH. Diagnosis and management of low back pain and sciatica. Am Fam Physician 1995;52: 1333–1341.

8. Von Korff M, Deyo RA, Cherkin D, Barlow W. Back pain in primary care: outcomes at 1 year. Spine 1993;18:855–862.

9. Carey TS, Evans A, Hadler N, Kalsbeek N, McLaughlin C, Fryer J. Care-seeking among individuals with chronic low back pain. Spine 1995;20:312–317.

10. Klenerman L, Slade PD, Stanley M, et al. The prediction of chronicity in patients with an acute attack of low back pain in a general practice setting. Spine 1995;20:478–484.

11. Deyo RA, Diehl AK. Psychosocial predictors of disability in patients with low back pain. J Rheumatol 1988;15:1557–1564.

12. Lacroix JM, Powell J, Lloyd GJ, Doxey NC, Mitson GL, Aldam CF. Factors of value in predicting outcome. Spine 1990;15:210–213.

13. Lanier DC, Stockton P. Clinical predictors of outcome of acute episodes of low back pain. J Fam Pract 1988;27: 483–489.

14. Murphy KA, Cornish RD. Prediction of chronicity in acute low back pain. Arch Phys Med Rehabil 1984;65: 334–337.

15. Deyo RA, Rainville J, Kent DL. What can the history and physical examination tell us about low back pain? JAMA 1992;268:760–765.

16. van der Hoogen JM, Koes BW, van Eijk J, Bouter LM. On the accuracy of history, physical examination, and erythrocyte sedimentation rate in diagnosing low back pain in general practice. In: van Tulder MW, Koes B, Bouter LM, eds. Low Back Pain in Primary Care: Effectiveness of Diagnostic and Therapeutic Interventions. The Hague (Netherlands): EMGO Institute, 1996.

17. Kerr RSC, Cadous-Hudson TA, Adams CBT. The value of accurate clinical assessment in the surgical management of the lumbar disc protrusion. J Neurol Neurosurg Psychiatry 1988;51:169–173.

18. Anderson GBS, Deyo RA. History and physical examination in patients with herniated lumbar discs. Spine 1996;21:105–185.

19. Hudgins WR. The crossed straight leg raising test: a diagnostic sign of herniated disc. J Occup Med 1979; 21:407–408.

20. Den Hoogen HJM, Koes BW, Deville W, van Eijk JTM, Boute RLM. The interobserver reproducibility of Lasègue's sign in patients with low back pain in general practice. Br J Gen 1996;46:727–730.

21. Dvorak J. Neurophysiologic tests in diagnosis of nerve root compression caused by disc herniation. Spine 1996;21:39S–44S.

22. van Tulder M. Diagnostics and treatment of chronic low back pain in primary care. Amsterdam (Netherlands): Thesis Publishers, 1996.

23. Curtis P. Low back pain. In: Sloane P, Slatt L, Curtis P, eds. Essentials of Family Medicine, 2nd ed. Baltimore: Williams & Wilkins, 1993.

24. Weber H. Lumbar disc herniation. A controlled, prospective study with ten years of observation. Spine 1983;8(2):131–140.

25. Clinical Standards Advisory Group. Epidemiology Review: The Epidemiology and Cost of Back Pain. London: HMSO, 1994.

32. Menstrual Syndromes

BARBARA SUPANICH

Key Clinical Questions

1. How do you evaluate and manage dysmenorrhea and premenstrual syndrome (PMS)?
2. How do you classify abnormal uterine bleeding?
3. Is vaginal ultrasonography useful in the diagnosis and management of abnormal uterine bleeding?
4. What are the appropriate treatments for abnormal uterine bleeding?

Abnormal menstrual syndromes can be categorized as chronic pain syndromes or abnormal uterine bleeding disorders. The most common chronic pain syndromes associated with the menstrual cycle are dysmenorrhea and the premenstrual syndrome (PMS), occurring in about 10 to 15% of menstruating women in the United States (1, 2). Abnormal uterine bleeding disorders are also very common, with a prevalence of 9 to 14% in healthy menstruating women (3).

The diagnosis of abnormal menstrual syndromes is an example of the blending of the art and science of medicine. Women are understandably very concerned when their menstrual cycles are irregular or when they have abnormally long or unexpected bleeding cycles. Depending on the age of the woman and her gynecologic history, these symptoms could mean that she is pregnant, has a gynecologic cancer, has uterine fibroids or an ovarian hormonal imbalance, or may have a pelvic infection. For many younger women, dysmenorrhea can range in severity from merely annoying to severely disabling and accounts for a significant number of lost hours from school or work.

Painful Menses

PATHOPHYSIOLOGY

When evaluating the patient with painful menses or *dysmenorrhea*, it is important to distinguish between primary and secondary causes. *Primary dysmenorrhea* is defined as menstrual pain with normal pelvic anatomy; the usual onset is from menarche to age 19. The onset of the pain is typically 24 to 36 hours before the onset of menses and can continue for 24 to 72 hours into the menses. *Secondary dysmenorrhea* is defined as menstrual pain with pelvic organ pathology on physical examination or at laparoscopy. The usual onset is in women over 20 years of age; the pain is usually progressive with age; and it is not always synchronized with the menses.

Primary and secondary dysmenorrhea have different pathophysiologies. Primary dysmenorrhea is thought to be due to increased prostaglandin activity in the uterus, which results in increased uterine contractility. There appears to be increased production of prostaglandins (most likely PGI_2) and an increased secretion of vasopressin (2, 4, 5). Studies have shown that the normal hormonal changes of the menstrual cycle result in progressive differentiation of the arterioles of the uterine vascular tree up to the premenstrual state. Hormonal factors also influence the innervation of the uterine arteries (cholinergic, adrenergic, and peptidergic), regulate the spontaneous contractile activity of the smooth muscle of vessel walls, and affect the motor responses of these tissues to different vasoactive substances (6). Of the vasoactive substances, vasopressin, oxytocin, endothelin, and noradrenaline have the most pronounced effect on blood vessels. Women with primary dysmenorrhea have an increased secretion of vasopressin. By an action on type VI vasopressin receptors of the uterus, vasopressin causes myometrial hyperactivity and vasoconstriction with resultant uterine ischemia and pain (6).

The pathophysiology of secondary dysmenorrhea varies with the underlying cause. Common causes for secondary dysmenorrhea include endometriosis, leiomyomas, endometrial cancer, intrauterine devices (IUD), polyps of the cervix or uterus, pelvic inflammatory disease (PID), cervical stenosis, ovarian cysts, imperforate hymen, and uterine synechiae (2).

DIFFERENTIAL DIAGNOSIS

Approximately 80% of dysmenorrhea is primary dysmenorrhea. The differential diagnosis for secondary dysmenorrhea is shown in Table 32.1. The differential diagnosis for a particular patient depends on her age, historical information, and physical examination findings. For example, endometriosis should be considered in women less than 30 years of age who have dysmenorrhea and pelvic pain at the time of ovulation. Cervical stenosis, leiomyomas, and endometrial cancer should be considered for perimenopausal, menopausal, and postmenopausal women. Imperforate hymen is possible in younger women who have not had any menses and present with severe pelvic pain. Finally, you should consider pelvic inflammatory disease (PID) in any sexually active woman who presents with pelvic pain, with or without vaginal discharge.

CLINICAL EVALUATION

When you evaluate a woman with dysmenorrhea, your history should be guided by the woman's age, sexual history, and the timing of her menstrual cycle events with her pelvic pain. If the woman describes moderate to severe menstrual cramps within 48 hours of the onset of her menses and has a normal abdominal and pelvic examination, then primary dysmenorrhea is the most likely diagnosis. However, if she is older than 20 years and her pelvic pain is not always synchronous with her menses, then secondary causes should be more aggressively explored.

The diagnosis of secondary dysmenorrhea is made when a woman with menstrual pain has pelvic pathology identified at the time of the physical examination, following appropriate laboratory studies, or at laparoscopy. Women with secondary dysmenorrhea are usually older than 20 years of age, their symptoms progress with age, and symptoms are not always synchronous with their menstrual cycle.

One of the most common causes of secondary dysmenorrhea is endometriosis. Several good case-control studies (7–10) have concluded that the following factors are associated with a higher risk for endometriosis in relative order of the strengths of the association: Asian race, tampon use for at least 14 years, a long duration of IUD use, heavy menstrual flow, severe menstrual cramps, one live birth, age over 30 years, long cycle length and long duration of menstruation.

Table 32.1.
Differential Diagnosis of Menstrual Problems

Diagnosis	Frequency in Primary Care
Dysmenorrhea	
Primary dysmenorrhea	Very common
Secondary dysmenorrhea	
Cervical stenosis	Common
Cervical polyps	Common
Ovarian cysts	Common
Pelvic inflammatory disease	Common
Endometriosis	Common
Leiomyomas/fibroids	Common
IUD complications	Uncommon
Endometrial cancer	Uncommon
Imperforate hymen	Rare
Uterine synechiae	Rare
Abnormal uterine bleeding	
Hormonal dysfunctional uterine bleeding	Common
Pregnancy states	
Intrauterine	Common
Spontaneous abortion	Common
Ectopic	Uncommon
Molar pregnancy, placenta previa, placenta abruptio	Rare
Inflammatory/infectious conditions	
Vaginitis	Common
Cervicitis	Common
Pelvic inflammatory disease	Common
Endometritis	Uncommon
Vulvitis	Rare
Trauma	
Foreign body	Fairly common
Direct trauma	Uncommon
Systemic diseases	
Thyroid disease	Fairly common
Coagulopathies, blood dyscrasias, drug effects, adrenal disease	Rare
Neoplasia	
Cervical	Uncommon
Uterine	Uncommon
Ovarian, fallopian tube, vaginal, vulvar	Rare
Premenstrual syndrome	
Major depressive and anxiety disorders	Common
Dysmenorrhea	Common
Mittelschmerz	Common
Endometriosis	Uncommon
Tubo-ovarian abscess	Rare

Adapted from Johnson CA. Making sense of dysfunctional uterine bleeding. Am Fam Physician 1991;44:149–157.

See Chapter 14 (Abdominal Pain) for a more detailed discussion of the diagnosis and management of endometriosis. Table 32.2 lists the key elements of the history and physical examination for dysmenorrhea. Table 32.3 lists the "red flags" suggesting progressive or life-threatening disease.

History

Important elements of the history and physical examination include a current and past menstrual history, a description of the pain and timing of the pain in relation to the menstrual cycle, the level of disability experienced by the patient due to the dysmenorrhea, the patient's perception of her pain and disability, and the effect of the pain on her life. Other helpful information includes a sexual history, a history of past sexually transmitted diseases (STDs), contraceptive use, endometriosis, family history of gynecologic cancers, and any history of gynecologic surgeries or procedures. Primary dysmenorrhea is very likely (>90%) if a woman is less than 20 years old and the onset of her pain occurs 24 to 48 hours before the onset of her menses.

Certain symptom patterns may suggest a specific cause of secondary dysmenorrhea. If your patient has severe dysmenorrhea that is particularly intense at the time of ovulation and her menses, you should consider a diagnosis of endometriosis. Associated back pain and diarrhea suggest the possibility of endometrial bowel

Table 32.2.
Key Elements of the History and Physical Examination for Dysmenorrhea and Abnormal Uterine Bleeding

Question/Maneuver	Diagnosis
Dysmenorrhea	
Information about age, duration and description of symptoms, prior history of dysmenorrhea, prior treatments and response to treatments, previous prescribed and OTC medications for dysmenorrhea, other key medical conditions, general health	Assist in creating and narrowing the differential diagnosis
Look for "red flags" (see Table 32.3)	Screen for pelvic inflammatory disease (PID), endometrial cancer, ectopic pregnancy, and tubo-ovarian abscess
Dysmenorrhea that is more intense at the time of ovulation and menses	Endometriosis
Obtain sexual history, history of STDs	PID, dyspareunia
History of gynecologic surgery	Pelvic adhesions, cervical stenosis
Psychosocial history	Assist in understanding the patient's perception(s) of pain, coping skills, and formulation of a treatment plan
Temperature	Infectious causes
Focused abdominal and pelvic examinations	
Palpable/enlarged uterus	Leiomyomas, pregnancy, malignancy
Cervical stenosis on speculum examination	Cervical stenosis
Thick purulent cervical discharge	Cervicitis, PID
Tender and enlarged adnexal area	PID
Bleeding from cervical os in postmenopausal woman	Malignancy
Abnormal uterine bleeding	
Determine if woman is ovulatory	Determines which diagnostic pathway to follow (Figs. 32.3 and 32.4)
Information about age, ob/gyn history, menstrual history, description of symptoms, rating of pain, response to prior treatments, and general health	Assist in creating and narrowing the differential diagnosis
Look for "red flags" (see Table 32.3)	Screen for uterine cancer, ectopic pregnancy, threatened or missed abortion
Medications	Warfarin sodium or aspirin
Focused physical examination:speculum and bimanual examination, observe for petechiae, palpate thyroid	If abnormalities are elicited, focuses examiner on particular differential diagnosis

Table 32.3.
"Red Flags" Suggesting Progressive or Life-Threatening Disease in Patients with Pelvic Pain or Abnormal Uterine Bleeding

Diagnosis	"Red Flags" Suggestive of the Disease
Uterine cancer	Any vaginal bleeding in a postmenopausal woman or intermenstrual bleeding in a perimenopausal woman, >4 mm of thickness of endometrium on transvaginal ultrasound, palpable pelvic mass, or endometrial cells on Pap smear
Ectopic pregnancy	Missed period, or abnormal previous period, with unilateral pelvic pain; may have vaginal bleeding; may have adnexal fullness palpated on pelvic examination
Missed or threatened abortion	Missed or abnormal previous period, with severe pelvic cramping/pain and vaginal bleeding
Pelvic inflammatory disease (PID)	Fever, purulent vaginal discharge, abdominal or pelvic pain, exquisitely tender on palpation of pelvic organs, malaise, septic appearance
Tubo-ovarian abscess	Fever, malaise, septic appearance, palpable fullness in the adnexa, or exquisite tenderness on pelvic examination

implants. If your patient relates a history of multiple colposcopies for severe cervical dysplasia and has had her cervix frozen multiple times, consider cervical stenosis. Finally, if she is postmenopausal and is having menometrorrhagia, endometrial cancer must be ruled out before proceeding with any other evaluations. Fever and malaise suggest PID or tubo-ovarian abscess.

Physical Examination

Physical examination should begin with an abdominal examination to evaluate for an enlarged uterus or large ovarian masses. You should also perform a complete pelvic examination, which includes a rectovaginal examination in order to evaluate the uterus and adnexal areas for size, masses, and areas of tenderness. The physical examination is performed to rule out any abnormal pelvic pathology that could be associated with secondary dysmenorrhea.

Unfortunately, the physical examination is not very sensitive or specific in the evaluation of the patient with secondary dysmenorrhea. For example, although uterosacral pain, cervical motion tenderness, uterosacral nodularity, limited uterine mobility, and a fixed uterus are all highly specific findings for the presence of endometriosis (>94%), their sensitivity is poor (≤ 7%) (11, 12). The family physician should therefore use the historical and physical findings of women with suspected secondary dysmenorrhea to guide the selection of appropriate laboratory and imaging studies.

Laboratory Tests

Because the diagnosis of primary dysmenorrhea is based largely on an accurate history, there is no need to obtain any confirmatory tests. For secondary dysmenorrhea, the choice of laboratory test(s) is guided by the historical findings. Cultures for gonorrhea and chlamydia should be obtained in women with a history of vaginal or cervical discharge, those with a history of multiple partners and unprotected intercourse, and those with a duration of symptoms between 4 and 14 days. These women are also at higher risk for HIV infection and therefore should receive appropriate HIV test counseling. Postmenopausal women with heavy or irregular bleeding and premenopausal women over age 40 with chronic anovulatory cycles, obesity, hypertension, diabetes mellitus, or long-term use of unopposed estrogens are at higher risk for endometrial cancer and should receive an endometrial biopsy. Patients with pain at the time of ovulation should receive an ultrasound to evaluate for possible endometriosis or ovarian cysts. Table 32.4 lists characteristics of diagnostic tests.

MANAGEMENT

The evaluation and management of dysmenorrhea is summarized in Figure 32.1. Central to the evaluation is the distinction between primary and secondary causes, based on the history and physical examination. The level of evidence for different interventions is summarized in Table 32.5.

Table 32.4.

Characteristics of Diagnostic Tests Useful in Patients with Dysmenorrhea and Abnormal Uterine Bleeding

Diagnosis	Test	Sensitivity	Specificity	LR+	LR−
Hypothyroidism	TSH	0.93	0.70	3.1	0.23
Cervical cancer	Pap	0.90	0.92	11.3	0.11
Uterine cancer	Endometrial biopsy	0.98	0.97	32.6	0.02
	Transvaginal ultrasound	0.96	0.89	9.1	0.04
Menorrhagia	Endometrial biopsy	0.98	0.99	98	0.02
	Transvaginal ultrasound	0.79	0.93	14.1	0.22
Pregnancy	Urine HCG	0.98	0.97	32.6	0.02
Von Willebrand's disease	Bleeding time	0.2	0.85	1.3	0.94

Adapted from Dodson MG. Use of transvaginal ultrasound in diagnosing the etiology of menometrorrhagia. J Reprod Med 1994;39:362–372; Emanuel MH, Verdel MJ, Wamsteker K, Lammes F. A prospective comparison of transvaginal ultrasonography and diagnostic hysteroscopy in the evaluation of patients with abnormal uterine bleeding: clinical implications. Am J Obstet Gynecol 1995;172:547–552; Dijkhuizen FP, Brolmann HA, Potters AM, Bongers MY, Heintz AP. The accuracy of transvaginal ultrasonography in the diagnosis of endometrial abnormalities. Obstet Gynecol 1996;87:345–349; Schectman JM, Paulson LG. The cost-effectiveness of three thyroid function-testing strategies for suspicion of hypothyroidism in a primary care setting. J Gen Intern Med 1990;5(1):9–15; Martin D, Umpierre SA, et al. Comparison of the endocervical brush and endocervical curettage for evaluation of the endocervical canal. P R Health Sci J 1995;14(3):195–197; Stovall TG, Photopeloz GJ, et al. Pipelle endometrial sampling in patients with known endometrial cancer. Obstet Gynecol 1991;77(6):954–956; Chard T. Pregnancy tests: a review. Hum Reprod 1992;7:701–710; Parkin JD, Smith IL, et al. Mild bleeding disorders: a clinical and laboratory study. Med J Aust 1992;156:614–617.

Primary Dysmenorrhea

For primary dysmenorrhea, the most common primary treatment is nonsteroidal anti-inflammatory drugs (NSAIDs) (see doses in Table 32.6). The NSAIDs should be initiated 3 days before the onset of menses and continued through at least day two or three of menstrual flow. The effectiveness of this treatment plan should be reevaluated after two or three cycles; if ineffective, the patient can be started on an NSAID from a different class, or you can consider prescribing an oral contraceptive (OC). The low-dose, triphasic OCs are usually well tolerated and effective in relieving dysmenorrhea. The woman should be reevaluated if her symptoms occur, and the physician should assess the effectiveness of the current treatment with the patient at the time of her annual health maintenance examination.

Secondary Dysmenorrhea

When evaluating a patient for secondary dysmenorrhea, you must keep in mind the secondary causes of dysmenorrhea (see Fig. 32.1). Also, the severity of the pelvic pain varies by diagnosis and by the individual patient's perception of pain. Some patients are in excruciating pain with very small endometrial implants, whereas other pa-

tients complain of very little pain and have multiple large implants. The same variability in pain perception is observed in patients with ovarian cysts; the size of the cyst may have no correlation to the severity of pain that the patient is experiencing. The overall goals of management are to identify the cause of the patient's dysmenorrhea, relieve her symptoms, and help the patient return to normal function as soon as possible.

Therapy must be individualized, taking into account the patient's current and past symptoms, sexual and menstrual history, and her desire for future pregnancy. If the pain is structural in nature, you should consider diagnoses such as ovarian cysts, cervical or endometrial polyps, or tubo- ovarian abscess. Nonstructural causes that should be considered include endometriosis, PID, and leiomyomas (see Chapter 14, Abdominal Pain, for additional discussion of the diagnosis and management of PID and endometriosis).

Ovarian Cysts and Cervical Polyps

If the ovarian cysts are small (less than 4 cm on ultrasound), the patient can be treated with NSAIDs or OCs. If the cysts are larger than 6 cm, you should refer the patient to a gynecologist for further evaluation and possible laparoscopy to remove the cyst(s). Ovarian cysts between 4 and

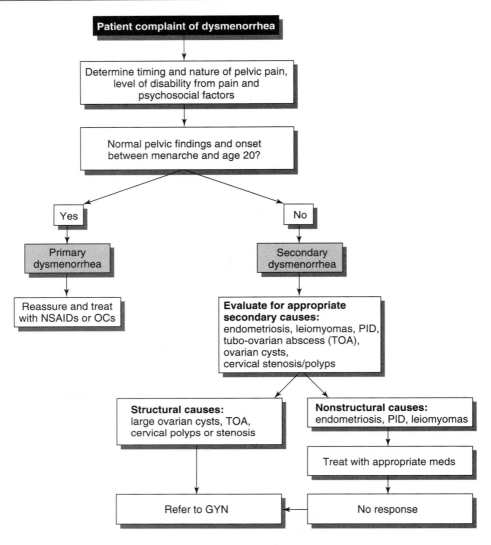

Figure 32.1. *General approach to the patient with dysmenorrhea.*

6 cm can usually be carefully followed clinically by the family physician and treated medically; if symptoms worsen, you should refer the patient to a gynecologist for probable laparoscopy. If cervical or endometrial polyps are the cause of the pelvic pain, referral to a gynecologist is appropriate if the family physician has not received training in cervical curettage or hysteroscopy.

Tubo-ovarian Abscess

Tubo-ovarian abscess is characterized by fever, malaise, a septic appearance, and exquisite pain on palpation of an adnexal mass or area of full-

ness (see Table 32.3 for other diagnostic "red flags"). This is a medical emergency, and the patient should be immediately stabilized with IV fluids and antibiotics and referred to a gynecologist. If the patient is cardiovascularly stable and not septic, you can consider obtaining an ultrasound first to confirm your diagnosis.

Pelvic Inflammatory Disease

Pelvic inflammatory disease (PID) is characterized by fever, malaise, purulent vaginal discharge, and exquisite tenderness on palpation of the pelvic organs. Most patients can be treated as

Table 32.5.

Management of Dysmenorrhea, Premenstrual Syndrome, and Abnormal Uterine Bleeding

Treatment Strategy	Level of Evidence for Effectiveness[a]	Comment
Dysmenorrhea		
Nonsteroidal anti-inflammatory drugs (NSAIDs)	A	Most studies have used ibuprofen (Motrin, others) and mefenamic acid (Ponstel) and found that both are better than placebo. Mechanism of action is prostaglandin inhibition.
Oral contraceptives	A	For control of dysmenorrhea[b, c] and endometriosis; [d, e] also has contraceptive benefits if desired
Danazol	A	Endometriosis [d, e]
Medroxyprogesterone acetate	A	Endometriosis[d, e]
GnRH analogues	A	Endometriosis[d, e]
Abnormal uterine bleeding		
Oral contraceptives	C	Works very well for all types of abnormal uterine bleeding; need to counsel patients on adverse effects and that OCs may take two or three cycles to be effective
Hormone replacement therapy	C	For perimenopausal women who have been amenorrheic for at least 6 months and for postmenopausal women; need to counsel women on the adverse effects and that HRT may take up to 4–6 months to regulate the abnormal uterine bleeding
Premenstrual syndrome		
Fluoxetine (Prozac)	A	Several good randomized trials supporting the use of Prozac for dysphoria in PMS[f]
Premenstrual assessment form and diary	C	Assists the woman and the physician in understanding the woman's particular constellation of symptoms and possible treatment approaches[g]
Dietary measures	C	
Reassurance and patient education	C	

[a]Level of evidence for effectiveness: A, strong or moderate research-based evidence (consistent across several studies, including at least two randomized controlled trials); B, limited research- based evidence (less consistent or extensive evidence, but preponderance of evidence supports use of treatment; C, common practice with little or no research-based evidence; X, moderate or strong evidence suggesting that this treatment is not effective.

[b]Ory HW. The noncontraceptive health benefits from oral contraceptive use. Fam Plann Perspect 1982;14:182–183.

[c]Speroff L, Glass RH, Kase NG. Clinical Gynecologic Endocrinology and Infertility, 3rd ed. Baltimore: Williams & Wilkins, 1983.

[d]Lu PY, Ory SJ. Endometriosis: current management. Mayo Clin Proc 1995;70:453–463.

[e]Olive DL, Schwartz LB. Endometriosis. N Engl J Med 1993;328:1759–1769.

[f]Steiner M, Steinberg S, Stewart D, et al. Fluoxetine in the treatment of premenstrual dysphoria. Canadian Fluoxetine/Premenstrual Dysphoria Collaborative Study Group. N Engl J Med 1995;332:1529–1534.

[g]Klein T. Office gynecology for the primary care physician, part II; pelvic pain, vulvar disease, disorders of menstruation, premenstrual syndrome, and breast disease. Med Clin North Am 1996;80:321–336.

Table 32.6.

Drug Therapy of Dysmenorrhea and Abnormal Uterine Bleeding

Drug (Common/Trade Name)	Common Dosing Range (mg/day)	Type of Drug
Ibuprofen (Motrin)	600–800	NSAID
Mefenamic acid (Ponstel)	500	NSAID
Naproxen (Naprosyn)	500	NSAID
Conjugated estrogen (Premarin, Ogen)	0.625–1.25	Synthetic hormone
Medroxyprogesterone acetate (Provera, Aygestin)	2.5–10.0	Synthetic hormone
Ethinyl estradiol/norethindrone (Demulen, Demulen 1/35, Ortho-Novum 1/35, 7/7/7, 10/11)	One pill/day	OC
Ethinyl estradiol/levonorgestrel (Triphasil, Tri-Levlen, Lo/Ovral)	One pill/day	OC

outpatients. If the patient appears septic, however, or will not be able to make follow-up appointments, she should be admitted for IV antibiotic treatment of her PID. PID is a serious disease, and prompt diagnosis and treatment is of paramount importance because PID is a leading cause of sterility in young women.

Endometriosis

Endometriosis can be initially managed by the family physician with OCs and NSAIDs. When these are not successful, it is appropriate to refer the patient to a gynecologist for laparoscopic evaluation and possible ablation of lesions as well as discussion of other forms of medical management such as danazol and GnRH agonists.

Premenstrual Symptoms

PATHOPHYSIOLOGY AND DIFFERENTIAL DIAGNOSIS

Premenstrual syndrome (PMS) is a constellation of physical, emotional, and/or behavioral symptoms that occur during the second half of the menstrual cycle (the luteal phase), approximately 7 to 10 days before the menses, with resolution of symptoms soon after flow begins. Women with PMS must, by definition, be symptom-free during the first half of the menstrual cycle (the follicular phase) (1). PMS affects about 10% of menstruating women in the United States (1), is most common in women in their late twenties to thirties, and has no racial, socioeconomic, or other demographic predilection.

The nature and severity of symptoms can vary from cycle to cycle for a particular woman, and symptom combinations and intensity of symptoms vary from woman to woman. The most common and distressing symptoms are emotional lability, anxiety, and depression. Other common symptoms include fluid retention, edema, craving of certain foods (primarily chocolate and salty foods), and pelvic and abdominal pain of variable intensity (13).

The diagnosis of PMS is one of exclusion. The family physician must therefore rule out other significant disorders such as major depressive and anxiety disorders, dysmenorrhea, ovulation pain (Mittelschmerz), tubo-ovarian abscess, and endometriosis before making the presumed diagnosis of PMS. Although almost all ovulating women have some degree of premenstrual discomfort or mood change, those in whom the symptoms interfere with normal work, personal activities, or relationships are considered to have PMS (13).

CLINICAL EVALUATION

You should ask about pain at the time of ovulation (Mittelschmerz), fevers, malaise, and purulent cervical or vaginal discharge. If none of these are present, a diagnosis of PMS can be considered. If PMS is suspected, you should also explore variation from cycle to cycle, any relationship to past pregnancies and postpartum periods, and any past psychiatric treatments (13). A standard PMS symptom chart developed jointly by the American Psychiatric Association and by the National Institute of Mental Health (Fig. 32.2) should be administered to the patient (13). This chart should be completed by the patient for at least two consecutive menstrual cycles due to the possible variability of symptoms in each cycle. Whether the patient records her symptoms on a standard chart or records her symptoms in her own diary, she should rate each symptom on a scale of one to four (four being most severe) during both the follicular and luteal phases of her menstrual cycle. In PMS, the scores during the luteal phase should be at least three times those in the follicular phase, and there should be little if any follicular phase discomfort (13). The follow-up appointment should allow sufficient time to review your patient's symptom chart results and explore her symptoms.

There are no characteristic findings on the physical examination for a woman with PMS. If you detect abnormalities on the abdominal and/or pelvic examinations, they should be properly evaluated before proceeding with a diagnosis and treatment of PMS. There are no laboratory or imaging tests that confirm the diagnosis of PMS.

MANAGEMENT

Many interventions have been suggested in the literature that claim to be effective in the treatment of PMS; unfortunately, many of these studies are methodologically flawed (14). Because there is not one proven therapy for all patients with PMS, you should focus your attention on the symptoms that are most severe and debilitating for your particular patient. The level of evi-

Premenstrual Symptom Calendar: Depression

Name: _____   Month/Year: _____

Instructions: On the date lines below, please mark your mood each **evening.** The numbers below the lines refer to the days of the month. **Please circle the days of the month you are menstruating.** Refer to the following example. Please call your physician if you have any questions about completing this symptom chart.

Example:

Most Depressed Ever	Most Happy Ever
X	
(4th)	

Most Depressed Ever	Most Happy Ever	Most Depressed Ever	Most Happy Ever	Most Depressed Ever	Most Happy Ever
1st		2nd		3rd	
4th		5th		6th	
7th		8th		9th	

Figure 32.2. Sample premenstrual symptoms chart for depression. A similar chart can be made for anxiety and irritability. The patient should complete both charts for two consecutive months.

dence to support treatment recommendations for PMS is summarized in Table 32.5.

Initial

Educational and supportive measures are central in the management of PMS and should be offered initially. After reviewing the patient's symptom chart, the family physician can identify with the patient which symptoms are most severe on which days and then design specific treatment approaches and coping mechanisms. After making your initial recommendations, have the patient continue her diary entries and follow-up in 2 months to review her progress and reevaluate your strategy. For example, if your patient's main symptoms are irritability and a craving for chocolate, you should recommend that she avoid chocolate and salty foods during the luteal phase and watch for any changes in the level and intensity of her irritability. If the woman is experiencing increased levels of stress and mood swings and leads a basically sedentary lifestyle, you should suggest increased exercise activity on a daily basis and especially during the luteal phase (13). If the patient has moderate-to-severe psychiatric symptoms, you should initiate appropriate treatment including medication, psychologic counseling services, and psychiatric referral as appropriate.

Long Term

If initial conservative measures do not give the patient appropriate relief from her symptoms, drug therapy is often beneficial. The best documented treatments to date are vitamin B_6 throughout the month, NSAIDs for pain relief, and fluoxetine (Prozac), a serotonin-specific reuptake inhibitor (see Table 32.6). Vitamin B_6 deficiency is thought to be one of the etiologies of PMS, and for some women administration of vitamin B_6 is very helpful in reducing PMS symptoms. NSAIDs for pain relief given for the 10 days preceding menses and for the first 2 days of the menses have been shown to be effective (see Table 32.6 for details) (1, 13). In a very well-designed study, Prozac 20 mg taken orally every day was shown to be effective for the treatment of PMS dysphoria (15). However, doses larger than 20 mg per day only increased the likelihood of adverse effects and did not improve efficacy.

Abnormal Uterine Bleeding

PATHOPHYSIOLOGY

Normal uterine bleeding in women of childbearing age is bleeding that lasts 2 to 6 days with a blood loss of 20 to 60 mL, at intervals of 21 to 35 days. Flow lasting longer than 7 days, blood loss of 80 mL or more, or irregular menstrual intervals (less than 21 days or more than 35 days) are considered to be *abnormal* bleeding patterns (5). The following descriptions of abnormal uterine bleeding facilitate consistent communication among professionals:

- *Menorrhagia:* prolonged or excessive bleeding occurring at regular intervals
- *Metrorrhagia:* uterine bleeding occurring at irregular but frequent intervals, the amount being variable
- *Menometrorrhagia:* prolonged uterine bleeding occurring at irregular intervals
- *Intermenstrual bleeding:* bleeding of variable amounts occurring between regular menstrual periods
- *Polymenorrhea:* uterine bleeding occurring at regular intervals of less than 21 days
- *Oligomenorrhea:* uterine bleeding in which the interval between bleeding episodes varies from 35 days to 6 months
- *Amenorrhea:* no uterine bleeding for at least 6 months (5)
- *Dysfunctional uterine bleeding (DUB):* abnormal uterine bleeding whose etiology is hormonal; it accounts for 80% of cases of menorrhagia (5, 16)

There are five types of hormonal dysfunction associated with dysfunctional uterine bleeding: progesterone and estrogen withdrawal, estrogen withdrawal, progesterone withdrawal, estrogen breakthrough, and progesterone breakthrough.

Progesterone and estrogen withdrawal is the mechanism for bleeding in the normal menstrual cycle, in perimenopausal patients who take cyclic hormone replacement therapy, and in patients taking combined oral contraceptives (OCs). Estrogen-withdrawal bleeding can result from destruction of the ovaries with radiation therapy, from oophorectomy, and when estrogen replacement therapy is only taken for 25 days of the month. It can also cause midcycle spotting in an ovulating patient, because the estrogen level decreases slightly just before ovulation (5). Progesterone-withdrawal bleeding occurs whenever progestins are initiated and then stopped, as in a progestin challenge test for diagnostic purposes. Breakthrough bleeding may also accompany both low- and high-estrogen states. Use of low-dose OCs may result in prolonged light bleeding because the amount of estrogen is insufficient to build up a stable endometrial lining, whereas in high-estrogen states, heavy bleeding often occurs as a result of excessive buildup of the endometrium. Progesterone breakthrough is less common and usually results from continuous administration of progestins alone for contraception (the "minipill" or Depo-Provera injections). It can also occur with the use of OCs that contain a higher proportion of progestin-to-estrogen component.

The etiology of dysfunctional uterine bleeding is often related to the patient's reproductive phase. The postpuberty phase includes girls who have recently reached puberty, are not sexually active, and whose menstrual cycles are not yet regular. Their cycles may be anovulatory, resulting in irregular menses; full maturation of the hypothalamic-pituitary-ovary axis usually occurs within 18 months of menarche (5). The reproductive phase includes all postpubertal women who do not yet have perimenopausal menstrual irregularities. They often have dysfunctional uterine bleeding due to hormonal contraception or may be anovulatory as a result of polycystic ovary syndrome, stress, weight change, or exercise. Intervention for this group depends upon the woman's desire to maintain her fertility and her desire for pregnancy. Finally, the perimenopausal group has dysfunctional uterine bleeding as a result of anovulatory cycles or short ovulatory cycles.

If your patient is under 30 years of age and sexually active, you should consider pregnancy-related conditions such as spontaneous abortion or placenta previa, and if the patient also has abdominal pain, you should consider ectopic pregnancy and placenta abruptio. You should also consider sexually transmitted diseases (STDs) in this age group, especially in women with multiple partners and those who have unprotected intercourse. For women over 40 years of age with abnormal uterine bleeding, you must consider uterine neoplasm in the differential diagnosis. Cervical and vaginal cancers are very rare causes of uterine bleeding in this age group. Other than

age, risk factors for endometrial cancer include chronic anovulation, obesity, hypertension, diabetes mellitus, and exposure to unopposed estrogen. The differential diagnosis of abnormal uterine bleeding is summarized in Table 32.1.

CLINICAL EVALUATION

History

When a woman comes to the family physician complaining of abnormal vaginal bleeding, the physician has two initial tasks: to determine the amount and chronicity of menstrual or intermenstrual bleeding and to determine whether the bleeding is ovulatory or anovulatory. Once these tasks have been completed and after an appropriate physical examination, the need for ultrasound and laboratory tests can be determined. Bleeding that occurs at regular intervals and is preceded by premenstrual symptoms such as breast tenderness, water weight gain, mood swings, or abdominal cramping is likely ovulatory in nature. Anovulatory bleeding is characterized by prolonged bleeding that occurs at irregular intervals and usually follows several months of amenorrhea. Bleeding abnormalities associated with ovulatory cycles include menorrhagia and intermenstrual bleeding, whereas abnormalities associated with anovulatory cycles may include irregular, heavy menses (menometrorrhagia) or frequent bleeding and spotting (polymenorrhea) (16).

The evaluation of the patient with abnormal uterine bleeding is summarized in Figures 32.3 through 32.5, and the key elements of the history and physical are summarized in Table 32.2 (16). Begin by obtaining a screening history for the major causes of menorrhagia. It should include a careful history from the woman concerning bleeding disorders: bleeding problems with dental work and extractions, a family history of bleeding disorders (von Willebrand's), a history of heavy bleeding since menarche, or bleeding that required transfusions should all raise your suspicion of serious inherited bleeding coagulopathies. Patients who present with menorrhagia and a low platelet count may have immune thrombocytopenic purpura. Subclinical hypothyroidism can be an underlying cause of menorrhagia. You should also inquire if any physician has made a diagnoses of uterine fibroids or endometriosis in the past, since these conditions can cause abnormal uterine bleeding. A review of the patient's medication history should be done with particular attention to medications such as aspirin or warfarin sodium (Coumadin), which can impair coagulation.

Physical Examination

The physical examination should be directed at detecting signs of thyroid disease (palpable thyroid), bleeding abnormalities (bruising, petechiae), and/or severe liver disease (tender and enlarged liver, petechiae, jaundice). A pelvic examination should be performed to evaluate the patient for an enlarged uterus (pregnancy, uterine malignancy, or fibroids), cervical infection, cervical polyps, and adnexal tenderness. Although the sensitivity of the pelvic examination to accurately diagnose uterine pathology is only about 33% (17), etiologies such as cervical polyps, purulent cervical discharge, vaginal lesions, and gross lesions of cervical malignancy are readily identifiable by the skilled clinician.

Laboratory Tests

Women over 40 with abnormal uterine bleeding should have an endometrial biopsy to rule out endometrial cancer. A Papanicolaou (Pap) test should be ordered for any woman who has postcoital bleeding to evaluate for cervical cancer. Gross lesions should be biopsied in the office because the Pap test is not accurate in the evaluation of gross cervical lesions.

You should only order laboratory tests when the findings from the history and physical examination increase the probability that the patient has an underlying disease or disorder. For instance, if the woman is complaining of very heavy bleeding with menses, appears pale, and is tachycardic, you should suspect an anemia and order a complete blood count (CBC). If she has a family history of bleeding coagulopathies, you should order appropriate coagulation studies. Thyroid, serum prolactin, and androgen studies should be reserved for those women who have chronic anovulation of over 6 months and associated systemic symptoms.

Several recent studies have considered the use of transvaginal ultrasound (TVU) and diagnostic hysteroscopy in the evaluation of abnormal uterine bleeding (17–20). These studies concluded that TVU is an effective procedure to exclude endometrial and intrauterine abnormalities in women with abnormal uterine bleeding. When TVU was compared with diagnostic hysteroscopy and histologic examination, it had a sensitivity of 0.96 and a specificity of 0.89 for abnormal uterine bleeding (LR+ 9.1 and LR− 0.04). TVU is a helpful first test to evaluate a woman with DUB or abnormal uterine bleeding prior to referral for hysteroscopy, dilatation and curettage, or hysterectomy. However, TVU is not a definitive diagnostic test and is incapable of distinguishing between hyperplasia and neoplasia. Therefore, patients with an endometrial thickness greater than 4 mm should be considered for endometrial biopsy (19, 21).

MANAGEMENT

First determine whether the bleeding pattern is ovulatory or anovulatory (Fig. 32.3). If the woman is having ovulatory cycles with heavy bleeding or menorrhagia, you should consider anemia, hypothyroidism, coagulopathies, structural lesions, and medications such as warfarin sodium and NSAIDs. If no abnormalities are discovered, you should reassure her or consider a trial of OCs to regulate her abnormal bleeding pattern. It is important for the family physician to understand the relative potencies of the estrogenic and progestin agents and the different types of formulations (e.g., monophasic, biphasic, or triphasic) in order to both treat the woman's symptoms and minimize adverse effects (Table 32.7).

If the patient has mild iron-deficiency anemia and an otherwise normal evaluation, you should treat her with OCs or NSAIDs. If she does not respond to this therapy within 3 months, you should consider a referral to a gynecologist. If you discover a structural lesion on either physical examination or ultrasound in a patient with severe anemia, a referral to a gynecologist is appropriate. If the patient is having anovulatory bleeding (Fig. 32.4), you should perform a focused history and physical examination and appropriate laboratory studies to rule out pregnancy, hypothyroidism, anemia, prolactinoma, and structural lesions such as leiomyomas.

If no abnormalities are found, the patient has dysfunctional uterine bleeding. The treatment of dysfunctional uterine bleeding is based on the age of the woman and the presence of risk factors for endometrial cancer. If the patient is a woman less than 35 years of age with no risk factors for endometrial cancer (such as chronic anovulation, obesity, hypertension, and diabetes mellitus) or is an adolescent, you can treat her with OCs or cyclic oral progesterone. The medication can be

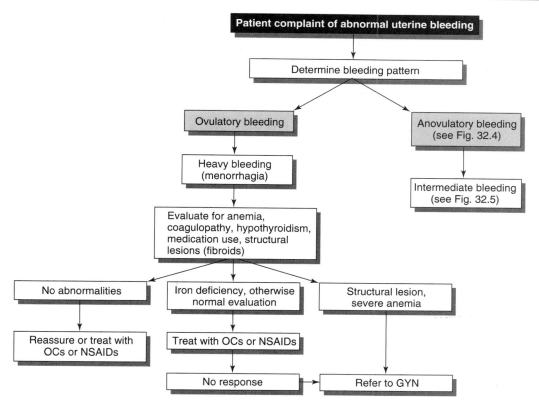

Figure 32.3. *General approach to the patient with abnormal uterine bleeding.* (Reprinted with permission from Wathen PI, Henderson MC, Witz CA. Abnormal uterine bleeding. Med Clin North Am 1995;79: 329–344.)

discontinued if the patient resumes normal cycles after 3 to 6 months of treatment. If she continues to have abnormal uterine bleeding, you should resume treatment and consider referral if pregnancy is desired. If the woman continues to bleed abnormally after you initiate treatment with OCs or oral progesterone, you should refer her to a gynecologist for hysteroscopy.

If the patient is older than 35 years of age and has risk factors for endometrial cancer, you should perform an endometrial biopsy in the office. If the biopsy report reveals no endometrial cancer or hyperplasia, you should treat her with OCs, oral progesterone, or hormone replacement therapy (HRT). If the biopsy report reveals endometrial neoplasia, you should refer her to a gynecologist for appropriate management and care of her uterine cancer.

If the patient is having intermenstrual (ovulatory) bleeding, you should perform a urine pregnancy test (Fig. 32.5). If the test is positive, the di-

agnoses of ectopic pregnancy and threatened abortion need to be considered and appropriately managed. If it is negative, further management depends upon whether or not the patient is taking OCs.

If the patient is taking OCs, your management should include advising her about additional contraceptive methods for this cycle, encouraging her to take her OCs daily and at approximately the same time each day, and asking her about the use of medications that could cause breakthrough bleeding such as certain antibiotics. If these initial management steps fail, you should consider changing her OC formulation, and if she continues to have intermenstrual bleeding after two cycles of the new OC formulation, you should refer her to a gynecologist for hysteroscopic endometrial sampling.

If the patient is not taking OCs, she should be evaluated for structural lesions such as cervicitis, cervical polyps or cancer, vaginal lacerations,

Table 32.7.
Relative Estrogenic and Progestogenic Content of Oral Contraceptives (OCs)

Type	Preparation	Estrogen (µg)	Progestin (mg)	Pills Taken per Phase of Cycle (21 Days Total)
Combination monophasic				
Ethinyl estradiol/norethindrone	Loestrin 1/20	20	1	21
	Loestrin 1.5/30	30	1.5	21
	Brevicon	35	0.5	21
	Ortho-Novum 1/35	35	1	21
	Ovcon - 35	35	0.4	21
	Ovcon - 50	50	1	21
Ethinyl estradiol/norgestrel	Lo/Ovral	30	0.3	21
	Ovral	50	0.5	21
Ethinyl estradiol/ethynodiol diacetate	Demulen 1/35	35	1	21
	Demulen 1/50	50	1	21
Combination biphasic and triphasic				
Ethinyl estradiol/norethindrone	Ortho-Novum 10/11	35	0.5	10
		35	1	11
Ethinyl estradiol/norethindrone	Ortho-Novum 7/7/7	35	0.5	7
			0.75	7
			1.0	7
Ethinyl estradiol/levonorgestrel	Tri-Levlen, Triphasil	30	0.05	6
		40	0.075	5
		30	0.125	10
Progestin only				
Norethindrone	Micronor	None	0.35	Continuous
Norgestrel	Ovrette	None	0.075	Continuous

Adapted from Facts and Comparisons. Facts and Comparisons, St. Louis, MO.

and fibroids. If no obvious cause is found during your initial evaluation, you should refer her to a gynecologist for hysteroscopic endometrial sampling. Management of the other causes of dysfunctional uterine bleeding (pregnancy, hypothyroidism, prolactinoma, anemia, cervical polyps, or gynecologic cancers) needs an individualized management approach. Please refer to the appropriate chapters in this text for a more detailed discussion of diagnostic and management strategies.

CASE STUDY 1

Ms. M. is a 20-year-old African-American woman who relates a 5-year history of terrible cramps at the onset of her menses. The pain is so severe that she regularly misses 2 to 3 days of work per month; she missed the same amount of high school when she was younger. Since her menarche at age 10, her menses have been reg-

ular and occur every 29 days with a flow of 6 days. The first two days of her menses are very heavy with passage of several quarter-sized clots, and during the remaining 4 days she has a moderate flow that decreases to only spotting by day 5. She describes the pain as very intense, colicky in nature, and a level nine out of 10 on days 1 and 2. Upon further questioning, she informs you that she has moderate cramping about 3 days before her period starts. She has tried acetaminophen in the past with poor resolution of her symptoms. Her basic health history is otherwise unremarkable. She is quite concerned about the source of her pelvic pain and does not want to lose any more days from work. She is also very active in sports (volleyball and tennis) and wants to remain active all month. She has been sexually active since age 16, has had one sexual partner (her present boyfriend), and is G_0P_0. She has not had any STDs. Her affect in the office is appropriate and pleas-

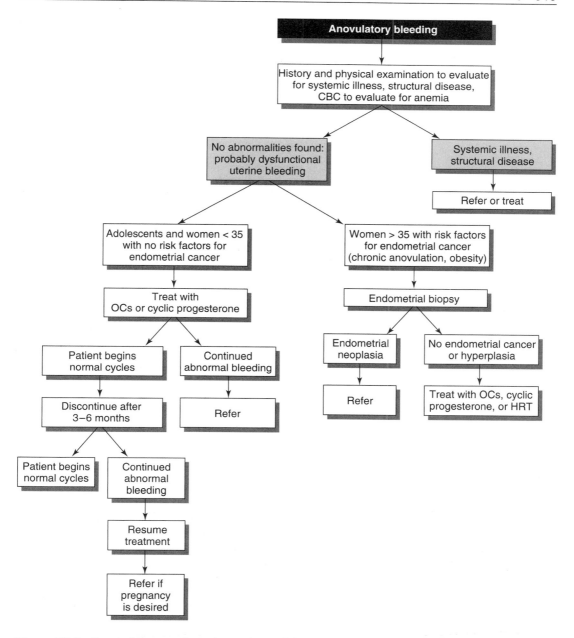

Figure 32.4. *General approach to the patient with anovulatory bleeding.* (Adapted from Wathen PI, Henderson MC, Witz CA. Abnormal uterine bleeding. Med Clin North Am 1995;79:329–344.)

ant, and a physical examination including a pelvic is normal. Because she had a Pap smear performed 3 months ago, you do not repeat the study.

QUESTIONS

1. What should you tell Ms. M. about the etiology of her pain?

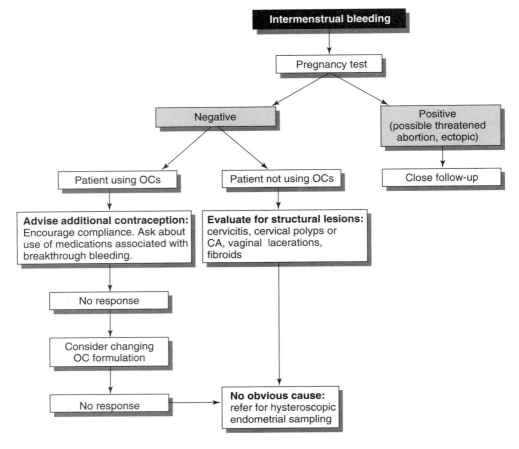

Figure 32.5. *General approach to the patient with intermenstrual bleeding.* (Adapted from Wathen PI, Henderson MC, Witz CA. Abnormal uterine bleeding. Med Clin North Am 1995;79:329–344.)

2. Should you order any laboratory tests or radiologic studies?
3. What is the best course of treatment for Ms. M.'s symptoms, and what is her prognosis?

DISCUSSION

The history of Ms. M.'s menstrual and premenstrual cramps, her negative ROS, and her completely negative physical examination confirm that this is a case of primary dysmenorrhea. She has no findings in her history to make you consider any secondary causes of dysmenorrhea seriously because she does not have any signs of pelvic infection, nor does she have any risk factors for endometriosis (age > 30, Asian race, having one live birth, or excessively long periods) (7). Therefore, there is no reason to order any laboratory or radiologic testing.

The best course of treatment would be an NSAID such as ibuprofen 800 mg taken orally three times a day, given 48 hours before her menses begins and continued through the first 2 to 3 days of her menses. In the case of individuals with severe cramping, a follow-up phone call after one month of treatment is helpful to confirm the efficacy of the treatment and, if appropriate, to discuss other treatment options and the need for office reevaluation.

CASE STUDY 2

Ms. E. is a 50-year-old white woman ($G_3P_3A_0L_3$) who presents to your office concerned about the changes in her menstrual pattern. For the past 6 months, she has had one of two menstrual patterns: either very heavy menstrual flow for up to 10 days at the time of each menses or very light spotting at the time of her menses. Over the past 2 months, she has had no menstrual flow. All of her pregnancies were normal and she had three normal vaginal deliveries. She is presently divorced and has had no sexual activity for the past 6 months. Her past medical history reveals no major medical illnesses and no surgeries. Her menses began at age 12 and were always regular. Her weight has been stable over the past 10 years and is normal for her height and build at 136 pounds. She has no drug allergies and takes no chronic medications. Her mother had her menopause at age 55. There is no family history of cancers, thyroid disease, or diabetes, and her ROS is completely normal. Given the information revealed in her history, you explain to Ms. E. the need to obtain an endometrial biopsy.

Her physical examination is completely normal; her pelvic examination revealed no evidence of vaginal, cervical, or uterine abnormalities. Because of her abnormal uterine bleeding and age, you performed an endometrial biopsy at the time of the pelvic examination. The endometrial biopsy report states that the endometrium shows simple hyperplasia.

QUESTIONS

1. What do you need to tell Ms. E. about the reason for her abnormal uterine bleeding?
2. Are there any serious diagnoses that need to be considered and explained to Ms. E.?
3. What are the next appropriate management steps?

DISCUSSION

Ms. E. presents with menstrual flow that is either very heavy, very light, or nonexistent. All of these patterns began about 6 months ago. She has no evidence for any serious systemic diseases in her medical history. Her sexual history reveals no risks for serious illness. Her physical examination was normal, and her endometrial biopsy revealed simple hyperplasia. You can tell Ms. E. that her present menstrual experience is quite typical for a woman in her late forties to early fifties. Because she is basically a healthy woman without any significant risk factors for endometrial cancer, and given the results of her endometrial biopsy, you would recommend that she start on a course of medroxyprogesterone acetate (Provera) or an OC. The use of medroxyprogesterone acetate or OCs will help to restore the lining to a healthier state and her bleeding to a more normal pattern. If the patient begins normal cycles on the treatment, it should be continued for at least 6 months. After 6 months of treatment, the medicine can be discontinued and the patient's menstrual pattern observed. If it is normal, then nothing further needs to be done. If abnormal bleeding resumes, treatment should be restarted.

REFERENCES

1. Talley P. Dysmenorrhea. In: Levy B, et al, eds. Mosby-University of Iowa Family Practice Handbook. St. Louis: Mosby-Yearbook, 1997.
2. Talley P. Premenstrual syndrome. In: Levy B, et al, eds. Mosby-University of Iowa Family Practice Handbook. St. Louis: Mosby-Yearbook, 1997.
3. Rosenfeld JA. Treatment of menorrhagia due to dysfunctional uterine bleeding. Am Fam Physician 1996; 53:165–172.
4. Koike H, Ikenoue T, Mori N. Studies on prostaglandin production relating to the mechanism of dysmenorrhea in endometriosis. Nippon Naibunpi Gakkai Zasshi 1994;70:43–56.
5. Johnson CA. Making sense of dysfunctional uterine bleeding. Am Fam Physician 1991;44:149–157.
6. Akerlund M. Vascularization of the human endometrium; uterine blood flow in healthy condition and in primary dysmenorrhea. Ann NY Acad Sci 1994; 734:47–56.
7. Sangi-Haghpeykar H, Poindexter AN. Epidemiology of endometriosis among parous women. Obstet Gynecol 1995;85:983–992.
8. Darrow SL, Vena JE, Batt RE, Zielezny MA, Michalek AM, Selman S. Menstrual cycle characteristics and the risk of endometriosis. Epidemiology 1993;4:135–142.

9. Han M, Pan L, Wu B, Bian X. A case control study epidemiologic study of endometriosis. Chin Med Sci J 1994;9:114–118.
10. Matorras R, Rodriguez F, Perez C, et al. Infertile women with and without endometriosis: a case control study of luteal phase and other infertility conditions. Acta Obstet Gynecol Scand 1996;75:826–831.
11. Mattoras R, Rodriguez F, Pijoan JI, et al. Are there any clinical signs and symptoms that are related to endometriosis in infertile women? Am J Obstet Gynecol 1996;174:620–623.
12. Lu PY, Ory SJ. Endometriosis: current management. Mayo Clin Proc 1995;70:453–463.
13. Klein T. Office gynecology for the primary care physician, part II; pelvic pain, vulvar disease, disorders of menstruation, premenstrual syndrome, and breast disease. Med Clin North Am 1996;80:321–336.
14. Rubinow DR, Roy-Byrne P. Premenstrual syndromes: overview from a methodological perspective. Am J Psychiatry 1984;141:29–38.
15. Steiner M, Steinberg S, Stewart D, et al. Fluoxetine in the treatment of premenstrual dysphoria. Canadian Fluoxetine/Premenstrual Dysphoria Collaborative Study Group. N Engl J Med 1995;332:1529–1534.
16. Wathen PI, Henderson MC, Witz CA. Abnormal uterine bleeding. Med Clin North Am 1995;79:329–344.
17. Dodson MG. Use of transvaginal ultrasound in diagnosing the etiology of menometrorrhagia. J Reprod Med 1994;39:362–372.
18. Emanuel MH, Verdel MJ, Wamsteker K, Lammes F. A prospective comparison of transvaginal ultrasonography and diagnostic hysteroscopy in the evaluation of patients with abnormal uterine bleeding: clinical implications. Am J Obstet Gynecol 1995;172:547–552.
19. Dijkhuizen FPHLJ, Brolmann HAM, Potters AME, Bongers MY, Heintz APM. The accuracy of transvaginal ultrasonography in the diagnosis of endometrial abnormalities. Obstet Gynecol 1996;87:345–349.
20. Conoscenti G, Meir YJ, Fischer-Tamaro L, et al. Endometrial assessment by transvaginal sonography and histological findings after D&C in women with postmenopausal bleeding. Ultrasound Obstet Gynecol 1995;5:108–115.
21. Shelly Schirch M. Endometrial biopsy. Am Fam Physician 1997;55:1731–1736.

33. Neck Pain

PETER CURTIS

Key Clinical Questions

1. What type of evaluation is needed for a patient who has severe neck pain that radiates down the arm?
2. When should a patient who has neck pain be referred for surgical evaluation?

Neck pain has a lifetime prevalence of 50%, and in some industries leads to as much work loss as low back pain. The two major symptoms associated with neck diseases are pain and limited motion. The pain may be located only in the neck or radiate either up into the head or to the shoulder and down the arm. The most common cause, considering all age groups, is myofascial syndrome, a condition of localized muscle spasm. Degenerative arthritis in the cervical vertebrae is the other common cause of neck pain, particularly in the older patient, and is known as cervical spondylosis (1, 2). Trauma, particularly motor vehicle accidents, can lead to whiplash and other neck injuries. In the United States, there are 11 million new vehicle-related whiplash injuries each year, of which approximately 20% lead to chronic pain. In Canada, the incidence of whiplash is between 1 and 7 per 1000 population. The threshold of injury is an impact of between 6 and 8 mph, exerting up to 4.5 G (gravitational force) to the neck (3). Sedentary occupations (e.g., desk work and driving motor vehicles) are often associated with neck pain, but the precise anatomic cause of pain is in many cases uncertain.

When approaching the problem of neck pain, the clinician should pose these "internal" questions: Can I make an accurate diagnosis? What is the anatomic level of the problem? Are there several vertebral levels involved? How well do I know the patient? (Neck pain can be modified by personality or stress.) What is the patient's functional limitation? Is it produced by pain or specific damage? Together, answers to these questions form the basis for management and remediation.

Most acute neck pain is caused by mechanical problems of the musculoskeletal system, such as muscle spasm, traumatic ligament sprains, and myofascial syndrome. The latter consists of scattered areas of localized muscle tenderness produced by local spasm of muscle fibers (trigger points) (2). Diagnosis of these common conditions is clinical, relying entirely on the history and physical examination. Causes of subacute and chronic neck pain are also most commonly structural, with degenerative arthritis becoming more likely with increased age. Stress and biomechanics (e.g., positioning at work) are often important contributing factors to both acute and chronic neck pain, so they should be evaluated by the clinician (4). Less common but serious conditions must also be considered in developing a differential diagnosis. The causes of neck pain are listed in Table 33.1.

CLINICAL EVALUATION

History

Ask about the following: the patient's occupation; daily postural habits; stresses at work and at home; the onset of pain (sudden or gradual); the main focus and character of the pain (sharp, dull, or aching); and whether there has been weakness or tingling in the arms. Also ask about gait and bladder function to screen for possible spinal cord injury in the cervical region.

There are certain trajectories of symptoms, depending on the cause and age of the patient.

- Acute pain with limited motion can follow trauma or persistent, out-of-the-ordinary activity, such as house painting or chopping wood. This often occurs in younger patients and is associated with tender neck muscles.

- Recurrent or persistent pain is common in middle-aged patients and is sometimes associated with tingling in the arms and/or fingers. There may also be pectoral pain from an affected C-6 nerve root that can simulate angina.

- Severe persistent neck pain with weakness and radiating pain down one arm is often the result of a nerve root impingement by an osteophyte or a damaged cervical disc. Pain

519

Table 33.1.
Causes of Neck Pain

Structural	Nonstructural	Other
Myofascial syndromes (++)	Ankylosing spondylitis	Stress (++)
Facet joint asymmetry (+)	Rheumatoid arthritis	Occupation (++)
Osteoarthritis (+)	Bone infection	
Muscle spasm (++)	Neoplasia—primary metastasis	
Fracture	Lymphadenitis	
Disc prolapse		
Outlet compression syndrome		

(+), frequent cause of neck pain; (++), very frequent cause of neck pain.

over the lower pole of the scapula and posterior aspect of the shoulder, radiating into the neck, is usually caused by myofascial syndromes and is often associated with stress or poor posture.

- A persistent aching or piercing pain down the arm suggests nerve root compression. Pain with gradual onset that gets worse even with rest is particularly worrisome; it may be caused by infection or malignancy in a vertebra.

Whiplash injuries have a different presentation. In minor to moderate crashes, onset of stiffness and headache is usually delayed for 24 to 48 hours. There may be obvious swellings (hematomas) in the neck area because of the flexion-extension shearing forces. It is postulated that important functional elements in the neck (proprioception, ligaments, nerves, and the sympathetic chain) are stretched and injured (3). This leads to a number of unusual symptoms that cluster into certain patterns of presentation that may persist for a long time (Table 33.2). Facet joint pain is the most common basis for chronic pain after whiplash, with headache arising mainly from the C-2 to C-3 joints.

What do patients think and say about their pain? Quite often they will complain of clicking or grinding on turning the head. This is not a pathologic noise unless it is associated with rheumatoid disease of the cervical spine, when it can represent instability of the vertebrae. Instead, the noise comes from normal mechanical motion of the vertebrae. Patients may become more aware of these sounds or feelings, by either focusing on their pain or being more aware of their bodies when depressed or under stress. Neck pain can be quite variable throughout the day, depending on activity and mood.

Psychologic features may be closely linked to neck pain. Some persons who suffer from high anxiety or tension states present with muscle trigger points in the neck and shoulder, "cracking" joints, and overreactive behavior. A patient with an anxiety or depressive state and neck pain will often exaggerate symptoms.

Physical Examination

During the physical examination, focus your attention on the neck, occiput, and arms. Test the range of neck motion in flexion, extension, rotation, and side-bending, to establish the degree of limitation and the movements that cause pain. Press the top of your patient's head gently down into the shoulders; increased pain down an arm suggests root compression. Then carefully palpate the neck anteriorly and posteriorly, check-

Table 33.2.
Pattern Groups of Whiplash Symptoms

Neck and Head Pattern	General Pattern	Lower Cervical Pattern
Headache	Irritability	Neck pain
Tiredness	Hearing problems	Tiredness
Dizziness	Forgetfulness	Arm pain
Vision problems	Anxiety	Paresthesia

ing for lymphadenitis, muscle spasm, and tender areas of muscle or bone. Palpate the region of each cervical facet joint, approximately 1 inch lateral to the cervical spinous process. Facet joint tenderness suggests injury, instability, or arthritis involving the facet.

Next examine both arms for neurologic deficits that would indicate injury to one or more cervical nerve roots. Check the power of major muscle groups and the sensation in each dermatome. Test the biceps (C-5 and C-6) and triceps (C-7) reflexes. Many patients have subjective pain or paresthesias in root distributions, but relatively few have objective neurologic findings. Subjective neurologic symptoms with a normal examination reflect referred pain from damaged soft tissue such as ligaments, facet joint capsules, or muscle. True radiculopathy, on the other hand, is confirmed clinically by specific neurologic deficits such as muscle weakness, atrophy, diminished tendon reflexes, and sensory loss (Table 33.3). Such findings suggest nerve root compression or myelopathy but can also occur transiently in severe sprains.

Rarely, spinal cord compression caused by a prolapsed disc or narrow spinal canal in the elderly will affect descending tracts. This causes upper motor neuron findings in the legs and, sometimes, neuropathy in the arms. In this case, there is spasticity in the legs with increased muscle tone, instead of flaccidity, and heightened rather than decreased deep tendon reflexes. There may be bladder or rectal dysfunction.

Another unusual but important condition is the thoracic outlet syndrome. This involves compression of the neurovascular bundle (brachial plexus, subclavian vessels) as it passes out

through the narrow space between the clavicle and first rib. Symptoms consist of pain and numbness down the arm as well as weakness. The syndrome occurs predominantly in women in their 20s and 30s. The symptoms can often be replicated by the following simple clinical maneuvers:

1. Have the patient sit upright and thrust the shoulders backward with hands on thighs; or
2. Abduct the arm to 180° and rotate it externally while the patient sits upright.

During both of these maneuvers, monitor the radial pulse and listen with a stethoscope over the supraclavicular area. A positive result is indicated by a reduced or absent pulse and/or a bruit heard in the clavicular area.

Laboratory Tests

Laboratory studies are indicated only when the history and physical examination suggest systemic disease, inflammatory arthritis or bone damage (e.g., fever, symptoms in other organs, or severe trauma). As most problems (including prolapsed intervertebral disc) improve within 4 weeks, expensive tests are not worth doing in the initial evaluation phase unless surgery is being considered. However, if there is deterioration, persistent pain, disability, or weakness for more than 3 weeks in a patient over age 40, erythrocyte sedimentation rate, blood count, radiographs, and possibly calcium studies should be ordered. Radiographs are useful for detecting bony metastases, Paget's disease, myeloma, and ankylosing spondylitis. Computed tomography (CT) scanning and magnetic resonance imaging (MRI) are much more useful but costly tools in diagnosing nerve root compression, disc disease, and other soft tissue pathology in the neck. MRI is the study of choice in evaluating disc prolapse, but an additional CT scan or myelogram may be needed to clarify a difficult diagnosis.

Radiographs of the neck area should include anteroposterior, lateral, and oblique views to show the foramina of the vertebrae. It is useful to request views in flexion and extension to show how vertebra are positioned relative to each other. These views can sometimes show considerable sliding of one vertebra on another. However, because of the quite rapid process of spine degeneration, even in healthy people, the results of these studies are often nonspecific with the same

Table 33.3.
Neurologic Findings Associated with Cervical Nerve Root Lesions

Roots	Motor Weakness	Sensory Loss
C-4	Shoulder abductors	Shoulder
C-5	Elbow flexors	
	Diminished biceps/ brachioradialis reflex	Lateral arm
C-6	Wrist extensors	Thumb/index fingers
C-7	Elbow extensors	Middle ring finger
C-8	Intrinsic hand muscles	Little finger
T-1	Finger flexors	Medial arm

problems of sensitivity and specificity noted for low back pain (Chapter 31, Low Back Pain). For example, at age 50, half of the population has radiologic evidence of degenerative arthritis. This increases to 85% at age 65. In whiplash injuries, studies show that radiographs have a low yield if the patient is alert and has only moderate pain immediately after the crash (5). However, medicolegal concerns tend to pressure clinicians to order imaging studies early in the process.

If entrapment neuropathy (e.g., carpal tunnel syndrome) is suspected as the cause of arm pain or sensory disturbance, the results of electromyogram and nerve conduction studies may be abnormal. These tests can also help to confirm nerve root compression syndromes, although their sensitivity is poor.

MANAGEMENT

A number of simple therapeutic modalities, such as ice or heat, analgesics, and rest, are used to manage the majority of neck pain problems. Because the most common conditions causing pain (degenerative arthritis of the cervical spine, muscle spasm, and minor trauma) are usually self limited, therapy is directed toward reassuring and supporting the patient, relieving pain, reducing mechanical stresses, and relieving muscle spasm. There are few data from clinical trials that help the clinician identify the most effective treatments (6). Therefore, you should try various approaches, based on the severity and chronicity of the pain, patient preferences, and the cost of treatment. Recommendations for the management of common neck problems are outlined in Table 33.4. Findings of persistent or progressive neurologic deficit, systemic bony disease or bony destruction on physical evaluation should lead to neurologic, orthopedic, or neurosurgery consultation.

Initial Care

Acute injuries should be treated with ice every 4 hours and rest for 24 to 48 hours, followed by a gentle exercise/mobilization program. Subsequently, supportive management, such as moist heat, helps promote muscle relaxation. Heat can be applied with a heating pad, by taking a warm bath (15 to 20 minutes), or with a Hydrocollator pack. A soft collar, positioned round the neck to produce the least pain, allows the cervical muscles to relax by limiting head motion by 20%, although no data exist to support its effectiveness. For patients with chronic severe neck pain or injury, a molded plastic collar (Philadelphia brace) may be necessary. It can decrease neck motion by 75% and can be worn for several months (4).

For relief of pain and inflammation, a variety of drugs can be used (see Chapter 18, Arthritis and Rheumatism). Aspirin or acetaminophen is usually sufficient for pain relief. For severe pain, particularly at night, an opiate such as codeine or oxycodone may be necessary. Any of the nonsteroidal anti-inflammatory drugs (NSAIDs) may also be tried. Muscle relaxants have no proven benefit beyond their sedative effects, and these agents have side effects. Patients taking muscle relaxants should take extra care when they drive.

For whiplash injuries, evaluation and treatment can be based on the grade of the injury (Table 33.5). There is no close relationship between symptoms and the degree of impact in minor to moderate crashes (up to 25 mph). One should follow clinical findings in planning evaluation and treatment. Patients with neurologic signs need adequate pain relief and intensive rehabilitation.

Table 33.4.
Management of Common Neck Problems

	Physical Measures	Medication
Degenerative disc and joint disease	Heat, exercises	Aspirin, NSAID[a]
Muscle spasm	Relaxation techniques, massage, heat, stress management	Aspirin, acetaminophen, muscle relaxants
Traumatic sprain	Rest, ice, cervical collar	Aspirin, acetaminophen
Myofascial syndromes	Deep massage, injection therapy, relaxation techniques	Muscle relaxants
Facet joint asymmetry	Rest, mild traction, spinal manipulation	Aspirin, acetaminophen, NSAID

[a]A nonsteroidal anti-inflammatory drug.

Table 33.5.
Management of Whiplash

Grades	Radiograph	CT Scan	Average Time to Full Activity	Analgesics	PT/Exercises
Grade 1: neck pain, stiffness tenderness, no physical signs	−	−	Immediate	None	Self Home care
Grade 2: neck pain and musculoskeletal signs	+	−	1wk	NSAID Nonnarcotics	Self-care/referral
Grade 3: neck pain and neurologic signs	+	±	3+ wk	Narcotics	Referral to physical therapy
Grade 4: neck pain and fracture/dislocation	+	+	6+ wk	Narcotics	Long-term management; neurosurgery referral

Persistent Neck Pain

In treating persistent or chronic neck pain, intermittent traction is sometimes helpful. Its potential value as treatment can be assessed clinically by anchoring the mandible with both hands and stretching the head upward on the neck, trying out different angles for optimal relief. If this maneuver relieves the pain, a course of standard traction therapy may be useful. This can be done in a physical therapy department or, more economically, using a home traction kit obtainable from the local drug store. The traction force should start at approximately 10 lbs., moving up to between 15 and 20 lbs. for 15 minutes three times daily. In a few patients, traction makes the pain worse and should be discontinued after a brief trial. Continuous traction is rarely indicated but is given to some patients suffering from intractable pain. This must be done in the hospital, and then only for a period of 3 to 4 days. Again, this treatment is empiric, and the mechanism is unknown, but some patients will respond well.

Increasingly, mobilization and spinal manipulation are being used to treat chronic neck pain and prevent recurrence of symptoms. Mobilization involves careful and gentle movement of the neck through its physiologic range of motion, often using gentle traction with the hands. Manipulation moves a specific joint to its anatomic limits, with the final movement being a short, high-velocity thrust. It is performed by many different kinds of health providers; osteopaths and chiropractors are most commonly trained in this procedure. Although its efficacy is not well supported by controlled studies, patients often report that manipulation relieves pain and spasm. Neurologic symptoms, including stroke, can occur but are rare following manipulation; they usually result from injury to the vertebrobasilar artery.

Early mobilizing exercises have been shown in randomized studies to be of benefit in speeding recovery. Stretching and strengthening exercises are also helpful, particularly in the late recovery phase. To prevent recurrence, exercise should be included in most neck rehabilitation programs. Figure 33.1 outlines several neck exercises.

Local injections of lidocaine and/or steroids (see Chapter 18, Arthritis and Rheumatism) are also commonly used to treat acute neck pain, particularly if a muscle trigger point is identifiable. If the procedure is directed to the facet joint, it should only be undertaken below the third cervical disc level to avoid the vertebrobasilar artery as it winds up to the occiput.

Despite a wide array of interventions for neck pain, a recent meta-analysis of 24 randomized controlled studies reviewing manipulation, medication, physical therapy, acupuncture, and patient education interventions showed almost no evidence to support single or multiple modalities in treatment (6). Thus, the clinician is currently left with little scientific data to guide management strategies. When counseling the patient about management options it is best to try the most economic and easily accessible empiric remedies first.

CHRONIC NECK PAIN SYNDROMES

Some patients develop chronic neck pain syndromes that do not respond to the usual therapeutic modalities. These syndromes are often

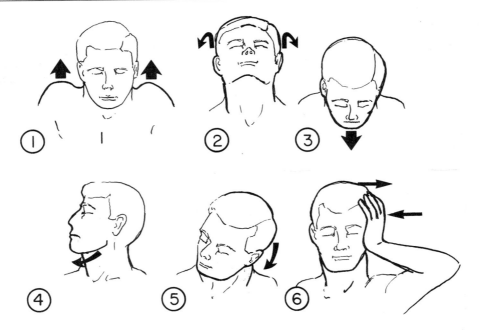

Figure 33.1. *Neck exercises.* **1.** For relaxation, hunch your shoulders up high. **2.** Bend your head backward as far as you can, so you can see the ceiling directly above your head. **3.** Gradually bend your head forward to touch your chin to your chest. **4.** Turn your head to the right, trying to bring your chin over your right shoulder. **5.** Try to bring your left ear down to your left shoulder. **6.** Place your left hand against the left side of your head. Push your head against the heel of your palm without allowing it to move. Hold.

associated with environmental stress, emotional illness, or personality disorders, and are very difficult to manage. They may require alternative methods of pain relief such as transcutaneous nerve stimulation, biofeedback, acupuncture, hypnosis, or referral to a psychologist, psychiatrist, or pain clinic. A small number of patients with intractable pain or progressing neurologic deficits may be considered for surgery, but this is usually considered only after medical management has failed and symptoms have persisted for approximately 6 weeks. Surgical approaches include anterior and posterior discectomy, with or without fusion. This usually requires postoperative stabilization in a Philadelphia brace for about 6 weeks.

ASSESSING IMPAIRMENT

A number of patients with neck pain will have symptoms and dysfunction that prevent their return to work. In such cases, their primary care physician may become involved in the complicated and protracted process of disability assess-

ment. Disability is awarded by the Department of Health and Social Services based on evidence from the primary care physician, together with evaluations by orthopedists, neurosurgeons, and physicians specializing in disability assessment. If approved, disability payments are awarded based on the degree of dysfunction experienced by the patient, without taking into account the amount of pain suffered by the patient. There is a large official text that identifies, in great detail, the extent of disabilities (7). For example, neck dysfunction is generally assigned a 10 to 15% disability rating.

CASE STUDY

Ms. J, aged 22 years, was rear-ended while her automobile was stationary at a traffic light. The impact was mild (15 mph), and she did not go to the emergency room. Two days later she came to her physician's office because of severe neck stiffness, difficulty sleeping, and pain down the right arm. There was no previous history of neck problems. Examination revealed marked limitation of motion, very tender trapezius and sternomastoid muscles, but no obvious weakness. However, the biceps reflex was reduced in the right arm.

QUESTIONS

1. How should Ms. J be managed?
2. What is the probable diagnosis?

DISCUSSION

The details of the accident indicate that this was a mild whiplash injury, although the neurologic deficit is of concern. The clinical indication for imaging is weak, but it will probably be to Ms. J's advantage legally to have a baseline neck radiograph in the event that she develops arthritic changes later on. No other tests are worth doing at this stage. The pain can be managed by regular icing and analgesics such as acetaminophen or NSAIDs. Oxycodone could be used for 2 to 3 days if the pain is very severe. Ms. J may require 2 to 4 days off from work. She should be given a gentle home exercise program to start mobilizing the neck. If the situation is not greatly improved after 5 days, referral to a physical therapist would be helpful, with the express intent of the patient returning to work even with some continued pain. De-

layed return to work may lead to chronic illness behavior. Rechecking the patient in 2 to 5 days after the first visit is important to monitor the adequacy of pain relief, change in mobility, and neurologic findings. Referral to a neurosurgeon would be indicated only if the pain was unresponsive to treatment or there was a progressive weakness and sensory loss in the right arm. The patient should be told that the chances for full recovery are good, but that approximately 10 to 15% of persons may experience persistent symptoms for several months.

REFERENCES

1. Bland JH. Disorders of the Cervical Spine. Diagnosis and Medical Management. Philadelphia: WB Saunders, 1987.
2. Bonica JJ, Caillet R, Sola AE. General considerations of pain in the neck and upper limb. In: Bonica JJ, ed. Management of Pain. Philadelphia: Lea & Febiger, 1990: 812–847, 848–867.
3. Curtis P, Spanos A, Reid A. Persistent symptoms after whiplash injuries. Implications for prognosis and management. J Clin Rheumatol 1995;1:149–157.
4. Camins MB, O'Leary PF, eds. Disorders of the Cervical Spine. Baltimore: Williams & Wilkins, 1992.
5. Quebec Task Force. Scientific monograph of the Quebec task force on whiplash-associated disorders. Spine 1995;20:2S–68S.
6. Aker PD, Gross AR, Goldsmith H, Peloso P. Conservative management of mechanical neck pain: systematic overview and meta-analysis. Br Med J 1996; 313:1291–1296.
7. American Medical Association. Guide to the Evaluation of Permanent Impairment, 3rd ed. Chicago: American Medical Association, 1990.

34. Prostate Diseases

JOHN M. HICKNER AND JULIE P. GRUBB

Key Clinical Questions

1. Does screening for prostate cancer reduce morbidity and mortality?
2. Does treatment of localized prostate cancer improve survival?
3. What factors should you take into consideration when making benign prostatic hyperplasia (BPH) treatment decisions?
4. Describe the diagnosis and treatment of each of the four types of prostatitis.

Although prostate disease is a common cause of morbidity and mortality among older men, it is not clear that screening for disease improves the quality or quantity of patient's lives. Similarly, treatment of conditions such as prostate cancer and benign prostatic hyperplasia (BPH) may not result in reduced morbidity and mortality, or it may involve a tradeoff of one for the other. Therefore, a careful discussion of the patient's goals is integral to the evaluation and management of prostate disease.

Prostate Cancer

Prostate cancer is the most common cancer in American men and the second leading cause of death from cancer, accounting for about 41,000 deaths in 1996 (1). Prostate cancer is more prevalent in black men than in white men and is diagnosed at later stages in black men. The prevalence of prostate cancer increases directly with age; it is rarely diagnosed in men under age 50. Whereas the cause of prostate cancer is unknown, tumor growth is under hormonal influence. In general, prostate cancer is a slow-growing tumor, with an average doubling time of 4 to 5 years. Autopsy studies of men dying from other causes reveal asymptomatic prostate cancer in 15 to 25% of men aged 50 to 59 years old, 20 to 30% in men aged 60 to 69 years old, 30 to 45% in men aged 70 to 79 years old, and more than 50% in men over 80 (2). A man's lifetime risk of having any form of prostate cancer (including asymptomatic) is

40%; the risk of developing clinical disease is 10%; and the risk of dying from prostate cancer is 3% (2). Therefore, only one of 15 men who have any form of prostate cancer will die from it. Nonetheless, because of its high prevalence, prostate cancer is still a major cause of morbidity and mortality. The challenge of effective screening is therefore to develop protocols that will identify those at high risk of dying and treat them appropriately, to avoid subjecting those who have benign disease to medical and surgical interventions that may cause injury, and to do both in a cost-effective manner.

The prognosis from prostate cancer varies inversely with the stage at which it is detected and with the degree of cellular atypia (or "grade") as rated by the Gleason system (3). The TNM system (tumor, nodes, metastases) is commonly used to stage many cancers including prostate cancer. Definitions for the Gleason system for histology and the TNM system for staging prostate cancer are given in Table 34.1. Alternative and commonly used methods of classifying stage (A to D), and tumor grade (1, 2, or 3) are noted as well. The 10-year disease-specific survival rate[1] for men with prostate-confined tumors (T0 or T1) with grade 1 histology (Gleason 2 to 4) is above 90% regardless of treatment, including expectant management. Survival for men with prostate-confined grade 2 (Gleason 5 to 7) tumors is about 80%, but survival for prostate-confined grade 3 (Gleason 8 to 10) tumors is only 45 to 65% (4). The average 10-year disease-specific survival for locally invasive tumors of all histologic grades is about 60% (4).

Prostate cancer is asymptomatic in its early stages. Larger tumors may cause obstructive symptoms indistinguishable from benign

---

[1]Patients dying of all causes are included in overall mortality rates, whereas only those dying of the disease, prostate cancer in this case, are included in the disease-specific rate. Disease-specific mortality is always less than overall mortality, and there can be a significant difference between the two. For example, one investigator found the 10-year disease-specific mortality for localized prostate cancer to be 15%, whereas the overall mortality was 62%. Overall mortality is the more important of the two outcomes *for patients*, although disease-specific mortality more directly compares the effectiveness of treatments.

Table 34.1.
Staging Classifications for Prostate Cancer

Alphabetic Staging System (American Urological Association)

A Tumor clinically unsuspected
B Palpable prostate nodule
C Locally invasive tumor
D Metastatic

American Joint Committee on Cancer Staging[a]

(TNM system—tumor has a descriptor for each numeral)

T0 Tumor discovered incidentally at prostatectomy
T1 Nodule with surrounding normal prostate tissue
T2 Large or multiple nodules, limited to prostate
T3 Tumor invasion through the prostate capsule
T4 Tumor invasion into surrounding tissue

N0 No positive pelvic lymph nodes
N1 Single positive pelvic lymph node (2 cm or less)
N2 Single large pelvic node (>2 cm but <5 cm) or multiple positive nodes
N3 Positive pelvic nodes greater than above

M0 No distant metastases
M1 Distant metastases or positive lymph nodes outside the pelvis

Histologic grading of prostate cancer[b]

Grade 1 Gleason score 2–4, low grade
Grade 2 Gleason score 5–7, moderate grade
Grade 3 Gleason score 8–10, high grade

[a]American Joint Committee on Cancer. Manual for Staging of Cancer, 4th ed. Philadelphia: JB Lippincott, 1992.

[b]Gleason DF, Mellinger GT. Prediction of prognosis for prostatic adenocarcinoma by combining histologic grading and clinical staging. J Urol 1974;111:58–64.

prostatic hyperplasia. The most common sites for metastases include bone and pelvic lymph nodes. In fact, the first symptom of prostate cancer may be bone pain from bony metastases or unilateral lymphedema of the leg from pelvic lymph node metastases. About 30% of men will have distant metastases at the time of diagnosis, whereas another 30% will have tumor spread to lymph nodes or locally invasive disease. The lack of symptoms in patients with early prostate cancer and the poor prognosis for advanced stages of disease make the arguments to screen for early disease compelling. The majority of prostate cancers detected in screening programs are clinically localized tumors. However, because of the slow growth rate of prostate cancer, the morbidity and mortality of aggressive treatment, and the lack of an ideal test, screening for prostate cancer is controversial.

SCREENING FOR PROSTATE CANCER

Tests currently used to screen for prostate cancer include the digital rectal examination (DRE), prostate-specific antigen (PSA), and transrectal ultrasound (TRUS). Some proponents advocate yearly PSA and DRE as the initial screening tests in men age 50 and over, followed by transrectal ultrasound-guided multiple-needle biopsies for patients with positive results. Although each of these tests can detect asymptomatic prostate cancer, none are proven to fulfill generally accepted criteria for an effective screening test (5). It is important to be familiar with the empiric evidence regarding accuracy of these screening tests in order to offer patients an informed choice.

Estimates of likelihood ratios for DRE and PSA are given in Table 34.2 (6). The true test characteristics are unknown. Calculation of the true sensitivity, specificity, and negative predictive value requires that the outcome (disease or no disease) be known for all screened individuals. For prostate cancer, that would require multiple prostate biopsies and histologic examination on all men screened; such a trial has not been done and is not likely to occur. Therefore, estimates of sensitivity, specificity, and negative predictive value for DRE and PSA vary widely depending

Table 34.2.

Test Characteristics of the PSA and Digital Rectal Examination for the Detection of Prostate Cancer[a]

	Sensitivity	Specificity	LR+	LR−
Digital rectal examination				
Intracapsular tumor	0.21	0.88	1.7 (1.5–2.0)	0.89 (0.83–0.96)
Extracapsular tumor	0.45	0.92	5.6 (2.7–8.6)	0.62 (0.53–0.72)
Prostate-specific antigen				
Intracapsular tumor				
<4.0 ng/mL	—	—	—	0.84 (0.70–0.98)
4.1–10	0.26	0.88	2.2 (1.4–3.0)	—
>10	0.33	0.81	1.7 (0.4–3.0)	—
Extracapsular tumor				
<4.0 ng/mL	—	—	—	0.30 (0.09–0.50)
4.1–10	0.76	0.82	4.1 (3.2–5.1)	—
>10	0.73	0.98	36 (23.7–49.6)	—

[a]The likelihood ratios are from Coley, et al. Early detection of prostate cancer, Part 1: prior probability and effectiveness of tests. Ann Intern Med 1997;126:394–406. They are based on Coley's review of the literature. Midpoints of the range they report are shown. The sensitivities and specificities are "back-calculated" from the likelihood ratios, using the midpoints of the likelihood estimates. Therefore, the sensitivities and specificities should be considered rough estimates.

on study methods, the population screened, and the method of ascertaining disease.

Positive predictive value (PPV) is the proportion of those individuals screening positive who have the disease. Because patients with positive screening tests are subjected to biopsies, estimates of PPV are likely to be reasonably stable and accurate. However, even needle biopsy may give false-negative results. One study noted that 19% of patients with an abnormal screening test had an initial negative needle biopsy and a subsequent positive biopsy (7).

Digital Rectal Examination (DRE)

Abnormal findings on digital rectal examination of the prostate that suggest prostate cancer include significant asymmetry and hard nodules. Estimates of the sensitivity of DRE for detecting prostate cancer in asymptomatic men vary widely from 18 to 68% (5). The reported positive predictive value ranges from 6 to 33% (5). In a urologic clinic case series, 4,160 DREs were performed on 2,131 men over 45 years old during a 6-year period (8). A prostate biopsy for abnormal findings was performed on 144 men, and 36 malignant tumors were detected, a positive predictive value of 25%. The estimate of sensitivity of 26% used transrectal ultrasound as the diagnostic standard. True sensitivity has not been determined for reasons noted previously and is probably somewhat lower.

Prostate-Specific Antigen (PSA)

Prostate-specific antigen is a glycoprotein produced by normal, hyperplastic, and cancerous prostate tissue. Normal levels of serum PSA are below 4.0 ng/mL, and there is a slight age-related increase in men without prostate cancer or prostatitis (9). Whereas serum PSA is not significantly affected by digital rectal examination of the prostate (10), benign prostatic hyperplasia, prostatitis, and prostate cancer all can cause significant serum elevations of PSA. Despite considerable overlap, mean PSA values are generally greater for prostate cancer, and several studies have demonstrated the ability of PSA to identify asymptomatic men at high risk of prostate cancer. Estimates of the sensitivity of PSA range from 30 to 80%, but these values come from urologic clinics and volunteer screening programs, and their applicability to a general population is not known (11–15). The best current estimates of PSA test characteristics are derived from the longitudinal Physicians Health Study (11). The sensitivity of a single abnormal PSA measurement (>4.0 ng/mL) was 73% for a 4-year follow-up period, and the specificity was 91%. Further refinements of PSA testing have been proposed, including age-adjustment (9), change in PSA value with time (PSA "velocity") (13), PSA corrected for prostate volume as judged by TRUS (PSA "density") (12–14), and free PSA measurement for PSA values of 2.6 to

4.0 ng/mL (14). A recent study suggested that if you choose to use PSA for screening, the appropriate interval is 2 years rather than annually, at least for men with a PSA value less than 2.0 (14).

Transrectal Ultrasound (TRUS)

Transrectal ultrasound has been evaluated in several case series, usually in combination with DRE and/or PSA (15–19). Because of the cost, inconvenience for the patient, and very low positive predictive value when PSA and DRE are negative, TRUS is not recommended as an initial screening test. It is used as a second-line test to guide prostate biopsies when the PSA is abnormal and to enhance the accuracy of PSA by determining the PSA density (12, 14).

Limitations of Screening Tests for Prostate Cancer

Prostate cancer diagnosed by screening with PSA and DRE is discovered at an earlier stage than in unscreened patients (19), but although early detection is intuitively attractive, its value to patients is unknown. Because of the many possible sources of bias in uncontrolled studies, conclusive evidence that screening reduces mortality or morbidity (i.e., helps patients live longer or better) requires a randomized trial. Such trials are underway, but results will not be available until approximately the year 2005.

Evidence for Screening

Proponents for screening argue that prostate cancer is common, the prognosis for advanced disease is poor regardless of treatment, and the prognosis is much better for small, localized tumors. Screening with PSA does detect small tumors that are potentially curable. Moreover, because current screening tests are not sensitive enough to detect small, clinically insignificant tumors (such as those discovered incidentally at autopsy), most of the tumors detected will be clinically significant. Although some men will have tumors detected and treated unnecessarily, on balance deaths will be prevented by screening. Although proponents concede that only a randomized trial will prove the benefit or lack of benefit of screening, they believe there is sufficient evidence to recommend screening at this time. Although there are significant side effects of treatment such as incontinence and impo-

tence, proponents argue that techniques for surgical and radiation therapy for prostate cancer are improving steadily, lowering the morbidity and mortality of treatment.

Evidence Against Screening

Skeptics of screening argue that there is no conclusive evidence that screening will do more good than harm. Although the lifetime risk of developing prostate cancer is about 40%, only 3% of men die of the disease. Even assuming that most prostate cancers would be diagnosed at an early stage by screening and assuming a favorable prognosis with treatment for 90% of these men, less than one in 10 would have improved survival from early detection. In fact, when the investigation and treatment that follow a positive test are considered, a policy of screening may actually increase morbidity and mortality. Two decision analyses that considered quality-adjusted survival in a screened versus an unscreened cohort of men found no advantage for the screened group (20, 21). One commentator has compared the current situation regarding prostate cancer screening to the early enthusiasm for lung cancer screening with chest radiography: despite early enthusiasm, subsequent randomized trials showed no benefit (22). On the other hand, breast cancer screening with mammography was initially unproven but has ultimately been shown to save lives.

Current Screening Recommendations

In 1997, the American Cancer Society and the American Urological Society recommended annual screening for prostate cancer of men 50 and older with DRE and PSA. In 1996, the American Academy of Family Physicians recommended that physicians counsel men age 50 to 65 about the "known risks and uncertain benefits of screening for prostate cancer" (25). The U.S. Preventive Services Task Force (USPSTF) and the American College of Physicians (24) currently do not recommend routine screening for prostate cancer. In its summary statement, the USPSTF (5) states:

Routine screening for prostate cancer with DRE, serum tumor markers (e.g., PSA), or TRUS is not recommended ("D" recommendation). Patients who request screening should be given objective information about the potential benefits and harms of early de-

tection and treatment. Patient education materials that review this information are available. If screening is to be performed, the best-evaluated approach is to screen with DRE and PSA and to limit screening to men with a life expectancy greater than 10 years. There is currently insufficient evidence to determine the need and optimal interval for repeat screening or whether PSA thresholds must be adjusted for density, velocity, or age.

Because of the lack of conclusive evidence for screening, testing for prostate cancer should only take place in situations that allow adequate discussion of the possible risks and benefits. This is best accomplished in a clinical consultation with a physician knowledgeable in prostate cancer screening such as a family physician, internist, or urologist.

TREATMENT OF PROSTATE CANCER

Localized Prostate Cancer

The dilemma of screening is compounded by uncertainty regarding the best treatment for early prostate cancer when it is discovered. Although a large randomized trial is underway (30), only epidemiologic data and comparisons of case series are currently available to guide decision making (4, 25–29). Three treatment regimens are available for localized prostate cancer: surgery, radiation therapy, and expectant management (expectant management or "watchful waiting" includes monitoring tumor progression and treating only in cases of advancing disease.) No experimental trials have directly compared these three strategies.

Table 34.3 lists 10-year survival rates for localized prostate cancer treated by prostatectomy, radiation therapy, and conservative management from the Surveillance, Epidemiology, and End Re-

Table 34.3.

Ten-Year Disease-Specific Survival in Patients with Clinically Localized Prostate Cancer (by Histologic Grade and by Treatment)

	% Survival (95% Confidence Interval [CI])		
	SEER[a]	PORT[b]	AUA[c]
All Grades			
Radical prostatectomy	83 (81–84)	91 (88–93)	90 (88–92)
Radiation therapy	76 (74–78)	79 (74–90)	67 (59–67)
Conservation management	82 (81–84)	91 (87–94)	87 (81–93)

	N	% Survival (95% CI)	
Grade 1			
Prostatectomy	3,854	94 (91–95)	
Radiotherapy	4,065	90 (87–92)	
Conservative	9,804	93 (91–94)	
Grade 2			
Prostatectomy	14,287	87 (85–89)	
Radiotherapy	7,939	76 (72–79)	
Conservative	6,198	77 (74–80)	
Grade 3			
Prostatectomy	5,133	67 (62–71)	
Radiotherapy	2,596	53 (47–58)	
Conservative	2,236	45 (40–51)	

[a]SEER Database. Data are from Lu-Yao GL, Yao SL. Population-based study of long-term survival in patients with clinically localised prostate cancer. Lancet 1997;349:906–910.

[b]Prostate Disease Patient Outcomes Research Team. Data are from Fleming C, Wasson JH, Albertsen PC, et al. A decision analysis of alternative treatment strategies for clinically localized prostate cancer. JAMA 1993;269:2650–2658.

[c]American Urological Association. Data are from Wasson JH, Reda DJ, Bruskewitz RC, Elinson J, Keller AM, Henderson WG. A comparison of transurethral surgery with watchful waiting for moderate symptoms of benign prostatic hyperplasia. N Engl J Med 1995;332:75–79.

sults (SEER) database (59,876 patients), and from two meta-analyses (4, 25, 30). Survival for prostatectomy and conservative management appear nearly the same. Survival with radiation therapy appears worse, but this probably reflects the fact that less-healthy patients were more likely to receive radiation. As summarized in Table 34.3, survival is highly dependent on histologic grade. Men with grade 1 tumors (Gleason 2 to 4) have excellent 10-year survival regardless of treatment; men with grade 2 histology (Gleason 5 to 7) appear to have better survival with prostatectomy; and men with grade 3 histology have a worse prognosis overall but better survival with prostatectomy compared to radiation therapy and conservative management. However, a decision analysis that considered the adverse outcomes as well as the benefits of treatment found that prostatectomy or radiation therapy may benefit only younger men with high-grade tumors (31).

Until the results of randomized trials are available, treatment decisions must be individualized after a careful discussion of the potential risks and benefits. Currently available data suggest that for localized grade 1 prostate cancer, no strategy is clearly the best; patient preference must guide therapy. For grade 2 tumors, surgery or radiation therapy may have a slight advantage over watchful waiting. For grade 3 tumors, surgery appears to have clear advantage. All of these recommendations may change with better data from randomized trials.

Advanced Prostate Cancer

Survival from prostate cancer that has spread beyond the capsule is worse than survival from localized prostate cancer of a similar histologic grade. Estimated 10-year disease-specific survival is about 40% with lymph node involvement (2). However, even metastatic disease may have a fair prognosis if the histologic grade is low. Hormonal therapy is used for palliation of metastatic disease, and radiation therapy can be useful for palliation of bony metastases.

Benign Prostatic Hyperplasia

PATHOPHYSIOLOGY AND DIFFERENTIAL DIAGNOSIS

Benign prostatic hyperplasia (BPH) is benign enlargement of the prostate, which occurs as a part of the normal aging process. As the prostate grows in size, it puts pressure on the urethra and thereby creates resistance to urine flow. Although the cause of BPH is largely unknown, we do know that prostate growth is influenced by the presence of androgens and occurs in males as they age (32). Symptoms of BPH tend to wax and wane, and potential complications include acute and chronic urinary retention, renal failure, serious urinary tract infection, and bladder decompensation. It is not known whether there is a chance of spontaneous improvement or stabilization of symptoms with time, but this is an important question.

BPH is a common condition in men of all races and cultures, and it is responsible for the majority of urinary symptoms in men over age 50. A meta-analysis of autopsy data showed that by age 60, over 50% of men had pathologic BPH and by age 85, the prevalence was 90% (33). The differential diagnosis of BPH includes prostatitis, bladder tumor or calculus, neurogenic bladder, urethral stricture, and urethritis.

CLINICAL EVALUATION

History

Conditions that may simulate BPH must be considered. You should therefore ask the patient what medications he is taking and whether he has a history of UTI, prostatitis, or other urologic disease. If the patient reports painless hematuria or if pain is localized to the bladder or penis, consider bladder tumor or calculus. Consider the possibility of a neurogenic bladder if there are neurologic symptoms and if there is a history of recent sexual dysfunction. If your patient has urinary obstructive symptoms, be alert to a history of anticholinergic medications such as tricyclic antidepressants or older antihistamines (e.g., diphenhydramine). Finally, consider the possibility of urethral stricture if there is a history of urethral trauma, if the man has had prior urethral instrumentation, or if he has had gonorrhea.

BPH causes both obstructive and irritative symptoms. Common signs and symptoms include:

- Decreased force and caliber of urinary stream secondary to urethral compression;

- Hesitancy getting urinary stream started because the detrusor takes longer to generate the increased pressure needed to overcome the urethral resistance;

- Terminal dribbling and incomplete emptying because the detrusor is unable to sustain the increased pressure needed to fully empty the bladder;

- Urinary frequency because incomplete emptying results in shorter intervals between each void;

- Nocturia because the symptoms of frequency become more pronounced;

- Incontinence (not a common symptom) can occur in severe BPH when there may be overflow incontinence; and

- Hematuria at the initiation of the urinary stream is also sometimes associated with BPH.

The American Urological Association (AUA) Symptom Index is a checklist of seven simple questions and is the best available method of evaluating the severity of your patient's BPH (Table 34.4). In primary care, the AUA Symptom Index can be used to document whether your patient's BPH is getting worse over time, help you make management decisions, show your patient how severe his symptoms are compared with other men who have the condition, and monitor treatment effectiveness.

Table 34.4.
American Urological Association Symptom Checklist[a]

(CIRCLE THE ONE BEST ANSWER TO EACH QUESTION)

Questions	Never	<1 Time in 5	<1/2 the Time	About 1/2 the Time	>1/2 the Time	Almost Always
Over the past month, how often have you had the feeling that you didn't empty your bladder completely after you finished urinating?	0	1	2	3	4	5
Over the past month, how often have you had to urinate again less than 2 hours after you finished urinating?	0	1	2	3	4	5
Over the past month, how often have you found you stopped and started again several times when you urinated?	0	1	2	3	4	5
Over the past month, how often have you found it difficult to postpone urination?	0	1	2	3	4	5
Over the past month, how often have you had a weak urinary stream?	0	1	2	3	4	5
Over the past month, how often have you had trouble getting your urine stream started?	0	1	2	3	4	5
Over the past month, how many times have you averaged getting up to urinate from the time you went to bed at night until the time you got up in the morning?	None	One time	Two times	Three times	Four times	Five times

Total score: _____ (sum of 7 circled numbers)[b]

Modified from Barry MJ, et al. The American Urological Association Symptom Index for benign prostatic hyperplasia. J Urol 1992;148: 1549–1557.

[a]This checklist can be used to quantitate the severity of BPH symptoms and to follow patients over time. It is suggested that you date it and insert it in the patient's medical record.

[b]Key: 0–7, absent/mild symptoms; 8–19, moderate symptoms; 20+, severe symptoms.

Physical Examination

A directed physical examination for suspected prostatic hyperplasia should include the abdomen and rectum. On the abdominal examination, check for bladder distention due to outlet obstruction by palpating and percussing the lower abdomen. During the rectal examination, note the size, consistency, and shape of the prostate. Any area of firm induration is suggestive of malignancy. In BPH, the prostate typically feels large and rubbery. However, the size of the prostate does not necessarily correlate with the severity of the patient's BPH symptoms. Finally, assess the anal sphincter tone; this is decreased with a neurogenic bladder.

Laboratory Tests

Two laboratory tests are recommended for suspected BPH: urinalysis and serum creatinine. If there are greater than 4 WBC/HPF, you should consider cystitis or prostatitis in your differential diagnosis. If there are greater than 3 to 5 RBC/HPF, you should consider referring the patient for cystoscopy to rule out bladder cancer (see Chapter 25, Dysuria, for more information on the diagnosis and management of urinary tract infections). Serum creatinine is used to determine whether there is any renal insufficiency as a result of obstructive uropathy. If the serum creatinine is elevated, imaging studies of the upper urinary tract are recommended. There is insufficient evidence to recommend routine use of the serum PSA in men with BPH. PSA values are often similar in men with BPH and in those with organ-confined prostate cancer (34).

MANAGEMENT

Treatment of BPH is tailored to the AUA symptom severity score. Current management of BPH is in a period of transition away from surgery and toward medical management. Therefore, primary care physicians are now more involved in the decisions their patients with BPH face. Because treatment decisions in BPH are often unclear, you must be prepared to educate and support your patients through an often prolonged and/or repeated decision-making process. An algorithm for the management of BPH is shown in Figure 34.1, and the outcomes of the most common therapies are shown in Table 34.5.

The three general treatment options are watchful waiting, medical therapy, and surgery. Watchful waiting is recommended for men with mild symptoms, because 30 to 50% of men will experience spontaneous symptomatic improvement (35). It is important to remember that watchful waiting implies ongoing monitoring of symptoms; another assessment (including history, examination, urinalysis, creatinine) should be repeated in 1 year. A randomized controlled trial comparing watchful waiting with transurethral resection of the prostate (TURP) in patients with moderate symptoms found that 24% of men in the watchful waiting group had surgery within 3 years, and that there were fewer treatment failures in the TURP group after 3 years of follow-up (relative risk 0.48, 95% confidence interval [CI] 0.30 to 0.77). At the same time, more than two-thirds of the men in the watchful waiting group did well with that strategy (36).

If further intervention is being considered because of symptom progression as measured by the AUA Symptom Index, measurement of peak urine flow rate and bladder ultrasound for residual urine may help quantify the degree of obstruction (a flow rate of >15 mL/sec is normal, 10 to 15 mL/sec is borderline, and <10 mL/sec suggests significant obstruction). Most important, though, is the effect of symptoms on the patient's life; an improvement in the urinary flow rate without a concomitant improvement in symptoms is of little value.

Medical therapy is recommended for patients with moderate-to-severe symptoms. The choices are α-adrenergic blockers and 5-α-reductase inhibitors (37). α-Adrenergic blockers such as terazosin are also antihypertensive agents and are especially useful in men who have both BPH and hypertension. Avoid adverse side effects by starting with the lowest dose given at bedtime, then slowly titrate upward as needed for symptom relief.

Finasteride (Proscar), a 5-α-reductase inhibitor, prevents the production of the major intracellular androgenic metabolite within the prostate (38). This leads to gradual shrinkage of the prostate by an average of 20 to 30%; however, it may take 3 to 6 months before its effect is realized (36). Although approximately 50% of patients will have symptomatic improvement, recall that spontaneous improvement in symptoms occurs in 30 to 50% of patients. A double-blind, randomized, placebo-controlled trial showed no significant difference between finasteride and placebo (39). Table 34.6 lists the medications commonly used in BPH.

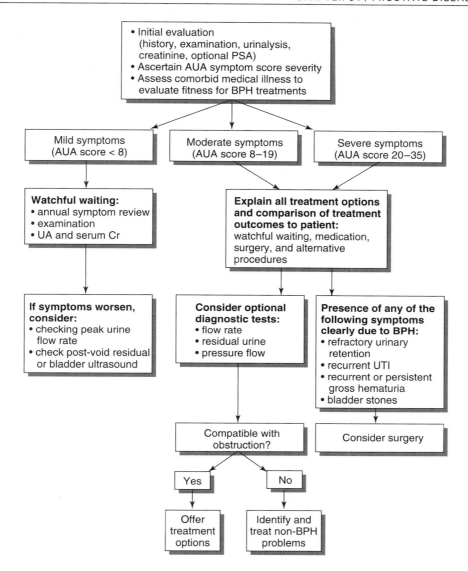

Figure 34.1. *Algorithm for management of benign prostatic hyperplasia.* (Modified from McConnell JD, et al. Benign Prostatic Hyperplasia: Diagnosis and Treatment. Clinical Practice Guideline, no. 8. AHCPR publication no. 94–0582. Rockville, MD: Agency for Health Care Policy and Research, Public Health Service, US Department of Health and Human Services, 1994.)

Surgery is also an option for patients with moderate-to-severe symptoms. Transurethral resection of the prostate (TURP) is the "gold standard" surgical procedure for BPH, and remains one of the most common surgeries reimbursed by Medicare. Good resolution of urinary symptoms occurs in 80 to 90% of patients at 1 year, although it decreases to 60 to 75% by 5 years, and 25% require repeat TURP within 10 years (36). Transurethral incision of the prostate (TUIP) and

open prostatectomy are other surgical options. Surgical complications include the risk of anesthesia, postoperative bleeding, inability to void, infection, pain, and possible sexual dysfunction.

Surgery may be indicated when BPH patients have:

- Refractory urinary retention and have failed at least one attempt at catheter removal

- Recurrent urinary tract infections due to BPH

Table 34.5.

Outcomes of Common Interventions for Benign Prostatic Hyperplasia

Treatment Outcomes	Nonsurgical Options			Surgical Options		
	Watchful Waiting	α Blockers	Finasteride	TURP	Open Surgery	TUIP
Chance that symptoms will improve	31–35%	59–86%	54–78%	75–96%	94–99.8%	78–83%
Expected amount of symptom improvement (for patients who improve)	Unknown	51%	31%	35%	79%	73%
Complications of treatment (20% of all complications assumed to be significant)	1–5% complications from BPH progression	3–43%	14–19%	5–31%	7–43%	2–33%
Likelihood of total urinary incontinence due to treatment	Incontinence associated with aging	0	0	0.7–1.4%	0.34–0.74%	0.06–1.1%
Likelihood of need to reoperate due to surgical complication	0	0	0	0.7–10.1%	0.6–14.1%	1.3–2.7%
Likelihood of impotence	About 2% of men over age 67 become impotent per year	Long-term data on α blockers not available	2.5–5.3% (also decreased volume of ejaculate)	3.3–34.8%	4.7–39.2%	3.9–24.5%
Likelihood that a patient will experience retrograde ejaculation following treatment	0	4–11%	0	25–99%	36–95%	6–55%
Number of days lost from work (estimated)	1	3.5	1.5	7–21	21–28	7–21
Hospitalized days (estimated)	0	0	0	3–5	5–10	1–3

Adapted from McConnell JD, et al. Benign Prostatic Hyperplasia: Diagnosis and Treatment. Clinical Practice Guideline, no. 8. AHCPR publication no. 94–0582. Rockville, MD: Agency for Healthcare Policy and Research, Public Health Service, US Department of Health and Human Services, 1994.

- Recurrent gross hematuria due to BPH
- Renal insufficiency due to BPH
- Bladder stones due to BPH

There is little evidence that other treatments are beneficial in relieving these complications. Alternative therapies should be considered if the patient refuses surgery or has an unacceptable surgical risk: these include prostatic balloon dilation, intraurethral stent, microwave thermopathy, and laser ablation. Although they are associated with less operative risk than TURP, they have unknown long-term efficacy. These interventions may be an option for men who are poor surgical risks and fail to respond to other methods.

Patient Education

You should educate your patient about BPH and the inherent medical uncertainties. Individual patients will vary both in their perception of treatment risk and how bothered they are by their symptoms. You can help your patient sort through the available therapies by taking account of the timeline of the patient's symptoms, their overall health status, and any relevant psychosocial issues. You should discuss the potential benefits and harms of each treatment option as well as the range of uncertainty associated with each. Reassessment of the AUA Symptom Index over time may be the best initial approach

Table 34.6.

Medications Commonly Used to Treat Benign Prostatic Hyperplasia

Medication	Dosage Range			Common Adverse Effects	Comment
	Starting	Maintenance	Maximum		
Terazosin (Hytrin)	1 mg hs	2–5 mg hs	10 mg hs	Orthostatic hypotension, dizziness, weakness, headaches	Dosing qd
Doxazosin (Cardura)	1 mg hs	2–4 mg qd	16 mg qd	As above	Dosing qd
Prazosin (Minipress)	1 mg hs	1–2 mg tid	5 mg tid	As above	Generic available
Finasteride (Proscar)	5 mg qd	5 mg qd	10 mg qd	Impotence, decreased libido	Shrinks prostate

for men with mild-to-moderate symptoms because many men with BPH do not experience worsening of symptoms, and some experience symptom improvement. Absolute indications for treatment of BPH include severe obstruction and urinary retention or renal insufficiency due to obstruction (40). In general, men with the most severe symptoms and the best overall health experienced the greatest benefit of TURP (41).

If a patient experiences symptom progression with medical therapy, it may be appropriate to reconsider surgical options. However, failure to respond to medical or alternative strategies is not an automatic indication for surgery. Some patients will elect to resume watchful waiting rather than accept the risks of surgery. Unfortunately, the medical literature lacks large randomized, controlled trials with long-term follow-up that compare medical and surgical therapy in similar patient populations. See Table 34.5 for a comparison of BPH treatments.

Prostatitis and Prostatodynia

Prostatitis is a relatively common complaint among men, and approximately 25 to 50% will have symptoms of prostatitis during their life (42). Four types of prostatitis are now recognized: acute bacterial prostatitis, chronic bacterial prostatitis, nonbacterial prostatitis, and prostatodynia. Men with acute bacterial prostatitis and chronic bacterial prostatitis have evidence of infection. In nonbacterial prostatitis, men have evidence of inflammation without infection, while with prostatodynia, men have prostatic symptoms but no evidence of inflammation or infection. Acute bacterial prostatitis is much less com-

mon than the other three types of prostatitis; however, the true incidence of the four types is not known (43).

Bacterial prostatitis is either acute or chronic. Either type is always associated with a urinary tract infection and is usually caused by the same type of gram-negative organisms responsible for urinary tract infections. *Escherichia coli* infections predominate, although *Pseudomonas aeruginosa*, *Klebsiella pneumoniae*, *Proteus mirabilis*, or the gram-positive organisms *Streptococcus faecalis* and *Staphylococcus aureus* are also known pathogens (44, 45). Bacterial prostatitis is thought to result from:

- Ascending urethral infection,
- Reflux of infected urine into the prostatic ducts,
- Direct invasion or lymphatic spread of rectal bacteria, or
- Hematogenous infection

A major difficulty of prostatitis syndromes is the lack of good randomized controlled studies and the relative paucity of good evidence to support the diagnosis and management of prostatitis. Table 34.7 summarizes prostatitis syndromes and their management.

ACUTE BACTERIAL PROSTATITIS

Acute bacterial prostatitis typically has a sudden, dramatic onset characterized by fever, chills, low-back or perineal discomfort, suprapubic discomfort, dysuria, urinary frequency or urgency, and in some cases, urinary retention. The pathogen in acute bacterial prostatitis is identified by urine culture. Treatment for 4 to 6 weeks with an oral

Table 34.7.

Features of the Four Prostatitis Syndromes

Diagnosis	Symptoms	Physical Examination	Laboratory Tests	Management
Acute bacterial prostatitis (least common)	Acute onset of fever, chills, dysuria, low frequency, low back, suprapubic, or perineal discomfort Possible urinary retention Sepsis possible	Prostate tender, boggy, often warm Avoid prostatic massage (risk of bacteremia)	Leukocytosis Pyuria Bacteriuria Occasional hematuria Positive urine culture Get blood cultures if suspect sepsis Consider doing gonorrhea/ *Chlamydia* cultures	Avoid urethral catheter. If systemically ill, hospitalize. Initial medication: ampicillin/ sulbactam (Unasyn) or ampicillin plus gentamycin Oral medications: TMP/SMX DS bid, or a fluoroquinolone (e.g., ciprofloxacin, ofloxacin); treat for 4–6 wks to prevent chronic bacterial prostatitis
Chronic bacterial prostatitis	More gradual onset Mild/moderate voiding symptoms Pain/discomfort in low back, lower abdomen, perineum, scrotum, penis, or thighs Hematospermia Painful ejaculation May complicate acute bacterial prostatitis	Prostate often minimally tender/ boggy, but can be normal Differential diagnosis: BPH, urethral stricture, bladder CA	Relapsing UTI Obtain urinalysis and urine culture Consider doing gonorrhea/ *Chlamydia* cultures Consider checking BUN/ creatinine	TMP/SMX DS Fluoroquinolones Medicate for up to 3 mo If symptoms recur, consider suppressive antibiotic therapy of TMP/SMX DS 1 tablet qd, or doxycycline 100 mg qd
Nonbacterial prostatitis	Similar to chronic bacterial prostatitis	Prostate normal or minimally tender May have mucoid penile discharge	Pyuria No bacteriuria Negative urine culture Consider getting gonorrhea/ *Chlamydia* cultures	If suspect chlamydia or ureaplasma, use doxycycline 100 mg bid × 2–4 wks, or erythromycin 500 mg qid × 2–4 wks Otherwise, use ibuprofen 600 mg qid Sitz baths, oxybutynin 2.5–5.0 mg tid or allopurinol 300–600 mg qd × 3 mo[a]
Prostatodynia	Pain/discomfort in penis/urethra or perineum, groin, testicles, low back, or suprapubic region May have frequency, urgency, or nocturia	Prostate can be normal or tender May have "tight" anal sphincter or tender periprostatic tissue	Normal UA and culture Consider doing gonorrhea/ *Chlamydia* cultures	Prazosin 1 mg hs × 1 wk then 1 mg bid × 1 wk, up to 2 mg bid to control symptoms Continue indefinitely for responders Sitz baths Treat anxiety and depression

(handwritten margin note: prostatitis symptoms s̄ evidence of infection or inflammation)

TMP/SMX, trimethoprim/sulfamethoxazole.

[a]Persson BE, Ronquist G, Ekblom M. Ameliorative effect of allopurinol on nonbacterial prostatitis: a parallel double-blind controlled study. J Urol 1996;155:961–964.

antibiotic is recommended to prevent the development of chronic bacterial prostatitis. Rarely, the patient may be systemically ill enough to require parenteral antibiotics; however, this is not a common presentation in primary care.

CHRONIC BACTERIAL PROSTATITIS

Chronic bacterial prostatitis is more subtle than acute prostatitis. Symptoms are similar but less dramatic; relapsing urinary tract infections are a characteristic finding. Most patients have mild-to-moderate voiding symptoms and/or pain or discomfort involving the low back, lower abdomen, perineum, scrotum, penis, or inner thighs. Hematospermia or painful ejaculation may be present. Chronic bacterial prostatitis can occur without there ever having been an episode of acute bacterial prostatitis. The pathogen in chronic bacterial prostatitis is thought to sustain itself in small, deep nests within the prostate, only to reemerge once the antibiotic is stopped. Once the urine is reinfected, the patient experiences recrudescence of his symptoms. Chronic suppressive therapy can be useful if symptoms continue to recur despite long antibiotic courses. In such cases, discontinuation of the suppression often leads to recurrence (45).

NONBACTERIAL PROSTATITIS

Nonbacterial prostatitis is probably the most common of the four types of prostatitis. It is an inflammatory condition of unknown etiology. There is controversy about whether *Chlamydia trachomatis* or *Ureaplasma urealyticum* may play a role in nonbacterial prostatitis. Men with nonbacterial prostatitis have symptoms that are much like chronic bacterial prostatitis with pyuria, but they do not have a documented urinary tract infection (UTI). The urologic literature focuses on the evaluation of prostatitis through the microscopic examination of expressed prostatic secretions and the first 10 mL of urine collected after prostatic massage. However, be forewarned that it is not unusual to be unsuccessful in your efforts to obtain prostatic secretions (40). One small randomized, double-blind controlled study showed an improvement in symptoms among patients with nonbacterial prostatitis given allopurinol, which reduces uric acid levels (46).

PROSTATODYNIA

Men with prostatodynia have prostatitis symptoms without evidence of infection or inflammation. The typical patient is young to middle-aged. They describe discomfort and pain that is often prominent in the penis and urethra but may also be perceived in the pelvic, perineal, and low-back regions. Some studies suggest that this may be a bladder neck/urethral spasm syndrome. α-Adrenergic receptors are present in the smooth muscle of the bladder neck and prostate. Accordingly, α-blockers can be effective in controlling prostatodynia symptoms (47). Chronic bacterial prostatitis, nonbacterial prostatitis, and prostatodynia can be more difficult to treat than acute bacterial prostatitis.

CASE STUDY

Mr. P. is 74 years old and complains that he has to urinate frequently during the day and usually awakens several times during the night to void. Despite having a strong urge to urinate, he finds it difficult to get his stream started and sometimes feels that he is not completely emptying his bladder. His symptoms interrupt his daily activities and prevent him from getting adequate rest at night. Mr. P.'s history, physical examination, urinalysis, and serum creatinine are otherwise normal. His AUA symptom score is 18 (moderate severity).

QUESTIONS

1. How bothered is Mr. P. by his BPH symptoms?
2. Which treatment options would you discuss with Mr. P?
3. How do you decide when you want Mr. P. to follow-up?

DISCUSSION

With an AUA symptom score of moderate severity, it would be best to describe all of the treatment options to Mr. P. You explain the waxing and waning nature of BPH symptoms and uncertainty about the potential for reversal vs. progression of symptoms. You also do your best to make sure Mr. P. has the information he needs to make his own best decision about what to do next. Although clearly bothered by his symptoms, he is glad to know where he fits on the continuum compared to other men and decides he would like a trial of an α-blocker at a low dose.

Next, you will have to decide how to titrate his α-blocker upward until symptoms are more livable for Mr. P. You should also educate him about possible medication adverse effects and what he should do if he develops one. For follow-up, you arrange to have him call you in 7 to 10 days to discuss whether to advance the dose of the α-blocker and plan for the next office visit. If Mr. P has a satisfactory result, you should set regular intervals for an interval history, physical examination, urinalysis, serum creatinine, and reassessment of his treatment options.

REFERENCES

1. Parker SL, Tong T, Bolden S, Wingo PA. Cancer Statistics, 1996. CA Cancer J Clin 1996;46:5–27.
2. Scardino, PT. Early detection of prostate cancer. Urol Clin North Am 1989;16:635–655.
3. Gleason DF, Mellinger GT. Prediction of prognosis for prostatic adenocarcinoma by combining histological grading and clinical staging. J Urol 1974;111:58–64.
4. Lu-Yao GL, Yao SL. Population-based study of long-term survival in patients with clinically localised prostate cancer. Lancet 1997;349:906–910.
5. US Preventive Services Task Force. Screening for prostate cancer. In: Guide to Clinical Preventive Services. Report of the US Preventive Services Task Force, 2nd ed. Baltimore: Williams & Wilkins, 1996:119–134.
6. Coley CM, Barry MJ, Fleming C, Mulley AG. Early detection of prostate cancer. Part 1: prior probability and effectiveness of tests. Ann Intern Med 1997;126:394–406.
7. Keetch DW, Catalona WJ, Smith DS. Serial prostatic biopsies in men with persistently elevated serum prostate-specific antigen values. J Urol 1994;151:1571–1574.
8. Chodak GW, Keller P, Schoenbert HW. Assessment of screening for prostate cancer using the digital rectal examination. J Urol 1989;141:1136–1138.
9. Oesterling JE, Jacobsen SJ, Chute CG, et al. Serum prostate-specific antigen in a community-based population of healthy men. JAMA 1993;270:860–864.
10. Crawford ED, et al. The effect of digital rectal exami-

nation on prostate-specific antigen levels. JAMA 1992;267:2227–2228.
11. Smith DS, Catalona WJ. The nature of prostate cancer detected through prostate-specific antigen-based screening. J Urol 1994;152:1732–1736.
12. Benson MC, Whang IS, Pantuck A, et al. Prostate-specific antigen density: a means of distinguishing benign prostatic hyperplasia and prostate cancer. J Urol 1992; 147:815–816.
13. Benson MC, Whang IS, Olsson CA, et al. The use of prostate-specific antigen density to enhance the predictive value of intermediate levels of serum prostate-specific antigen. J Urol 1992;147:817–821.
14. Catalona WJ, Smith DS, Ornstein DK. Prostate cancer detection in men with serum PSA concentrations of 2.6 to 4.0 ng/mL and benign prostate examination. JAMA 1997;277:1452–1455.
15. Chodak GW, Wald V, Parmer E, et al. Comparison of digital examination and transrectal ultrasonography for the diagnosis of prostatic cancer. J Urol 1986;135:951–954.
16. Lee F, Littrup PJ, Torp-Pedersen ST, et al. Prostate cancer: comparison of transrectal US and digital rectal examination for screening. Radiology 1988;168:389–394.
17. Babaian RJ, Mettlin C, Kane R, et al. The relationship of prostate-specific antigen to digital rectal examination and transrectal ultrasonography. Cancer 1992;69:1195–1200.
18. Mettlin C, Lee F, Drago J, et al. The American Cancer Society National Prostate Cancer Detection Project. Cancer 1991;67:2949–2958.
19. Catalona WJ, Smith DS, Ratliff TL, et al. Detection of organ-confined prostate cancer is increased through prostate-specific antigen-based screening. JAMA 1993;270:948–954.
20. Krahn MD, Mahoney JE, Eckman MH, et al. Screening for prostate cancer. JAMA 1994;272:773–780.
21. Cantor SB, Spann SJ, Volk RJ, et al. Prostate cancer screening: a decision analysis. J Fam Pract 1995;41:33–41.
22. Collins MM, Barry MJ. Controversies in prostate cancer screening. JAMA 1996;276:1976–1979.
23. American Academy of Family Physicians. Summary of policy recommendations for periodic health examination. Reprint no. 510. Kansas City: American Academy of Family Physicians, 1996.
24. American College of Physicians. Screening for prostate cancer. Ann Intern Med 1997;126:480–484.
25. Wasson JH, Cushman CC, Bruskewitz RC, et al. A structured literature review of treatment for localized prostate cancer. Arch Fam Med 1993;2:487–493.
26. Chodak GW, Thisted RA, Gerber GS, et al. Results of conservative management of clinically localized prostate cancer. N Engl J Med 1994;330:242–248.
27. Albertsen PC, Fryback DG, Storer BE, et al. Long-term survival among men with conservatively treated localized prostate cancer. JAMA 1995;274:626–631.
28. Gerber GS, Thisted RA, Scardino PT, et al. Results of radical prostatectomy in men with clinically localized prostate cancer. JAMA 1996;276:615–619.
29. Johansson JE, Holmberg L, Johansson S, et al. Fifteen-year survival in prostate cancer. JAMA 1997;277:467–471.
30. Middleton RG. The management of clinically localized

prostate cancer: guidelines from the American Urological Association. Ca Cancer J Clin 1996;46:249–253.

31. Fleming C, Wasson JH, Albertsen PC, et al. A decision analysis of alternative treatment strategies for clinically localized prostate cancer. JAMA 1993;269:2650–2658.

32. Ekman P. BPH epidemiology and risk factors. Prostate 1989;2(suppl):23–31.

33. Berry SJ, Coffey DS, et al. The development of human benign prostatic hyperplasia with age. J Urol 1984;132: 474–479.

34. Carter HB, et al. Longitudinal evaluation of PSA levels in men with and without prostate disease. JAMA 1992; 267:2215–2220.

35. Grayhack JT. Benign prostatic hyperplasia: the scope of the problem. Cancer 1992;70:275–279.

36. Hicks RJ, Cook JB. Managing patients with benign prostatic hyperplasia. Am Fam Physician 1995;52:135–142.

37. Monda JM, Oesterling JE. Medical treatment of benign prostatic hyperplasia: 5-α-reductase inhibitions and α-adrenergic antagonist. Mayo Clin Proc 1993:68;670–679.

38. Wilson JD. The intranuclear metabolism of testosterone in the accessory organs of reproduction. Recent Prog Horm Res 1970:26;309–336.

39. Lepor H, Williford WO, Barry MJ, et al. The efficacy of terazosin, finasteride, or both in benign prostatic hyperplasia. N Engl J Med 1996;335:533–539.

40. Hollander JB, Diokno AC. Prostatism: benign prostatic hyperplasia. Urol Clin North Am 1996;23:75–86.

41. Doll HA, Black NA, McPherson K. Transurethral resection of the prostate for benign prostatic hyperplasia: factors associated with a successful outcome at 1 year. Br J Urol 1994;73:669–80.

42. Lipsky BA. Urinary tract infections in men. Ann Intern Med 1989;110:138–150.

43. Brunner H, et al. Studies of the role of *Ureaplasma urealyticum* and *Mycoplasma hominis* in prostatitis. J Infect Dis 1983;147:807–813.

44. Weidner W. Prostatitis: diagnostic criteria, classification of patients, and recommendations for therapeutic trials. Infection 1992;20:S227-S231.

45. Meares EM Jr. Prostatitis. Med Clin North Am 1991; 75(2):405–425.

46. Persson BE, Ronquist G, Ekblom M. Ameliorative effect of allopurinol on nonbacterial prostatitis: a parallel double-blind controlled study. J Urol 1996;155: 961–964.

47. Meares EM Jr. Prostatitis: review of pharmacokinetics and therapy. Rev Infect Dis 1982;4:475–483.

35. Respiratory Tract Infections

PETER CURTIS

Key Clinical Questions

1. What upper respiratory problems among children and adults are most frequently seen in the office setting?
2. What are the indications for using antibiotics in upper respiratory disease?
3. What clinical factors indicate serious lower respiratory infection?

Infections of the respiratory tract are the leading cause of illness among children and adults. Upper respiratory tract infections are the most common acute problem seen by family physicians and cause the most days lost from school and work (1). Colds, upper respiratory infections (URI) and bronchitis account for 21 million office visits and 12 million antibiotic prescriptions each year (2, 3). One of the major challenges in current management is the often-unjustified prescribing of antibiotics for these infections and the development of drug-resistant organisms (4, 5). This chapter reviews the common infections of the upper and lower respiratory tract.

PATHOPHYSIOLOGY

The respiratory epithelium, along with the skin and the lining of the gastrointestinal tract, comprise a major interface between the human body and the external environment. The warm, humid environment of the respiratory tract is relatively hospitable to the growth of viruses and bacteria. Although respiratory infections are common, our body defenses, particularly the lymphatic system, usually keep them localized and self-limited.

The respiratory tract includes the mucosal surfaces of the nose, the paranasal sinuses, pharynx, eustachian tube, middle ear, epiglottis, larynx, trachea, bronchi, bronchioles, and alveoli. Clinically, we usually differentiate between the upper respiratory tract—all respiratory structures above the larynx—and the lower respiratory tract. Each of these areas, when inflamed or infected, presents with a clinical syndrome. However, there can be considerable overlap in symptoms and signs, all of which are the result of the inflammatory response, producing mucosal swelling, discharge (often purulent) and local pain.

CLINICAL EVALUATION

Patients with upper respiratory disorders need a brief focused history that should include details of prior episodes and treatment, other family members affected, risk factors, and smoking history. Awareness of "epidemics" of URI, influenza, and "strep" throat is useful in making decisions about testing and treatment. Presenting signs and symptoms by anatomic site are shown in Table 35.1.

History

Each of the common symptoms of respiratory disease is discussed briefly below:

- Fever is a nonspecific sign. However, both the level of fever and the pattern of its development can give clues to diagnosis. For example, upper respiratory infections ("colds") generally cause little or no fever. A patient with rhinitis who after several days develops a high fever probably has developed sinusitis, a secondary bacterial infection.

- Rhinorrhea is nasal discharge, either watery or purulent. It can be either infectious or noninfectious, since nasal respiratory epithelia produce mucus in response to any insult. Thus, hay fever (an allergy to airborne allergens), a foreign body in the nose, the common cold, and sinusitis can all present with rhinorrhea.

- Headache can arise from respiratory and nonrespiratory structures. Frontal headache, particularly if it is worsened by bending over, suggests sinusitis. Facial pain is another symptom of paranasal sinus disease, since portions of the sinuses, the ear, and the skin of the face are all supplied by the trigeminal nerve.

Table 35.1.
Presenting Signs and Symptoms of Respiratory Infections

Anatomic Site	Typical Presenting Signs and Symptoms	Common Diagnoses
Nose	Sneezing, rhinitis, nasal stuffiness, mild headache; fever (rare)	Common cold
Paranasal sinuses	Headache (either frontal or on top of the head), facial pain, dental pain; nasal discharge, fever; tenderness on percussion over the affected sinus	Sinusitis
Pharynx	Sore throat; swollen anterior cervical lymph nodes; redness, swelling, and exudate on examination; fever	Pharyngitis
Middle ear/eustachian tube	Earache, ear stuffiness, hearing loss, fever; bulging and loss of normal landmarks of tympanic membrane	Otitis media
Epiglottis	Abrupt onset of high fever, chills, sore throat, loss of voice, stridor, drooling	Epiglottitis
Larynx	Inspiratory stridor (children), hoarseness or loss of voice (adults), mild fever	Laryngitis
Trachea	Cough, low-grade fever (most infections are viral), tenderness on palpation of the trachea	Tracheitis
Bronchi	Cough, sputum production, wheezes and rhonchi, low-grade fever	Bronchitis
Bronchioles	Cough, dyspnea, wheezing, fever	Bronchiolitis
Alveoli	Cough, fever, dyspnea, chest pain, chills	Pneumonia

- Pain in the upper teeth and the eye can result from infection in the maxillary sinus, since the superior alveolar nerve passes through that sinus.

- Sore throat indicates pharyngitis. To review this symptom and its differential diagnosis, see Chapter 40.

- Earache can be caused by a variety of problems, some of which are respiratory in origin. In office practice, acute ear pain is common, and the differential diagnosis is often between otitis externa and otitis media. Ear pain can also be referred because the pharynx and portions of the external and middle ear are all supplied by the vagus nerve. Other causes of ear pain include inflammation of the preauricular or postauricular regional lymph nodes (usually secondary to a skin infection on the scalp or face), parotitis, and temporomandibular joint disorders.

- Cough is the cardinal symptom of lower respiratory tract disease (see Table 35.1). Any inflammatory disorder of the trachea, bronchi, bronchioles, or alveoli can cause cough because of inhibition of the mechanism for clearing secretions from the tracheobronchial tree and increased mucus (sputum) production. Cough also can occur in the absence of sputum production because the cough reflex is activated by any irritation of the trachea or bronchi. Influenza, mycoplasma, and viral infections are typified by nonproductive ("dry") cough. Degree of cough provides little indication of disease severity; many viral respiratory infections cause severe, persistent cough even when they are largely healed.

- Dyspnea is generally a sign that pulmonary gas exchange (and, consequently, blood oxygenation) is inadequate. Cardiac and respiratory disorders are the most common causes of dyspnea. The mechanism, in pneumonia for example, involves the filling of alveoli by purulent exudates, preventing gas exchange. The general rule is that the more severe the dyspnea, the more severe the pathology.

- Hoarseness generally indicates narrowing of the airway in the region of the larynx. Typically, the cause is inflammation of the vocal cords due to laryngitis. In small children, narrowing of the same air passage leads to stridor.

- Chest pain is not usually caused by respiratory infection. Cough can lead to chest pain by straining or otherwise injuring the muscles and bones of the chest wall or by irritating an inflamed trachea or bronchi. Pleuritic chest pain can be caused by pneumonia adjacent to the pleura. In general, however, the differential diagnosis of chest pain extends beyond respiratory disease. (For a detailed discussion of chest pain, see Chapter 21.)

Physical Examination

In patients with respiratory tract disease, a careful physical examination often establishes the diagnosis. Elements of the respiratory examination include:

- Ability to interpret cues from inspection of the patient, particularly infants and children, e.g., the degree of anxiety or irritability of the patient
- Vital signs; temperature, respiratory rate, pulse
- Percussion of the paranasal sinuses
- Visualization of the nasal cavity using an otoscope
- Examination of the mouth and throat, sputum, and rhinorrhea
- Physical examination of the ear, including use of the pneumatic otoscope
- Office laryngoscopy
- Palpation of the structures of the anterior neck
- Inspection, palpation, percussion, and auscultation of the chest

DIFFERENTIAL DIAGNOSIS

Physical findings are often the key to resolving several common diagnostic dilemmas involving respiratory infections. The most common dilemmas are:

- Differentiating otitis media from otitis externa—a diagnosis of otitis externa is supported by (a) tenderness of the ear canal on movement of the pinna or gentle insertion of the otoscope speculum, and (b) an inflamed external canal, often covered by friable cerumen. In otitis media, the external canal is normal and the tympanic membrane is bulging and red, often with distorted or absent landmarks.
- Differentiating sinusitis from the common cold—patients frequently present to primary care physicians with rhinitis and low-grade fever, wondering if they have a "sinus infection." Physical examination can help identify

paranasal sinus disease, as these are generally accompanied by tenderness to percussion over the involved sinus and occasionally by eye pain and skin edema over the sinus (Table 35.2).

- Differentiating bronchitis from pneumonia—cough, malaise, and fever are common presenting complaints of both diseases. Physical findings consistent with bronchitis include absent or low-grade fever, a normal respiratory rate (unless the patient has chronic lung disease), and rhonchi and wheezes on auscultation. In pneumonia, dyspnea and an elevated respiratory rate are common, moderate-to-high fever is generally present, localized inspiratory rales can be heard on auscultation, and dullness to percussion over the affected area is occasionally present.
- Persistent cough—may occur for weeks or months after a respiratory illness (6). The quest for the cause can be frustrating, but it is necessary to exclude serious pathology. The causes include:

  1. URI
  2. Postnasal drip (rhinosinusitis)
  3. Asthma (often nocturnal cough)
  4. Chronic bronchitis
  5. Emphysema, chronic obstructive pulmonary disease (COPD)
  6. Gastroesophageal reflux
  7. Angiotensin-converting inhibitors (ACE)
  8. Lung tumors
  9. Foreign body in lung
  10. Cardiac failure, pulmonary infarct

Table 35.2.
Differentiating Sinusitis from Upper Respiratory Tract Infections (URIs)

Symptoms/Signs	URI	Sinusitis
Duration	5–10 days	>10 days
Rhinorrhea	Watery, thin	Serous, mucoid, purulent
Cough	Nonspecific	Often worse at night
Breath	Normal	Malodorous
General	Myalgias, headache	Headache, often over sinus
Facial pain	Absent, mild	Present, and referred to cheek/teeth (maxillary sinus), nose/eyes (ethmoid sinus), head/occiput (frontal sinus)

DIAGNOSTIC TESTS

Laboratory tests are not very useful in the evaluation of respiratory infections in family practice (7). Cultures are unreliable or contaminated, and, for certain problems, radiographs are often of limited value because of low sensitivity and specificity. Empiric treatment is often the most cost-effective strategy (1, 8).

The most commonly used test is the "rapid strep" test (see Chapter 40, Sore Throat), which can identify streptococcal pharyngitis. The white blood cell (WBC) count may sometimes be helpful to the clinician to determine the probability that a bacterial or viral etiology is present in lower respiratory infections. In patients with suspected pneumonia, a sputum Gram stain is often used to identify the probable organism, but most infections are treated empirically.

The chest radiograph will often identify a pneumonia (e.g., mycoplasma) that is not readily apparent on physical examination. For this reason, radiographs should be obtained on all patients with lower respiratory symptoms in whom you suspect but cannot clinically diagnose pneumonia. Chest radiographs are also ordered to rule out occult disease (e.g., a foreign body, a mediastinal mass, or a pulmonary infiltrate) in the patient who has a persistent cough. Appropriate laboratory tests will be reviewed in the discussion of the management of specific respiratory syndromes described below.

TREATMENT

Approach to the Patient

There are three general issues in the management of respiratory disorders that are particularly relevant to how your treatment is organized.

Patient Expectations

Your patient may present with a minor respiratory infection, but the actual reason for coming (ARC) may be something very different. A common ARC is the need for a written work excuse from a physician. Anxiety, depression, or stressful situations (e.g., marital discord) can underlie a seemingly minor medical complaint. Thus, uncovering the patient's concerns is often as important as making the diagnosis.

Demands for antibiotics in the treatment of apparent viral infections are common. Such demands usually occur either because a previous physician was liberal with antibiotics or because the patient had a personal experience in which antibiotics appeared to be quite effective. In working with patients who demand antibiotics, you should develop a patient-centered way of explaining the real indications and drawbacks of treatment in the hope of changing their beliefs.

Telephone Management

People with respiratory infections frequently telephone the office for advice. Usually, the decision that needs to be made by the receptionist or nurse is whether to reassure the patient over the phone, arrange an office visit, or set up an early appointment. Here are a few general principles:

- Know what infections are prevalent in the local community.
- Fever, malaise, and other constitutional symptoms suggest a more severe infection.
- Because the likelihood of bacterial infection is highest in young children and in the very old, these groups should be seen most frequently.
- Printed patient education materials about common respiratory complaints can be helpful in reducing telephone calls and office visits. Your office staff should be similarly educated, as they usually screen the calls.
- If the patient has a typical "cold," telephone reassurance and symptomatic management is generally all that is needed.
- In speaking with patients with cold symptoms, be aware that worsening of symptoms several days after the onset of illness suggests a secondary bacterial infection (e.g., otitis media or sinusitis).
- Some patients call because they want to know whether or not they have a "strep" throat. Most offices allow such patients to have a rapid strep test or a throat culture performed without seeing the physician. If your office has such a policy, be sure that the nurse who performs the culture instructs each patient to return for a formal physician visit if the sore throat persists for longer than 3 or 4 days, if symptoms become very severe, or if breathing difficulty develops.

Epidemics

Most common respiratory infections are viral and highly contagious, often resulting in epidemics. When an epidemic is forecast or occurs, the family physician should work to institute preventive measures, often in collaboration with the local health department. Such preventive measures can be designed to (a) reduce contagion (e.g., hand washing), (b) identify and treat cases early (e.g., streptococcal pharyngitis during an epidemic of scarlet fever), or (c) enhance herd immunity (e.g., influenza vaccine). Common respiratory epidemics that can be targeted for preventive measures include upper respiratory infections in day-care centers; streptococcal pharyngitis in elementary schools, mycoplasma among military recruits, and influenza among nursing home patients.

Upper Respiratory Infections

THE COMMON COLD

The common cold is the leading upper respiratory tract infection in both adults and children. Adults average two to four colds per year with the incidence rising in the fall, peaking in the winter, and declining significantly in the early to late spring. Children on average have between six and eight colds per year and are a major reservoir of cold viruses, as evidenced by an increased incidence of colds among adults who have children in their household (1, 3, 8). The rhinovirus, with more than 100 antigenic serotypes, is responsible for 25 to 40% of colds. The corona virus, parainfluenza virus, respiratory syncytial virus, influenza virus, adenovirus, and enteroviruses cause another 10 to 40% of infections (7). Less commonly, *Mycoplasma pneumoniae* and other agents may cause cold symptoms. Transmission primarily occurs by hand contact with the infectious agent. Symptoms usually develop within 2 days after exposure, with a range of 1 to 6 days.

History and Physical Examination

Usual symptoms include sneezing, nasal congestion, and a watery nasal discharge that becomes thick and yellow after several days. Some patients complain initially of malaise, headache, muscle aches, chills, and irritated eyes. If present, fever seldom exceeds 102°F. A scratchy or sore throat with pain occasionally referred to the ear, a nonproductive cough, and (less frequently) hoarseness are common associated symptoms. Impaired taste and smell along with pressure in the sinuses

and ears may also be present. Symptoms peak by the second or third day and subside within 7 to 10 days. Cough may persist for days to weeks after the resolution of other symptoms, particularly in young children and smokers.

Physical findings include mildly swollen and erythematous nasal and pharyngeal mucosa without exudate, nasal passage occlusion, postnasal discharge, and enlarged posterior pharyngeal lymphoid tissue. Cervical lymph nodes may or may not be enlarged and tender. Tympanic membrane dysfunction with transient impaired hearing may accompany eustachian tube obstruction secondary to mucosal edema.

Secondary bacterial infections can occur as complications of the common cold. These secondary infections include acute otitis media, sinusitis, tonsillitis, pharyngitis, cervical adenitis, laryngitis, tracheobronchitis, bronchiolitis, and pneumonia. They usually present between 3 and 10 days after onset of cold symptoms as an increase in fever (above 102°F), localized pain, and/or pronounced cough.

Anterior nosebleeds occasionally occur as complications of the common cold as a result of cracking of the mucosa. Frequent nose blowing and wiping can traumatize the area, increasing the likelihood of a bleed. Pinching the nostrils for 5 to 10 minutes usually stops nosebleeds associated with the common cold. Gentle topical application of petroleum base products can often prevent recurrences by protecting the mucosa from drying out.

Treatment

The main objective is to relieve symptoms. Recently zinc preparations have been shown by randomized trials to shorten the duration of cold symptoms by about 3 days (8). Zinc probably inhibits viral replication. The dose is 13 to 23 mg of zinc gluconate every 2 hours for 3 to 5 days (effectiveness rating A).

In treating adults, oral pseudoephedrine 60 mg every 6 hours singularly or in combination with an antihistamine is more effective in relieving nasal congestion than placebo or antihistamines alone (effectiveness rating A). Antihistamines may cause drowsiness and should be avoided in situations that require alertness. Phenylpropanolamine is frequently found in over-the-counter preparations, but it must be used judiciously or not at all in hypertensive patients because it may elevate blood pressure.

Topical nasal decongestants may avoid the systemic effects of oral decongestants/antihistamines but should be limited to 3 days of use because of their potential to cause rebound persistent congestion. Although evidence is inconclusive, topical nasal decongestion may prevent secondary sinus or ear infections. Xylometazoline hydrochloride (Otrivin), 0.05% spray or drops, is preferred because of its prolonged duration of action, allowing an every 8-to-10-hour application of two to three sprays or drops. Topical nasal decongestants are not recommended for infants and toddlers; however, saline nasal drops and suction with a bulb syringe may be effective in alleviating nasal congestion. Drinking warm liquids and inhalation of steam or cold water vapor from a vaporizer offer some relief (effectiveness rating C). Antibiotics do not have a role in treating the common cold and should be used only in the case of secondary bacterial infections.

Cough in young children should generally not be treated. Traditional treatments such as expectorants (guaifenesin) and cough suppressants (codeine, dextromethorphan) have no proven value by clinical trials but are still widely used. Persistent cough in older children and adults may be relieved with products containing dextromethorphan in an equivalent dose of 10 to 20 mg every 6 hours for adults; 5 mg 4 times a day for children 3 to 6 years, and 10 mg 4 times a day for children over 6.

In adults with severe coughs, codeine 30 mg every 6 hours is recommended, but it should be used with caution because of the potential of abuse and constipation. Benzonatate (Tessalon Perles) is effective but expensive (effectiveness rating B). Mild sore throat can be relieved with lozenges, sprays, or gargles that contain topical anesthetics such as benzocaine or phenol. Gargles with warm salt water (1 teaspoon in 1 quart of water) may be as effective. Antiseptic mouthwashes are generally not beneficial.

Fever and muscle aches are usually relieved with aspirin or acetaminophen in doses of 650 to 975 mg every 4 to 6 hours for adults and acetaminophen 10 to 12 mg/kg every 3 to 4 hours for children. Because of its association with Reye's syndrome, aspirin should not be used in children.

Prevention of the common cold is generally focused on limiting transmission by frequent hand washing, use of disposable tissues, and limiting human contact with symptomatic individuals during the peak of nasal discharge. Studies on the preventive effects of vitamin C have failed to demonstrate efficacy.

PHARYNGITIS

Pharyngitis is most frequently caused by the following viruses:

- Adenovirus infections typically present with sore throat, conjunctivitis, fever, and often rhinitis; the infection usually lasts around 5 days. Adenovirus infections occur primarily during summer months; transmission has been associated with contaminated swimming pools.

- Coxsackie virus causes herpangina, an acute pharyngitis with small, tender blisters (vesicles) on the soft palate, uvula, and tonsillar pillars that rupture and leave a shallow, grayish ulcer with an erythematous halo. Outbreaks are prevalent in summer months. Occasionally the herpes simplex virus causes a similar clinical syndrome. Distinguishing features are that herpes ulcers are fewer and larger; that coxsackie infections are often accompanied by ulcerations of the hands and feet ("hand, foot, and mouth disease"); and by abdominal symptoms (vomiting, pain, or diarrhea).

- Infectious mononucleosis frequently presents with pharyngitis, tonsillar exudate, fever, prominent lymphadenopathy, and fatigue.

Diagnosis and Treatment

Treatment for these virus infections is symptomatic. Of bacterial infections, streptococcal pharyngitis is by far the most common. It classically presents with severe sore throat, tonsillar or pharyngeal exudate, anterior cervical adenopathy, fever to 104° F, lethargy, myalgias, and anorexia. However, 40% of patients have symptoms indistinguishable from the common cold and other causes of pharyngitis. It is most prevalent between the ages of 5 and 17 years. The importance of diagnosing and treating this infection is to prevent the severe complications of rheumatic fever and glomerulonephritis, and the local suppurative complications of peritonsillar and retropharyngeal abscess, cervical lymphadenitis, otitis media, and septicemia. Rarer bacterial causes of pharyngitis include group G streptococci, *Neisseria gonorrhoeae*, anaerobic and spirochetal organisms (Vincent's angina), *Staphylococcus aureus*, and, rarely, diphtheria. In adolescents and young adults, mycoplasma infections can also cause pharyngitis. For details on the diagnosis and management of patients with sore throat, see Chapter 40.

SINUSITIS

Sinusitis is caused by viral, bacterial, or fungal infection of the paranasal sinuses. The most common bacteria include *Streptococcus pneumoniae, Moraxella catarrhalis, and Hemophilus influenzae.* Anaerobes are found mostly in chronic cases. Allergic fungal sinusitis occurs in 5 to 10% of chronic sinusitis (9). Sinusitis in adults may be classified as acute, subacute, or chronic, based on the length of symptoms (less than 3 weeks, 3 weeks to 3 months, and longer than 3 months, respectively). Children can also suffer from sinusitis because maxillary sinuses are developed by 3 years and frontal sinuses by 8 to 10 years (10–12). The most common predisposing factors are allergies (asthma, seasonal rhinitis), nasal polyps, large adenoids, and smoking.

History and Physical Examination

The presentation of acute sinusitis includes a range of symptoms that have poor sensitivity and specificity for the disease. Many cases of sinusitis do not produce classic symptoms. These include:

- Pain located over the affected sinus, which increases as the day progresses and with bending

- Pain may be referred to structures contiguous to the affected sinuses (see Table 35.2), presenting as headache

- Nasal congestion, often with purulent nasal discharge; colored discharge has a sensitivity of 80% and a specificity of 52% for detecting sinus infection

- Fever

- Symptom onset 3 to 10 days into a "cold"

Sinusitis in children presents with cold symptoms lasting longer than 10 days, nasal discharge, and a daytime cough (44% sensitivity). Children may also present acutely with high fever, periorbital swelling, facial pain, headache, and copious purulent nasal discharge.

Children and adults will generally reveal tenderness over the affected sinus (sensitivity 45%, specificity 65%), an edematous nasal mucosa, and nasal discharge that may or may not be purulent.

Laboratory Tests

Transillumination of the sinuses has very low efficacy in diagnosing infection and should not be used (sensitivity 48%, specificity 65%; LR+ 1.6, LR− 0.5). Similarly, cultures of nasal discharge do not reliably aid in the diagnosis of sinusitis because the results do not correlate with culture of material directly aspirated from the affected sinus.

Radiographs of the sinuses may be helpful in detecting air-fluid levels or densities in the sinuses, but can be abnormal in other upper respiratory disorders (34% false-positive, 43% false-negative findings) (10). Limited axial or coronal computed tomography (CT) scans of the sinuses cost about the same as radiographs and are much more accurate. Compared to a standard high-cost CT, limited views still have 93% sensitivity and 89% specificity (10). Imaging should be reserved for failure of response to treatment, chronic sinusitis, or high-risk patients (i.e., diabetics).

A complete blood count (CBC) can be useful to identify eosinophilia, if allergy is suspected, or to evaluate the white blood count in the event of severe symptoms or high fever. Other tests, usually undertaken by the specialist, include nasal/sinus endoscopy and nasal allergy challenge.

The physician's overall clinical impression of sinusitis is superior in accuracy than any historical or physical finding, although toothache, purulent nasal discharge, and poor response to decongestants are important predictors (13).

Treatment

An algorithm showing the management options for treating acute and chronic sinusitis is shown in Figure 35.1. The decision to treat is often not clear cut, but strong indications include facial pain, purulent nasal discharge, fever, and opacified maxillary sinuses on radiograph or CT (effectiveness rating B). The patient should be advised to avoid smoking and take oral decongestants to aid sinus drainage. Locally applied decongestants (for up to 4 days only), in spray or drops, followed 15 minutes later by inhalation of steam, may offer symptomatic relief (effectiveness rating C).

Choice of antibiotics is not clear-cut because of the many possible pathogens and the unreliability of cultures. *Haemophilus influenzae* (35% of strains) and *Moraxella catarrhalis* (90% of strains) are often resistant to erythromycin

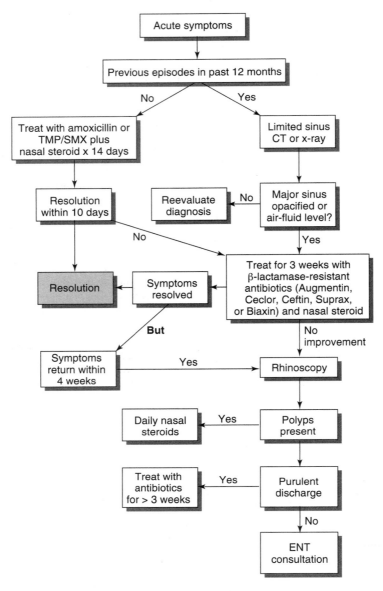

Figure 35.1. *Algorithm for treatment of sinusitis.* (Adapted from Wagner W. Changing diagnostic and treatment strategies for chronic sinusitis. Cleve Clin J Med 1996;53:396–405.)

and trimethoprim/sulfamethoxazole (TMP/SMX), whereas 50% of *Streptococcus pneumoniae* are resistant to erythromycin and TMP/SMX (5, 7, 11). Initial treatment selections for acute sinusitis in adults include amoxicillin 250 to 500 mg 3 times a day, double-strength (DS) TMP/SMX one tablet twice a day, or cefuroxime axetil 250 mg 4 times a day for at least 14 days. If there is evi-

dence of significant penicillin resistance, a cephalosporin or clindamycin are indicated.

Clarithromycin (Biaxin), an agent with 4 to 8 times more activity than erythromycin against *H. influenzae,* is an option for patients with sensitivity to penicillin and covers a wide range of pathogens. Erythromycin or clarithromycin should not be taken with the antihistamines terfenadine (Seldane) or astemizole (Hismanal) because of serious drug interactions causing cardiac arrhythmias. There have been no controlled studies on the appropriate duration of antibiotics for sinusitis.

For children with sinusitis, the drug of choice is amoxicillin, 40 mg/kg /day because of low cost, safety, and effectiveness (failure rate 10 to 15%) (11); TMP/SMX based on 8 mg/kg trimethoprim or 40 mg/kg sulfamethoxazole twice a day; the β-lactamase-resistant antibiotics, cefaclor 15 mg/kg/day, and amoxicillin-clavulanate (Augmentin) are appropriate for children. All should be treated for at least 10 days.

Adults or children with severe sinus or orbital pain, facial cellulitis, and fever may require hospitalization, parenteral antibiotics, and direct drainage of the sinuses. Referral to the otolaryngologist should occur for treatment failures, chronic infection, or the suspicion of complications (14). Three- to 4-day use of topical sympathomimetic decongestants in spray or drops, inhalation of steam, and oral analgesics offer symptomatic relief (effectiveness rating C).

RHINITIS

An estimated 40 million Americans have nasal problems leading to costs of $15 billion annually for medication and $60 billion for surgery (10, 14).

History and Physical Examination

Most symptoms related to structural problems of the nose (deviation of the septum, polyps, foreign bodies, tumors) are unilateral. The presence of nasal discharge (rhinorrhea) commonly occurs with allergic and nonallergic rhinitis, vasomotor rhinitis, and infections.

- Allergic rhinitis—occurs seasonally or continuously (perennial). Patients are sensitive to specific allergens (pollens, molds, animal dander, feathers, dust mites). Symptoms include nasal obstruction, sneezing, itching of the nose and eyes, and postnasal drainage. The nasal mucosa is pale and boggy, the conjunctivae inflamed. There may be loss of the sense of smell.

- Vasomotor rhinitis—this can be triggered, particularly in the elderly, by a range of stimuli (cold water, spicy food ["salsa snuffles"], rain, tobacco smoke, wine, etc). Symptoms in-

clude nasal obstruction and postnasal drainage without itching or sneezing. There is no eosinophilia.

- Nasal polyps—the etiology of these gelatinous grape-like masses that develop in the posterior nasopharynx is unclear. They cause obstruction of the nose and sinuses and are often associated with asthma, sinusitis, and cystic fibrosis in children.

Unilateral bleeding (epistaxis) or obstruction may be due to polyps, a foreign body (i.e., a peanut), or tumor. An illuminated speculum only provides access to the anterior third of the nasal cavity but can reveal changes in the mucosal color and structural deformities.

Laboratory tests

Laboratory testing is usually not helpful in diagnosis or guiding treatment except for the following:

- Nasal cytology can be useful in showing neutrophils (infection) or eosinophils (allergy). However, this is time consuming and most clinicians will use a trial course of intranasal corticosteroids first.

- Intradermal skin testing for specific IgE antibodies to allergens has good sensitivity (70%) but low specificity (50%). It is costly to perform and must be correlated with clinical findings.

- Fiberoptic endoscopy is effective in identifying posterior nasal structures. This technique is performed by specialists using topical anesthesia.

Treatment

If a specific cause for rhinitis can be found, management is usually more successful, but usually this is difficult because of the wide overlap of symptoms. The most commonly used medications include the following:

- Antihistamines—the primary role is to control itching, rhinorrhea, sneezing, and watery eyes. Traditional agents (i.e., Benadryl) have a significant sedating effect. The newer, nonsedating agents astemizole (Hismanal; 10 mg daily), loratadine (Claritin; 10 mg daily), cetirizine (Zyrtec; 5 to 10 mg daily) and fexofenadine (Allegra; 25 mg TID) are metabolized by the liver. Hismanal and Claritin can produce ventricular arrhythmia in the event of hepatic dysfunction, electrolyte imbalance, and bradycardia (15). Similar problems occur when taking these antihistamines with systemic antifungal agents (itraconazole, ketoconazole, etc.), erythromycin, and clarithromycin.

- Anticholinergics—in patients with rhinitis, the mucosa is overly sensitive to cholinergics, producing a lot of fluid. Topically applied anticholinergics (ipratropium bromide [Atrovent] nasal 0.03% or 0.06%, 2 sprays in each nostril twice a day) are useful for watery rhinorrhea occurring in allergic and vasomotor rhinitis and in the common cold.

- Vasoconstrictors—by acting on the sympathetic nerves in the mucosa, vasoconstrictors (e.g., pseudoephedrine, 30 mg 4 times a day) reduce nasal blockage but do little to help sneezing and discharge. Nasal use for more than 3 to 4 days can produce rebound vasodilatation and congestion. Oral agents can produce wakefulness, irritability, tachycardia, raised blood pressure, and night terrors in children.

- Cromolyn sodium (1 spray [5 mg] 4 times a day)—inhibits mast cell activity and blocks the allergic response. It is used prophylactically before allergen exposure. It is available as a nasal spray, eye drops, and metered dose inhalation for asthma. Dosage is every 4 to 6 hours.

- Intranasal corticosteroids—these are more effective for allergic rhinitis and polyposis than other medications, but they have a slower onset of action (evidence rating A) (10, 16). A 1-month trial of therapy will establish whether the patient will respond. Adverse effects include nasal irritation (10%) and bloody discharge (2%). Agents include beclomethasone (2 sprays twice a day), triamcinolone (two sprays every day), flunisolide (2 sprays twice a day), and fluticasone, usually 2 to 4 puffs three times a day into each nostril.

- Systemic corticosteroids may be needed to treat severe obstructive polyposis or rhinoconjunctivitis (e.g., prednisone 40 mg per day for 4 to 5 days, tapering off over 7 to 10 days).

- Immunotherapy—skin testing can clearly identify the allergens in allergic rhinitis in about 50% of cases (17). A vaccine can then be prescribed designed to desensitize the patient. This requires frequent injections starting at very small doses over several months, followed usually by a monthly maintenance dose over about 3 years. The effect can last for up to 5 years. Polysensitized patients do not respond. This is a very costly approach to treatment and its effectiveness is not clearly established by controlled studies. Allergic reactions and life-threatening anaphylaxis are fairly common (16). Decision factors in considering immunotherapy include demonstrating IgE-mediated allergy, evidence that the allergen cannot be avoided, severity of symptoms, and the availability and cost of high-quality standard extracts.

Specific treatment includes the following approaches:

- Allergic rhinitis—exposure avoidance and control, medication for congestion, and possibly immunotherapy.

- Vasomotor rhinitis—avoidance of specific stimulants, symptomatic therapy with decongestants and antihistamines, and if not improved, a trial of an intranasal corticosteroid (17, 18).

- Nasal polyps—intranasal corticosteroids are quite effective (effectiveness rating A), but surgery is often indicated (16). Recurrences are common.

OTITIS MEDIA (OM)

Otitis media occurs most frequently in young children and is the most common reason for prescribing antibiotics (11, 19) (see Chapter 27, Fever in Infants and Preschool Children). It also occurs in older children and in adults, although less frequently, presenting as acute ear pain, often at night, with or without decreased hearing. However, earache and fever are frequently absent in children with OM. Earache predicts OM in 80% of cases (20).

Clinical Evaluation

Direct observation of the tympanic membrane is required to make the diagnosis. A pneumatic otoscope is recommended that will allow direct visualization and determination of the mobility of the tympanic membrane. Removal of cerumen may be necessary to visualize the tympanic membrane, or cerumen softeners can be used (Cerumenex, Colace drops). A bulging, cloudy, or immobile tympanic membrane predicts OM and middle ear effusion in 80% of cases (21).The impedance tympanometer is sensitive (90%) and reliable in determining the presence of middle ear fluid and is frequently used in office practice. However, specificity is 70 to 80%.

Treatment

Antibiotics may not significantly change the clinical course of uncomplicated otitis media, but they do help reduce recurrences and prevent suppurative complications, such as chronic otitis media, cholesteatoma, and mastoiditis (20). Meta-analysis of 250 clinical trials show that antibiotics produce only moderate improvement (14%) in the prevention and treatment of OM. Amoxicillin is preferred in children and adults. The antibiotics and dosages listed for sinusitis are similarly effective for OM. Oral and nasal decongestants as well as antihistamines have no proven benefit (19). Auralgan (a combination product containing benzocaine, antipyrine, and cryconin) is useful as a topical anesthetic (effectiveness rating B). Acetaminophen in children and aspirin in adults provides effective analgesia for mild-to-moderate pain; opioids may be necessary for up to 48 hours to relieve severe pain.

Lower Respiratory Infections

Lower respiratory infections occur at or below the level of the larynx. Differentiating between viral and bacterial causes is useful because viral infections generally only need supportive care. Most lower respiratory tract infections (LRIs) in children between the ages of 2 months and 12 years are caused by viruses, including the respiratory syncytial virus, parainfluenza viruses, and the adenovirus. Of all infants visiting the physician, 30% have an LRI but only 1% will be admitted to hospital (22).

In adolescents and adults, bacterial causes are relatively more frequent, and *Mycoplasma* is a common cause of pneumonia and bronchitis. In the elderly, gram-negative organisms and *Legionella* become prominent as causes of LRIs. Smokers have a particularly high incidence of lower respiratory tract disease, presumably because the protective mucociliary system is damaged. They are often colonized with gram-negative organisms such as *Klebsiella pneumoniae*, which explains why these organisms are more frequent LRI pathogens in smokers.

CROUP

Croup, seen in children between 3 months and 3 years of age, is generally caused by the parainfluenza virus. It presents with inspiratory stridor and a characteristic barking cough, a low-grade fever, and coryza. The infection is generally self-limited and is helped by humidification. Decongestants may also be of some value. In older children, it must be differentiated from epiglottitis, a severe illness that presents acutely with stridor and fever and is caused by *Haemophilus influenzae*.

LARYNGITIS

Laryngitis is the adult counterpart of croup. In adults, because the airway is larger, hoarseness is the only symptom produced by the laryngeal edema, and respiratory compromise does not occur. A viral illness usually preceded by pharyngitis and/or rhinitis, laryngitis is self-limited. Treatment is with acetaminophen, aspirin, or ibuprofen, with humidification and warm liquids. Resting the vocal cords speeds resolution of the hoarseness.

BRONCHIOLITIS

Acute bronchiolitis is a distinct syndrome occurring in infants under 2 years with a peak incidence at 6 months of age. It is usually caused by the respiratory syncytial virus (RSV), although other viruses can occasionally be responsible. RSV is the most important respiratory pathogen in childhood and the most common cause of bronchiolitis and pneumonia in children under 1 year. Typically, a minor respiratory illness in an older family member is passed to the infant, leading to bronchiolitis. The severity of symptoms results from the fact that the infant's bronchiolar airway is so small that wall edema caused by the infection significantly reduces airflow.

Bronchiolitis begins as an upper respiratory infection, but soon the patient develops a cough, audible wheezing, irritability, listlessness, dyspnea, and cyanosis. Chest x-ray films may reveal atelectasis, hyperinflation, or both. Untreated, infants with bronchiolitis can die from hypoxemia, dehydration, or apnea. Fewer than 1% of affected infants die, however. Most recover but suffer recurrent wheezing episodes, usually precipitated by viral infections, for 5 to 10 years following the infection.

Treatment

An antiviral agent, ribavirin, is effective against RSV, particularly if used early in the infection. Rapid antibody kits for RSV, similar to the rapid strep test kits, are now available; these can help identify infants who may merit hospitalization because of increased risk for severe lower respiratory disease. Other treatment includes adequate fluid intake (oral or intravenous), humidification, and oxygen supplementation, if necessary. β-Agonists may be used for a limited period to dilate the airways.

BRONCHITIS

Acute Bronchitis

Bronchitis is seen at all ages beyond 6 months. In children, it is usually the result of a viral infection that initially affected the nasopharynx and progressed to involve the trachea and bronchi. However, bacteria (*H. influenzae, Mycoplasma, Pneumococcus*) can be the cause in about 25% of cases. Symptoms include low-grade fever (101°F), mild cough, wheezing, rhonchi, and, occasionally, rales.

In adults, acute bronchitis is the most frequent lower respiratory infection. It is most prevalent in winter and is primarily caused by the rhinovirus, coronavirus, adenovirus, or influenza virus. The typical presentation includes:

- Being preceded by an upper respiratory tract infection
- An initially nonproductive cough that becomes productive of mucopurulent sputum
- Chest pain brought on by coughing, deep breathing, and movement
- Absent or mild fever

On auscultation, there is often little to find except some rhonchi or wheezes that shift with cough.

Antitussives should be used sparingly for cough (see section on the common cold) and acetaminophen for fever. Antibiotics are used to treat bronchitis in smokers because their lungs are often colonized with pathogenic bacteria. Erythromycin, amoxicillin, and TMP/SMX are commonly used. There is continued controversy regarding the routine use of antibiotics for bronchitis (23). The most cost-effective approach appears to be treatment with antibiotics only for patients who have bronchitis and a persistent cough. Complete smoking cessation may be necessary to clear the cough and prevent recurrence in smokers.

Chronic Bronchitis

Chronic bronchitis is seen primarily in older adults with a history of smoking and/or exposure to air pollutants. It results from permanent inflammatory changes in the lower respiratory tract. Superimposed infection occurs frequently and presents as increased sputum production, cough, wheezing, and respiratory distress. *S. pneumoniae, H. influenzae,* α-hemolytic Streptococci, and *Moraxella catarrhalis* are common pathogens. Antibiotics are generally indicated, with the recommended agents being the same as those used in acute bronchitis. Adequate hydration, supplemental oxygen, and bronchodilation are important.

INFLUENZA

Several related viruses cause the "flu." Classic epidemic influenza is caused by influenza virus type A (80% of epidemics) or influenza virus type B (20% of epidemics). Its onset is abrupt, with severe myalgias, prominent headache, a nonproductive cough, and fever in the range of 102 to 103° F. The illness is generally self-limited and subsides within a few days. In some individuals, however, pneumonia results. This pneumonia can be caused either by the influenza virus or by a secondary bacterial pathogen, most commonly *H. influenzae, S. pneumoniae,* or *Staphylococcus aureus.*

Influenza should be prevented in high-risk patients (adults with chronic pulmonary or cardiovascular diseases, nursing home residents, age greater than 65, those with diabetes or renal or marrow dysfunction, and the immunocompromised). Flu injections are made available annually in October or November, and each office should have a plan for getting as many patients as possible immunized. Early use of amantadine 200 to 300 mg per day during an acute infection with influenza A may be beneficial (effectiveness rating B). Supportive care consists of rest, fluids, and acetaminophen.

PNEUMONIA

In the United States, pneumonia in adults is the sixth leading cause of death (24). It is common among the elderly and patients with chronic diseases. A variety of organisms causing the disease can coexist in the sputum, and diagnostic testing is often of little value. People with HIV infection and patients in hospitals and nursing homes are prone to unusual causes of pneumonia (*Pneumocystis*, tuberculosis, fungal infections, etc.).

Community-acquired pneumonia generally presents as "typical" and "atypical" forms. Table 35.3 outlines the differences between these pneumonia syndromes. In general, atypical pneumonias are milder and slower in onset, whereas typical pneumonias are more severe and abrupt in onset. Most pneumonias in adults under age 40 are atypical, with *Mycoplasma pneumoniae* being the predominant pathogen. As adults become older and as the prevalence of chronic disease rises, the relative frequency of typical pneumonias rises.

S. pneumoniae is the most common community-acquired pneumonia. It is rapid in onset ("typical"), presenting with shaking chills or rigor, high fever, a cough producing rusty blood-tinged sputum, pleuritic chest pain, and dyspnea. Occasionally, it can present as upper abdominal pain accompanied by fever and chills. Auscultatory examination of the chest may reveal signs of consolidation and/or a friction rub. Chest x-ray films will show a lobar consolidation with or without effusion. There is prominent leukocytosis.

Mycoplasma pneumonia tends to occur in epidemics in late summer and early fall among closed groups such as families, college students, summer camps, and military recruits. It presents with a dry hacking cough, low-grade fever, headache, sore throat, and myalgias. Patients usually do not appear very ill and are ambulatory. Physical findings may be nonspecific, but in advanced cases, rales and signs of consolidation will be evident. A chest x-ray film usually looks worse than the patient appears, revealing one or more infiltrates. Rash, otitis media, and joint symptoms may be present. There is not a prominent leukocytosis. Cold agglutinins may be present, but are positive in only about half of cases and are not clinically useful.

In clinical practice, the categorization of "typical" and "atypical" pneumonia is often unclear with considerable overlap and does not greatly affect treatment decisions.

In children, most pneumonias are viral and require symptomatic treatment. Predominant bacterial pathogens vary by age:

- In the newborn, *Escherichia coli, S. aureus,* group B streptococci, and *Chlamydia* are the most common pathogens.

- Between 3 months and 8 years of age, *S. pneumoniae* and *H. influenzae* predominate.

- In older children, *Mycoplasma pneumonia, S. pneumoniae,* and *Neisseria meningitidis* are common pathogens.

Clinical Evaluation

The diagnosis of pneumonia is based on the history and demonstration of either (a) rales or signs of consolidation on physical examination, or (b) an infiltrate on chest x-ray films.

Presentation may vary, being either secondary to a prior viral syndrome (slow onset) or occurring acutely (probably bacterial). The infant or child may have trouble feeding, seem anxious, and present with a cough, wheezing, rapid respirations, congestion, hoarseness, or stridor. Findings include fever and tachypnea (count for 60 seconds), often indrawing of the costal margins, and rales and rhonchi may be heard. Auscultation is somewhat unreliable in infants. The best finding to rule out pneumonia

Table 35.3.
Characteristics of "Typical" and "Atypical" Pneumonias

Characteristic	"Typical" Pneumonia	"Atypical" Pneumonia
Onset	Rapid	Gradual
Chills	Common	Rare
Cough	Productive	Nonproductive
Pleuritic pain	Common	Rare
Fever	>38.9°C (102°F)	<38.9°C (102°F)
Usual distribution	One lobe or segment	Multiple lobes or segments
Most common pathogen	*Streptococcus pneumoniae*	*Mycoplasma pneumoniae*

Adapted from Rodnick JE, Gude JK. Diagnosis and antibiotic treatment of community-acquired pneumonia. West J Med 1991;154:405–409.

is the absence of tachypnea. Respiratory rate elevation is >60 per minute at less than 2 months of age, >50 per minute for 2 to 12 months; and >40 per minute for over 12 months (25). Increased accessory muscle use, lethargy, pale color, poor attentiveness, and poor consolability are highly predictive of hypoxemia and the need for admission to hospital (26). The presence of two of these findings gives a positive likelihood ratio (LR) of 8.9, whereas four findings give a positive LR of 34.4.

A chest radiograph is often negative early in the disease and has a sensitivity of 75% and specificity of 100% (22). The white blood count (>15,000) has a sensitivity of 65% and specificity of 75% for bacteremia (27). Clinical symptoms and laboratory findings that suggest bacterial pneumonia include sudden onset, high fever (>102°F), tachypnea, tachycardia, cough, consolidation on x-ray films, leukocytosis, and, in older children, chest pain, sputum production, and shaking chills. Symptoms associated with viral pneumonias and *Mycoplasma pneumoniae* are gradual onset, prominent nonproductive cough, and low-grade fever without significant laboratory findings.

Laboratory Tests

Specificity and sensitivity are poor for both sputum culture and Gram stain. However, culture may reveal resistant or unusual organisms that may modify treatment decisions. Routine laboratory tests such as complete blood count and electrolytes may provide useful evidence when considering hospitalization for seriously ill patients. Extensive diagnostic testing is of little value in establishing the etiology (27). Chest radiograph is the most important diagnostic test.

Management

In office practice, pneumonia in otherwise healthy adults, without respiratory compromise, can be managed on an outpatient basis with appropriate antibiotics, hydration, and symptom relief. Patients with chronic illness or debilitating or immunocompromised conditions generally require hospitalization, more aggressive management, and a search for less common pathogens.

Ideally, a sputum should be obtained and Gram stained to help guide therapy. Sputum cultures are unreliable and are not worth obtaining in the office setting. In practice, many uncomplicated community-acquired pneumonias are treated empirically, either because the patient cannot produce sputum or because the Gram stain is nondiagnostic. Current antibiotic usage for certain patients and organisms is shown in Table 35.4. Empiric therapy for nonaspiration pneumonia is erythromycin 250 mg 4 times a day or azithromycin 500 mg immediately, then every day for 4 days. For aspiration pneumonia, you can use clindamycin 300 mg three times a day or amoxicillin-clavulanate 500 mg three times a day. If the etiology is known (based on Gram stain), penicillin is used for gram-positive cocci, and cefuroxime 250 mg twice a day, TMP/SMX DS twice a day, or ciprofloxacin 500 mg twice a day are used for gram-negative organisms.

An important treatment decision is whether or not to manage the patient with pneumonia at home. Patients who can take medication and fluids by mouth, who have a family member or other caretaker to look after them, and who are not gravely ill can be considered for home treatment. Easy access to the physician and the patient's ability to comply with the prescribed regimen (and follow-up) are other factors favoring outpatient treatment. Certain risk factors predict serious morbidity and the need for admission. These include:

- Chronic disease—diabetes, COPD, renal failure, congestive heart failure, suspected aspiration, alcohol abuse
- Clinical findings—respiratory rate > 30/min, hypotension, fever > 38.3°C, mental confusion
- Laboratory findings—low or high WBC, PaO_2 < 60 mmHg or $PaCO_2$ > 50 mmHg on room air, abnormal renal function, hematocrit < 30%, radiographic evidence of widespread infection, metabolic acidosis.

Follow-up is important in pneumonia. Patients can fail to respond to antibiotics because of noncompliance or because the pathogenic organism was not susceptible to the drug used. Occasionally, tuberculosis will present as pneumonia and will only be identified when the patient does not get better. Complications such as parapneumonic effusions, empyema, and secondary infections can occur. Finally, pneumonia can be the presentation of an occult carcinoma of the lung.

Table 35.4.

Selecting an Antibiotic for Empiric Treatment of Adults with Community-Acquired Pneumonia (When a Sputum Gram Stain Is Unavailable or Is Not Helpful)

If the patient is . . .	The most likely organism is . . .	Other likely pathogens include . . .	The antibiotic(s) of choice include . . .
A healthy adult with "typical" pneumonia	*Streptococcus pneumoniae*	*Haemophilus influenzae*	Penicillin G, amoxicillin, a second generation cephalosporin (e.g., cefuroxime axetil)
A healthy adult with "atypical" pneumonia	*Mycoplasma pneumoniae*	Viruses	Erythromycin, doxycycline, or extended spectrum microlides (azithromycin, clarithromycin)
A geriatric patient without suspected aspiration	*S. pneumoniae*	*H. influenzae*, mixed flora, *Legionella*	A second-generation cephalosporin or TMP/SMX
A geriatric patient with suspected aspiration	Oral anaerobes	Bacteroides, mixed flora, *Staphylococcus aureus*	Penicillin, clindamycin
A smoker or with chronic lung disease	*S. pneumoniae*	*H. influenzae*, *Moraxella catarrhalis*	A second-generation cephalosporin, TMP/SMX, or extended spectrum macrolides

Adapted from McFarlane JT. Treatment of lower respiratory infections. Lancet 1987;ii:1446–1449; Norman DC. Pneumonia in the elderly: empiric antimicrobial therapy. Geriatrics 1991;46:26–32; Perlman PE, Ginn DR. Respiratory infections in ambulatory adults: choosing the best treatment. Postgrad Med 1990;87:175–184; Rodnick JE, Gude JK. Diagnosis and antibiotic treatment of community-acquired pneumonia. West J Med 1991;154:405–409.

TMP/SMX, trimethoprim/sulfamethoxazole.

For these reasons, patients with pneumonia should return frequently for reassessment until they are clinically better. All patients over 40 should have a follow-up chest radiograph in 3 to 6 weeks to confirm resolution of the infiltrate. If the patient has not previously received one, a pneumococcal vaccine should be administered as soon as he or she has recovered from the pneumonia.

CASE STUDY

A 66-year-old retired mechanic comes to the office in November, complaining of increasing cough over a few days. He has no other upper respiratory symptoms. He is a 1-pack/day smoker and has recently made a good recovery from a mild stroke. Clinical evaluation reveals a respiratory rate of 26/minute, normal vital signs apart from a temperature of 100°F, and yellow-stained sputum. There are scattered rhonchi at the bases of both lung fields.

QUESTIONS

1. What is the likely diagnosis?
2. What tests would you perform to confirm the diagnosis and guide treatment?
3. Are there any preventive measures on which you should advise the patient?

DISCUSSION

The history is nonspecific in this patient, but together with the clinical findings, they suggest either acute bronchitis or early pneumonia. Laboratory tests would not be particularly helpful at this stage, although a white cell count might help in determining which antibiotic to use. A chest radiograph is not really justified at this time.

Empiric treatment with antibiotics are ~~indicated because of his age,~~ smoking history, ~~recent stroke, and the winter sea-son, when~~ respiratory infections are more prevalent. There should be close follow-up if improvement does not occur within 2 to 3 days. The patient should be ~~advised~~ to stop ~~smoking during the illness,~~ return in 2 weeks to start ~~cessation counseling, and~~ review the need for pneumococcal vaccine.

REFERENCES

1. Bamberger DM, Jackson MA. Introduction: overview of upper respiratory infections. Semin Respir Infect 1995;10:1–2.
2. Schappert SM. National Ambulatory Medical Care Survey: 1993 summary. Vital and Health Statistics. Series 16, no. 270. DHHS publication no. 96–1886. Hyattsville, MD: US Department of Health and Human Services, PHS, Centers for Disease Control and Prevention, 1996.
3. Dixon RE. Economic costs of respiratory infections in the United States. Am J Med 1985;78 (suppl 6B):32–37.
4. Neu HC. The crisis in antibiotic resistance. Science 1992;257:1064–1073.
5. Tenover FC, Hughes JM. The challenge of emerging infectious diseases: development and spread of multiply resistant bacterial pathogens. JAMA 1996;275:300–304.
6. Chung KE, Lalloo VG. Diagnosis and management of chronic persistent cough. Postgrad Med J 1994;72:594–598.
7. Carroll K, Reimer L. Microbiology and laboratory diagnosis of upper respiratory tract infections. Clin Infect Dis 1996;23:442–448.
8. Mossad SB, Macknin ML, Medendorp SV, Mason P. Zinc gluconate lozenges for treating the common cold. Ann Intern Med 1996;125:81–88.
9. Morpeth JF, Rupp NT, Dolen WK, et al. Fungal sinusitis: an update. Ann Allergy Asthma Immunol 1996;76:128–140.
10. Wagner W. Changing diagnostic and treatment strategies for chronic sinusitis. Cleve Clin J Med 1996;53:396–405.
11. Mason WH. The management of common infections in ambulatory children. Pediatr Ann 1996;25:620–629.
12. Gungor A, Corey JP. Pediatric sinusitis: a literature review with emphasis on the role of allergy. Otolaryngol Head Neck Surg 1997;116:4–15.
13. Williams JW Jr, Simel DL, Roberts L, Samsa GP. Clinical evaluation for sinusitis. Making the diagnosis by history and physical examination. Ann Intern Med 1992;117:705–710.
14. Chester A. Chronic sinusitis. Am Fam Physician 1996;53:877–887.
15. Ament PW, Paterson A. Drug interactions with the nonsedating antihistamines. Am Fam Physician 1997;56:223–230.
16. Ruhno J, Andersson B, Denburg J, et al. A double-blind comparison of intranasal budesonide with placebo for nasal polyps. J Allergy Clin Immunol 1990;86:946–953.
17. Bousquet J, Michel F-B. Specific immunotherapy in allergic rhinitis and asthma. In: Busse WW, Holgate ST, eds. Asthma and Rhinitis. Boston: Blackwell Scientific, 1995:1309–1324.
18. Mygind N. Effects of corticosteroid therapy in nonallergenic rhinosinusitis. Acta Otolaryngol (Stockh) 1996;116:164–166.
19. Rosenfeld RR. An evidence-based approach to treating otitis media. Pediatr Clin North Am 1996;43:1165–1181.
20. Weiss JC, Yates GR, Quinn LD. Acute otitis media: making an accurate diagnosis. Am Fam Physician 1996;53:1200–1206.
21. Simons FER. New medications for rhinitis. In: Busse WW, Holgate ST, eds. Asthma and Rhinitis. Boston: Blackwell Scientific, 1995:1325–1336.
22. Margolis PA, Ferkol TW, Marsocci S, Super DM, Keyes LL, McNutt R, Harrell FE Jr. Accuracy of the clinical examination in detecting hypoxemia in infants with respiratory illness. J Pediatr 1994;552–560.
23. Hueston WJ. Antibiotics: neither cost-effective nor "cough"-effective. J Fam Pract 1997;44:261–265.
24. American Thoracic Society. Guidelines for the initial management of adults with community-acquired pneumonia: diagnosis, assessment of severity, and initial antimicrobial therapy. Am Rev Respir Dis 1993; 148:1418–1436.
25. World Health Organization (WHO). Acute respiratory infections in children: case management in small hospitals in developing countries. In: Programme for the Control of Acute Respiratory Infections. Geneva, Switzerland: World Health Organization, 1991.
26. Margolis PA, Gadomski A. Does this infant have pneumonia? In press. JAMA
27. Baraff LJ, Bass JW, Fleisher GR, Klein JO, McCracken GH Jr, Powell KR, Schriger DC. Practice guidelines for the management of infants and children 0–36 months of age with fever without source. Pediatrics 1993;92: 1–10.

36. Sexually Transmitted Diseases

MARGARET R. H. NUSBAUM

Key Clinical Questions

1. Which of your patients are at increased risk for acquiring sexually transmitted diseases (STDs)?
2. For your patient at increased risk, what testing or treatment should you recommend?
3. What health education can you provide to help reduce your patient's risk for STDs?

Sexually transmitted diseases (STDs) are most commonly asymptomatic; therefore, deciding what patients to screen is the most important job for the primary care clinician. Other common presentations include urethritis, epididymitis, cervicitis, pelvic inflammatory disease, pelvic pain, genital ulcers, and proctitis.

STDs are hidden epidemics of tremendous health and economic consequence in the United States (1). They are hidden from public view because of society's reluctance to address sexual health issues in an open way and because of the biologic and social factors associated with these diseases.

Biologic factors associated with STDs include gender; other preexisting or concurrent STDs, including human immunodeficiency virus (HIV); lack of conspicuous signs and symptoms; long lag time from initial infection to signs of severe complications; young women and adolescents infected more often than men; and other factors, such as male circumcision, vaginal douching, use of hormonal and intrauterine contraceptive devices (IUDs), and cervical eversion (1).

Social factors associated with STDs (1) include poverty; inadequate access to health care; substance abuse; lack of education; social inequities indirectly increasing the prevalence of STDs in certain populations; sexual abuse and violence; disenfranchised populations (commercial sex workers, homeless persons, adolescents, and persons in detention); and mixed messages and secrecy regarding sexual health. Secrecy regarding sexual health impedes a person's willingness or ability to communicate regarding sex and has a negative effect on sexual behavior and the ability to take protective measures against STDs.

The diagnosis of an STD is a sentinel event indicating sexual health risk, because one STD facilitates the transmission and acquisition of other STDs. Although the incidence of gonorrhea and syphilis appears to be decreasing, incurable viral STDs, such as human papillomavirus (HPV), human immunodeficiency virus (HIV), and herpes simplex virus (HSV), are increasing (1).

Surveillance and other information systems for STDs, coordinated by the Centers for Disease Control and Prevention (CDC), monitor and evaluate a national system for prevention. Each of the 50 states has the authority to declare that certain diseases or health conditions must be reported by clinicians and laboratories. Syphilis, gonorrhea, and acquired immunodeficiency syndrome (AIDS) are reportable in all 50 states; 48 states also require *Chlamydia* reporting (1). Other bacterial and viral STDs are inconsistently reportable state to state. This is a passive system, in that reports are brought to the attention of public health officials by clinicians or laboratories. Public health officials do not actively seek out cases. Reporting from publicly funded clinics tends to be more complete than from private practices. It is believed that true STD incidence is under reported by 50% or greater. Figure 36.1 is an example of a reporting card.

Treatment for viral STDs is limited, so the control strategy that must be emphasized is primary prevention through reducing exposure. Control programs for bacterial STDs emphasize case detection and treatment. Control programs for STDs include modification of risk behavior, promotion of barrier contraceptive use, treatment of symptomatic patients, detection of asymptomatic infections, and the tracing of sexual contacts of infected persons. It is important not only to treat the individual but to treat partners, to immunize for hepatitis B, and to provide sexual health counseling.

PATHOGENESIS

It is helpful to think in terms of acute disease presentation, maternal-child health impact, and long-term consequences. Women and children

☐ Surveillance Form Required   **PLEASE ENTER CODE NUMBER IN BLOCK ON FRONT OF CARD**   *Add'l Information Required on Other Side of Card

GENERAL		TUBERCULOSIS	SEXUALLY TRANSMITTED DISEASES

GENERAL

REPORT WITHIN 24 HOURS		REPORT WITHIN 7 DAYS	
ANTHRAX	3	ACQUIRED IMMUNO-DEFICIENCY SYN. (AIDS)	1
BOTULISM	10		
CAMPYLOBACTER INFEC.	50	MENINGITIS, PNEUMOCOCCAL	*25
CHOLERA	6	AMEBIASIS	2
DIPHTHERIA	8	MENINGITIS, VIRAL	*26
E. COLI O157:H7 INFECTION	53	BLASTOMYCOSIS	4
FOOD BORNE DISEASE:		MUMPS	28
C. perfringens	11	BRUCELLOSIS	5
STAPHYLOCOCCAL	12	PSITTACOSIS	31
OTHER or UNKNOWN	*13	DENGUE	7
HEMOPHILUS INFLUENZAE, INVASIVE DISEASE	*23	Q FEVER	32
		ENCEPHALITIS	*9
HEPATITIS A	14	REYE'S SYNDROME	34
HEPATITIS B, ACUTE	15	HEPATITIS B CARRIER	115
MEASLES (rubeola)	22	ROCKY MOUNTAIN SPOTTED FEVER	35
MENINGOCOCCAL DISEASE	*27	HEPATITIS, NON-A, NON-B	16
PLAGUE	29	RUBELLA CONGENITAL SYNDROME	37
POLIO, PARALYTIC	30	HIV INFECTION	101
RABIES, HUMAN	33	(1. Repeatedly reactive EIA and positive confirmatory test; or	
RUBELLA	36	2. Positive virus culture; or	TETANUS	40
SALMONELLOSIS	*38	3. Positive PCR)	TOXIC SHOCK SYNDROME	41
SHIGELLOSIS	39	KAWASAKI SYNDROME	52
TULAREMIA	43	LEGIONELLOSIS	18	TRICHINOSIS	42
TYPHOID, ACUTE	44	LEPROSY	19	TYPHOID CARRIER	144
WHOOPING COUGH	47	LEPTOSPIROSIS	20	TYPHUS, EPIDEMIC (louse-borne)	46
		LYME DISEASE	51	YELLOW FEVER	48

MALARIA 21

TUBERCULOSIS

REPORT WITHIN 24 HOURS — Bacteriologic Status

	POS. SMEAR	POS. CULTURE	NEGATIVE	NOT DONE OR UNKNOWN
PULMONARY	601	701	801	901
PLEURAL	602	702	802	902
LYMPHATIC	603	703	803	903
BONE-JOINT	604	704	804	904
G.U.	605	705	805	905
MILIARY	606	706	806	906
MENINGEAL	607	707	807	907
PERITONEAL	608	708	808	908
OTHER*	609	709	809	909

SEXUALLY TRANSMITTED DISEASES

REPORT WITHIN 24 HOURS

SYPHILIS

PRIMARY (lesion present)	211
SECONDARY (skin or mucosal lesions)	221
EARLY LATENT (< 1 yr)	232
LATE LATENT (> 1 yr)	243
LATE	*277
CONGENITAL	284
EPIDEMIOLOGIC Rx	200

GONORRHEA

GENITO-URINARY (non-PID)	*315
GONOCOCCAL PID	*385
OPHTHALMIA NEONATORUM	345
OTHER	*395
EPIDEMIOLOGIC Rx	300

| CHANCROID | 466 |
| GRANULOMA INGUINALE | 576 |

OTHER STD — REPORT WITHIN 7 DAYS

CHLAMYDIA			Other than lab-confirmed	
Lab confirmed	*500		CHLAMYDIA:	
EPIDEMIOLOGIC Rx	515		NONGONOCOCCAL URETHRITIS (NGU)	365
LYMPHOGRANULOMA VENEREUM	686		EPIDEMIOLOGIC Rx	400

FOR STD ONLY: ☐ VOL. ☐ EPI. ☐ SCREEN   N.C. Department of Environment, Health, and Natural Resources — Division of Epidemiology

NORTH CAROLINA COMMUNICABLE DISEASE REPORT CARD

USE FOR ALL REPORTABLE DISEASES EXCEPT CANCER—REPORT ONLY ONE DISEASE PER CARD

Patient's Name — Last — First — Middle/Maiden   Sex ☐ M ☐ F   SSN

Date of Report ___/___/___   Date of Onset ___/___/___   Was this Disease Fatal? ☐ Yes ☐ No   Hospitalized For this Disease? ☐ Yes ☐ No

▲ ENTER CODE FOR DISEASE REPORTED (see other side)

Race ☐ White ☐ Black ☐ American Indian or Alaska Native ☐ Asian or Pacific Islander   Ethnic Origin ☐ Hispanic ☐ Non-Hispanic

Patient's Address: Street or RFD No.   Phone

City   Zip   County

Birthdate ___/___/___   Age ____ Years OR ____ Months   Site of Care: ☐ Active Military ☐ Public ☐ Private   Location Where Acquired (if other than county of residence)   ☐ SAME

*Complete this Section for Codes 9, 13, 23, 25, 26, 27, 38, Other TB, Chlamydia, Late Syphilis, Gonorrhea (if known)

Encephalitis (9), Viral Meningitis (26), Other Foodborne Disease (13) Causative Organism:

Hemophilus Influenzae (23), Meningococcus (27), Salmonella (38) Serotype:

Hemophilus Influenzae (23), Meningococcus (27), Other TB, Late Syphilis, Chlamydia Site of Infection:

Hemophilus Influenzae (23), Meningococcus (27), Gonorrhea Antibiotic Resistance: ☐ SENS.

COMMENTS:

Parent or Guardian (of minors)

Reported By (Full Name and Title)

Agency and Address

Attending Physician (if not individual reporting case)

Address   Phone

Patient is: ☐ Child or Worker in Day Care ☐ Parent of Child in Day Care ☐ Foodhandler ☐ Health Care Worker ☐ None of Above

State/LHD Use Only: outbreak related: ☐ no ☐ yes; specify:

Surveillance Form ☐ Completed ☐ Not Required   Case Investigation No.

Local Health Director's Signature or Stamp   Clinic No.

DEHNR 2124 (Revised 12/94) EPIDEMIOLOGY (Review 12/97)

Figure 36.1. Sample reporting card for communicable diseases.

bear the disproportionate burden of STD-associated complications. Table 36.1 presents the acute, chronic, and maternal-child impact of common STDs.

The main STD pathogens that are seen in the primary care setting are *Chlamydia*, *Neisseria gonorrhoeae* (GC), *Trichomonas*, HSV, *Treponema pallidum*, HPV, *Haemophilus ducreyi*, molluscum contagiosum, scabies, and lice. Each is discussed in the following text.

Chlamydia trachomatis is an obligate intracellular bacterium whose primary target cells are columnar epithelial cells that line the conjunctiva, urethra, endocervix, endometrium, and fallopian tubes. Its incubation period ranges from 1 week to more than 1 month. In men, the acute presentation of *Chlamydia* includes urethritis, epididymitis, and proctitis. *Chlamydia* causes 30 to 50% of cases of nongonococcal urethritis, an even higher portion of postgonococcal urethritis, and most cases of epididymitis in sexually active men younger than age 35 (2). Physical symptoms include dysuria, urethral discharge, anorectal pain and discharge, and perineal, pelvic or testicular pain. Chronic

Table 36.1.
Health Effects of Common Organisms Causing STDs

Organism	Acute Disease (Often Asymptomatic)	Effect on Maternal Child Health	Chronic Disease
Neisseria gonorrhoeae (GC)	Urethritis Cervicitis Salpingitis Epididymitis Proctitis Pharyngitis Disseminated infection	Premature rupture of membranes Prematurity Low birth weight Septic abortion Neonatal conjunctivitis Postpartum endometritis Perihepatitis	Infertility Ectopic pregnancy Pelvic adhesive disease (PAD)
Chlamydia trachomatis (chlamydia)	Urethritis Cervicitis Salpingitis Epididymitis Proctitis Pharyngitis	Premature rupture of membranes Prematurity Low birth weight Septic abortion Neonatal conjunctivitis Neonatal pneumonia Postpartum endometritis Perihepatitis	Infertility Ectopic pregnancy PAD Reiter's syndrome
Treponema pallidum (syphilis)	Primary (oral or anogenital ulcers) Secondary syphilis Tertiary syphilis	Spontaneous abortion Stillbirth Congenital syphilis	Neurosyphilis Cardiovascular syphilis Gumma
Haemophilus ducreyi (chancroid)	Anogenital ulcer	None known	? Phimosis
Human immunodeficiency virus (HIV)	Mild fever, malaise, and lymphadenopathy	Prematurity Stillbirth Perinatal HIV	AIDS
Human papillomavirus (HPV)	Oral, anal, and urogenital warts	Condyloma acuminatum Laryngeal papillomatosis	Anogenital cancer (cervical, vaginal, vulvar, anal, penile carcinoma)
Herpes simplex virus (HSV)	Oral, anal, and urogenital ulcers Pharyngitis Proctitis Meningitis	Neonatal HSV Prematurity	Vestibulitis (?)
Hepatitis B virus (HBV)	Acute hepatitis	Perinatal HBV	Chronic hepatitis Cirrhosis Hepatocellular carcinoma Hepatoma Vasculitis

Data are from Eng TR, Butler WT, eds. The Hidden Epidemic: Confronting Sexually Transmitted Disease. Committee on Prevention and Control of Sexually Transmitted Disease: Executive Summary (Appendix A). Institute of Medicine, Division of Health Promotion and Disease Prevention. Washington, DC: National Academy Press, 1996:1–15, 2–1, 2–38, 3–1, 3–48; and Brunham RC, Plummer FA. A general model of sexually transmitted disease epidemiology and its implications for control. Med Clin North Am 1990;74(6)1339–1352.

disease for men includes infertility after bilateral epididymitis and Reiter's syndrome. In women, chlamydial infection occurs acutely as urethritis, cervicitis, pelvic inflammatory disease (PID), and proctitis. Physical symptoms include dysuria, vaginal discharge, dyspareunia, anorectal pain and discharge, and pelvic pain. Chronic disease for women includes infertility, ectopic pregnancy, chronic pelvic pain, and Reiter's syndrome. In infants, *Chlamydia* manifests as conjunctivitis and pneumonia. Table 36.1 describes the acute and chronic effects as well as the effect on maternal-child health of chlamydial infections.

Neisseria gonorrhoeae is a bacterium capable of infecting and colonizing a very wide range of columnar or transitional epithelial mucous membranes. These include the urethra of both sexes, genital glands such as Tyson's in men and Bartholin's in women, the uterine cervical canal and tubes; the epididymis (leading to the male counterpart of salpingitis); the anal canal and distal rectum; and the conjunctiva and pharynx. The majority of anal canal and pharyngeal infections have no or nonspecific symptoms, and the natural histories are not well understood. Disseminated infections include skin (rash), joint (tenosynovitis, septic arthritis), cardiac (endocarditis), and central nervous system (meningitis) involvement.

GC manifests similarly to *Chlamydia*, but with a shorter incubation period of approximately 4 days. Table 36.1 lists the acute and chronic disease manifestations of GC. Patients present with complaints of dysuria, discharge, and testicular or pelvic pain. In infants, GC manifests as conjunctivitis, which if left untreated results in severe conjunctivitis, corneal scarring, abscess, eye perforation, and blindness.

Trichomonas vaginalis, a flagellated ameboid organism, usually elicits an acute inflammatory response that results in profuse vaginal discharge. Transmission is usually during sexual activity, but transmission via sheets and towels has been reported. The vagina and cervix in women, and the urethra and bladder in men, are the most common sites of infection. Symptoms for women include dysuria, urinary frequency, pelvic or lower abdominal pain, vaginal discharge, and pruritus. Physical findings include vulvar edema and erythema, vaginal discharge, erythematous vaginal walls, and punctate hemorrhages on the cervix (strawberry cervix). The majority of men are asymptomatic except for occasional urethritis.

Herpes simplex virus (HSV) tends to infect mucocutaneous sites and neuronal nuclei within the sensory ganglia. Both HSV-1 and HSV-2 cause similar infections and can infect mucous membranes and abraded skin at any site (3). Cell-mediated immune response appears more important than humoral immune response in controlling the severity of mucocutaneous HSV, so immunocompromised patients have episodes that are severe and prolonged.

By far the most common form of HSV infection in primary care is recurrent genital herpes, a relatively mild but recurrent outbreak of vesicles that ulcerate and then heal within 10 days. Approximately 50% of recurrences are preceded by a prodrome 1 to 48 hours beforehand, which is variously described as a tingling sensation, mild itching, or pain in the affected locations. Lesions of recurrent genital herpes tend to be unilateral and well localized.

Although most cases of genital HSV are recurrent, asymptomatic, and unrecognized, symptomatic first-episode infection is often a severe disease. Multiple bilateral lesions, moderate to severe local pain and dysuria, sacral paresthesia, tender inguinal adenopathy, fever and malaise are typically present. Lesions begin as vesicles or pustules and progress through stages of ulcer formation, crusting, and healing. The initial crop of lesions is often extensive, and adjacent pustules often coalesce to form larger areas of ulceration, sometimes into deep necrotic ulcers. Without treatment, most patients form crops of new lesions in the second week and heal all lesions by the end of the third week of illness. Complications of first-episode genital herpes include HSV pharyngitis, extragenital cutaneous lesions acquired by autoinoculation, aseptic meningitis, and urinary retention from local pain or autonomic nervous system dysfunction. Women are twice as likely as men to have systemic symptoms. Herpes simplex proctitis usually involves fever, malaise, severe rectal pain, tenesmus, constipation, and discharge.

The primary lesion of **syphilis** (*Treponema pallidum*), the chancre, is a painless, solitary ulcer with raised, well-defined borders and a clean, indurated base, usually associated with nontender regional lymphadenopathy and healing spontaneously in 3 to 6 weeks (4). Systemic dissemination of spirochetes begins during the primary stage, and in 60 to 90% of patients, clinically apparent secondary syphilis develops. Clinical manifestations of secondary syphilis typically occur 4 to 10 weeks after primary syphilis and include a broad array of clinical findings: myalgia, arthralgia, malaise, low-grade temperature, generalized lymphadenopathy, and rash. The rash is the most prominent feature; it is present in 10 to 75% of patients—a nonpruritic, maculopapular eruption affecting the trunk and limbs, including palms and soles. Condylomata lata—broad-based, flat or raised, fleshy lesions, usually on the anogenital, oral, or other mucous membranes—are also common in secondary syphilis. In 18 to 34% of patients who have secondary syphilis, the primary chancre is still present at the time of diagnosis (5).

Without treatment, clinical manifestations of secondary syphilis resolve spontaneously in 3 to 12 weeks, but symptomatic relapses occur for as long as 4 years after primary infection. After resolution of secondary syphilis, untreated individuals are referred to as having latent syphilis, during which there are no readily apparent clinical findings. Without therapy, approximately one third of partners develop tertiary syphilis, manifested as gummatous syphilis, cardiovascular syphilis, or neurosyphilis (5). Tertiary disease typically arises 10 to 30 years after initial infection. Sexual contact with persons who have early disease is associated with the highest risk of developing disease, whereas sexual contact in the latent phase has a lower risk of transmission.

Human papillomavirus plays a role in the development of anogenital malignancies in women and men. The most common manifestation of HPV in primary care is subclinical disease. Whether subclinical or clinical disease has greater infectivity is unknown, and treatment of clinical disease leads to subclinical disease rather than cure. Often HPV is first detected on routine cervical smears, manifesting as koilocytosis, atypia, and multinucleation, also known as low-grade squamous intraepithelial lesions (LGSIL). Some HPV DNA types are more likely to progress from LGSIL to high-grade squamous intraepithelial lesions (HGSIL). LGSIL will spontaneously regress in 80 to 90% of patients, whereas HGSIL are considered premalignant and are more likely to progress to cancer.

HPV probably gains entry through microabrasions occurring during sexual activity, infecting the internal and external genitalia, perineum, and anorectal areas. The most obvious clinical manifestation of HPV infection is overt genital warts, or condyloma acuminata. Genital lesions usually appear after an incubation period of approximately 3 months, with a range of 3 weeks to 8 months. Spontaneous regression of HPV occurs in 80 to 90% of exposed persons. Trauma or surgical manipulation of warts may lead to regression. Immunocompromised individuals have higher incidence of warts, genital dysplasia, and neoplasia. Existing HPV infections often worsen during pregnancy.

HPV lesions are either soft, sessile papules or fine, fingerlike projections. Perianal condylomata acuminata are usually rough and cauliflower-like, whereas penile lesions are usually smooth and papular. Although usually asymptomatic, some patients complain of pruritus, irritation, or bleeding of HPV lesions. Subclinical HPV infection is detected by application of dilute acetic acid followed by colposcopic or androscopic examination; the areas of HPV infection turn white.

Chancroid is a rare disease caused by *Haemophilus ducreyi*, most commonly seen in those who travel and have high-risk sexual exposure. The initial lesion is a small, often unnoticed, papule with surrounding erythema. This ulcerates and is covered by a gray-yellow necrotic exudate. The ulcer is typically painful, with ragged edges that are undermined, and a base that is friable, rough, and bleeds easily. Men most frequently have two to three ulcers that involve the frenulum, coronal sulcus, prepuce, or penile shaft. Left untreated, the ulcers coalesce to form giant ulcers that can erode through tissue planes, causing fistula formation. Concurrent inguinal adenitis occurs in 20 to 40% of patients and is often unilateral. Adenitis of 5 cm or more in diameter will often progress to suppuration that either ruptures spontaneously or requires aspiration.

Molluscum contagiosum, an unclassified member of the Poxviridae, is spread by person-to-person contact, auto-inoculation, and by sheets and towels. The infectious presentation is small, firm, smooth papules that are occasionally pruritic and usually pearly or flesh-colored with an erythematous base around an umbilicated center. They usually enlarge for approximately 1 month, persist for a few more months, and then spontaneously resolve.

Scabies, an infestation by the human itch mite, *Sarcoptes scabiei*, is transferred directly by skin-to-skin contact or in nits dislodged onto sheets and towels. Mites can survive off the host at normal temperature and humidity. Immunity to scabies does not develop and reinfection is possible. Social conditions that promote transmission include multiple sexual partners, overcrowding, and increased population mobility. There is a 4- to 6-week latent period as the mite burrows in the skin and sets off the host immune response. Symptoms develop much quicker with subsequent infections, as the immune response has already been prompted. The greatest number of nits are found in areas of skin folds and skin-to-skin contact, plus wrist folds, navel, nipples, and genitalia. The rash and burrows are rare above the neck and on the palms and soles. Usually the patient is continually scratching unless immunosuppressed.

Lice consist of crab louse (*Phthirius pubis*), body louse (*Pediculus humanus*), and head louse (*Pediculus humanus capitis*). Pubic lice can be found in any haired areas of the body; whereas head lice seem adapted to grasp scalp hair and are difficult to transplant to other areas of the body. Crab lice attach their eggs to hair follicles with a cementlike material secreted by the female; even after hatching, the empty nits stick to hair for a period of time. Washing, shampooing, vinegar, and even organic solvents do not always remove the empty egg cases; removal requires a fine-toothed comb or hair growth or cutting.

Lice are transmitted by intimate contact, sharing of clothing and hair brushes, toilets seats, and beds. Head lice are more common in children 6 years and younger, whereas pubic lice are more common in 15 to 25 year olds. Patients can be asymptomatic, mildly symptomatic, or have significant itching, erythema, and inflammation. It takes approximately 5 days before sensitization occurs. Many bites over a short period lead to fever, malaise, and irritability, whereas with long periods of infestation people become oblivious to the lice. Excessive scratching leads to superinfection.

GENERAL PRINCIPLES OF STD EVALUATION

History taking, particularly sexual history, and physical examination are key components to evaluating your patient's risk for acquiring an STD. In taking a sexual history, try to be very professional, sensitive, and nonjudgmental. Although sexual behavior and choice of partner are crucial factors, individual physiologic and sociologic characteristics also increase the risk for acquiring an STD (Table 36.2). Fear of AIDS has had a powerful motivating effect on sexual behavior, but people often underestimate their risk for exposure to HIV and other STDs and lack knowledge of safe-sexual practices. This makes a sexual history not always reliable. You should screen for STDs based on your patient's risk factors and the epidemiology of STDs in your patient population. Because self-reported sexual history is often an unreliable indicator of actual risk of infection, consider broader screening of populations in which prevalence of STDs is high.

STDs are more prevalent among persons in lower socioeconomic status (SES), and in African-American and Latino-American ethnic and racial groups (1). Race and ethnicity in the United States are risk markers that correlate with other more fundamental determinants of health status, such as poverty, access to quality medical care, health care-seeking behavior, drug use, and living in communities of higher STD prevalence (6). Sociologic factors that increase the risk for acquiring STDs are limited access to quality medical care; reduced priority for seeking health care in order to meet other needs, such as food and shelter; limited sources of income; and choosing a partner who lives in a community with a higher STD prevalence and who is in a lower SES.

Table 36.2.
Epidemiologic Factors Increasing the Risk for Acquiring STDs[a]

Physiologic	Sociologic	Behavioral
Adolescents	Commercial sex workers	Inconsistent use of condoms
Women age 25 and younger	Incarceration	New sex partner
Pregnant women	African-American	More than one sex partner within the past 3 mo, or more than two in the past year
STD	Latino-American	
Oral contraceptives	Lower socioeconomic status	Drug and alcohol use
Physical findings of cervicitis, urethritis, proctitis, testicular pain	Inner city neighborhood	Exchange of sex for money or drugs
Intact penile foreskin	Living where prevalence of STDs is higher	Unprotected oral, vaginal, or rectal intercourse
Uncircumcised patient or partner	Women undergoing elective termination of pregnancy	
Intrauterine contraceptive device (IUD)	Previous STD	
Vaginal douche use		

[a]Data in this table are based on the assumption that the individuals are sexually active.

Behavioral factors put your patients at the highest risk for acquiring STDs. Persons at high risk for STDs are those who have unprotected oral, vaginal, or rectal intercourse or inconsistently use condoms; have a new sex partner, more than one sex partner within the past 3 months or more than two partners in the past year; engage in sex for money or drugs; use parenteral or nonparenteral drugs; use drugs or alcohol during sexual activity, because they are less likely to practice safe sex; and have sexual partners who have any of the aforementioned risk factors.

SCREENING

The majority of STDs are asymptomatic, so the major role for the primary care clinician is to decide who to screen, when to screen, and how to screen. In general, all patients with one STD should be considered to be tested for others, and all patients at risk for STDs should be offered testing in accordance with recommendations on screening for syphilis, gonorrhea, HIV infection, and chlamydial infection and should receive hepatitis B vaccine.

The predictive value of STD testing increases within populations of higher prevalence of STDs, symptomatic persons, and persons at increased sexual risk. In asymptomatic persons, where prevalence is low and sexual health risk is low, very sensitive nonculture tests, such as enzyme immunoassay (EIA) or direct fluorescent antibody (DFA) for *Chlamydia,* are often false positive. Table 36.3 describes properties of available tests for several STD pathogens and the recommended screening guidelines. Where data are unavailable for sensitivities and specificities, comments are made in the chart and likelihood ratios are not reported.

You should check with your supporting laboratory as to the preferred method of testing. Culture is often a preferred test for sexual assault and abuse cases. The most common screening and confirmation test for each pathogen are as follows:

- GC screening: Gram's stain; confirmation: culture

- Chlamydia screening: EIA; confirmation: culture

- Syphilis screening: nontreponemal tests; confirmation: treponemal tests

- HPV screening: cytology; confirmation: where available, hybrid capture system, Southern blot or HPV/DNA

- HSV screening: DFA or EIA; confirmation: culture

COMMON PRIMARY CARE PROBLEMS INVOLVING STDS

In the primary care office and urgent care settings, STDs generally present as symptoms rather than with a diagnosis already identified. Common complaints consist of urethral discharge or burning; testicular pain; vaginal discharge or pelvic pain; genital lesions or itching; and concern about possible exposure to STDs. Signs and symptoms of cervicitis, proctitis, testicular pain, or undesired conception indicate a higher risk of the patient having acquired an STD.

Urethritis/Epididymitis

Painful urethral discharge and testicular swelling are the most common presentations of symptomatic STDs in men. The urethra is the site infected by the most treatable genital pathogens in men, and it is the reservoir for spread of infection to sexual partners. Ascending infection to the epididymis in men is infrequent; however, the majority of epididymitis in young men is secondary to STDs. Complications of urethritis include epididymitis and Reiter's syndrome. If the patient has testicular pain, you should consider testicular torsion in your differential diagnosis. Clues to the presence of testicular torsion include younger age; prior history of scrotal pain or torsion; a rotated or high-riding testicle; and absence of pyuria on urinalysis.

PATHOPHYSIOLOGY AND DIFFERENTIAL DIAGNOSIS

Classically urethritis is divided into gonococcal and nongonococcal. Gonococcal urethritis is diagnosed when gram-negative intracellular diplococci (GNIDs) are demonstrated on Gram's stain or by culture. *Trichomonas* also commonly infects the bladder and urethra and can cause complaints of dysuria and urethral discharge. *Chlamydia* causes many of the cases of nongonococcal urethritis and postgonococcal urethritis in men. *Ureaplasma urealyticum* appears to be causative in the remaining cases. The cause is unknown in approximately one third of men who have nongonococcal urethritis. Chlamydial urethritis cannot be distinguished on clinical ground from other

Table 36.3.
Properties of Commercially Used Screening Procedures for STDs[a]

STD	Laboratory Tests	Sensitivity	Specificity	LR+[b]	LR−[b]	Whom to Screen: Level of Evidence for Effectiveness[c,d]
GC	1. Culture	1. Endocervical culture 80–95%[d]				Ocular prophylaxis of newborns: A All high-risk women: B
	2. Gram stain	2. Male urethra 70–99%[d]; cervix 30–65%; pharyngeal and rectal not useful	2. Men 97–99%; women 90–97%[d]	2. Men 99; women 21.66	2. Men .01; women .36	High-risk pregnant women: B All pregnant women: C
	3. EIA[e]	3. 95%[d] male urethra; 60–100% endocervical	3. 95% male urethra[d]; endocervical 70 to 98%	3. Men 19; women 49.50	3. Men .05; women .01	General screening: X
	4. Urine LE[e]	4. 46–60%[e]	4. 93–96%[d]	4. 15	4. 41	
	5. DNA probe	5. 97–99%[e]	5. 97–99%[d]	5. 99	5. 01	
Chlamydia	1. Culture	1. 70–90%[d]	1. 100%[d]	1. 90	1. 10	All sexually active adolescents and high-risk women: B
	2. EIA[e]	2. 70–90%[d]; urine EIA 77–91%[d]	2. 97–99%[d]; urine EIA 97–100%[d]	2. 90; urine .92	2. .10; urine .09	All pregnant women: C High-risk pregnant women/high-risk men: C
	3. DFA[e]	3. 70–90%[d]	3. 97–99%[d]	3. 99	3. 99	Ocular prophylaxis of newborn: C
	4. Urine LE[e]	4. 40–100%[d]				General screening: X
	5. Pap[e]	5. 10%[f]	5. 4.5%[f]	5. 11	5. 20	
	6. PCR[e]	6. Vaginal, cervical or urethral specimens 60–95%[d]; urine specimens 95 to 99%[d]	6. 95%[d]	6. 19	6. 05	
	7. LCR[e]	7. Vaginal, cervical or urethral 95%[d]; urine 95–99%[d]	7. Vaginal, cervical urethral 95%[d], urine 95–99%	7. 19	7. 05	
	8. DNA probe	8. 60–95%[d]	8. Vaginal, cervical, urethral 95%[d]; urine 95–99%[d]	8. 19	8. 05	
Syphilis	1. Nontreponemal tests: a. RPR[e] b. VDRL[e]	1. Early, primary 62–76%[d]; secondary 100%; late 70%[d]	1. 75–85% with concomitant illness and 100% without concomitant illness[d,g]	1. Primary 76; secondary .24; late 99	1. Primary .01; secondary 70; late .30	All high-risk persons: A Pregnant women at first visit: A Repeat testing for high-risk pregnant women in third trimester and at delivery: A

	2. Treponemal tests: a. FTA-ABS^e b. MHA-TP^e	2. Primary 84%, 100% other stages^d	2. 96%^{d,g}	2. Primary 21; other 24.75	2. Primary: .17; other: .01	Persons with other STDs (including HIV): A Sexual contacts of persons with syphilis: A
	3. Dark-field microscopy	3. Primary syphilis: approximately 80%	3. Primary syphilis: specificity "fairly high"			
HPV	1. Histology	1. 15–36%^h "probably equivalent to cytology"	1. Koilocytosis felt to be highly specific but subjective; operator dependent			Routine screening: C
	2. Cytology	2. 15–36%^h	2. Same as #1 above			
	3. HPV DNA	3. Possibly 100%	3. 90%			
	4. Southern blot	4. "Sensitive"	4. "Specific;" sometimes used as confirmatory			
	5. PCR^e	5. 90%^i	5. Sometimes used as confirmatory; false positives			
	6. HCS^e	6. "Very sensitive"	6. 100% considered by some to be the new gold standard			
HSV	1. Viral culture	1. 43% for recurrent lesions; 82% primary lesions; vesicles 93%, ulcers 72%, crusted lesions 27%,^d				Routine screening in asymptomatic persons: X Routine screening in asymptomatic pregnant women; clinicians should take a complete sexual history on all adult and adolescent patients: X
	2. Tzanck smear	2. 65%	2. 85% (does not differentiate HSV-1, HSV-2, and VZV)	2. 4.33	2. 0.41	
	3. Serology	3. Does not differentiate HSV-1 and HSV-2	3. Does not differentiate HSV-1, HSV-2, and VZV			Recommending abstinence or condoms during intercourse for pregnant women with HSV-positive partners: C
	4. Cytology	4. 30–80%	4. Does not differentiate HSV-1, HSV-2, and VZV			Examining pregnant women for signs of active genital lesions and performance of cesarean section on those with lesions present: C
	5. DFA^e	5. 70–90%^g				
	6. EIA^e	6. 59–93%^d				

continued

Table 36.3. (continued)
Properties of Commercially Used Screening Procedures for STDs[a]

STD	Laboratory Tests	Sensitivity	Specificity	LR+[b]	LR−[b]	Who to Screen: Level of Evidence for Effectiveness[c, d]
	7. PCR[e]	7. 93–100%[d]				Use of systemic acyclovir in pregnant women with recurrent herpes to prevent reactivation near term: C
Trichomonas	1. Wet prep	1. 50–75%[h]	1. 70–98%[h]	1. 37.50	1. 25	
	2. DFA[e]	2. 80–86%[h]	2. 98%[h]	2. 43	2. 04	

[a]Many testing techniques are reader dependent, and it would be valuable to check with your supporting laboratory to obtain local sensitivity, specificity, as well as prevalence data.

[b]Where ranges are given for sensitivity and specificity, the highest reported value is used for likelihood ratios, except 99% is used for any values of 100%.

[c]See chapter section on General Principles of STD Evaluation for defining high risk. Abbreviations used with level of evidence for effectiveness: A, strong or moderate research-based evidence (consistent across several studies, including at least two randomized controlled trials); B, limited research-based evidence (less consistent or extensive evidence, but preponderance of evidence supports use of treatment); C, common practice with little or no research-based evidence; X, moderate or strong evidence suggesting that this treatment is not effective.

[d]Data are from Guide to Clinical Preventive Services. Report of the US Preventive Services Task Force, 2nd ed. Baltimore: Williams & Wilkins, 1996;287–302; 325–346.

[e]EIA, enzyme immunoassay; LE, leukocyte esterase; DFA, direct fluorescent antibody; PCR, polymerase chain reaction; LCR, ligase chain reaction; RPR, rapid plasma reagin; VDRL, Venereal Disease Research Laboratory; MHA-TP, microhemagglutination assay for antibodies to *Treponema pallidum*; FTA-ABS, fluorescent treponemal antibody absorption test; HCS, hybrid capture system.

[f]Data are from Caudill JL, Humphrey SK, Goeller JR. Cervicovaginal cytology and the diagnosis of *Chlamydia trachomatis*: a comparison with immunofluorescent results. Diagn Cytopathol 1994;11(1):20–22.

[g]HIV infection may reduce the specificity of syphilis testing. Nontreponemal test results may remain persistently positive after treatment, thus making treatment difficult to assess; and treponemal test results may become nonreactive after treatment, thus making documentation of past infection difficult.

[h]Data are from Bickley LS. Acute vaginitis. In: Panzer RJ, Black ER, Griner PF, eds. Diagnostic strategies for common medical problems. Philadelphia: American College of Physicians, 1991:249–259.

[i]Data are from Eng TR, Butler WT, eds. The Hidden Epidemic: Confronting Sexually Transmitted Disease. Committee on Prevention and Control of Sexually Transmitted Disease: Executive Summary (Appendix A). Institute of Medicine Division of Health Promotion and Disease Prevention. Washington, DC: National Academy Press, 1996;1–15; 2–1, 2–38, 3–1, 3–48.

nongonococcal urethritides. *Chlamydia* appears to be the cause of epididymitis in the majority of cases of sexually active men younger than age 35. Epididymitis tends to be caused by urinary tract pathogens, such as *Escherichia coli* and *Pseudomonas,* in men who are older, have structural abnormalities of the urethra, have recently undergone a urinary tract procedure or manipulation, or men who practice anal intercourse.

CLINICAL EVALUATION

The patient has symptoms of urethral discharge, dysuria, or even urethral itching. The urethral discharge varies from a slight increase in urethral secretions noted only in the morning to a florid and spontaneously present yellow or green discharge. The more pronounced the discharge, the more acute the symptoms, the greater the likelihood of GC. GC incubation is often less than a week versus nongonococcal urethritis (NGU), which peaks at 2 to 3 weeks. NGU discharge is often slight, not apparent without stripping the urethra, and tends to be gray, white, or mucoid rather than yellow. Patients with epididymitis often have acute onset of unilateral testicular pain and swelling; tenderness of the epididymis and vas deferens; erythema and edema of the overlying scrotal skin; and urethral discharge and dysuria. Most epididymitis is secondary to urethritis or prostatitis; when accompanied by urethritis, it is probably sexually acquired. Differential diagnosis should include noninfectious causes, such as trauma, torsion of the testicle, and tumor.

Be sure to take a careful history of sexual activity, genital or urinary tract symptoms, recent history of trauma or genitourinary (GU) tract manipulation, or known or suspected structural or functional abnormalities of the urinary tract.

Do a gentle, careful GU examination to look for urethral discharge and to examine the scrotal contents. When urethral discharge is not obvious on genitourinary examination, have the patient milk his urethra from the base to the meatus three or four times. If no discharge can be obtained at the initial examination, consider having symptomatic patients return for reexamination at least 4 hours after they have voided. Early in epididymitis the swelling and tenderness is localized to one area of the epididymis, but in time swelling usually extends to involve the whole epididymis and surrounding areas such that the epididymis is not discernible

in the inflammatory mass. Gentle elevation tends to relieve the pain of testicular torsion, whereas it increases the pain of epididymitis. Testicular torsion is a surgical emergency. A nontender, rock-hard scrotal mass should make you concerned about cancer.

Laboratory Tests

Obtain a urethral swab, culture it for GC, and test for *Chlamydia;* also look for GNIDs on Gram's stain. Obtain a midstream urine for urinalysis and culture (red blood cells may be present, secondary to urethral trauma from urethral swab, but do the urethral swabs first). Positive leukocyte esterase (LE) on urinalysis can indicate the presence of *Chlamydia,* GC, or urinary tract pathogens.

MANAGEMENT

If *Chlamydia* and GC are suspected by history, physical, and preliminary laboratory test results, presumptively treat for both, while awaiting laboratory culture results (see Tables 36.3 and 36.4). If *Trichomonas* appears to be the etiologic pathogen, treat while awaiting GC and *Chlamydia* test results. Patients need to be informed that they have a sexually transmitted infection and that their sexual contacts need to be treated. This is a good opportunity to provide patient education on safe sexual practices (see patient education section). If the urine looks suspicious for UTI, treat for urinary pathogens. Table 36.5 summarizes the diagnosis and management of common symptomatic STDs in men.

Cervicitis, Pelvic Inflammatory Disease (PID), and Pelvic Pain

In contrast to men, where STDs tend to remain confined to the urethra, lower genital tract pathogens in women frequently and rapidly ascend to the endometrium and adnexa. PID is a spectrum of upper genital tract disorders that includes endometritis, salpingitis, tubo-ovarian abscess, and pelvic peritonitis, and which can lead to infertility, ectopic pregnancy, and chronic pelvic pain. Because of potential significant damage to the reproductive health of women (see Table 36.1), you should have a low threshold for diagnosis and treatment.

Table 36.4.
Summary of STD Treatment

STD (Etiology)	Primary Treatment	Alternative Treatment	Comments
Anogenital warts (HPV)	(1) 10–25 % podophyllin: apply to lesions, have patient wash off lesions in 1–4 h; apply weekly for 6 wk (2) Podofilox: patient can self-apply; twice a day for 4 d, off 4 d, then reapply for 4 d for a total of 4 cycles	(1) Liquid nitrogen; bichloroacetic or trichloroacetic acid; applied weekly for 6 wk (2) Electrodesiccation (3) Surgical removal (4) Imiquimod 5% cream applied three times a wk for up to 6 wk	Women should have annual Pap smear; no podophyllin in pregnant women; caution with podophyllin application to mucosal areas, it is a caustic agent
Chlamydia (Chlamydia trachomatis)	(1) Doxycycline 100 mg po bid × 14 d (2) Tetracycline 250/500 bid for 14 d (3) Azithromycin 1.0 g po single dose	(1) Erythromycin base 500 mg qid for 7 d (2) Erythromycin ethylsuccinate 800 mg qid for 7 d (3) Ofloxacin 300 mg bid for 7 d	Most have concomitant GC—treat for both; use erythromycin and azithromycin if breast feeding or pregnant
Gonorrhea (*N. gonorrhea*)	(1) Ceftriaxone 125 mg IM (2) Cefixime 400 mg po single dose	(1) Spectinomycin 2 g IM (2) Cefotaxime 500 mg IM single dose (3) Ciprofloxacin 500 mg po single dose (4) Ofloxacin 400 mg po single dose	Most have concomitant *Chlamydia*—test and treat for both; fluoroquinolones contraindicated in pregnant, lactating women, and children and adolescents 17 years and under
Nonspecific urethritis or cervicitis (*Mycoplasma hominis, Ureaplasma, Mycoplasma genitalium*)	(1) Doxycycline 100 mg bid for 7 d (2) Azithromycin 1.0 g po as single dose	(1) Erythromycin base 500 mg qid po for 7 d (2) Ofloxacin 300 mg bid po for 7 d	Test for Chlamydia—use erythromycin or azithromycin in pregnant women
HSV (herpes simplex virus 1 or 2)	Primary HSV (1) Acyclovir 200 mg 5 times a day for 7 to 10 d, or 400 mg tid for 10 d	Recurrent HSV (1) Acyclovir 400 mg po tid for 5 d; 200 mg five times a day for 5 d; 800 mg bid for 5 d (2) Famciclovir 125 mg bid for 5 d (3) Valacyclovir 500 mg po bid for 5 d	Proctitis: 400 mg 5 times a day for 10 d Daily suppressive RX (for 6 or more episodes a year): acyclovir 400 mg bid or 200 mg 3 to 5 times a day; reassess after 1 y

Disease	Treatment	Alternative	Comments
Syphilis (Treponema pallidum): early, primary, secondary, latent < 1 y	Benzathine penicillin G (2.4 million U IM) once	(1) Doxycycline 100 mg bid for 14 d (2) Tetracycline 500 mg qid po for 14 d (3) Ceftriaxone 125 mg qd IM for 10 d or 250 mg qod IM for 5 doses or 1 g IM qod for 4 doses	For late latent, unknown duration, or tertiary, benzathine penicillin G 2.4 million U IM weekly for 3 wk, or ceftriaxone for 4 wk duration; serologic testing should decrease by 3 mo after treatment; if not, consider a lumbar puncture to rule out CSF involvement
Trichomonas (Trichomonas vaginalis)	(1) Metronidazole 2 g single dose (2) Metronidazole 500 mg bid for 7 d		First-trimester pregnancy, clotrimazole tablets vaginally 100 mg at bedtime for 7 to 14 d; treat with metronidazole after first trimester
Molluscum contagiosum	(1) Curettage (2) Liquid nitrogen (3) Trichloroacetic acid (4) Cantherone 0.7% (5) Salicylic acid 16%	(1) Retin A	"Tincture of time" can sometimes be used
Lice (Phthirus pubis)	(1) Permethrin 1% (Nix) rinse—wash off after 10 min (2) Lindane 1% shampoo—apply for 4 min, then wash off	(1) Pyrethrins with piperonyl butoxide—wash off after 10 min	Wash all bedding and clothing—machine wash or machine dry; no lindane in pregnant women or children under age 2
Scabies (Sarcoptes scabiei)	(1) Permethrin 1% (Nix)—apply from neck down; wash off after 8 h (2) Lindane (Kwell)—apply from neck down; wash off in 8 h (3) Pyrethrin with piperonyl butoxide (RID)		Wash all bedding and clothing with pyrethrins (e.g., RID Spray)—machine wash or machine dry; no lindane in pregnant women or children under age 2
Chancroid (Haemophilus ducreyi)	(1) Azithromycin 1.0 g single dose (2) Ceftriaxone 250 mg IM in single dose	(1) Erythromycin 500 mg qid for 7 d (2) Augmentin 500 mg tid for 7 d (3) Ciprofloxacin 500 mg bid for 3 d	

Table 36.5.
Diagnosis and Management of Common Symptomatic STDs in Men

Diagnosis	Symptom	Sign	Laboratory Findings	Management[a]
GC urethritis	Urethral discharge (with or without epididymal pain)	Purulent discharge	GNID on Gram's stain PMNs and LE on UA	Test and treat for both GC and *Chlamydia*; treat partner; patient education
NGU	Urethral discharge (with or without epididymal pain)	Minimal, mucoid discharge	No GNID on Gram's stain PMNs and LE on UA	Test and treat for both GC and *Chlamydia*; treat partners; remember other pathogens[b]; patient education
Trichomonal urethritis	Dysuria, urethral discharge	Minimal, mucoid, to frankly purulent discharge	PMNs and *Trichomonas* rich on UA or wet prep	Test for GC and *Chlamydia*; treat for *Trichomonas*; consider presumptive treatment for GC and *Chlamydia* while awaiting cultures; treat partners; patient education
Epididymitis	Testicular pain	Tender epididymis and vas deferens, erythema and edema of overlying skin, testicular pain and swelling, testes in usual position	PMNs and LE on UA	Test for GC and *Chlamydia*; presumptively treat for *Chlamydia*; Ice, NSAIDs, scrotal support, rest; treat first partners; patient education

[a]See Table 36.4 for treatment options.
[b]*Ureaplasma urealyticum, Mycoplasma hominis, Mycoplasma genitalium,* and HSV cause NGU, and often coexist with *Chlamydia.*

PATHOPHYSIOLOGY AND DIFFERENTIAL DIAGNOSIS

The endocervix is the most common female organ infected by STD pathogens; causes of cervicitis include *Trichomonas*, *Chlamydia*, HSV, and GC. More than half of endocervical infections do not cause sufficient inflammation to result in clinical signs. GC, *Chlamydia*, anaerobic bacteria, gram-negative rods (*E. coli*), and other organisms can ascend and cause significant inflammation (PID) and scarring (pelvic adhesive disease [PAD]) of the female reproductive organs; *Trichomonas* and HSV do not.

Some women who have PID present as medical emergencies because they are very ill. If you suspect PID, you should rule out surgical emergencies such as ovarian torsion, ectopic pregnancy, and appendicitis.

CLINICAL EVALUATION

Patients with cervicitis and PID represent a continuum from minimally symptomatic to very ill. Differential diagnosis of pelvic pain should include PID, appendicitis, endometriosis, uterine fibroids, adnexal or ovarian masses, depression, and history of abuse or presently abusive relationship.

History

With acute cervicitis or PID, physical symptoms involve:

- Perineal and urethral complaints—itching or burning

- Vaginal complaints—discharge, odor, or insertional dyspareunia

- Cervical symptoms—deep dyspareunia, pelvic pain, and spotting after intercourse

- Menstrual and abdominal complaints—pelvic pain, deep dyspareunia, constant abdominal pain or abdominal pain worse at time of or just after menses, worsening dysmenorrhea, or heavier menses, and/or

- Systemic symptoms—fever, chills, myalgia, and malaise

With chronic PID or PAD, complaints include infertility, dysmenorrhea, or deep dyspareunia.

Your sexual history should ask about any specific sexual concerns the patient might have as well as any history of sexual trauma or assault.

When you are inquiring about possible sexual trauma, such as rape or sexual abuse, you can make this less threatening by using unloading techniques, such as saying, "Sometimes women with pelvic pain have had sexual trauma or abuse. Have you been hurt or abused in any way?" Being aware of previous sexual trauma alerts you to the need to perform a much slower, and even more gentle examination.

Physical Examination

In doing the pelvic examination, look for

- Vulvar and labial erythema and swelling, which is indicative of trichomonal or HSV infection

- Perineal swelling, vesicles, or ulcers, which suggest HSV infection

- Swelling, tenderness, and drainage in Bartholin's gland sites, which suggest GC infection

- Inflammation at the opening of Bartholin's or Skene's glands, or tenderness in the vestibule, which are indicative of vestibulitis, possibly from HPV or HSV

Vulvar findings of *Trichomonas* include diffuse erythema, copious profuse vaginal discharge, and edema of the labia. The discharge is usually yellow-green and frothy, sometimes gray, and the vaginal walls are often erythematous and granular appearing, while punctate hemorrhages of the cervix give it a strawberry appearance. Increased polymorphonuclear neutrophils (PMNs) are seen in the wet prep. Cervicitis appears as a red, "angry" cervix that bleeds easily (friable), with mucopurulent drainage coming from the os. Vesicles on the cervix are consistent with HSV. Mucopurulent discharge is seen with GC and chlamydial cervicitis or PID. Vaginal HPV lesions are associated with vaginal discharge, pruritus, and postcoital bleeding, although most are asymptomatic. Cervical motion tenderness on bimanual pelvic examination indicates PID. An adnexal mass may indicate an enlarged, swollen, inflamed fallopian tube, a tubo-ovarian abscess, or an ectopic pregnancy. The Fitz-Hugh-Curtis syndrome reveals the same physical signs and symptoms as PID, plus right upper quadrant pain and tenderness to palpation of the liver.

When no vaginal or cervical discharge or inflammation is noted, and the patient's main complaint is infertility or chronic pelvic pain, you should examine the cervix, uterus and adnexa for mobility and tenderness. A fixed or not freely mobile uterus, or adnexal masses are indicative of pelvic adhesive disease.

Look for fever, increased pulse rate and blood pressure, particularly if the patient is in significant pain. Enlarged, painful inguinal lymph nodes can be present. When lower abdominal pain is present, you should do a careful abdominal examination to rule out an acute abdomen from other etiology such as appendicitis, ruptured ectopic, ruptured ovarian cyst, kidney stones or pyelonephritis. Abdominal examination should include examination for suprapubic pain and costovertebral angle pain, which indicate a urinary etiology for the pain and fever. Examine Skene's and Bartholin's glands for swelling, tenderness, and drainage. Any external genital, perineal, and perianal lesions or drainage should be noted.

A gentle, careful vaginal speculum examination should be done. The patient may be very tender and the inflamed cervix bleeds easily from trauma. Examine the cervix for friability, discharge, vesicles, or other lesions. Perform a gentle pelvic examination for cervical motion tenderness, adnexal masses or fullness, and mobility of the uterus and adnexa.

Laboratory Tests

Women who have mucopurulent vaginal discharge, drainage from the cervix, cervicitis, or a friable cervix that cannot be easily explained by increased ectropion from pregnancy or oral contraceptives (OCPs) should be tested for GC, chlamydial, trichomonal, and bacterial vaginosis. Cervical ulcerative lesions should be tested for HSV. Definitive diagnosis of *Trichomonas* requires identifying the organism on wet prep. Elevated complete blood count and erythrocyte sedimentation rate will help you diagnose PID. If pregnancy is likely and ectopic pregnancy must be ruled out, you should obtain an HCG titer.

MANAGEMENT

Table 36.6 presents the diagnosis and management of common symptomatic STDs in women. Admission, for intravenous management of antibiotics, fluid, and pain, should be considered for the very ill-appearing woman. Patient education should be provided.

Genital Ulcer Disease

Herpes simplex virus is the most common single cause of genital ulcers in patients seen in gynecology and STD disease clinics in the United States, but you should also consider syphilis, chancroid, and noninfectious cause of such as trauma, contact dermatitis, or Behçet's syndrome.

PATHOPHYSIOLOGY AND DIFFERENTIAL DIAGNOSIS

Noncircumcised men have an increased rate of genital ulcerative disease (GUD). Ulcers appear on the foreskin, coronal sulcus, glans, shaft, and anorectal area in men. In women ulcers appear on the external genitalia, in the vagina, on the cervix, and in the anorectal area. Ulcers of the perianal area and female genitalia tend to be easily overlooked unless symptomatic.

Physical examination is helpful but cannot always establish the cause of genital ulcers. Knowing the disease prevalence in the practice area is very helpful, as prevalence is the best predictor of etiology. A minority of ulcers, usually less than 10%, are the result of more than one etiologic agent, and these cannot be diagnosed except by laboratory investigation. Remember that the clinical features of ulcers are altered in the individual with immunosuppressive illness.

Some tips on establishing a differential diagnosis of genital ulcers are as follows:

- Superficial erosion can result from contact dermatitis, trauma, candidal balanitis, or intertrigo.

- Herpes zoster affects the anogenital region as multiple ulcers in a single, unilateral dermatomal distribution.

- Lichen sclerosis can result in anogenital ulcerations.

- Contact dermatitis from any agent in contact with this area, including sexual toys, aids, and lubricants, can present as a rash with ulceration.

- Traumatic lesions may result from sexual intercourse, masturbation, or accidental injury.

- Allergic or traumatic ulcers tend to be shallow, surrounded by erythema, with a clear, weeping discharge, and accompanying local swelling and erythema.

Table 36.6.
Diagnosis and Management of Common Symptomatic STDs in Women

Diagnosis	Symptom	Sign	Laboratory Findings	Management[a]
Vaginitis or cervicitis	Vaginal discharge, pain or spotting with intercourse	Vaginal discharge; vulvar or labial erythema or edema; friable, inflamed cervix; perineal, vaginal, or cervical vesicles or ulcers	PMNs and/or *Trichomonas* on wet prep	Test βHCG if warranted; culture for *Chlamydia* and GC; test for HSV if suspicious; treat *Trichomonas* if present; consider presumptively treating for GC and *Chlamydia* until cultures return; treat partners; patient education
PID	Pelvic pain; ± vaginal discharge; lower abdominal pain, worse with menses	Fever; ± lower abdominal pain; ± vaginal discharge; ± friable cervix; cervical motion tenderness; adnexal tenderness	Elevated WBC; elevated sedimentation rate; PMNs and/or clue cells on wet prep	Test βHCG if warranted; culture for *Chlamydia* and GC and treat presumptively; treat *Trichomonas* if present; treat for pain; consider hospitalization; treat partners; patient education
PAD	Pelvic pain, deep dyspareunia; ± history of STD	Normal or tender examination; ± sense of nonmobility to uterus or thickness in rectovaginal septum or fullness to adnexa	Negative HCG; normal wet prep, WBC, and sedimentation rate	Consider culture and presumptive treatment for PID; consider ultrasound to rule out pelvic adhesive disease from PID or endometriosis or adnexal masses (hydrosalpinx or ovarian mass); patient education
Chronic pelvic pain	Pelvic pain; dyspareunia; sexual concerns	Normal or highly tense pelvic examination; pain at introitus or opening of Bartholin's or Skene's glands	Normal laboratory findings	Explore for sexual or psychic trauma; explore for depression; if pain at introitus or opening of Bartholin's or Skene's glands, consider vestibulitis; patient education

[a]See Table 36.4 for treatment options.
[b]PID is an unusual complication in pregnancy but can occur. An ultrasound should be done to rule out ectopic pregnancy.

Abbreviations: βHCG, β-human chorionic gonadotropin; GC, *Neisseria gonorrhoeae*; HCG, human chorionic gonadotropin; HSV, herpes simplex virus; PAD, pelvic adhesive disease; PID, pelvic inflammatory disease; PMN, polymorphonuclear neutrophils; WBC, white blood cells.

CLINICAL EVALUATION

Patients may simply complain of a lesion on the genitals, or they have symptoms of pain, dysuria, or discharge. After taking a careful history, you should perform a genitourinary examination to characterize the ulcer and to identify any accompanying signs, such as urethral or vaginal discharge, inguinal adenopathy or any associated skin lesions.

syphillis = painless

MANAGEMENT

Patients with painless ulcers, with or without accompanying painless inguinal adenopathy, should be tested for syphilis. HSV, chancroid, herpes zoster, contact dermatitis, or trauma all tend to produce painful ulcers. If HSV is suspected, you should consider treating your patient presumptively pending test results.

Dysuria from urine hitting sensitive ulcers, is managed by having patients empty their bladders while sitting in a tub of warm water. Safe sexual practices should be reiterated to the patient. Because acquisition of HSV is more commonly asymptomatic, be careful not to implicate your patient's most recent partner. Table 36.7 summarizes the presentation and management of common STD pathogens associated with genital ulcer disease.

SUSPECTED STD EXPOSURE

Patients sometimes have concerns about possibly having acquired an STD in one of the following situations: unprotected sex or casual sex with a new, not well-known partner; having the condom break; having been a victim of sexual violence, including coercion; having been informed by sexual partners or public health authorities that they have come in contact with an STD; or having discovered that their usual sexual partner has had a sexual relationship with someone outside their relationship. Such situations often lead to a great deal of anxiety. You should handle these situations very professionally and with sensitivity, expecting the full range of emotional feelings to the possible diagnosis of an STD.

Obtaining as much historical data as possible from the patient is helpful in guiding your evaluation and approach. If the partner was truly anonymous or casual, test for *Chlamydia*, GC, syphilis, and HIV, and offer hepatitis B vaccination. Presumptive treatment, although controversial, helps alleviate patients' fears as they await cultures. For patients anxious over the discovery of their partners having other sexual partners, consider offering them an STD work up to help alleviate their anxiety. Counsel them about hepatitis B to determine if they are candidates for the immunization. You should also assess risk for

Table 36.7.
Common STD Pathogens Associated with Genital Ulcerative Disease

Etiology	Ulcer	Other Signs or Symptoms	Management[a]
Syphilis	Painless, smooth margins, firm, raised borders, clean indurated base, serous exudate	Rubbery, nontender adenopathy	RPR or VDRL; confirm positive results with FTA-ABS; dark-field examination if available, report positive results for contact tracing; patient education
HSV	Blisters on erythematous base or shallow ulcers	Prodrome: fever, malaise, myalgias, headache, dysuria	Culture; Tzanck smear; treat pending results; patient education
Chancroid	Starts as small papule surrounded by erythema, ulcerates into a painful, deep, raw, purulent, irregular, undermined border, bleeds easily	Painful lymphadenopathy, lymphadenitis, lymph nodes can be fluctuant	Test for syphilis, culture, Gram's stain of colonies (gram-negative coccobacillus in parallel rows ["school of fish"]), treat results of pending cultures; patient education

[a]See Table 36.4 for treatment options.

Abbreviations: FTA-ABS, fluorescent treponemal antibody absorption; RPR, rapid plasma reagin; VDRL, Venereal Disease Research Laboratory.

pregnancy and offer emergency contraception if indicated. Table 36.8 summarizes the approach to patients who have suspected STD exposure.

Genital Itching

Anogenital or perineal itching is a common reason for seeking health care. It occurs alone as a symptom or in combination with other genitourinary or perianal symptoms. As with other genital complaints, patients may be very embarrassed to disclose their symptoms and concerns to the health care provider for fear of judgment.

PATHOPHYSIOLOGY AND DIFFERENTIAL DIAGNOSIS

Scabies, HPV, lice, vaginal discharge from *Trichomonas,* bacterial vaginosis, *Candida, Chlamydia,* and GC can cause genital itching and should be considered in the differential diagnosis. Molluscum contagiosum can occasionally be pruritic. Scabies develops a severe itch secondary to the allergic reaction to the itch mite. Itching is the prominent feature in all louse infections. HPV, especially subclinical, tends to be pruritic. Itching may also be secondary to contact dermatitis or other dermatologic conditions such as psoriasis, eczema, lichen sclerosis, or atrophy. Local allergic reaction to cleansing agents (hygiene sprays), hygienic products (deodorant tampons, pads, or panty liners), sexual aids (spermicide or lubricants), as well as alteration in normal physiology or pH (douches) or trauma (abrasions from rough sex play) can all result in genital itching. Changes from over-the-counter or home remedies your patient has tried often further confuse the diagnosis.

CLINICAL EVALUATION

Patients may present with complaints of itching, irritation, or even having seen something jump around in the hairy areas of their genitals. Itching can be associated with vaginal or urethral discharge, or clearly follow exposure to a potential allergen (e.g., new soap).

Table 36.8.
Approach to Patient with Suspected or Known STD Exposure

Situation	Management
Known pathogen exposure	Consider testing for other pathogens; treat for known pathogen while awaiting other test results; offer hepatitis B vaccine; assess for possible pregnancy; supportive counseling; patient education
Casual, unsafe sexual exposure	Consider testing for all STDs from all sites of contact; consider treating if symptomatic; offer hepatitis B vaccine; assess for possible pregnancy; supportive counseling and patient education; consider syphilis/HIV serology in 12 wk
Victim of sexual assault, no condom used, known low-risk partner	Consider testing for all STDs from all sites of contact; assess risk as to whether to treat presumptively; offer hepatitis B vaccine; give morning-after pill if risk of undesired pregnancy[a]; supportive counseling; patient education
Victim of sexual assault, no condom used, unknown risk or known high risk	Test for all STDs from all sites of contact, including hepatitis A,B,C; consider presumptive treatment for *Chlamydia,* GC, and *Trichomonas*[b]; offer hepatitis B vaccine; give morning-after pill if risk of unwanted pregnancy[a]; supportive counseling; patient education[c]; consider repeating examination in 2 wk and syphilis/HIV serology 12 wk after assault[d]

[a]Common morning-after pill regimens: two doses of 2 Ovral ts orally, 12 hours apart; or two doses of 4 ts, 12 hours apart of Lo/Ovral, Nordette, Levlen, Triphasil, or Tri-Levlen; or RU 486 single 600 mg dose; or Alesse, two doses of 5 pink tablets, 12 hours apart. Treatment must be given within 72 hours after unprotected intercourse. Anticipate having to treat for nausea.

[b]Ceftriaxone 125 mg IM plus metronidazole 2 g po plus doxycycline 100 mg po bid for 14 days

[c]The risk of acquiring HIV is <0.1% for mucous membrane exposure to blood.

[d]On initial testing, the pathogen may not be present in high-enough quantities.

You should do a GU examination to look for skin changes and urethral or vaginal discharge, and note any movement (lice) or whitish debris (nits). HPV lesions include condyloma or minimal skin changes with erythema from scratching. HPV-exposed areas will turn white on application of 2 to 3% acetic acid (vinegar). Erythema, swelling, excoriation, and ulcerative changes can result from scratching.

MANAGEMENT

Management entails identifying the etiology, breaking the itch-scratch cycle, and providing patient education. Often a presumptive diagnosis is made, and treatment instituted, with follow-up in a week or 10 days.

Treatment of STDs

Table 36.4 summarizes treatment for STDs. You should stress the importance of completing the entire course of antibiotics to reduce the chance of recurrent infection and decrease the likelihood of antibiotic resistance developing. Remember that sexual partners need to be treated to prevent reinfection of the patient and spread of the disease. Treatment failures are usually due to reinfection, failure to treat sexual partners, or noncompliance with therapy.

PATIENT EDUCATION

Patient and public education is crucial in reducing transmission of STDs. Sexual health concepts important for individuals to understand include safe sexual practice, sexual health risks, and risks inherent in choice of sexual partners. You should help your patients to feel empowered to negotiate what type of sexual activity they are willing to participate in and to negotiate safe sexual practices with their partners.

Latex condoms and spermicide reduce transmission for several STD pathogens. Latex condoms should be used during vaginal, anorectal, and oropharyngeal sexual activities. You should be prepared to teach patients the correct use of condoms. Petroleum-based lubricants should not be used because they reduce effectiveness of condoms, but use of water-based lubricants (Astroglide, KY Jelly, Slippery Stuff) should be encouraged to reduce the possibility of microabra-

sions that enhance transmission of STDs. The female condom should be used when the male condom will not be used. Spermicide should be used for its bactericidal and viricidal properties. The only exception is for individuals who have a sensitivity to nonoxynol-9, in whom the risk of acquiring STDs is increased through the inflammatory reaction caused by the local allergic reaction. HIV testing should be done before the initiation of sexual activity with a new partner, and condoms should be used until another HIV test at least 6 months into a mutually monogamous relationship reveals both partners to be seronegative.

Availability of condoms has been shown to increase the likelihood of condom use. There are no data showing that condoms' availability or sexual health education promotes increased sexual activity.

When informing patients about an STD diagnosis, make sure they understand how the disease is transmitted, why medication is needed, exactly how to take it, and the importance of notifying partners. Patients are often afraid or ashamed to notify partners; you can help by offering role playing to practice informing their partners. Safe sexual practices should be reviewed with the patient to ensure understanding; handling this in a professional and empathic manner is imperative for patient confidence and compliance.

Dealing with patients' emotional response is extremely important. Persons with STDs often have to deal with feelings of guilt, anxiety, anger, tension, and preoccupation. The diagnosis of a STD can be very traumatic, alter self-image, and affect the present relationship dynamics as well as the dynamics of future relationships.

CASE STUDY 1

Ms. M. is a single, unemployed 18-year-old who is 26 weeks pregnant. Today she is accompanied by Mr. B., whom she introduces as her new boyfriend. They have read that it is normal to get increased vaginal discharge during pregnancy but are concerned because she is also having vaginal spotting. She has had no uterine contractions, fever, or symptoms suggestive of urinary tract infection. After the abdominal examination, and listening to the heartbeat, you inform them that because of the vaginal spotting and discharge, a pelvic examination needs to be done. You ask the boyfriend to step out, and once Ms. M. is alone, you take her sexual history. She reveals that she has been sexually active with Mr. B. for the past 9 weeks. She has not been sexually active with the father of the baby since the positive pregnancy test result at 6 weeks of pregnancy. She has not had any other partner outside of Mr. B. for the past 20 weeks. She doesn't think he has any other partners but has been afraid to ask for fear that he won't be there to support her during her pregnancy. She confirms that he has been very supportive and denies any history of abuse. They have never used condoms because she was already pregnant. Her chlamydial, GC, RPR, hepatitis B, and HIV test results were all negative on her initial prenatal visit.

On examination you note a physiologic-appearing vaginal discharge and a cervix that bleeds easily upon swabbing. Her cervix is closed and long. She has no tenderness on bimanual examination.

QUESTIONS

1. What should you tell Ms. M. about the cause of her vaginal spotting?
2. What tests should you do?
3. What is the best treatment for Ms. M.?
4. What are you concerned about in respect to her pregnancy and sexual health?

DISCUSSION

Ms. M.'s sexual history, her age, and her pregnancy put her at an increased risk for acquiring an STD. Her friable cervix is suspicious for *Chlamydia*, GC, *Trichomonas*, or bacterial vaginosis. Therefore, you should do a chlamydia test, GC test, and a wet prep. Treat for any trichomonal or bacterial vaginosis seen on wet prep. You can use metronidazole after the first trimester. If you are highly suspicious, presumptively treat for GC and/or *Chlamydia*. The easiest medications for compliance for both the patient and her partner would be ceftriaxone and azithromycin.

Inform her that she may have a cervical infection, possibly an STD. Be prepared for the whole range of normal emotional responses to your news. Inquire about any symptoms Mr. B. may have. Ask her how she would discuss this with Mr. B. if she tests positive, and offer to either help her practice speaking with him or to meet with them both. Remember to maintain patient confidentiality and neutrality. Remember that all sexual partners would need to be treated.

Educate both Ms. M. and Mr. B. about safe sexual practices and cervical infections in pregnancy. If she has untreated *Chlamydia* or GC, she will be at increased risk for premature rupture of membranes, preterm labor, preterm delivery, and endometritis, and her baby will be at increased risk for neonatal conjunctivitis and pneumonia. Consider retesting at her next prenatal visit and follow up on compliance with condom usage.

CASE STUDY 2

Mr. J. is a 33-year-old single businessman who presents with scrotal pain and mild dysuria of 24 hours' duration. He denies recent GU trauma or manipulation or any prior history of GU problems. He has had no fever or chills. On sexual history he describes himself as practicing "serial monogamy," which he defines as having exclusively one sexual partner for the duration of the relationship. He has had both male and female sexual partners over the years but has been exclusively sexually active with a female partner for the past 3 months. His sexual practice includes oral, genital, and anal intercourse. He has used condoms with all his male partners. With female partners, he usually uses condoms for a couple of months and then relies on their use of oral contraception. He had HIV testing at the onset of this relationship, and after both tested negative, they used her oral contraceptives. He has had GC in the past. He denies use of any illicit drugs and uses alcohol only occasionally during sex to "heighten sensitivity." He is otherwise very healthy.

His examination findings reveal a tender epididymitis on the right side. The testes are in their normal position in the scrotum. There is mild exacerbation of pain with elevating the scrotum. There is no inguinal adenopathy. He is noncircumcised and his foreskin easily retracts. He last voided 4 hours ago and is unable to express any urethral discharge. You note several broad-based fleshy lesions in the genital and perianal area. There are no ulcerative lesions noted on GU, perirectal, or oral examination. His skin examination is otherwise normal.

QUESTIONS

1. What is your working diagnosis?
2. What tests do you want to perform on Mr. J.?
3. What prevention measures would you recommend for Mr. J.?
4. What education do you consider to be appropriate for Mr. J.?

DISCUSSION

Mr. J.'s history and examination suggest his chief complaint is related to epididymitis. With his sexual history, his epididymitis could most likely be the result of Chlamydia or Escherichia coli. His history of having had GC indicates that he is not consistently practicing safe sex. He also has skin lesions suggestive of either condyloma acuminatum (HPV) or condyloma latum (syphilis).

You should do urethral swabs for Chlamydia and GC. Look for Trichomonas, white blood cells, and LE on urinalysis, and culture the urine for pathogens if it looks suspicious. Obtain a serologic test for syphilis.

You should offer hepatitis B vaccine to Mr. J. and counsel him on safe sex practices. He has some misunderstanding of his risk between male and female partners, the use of HIV testing, and what constitutes safe sex. He needs to be aware that he is at increased risk for STDs based on his lack of safe sex practices, his use of alcohol during sexual activity, his new and frequent sexual partners, and his noncircumcised status.

Circumcision does not need to be recommended—just attention to hygiene, use of condoms, and appropriate and adequate lubrication during intercourse. Let him know that he appears to have at least one STD as evidenced by condyloma, and probably has chlamydial or E. coli epididymitis. He should abstain from intercourse until all his tests have returned and he will need to notify his partners. He and his partner should be presumptively treated for Chlamydia until test results return. Anticipate that he may express the full range of normal emotions to the diagnosis of an STD.

REFERENCES

1. Eng TR, Butler WT, eds. The Hidden Epidemic: Confronting Sexually Transmitted Disease. Committee on Prevention and Control of Sexually Transmitted Disease: Executive Summary (Appendix A). Institute of Medicine, Division of Health Promotion and Disease Prevention. Washington, DC: National Academy Press, 1996:1–15, 2–1, 2–38, 3–1, 3–48.
2. Martin DH. Chlamydial infections. Med Clin North Am 1990;74(6):1367–1388.
3. Mertz GJ. Genital herpes simplex virus infections. Med Clin North Am 1990;74(6):1433–1454.
4. Hutchinson CM, Hook EW. Syphilis in adults. Med Clin North Am 1990;74(6):1389–1416.
5. Caudill JL, Humphrey SK, Goeller JR. Cervicovaginal cytology and the diagnosis of Chlamydia trachomatis: a comparison with immunofluorescent results. Diagn Cytopathol 1994;11(1):20–22.
6. Centers for Disease Control and Prevention, Division of STD Prevention. Sexually Transmitted Disease Surveillance 1995. US Department of Health and Human Services, Public Health Service. Atlanta: Centers for Disease Control and Prevention, September 1996:1–7.
7. Hatcher RA, Trussell J, Stewart F, et al. Contraceptive Technology, 16th rev. ed. New York: Irvington Publishers, 1994:415–432.

37. Shoulder Pain

SCOTT H. GRINDEL AND DOUG MCKEAG

Key Clinical Questions

1. What are important common causes of shoulder pain in the primary care setting?
2. How can the history and physical examination help to isolate the diagnosis, and when are imaging studies indicated?
3. Which causes of shoulder pain can the family physician manage, and which problems require consultation?

Shoulder pain is a common complaint in the primary care physician's office and is responsible for 1.2 to 2.5% of office visits (1). High rates of injury are due to the extreme mobility of the shoulder joint, making it inherently less stable and more susceptible to injury. Shoulder problems are not confined to athletes; in fact, a population-based survey revealed that approximately 20% of the elderly have shoulder pain (2).

Injury can be categorized as traumatic, chronic overuse, or atraumatic. The diagnosis can usually be identified by a careful history and thorough physical examination, supplemented with appropriate radiologic and laboratory investigations. In patients with shoulder pain, 23% have complete recovery by 1 month, and 59% have complete recovery by 12 months (3). Factors associated with early recovery are mild trauma, acute onset, overuse problems, and early presentation. Concurrent problems that are related to prolonged recovery are diabetes mellitus, cervical spondylolysis, radicular symptoms, advancing age, and involvement of the dominant extremity (2–5).

PATHOPHYSIOLOGY AND DIFFERENTIAL DIAGNOSIS

Pathophysiology

Important areas of shoulder anatomy are the musculotendinous units of the rotator cuff and biceps, the bony landmarks of the humerus, scapula, and clavicle, and the four joints of the shoulder (Fig. 37.1). The rotator cuff is comprised of four muscles: the subscapularis is located an-teriorly on the scapula, whereas the supraspinatus, infraspinatus, and teres minor are located posteriorly (Fig. 37.2). Their tendons form the rotator cuff and are closely associated with the glenohumeral capsule, as is the biceps tendon. The primary function of the rotator cuff is to position the humeral head to allow larger muscles to provide power. The glenohumeral joint lacks the bony and ligamentous stability of other joints and relies on the musculotendinous complex of the rotator cuff, a cartilaginous lip (the labrum), and the joint capsule to maintain stability.

One of the important bony landmarks of the humerus is the greater tuberosity. This is the insertion site of the supraspinatus, infraspinatus, and teres minor and is often associated with impingement. The bicipital groove is a palpable indentation immediately medial to the greater tuberosity and slightly inferior to the acromioclavicular joint. It houses the tendon of the long head of the biceps. The area around the bicipital groove may be tender with tendonitis or if there is subluxation of the long head of the biceps. The lesser tuberosity is the insertion site of the subscapularis and is located anterior and slightly inferior to both the greater tuberosity and the bicipital groove.

The glenohumeral joint, acromioclavicular joint, and the sternoclavicular joint are the three true joints of the shoulder; they are therefore susceptible to arthritides and trauma. All three may have a fibrocartilaginous disc present within the articulation. The fourth joint of the shoulder, the scapulothoracic joint, is a physiologic joint and may be associated with pain syndromes, bursitis, and neuropathies. The clavicle and its attachments with the sternum, acromion process, and coracoid process are especially susceptible to injuries. This is because the clavicle is the only bony connection of the shoulder to the thorax and absorbs a large portion of the traumatic stresses to the upper extremity.

There are three important bursae in the shoulder. The subacromial bursa is located immediately inferior to the acromioclavicular joint and superior to the glenohumeral joint. It often is involved in impingement syndrome. Injection into

581

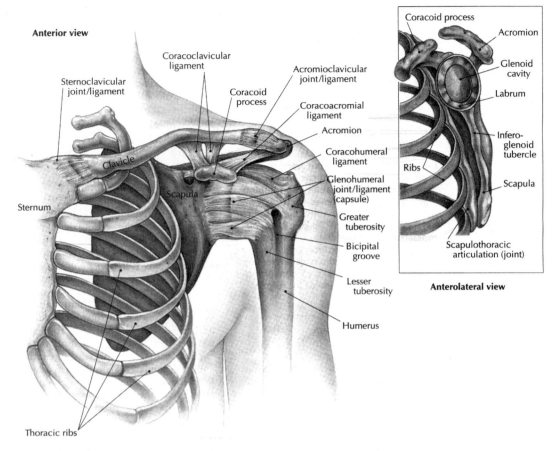

Anterior view

Sternoclavicular joint/ligament

Coracoclavicular ligament

Acromioclavicular joint/ligament

Coracoid process

Coracoacromial ligament

Acromion

Coracohumeral ligament

Glenohumeral joint/ligament (capsule)

Greater tuberosity

Bicipital groove

Lesser tuberosity

Clavicle

Scapula

Sternum

Humerus

Thoracic ribs

Coracoid process

Acromion

Glenoid cavity

Labrum

Infero-glenoid tubercle

Ribs

Scapula

Scapulothoracic articulation (joint)

Anterolateral view

Figure 37.1. *Anatomy of the shoulder showing four joints: sternoclavicular, acromioclavicular, glenohumeral, and scapulothoracic (physiologic) joint.* (Reprinted with permission from Glockner SM. Shoulder pain: a diagnostic dilemma. Am Fam Physician 1995;51:1678.)

this bursa to eradicate symptoms is the basis of the impingement test. The subdeltoid bursa is located inferior to the deltoid tendon on the lateral shaft of the humerus; it may become inflamed with repetitive overhead activities. Finally, the subscapular bursa is located between the scapula and the thoracic wall and may become inflamed with overuse.

The brachial plexus is a complex array of roots, trunks, divisions, cords, and branches. Any of these areas may be injured with stretching of the brachial plexus. The most likely peripheral nerve to be damaged is the musculocutaneous nerve because of the high incidence of anterior dislocations. Other nerves that may be damaged include the axillary, suprascapular, and long thoracic. In addition, the cervical spine is often a

source of referred pain to the shoulder. Finally, in the pediatric and young adult patient, epiphyseal injury is an important consideration.

Differential Diagnosis

In the ambulatory practice setting, the most common shoulder conditions encountered are acute or subacute rotator cuff tendonitis (52%), chronic rotator cuff tendonitis or tear (13%), pericapsular soft-tissue lesions (11%), and acromioclavicular joint pain (10%). Because these four conditions account for over 80% of patients with shoulder pain in the primary care setting, the family physician should be familiar with their evaluation and management. Referred pain from the cervical spine accounts for only 5% of symptoms, whereas

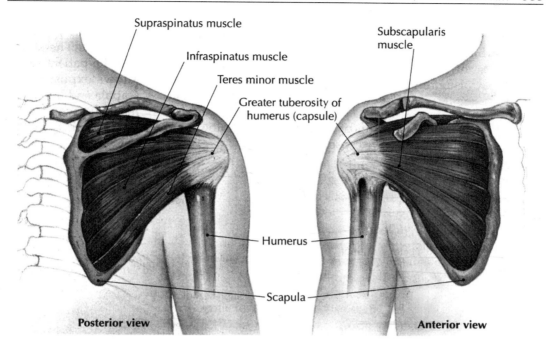

Figure 37.2. *Anatomy of the rotator cuff.* (Reprinted with permission from Glockner SM. Shoulder pain: a diagnostic dilemma. Am Fam Physician 1995;51:1679.)

glenohumeral osteoarthritis, fibromyalgia, frozen shoulder, and fracture are each responsible for 3% or less (1). Rotator cuff problems are also common in the elderly and are responsible for symptoms in 70% of older patients with shoulder pain (2). See Table 37.1 for a summary of the differential diagnosis of shoulder pain in the primary care setting.

CLINICAL EVALUATION

History

The key to developing an effective differential diagnosis for the patient with shoulder pain is a thorough history. Key questions in the evaluation are:

- What is the predominant symptom? Chief complaints may range from pain to instability to weakness. If pain is the predominant symptom, have the patient describe and quantify the pain on a scale from 1 to 10. This helps you assess the results of treatment.

- How long have the symptoms been present? How did they develop or how have they changed? Have you had similar symptoms in

the past? Was there a history of trauma? These questions help to determine whether the problem is chronic or acute in onset. If trauma was involved, the exact mechanism may help to determine the diagnosis. A history of dislocation or recurrent subluxations may be a clue to instability. Chronic pain with overhead activities may be due to impingement.

- Where did the pain begin and has it changed in its location? Does the shoulder hurt at night? Are there certain positions or activities that bother it more than others? These questions attempt to localize the problem. Night pain or pain with overhead activities may signify impingement, whereas pain with lifting, pushing open a car door, or carrying luggage may be due to instability.

- What is your job? What are your hobbies or sports activities? What hand do you use to perform the inciting activity? Injuries due to overuse are often seen in workers whose jobs required overhead lifting often, because lifting the arm over the head provokes impingement syndrome, subacromial bursitis, and acromioclavicular problems. Certain

Table 37.1.

Differential Diagnosis of Shoulder pain, in order of Likelihood among Primary Care Patients Presenting with Shoulder Pain

Diagnosis	Frequency (%) in Primary Care
Acute or subacute rotator cuff tendonitis	52
Chronic rotator cuff tendonitis or tear	13
Impingement syndrome	
Rotator cuff tears	
Pericapsular soft tissue lesions	11
Chronic instability of the glenohumeral joint	
Biceps tendonitis (including calcific tendonitis)	
Adhesive capsulitis	
Glenohumeral dislocations	
Biceps tendon rupture	
Biceps tendon dislocation	
Rheumatologic disorders	
Acromioclavicular joint pain	10
Acromioclavicular degenerative joint pain	
Acromioclavicular joint separations	
Other	14
Clavicular, scapular, and humeral fractures	
Septic arthritis	
Reflex sympathetic dystrophy	
Osteonecrosis	
Thoracic outlet syndrome	
Cervical radiculopathy	
Referred pain (angina, cholelithiasis)	
Tumors of the shoulder girdle	

sports have an increased incidence of shoulder injuries, especially volleyball, swimming, overhead-throwing sports, racquet sports, hockey, and wrestling.

- What has been done for treatment? Have there been any previous injuries to either of the shoulders? This is important to know because it may change the examination or the comparison with the opposite shoulder.

- Do you have problems with neck pain? Is there pain that radiates into the shoulder or down the upper extremity? Determining whether pain is referred from the cervical spine may prevent an expensive and inappropriate workup.

Problems that occur acutely with rapid onset include trauma, acute overuse, and cervical nerve

root compression. Progressive pain and decreased motion may occur over days to a few weeks with any of these problems. Degenerative problems occur over a prolonged period and may wax and wane over weeks to months. Knowing the age and chief complaint can often narrow the differential significantly. Patients below the age of 45 often have a biomechanical cause to their problem, such as instability or tendonitis, whereas those older than 45 are more likely to have degenerative conditions such as osteoarthritis or rotator cuff tears. Barring significant trauma, young patients rarely have rotator cuff tears. If there is a history of diabetes mellitus, progressive pain, and loss of motion, evaluate the patient for adhesive capsulitis. "Red flags" for the patients with shoulder pain are summarized in Table 37.2.

Physical Examination

The most important aspect of the physical examination is inspection. Every evaluation for shoulder pain should begin with having the patient change into a patient gown (bras may be left in place as long as adequate visualization of the shoulders, including the shoulder blades, can be accomplished). Begin with an evaluation for referred pain; at the very least, a screening evaluation for cervical spine and cardiopulmonary and abdominal pathology should be performed. This should be followed by observation for any atrophy of the muscles of the shoulder. Atrophy of the biceps suggests musculocutaneous nerve dysfunction, whereas scapular winging could be due to long thoracic nerve pathology. Asymmetry of the biceps muscles could be due to a biceps tendon rupture ("Popeye defect"). Prominence of the scapular spine may be due to a nerve palsy in a younger patient or to a long-standing rotator cuff tear in the older patient.

Range of Motion

There are nine movements described in the shoulder: abduction (normal 180°), adduction (normal 45°), flexion (normal 180°), extension (normal 45°), internal rotation and external rotation (normal 75°), protraction, retraction, and elevation. You should assess the smoothness of the scapulohumeral and scapulothoracic rhythm and test for a painful arc that may suggest impingement, rotator cuff problems, or labral tears. Impingement usually occurs between 90° and

Table 37.2.
"Red Flags" Suggesting Progressive Life-Threatening Disease in Patients with Shoulder Pain

"Red Flag"	Diagnosis Suggested
Shortness of breath, nausea, palpitations	Cardiac disease
Fever	Septic arthritis
Right upper-quadrant abdominal pain, nausea, vomiting	Cholelithiasis or cholecystitis
Progressive pain and/or neurologic abnormality	Spinal stenosis or cervical disk lesion
Shortness of breath, pleuritic pain, with or without history of trauma	Pneumothorax
Pulseless, cold extremity	Vascular disease or obstruction (including thoracic outlet syndrome)
Fever, weight loss, progressive pain, pulmonary symptoms	Shoulder/thoracic neoplasm

120° of abduction. Restricted or painful internal rotation at 90° of abduction may signify shoulder impingement. This is best observed with the "behind the back" scratch test, also known as the Apley scratch test. The patient is asked to touch the bottom of the opposite scapula from below and the top of the opposite scapula from above. At least 55° of internal rotation is required to perform this maneuver, and you can quantitate the range of motion according to the level of the thoracic spine they can reach (T7 is at the inferior angle of the scapula).

Palpation

Localize the point of maximum tenderness only after the remainder of the examination is complete. If the patient feels discomfort and guards the joint during examination, you may miss an important finding. Bony palpation of the shoulder should include the suprasternal notch, sternoclavicular joint, clavicle, coracoid process, acromioclavicular joint, acromion, greater tuberosity of the humerus, bicipital groove, spine of the scapula, and medial border of the scapula. Palpation of the soft tissues should include the rotator cuff, subacromial and subdeltoid bursa, axilla, and the major muscles of the shoulder (see Fig. 37.1) (6).

Special Maneuvers

Many of the tests used to help narrow the differential diagnosis have never been validated. A review of the evidence to support use of these maneuvers is summarized in Table 37.3, but you should be aware that some of the studies had sig-

nificant flaws in their design (7). The maneuvers are described below.

Tests of Glenohumeral Joint Stability

Anterior Apprehension Test (Fulcrum Test). With the scapula stabilized, the arm is passively moved to 90° of abduction and gently externally rotated until there is apprehension and the patient resists further external rotation. Apprehension or the feeling that the joint is going to dislocate constitute a positive test. Pain alone does not necessarily signify instability. Caution should be exercised not to completely dislocate the joint with this maneuver.

Relocation Test. The patient is in the apprehension position as described above. With a positive test, a posterior force placed on the anterior humerus will relieve the apprehension. Further external rotation may then be possible. If the posterior force is removed, apprehension returns (augmentation test).

Posterior Apprehension Test. The arm is passively moved to 90° of abduction and gently internally rotated until the patient is apprehensive and resists further internal rotation. A posteriorly directed force placed upon the humeral shaft may intensify the feeling of instability.

Sulcus Sign. The arm is passively at the side in the standing or sitting position. The humerus is distracted inferiorly. The sulcus sign is an indentation seen immediately inferior to the acromioclavicular joint; normal is less than 1 cm.

Table 37.3.
Characteristics of Physical Examination Maneuvers for the Diagnosis of Shoulder Disorders

	Sensitivity	Specificity	LR+	LR−
Instability tests				
Relocation test[a]	57	100	57	0.43
Augmented relocation test[a]	68	100	68	0.32
Rotator cuff tears				
Posterior superior tears				
Empty can test[b, c]	85	58	2.1	0.26
External rotation lag sign[b]	70	100	70	0.30
Drop sign[b]	21	100	21	0.80
Subscapularis tears				
Lift off test[b]	62	100	62	0.38
Internal rotation lag sign[b]	97	96	24	0.03
Impingement tests				
Neer's test[c]	89	NA		
Hawkins' test[c]	87	NA		
Yocum's test[c]	78	NA		

[a]Speer KP, Hannafin JA, Altchek DW, Warren RF. An evaluation of the shoulder relocation test. Am J Sports Med 1994;22:177–183.

[b]Hertel R, Ballmer FT, Lombert SM, Gerber C. Lag signs in the diagnosis of rotator cuff rupture. J Shoulder Elbow Surg 1996;5:307–313.

[c]Leroux JL, Thomas E, Bonnel F, Blotman F. Diagnostic value of clinical tests for shoulder impingement syndrome. Rev Rhum Engl Ed 1995;62:423–428.

TESTS FOR IMPINGEMENT OF THE
SUBACROMIAL BURSA
(IMPINGEMENT SYNDROME)

Neer's Test (Impingement Sign). This test attempts to force the greater trochanter under the acromioclavicular joint to compress the bursa, rotator cuff, and biceps tendon. The arm is placed into maximum forward flexion and internal rotation ("Heil Hitler" sign) while stabilizing the scapula. The test is positive if pain is experienced.(8)

Hawkins' Test. With the elbow flexed at 90° and the shoulder forward-flexed at 90°, the humerus is progressively internally rotated in order to grind the proximal humerus against the acromioclavicular joint. The test is positive if pain is experienced (9).

Impingement Test. The impingement test involves the injection of a 1% lidocaine solution into the subacromial space. Resolution of the pain with repeat testing for impingement signs is a positive test and suggests impingement syndrome.

TESTS FOR CUFF INJURY

Drop Arm Test. With the arm straight and the shoulder abducted past 90° and then forward-flexed to 30°, the patient is asked to slowly lower it to the side. With a supraspinatus tear, the patient is unable to lower the arm slowly, and the arm drops to the side.

Empty Can Test (Jobe's Maneuver). With the arm straight and the shoulder abducted to 90° and horizontally adducted to 30°, the humerus is internally rotated to 45° (as if emptying a beverage can). With a supraspinatus tear, the patient is unable to maintain the position against resistance. The shoulder must be compared to the opposite side (10). A study using electromyography calls the position of pronation into question and suggests that supination (full-can position) provides improved isolation of the supraspinatus (11).

Lift Off Test (Gerber's Test). With the dorsum of the hand placed over the sacrum, the patient is asked to push away from the back against resistance. With subscapularis weakness or tear, the patient is weaker on the affected side compared to the contralateral side (12).

External Rotator Test. With the elbows at their side and at 90° of flexion and the humerus in 45° of internal rotation, patients are asked to externally rotate the humerus against resistance. With infraspinatus weakness, the patients are weaker on the affected side as compared to the contralateral side.

External Rotation Lag Sign. This tests infraspinatus and supraspinatus integrity. The patient is seated with his or her back to the examiner. The elbow is passively flexed to 90°, and the shoulder is held at 20° of abduction and near maximal external rotation (maximal external rotation minus 5° to avoid elastic recoil). The patient is then instructed to maintain this position as the examiner releases the arm, supporting only the elbow. The sign is positive when a lag or angular drop is seen (13).

Drop Sign. This tests mainly the infraspinatus integrity. The patient is seated with the back to the examiner. The affected arm is held at 90° of abduction and almost full external rotation, with the elbow flexed at 90°. The patient is then asked to maintain this position as the examiner releases the hand and supports only at the elbow. The sign is positive if a lag occurs (13).

Internal Rotation Lag Sign. This tests the subscapularis integrity. The patient is seated with his or her back to the examiner. The affected arm is held behind the back. The elbow is flexed to 90°, and the shoulder is held at 20° of abduction and 20° of extension. The patient's hand is then pulled away from the back until it is in almost maximal internal rotation. The patient is then asked to maintain this position as the examiner releases the hand and supports only at the elbow. The sign is positive if a lag occurs (13).

TEST FOR PAIN IN THE
ACROMIOCLAVICULAR JOINT

Crossover Test. With the elbow extended, the arm is brought across the chest, stressing the acromioclavicular joint. Tenderness is felt in the lateral shoulder if the test is positive.

MANEUVERS TO ELECT BICEPS PAIN

Yergason's Test. With the elbow at 90° and the wrist held in pronation, the patient will experience pain if he attempts to supinate the wrist against resistance.

Speed's Test. With the elbow flexed at 30°, the humerus at 60° of flexion, and the wrist supinated, the patient will experience pain if the arm is flexed against resistance (i.e., the position your arm may take if you are upset with someone who "speeds" past you).

MANUEVERS TO DETECT TEARS OF
THE GLENOHUMERAL JOINT CAPSULE
(LABRAL TEARS)

Clunk Test. While applying gentle axial pressure to the humerus with the elbow at 90°, rotate the humerus internally and externally while simultaneously abducting the arm. If the examiner's opposite hand is placed under the humeral head, a clunk, pop, or snap may be felt if a labral tear is present (14).

Crank Test. With the patient in the sitting or standing position, the arm is elevated to 160° in the scapular plane. An axial load is applied to the humerus while simultaneously internally and externally rotating the humerus. Pain or reproduction of the patient's symptoms (usually pain or catching) is considered a positive test.

Diagnostic Tests

Test characteristics of imaging studies are summarized in Table 37.4. Many of the techniques are highly dependent upon the experience of the investigators and the sophistication of the equipment. Special views useful for the evaluation of specific syndromes are summarized below.

Plain Radiographs

The standard 3-view series of the shoulder consists of a true scapular anteroposterior view, the supraspinatus outlet view, and the axillary lateral view. The transscapular lateral view (scapular Y view or supraspinatus outlet view) evaluates anterior and posterior dislocations. It allows better visualization of the inferior acromion, the subacromial space, and the supraspinatus outlet. This allows assessment of acromioclavicular joint pathology, impingement, and rotator cuff tears, respectively. It is also useful in demonstrating proximal humerus fractures and evaluates the scapula well. The axillary lateral view shows glenohumeral joint displacement (especially posterior dislocations) and assists in the visualization of degenerative arthritis and bony spurs.

The Stryker notch view demonstrates the superior and posterior portion of the humeral head.

Table 37.4.
Characteristics of Imaging Studies for the Diagnosis of Shoulder Disorders

	Sensitivity	Specificity	LR+	LR−
MRI (unenhanced)				
Anterior labrum[a, b, c]	95	97	32	0.05
Superior labrum[b, c]	80	100	80	0.20
Posterior labrum[b]	74	95	14.8	0.27
Multiple labrum tears[b]	94	NA		
Overall[a, b, d]	86	96	21.5	0.15
MRI (enhanced)				
Rotator cuff tears				
Partial[d]	100	95	19.8	0.01
Complete[d]	82	85	5.5	0.21
Overall[e]	92	100	92	0.08
Tendonitis[d]	93	87	7.1	0.08
Impingement syndrome[d]	93	87	7.1	0.08
MRI arthrography				
Rotator cuff tears				
Overall[f, g]	90	95	18	0.10
Plain arthrography				
Rotator cuff tears				
Partial[h]	70	NA		
Complete[h]	90	NA		
CT arthrography (double-contrast)				
Rotator cuff tears				
Partial[h]	95	NA		
Complete[h]	70	NA		
Overall[e]	92	100	92	0.08
Ultrasound				
Rotator cuff tears				
Partial[h]	80	NA		
Complete[h]	90	NA		

[a]Green MR, Christensen KP. Magnetic resonance imaging of the glenoid labrum in anterior shoulder instability. Am J Sports Med 1994;22:493–498.

[b]Gusmer PB, Potter HG, Schatz JA, et al. Labral injuries: accuracy of detection with unenhanced MR imaging of the shoulder. Radiology 1996;200:519–524.

[c]Legan JM, Burkhard TK, Goff WB II, et al. Tears of the glenoid labrum: MR imaging of 88 arthroscopically confirmed cases. Radiology 1991;179:241–246.

[d]Iannotti JP, Zlatkin MB, Esterhai JL, Kressel HY, Dalinka MK, Spindler KP. Magnetic resonance imaging of the shoulder. Sensitivity, specificity, and predictive value. J Bone Joint Surg [Am] 1991;73:17–29.

[e]Burk DL Jr, Karasick D, Kurtz AB, et al. Rotator cuff tears: prospective comparison of MR imaging with arthrography, sonography, and surgery. Am J Roentgenol 1989;153:87–92.

[f]Palmer WE, Brown JH, Rosenthal DI. Labral-ligamentous complex of the shoulder: evaluation with MR arthrography [comments]. Radiology 1994;190:645–651.

[g]Tirman PF, Stauffer AE, Crues JV III, et al. Saline magnetic resonance arthrography in the evaluation of glenohumeral instability. Arthroscopy 1993;9:550–559.

[h]Farin PU, Kaukanen E, Jaroma H, Vaatainen U, Miettinen H, Soimakallio S. Site and size of rotator cuff tear. Findings at ultrasound, double-contrast arthrography, and computed tomography arthrography with surgical correlation. Invest Radiol 1996;31:387–394.

The West Point lateral view evaluates the anteroinferior glenoid rim. Finally, Zanca's view is useful in evaluating the acromioclavicular joint and distal clavicle, whereas the reduced voltage view (routine anteroposterior [AP] view with about 50% of the power) evaluates the acromioclavicular joint well.

Plain Film Arthrography

Although a single contrast study may be useful for identifying full-thickness rotator cuff tears and adhesive capsulitis, it is an invasive procedure and involves the use of radioactive material. Double-contrast studies involve the injection of contrast into the joint and then replacing the contrast with air. This procedure may allow the evaluation of some labral tears.

Computed Tomography (CT)

Plain CT may be useful for identifying proximal humeral fractures, glenoid rim fractures, and humeral head fractures and abnormalities. A CT arthrogram is useful in evaluating full-thickness rotator cuff tears but fails to identify 30% of the partial-thickness tears (15). It is abnormal in 80 to 100% of patients with large labrum lesions, but it is less accurate in evaluating small labral tears (16). Double-contrast CT arthrography may be more precise but has not been extensively evaluated (17, 18).

Ultrasound

In some studies, ultrasound accuracy approaches that of arthrography for full-thickness rotator cuff tears, and it may even exceed arthrography in partial-thickness rotator cuff tears (sensitivity of 60 to 94%) (19–23). The results of these studies have not been reproduced by other investigators, and sonography appears to be highly operator dependent.

Magnetic Resonance Imaging

MRI is most useful for evaluation of suspected impingement syndrome and rotator cuff pathology. It may also be useful in the evaluation of biceps tendon pathology, avascular necrosis, inflammatory processes, osteoporosis, and tumors. Its value in the diagnosis of glenoid labrum tears is dependent upon the location of the tear and the skill of the radiologist; it is imperative to provide as much clinical information as possible when ordering the study (24). The use of MRI may allow conservative management of nonsurgical problems if used appropriately.

GENERAL MANAGEMENT

The general management of shoulder pain, like many musculoskeletal conditions, is summarized using the RICE acronym: Rest (protection), Ice, Compression, and Elevation (the latter two are generally not possible in shoulders, though). Range-of-motion and strengthening exercises should be encouraged, and nonsteroidal anti-inflammatory drugs (NSAIDs) may also be of benefit in select cases.

Rest includes refraining from all activities and movements that aggravate the problem, with a gradual return as tolerated to full activity. A sling can help provide complete rest to shoulder muscles. If one is used, it should be removed at least twice daily with gentle range of motion to prevent adhesive capsulitis, and it is rarely needed for more than 10 days. Aggressively icing the area of discomfort for 20 minutes, three to four times per day, will help alleviate both pain and inflammation.

Range-of-motion exercises are extremely important in most cases of shoulder pain; otherwise a stiff shoulder may result. Exercises should begin as soon as tolerated, (i.e., when they cause no more than minor discomfort), and they should be performed at least twice a day. Begin by having the patient perform pendulum exercises. These are accomplished by allowing the arm to hang limp at the side and leaning slightly forward at the hip. The arm is then actively or passively moved in circles like a pendulum. Start with small circles and gradually make bigger and bigger circles as tolerated. Next, the towel method may be used. This is done by holding a towel by both its ends, one in each hand. Gently move the affected shoulder through its range of motion, leading it by moving the towel with the unaffected hand and shoulder. This allows broader range of motion and some stretching.

Next, strengthening exercises should be added. They should concentrate at first on the rotator cuff and then progress to the larger muscle groups. The goal is not to build bulk, but rather to tone and strengthen the muscles to allow more stability and protect against injury. Encourage the patient to use light weights, with the gradual addition of more repetitions as needed. Although some patients may require a course of formal physical therapy to ensure compliance or to instruct them in home programs of exercise, this is not necessary for all patients with shoulder pain.

NSAIDs may be of use for chronic inflammation but are of limited benefit for acute injuries other than for their analgesic effects (25). Use of NSAIDs for at least 7 days is usually necessary to maximize their anti-inflammatory effects.

EVALUATION AND MANAGEMENT OF COMMON SHOULDER SYNDROMES

This section describes some common causes of shoulder pain in the primary care setting and discusses their evaluation and management. See Table 37.5 for a summary of the level of evidence to support the interventions discussed and Figure 37.3 for a general approach to the management of shoulder conditions.

Table 37.5.
Treatment Interventions for Common Shoulder Complaints[a]

Intervention	Level of Evidence for Effectiveness[b]
Glenohumeral instability	
Physical therapy	A
Surgery	A
NSAIDs	B
Steroid injection	X
Rotator cuff tendonitis (impingement syndrome)	
NSAIDs	A
Physical therapy	A
Injection of steroids	A
Surgery	A
Rotator cuff tears	
Physical therapy	A
Surgery	A
NSAIDs	B
Steroid injection	X
Biceps tendonitis	
NSAIDs	A
Physical therapy	A
Steroid injection	X
Surgery	X
Acromioclavicular degenerative joint disease	
NSAIDs	A
Steroid injection	A
Surgery	A
Physical therapy	B
Adhesive capsulitis	
Physical therapy	A
Surgery	A
NSAIDs	B
Immobilization	X
Steroid injection	X
Clavicle fracture	
Physical therapy	A
NSAIDs	B
Surgery (complicated)	B
Surgery (uncomplicated)	X

[a]The indication for a particular patient depends on the severity of the condition and other patient-specific factors.

[b]Level of evidence for effectiveness: A, strong or moderate research-based evidence (consistent across several studies, including at least two randomized controlled trials); B, limited research-based evidence (less consistent or extensive evidence, but preponderance of evidence supports use of treatment; C, common practice with little or no research-based evidence; X, moderate or strong evidence suggesting that this treatment is not effective.

Rotator Cuff Tendonitis (Impingement Syndrome)

Rotator cuff tendonitis is an overuse injury to the shoulder that results in the impingement of the rotator cuff between the greater tuberosity of the humerus and the acromion, coracoid, and/or coracoacromial ligament (Fig. 37.1). The three stages of impingement as described by Neer (8) are:

Stage I: edema and hemorrhage
Stage II: fibrosis and tendonitis
Stage III: bone spurs and tendon rupture.

The typical case (Stage I) has inflammation in the subacromial bursa and the supraspinatus tendon that leads to edema and decreased relative space between the acromion and the humeral head. It is most often seen with overuse of the shoulder or in chronic instability in patients under age 25. Joint instability may accentuate an impingement syndrome because the humeral head is allowed to migrate superiorly. Increased mechanical irritation on the bursa and rotator cuff over time leads to increased fibrosis, partial-thickness rotator cuff tears, and partial-thickness biceps tendon tears (Stage II). This may eventually lead to full-thickness rotator cuff and biceps tendon tears. If degeneration of the collagen fibers of the tendons of the rotator cuff does occur, calcium salts may infiltrate the substance of the tendon and cause inflammation. This condition is termed calcific tendonitis and may be associated with acute or chronic symptoms. The most common site of involvement is the supraspinatus tendon, but it may also involve the biceps tendon, infraspinatus, or subscapularis. Pain is often severe, and if calcification is chronic, the patient may present much like an impingement syndrome.

Impingement syndrome may also result from direct trauma (such as a fall onto an elbow or an outstretched hand), muscular imbalances, posterior capsule tightness, or anatomic overgrowth of the acromion process. Impingement is rarely seen in patients under 40 years of age unless there is trauma involved or they are athletes. Athletes at particular risk include those involved in pitching, swimming, tennis, weight lifting, and golf, especially if the patient is overtraining or has poor technique. In Stage III, there are radiographic changes and pathologic ruptures; patients suffer progressive disability and often require surgical repair.

The onset of pain in rotator cuff tendonitis is

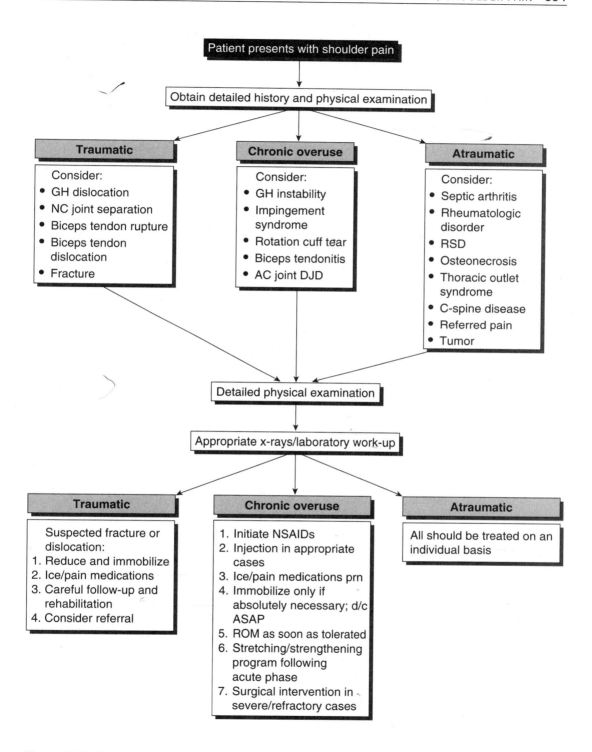

Figure 37.3. *General approach to shoulder problems.* AC, acromioclavicular; DJD, degenerative joint disease (osteoarthritis); GH, glenohumeral; ROM, range-of-motion exercises; RSD, reflex sympathetic dystrophy.

usually gradual but occasionally follows a specific activity. The pain is usually located in the lateral deltoid just distal to the tip of the acromion, but it may also be present in the biceps down to the elbow. Pain is usually worsened with overhead activities and when lying on the involved side; it is often worse at night. The patient may complain of popping, snapping, or grinding.

Patients with rotator cuff tendonitis typically have pain between 90° and 120° of abduction (painful arc). There may be tenderness with internal and external rotation while the shoulder is at 90° of abduction. Hawkins' test and Neer's test may be positive, and the impingement test is usually positive. There may also be signs of rotator cuff and biceps tendon irritation as well as frank weakness due to pain. This must be reevaluated after treatment to rule out a complete or partial tear.

Radiographic evaluation is rarely indicated; it is usually normal unless there is acromial overgrowth or degenerative joint disease (Stage III). Treatment involves rest, range-of-motion exercises, and strengthening of the scapula and thorax. Injection of steroids across (but not into) the superior aspect of the rotator cuff may be of benefit to some patients. If conservative measures fail after 6 weeks or if partial or complete tears are present, surgical intervention should be considered. Prevention is by avoidance of improper techniques used in overhead sport activities and minimizing offending activities. Exercises to strengthen the deltoid muscle help prevent recurrences.

Rotator Cuff Tears

Rotator cuff tears occur when there is a complete separation of the tendinous fibers. It is usually seen in patients over 40 years of age who have had long-standing impingement symptoms. Half of cases involve an acute traumatic event, usually a fall onto an abducted arm or a direct blow to the lateral shoulder. The first tendon to be affected is usually the supraspinatus; the tear may then extend to the infraspinatus, and in severe cases, it may involve the teres minor and biceps tendon.

The patient usually presents with weakness and poorly localized pain that radiates to the humerus. Pain is worsened with overhead activities. Inspection may demonstrate wasting of the supraspinatus and infraspinatus if the problem has been long-standing. The rotator cuff is often tender to palpation or associated with crepitus in the subacromial bursa. Direct testing of the mus-

cles of the rotator cuff will find weakness when compared with the unaffected side. The ability to externally rotate the shoulder decreases with the extent of the tear owing to involvement of the infraspinatus. Patients usually have less tenderness with passive than with active range of motion. Resisted adduction from the point of impingement may decrease the tenderness because the latissimus dorsi and the pectoralis major pull the humeral head down and away from the acromioclavicular joint and the coracoacromial ligament. Tests for impingement are often positive.

Plain films may only identify acromial overgrowth. The gold standard had always been the arthrogram, but MRI is gaining favor as a noninvasive replacement (19). Although MRI is more expensive, it can differentiate complete and partial tears and even visualize other shoulder conditions such as cartilage damage or tears of the glenoid labrum. CT provides less information. Neither CT, arthrogram, nor MRI is indicated unless surgery is being contemplated, a complete rotator cuff tear is suspected, or the patient has failed 6 to 8 weeks of conservative therapy.

Treatment of a rotator cuff tear involves rest, protection, and avoidance of overhead activities. A formal physical therapy program may be of benefit. Subacromial injections have not been proven to be effective and may impede tendon repair (26). Use in patients over 40 should be done with great caution. If symptoms persist for more than 6 to 8 weeks, patients should be referred to an orthopedic surgeon for debridement of partial-thickness tears or repair of full-thickness tears.

Biceps Tendonitis

Biceps tendonitis is characterized by pain and inflammation of the long head of the biceps tendon within the bicipital groove. Patients are usually young or middle-aged, and this condition is associated with occupations that require reaching and overhead lifting or with recreational activities such as tennis, swimming, golf, or throwing sports. It is often associated with impingement syndrome and rotator cuff tears. The patient typically presents with diffuse pain in the anterior shoulder that is worse during and directly after offending activities and improves with rest. Unlike rotator cuff tendonitis, there is usually no pain at night.

On physical examination, the patient usually has tenderness with flexion of the elbow and supination of the wrist. There may also be tenderness to palpation within the bicipital groove and along the long head of the biceps tendon and limitation of the extremes of abduction, internal rotation, and external rotation. Speed's and Yergason's tests are typically positive; there may be weakness secondary to pain. Radiographs are usually normal. MRI is not warranted unless you suspect a surgically repairable rotator cuff tear.

Treatment is with rest, ice, local heat, and protection. A gentle stretching and exercise program should be initiated. The patient may benefit from a formal physical therapy program if a quick return to activities is important. Oral anti-inflammatories may be of benefit. Although injection of the tendon with corticosteroids is not recommended, subacromial injection may be of benefit.

Acromioclavicular Degenerative Joint Disease

All three true joints of the shoulder are susceptible to osteoarthritis. Degenerative joint disease of the acromioclavicular joint is common and develops much earlier than that of the glenohumeral or sternoclavicular joint. Problems with the acromioclavicular joint are usually associated with trauma or overuse injuries. Degenerative joint disease often occurs in patients in their thirties or older but may be seen in the early teens.

On examination, the patient is usually tender over the superior and anterior aspect of the acromioclavicular joint. There may be a prominence to the acromioclavicular joint on inspection. Radiologic evaluation can often make the diagnosis; the acromioclavicular joint is best seen with a "Zanca's view." Diagnosis can be verified by injection of lidocaine into the joint. If there is resolution of the pain, this supports the diagnosis.

Treatment is usually symptomatic with NSAIDs. Injection with a steroid solution may be of benefit. Surgical intervention consists of resection of the distal clavicle and removal of the intra-articular disc, if present.

Acromioclavicular Joint Separations

Acute acromioclavicular sprains are a common traumatic injury usually resulting from a fall on the point of the shoulder. Palpation over the acromioclavicular joint may elicit tenderness if there is any degree of separation. Some patients, however, may only sense instability. Grading is accomplished primarily by radiologic comparison:

- Type 1—a mild sprain to the acromioclavicular ligaments, with no difference in the separation of the acromioclavicular joint as compared to the unaffected side.
- Type 2—rupture of the acromioclavicular ligament. The coracoclavicular ligament is intact, and displacement of the acromion from the clavicle is less than 1 cm.
- Type 3—complete rupture of both acromioclavicular and coracoclavicular ligaments with complete displacement of the acromion from the clavicle, usually associated with gross deformity.

Although once recommended, weighted radiographs are no longer considered necessary (27). "Reduced voltage" films usually are adequate when compared to the unaffected shoulder.

Treatment is primarily symptomatic. The shoulder should be immobilized for a short period of time (1 to 2 days for a type 1 injury and 5 to 7 days for a type 2 or 3 injury). Braces and long-term slings are not recommended, and range-of-motion exercises should be started immediately as tolerated. Start with pendulum exercises and progress to walking the fingers up a wall. Light weights can then be added as tolerated with gradual progression to full activity. Concentrate on strengthening of the trapezius and deltoid for successful return to heavy labor and sports. Surgical stabilization is only indicated for chronic pain, instability, or for aesthetic reasons (28, 29).

Chronic Instability of the Glenohumeral Joint

Instability is defined as the pathologic inability to maintain the humeral head centered in the glenoid fossa, leading to pain or an unstable feeling in the shoulder. Instability may be due to an acute dislocation, chronic subluxation, or both. Due to the high mobility of the joint, a small injury may cause significant instability. Chronic instability is often heralded by an acute dislocation. Because of the greater incidence of anterior dislocations and the intrinsic weakness of the anterior capsule, anterior instabilities are seen more frequently.

Some patients may present with pain and mildly positive instability signs but no history of trauma. This is often seen with repetitive throwing and overhead work, which can cause small labral or capsular tears and place extra stress on the rotator cuff muscles. This recurrent microtrauma may lead to impingement syndrome or osteoarthritis. Larger lesions may result from acute dislocations.

Patients with anterior instability typically have

a positive apprehension sign, relocation test, and possibly an anterior load and shift test. In posterior instability, they will have a positive posterior apprehension sign, and perhaps a positive posterior load and shift test. Having the patient do a pushup against the wall may reproduce symptoms, as can carrying weights or suitcases. Inferior instability may show up on examination as a positive sulcus sign. Routine radiographs may show signs of chronic subluxation such as erosion of the glenoid rim. An MRI may be useful in diagnosing small labral tears but adds little unless a rotator cuff tear is suspected.

Rehabilitation alone is usually adequate for treatment. Only about one third of patients, usually those with an initial dislocation that occurred before the age of 30, need operations. If attenuated ligaments or a torn labrum are present, physical therapy will not likely resolve the problem. Nontraumatic instabilities respond well to physical therapy, but do poorly with surgical intervention.

Adhesive Capsulitis ("Frozen Shoulder")

Adhesive capsulitis is usually due to prolonged immobilization or disuse due to pain; the exact etiology is unclear. Women and patients with diabetes mellitus are at increased risk. The pain is usually gradual in onset and is located over the insertion of the deltoids. Patients may report difficulty sleeping on the affected side.

On physical examination, active and passive range of motion to abduction, internal rotation, and external rotation is limited by adhesions in the capsule. There is no specific point tenderness, but patients often have diffuse tenderness, especially with movement through the range of motion. Treatment is by extended aggressive physical therapy, and symptoms may take years to completely resolve. Surgical manipulation under anesthesia is occasionally required.

Glenohumeral Dislocation

Glenohumeral dislocation can be anterior, inferior, or posterior. Anterior dislocations are most common and account for over 90% of shoulder dislocations. They are classified from Grade I (less than 50% subluxation of the humeral head beyond the glenoid fossa) to Grade IV (complete translation past the glenoid rim, i.e., dislocation). Anterior dislocations occur when a patient lands

on the posterior aspect of the shoulder, forcing the humeral head anteriorly on the glenoid, or by forced external rotation while the upper extremity is abducted. This may disrupt the anterior stabilizers of the shoulder (the anterior inferior labrum and the inferior glenohumeral ligament). The force of the anterior glenoid on the posterior humerus during dislocation may also cause a small compression fracture or divot on the posterior humeral head ("Hill-Sachs lesion") seen to most chronic dislocators. While the humeral head is being forced anteriorly, the anterior capsule may tear the labral cartilage away from the underlying glenoid ("Bankart's lesion"), worsening the anterior instability.

With an acute anterior dislocation, patients usually have an obvious deformity on examination with a prominent acromioclavicular joint, and they will hold the arm in a partially abducted and externally rotated position. If such patients have autoreduced, they may have signs of instability. They often have a positive Speed's test. Diagnosis is made by history, physical examination, and if necessary, x-ray evaluation, particularly the scapular Y view. A thorough neurovascular examination should be documented in all cases to rule out brachial plexus injury.

Treatment is by immediate reduction. Prompt reduction improves the ease of reduction and decreases the likelihood of neurovascular injury. Surgical intervention after the first dislocation is controversial; it may be appropriate in the high-performance athlete at risk for repeated dislocations and worsening instability (in football, hockey, or other collision sport). Otherwise, treatment consists of immobilization for 5 to 10 days depending upon symptoms and aggressive physical therapy to stabilize the joint. If pain or instability remains despite physical therapy, surgery should be considered. Consider a rotator cuff tear in the first-time dislocator older than age 45; if a rotator cuff tear is suspected, immobilization should be avoided and range of motion encouraged.

Clavicle Fractures

Clavicle fractures are very common and typically result from a fall or direct blow to the clavicle. They are sometimes accompanied by a pneumothorax, and with severe displacement, the brachial plexus may be damaged. Evaluate the patient for swelling and deformity of the clavicle, any subcutaneous crepitation, and neurovascular deficits of the upper extremity. To determine the extent and location of the fracture, x-ray evaluation should include clavicular views and a posteroanterior (PA) view of the chest.

Because a significantly displaced fracture of the middle third of the clavicle usually heals well functionally, management of uncomplicated clavicular fractures is with a sling or figure-of-eight brace until comfortable, followed by range-of-motion exercises. Surgery is rarely necessary. Referral to an orthopedist is appropriate for comminuted fractures and fractures of the very proximal or very distal clavicle.

Rheumatologic Disorders

The most common rheumatologic disorders involving the shoulder are osteoarthritis and rheumatoid arthritis. Osteoarthritis is not as common in the shoulder as it is in the weight-bearing joints; laborers and athletes may be more susceptible than the general public. Osteoarthritis of the shoulder is often accompanied by osteoarthritis of the acromioclavicular or sternoclavicular joints. Treatment of osteoarthritis is with NSAIDs and encouragement of activity. In severe arthritic damage to the joints, referral for joint replacement is in order when conservative treatment fails and range of motion and pain are unacceptable.

Rheumatoid arthritis is rarely seen in the shoulder initially, so it is usually accompanied by symmetric hand and wrist joint arthritis. Pain and stiffness tend to be worse in the mornings but may also cause pain at night. Synovial fluid is inflammatory with many polymorphonuclear leukocytes. For further discussion of the management of arthritis, see Chapter 18.

Cervical Radiculopathy

Always consider the cervical spine in any evaluation of shoulder pain. Cervical radiculopathy typically causes deep burning pain that radiates from the shoulder to the fingertips and may be associated with paresthesias. It is often relieved by forward shoulder elevation or repositioning of the neck. Range of motion of the cervical spine should be tested. Deep tendon reflexes and sensation should be tested in the upper extremity. Motor function of the upper extremity, including fine movements of the hand, should also be evaluated. If any abnormalities are found, an appropriate cervical workup should precede a shoulder workup.

Other Causes of Shoulder Pain

Uncommon but usually obvious causes of shoulder pain in primary care practice include fractures of the proximal humerus and scapula, rupture of the biceps tendon (with resulting "Popeye" deformity), and anterior dislocation of the shoulder. For more information on the diagnosis and management of these traumatic injuries, see one of the textbooks of orthopedics or sports medicine suggested at the end of this chapter. Septic arthritis of the shoulder is rare and is most frequently seen in infants and children age 2 or younger. It represents a surgical emergency, and if left untreated, could lead to septic shock, arthritis, or a fused joint.

CASE STUDY

A 50-year-old, right-hand-dominant male house painter presents with progressive right shoulder pain over the past year. His pain initially started in his lateral shoulder only when he worked overhead. It is now present in the anterior, posterior, and lateral shoulder. It is present throughout the day, and he rates it an 8 on a scale of 10. It wakens him at night. He has recently noticed problems washing and combing his hair. He cannot perform any overhead activities at work. There is no history of injury to the shoulder or problems with his shoulders prior to this episode. He is not complaining of neck pain. He is taking ibuprofen, but it is no longer affecting his pain.

QUESTIONS

1. Which special maneuvers from the physical examination will help rule-in an impingement syndrome?
2. What is an appropriate course of treatment?

DISCUSSION

On examination the patient has tenderness with abduction at 90 to 100°. He cannot perform the back scratch test due to pain. Neer's and Hawkins' impingement signs are positive, as are Speed's and Yergason's tests for biceps function. Testing of supraspinatus, infraspinatus, and subscapularis muscle function show tenderness, but strength is intact. Lag signs are negative. Radiographs (scapular anteroposterior, supraspinatus outlet, and axillary lateral views) are normal. Injection of a 1%-lidocaine solution into the subacromial space resolved the patient's pain almost completely (rated 1 on a scale of 10) after 10 minutes.

The diagnosis is rotator cuff tendonitis with biceps tendon irritation. The patient was injected with a steroid solution in the subacromial space and started on gentle range-of-motion exercises. At his 2-week follow-up, he was doing well, without pain or weakness. He was given exercises to strengthen the rotator cuff, followed by exercises for the larger muscles of the shoulder. He was allowed to return to overhead activities as tolerated. He has remained symptom-free at 1-year follow-up.

REFERENCES

1. Vecchio P, Kavanagh R, Hazleman BL, King RH. Shoulder pain in a community-based rheumatology clinic. Br J Rheumatol 1995;34:440–442.
2. Chard MD, Hazleman R, Hazleman BL, et al. Shoulder disorders in the elderly: a community survey. Arthritis Rheum 1991;34:766–769.
3. van der Windt DA, Koes BW, Boeke AJ, et al. Shoulder disorders in general practice: prognostic indicators of outcome. Br J Gen Pract 1996;46:519–523.
4. Pollock RG, Duralde XA, Flatow EL, Bigliani LU. The use of arthroscopy in the treatment of resistant frozen shoulder. Clin Orthop 1994;304:30–36.
5. Yamanaka K, Matsumoto T. The joint side tear of the rotator cuff. A followup study by arthrography. Clin Orthop 1994;304:68–73.
6. Hoppenfeld S, Hutton R. Physical Exam of the Spine and Extremities. New York: Appleton-Century-Crofts, 1976.
7. Speer KP, Hannafin JA, Altchek DW, Warren RF. An evaluation of the shoulder relocation test. Am J Sports Med 1994;22:177–183.
8. Neer CS II. Anterior acromioplasty for the chronic impingement syndrome in the shoulder: a preliminary report. J Bone Joint Surg [Am] 1972;54:41–50.
9. Hawkins RJ, Kennedy JC. Impingement syndrome in athletes. Am J Sports Med 1980;8:151–158.
10. Jobe FW, Moynes DR. Delineation of diagnostic criteria and a rehabilitation program for rotator cuff injuries. Am J Sports Med 1982;10:336–339.
11. Kelley BT, Kadrmas WR, Speer KP. The manual muscle examination for rotator cuff strength. An electromyographic investigation. Am J Sports Med 1996; 24:581–588.
12. Gerber C, Krushell RJ. Isolated rupture of the tendon of the subscapularis muscle. Clinical features in 16 cases. J Bone Joint Surg Br 1991;73:389–394.
13. Hertel R, Ballmer FT, Lombert SM, Gerber C. Lag signs in the diagnosis of rotator cuff rupture. J Shoulder Elbow Surg 1996;5:307–313.
14. McMaster WC. Anterior glenoid labrum damage: a painful lesion in swimmers. Am J Sports Med 1986; 14:383–387.
15. Farin PU, Kaukanen E, Jaroma H, Vaatainen U, Miettinen H, Soimakallio S. Site and size of rotator-cuff tear. Findings at ultrasound, double-contrast arthrography, and computed tomography arthrography with surgical correlation. Invest Radiol 1996;31:387–394.
16. Green MR, Christensen KP. Magnetic resonance imaging of the glenoid labrum in anterior shoulder instability. Am J Sports Med 1994;22:493–498.
17. Ahovuo J, Paavolainen P, Jaaskinen J. Arthrotomography of the unstable shoulder. Acta Orthop Scand 1988; 59:681–683.
18. Callaghan JJ, McNiesh LM, DeHaven JP, Savory CG, Polly DW Jr. A prospective comparison study of double-contrast computed tomography (CT) arthrography and arthroscopy of the shoulder. Am J Sports Med 1988;16:13–20.
19. Burk DL Jr, Karasick D, Kurtz AB, et al. Rotator cuff tears: prospective comparison of MR imaging with arthrography, sonography, and surgery. Am J Roentgenol 1989;153:87–92.
20. Hodler J, Fretz CJ, Terrier F, Gerber C. Rotator cuff tears: correlation of sonographic and surgical findings. Radiology 1988;169:791–794.
21. Mack LA, Matsen FA 3d, Kilcoyne RF, Davies PK, Sickler ME. U.S. evaluation of the rotator cuff. Radiology 1985;157:205–209.
22. Middleton WD, Edelstein G, Reinus WR, Melson GL, Totty WG, Murphy WA. Sonographic detection of rotator cuff tears. Am J Roentgenol 1985;144:349–353.
23. Miller CL, Karasick D, Kurtz AB, Fenlin JM Jr. Limited sensitivity of ultrasound for the detection of rotator cuff tears. Skeletal Radiol 1989;18:179–183.
24. Iannotti JP, Zlatkin MB, Esterhai JL, Kressel HY, Dalinka MK, Spindler KP. Magnetic resonance imaging of the shoulder. Sensitivity, specificity, and predictive value. J Bone Joint Surg [Am] 1991;73:17–29.
25. Dupont M, Beliveau P, Theriault G. The efficacy of anti-inflammatory medication in the treatment of the acutely sprained ankle. Am J Sports Med 1987;15:41–45.
26. Withrington RH, Girgis FL, Seifert MH. A placebo-controlled trial of steroid injections in the treatment of supraspinatus tendonitis. Scand J Rheumatol 1985;14: 76–78.
27. Bossart PJ, Joyce SM, Manaster BJ, Packer SM. Lack of efficacy of "weighted" radiographs in diagnosing acute acromioclavicular separation. Ann Emerg Med 1988; 17:20–24.
28. Larsen E, Bjerg-Nielsen A, Christensen P. Conservative or surgical treatment of acromioclavicular dislocation. A prospective, controlled, randomized study. J Bone Joint Surg 1986;68:552–555.
29. Taft TN, Wilson FC, Oglesby JW. Dislocation of the acromioclavicular joint. An end-result study. J Bone Joint Surg 1987;69:1045–1051.

38. Skin Problems

RICHARD P. USATINE

Key Clinical Questions

1. Is the appearance of the lesion highly suggestive of a specific diagnosis?
2. When do you treat empirically, and when do you biopsy a skin problem?
3. What will you do if a patient fails to respond to your empiric treatment?

Pattern recognition plays a large role in the learning and practice of dermatology. Experts who have seen countless cases of skin conditions can look at most lesions and make an immediate and accurate diagnosis through pattern recognition.

How does the novice get to this point? The first step is to learn the basic patterns of the primary and secondary lesions listed in Table 38.1. This will give you the proper vocabulary and conceptual model to observe and describe what you are seeing. Then, if you combine keen observation of the lesions (including type and distribution) along with a careful history, you will be able to create an informed differential diagnosis. The information you acquire from observation and history can be taken to a dermatology atlas, textbook, or consultant to complete the diagnosis. Sometimes further testing such as a biopsy or culture may be needed; however, you need to know enough about the possible diagnoses to appropriately plan a biopsy or laboratory evaluation.

CLINICAL EVALUATION

Although we are taught in medical school to perform the history before doing the physical examination, this is not the most efficient way to approach the diagnosis of a skin condition. When the patient has a skin complaint, take a look at the skin right away and ask your questions while you have a look.

Physical Examination

The first step is to look carefully at the lesions. Try to determine the type of primary lesions and any secondary lesions (see Table 38.1). Next touch the lesions. Use gloves if you think the lesions may be transmissible, as in scabies. For some lesions, such as actinic keratosis with scaling or the sandpaper rash of scarlet fever, feeling the skin lightly gives you much information. For deeper lesions, such as nodules and cysts, deep palpation is needed.

Observe the distribution of the lesions. Look at the local distribution first to determine if the primary lesions are arranged in groups, rings, lines, or merely scattered over the skin. For example, the vesicles of herpes simplex are usually grouped together because they follow a sensory nerve, whereas the vesicles of chickenpox are often scattered because the virus is bloodborne. Then determine which parts of the skin are affected and which are spared.

Be sure to look at the remainder of the skin, nails, hair, and mucus membranes. Patients often only show you one small area and appear reluctant to show you the rest of their skin. With many skin conditions it is essential to look beyond the most affected area.

Think of yourself as a detective collecting clues. For example, it helps to look for nail pitting when considering a diagnosis of psoriasis. Patients may have lesions on their back or feet that they have not observed; for example, a patient may have an eruption on the hands that is an autosensitization to a fungal infection on the feet—if you don't look for the fungus on the feet you will miss the diagnosis. Some skin diseases (like lichen planus) have manifestations in the mouth; finding white patches on the buccal mucosa may lead you to the correct diagnosis of lichen planus. Don't be shy about asking patients to remove their shoes and clothing and to show you whatever areas of the body that are needed to make an accurate diagnosis. A magnifying glass is helpful to distinguish the morphology of many skin conditions.

History

Once you have started to look at the skin, your history will be more focused and directed toward zeroing in on the correct diagnosis. The fol-

Table 38.1.
Primary and Secondary Skin Lesions

Lesion Type	Description
Primary (basic) lesions	
Macule —Flat	Circumscribed flat discoloration
Papule — raised	Elevated solid lesion (up to 5 mm)
Plaque	Circumscribed superficially elevated solid lesion (>5 mm) (often, a confluence of papules)
Nodule	Palpable solid (round) lesion, deeper than a papule
Wheal (hive)	Pale-red edematous plaque—round or flat-topped and transient
Pustule	Elevated collection of purulence
Vesicle	Circumscribed elevated collection of fluid (up to 5 mm in diameter)
Bulla	Circumscribed elevated collection of fluid (>5 mm in diameter)
Secondary lesions (complications or progression of primary lesions)	
Scale (desquamation)	Excess dead epidermal cells
Crusts	A collection of dried serum, blood, or purulence
Erosion	Superficial loss of epidermis
Ulcer	Focal loss of epidermis and dermis
Fissure	Linear loss of epidermis and dermis
Atrophy	Depression in the skin from thinning of epidermis and/or dermis
Excoriation	Erosion caused by scratching
Lichenification	Thickened epidermis with prominent skin lines (induced by scratching)

Modified from Habif T. Clinical Dermatology: Color Guide to Diagnosis and Therapy, 3rd ed. St. Louis: Mosby, 1996; Fitzpatrick TB, Polano MK, Surmand D. Color Atlas and Synopses of Clinical Dermatology: Common and Serious Diseases, 2nd ed. New York: McGraw-Hill, 1996.

lowing information will help you make a diagnosis and plan the treatment:

- Onset and duration of skin lesions—continuous or intermittent?
- Pattern of eruption: Where did it start? How has it changed?
- Any known precipitants, such as exposure to medication (prescription and over-the-counter [OTC]), foods, plants, sun, topical agents, chemicals (occupation and hobbies)?
- Skin symptoms: itching, pain, paresthesia
- Systemic symptoms: fever, chills, night sweats, fatigue, weakness, weight loss
- Underlying illnesses: diabetes, human immunodeficiency virus (HIV)
- Family history: acne, atopic dermatitis, psoriasis, skin cancers, dysplastic nevi.

Prevention Examination

You should also learn to perform a competent, complete skin examination for cancer detection and prevention. In dermatology, primary prevention occurs when the clinician counsels the patient to avoid unnecessary sun exposure, and secondary prevention occurs when the clinician attempts to detect early skin cancer or precancer through examination of the skin. To do a complete skin examination:

- Look at the skin from head to toe—skin cancer can occur at any site.
- Focus on the highest risk areas for skin cancer: the face, neck, back, and arms (areas that receive the most sun exposure).

Patients at highest risk for skin cancer should get a complete skin examination regularly or yearly. These patients have fair skin, blond or red hair, blue eyes, or a family history of skin cancer. Previous skin cancer or evidence of sun damage (erythema, mottled hyperpigmentation, wrinkling, scaling) increases the risk significantly. When a person has had a basal cell carcinoma (BCC), the lifetime risk of a second BCC is 40%.

When doing a complete skin examination, be systematic. To protect the patient's privacy and modesty, you may have the patient show you one segment of the body at a time with the gown on, rather than asking the patient to stand or sit stark naked in front of you. Start with the head, looking at the face, ears, and scalp. Don't forget to look in the axillae, under the breasts, between the buttocks, and on the soles of the feet. This is a good time to discuss sun exposure, protective clothing, and use of sunscreens.

Laboratory Tests

The most important laboratory tests in dermatology are:

- *Microscopy:* in diagnosing a fungal infection, scrape some of the scale onto a microscope slide, add 10% KOH with DMSO, and look for the hyphae of dermatophytes or the pseudo-hyphae of yeast forms of *Candida* or *Pityrosporum* species.
- *Cultures:* may be useful for some suspected bacterial, viral, or mycologic infections.
- *VDRL/ANA (Venereal Disease Research Laboratory or antinuclear antibody) tests:* helpful in determining the etiology of unknown skin lesions.
- *Wood's light examination:* helpful in diagnosing tinea capitus and erythrasma. Tinea capitus caused by *Microsporum* species produce green fluorescence, but *Trichophyton* species do not fluoresce.
- *Surgical biopsy:* can be used as a diagnostic and treatment tool. Having a reasonable differential diagnosis will help you choose the appropriate biopsy type.

In most cases, the laboratory tests are used to confirm your clinical diagnosis based on history and physical examination.

THE FAMILY IN DERMATOLOGY

An understanding of the family is important in the diagnosis, treatment, and prevention of skin problems. A number of skin diseases have a strong genetic component, including acne, atopic dermatitis, psoriasis, skin cancers, dysplastic nevi, and some more rare conditions such as neurofibromatosis and tuberous sclerosis. Taking a family history may help when the diagnosis of these conditions is suspected. If other family members have a disease, it may help to explore the patient's or parents feelings about the impact this disease has had on the other individuals involved. For example, the "Heartbreak of Psoriasis" is the result of the patient's emotional response to a condition that is highly visible. If psoriasis has led to social limitations in a family member, it may help to work with your patient to maximize social function while at-tempting to keep the psoriasis under maximal control.

For children who have chronic skin disease, the parents must be well educated about the treatment of the condition. This is particularly important with atopic dermatitis because of the potential complexity of treating this condition. Parents also play an essential role in skin cancer prevention. Approximately 50% of our lifetime exposure to ultraviolet radiation occurs by age 18; therefore, parents should know how to protect their children from the sun. Although avoidance is most effective, parents should know how to allow their children to play in the sun safely. This involves using sunscreens and protective clothing. For example, most parents don't realize that the typical T-shirt has a sun protection factor of only 6, so a fair-skinned child would benefit from application of sunscreen underneath the shirt if going out in the midday summer sun.

TREATMENT PRINCIPLES

Treatment in dermatology can be divided into two categories, medical and surgical. Medical treatments include topical and systemic steroids, antibiotics, antifungal, and antiviral agents. Surgical treatments include shave, punch, elliptical, and scissor excisions. Cryosurgery and electrosurgery are also important surgical techniques.

Topical Corticosteroids

Topical corticosteroids work by at least three mechanisms:

- Reducing inflammation (useful for inflammatory processes and immunologic conditions)
- Decreasing mitosis in epidermal cells (useful for hyperproliferative conditions like psoriasis)
- Constricting small blood vessels (useful for erythema) (1)

Although the strength of topical steroids is measured by vasoconstrictor assays, their most beneficial effects occur from their anti-inflammatory and antimitotic activity. The topical steroids are most beneficial for the disorders that are classified under inflammatory processes. They also may be useful in treating some immunologic conditions and as adjunctive therapy with proper antimicrobial therapy for the inflammatory component of skin infestations and infections.

Local adverse effects of topical steroids are common with regular use over weeks to months. The most common adverse effect of topical steroids use over time is skin atrophy, in which the epidermis becomes thin and the superficial capillaries dilate. Atrophy can be accompanied by hypopigmentation, telangiectasias, and striae (1). Although the atrophy is usually reversible in months, striae are irreversible. When fluorinated steroids (the strongest steroids) are continuously applied to the face, perioral dermatitis, rosacea-like eruptions, and acneiform eruptions can occur (2).

Systemic adverse effects are rare and occur when large amounts of topical steroids are absorbed systemically. The risk of such absorption increases with stronger steroids, thinner skin, younger patients, longer duration of therapy, and the use of occlusion in therapy. Prescribing the minimum strength needed for the shortest duration of time required helps prevent adverse effects.

Choosing and Dispensing Topical Corticosteroids

The art and science of choosing a topical steroid is one of maximizing benefit and minimizing adverse effects. The factors that need to be considered involve:

- *Disorder:* as the severity or chronicity of the disorder increases, the need for higher-potency steroids increases directly. Thicker lesions (e.g., psoriatic plaques) need higher potency steroids.

- *Site:* the weakest potency steroids should be used on the face, genitals, and other intertriginous areas (skin folds) where skin is thin and/or moist and skin atrophy and striae occur most rapidly. It is best to avoid fluorinated steroids on the face or to use them for a few days only in the worst cases. In skin-fold areas, weaker steroids are suggested. The skin on the palms and soles is so thick that the most potent steroids may be needed.

- *Age:* avoid the use of high-potency topical steroids in infants and children, because they have greater surface area per body mass than adults and, therefore, greater risk and consequences of systemic absorption.

- *Steroid potency (strength and concentration):* There are more than 50 types and brands of steroids. It is not necessary to memorize these lists, but you should know the names of at least one steroid from each of four basic

strengths. Table 38.2 lists a few good choices. In order to save on costs, you can use generic agents from all the potency groups except the super-high-potency agents (which are newer and are not currently available in a generic form).

- *Vehicle:* The vehicle is the substance in which the steroid is dispersed. The most commonly used vehicles are creams, ointments, gels, solutions, and lotions (Table 38.3). The choice of vehicle is determined by the characteristics of the lesion (dry or moist), the site involved, and patient preference. Further, the vehicle affects the potency of the steroid because it determines the rate at which the steroid is absorbed through the skin (3).

Most skin preparations can be applied two times a day. This is convenient for working persons to do at home in the morning and evening. Try to estimate and prescribe an appropriate amount; many topical products are supplied in 15-, 30-, and 60-g sizes. To avoid adverse effects of steroid overuse, do not prescribe large quantities for small lesions, and specify a duration of use. On the other end of the spectrum, prescribing only 15 g of steroid for a large area of involvement will be frustrating to the patient when the steroid runs out before the prescribed treatment duration is completed.

Table 38.2.
Choosing Topical Corticosteroids

Vehicle
- If lesion is dry, use ointment or moisturizing lotion
- If moist or weeping, use cream (or gel)
- If in hair-covered area, consider lotion or liquid preparations

Strength (based on thickness of skin and severity and thickness of lesion)
- Face and genitals: thin skin—weakest strength, avoid atrophy
- Hands and feet: thickest skin—if lesion is severe and thickened (lichenified), may need most potent strength
- Other areas: use strength appropriate to severity and thickness of lesions

Examples
- Low potency: generic 1 or 2% hydrocortisone
- Moderate potency: generic 0.1% triamcinolone
- High potency: 0.05% fluocinonide (Lidex)
- Super-high-potency: 0.05% betamethasone dipropionate (Diprolene) or 0.05% clobetasol propionate (Temovate)

Table 38.3.
Commonly Used Vehicles for Steroids and Other Dermatologic Preparations

Creams
- Mixture of oil and water; may contain alcohol
- White color; may be somewhat greasy
- May cause stinging and irritation to broken skin
- May be drying; best for moist or exudative lesions
- Cosmetically most acceptable
- Better in skin folds than ointments

Ointments
- Base is frequently petroleum jelly (petrolatum)
- Translucent and very greasy
- Best for dry lesions; lubricating
- Greasy feeling persists after application
- May get on clothes and be transferred from hands to surfaces at work
- Cosmetically less acceptable in daytime (may be used at night and apply cream during the day)
- Increased absorption of steroid and therefore enhances potency of the steroid
- Too occlusive for exudative lesions and areas of skin folds (groin)
- Too messy for hair-covered areas.

Gels
- Greaseless mixtures of propylene glycol and water; may contain alcohol
- Clear and jelly-like
- Useful for exudative lesions; may be drying

Solutions and lotions
- Water and alcohol base
- Solutions usually clear; lotions have a milky appearance
- Best for scalp and other hair-covered areas: penetrates easily and doesn't make hair greasy
- May cause stinging and irritation to broken skin

Modified from Habif T. Clinical Dermatology: A Color Guide to Diagnosis and Therapy, 3rd ed. St. Louis: CV Mosby, 1996.

The duration of therapy should often be the time it takes for resolution of symptoms or lesions. To avoid adverse effects, the highest potency steroids should not be used for longer than 2 weeks continuously. However, they can be used intermittently for chronic conditions such as psoriasis in a pulse-therapy mode (e.g., apply every weekend, with no application on weekdays).

For dry lesions, liberal use of emollients between steroid applications can minimize steroid side effects while maximizing the benefits of therapy.

SKIN INFECTIONS

There are many infectious diseases that affect the skin. A helpful conceptual model divides skin infection into:

- *Primary infection:* skin lesions are caused by the pathogen itself (e.g., impetigo).

- *Secondary infection:* preexisting dermatitis becomes secondarily infected by a known skin pathogen (impetiginous flea bites, Color Plate Fig. 38.1).

- *Tertiary infection:* the skin lesions are the result of a systemic noncutaneous disease (measles).

Bacterial Infections

Bacterial skin infections can be classified by the portion of the skin involved (Table 38.4). Most bacterial skin infections are caused by group A β-hemolytic *Streptococcus* (GABHS) and/or *Staphylococcal aureus*. The characteristics, location, and depth of the lesion may make one of these two organisms more likely to be the causative agent, but together they account for almost all of the bacterial skin infections we see. Less common organisms may be seen in patients that are immunosuppressed or have HIV, diabetes, or a hospital-acquired infection.

Two antibiotics that cover *S. aureus* and GABHS well are dicloxacillin and cephalexin. These are both available in oral generic forms and are relatively inexpensive. If the patient has an allergy to both or a history of a severe allergy to penicillin, erythromycin can be used; however, some *S. aureus* in the community are resistant to erythromycin.

Topical antibiotics should only be used as monotherapy for the most mild and superficial bacterial skin infections. Mild cases of impetigo can be treated with Bactroban (mupirocin). Bacitracin, Polysporin, or Neosporin are not sufficiently effective to be used alone in the treatment of established skin infections. (Furthermore, you should avoid Neosporin because it is a fairly frequent cause of contact dermatitis.)

Impetigo

This condition is a superficial skin infection often characterized by translucent ("honey") crusts. It can be vesicular or bullous. Impetigo in children often occurs around the nose and mouth. Homeless adults and alcoholics are prone to getting

Table 38.4.
Bacterial Infections of the Skin

Site	Infection	Treatment
Epidermis	Impetigo Ecthyma (impetigo with ulceration) Bullous impetigo	Oral antibiotic[a] (topical mupirocin for small areas of mild infection)
Dermis	Erysipelas Cellulitis (dermis and subcutaneous tissue also)	Oral or intravenous antibiotic, based on severity
Dermal appendages (hair follicle, nail fold)	Folliculitis Carbuncle, furuncle Paronychia Abscess	Topical or oral antibiotic I&D I&D I&D
Subcutaneous tissue/fascia	Necrotizing fasciitis	Hospitalize; intravenous antibiotic; debridement

I&D, incision and drainage.

[a]Oral antibiotics must cover group A β-hemolytic streptococci and *Staphylococcus aureus:* first-line drugs—dicloxacillin or cephalexin; second-line drug—erythromycin.

impetigo (4). Impetigo should be treated for 7 to 10 days with antibiotics that cover GABHS and *S. aureus.* It also helps to remove the crusts with warm soaks and to apply dressings with or without antibiotic ointment, to keep the lesions clean and comfortable while the antibiotic is working.

Two variations of impetigo are ecthyma and bullous impetigo. Ecthyma has a ulcerated "punched-out" base. Bullous impetigo is more often caused by *S. aureus.* Staphylococcal-scalded skin syndrome (SSSS) is a life-threatening, more severe variation of bullous impetigo. The bullae are caused by exfoliating toxin, and the patient is systematically ill. Patients who have SSSS need emergent hospitalization for intravenous antibiotics, fluids, and supportive therapy.

Cellulitis

This condition is an acute infection of the skin that involves the dermis and subcutaneous tissues (5). Cellulitis is most often caused by GABHS and *S. aureus.* Erysipelas is a specific type of superficial cellulitis with prominent lymphatic involvement. It is almost always due to GABHS (5).

Cellulitis often begins with a break in the skin caused by trauma, a bite, or an underlying dermatosis (e.g., tinea pedis). It is most often seen on the legs and arms. The severity of the cellulitis, the systemic symptoms, and host factors determine whether oral or parenteral antibiotics are indicated.

Folliculitis

Folliculitis is an infection of the superficial portion of the hair follicle, usually caused by *S. aureus.* Its presentation can include perifollicular erythema, papules, or pustules. Magnification during the skin examination will reveal that the lesions are associated with hair follicles. Occlusion of hair follicles can cause folliculitis; treatment can range from avoidance of the external precipitating factors to the use of topical or oral antibiotics.

Abscess

An abscess is defined as a localized collection of pus; abscesses that occur in or directly below the skin include furuncles, carbuncles, and the abscesses around fingernails (acute paronychias). A furuncle or boil is an abscess that starts in a hair follicle or sweat gland. A carbuncle occurs when the furuncle extends into the subcutaneous tissue. External abscesses most often occur on the hands, feet, extremities, buttocks, and breast. Most skin abscesses are caused by *S. aureus.* Other organisms that can cause abscesses of the skin include *Streptococcus* species, gram-negative bacteria, and anaerobes (5, 6).

Incision and drainage (I&D) is the treatment of choice for all types of abscesses. The pus must be drained so that the lesion can heal. Systemic antibiotics, whether parenteral or oral, do not adequately penetrate an abscess to cure the infection. If there is significant surrounding cellulitis, systemic antibiotics may be needed as an adjunct to the I&D.

Diagnosis may be easy when the skin overlying the abscess is red, warm, tender, swollen, and fluctuant. When you are uncertain whether a red, warm, swollen area of the skin is cellulitis or an abscess, do a diagnostic needle aspiration. If you get pus from the aspiration, the abscess should be fully opened with a No. 11 scalpel.

Necrotizing Fasciitis

Necrotizing fasciitis, "flesh-eating bacteria," is a deep infection of the subcutaneous tissues and fascia. It often presents with diffuse swelling of the arm or leg, followed by the appearance of bullae with clear fluid that may become violaceous in color. The patient has marked systemic symptoms. There are two types of necrotizing fasciitis. Type 1 is caused by mixed anaerobes, gram-negative aerobic bacilli, and enterococci. Type 2 is caused by GABHS.

Predisposing factors for necrotizing fasciitis are varicella, penetrating injuries, minor cuts, burns, childbirth, and surgery (7). Necrotizing fasciitis can lead to cutaneous gangrene, myonecrosis, and shock. Necrotizing fasciitis may look like cellulitis at first. It is crucial to not miss necrotizing fasciitis because it is life- and limb-threatening and requires surgical debridement along with intravenous antibiotics.

Viral Infections

Warts

Warts are caused by more than 60 subtypes of human *Papillomavirus* (HPV) (8). Warts most commonly occur on the hands, feet, and genitals. The appearance of the wart is strongly related to its location. Warts on the hands (verruca vulgaris) are usually raised and hyperkeratotic. Warts on the soles of the feet (plantar warts) are flat, disrupt skin lines, have dark dots visible in them, and may be quite painful. Flat warts (verruca plana) are flat and usually seen in groups. Genital warts (condylomata acuminata) often have a cauliflower appearance, are transmitted sexually, and have been associated with cervical intraepithelial neoplasia and cervical cancer (9).

The natural history is for most warts to eventually regress; and there are many treatments for warts. Some warts do not respond to treatment, however, or recur within a short period of time. A comparison of treatment options for warts is found in Table 38.5. In office practice, the follow-

Table 38.5.
Comparison of Therapies for Human Papillomavirus Infection[a–c]

Treatment Modality	Average Number of Treatments	Success Rate[d] (%)	Recurrence Rate Within 6 Mo (%)	Estimated Cost to Patient ($)	Level of Evidence for Effectiveness[e]
Cryotherapy	1.9	83	28	375	A
Podophyllin resin	4.2	65	39	644	A
Podofilox (Condylox)	10.5 (patient applied)	61	34	325	A
Trichloroacetic acid	4	81	36	628	B
CO_2 laser	1.3	89	8	305	A
Electrocautery	1.4	93	24	317	B
LEEP	1	90	ND	270	B
Excision	1.1	93	24	282	A
Topical fluorouracil	6.6 (patient applied)	71	13	310	A

LEEP, loop electrosurgical excisional procedure; ND, no data or not recorded.

[a]This table is based on the author's best estimate as compiled from data from the available literature. Very small studies, studies with results that fell 2 standard deviations beyond the mean, and very poorly designed studies were excluded.

[b]Modified from Mayeaux EJ, Harper MB, Barksdale W, Pope JB. Noncervical human papillomavirus genital infections. Am Fam Physician 1995;52(4):1137–1147.

[c]Based on hypothetical patient with 6 initial warts and 2 re-treatment warts.

[d]Defined as clearance of all condylomata at the end of healing from therapy.

[e]Level of evidence for effectiveness: A, strong or moderate research-based evidence (consistent across several studies, including at least two randomized controlled trials); B, limited research-based evidence (less consistent or extensive evidence, but preponderance of evidence supports use of treatment); C, common practice with little or no research-based evidence.

ing treatments are generally considered "first line" for these conditions:

- Verruca vulgaris: salicylic acid, cryosurgery, or electrosurgery

- Plantar warts: salicylic acid, cryosurgery, or electrosurgery

- Flat warts: salicylic acid, topical tretinoin (Retin-A), or topical fluorouracil

- Condylomata acuminata: podophyllin resin, podofilox (Condylox), trichloroacetic acid, cryosurgery, or imiquimod (Aldura)

Herpesviruses

The major herpesviruses that affect the skin are herpes simplex (HSV) types 1 and 2 and varicella-zoster virus (VZV). A major characteristic of herpes infection is that the virus lies dormant in dorsal root ganglia, leading to recurrences. All herpetic skin infections are characterized by vesicular eruptions with surrounding erythema, which progress to ulcers, crust over, and then reepithelialize over days to weeks. Infections caused by herpesviruses include:

- *Herpes gingivostomatitis ("cold sores")*: caused by HSV (most commonly type 1, but sometimes type 2), a primary episode can affect the entire mouth and be accompanied by fever, chills, and malaise. Recurrent episodes often occur on the lips and are milder, sometimes asymptomatic, but accompanied by viral shedding (Color Plate Fig. 38.2).

- *Genital herpes*: caused by HSV (most commonly type 2, but sometimes type 1). This sexually transmitted disease presents as herpetic lesions on the genitals, anus, or buttocks. As in gingivostomatitis, first episodes are often more severe; subsequent episodes range from moderate to asymptomatic but are accompanied by viral shedding and the possibility of transmission to sexual partners.

- *Chickenpox*: this is the initial infection of VZV. It typically consists of a few days of fever and respiratory symptoms and the characteristic herpes rash lesions that begin on the trunk, and over several days spread more centrifugally.

- *Herpes zoster (shingles)*: this is a reactivation of dormant VZV along a skin dermatome (Color Plate Fig. 38.3).

Most infections with HSV and VZV are acutely painful, uncomplicated, and resolve sponta-

neously in 1 to 2 weeks. Complications include encephalitis and disseminated infections; these occur especially in infants or immunosuppressed individuals.

We do not have any curative antiviral agents for HSV or VZV; so the goals of therapy are to diminish pain, viral shedding, and duration of symptoms and to prevent recurrences. In HSV, treatment can prevent or reduce recurrences; in zoster, early antiviral treatment may prevent postherpetic neuralgia, a prolonged and painful after-effect of the infection.

Acyclovir (Zovirax) was the first antiviral agent with proven efficacy against HSV and VZV. Three newer agents now available are famciclovir (Famvir) and valacyclovir (Valtrex) and topical penciclovir (Denavir). The first three agents can be used to treat primary and recurrent herpes simplex and herpes zoster and to prevent recurrent herpes simplex. Penciclovir can be used topically to treat recurrent herpes labialis (cold sores). Acyclovir is also approved by the Food and Drug Administration to treat acute varicella (chickenpox). Preliminary data on both famciclovir and valacyclovir indicate that they are at least as effective for treatment of zoster and herpes simplex as acyclovir (10, 11). Both newer agents have the advantage of requiring fewer doses per day, and currently valacyclovir is priced less expensively than acyclovir and famciclovir (11). It remains to be seen if any one of these agents will be shown to be more effective than the others for any indication. Also, we now have the varicella vaccine for primary prevention.

Fungal Infections

Fungal infections of the skin occur at many sites and are most often caused by dermatophytes, *Candida*, or *Pityrosporum* species. The dermatophytes cause tinea infections that are commonly called "ringworm" (although no worm is involved in ringworm). The typical dermatophyte infection of the body (tinea corporis) has an annular appearance with central clearing, redness, and scaliness on the perimeter of this well-demarcated lesion (Color Plate Fig. 38.4). Tinea versicolor is caused by an inflammatory reaction to the yeast-like *Pityrosporum* species rather than a dermatophyte. *Candida* thrives on wet mucosal surfaces but also affects the skin; it causes thrush, balanitis, vaginitis, and rashes in areas such as the groin and under the breast.

Common dermatophyte infections are:

- *Tinea capitus* (tinea of the head) causes patchy alopecia (hair loss) with broken hairs and some scaling. Because the hair shaft and follicle are involved, topical antifungals are not effective. Oral griseofulvin for 4 to 8 weeks is still the treatment of choice.

- *Tinea corporis* (tinea of the body) can occur on almost any part of the body. Small areas may respond well to topical antifungals. Topical OTC antifungals (miconazole, clotrimazole) should be first-line agents. Large areas may require treatment with oral antifungals (griseofulvin, terbinafine, itraconazole) for 2 to 4 weeks.

- *Tinea cruris* (tinea of the groin) may be red and scaling without the central clearing seen in tinea corporis. It should also be differentiated from candidal infection (which tends to be redder and has satellite lesions) and erythrasma (a superficial bacterial infection that is more brown and has coral-red fluorescence under ultraviolet light). Topical or systemic antifungals may be used depending upon the severity of involvement. If you are uncertain if there is *Candida* involvement, it is best to choose an antifungal agent that covers both dermatophytes and *Candida* (not tolnaftate [Tinactin] or naftifine [Naftin]).

- *Tinea pedis* (tinea of the feet) may be seen as macerated white areas between the toes (Color Plate Fig. 38.5) or as dry red scaling on the soles or sides of the feet (moccasin distribution). It can be treated with the same topical or oral antifungals used for tinea corporis or cruris. Griseofulvin or the newer oral antifungals (terbinafine and itraconazole) may be used when the lesions are not responding to topical agents.

A skin scraping treated with KOH and analyzed with a microscope can be diagnostic when classic hyphae or yeast forms are detected. False-negative results are common when specimen collection is inadequate, when the patient has started OTC antifungals, or when the slide is read by an inexperienced viewer. Fungal cultures can be expensive and take a long time to grow, but they may provide the most definitive evidence of fungal infection while providing you with the identity of the fungus.

Onychomycosis is a fungal infection of the nails. Until the release of the newer oral antifungal agents (itraconazole, terbinafine), the success rate for eradication of nail fungus was poor. The newer agents can be given continuously for 3 months or as pulse therapy 1 week a month for 3 to 4 months; they are costly and have cure rates of approximately 72 to 84% (12). It is important to establish a definitive diagnosis of onychomycosis before starting treatment with oral antifungals, because there are other causes for dystrophic nails such as psoriasis, lichen planus, and trauma. When prescribing oral antifungal agents, you should go over the risks and benefits of these medications with your patients.

DERMATITIS

Dermatitis is a nonspecific term that means inflammation of the skin. There are many causes and patterns of skin inflammation including eczema, contact dermatitis, and atopic dermatitis. Eczema is the most common type of skin inflammation; it can occur in three stages: acute, subacute, and chronic (3). Color Plate Figure 38.6 provides an example of acute dermatitis, and Color Plate Figure 38.7 illustrates chronic eczema (lichen simplex chronicus). Common forms of dermatitis are described next:

- *Eczema* is frequently seen on the hands or feet but can occur on any part of the body. Acute eczema is typically vesicular and red, whereas subacute eczema lacks the vesicles and has prominent scaling and dry, cracking skin. Chronic eczema includes lichenification (thickened plaque with accentuation of the skin lines).

- *Nummular eczema* is coin-shaped (nummus = coin).

- *Contact dermatitis* is an allergic response to an allergen such as a chemical found in the poison ivy or poison oak plant (*Rhus* dermatitis). These lesions are often linear and vesicular. Other contact allergens include nickel in jewelry and belt buckles and chemicals in deodorants.

- *Atopic dermatitis* is a type of eczematous eruption that is itchy, recurrent, and symmetric and often found on flexural surfaces (3) (see Color Plate Fig. 38.6). These patients often have either a personal or a family history of asthma, allergic rhinitis, or conjunctivitis. In infancy, atopic dermatitis often appears on the face. After infancy, the dry, scaling, and red lesions are found in flexural areas such as the antecubital or popliteal fossa. Most atopic dermatitis is not due to specific allergens, but is set off by a number of trigger factors in patients who have a strong genetic predisposition to develop eczematous eruptions.

Treatment

Treatment for all types of dermatitis has basic principles. First, avoid skin irritants such as drying soaps and bathing in water that is too hot or for too long. This dries out the skin, increasing the pruritus and inflammation. Second, use emollients or moisturizers to moisten the skin. Third, treat inflammatory components with a topical steroid, choosing the strength and vehicle based on diagnosis, chronicity, and location.

Fourth, because itching is a prominent feature of many types of dermatitis, efforts should be made to stop the scratch-itch cycle. This is especially true for atopic dermatitis and lichen simplex chronicus. Lichen simplex chronicus often needs potent topical steroid ointments to penetrate the thick plaque and moisturize the cracked pruritic skin. The oral sedating antihistamines work well to stop itching, especially at night.

Finally, any type of dermatitis may develop a secondary bacterial infection. This may take the form of impetigo or just show weeping and crusting (see Color Plate Fig. 38.6). Signs of infection should lead to treatment with an antibiotic that covers GABHS and *S. aureus*.

Seborrhea

Seborrhea is a superficial inflammatory dermatitis. It is a common condition that is characterized by patches of erythema and scaling (Color Plate Fig. 38.8). The typical distribution of seborrhea includes the scalp (dandruff), eyebrows, eyelids, nasolabial creases, behind the ears, eyebrows, forehead, cheeks, around nose, under the beard or mustache, over the sternum, axillae, submammary folds, umbilicus, groin, and the gluteal creases. These areas are the regions with the greatest number of pilosebaceous units producing sebum.

The prevalence of seborrhea is approximately 3 to 5% in young adults. Its incidence increases with age, and it is especially common in persons with Parkinson's disease and in HIV-positive persons. Although the cause of seborrhea is not entirely clear, it is thought to involve an inflammatory hypersensitivity to epidermal, bacterial, or yeast antigens. Persons with seborrhea have a profusion of *Pityrosporum ovale* on the skin. Although this yeast can be a normal skin inhabitant, persons who have seborrhea appear to respond to its presence with an inflammatory reaction.

Seborrhea is characterized by remissions and exacerbations. The most common precipitating factors are stress, antibiotic use, and cold weather. The treatment of seborrhea should be directed at the inflammation and the *Pityrosporum*.

Seborrhea is highly responsive to topical steroids, so a low-potency steroid is usually adequate. To avoid atrophy, it is especially important to use a low-potency steroid for the treatment of seborrhea on the face; 1% hydrocortisone cream or lotion works well. Prescribe lotion for seborrhea in hair-covered areas because it is easier and less messy to apply than a cream. If scalp seborrhea is severe, you may prescribe a higher-potency steroid solution such as fluocinonide (Lidex) solution or clobetasol propionate (Temovate) scalp application, as the risk of atrophy on the scalp is less than on the face.

To reduce the profusion of *Pityrosporum*, you should direct the patient to apply antifungals to the affected areas. For seborrhea of the scalp, the antifungal shampoos that are most effective contain either selenium sulfide, zinc pyrithione, ketoconazole, or coal tar derivatives. For seborrhea of the skin, ketoconazole cream is the most effective antifungal preparation.

Patients need to understand that these treatments are not curative, and seborrhea may come back when they are under greater stress or they stop using the antiseborrhea shampoos. The antifungals can be used to prevent exacerbations, but the steroids should be applied only to active areas of inflammation.

PSORIASIS

Psoriasis is a chronic condition characterized by epidermal proliferation and inflammation. The lesions are well-circumscribed, red, scaling patches, with white thickened scales (Color Plate Fig. 38.9). Areas affected can include the scalp, nails, extensor surfaces of limbs, elbows, knees, the sacral region, and the genitalia. Psoriasis lesions may also be guttate as in water drops, inverse when found in intertriginous areas such as the inguinal and intergluteal folds, or volar when found on the palms or soles. Psoriatic nail changes occur in 10 to 40% of persons with psoriasis. These nail changes include pitting, onycholysis, subungual keratosis.

Treatment options for psoriasis include emollients, topical steroids, topical vitamin D, anthralin, topical tar and tar shampoo, intralesional steroids, ultraviolet light, methotrexate, and retinoids. The most common treatment of psoriasis involves topical steroids, with strong ointments being the most effective. Systemic steroids are contraindicated in psoriasis; they can precipitate severe flares and generalized pustular disease. When using potent topical steroids for chronic therapy in psoriasis (or eczema) it helps to use pulse therapy on weekends to avoid side effects and loss of efficacy.

ACNE

Acne is an inflammatory disease of the pilosebaceous unit (sebaceous glands and their associated small hairs). The glands produce sebum, which is a complex lipid mixture, to maintain hydration of the skin. Acne involves blockage of the pilosebaceous unit with sebum and desquamated cells, accompanied by an overgrowth of *Propionibacterium acnes* in the follicle.

Noninflammatory lesions of acne are open comedones (blackheads) and closed comedones (whiteheads). When there is disruption of the follicle wall, *P. acnes*, sebum, hair, and cells extrude into the dermis. This causes inflammation and leads to the formation of papules, pustules, nodules, and cysts. The causes or exacerbating factors for acne are genetics; androgens; stress; excessive friction on the skin (e.g., with sweat bands and helmet straps); cosmetics; and medications, including oral contraceptive pills (especially those with increased androgenicity, such as norgestrel and ethinyl estradiol [Ovral]), corticosteroids, lithium, and isoniazid.

Table 38.6 summarizes acne treatments. Mild acne responds to cleansing and benzoyl peroxides. Full combination therapy for acne consists of an oral antibiotic, tretinoin (Retin-A), topical antibiotic, and benzoyl peroxide. If this fails and acne is scarring, consider isotretinoin (Accutane). When prescribing topical tretinoin, explain to the patient that redness and scaling may occur and that the acne may worsen during the first 2 to 4 weeks. Because tretinoin increases sun sensitivity, the patient should be warned to use a sunscreen daily. For most patients, it helps to start with the mildest formulation, 0.025% cream. One may then increase to 0.05% to 0.1% cream if needed and tolerated. For oily skin and more severe acne, it may help to switch to the gel. Newer topical agents available to treat acne include adapalene (Differin), azelaic acid (Azelex), and tretinoin in microspheres (Retin-A micro).

SUN DAMAGE AND PRECANCERS

Sun damage to the skin can be seen in photoaging, which results in mottled hyperpigmentation and wrinkling. The sun damage can lead to precancers such as actinic keratosis and lentigo maligna.

Skin Cancers

The most common skin cancers are basal cell carcinoma (BCC), squamous cell carcinoma (SCC), and melanoma. Sun exposure is the most important risk factor; other risk factors include a positive family history and fair skin type. The incidence of these cancers increases with age, probably because of cumulative sun exposure.

BCCs are the most common skin cancer. They occur largely (85%) on the head and neck (3). There are three major morphologic types: nodular, superficial, and morpheaform (sclerosing). The typical nodular BCC is pearly and raised with telangiectasias (Color Plate Fig. 38.10). As it expands, its center may ulcerate and bleed and become crusted. Superficial BCCs look like SCC: red or pink, flat, scaling plaques that may have erosions or crusts. Sclerosing BCCs are rare (1% of BCCs), flat, and scar-like. SCCs can look like a superficial BCC or can be more elevated and nodular. SCCs are frequently hyperkeratotic and bleed easily (Color Plate Fig. 38.11).

Actinic keratosis (AK) are premalignant and have a 12% risk of becoming SCC if untreated (13). Recognizing and treating actinic keratoses is a method of skin cancer prevention (secondary prevention). Because there is a spectrum from actinic keratosis to Bowen's disease (SCC in situ) to SCC, it is sometimes necessary to biopsy a lesion that has features that appear more suspicious than a typical AK. Otherwise, AKs can be easily treated with cryotherapy by any trained physician.

Melanoma has been on the rise in the United States in the last few decades. Early detection and treatment can prevent deaths and morbidity (3). Table 38.7 presents "ABCDE" guidelines for the diagnosis of melanoma, and Color Plate Figure 38.12 provides an illustration of a melanoma. Many benign growths can resemble melanoma, so a suspicious growth should receive a full-depth biopsy to make a definitive diagnosis.

Benign Growths That Can Be Confused with Skin Cancers

Family physicians should have a working knowledge of the most common benign growths. Some benign pigmented lesions that may be confused with melanoma include nevi, congenital nevi, seborrheic keratoses, dermatofibromas,

Table 38.6.
Medications for Acne Therapy

Drug	Type	Typical Regimen	Comments
Topical			
Benzoyl peroxide (gel, cream, lotion)	Antimicrobial	Apply bid	
Clindamycin and erythromycin	Topical antibiotics		
• Erythromycin			Solution, gel, lotion
• Clindamycin (Cleocin-T)			Solution, gel, lotion
• Benzoyl peroxide/ erythromycin (Benzamycin)	Antimicrobial/antibiotic combination		Erythromycin 3%, benzoyl peroxide 5%; effects are synergistic
Retinoids			
• Tretinoin (Retin-A)	Comedolytic agents	Apply q hs	
• Adapalene (Differin)			
Weak acids			
• Azelaic acid (Azalex)	Antimicrobial and comedolytic agents		Newer agents
• α-Hydroxy acids	Comedolytic agents		
Systemic			
Tetracycline	Oral antibiotics	500 mg qd bid	Inexpensive, need to take on an empty stomach
Doxycycline (Vibamycin, others)		50–100 mg qd bid	Inexpensive, well tolerated, increases sun sensitivity
Minocycline (Minocin)		50–100 mg qd bid	Expensive, highly effective
Erythromycin		250–500 mg bid	Inexpensive; frequent gastrointestinal disturbances
Trimethoprim/sulfamethoxazole (Septra, Bactrim, others)			Highly effective but significant risk of adverse effects with prolonged use
Isotretinoin (Accutane)	Retinoid acid		For cystic and scarring acne unresponsive to other therapies

The usual agents used in the treatment of acne are selected by the severity of the condition, and the previous response (if any):

Comedonal acne: mild (comedonal)
  • Start with topical benzoyl peroxide bid
  • Use tretinoin at first or when acne is improving
  • Azalex and α-hydroxy acids as adjunctive therapy

Papulopustular acne: mild
  • Topical antibiotics and benzoyl peroxide
  • May add oral antibiotics if topical agents are not working
  • Add Retin-A as needed

Papulopustular or nodulocystic acne: moderate and inflammatory
  • May start with topical antibiotic, benzoyl peroxide, and oral antibiotic (doxycycline, erythromycin)
  • Oral Antibiotics are often essential at this stage
  • Add Retin-A when acne is improving (1 month)
  • Consider stopping oral antibiotics when topical agents are working well

Cystic or scarring acne: severe
  • When acne has not responded to the above treatments, consider:
    —Accutane (Isotretinoin)
    —Hormonal treatment for women (estrogens, spironolactone)
  • Dermabrasion

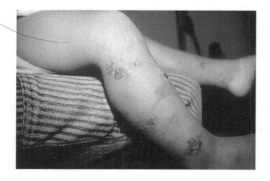

Color Plate Figure 38.1. *Impetiginous flea bites.*

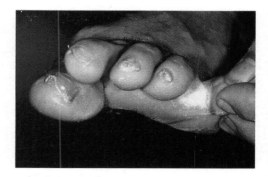

Color Plate Figure 38.5. *Tinea pedis and onycho-mycosis.*

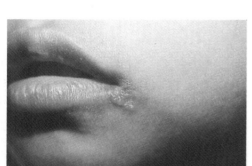

Color Plate Figure 38.2. *Herpes simplex virus.*

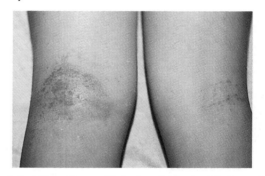

Color Plate Figure 38.6. *Atopic dermatitis (acute) in the popliteal fossa.*

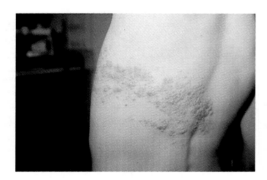

Color Plate Figure 38.3. *Herpes zoster.*

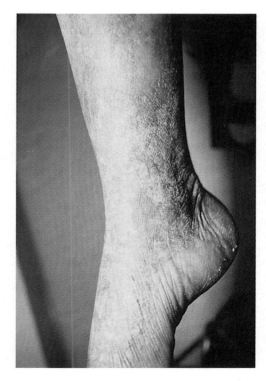

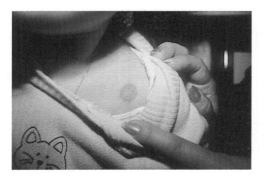

Color Plate Figure 38.4. *Tinea corporis.*

Color Plate Figure 38.7. *Chronic dermatitis (lichen simplex chronicus).*

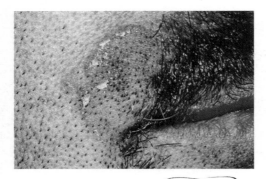

Color Plate Figure 38.8. *Seborrhea.*

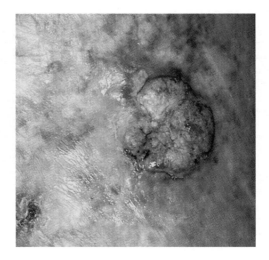

Color Plate Figure 38.11. *Squamous cell carcinoma.* (Reprinted with permission from Usatine R, Moy R, Tobinick E, Siegel D. Skin Surgery: A Practical Guide. St. Louis, MO: Mosby-Year Book, 1998.)

Look like BCC but more elevated & nodular

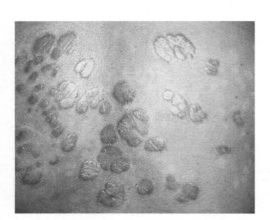

Color Plate Figure 38.9. *Psoriasis.*

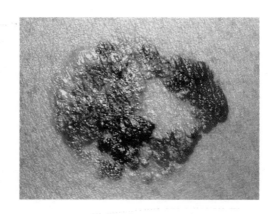

Color Plate Figure 38.12. *Melanoma.* (Courtesy of the Skin Cancer Foundation, New York, NY.)

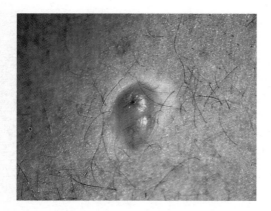

Color Plate Figure 38.10. *Basal cell carcinoma.* (Reprinted with permission from Usatine R, Moy R, Tobinick E, Siegel D. Skin Surgery: A Practical Guide. St. Louis, MO: Mosby-Year Book, 1998.)

Table 38.7.
ABCDE Guidelines for Diagnosis of Melanoma

Asymmetry
- Benign lesions are symmetrical.
- Melanomas tend to have pronounced asymmetry.

Border
- Benign lesions usually have smooth borders.
- Melanomas tend to have notched, irregular outlines.

Color
- Benign lesions usually contain only one color.
- Melanomas frequently have variegated color.

Diameter
- Benign pigmented lesions are usually smaller than 6 mm in diameter.

Elevation
- Malignant melanoma is almost always elevated, at least in part, so that it is palpable.

and lentigines. It is important to learn the appearance and characteristics of these benign lesions so that you can differentiate them from melanoma. When there is a reasonable suspicion that the lesion is malignant and not one of these benign lesions, a biopsy is in order.

Sebaceous hyperplasia can look like a basal cell carcinoma. These benign lesions are raised and can have pearly borders and telangiectasias like a BCC. When you are uncertain of the diagnosis, a shave biopsy can remove the lesion and determine whether it is malignant. Completely benign-appearing sebaceous hyperplasia is a cosmetic issue that can be treated electively if desired.

Seborrheic keratosis can mimic melanoma. These lesions develop with age and are often large and pigmented with irregular borders. Although they usually are verrucous and have a stuck-on appearance, they can be flat and irregular. When uncertain as to the diagnosis, get a consult or do a biopsy.

CONCLUSION

This chapter presented an approach to the diagnosis and treatment of common skin conditions. The focus of treatment has been medical rather than surgical. Because so much of the diagnosis of skin conditions involves learning patterns, we recommend that you spend time looking at pictures of skin conditions in the atlases and textbooks of dermatology. There are an increasing

number of dermatology sites and images on the Internet; use any search engine with the word dermatology to begin your search. Because there is often a lack of good evidence in the literature to make critical decisions, one must still rely on the experience and opinions of experts.

A skin biopsy can provide you with important information when you have some confidence in your differential diagnosis. It is not a good idea to biopsy a lesion if you have no idea what it might be. The biopsy type is determined by the suspected diagnosis. For example, a shave biopsy may not be deep enough for a suspected melanoma, and an elliptical excision may be unnecessarily large for a suspected BCC. When the lesion is benign, an experienced clinician may be able to diagnose an unknown case without a biopsy, thereby saving the patient from an invasive procedure.

Although the skin is the largest organ of the body, it is highly responsive to the psychologic state of the patient. Many skin conditions (acne, seborrhea, psoriasis, eczema) are worsened by stress. Therefore it is important to take into account the whole patient when treating many skin conditions. Some skin conditions are the results of sexually transmitted diseases or sun exposure, in such cases it is not enough to prescribe a medicine or cut out a cancer. Instead, you should address the lifestyle changes necessary to prevent recurrence.

Finally, optimal treatment and compliance depends on the patient having a good understanding of the diagnosis and treatment. Therefore, good health care to patients with skin conditions often requires a comprehensive approach to the patient, taking into account the principles of counseling for health education, prevention, psychosocial stressors, and attention to the role of the family.

CASE STUDY 1

History: A 2-year-old girl was brought to the doctor's office for a rash on her legs. The mother noted that the child had been scratching her legs for weeks and the sores were getting worse. Upon further questioning it was determined that the family had a cat and there are fleas in the house (see Color Plate Fig. 38.1).
Physical examination: There are crusting,

well-demarcated lesions with honey-colored crusts on the legs. There is no surrounding erythema or swelling. The crusts appear superficial.

Diagnosis: Flea bites with secondary impetigo infection.

Treatment: Cephalexin suspension by mouth three times daily for 10 days; warm soaks to remove the crusts atraumatically; ongoing flea treatment for the cat; and extermination of the house (if needed).

CASE STUDY 2

History: An 11-year-old girl came to the doctor's office with painful blisters around her mouth (see Color Plate Fig. 38.2). This was the second episode she knows of. On further questioning, she said she had just finished her final examinations in school. She denies sexual activity.

Physical examination: There is a group of vesicles at the corner of the mouth near the vermilion border.

Diagnosis: Recurrent herpes labialis.

Treatment: Options include (*a*) no treatment; (*b*) oral acyclovir, valacyclovir, or famciclovir; or (*c*) penciclovir cream.

Prevention: Use sunscreen, because sun exposure can precipitate a recurrence. Although "stress" is a known risk factor for recurrence, there is no evidence that "stress management" prevents recurrence. The severity and location of this case does not warrant the use of oral antiviral medications for prophylaxis (unlike severe recurrent herpes genitalis).

CASE STUDY 3

History: An 18-year-old boy came to the doctor's office with a painful rash on his trunk of 5 days' duration. He denies any

other health problems and has no HIV risk factors.

Physical examination: Groups of vesicles on an erythematous base covering a large dermatomal area on the trunk. Although the area involved is large, it represents one single dermatomal area on the left side (see Color Plate Fig. 38.3).

Diagnosis: Herpes zoster (shingles).

Treatment: No antiviral treatment is indicated because the lesions have been there for 5 days. Treatment has only proved to be effective if begun within 3 days of onset. Symptomatic treatment for pain or pruritus may be given as needed.

Prevention: None. This is unlikely to occur again for this patient, but if disseminated herpes zoster develops or there are risk factors for HIV, perform an HIV test.

CASE STUDY 4

History: A 6-year-old girl was brought to the office for a round, itchy rash on her body. It was first noted 2 weeks ago. No one else in the household has had such a rash. After seeing cat hair on the girl's shirt, the physician asked whether there was a cat in the home. The mother answered "yes," and stated that the cat did have some patches of hair loss (see Color Plate Fig. 38.4).

Physical examination: There is a well-demonstrated annular (ring-like) rash with scaling, erythema, and central clearing.

Diagnosis: Tinea corporis. Ultraviolet light showed green fluorescence. A skin scraping was done; KOH staining results were positive for branching hyphae. The main differential diagnosis is nummular eczema; central clearing and positive test results for fluorescence and hyphae make the diagnosis of tinea corporis certain.

Treatment: Apply an OTC antifungal cream (clotrimazole or miconazole) twice a day for

2 weeks or until lesion resolves. If initial topical treatment fails, try a second topical antifungal before considering an oral antifungal. (The area involved is too small to warrant systemic treatment.)
Prevention: Take the cat to the veterinarian for treatment.

REFERENCES

1. Amundson LH, Caplan RM. The skin and subcutaneous tissues. In: Taylor RB, ed. Family Medicine: Principles and Practice, 2nd ed. New York: Springer-Verlag, 1988.
2. Bondi EE, Brian V, Jegasothy, et al. Dermatology: Diagnosis and Therapy. Norwalk, CT: Appleton & Lange, 1991.
3. Habif T. Clinical Dermatology: A Color Guide to Diagnosis and Therapy, 3rd ed. St. Louis: CV Mosby, 1996.
4. Usatine RP. Skin diseases of the homeless. In: Wood D, ed. Delivering Health Care to Homeless Persons: A Guide to the Diagnosis and Management of Medical and Mental Health Conditions. New York: Springer-Verlag, 1992.
5. Mandell GL, Douglass RG, Bennett JE. Principles and Practice of Infectious Disease, 4th ed. New York: John Wiley & Sons, 1996.
6. Sanford JP, Gilbert DN, Moellering RC, Sande MA. The Sanford Guide to Antimicrobial Therapy 1997. Vienna, VA: Therapy Antimicrobial, 1997.
7. Bisno AL, Stevens DL. Streptococcal infections of skin and soft tissues. N Engl J Med 1996;334(4):240–245.
8. Mayeaux EJ, Harper MB, Barksdale W, Pope JB. Noncervical human papillomavirus genital infections. Am Fam Physician 1995;52(4):1137–1146.
9. Ferenczy A. Epidemiology and clinical pathophysiology of condylomata acuminata. Am J Obstet Gynecol 1995;172(4):1331–1339.
10. Famciclovir for herpes zoster. Med Lett 1994;36(934): 97–98.
11. Valacyclovir. Med Lett 1996;38(965):3–4.
12. Zaias N, Glick B, Rebell G. Diagnosing and treating onychomycosis. J Fam Pract 1996;42:513–518.
13. Olsen EA, Abernethy ML, Kulp-Shorten C, et al. A double-blind, vehicle controlled study evaluating masoprocol cream in the treatment of actinic keratoses on the head and neck. J Am Acad Dermatol 1991(5, pt 1):738–743.

39. Skin Wounds: Minor Lacerations, Contusions, and Abrasions

WAYNE A. HALE

Key Clinical Questions

1. Do the mechanism of injury or the examination findings suggest damage to vital structures or a likelihood of poor cosmetic outcome?
2. Is the wound at high risk for infection?
3. Do incongruities between the history of injury and examination findings suggest substance abuse by the patient or physical abuse by another?

Injuries to the skin are commonly treated in family practice settings. Although there are many different forms of skin wounds, this discussion is limited to contusions, abrasions, and lacerations.

APPROACH TO DIAGNOSIS

Wounds can present dramatically, but in all situations, you must initially focus on the basics of emergency care. Ensure a clear airway, control of bleeding, and adequate circulation before proceeding with a more specific evaluation of the wound.

Take a good history of how the injury happened to facilitate evaluation and treatment. An accurate examination is essential. Summarize this information for the medical record in a note that describes the age, size, shape, and extent of the wound and the amount of contamination. Descriptions of lacerations, such as linear, irregular, beveled, or flap, help clarify your approach to their repair. Drawings or photographs may be very useful for later comparison.

The key to evaluating skin wounds is to think carefully about the type of injury that occurred and the nearby structures that might be affected. Table 39.1 lists "red flags" suggesting that you are dealing with more than a minor wound. During your examination, palpate for a foreign body or fracture. Plain radiographs or xeroradiographs should be used if deeper foreign bodies are sus-

pected. Consider the possibility of injury to vital structures near the wound, such as nerves, tendons, or ducts (e.g., the parotid duct). Deep penetration by an injuring object or a high-pressure injection may make open exploration necessary. Wounds involving electrical, thermal, or chemical injury need special evaluation and care, as do bites and puncture wounds. In proximal limb injuries, consider and rule out injury to peripheral motor and sensory nerves.

Once your evaluation is complete, if the problem is indeed a minor skin wound, you can proceed to treatment, following the general principles outlined in this chapter. If the wound is complicated or if an optimum outcome is doubtful, obtain consultation after your preliminary evaluation and treatment.

Explore the possibility of substance abuse or physical harm by another if injuries have been recurrent or there are physical findings inconsistent with the history provided.

Any time you treat patients whose skin has been broken, remember to inquire about tetanus immunization status and to give any indicated immunization. Give a tetanus booster if the patient has not had one within 5 years for tetanus-prone wounds (contamination, devitalized tissue, puncture, muscle involvement, or more than 24 hours old), or 10 years for clean wounds. If the patient has not definitely had a primary tetanus immunization series, also administer tetanus immune globulin for tetanus-prone wounds. Advise those patients lacking previous immunization (as is true for some elderly) to have a tetanus booster in 1 month and again in 6 to 12 months (1).

CONTUSIONS

Clinical Evaluation

A contusion (also known as a bruise or ecchymosis) results from trauma that injures underlying soft-tissue structures while leaving the epidermis intact. Cellular, vascular, and lymphatic damage causes blood and other fluids to leak

613

Table 39.1.
Inspection Red Flags

Signs of possible bone fracture—deformity, severe swelling, increased pain on stressing bone
Penetration of bone, joint, ligament, or tendon
Altered nerve or muscle function
Difficulty controlling bleeding
Inability to visualize the extent of the wound

into the tissue, producing swelling and discoloration. If enough extravasated blood collects to produce a palpable "knot," a hematoma is said to have formed.

Large bruises can take weeks to resolve, particularly if there is accompanying hematoma formation. The area of ecchymosis will gradually change from a blue or purple color to yellow-brown as the blood is converted to hematin and reabsorbed. These ecchymoses may travel to more dependent areas. Thus, hematomas around the knee or calf will often lead to ecchymoses of the ankle or foot. Hematomas usually clot and become quite firm, then may become red, warm, and tender as the clot liquefies. At this stage they may appear to be infected, although this is seldom the case. Instruct patients about the sequential changes they can expect to reduce their concerns during the healing process.

Management

Direct initial treatment of contusions and hematomas at minimizing hemorrhage and edema by elevating the affected part and applying pressure and ice. Recommend over-the-counter acetaminophen 325 to 500 mg, 1 to 2 tablets every 4 hours when you anticipate that tissue cooling alone will not provide adequate anesthesia. For more painful injuries, prescribe codeine 30 to 60 mg (frequently prescribed in tablets also containing acetaminophen 300 mg) every 4 hours as needed. The total daily dose of acetaminophen should not exceed 4 g daily. Nonsteroidal anti-inflammatory drugs are usually avoided because of their inhibition of platelet function. In general, don't aspirate or otherwise drain hematomas because of the risk of infection and their tendency to recur. Consider an underlying hemostatic disorder if the amount of bleeding seems out of proportion to the injury, but remember that tissue fragility normally increases as people age.

Recommend the application of cold for 5 to 30 minutes several times daily until swelling has stopped increasing, usually for at least 48 hours after the injury. Depending on the area involved, give instructions on using an ice water bath, massaging with water frozen in a Styrofoam cup, or using an ice pack as appropriate. Refreezable chemical gel ice packs are commercially available, but bags of crushed ice or frozen vegetables may be more readily at hand.

After swelling stabilizes, have the patient apply heat to increase local blood flow and hasten resolution. Advise the patient that hematomas will generally be resorbed over several weeks if there is no reinjury, but those under perichondrium or periosteum may form scar tissue. Rarely, those in muscle will develop myositis ossificans with calcification of the involved tissue (2).

ABRASIONS

Clinical Evaluation

Abrasions are caused by scraping trauma that removes epidermis. Bicycle or motorcycle accidents, for example, which cause the rider to slide along the pavement, are frequent causes of severe abrasions. These injuries tend to be quite painful because many nerve endings are exposed. As in a second-degree burn, the loss of epidermis causes the skin to lose water through weeping and evaporation. These injuries are most often over joint surfaces, and the scab that forms tends to crack open when the joint moves.

Management

Adequate cleaning of abrasions usually requires good anesthesia. Apply topical anesthetic agents for superficial abrasions, but deep or dirty wounds generally require anesthetic injection. Next irrigate with sterile saline or a mild antiseptic solution. Using forceps, remove ground-in dirt as completely as possible to prevent tattoo formation.

Once the abrasion is clean, your goal is to keep the wound bed moist and free of infection until it is re-epithelialized. One method is to apply white petrolatum or Polysporin ointment under gauze or a nonstick absorbent dressing such as Telfa (3). Alternatively, synthetic semiocclusive transparent wound coverings (Tegaderm, Op-Site, Bioclusive) are available that hasten re-epithelialization by retaining moisture while allowing oxygen to reach the wound (4). If the abraded area is extensive, see the patient every day or two in follow-up until infection seems unlikely. Antibiotic prophylaxis is generally not indicated, but if the exudate becomes frankly purulent or there is spreading erythema, prescribe cephalexin, 500 mg twice a day; erythromycin, 333 mg three times a day; or dicloxacillin, 250 mg four times daily after obtaining cultures.

LACERATIONS

A laceration is a slice or tear in the skin or mucosa. Approximating the wound edges with sutures or adhesive strips minimizes scar formation and healing time. Superficial wounds may simply require cleansing and dressing. You can close lacerations whose edges are minimally separated with sterile adhesive strips or tissue adhesive (where available) (5). First clean the skin with ether or apply tincture of benzoin to improve adhesion of the sterile tape strips, but don't allow the chemical to contact the open wound. Use suture closure for larger lacerations and those located in areas of stretch.

Management

Anesthesia, Inspection, and Cleaning

Evaluation and treatment of larger lacerations requires adequate anesthesia. For patients such as young children or demented adults, you may need to premedicate 30 minutes before the procedure with a narcotic (morphine sulfate, 15 to 30 mg po, or 5 to 10 mg subcutaneously for adults, 0.2 mg/kg for children) and/or sedative (chloral hydrate, 50 mg/kg, maximum 1 g, po). Reassurance, explanation, and firm restraint usually make use of a local anesthetic sufficient. For small (<7 cm) wounds, TAC (0.5% tetracaine, 1:2000 adrenaline, 11.8% cocaine) or the less expensive LAT (4% lidocaine, 1:2000 adrenaline, 0.5% tetracaine) solution applied topically for 10 to 30 minutes will provide adequate anesthesia (6, 7). To lessen the pain of injection, use a 25- to 30-gauge needle inserted through the wound into the dermis (8). Lidocaine in 1 or 2% concentration is the most commonly used anesthetic solution. Before injection, it must be ascertained that the patient is not allergic to the medication. Although it is permissible to give up to 4.5 mg of lidocaine per kilogram of body weight (the 1% solution contains 10 mg/mL), use the minimum amount necessary to avoid toxicity. Preparations that combine lidocaine with epinephrine can be used to decrease bleeding and prolong anesthesia. Epinephrine must not be used in areas where its vasoconstrictive effects might cause gangrene by compromising circulation, such as the fingers, toes, earlobes, or penis. Adequate anesthesia is generally produced in 10 minutes.

In some areas, a nerve block may be more effective than local injection. Circumferential blocks work well for injuries of the ear and nose. Block of the mental nerve produces good anesthesia to the lower lip and chin. Most frequently used is a digital block of a finger or toe. This can be performed by anesthetizing the dorsal and ventral nerve branches on each side of the affected digit. Alternatively, anesthetic solution can be placed on each side of the digit's metacarpal head to block the digital nerves before they branch. To perform a digital block, you can insert the needle through either the dorsal or palmar surface, but remember that the nerve is closer to the palm and adjacent to the bone. Your patient may report a shooting sensation down the digit when your needle touches the nerve. Aspirate through the needle to be sure you are not in a blood vessel, inject 2 or 3 mL of anesthetic, then reposition the needle and inject the nerve on the opposite side of the digit.

Under adequate anesthesia, the wound can be inspected and cleaned. An antiseptic solution, such as povidone-iodine (Betadine) or chlorhexidine (Hibiclens) can be used for initial cleaning of the surrounding skin, but not in the wound. If significant contamination with bacteria or chemicals is suspected, flush the wound profusely with sterile saline. A 19-gauge needle can be used with a 30- to 50-mL syringe or an intravenous bag with a compression device to provide a high-pressure stream. Gross dirt and other materials may require removal by forceps or by scrubbing with a brush or sponge. Debride severely contaminated or nonviable tissue. This debridement must be done very judiciously on areas (such as the face) where significant tissue loss can result in deformity. Clipping hair from around the laceration can make suturing easier. Try to avoid shaving eyebrows, because regrowth may be abnormal.

The timing of wound closure is important. The risk of infection is lowest if a laceration is repaired within 6 hours, although very clean wounds generally do well if closed within 24 hours. Beyond these limits, the wound should simply be cleaned, inspected, and then dressed, because suturing would promote infection by introducing foreign material and preventing drainage. If there is no sign of infection by the third to fifth day and approximation of wound edges is desirable, then the wound may be sutured.

Preparing for Wound Repair

Having inspected and cleansed the wound and decided that it is appropriate for you to close the wound surgically, make certain that all potentially necessary instruments and supplies are at hand. Table 39.2 lists basic supplies for laceration repair. Table 39.3 suggests suture sizes for various body locations.

A number of suture materials are available, and each has its advantages:

- Monofilament nylon (Ethilon, Dermalon) or polypropylene (Prolene) sutures are more difficult to handle than silk and other braided suture materials, but they produce less skin reactivity and fewer infections.
- Braided sutures (Vicryl, Mersilene) cause less discomfort on mucosal surfaces (such as the lip or tongue) than the stiffer monofilaments.
- Absorbable materials (chromic gut, Vicryl, Dexon) are used for subsurface or mucosal repair.

Attached to the suture is a curved needle, whose size and shape is generally shown on the package. A reverse cutting needle is appropriate in most circumstances. Grip it with a needle holder not less than one third of the way from the blunt end. The proper grasp (Fig. 39.1), using the largest needle feasible, will minimize needle bending.

Before beginning the procedure, place the patient in a position that will be comfortable and allow optimal lighting and access to the wound. Seat yourself so that the wound and instrument tray can be reached easily. Have an assistant present who can obtain additional supplies and give surgical assistance if needed.

After the wound is anesthetized and cleaned, and you have positioned the patient and your instruments, you are ready to put on sterile gloves and drape the wound. When the wound involves the head or neck, take care that the drapes do not obstruct your patient's vision or breathing.

Next, examine the wound carefully and plan your repair. Trim wound edges so that they are parallel, if this can be done without removing essential tissue. When making an incision to straighten a wound margin, first mark the incision with the scalpel, then use scissors to cut perpendicular to the skin surface. Make excisions in hair-bearing skin parallel to the hair shafts, to avoid damage to the follicles. Because crushed tissue will not heal well, judiciously cut out crushed areas, using an elliptical incision whose length is three times its width. In areas like the nose, where there is no excess skin, it may be better to simply approximate the wound, planning later scar revision if necessary. After evaluating the wound, if you do not believe you can perform an optimum repair, consult a surgeon who has the necessary skills.

Table 39.2.
Basic Supplies for Laceration Repair

Equipment	Uses
Gauze sponges	Absorbing blood and dressing wounds
Sterile gloves	Protecting physician and patient from transfer of infectious organisms
Sterile drapes	Sterile field that sutures and instruments may contact
Adequate lighting	Complete visualization of wound
Toothed pickup forceps	Gentle grasp of tissues and foreign materials
Small hemostats (2)	Closing bleeding vessels
Smooth pickup forceps	Less traumatic grasp of tissues
Needle holder	Grasping the suture needle
Small curved scissors	Cutting and undermining tissue
Scalpel with blade (No. 15)	Cutting and undermining tissue
Suture material and needle	Drawing wound edges together
Hooks (optional)	Pulling wound edges without damaging the surface

Table 39.3.
Guidelines for Suture Selection and Timing of Suture Removal

Location	Suture Size for Skin Closure	Days to Removal
Face	5-0 or 6-0	3–5
Scalp	3-0 or 4-0	5–7
Trunk and extremities	4-0 or 5-0	7–10
Over joint surfaces	3-0 or 4-0	10–14

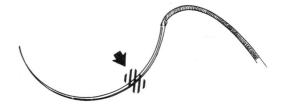

Figure 39.1. *Correct position to grasp a suture needle.* This position provides enough length to rotate the needle through soft tissues, but is far enough forward to minimize bending.

Suturing Techniques

Appropriate closure technique varies with the depth of the laceration and the body area involved. Single-layer closure is used for superficial wounds and in areas with little subcutaneous tissue, such as the digits and back of the hands. It is also useful in the scalp, where hemostasis can be a problem. Use layered repair for deeper wounds, particularly for lacerations in cosmetically sensitive areas such as the face.

Principles of proper suture placement are shown in Figure 39.2. Insert your needle vertically or angulated away from the wound, with the goal of making the loop wider at the bottom than near the skin surface. This placement is aided by pulling the deeper layers toward the wound. Then, rotate your wrist to bring the needle up through the opposite wound edge, again going wider in the deeper tissue. This is accomplished by scraping the needle point back before puncturing up through the dermis. Ideally, the suture's depth will be greater than its width. This technique produces good results because it approximates the wound edge with some eversion, an optimal situation for healing. Minor differ-

ences in elevation of wound edges can often be adjusted by pulling the suture knot from one side to the other.

Usually you will place sutures as far apart as they are wide. In areas of skin tension, however, place sutures closer together and closer to the wound edge. Figure 39.3 demonstrates this principle in the closure of an ellipse. Some surgeons like to close a wound by halving it, but it is probably better to start at one end and work toward the other, thereby reducing the tension on each suture.

A useful method in lacerations with widely separated edges is the vertical mattress suture (Fig. 39.4). Mattress sutures provide greater strength and better approximation of tissue. Because they tend to heal leaving visible suture marks, alternate them with simple sutures. The mattress sutures can then be removed early, leaving the simple sutures for support. Sterile adhesive strips are preferred by some physicians for surface closure, but they do not evert the wound edges and may not hold well in areas of skin movement.

The best technique for reducing tension on

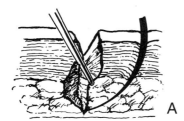
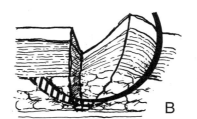
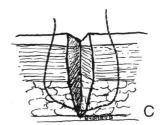

Figure 39.2. *Proper skin suture technique.* **A.** Perpendicular insertion of the needle is aided by traction at the fat-dermal layer. **B.** The needle point is dragged back along the undersurface of the dermis. **C.** Rotation of the needle while puncturing upward results in a suture wider at its base than at the surface.

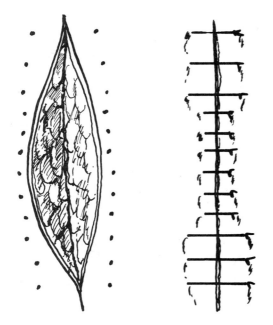

Figure 39.3. *Closure of an ellipse.* Suturing is begun at one end of the wound. As the middle is approached, sutures are placed closer to each other and closer to the wound edge, to minimize tension on each stitch.

surface sutures is layered closure (Fig. 39.5). Layers that hold sutures are the fat-fascial, the fat-dermal, and the dermal-epithelial interfaces. Placement of deep sutures is aided by undermining the tissue below the layer being closed. In part *A* of Figure 39.5, undermining has been done in the fatty layer. In this type of tissue it is best to use the curved scissors in a spreading motion to minimize vascular and nerve disruption. Invert subepithelial sutures so that the knots are buried. Most often, it is necessary only to suture the fat-dermal layer before final closure with

simple sutures or a running subcuticular stitch. Multiple layer closures have been associated with increased infection, so this risk must be balanced against the benefits of decreased tension on wound edges.

Special techniques are needed in certain situations. V-shaped lacerations are best repaired using the technique shown in Figure 39.6, which minimizes risk of compromise to the blood supply at the tip of the flap.

When closing any wound, it is important to separate sutures by equal distances on both sides. Despite efforts to do this, there will sometimes be more skin on one side than the other as the end of the wound is approached. The longer side tends to raise, making it difficult to approximate the edges without bunching on that side. Approach this "dog's ear" as follows (Fig. 39.7). Make the wound edges equal again by extending the wound with an incision at a 45-degree angle toward the side with excess length. After undermining, excise the overlapping dog's ear and suture the incision. If some excess still remains on that side, repeat the process.

Area-Specific Considerations

The character of skin and subcutaneous tissue varies greatly over the body. As a result, suturing techniques and materials vary from site to site, as shown in Table 39.2. Lacerations of the scalp are often caused by blows that split the skin to, and sometimes through, the galea. If the galea is lacerated, close it as a layer, after palpating to detect signs of skull fracture. The remaining closure is best performed as a single layer, using a large needle and 3–0 or 4–0 suture material. This generally provides adequate hemostasis if occasional large bleeders are clipped with a hemostat and coagulated or tied off (exercising care not to injure nerves or other vital structures). After the repair, rinse as much blood as possible out of the

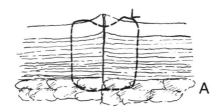 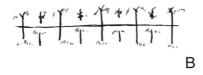

Figure 39.4. *Repair using vertical mattress sutures.* **A.** Placement of vertical mattress suture. **B.** Wound closure with simple sutures alternating with vertical mattress sutures.

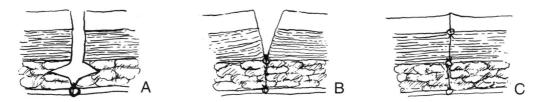

Figure 39.5. *Layered closure.* **A.** The fat-dermal junction is undermined after closure of the fat-fascial junction. **B.** The fat-dermal junction is sutured. **C.** The dermal-epithelial junction is closed with an inverted suture to bury the knot.

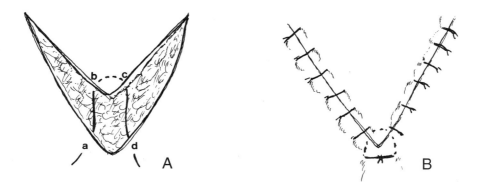

Figure 39.6. *Repair of a flap laceration.* **A.** The needle is inserted on one side of the wound apex (*a*), passed through the subcuticular tissue of the flap (*b–c*), and then brought out on the opposite side of the wound apex (*d*). **B.** Simple sutures are then placed far enough away from the apex to prevent compromise of circulation to the tip.

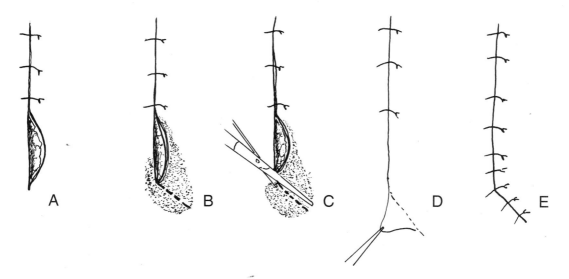

Figure 39.7. *Repair of the "dog ear."* **A.** Sometimes, as a wound is being sutured, one side ends up with more remaining tissue than the other, which creates an unsightly bulge called a "dog ear." **B.** To begin repair of a dog ear, a marking incision is made 45 degrees from the end of the wound toward the longer side. **C.** Scissors are used to cut along the marking, and then used to undermine the shaded area. **D.** The longer skin edge is pulled across the incision line, and the resulting triangle of skin is excised along the line of overlap. **E.** The even skin edges can now be easily sutured.

patient's hair, because it can be difficult to remove later.

Facial lacerations need particular care to minimize scarring. Trim the wound edges so they are smooth and follow natural skin lines, if this can be done by removing only a small amount of tissue. Use the layered skin closure shown in Figure 39.5, which will minimize tension on the surface. For surface suturing, use thin (6–0 or 7–0) monofilament sutures and remove them early, replacing them with adhesive strips (Steri-Strips).

Mark landmarks such as the vermilion border of the lips before they are obscured by injection of anesthetic. The first suture can then be placed to assure correct alignment. Lacerations of the tongue do not need to be repaired, unless they are very large or bleed persistently despite application of ice and pressure. Similarly, lacerations of the oral mucosa usually heal well without suturing. Lacerations that penetrate from the skin into the oral cavity should have repair of the skin and muscle only, unless the mucosal defect is large. Leaving the mucosal surface open to heal secondarily reduces the chance of infection.

Aftercare

Petrolatum or antibiotic ointment application promotes wound healing by keeping the epithelium moist. A semiocclusive transparent dressing (e.g., Tegaderm or Op-Site) may be applied if little drainage is expected. For draining wounds, apply a nonadherent material such as Telfa under a layer of cotton gauze.

Recommend keeping any sutured wound dry for 24 hours, after which showering is permitted. Support lacerations in areas of skin stretch by splinting the affected part until adequately healed.

Infection is the biggest threat to wound healing. As noted earlier, this is best prevented by aggressive wound cleaning and tetanus prophylaxis. Antibiotic coverage is advisable when a bone, tendon, or joint space has been penetrated and in some contaminated wounds. Bites and puncture wounds are particularly susceptible to infection if closed. Human bites require particularly careful cleaning and observation because of the large number of bacteria in saliva, and generally you should treat them as infected from the onset.

Whether antibiotics are used or not, inform the patient about signs of infection: progressive swelling, redness, heat or pain, and increased drainage. Closely follow-up wounds likely to become infected. Because infection typically takes 1 to 3 days to become apparent, recheck higher-risk lacerations at 48 to 72 hours. Written instructions regarding wound care can be quite helpful, because patients are often distressed and will remember little of the verbal advice they received.

Timing of suture removal varies with the location and type of wound. Table 39.3 lists suture removal times. The goal is to leave sutures in long enough to prevent wound dehiscence, but not so long as to cause suture marks. If infection occurs, you may need to remove some sutures early to allow drainage. To remove a suture, elevate the knot with forceps, cut one side of the loop near the skin, and then put gentle traction on the knot. Do not cut the knot off both sides of a loop, because the free ends may retract into the skin and be difficult to retrieve. To reinforce the wound during the next few days, apply sterile adhesive strips, preparing the wound edges with tincture of benzoin to promote adhesion. These strips come off when soaked; so advise the patient to keep them dry for a few days and then wash them off. Warn the patient about infection symptoms (Table 39.4) and that the natural healing process may cause the wound to look red and swollen over the first few months, but that it will have improved by 6 months.

Table 39.4.
Injury Care Instructions[a]

1. Keep the injured area raised above the heart as much as possible to decrease swelling.
2. Apply ice to sprains and deep bruises frequently for 2–3 days. For small areas, freeze water in a Styrofoam cup, then peel back the top edge. For larger areas, use an ice pack or a bag of frozen vegetables. A layer of cloth will prevent frostbite to the skin.
3. Inspect wounds daily for signs of infection (fever, swelling, or spreading redness and tenderness), and call for an earlier appointment if they develop or if the wound starts to pull apart.
4. Keep any splints or pressure dressings on until instructed to remove them.
5. Return to our office to have your wound(s) checked in ____ days.
   Return to our office for suture removal in _____ days.

[a] To be given to the patient.

CASE STUDY

Your 11-year-old patient, Billy G., is brought to your office by his mother shortly after his bicycle hit a tree root, which threw him over the handlebars. His helmet protected his head, and there are no indications of fractures or internal injuries. He does have a 4 × 5-cm V-shaped full-thickness laceration of the dorsum of his right hand, a 6 × 8-cm swelling of his left mid rectus femoris muscle, and abrasions of his left palm and both knees. All of the wounds contain some dirt and debris. Billy finished his primary tetanus immunization series with the last booster at age 5.

QUESTIONS

1. How would you anesthetize, clean, and dress his abrasions?
2. How should the hematoma be treated, and what warnings should be given about possible complications?
3. How would you anesthetize, clean, and repair the laceration?
4. Is a tetanus booster and/or tetanus immune globulin injection indicated?

DISCUSSION

Apply an ice pack and compression to the hematoma in the patient's anterior thigh. Use a topical solution of LAT or TAC to anesthetize the abrasions. Inject local anesthetic into areas remaining sensitive and also beneath the edges of the laceration. Flush all wounds profusely with normal saline solution, followed by mechanical debridement of any remaining foreign material. Then cover the abrasions with sterile petrolatum and nonstick gauze or a semipermeable synthetic occlusive dressing. You can close the laceration with single-layer sutures after determining that no underlying structures require repair. Take care at the apex of the V to avoid compromising blood supply to the tip.

Because Billy has had his primary immunization series, tetanus immune globulin is not indicated, but his dirty wounds make a tetanus booster necessary. Give instructions about wound dressings and signs of infection, and schedule a recheck in the office in 48 to 72 hours. Recommend that ice and pressure be repeatedly applied to the hematoma until that visit. If the wound appears to be under tension when the wrist is palmar flexed, a dorsiflexion splint may be beneficial. Warn the patient and his mother that the wounds will appear red for weeks and that some scar and possibly keloid tissue will develop. Pain in the area of the hematoma should gradually resolve if there is no further trauma, but if it persists reexamine him for signs of myositis ossificans.

REFERENCES

1. Recommendations of the Immunization Practices Advisory Committee (ACIP) on diphtheria, tetanus, and pertussis: recommendations for vaccine use and other preventive measures. MMWR 1991;40(suppl RR-10):1–28.
2. Smack DP, Harrington AC, Dunn C, et al. Infection and allergy incidence in ambulatory surgery patients using white petrolatum vs. bacitracin ointment. JAMA 1996;276:972–977.
3. Madden MR, Nolan E, Finkelstein JL, et al. Comparison of an occlusive and a semi-occlusive dressing and the effect of the wound exudate upon keratinocyte proliferation. JTrauma 1989;29:924–931.
4. Quinn JV, Drzewiecki A, Li MM, et al. A randomized, controlled trial comparing a tissue adhesive with suturing in the repair of pediatric facial lacerations. Ann Emerg Med 1993;22:1130–1135.
5. Hegenbarth MA, Altieri MF, Hawk WH, et al. Comparison of topical tetracaine, adrenaline, and cocaine anesthesia with lidocaine infiltration for repair of lacerations in children. Ann Emerg Med 1990;19:63–67.
6. Ernst AA, Marvex-Valls E, Nick TG, Weiss SJ. LAT (lidocaine-adrenaline-tetracaine) versus TAC (tetracaine-adrenaline-cocaine) for topical anesthesia in face and scalp lacerations. Am J Emerg Med 1995;13: 151–154.
7. Kelly AM, Cohen M, Richards D. Minimizing the pain of local infiltration anesthesia for wounds by injection into the wound edges. J Emerg Med 1994;12:593–595.
8. Common sports-related injuries and illnesses—generic conditions. In: McKeag DB, Hough DO, eds. Primary Care Sports Medicine. Dubuque, IA: Brown and Bookmark, 1993:227.

40. Sore Throat

MARK H. EBELL

Key Clinical Questions

1. Does this patient have an infectious or noninfectious cause of sore throat?
2. If infectious, is it streptococcal pharyngitis or infectious mononucleosis?

Sore throat is one of the most common symptoms evaluated in primary care and has been well studied as a model for clinical decision-making. Approximately 4.6% of patients seeing a family physician report "sore throat" as the primary reason for the visit, making it the second-most common reason for an office visit (1). Patients often present to the physician with the preconceived notion that they have a "strep throat" and expect antibiotic therapy. However, streptococcal pharyngitis is responsible for only a minority of cases of sore throat, and you should thoroughly consider all possible infectious and noninfectious causes of the symptom.

A variety of important rationales exist for the identification and treatment of streptococcal pharyngitis. For example, antibiotic therapy of streptococcal pharyngitis has been shown to (a) reduce the duration of symptoms; (b) reduce the incidence of complications such as abscess formation; (c) reduce the risk of spread to others; and, most importantly, to (d) reduce the incidence of rheumatic fever in U.S. children over the past 40 years by 90% if used appropriately. On the other hand, complications due to streptococcal pharyngitis are rare, with an incidence of any complication in untreated patients of approximately 4%, and overtreatment may increase the risk that resistant strains of the bacteria will develop. This chapter presents an approach to therapy that builds on our knowledge of the differential diagnosis for different ages, a rational approach to the history and physical examination, and judicious use of the laboratory.

PATHOPHYSIOLOGY

Infectious Causes

Sore throat can be caused by bacterial, viral, or fungal infection of the posterior pharynx and tonsillar tissue. Infection by group A β-hemolytic streptococcal (GABHS) bacteria is the most important cause of bacterial infection because of the rare but serious possible complications such as peritonsillar abscess, rheumatic fever, and acute glomerulonephritis. The incidence of rheumatic fever in particular has declined substantially over the past 40 years (since the widespread introduction of penicillin) from approximately 20 cases per million to 1.5 cases per million population (6). Other serotypes (notably group B and group C) are relatively common in the posterior pharynx but are not thought to cause sore throat.

The role of other bacterial pathogens such as *Chlamydia pneumoniae, Branhamella* species, *Haemophilus* species, and *Mycoplasma pneumoniae* remains controversial. These diagnoses should be considered in patients with lingering infections who do not have evidence of GABHS pharyngitis. *Mycoplasma pneumoniae* in particular is more common in patients who are older, less ill, and have less evidence of pharyngeal inflammation (7). Although uncommon in most settings, gonococcal pharyngitis should be considered in patients who are otherwise at higher risk for sexually transmitted disease.

Most episodes of pharyngitis are caused by viruses, including adenoviruses, influenza viruses, parainfluenza virus, and respiratory syncytial virus (8). However, it is not usually necessary or important to determine the specific virus responsible for an episode of viral pharyngitis. An exception is pharyngitis caused by Epstein-Barr virus (EBV) infection, also known as infectious mononucleosis, because of the protracted course and rare but potentially serious complications of this illness (such as splenic rupture and respiratory compromise due to severe tonsillar hypertrophy and cervical adenopathy) (9).

Another infectious cause of sore throat seen occasionally in the primary care setting is acute cytomegalovirus infection, and although it resembles infectious mononucleosis in some respects, it is associated with a greater degree of hepatic involvement in most patients. Candidiasis is a rare infectious cause of sore throat. It should be considered in immunosuppressed patients, especially those with Acquired Immune Deficiency Syndrome (AIDS), and in patients using nasal or inhaled steroid preparations.

Noninfectious Causes

A variety of noninfectious conditions can cause the symptom of "sore throat." Gastroesophageal reflux disease (GERD) causes pain by direct irritation of the pharyngeal tissue by stomach acid. Allergic rhinitis or sinusitis, with chronic posterior drainage from the nasopharynx, can cause pharyngeal irritation through a combination of chemical irritation and repeated drying. Persistent coughing (due to any of a variety of infectious and noninfectious stimuli) can cause sore throat without any direct infection of the pharynx. Acute thyroiditis causes anterior neck pain that may be mistaken for pharyngitis but is typically associated with more local tenderness to palpation. Other causes of throat pain include trauma (either external or internal, such as from a fish bone) and dental referred pain.

DIFFERENTIAL DIAGNOSIS

The differential diagnosis of sore throat in the primary care setting is summarized in Table 40.1.

No reliable estimates are available for the likelihood of noninfectious causes of sore throat. Depending on the age of the patient and the setting in which they present, the prevalence of GABHS pharyngitis varies from 5 to 36% (5, 10–15); estimates of the likelihood of streptococcal pharyngitis by age are shown in Table 40.2. GABHS pharyngitis in adults is more common in emergency departments, occurring in approximately 22% of patients with sore throat compared with 9% in the primary care setting (5, 13).

The likelihood of infectious mononucleosis is most strongly influenced by the age of the patient. The incidence peaks between the ages of 10 and 29 years and is rare in patients over age 40 or under age 10. Although the infection is thought to occur relatively often in younger children, it generally results in a mild or subclinical infection, so blood tests for infectious mononucleosis are only rarely ordered. Few data are available on the precise likelihood of mononucleosis in patients presenting to a family physician with a complaint of sore throat; estimates by age and setting are shown in Table 40.2 (15–19). These estimates were derived by combining incidence data (in cases/100,000 population) with reports of the likelihood of infectious mononucleosis among specific age groups.

Table 40.1.
Differential Diagnosis of Sore Throat[a]

Cause	Probability (%)
Infectious causes	
Viral	50–80
Streptococcal (group A)	5–36
Epstein-Barr virus	1–10
Chlamydia pneumoniae	2–5
Mycoplasma pneumoniae	2–5
Neisseria gonorrhoeae	1–2
Haemophilus influenzae type B	1–2
Candidiasis	<1
Noninfectious causes	
Gastroesophageal reflux disease	NA
Postnasal drainage due to allergic rhinitis and other upper respiratory conditions	NA
Acute thyroiditis	NA
Persistent cough	NA

[a]Data are from Komaroff AL, Pass TM, Aronson MD, et al. The prediction of streptococcal pharyngitis in adults. J Gen Intern Med 1986;1:1–7; Hoffman S. An algorithm for a selective use of throat swabs in the diagnosis of group A streptococcal pharyngo-tonsillitis in general practice. Scand J Prim Health Care 1992;10:295–300; Komaroff A, Aronson MD, Pass TM, Ervin CT, Branch WT. Serologic evidence of chlamydial and mycoplasmal pharyngitis in adults. Science 1983;222:927–928.

Table 40.2.
Likelihood of Group A β-Hemolytic Streptococcal (GABHS) Pharyngitis[a] and Infectious Mononucleosis in the Primary Care Setting by Age

Infection	Age (Years)	%
GABHS pharyngitis	0–4	15
	5–9	34
	10–19	16
	Adult	9
Infectious mononucleosis	0–4	<1
	5–14	1–2
	15–24	5–10
	25–34	1–2
	>34	<1

[a]Data are from Holmberg SD, Faich GA. Streptococcal pharyngitis and acute rheumatic fever in Rhode Island. JAMA 1983;250: 2307–2312; Komaroff AL, Pass TM, Aronson MD, et al. The prediction of streptococcal pharyngitis in adults. J Gen Intern Med 1986;1:1–7; Seppala H, Lahtonen R, Ziegler T, et al. Clinical scoring system in the evaluation of adult pharyngitis. Arch Otolaryngol Head Neck Surg 1993;119:288–291; Schachtel BP, Fillingim JM, Beiter DJ, Lane AC, Schwartz LA. Subjective and objective features of sore throat. Arch Intern Med 1984;144:497–500.

CLINICAL EVALUATION

When evaluating a patient with sore throat, be alert for "red flags" (summarized in Table 40.3). These patients need more rapid assessment and may require urgent referral. Otherwise, the key clinical questions for the patient with infectious sore throat are whether it is caused by GABHS pharyngitis or infectious mononucleosis.

In most cases, the history will help you determine whether the sore throat is due to an infectious or noninfectious cause. Noninfectious causes should be suspected in patients who are afebrile or who have no other signs of upper respiratory infection, have had symptoms longer than 1 to 2 weeks, and have associated symptoms such as heartburn or itchy eyes. Antacid use or a history of acid-peptic disease should alert the physician to the possibility of gastroesophageal reflux disease (GERD). Symptoms are typically worse late at night or early in the morning, and patients will often report a bitter or unpleasant taste in the back of the throat upon awakening.

The remainder of this section focuses on the history, physical examination, and laboratory testing for these diagnoses.

History

GABHS Pharyngitis

The three symptoms most strongly associated with GABHS pharyngitis are positive throat culture in the preceding year (LR+ 2.2), recent exposure to streptococcus (LR+ 2.1), and lack of cough (LR+ 1.5) (5, 14, 20, 21). Other symptoms associated with GABHS pharyngitis include pain with swallowing, a history of fever, and myalgias. Coryza and itchy eyes are less common in patients with streptococcal pharyngitis than in other causes of sore throat. The test characteristics for symptoms associated with streptococcal pharyngitis are shown in Table 40.4. Other symptoms that traditionally have been associated with streptococcal pharyngitis include sudden onset, headache, and gastrointestinal symptoms, but these associations have not been borne out in clinical epidemiologic studies (14, 21). No single symptom will rule in or rule out the diagnosis of streptococcal pharyngitis, but combinations of symptoms and signs have been used successfully in clinical prediction rules (see Table 40.6, Management).

A rare but serious complication of GABHS pharyngitis is peritonsillar abscess. These patients typically have a more toxic appearance, almost invariably have fever and chills, and may speak with a "hot-potato voice." The latter sounds like the patient is balancing a hot object in the back of the mouth.

Infectious Mononucleosis

Sore throat caused by infection with Epstein-Barr virus (infectious mononucleosis) typically follows a 30- to 50-day incubation period and a 3- to 5-day prodrome characterized by fever, malaise, myalgias, and headache. Although symptoms in general may be similar to those of streptococcal pharyngitis (sore throat, fever, chills, malaise, and headache) and the two coexist in 5 to 30% of patients, fatigue is a much more-prominent symptom in infectious mononucleosis and often interferes significantly with the patient's ability to function (9). Approximately 4% of patients have mild abdominal pain in the left upper quadrant; if this pain is severe, splenic rupture should be suspected and a surgical consultation obtained.

Physical Examination

Group A β-Hemolytic Streptococcal (GABHS) Pharyngitis

Signs in the physical examination strongly associated with GABHS pharyngitis include a severely

Table 40.3.
"Red Flags" Suggesting Progressive or Life-Threatening Disease in Patients with Sore Throat

Finding	Condition
Hot-potato voice, toxic appearance, altered mental status	Peritonsillar abscess
Splenic enlargement	Infectious mononucleosis with increased risk for splenic rupture
Increased respiratory rate, extremely enlarged tonsils, and significant cervical adenopathy	Respiratory compromise due to upper airway obstruction, rarely associated with GABHS pharyngitis and infectious mononucleosis

Table 40.4.
Key Elements of the History and Physical Examination for Sore Throat and Their Test Characteristics for the Detection of GABHS Pharyngitis

Symptom or Sign	Sensitivity	Specificity	LR+	LR−
History				
Positive throat culture in preceding year[a]	0.22	0.9	2.2	0.87
Recent exposure to strep[b]	0.25	0.88	2.1	0.85
Lack of cough[a–e]	0.58	0.67	1.8	0.63
Hearing loss[b]	0.14	0.92	1.8	0.93
Myalgias[a]	0.54	0.65	1.5	0.71
Lack of coryza[a–d]	0.52	0.62	1.4	0.77
Pain swallowing[a]	0.79	0.41	1.3	0.51
Fever history[c, d]	0.72	0.43	1.3	0.65
Lack of itchy eyes[a]	0.9	0.28	1.3	0.36
Physical examination				
"Severely red throat"	0.13	0.97	4.3	0.90
Pharyngeal/tonsillar exudate[a–d, f]	0.36	0.84	2.3	0.76
Enlarged/tender posterior cervical nodes[c]	0.17	0.91	1.9	0.91
Enlarged/swollen tonsils[a–c, g]	0.63	0.63	1.7	0.59
Enlarged/tender anterior cervical nodes[a–d, h]	0.76	0.53	1.6	0.45
Pharyngeal erythema[b, c]	0.97	0.17	1.2	0.18
Temperature > 38.2 (100.8°F)[a–c]	0.17	0.94	2.8	0.88
Temperature 37.2–38.2°C (99.0–100.8°F)[b]	0.31	0.74	1.2	0.93
Temperature <37.2° C (99.0°F)[b]	0.52	0.33	0.8	1.45

[a]Komaroff AL, Pass TM, Aronson MD, et al. The prediction of streptococcal pharyngitis in adults. J Gen Intern Med 1986;1:1–7.

[b]Walsh T, Bookheim WW, Tompkins RK. Recognition of streptococcal pharyngitis in adults. Arch Intern Med 1975;135:1493–1497.

[c]Centor RM, Meier FA, Dalton HP. Throat cultures and rapid tests for diagnosis of group A streptococcal pharyngitis. Ann Intern Med 1986; 105:892–899.

[d]Kreher NE, Hickner JM, Barry HC, et al. Do gastrointestinal symptoms accompanying sore throat predict streptococcal pharyngitis? An UP-RNet study. Upper Peninsula Research Network. J Fam Pract 1998;46:159–164.

[e]Reported range for sensitivity 0.37 to 0.82 and for specificity 0.48 to 0.78.

[f]Reported range for sensitivity 0.21 to 0.65 and for specificity 0.69 to 0.95.

[g]Reported range for sensitivity 0.37 to 0.87 and for specificity 0.39 to 0.88.

[h]Reported range for sensitivity 0.61 to 0.94 and for specificity 0.27 to 0.68.

red throat (LR+ 4.3), temperature > 100.8°F (LR+ 2.8), pharyngeal or tonsillar exudate (LR+ 2.3), enlarged posterior (LR+ 1.9) or anterior (LR+ 1.6) cervical nodes (LR+ 1.9), and enlarged tonsils (LR+ 1.7) (5, 14, 20, 21). Absence of any pharyngeal erythema makes GABHS pharyngitis considerably less likely (LR− 0.18), but it is a nonspecific finding. Therefore, the presence of pharyngeal erythema does not help rule in streptococcal infection (LR+ 1.2). Test characteristics for the physical examination in the diagnosis of GABHS pharyngitis are summarized in Table 40.4.

Patients with a more toxic appearance and those who have a muffled or "hot potato" voice should be carefully examined for peritonsillar abscess. This condition is usually unilateral; the tonsil on the affected side is often pushed out to the midline, giving the uvula, tonsil, and sur-

rounding structures an asymmetric appearance. Patients with peritonsillar abscess have fluctuance over the abscess and are extremely sensitive to direct palpation of the tonsillar tissue by a gloved hand.

Infectious Mononucleosis

Cervical adenopathy and fever are present in over 99% of patients with infectious mononucleosis (9, 23). In fact, if a patient does not have cervical adenopathy (either anterior or posterior) and fever (either by history or measured in the office), you can effectively rule out infectious mononucleosis. Because 90% of patients with mononucleosis have posterior cervical adenopathy, patients without this finding also have a very low probability of disease (6) unless they have other history or physical findings pointing strongly toward mononucleosis (e.g., recent exposure to someone with the disease, a protracted course, severe fatigue, or splenomegaly). Other signs found in patients with infectious mononucleosis include splenomegaly (present in 50%) (6), palatal petechiae (50%), jaundice (10%), and rash (3%) (9).

It is important to assess the size of the spleen in patients with suspected or confirmed infectious mononucleosis. Activity should be restricted during the acute phase of the illness to noncontact sports (no cheerleading, basketball, hockey, football, soccer, etc.) and continue to be restricted as long as the spleen is palpable. Although this recommendation is not supported by clinical trials, it seems prudent because splenic rupture is a rare but serious complication of infectious mononucleosis (23).

Laboratory Tests

GABHS Pharyngitis

A variety of rapid antigen tests and cultures are available to test for the presence of GABHS bacteria in the pharynx. Rapid antigen tests include enzyme immunoassays, latex agglutination tests, liposomal assays, and immunochromatographic assays. Their test characteristics vary considerably and are summarized in Table 40.5. You should know the type of test used in your office and its test characteristics in real clinical use.

Although the throat culture test is often considered a gold standard, a second throat culture taken simultaneously from a patient with an initial positive throat culture is only positive 90% of the time. Also, a small but significant percentage of sore throat patients with a positive throat culture for GABHS bacteria are actually carriers, in which a pathogen or mechanism other than GABHS bacteria is responsible for the sore throat.

Infectious Mononucleosis

Two types of laboratory tests are useful for confirming the diagnosis of infectious mononucleosis: the complete blood count (CBC) with differential and a variety of serologic tests. Most patients with infectious mononucleosis develop a lymphocytosis, which usually peaks 2 weeks after the onset of symptoms. Approximately 95% have more than 60% lymphocytes; therefore, a

relative lymphocytosis less than 60% at 10 to 14 days after the onset of symptoms largely rules out the diagnosis. The total white blood cell (WBC) count is also elevated in most patients, with a peak value greater than 10,000 cells/mm^3 in 77% of patients (9).

Atypical lymphocytes are also common in patients with infectious mononucleosis. In fact, in one study all patients with more than 40% atypical lymphocytes and clinically suspected infectious mononucleosis had serologic evidence of acute Epstein-Barr virus infection. In the same study, 69% of patients with 20 to 40% atypical lymphocytes had evidence of EBV infection (22). The likelihood ratios for different levels of atypical lymphocytosis are shown in Table 40.5.

Serologic tests are often negative in the first week of infection because they rely on the body's immune response. The traditional test is based on the fact that heterophil antibodies produced in patients with infectious mononucleosis agglutinate sheep erythrocytes; the "Monospot" test that is still widely used is a rapid latex agglutination test based on the same principle. However, up to 20% of patients may not produce this antibody (23). Viral capsid antigen (VCA) IgM antibodies are produced relatively early in infection and do not persist once the acute infection is over. This test is quite sensitive and specific, although like the Monospot test, the sensitivity improves during the second week of the illness. Other laboratory tests that are sometimes abnormal in patients with infectious mononucleosis include aspartate aminotransferase (>40 μmol/L in 76% of patients) and alkaline phosphatase (elevated in 71% of patients) (16). Characteristics of serologic tests are summarized in Table 40.5.

MANAGEMENT

The approach to management of sore throat is summarized in Figure 40.1. Viral pharyngitis is a self-limited condition, and only symptomatic treatment is indicated. Strategies for symptomatic treatment include nonsteroidal anti-inflammatory drugs (NSAIDs) for fever and throat pain, gargling with 2% viscous lidocaine for patients with severe throat pain, and topical sprays purchased over-the-counter. Gargling with salt water is also soothing and may reduce inflammation. Although none of these strategies have been evaluated in controlled clinical trials, they are safe and appear to be effective.

Table 40.5.

Characteristics of Tests Used to Detect Group A β-Hemolytic Streptococcal (GABHS) Pharyngitis and Infectious Mononucleosis

Test	Sensitivity	Specificity	LR +	LR−
GABHS pharyngitis				
Enzyme immunoassay[a–d]	0.60	0.89	5.5	0.45
Latex agglutination[e–g]	0.81	0.91	9.0	0.21
Liposomal method[h, i]	0.79	0.84	4.9	0.25
Immunochromatography[j]	0.97	0.97	32.3	0.03
Office culture[k]	0.89	0.95	17.8	0.11
Laboratory culture[k]	0.90	0.99	90.0	0.10
Infectious mononucleosis				
>40% atypical lymphocytes[l]			39	
36–40% atypical lymphocytes[l]			3.1	
31–35% atypical lymphocytes[l]			1.2	
20–30% atypical lymphocytes[l]			0.44	
>50% lymphocytes and >10% atypical cells[m]	0.39	0.99	39	0.61
Rapid slide agglutination (Monospot)[m]	0.86	0.99	86	0.14
1st week	0.69	0.88	5.7	0.35
2nd week	0.81	0.88	6.7	0.21
VCA-IgM[n]				
1st week	0.80	0.99	80	0.20
2nd week	0.85	0.99	85	0.15
3rd week	0.97	0.99	97	0.03
Anti-EBV ELISA (Biotest Anti-EBV recombinant)[o]	0.99	0.99	99	0.01

[a]Egger P, Siegrist CA, Strautmann G, Belli D, Auckenthaler R. Evaluation of two ELISA tests for the rapid detection of group A streptococci. Eur J Pediatr 1990;149:256–258.

[b]Macknin ML, Indich N, Easley KA, Imrie R. Comparison of two rapid diagnostic tests for group A streptococcus. Pediatr Infect Dis J 1988;7:735–736.

[c]Carey RD, Tilyard MW, Morris RW. Evaluation of a rapid diagnostic test for group A β-hemolytic streptococcus in general practice. N Z Med J 1991;104:401–403.

[d]Wegner DL, Witte DL, Schrantz RD. Insensitivity of rapid antigen detection methods and single blood agar plate culture for diagnosing streptococcal pharyngitis. JAMA 1992;267:695–697.

[e]Gerber MA, Spadaccini LJ, Wright LL, Deutsch L. Latex agglutination tests for rapid identification of group A streptococci directly from throat swabs. J Pediatr 1984;105:702–705.

[f]Taubman B, Barroway RP, McGowan KL. The diagnosis of group A, β-hemolytic streptococcal pharyngitis in the office setting. Am J Dis Child 1989;143:102–104.

[g]Reed BD, Huck W, French T. Diagnosis of group A β-hemolytic streptococcus using clinical scoring criteria, Directigen 1-2-3 group A streptococcal test, and culture. Arch Intern Med 1990;150:1727–1732.

[h]Hoffman S. An algorithm for a selective use of throat swabs in the diagnosis of group A streptococcal pharyngo-tonsillitis in general practice. Scand J Prim Health Care 1992;10:295–300.

[i]Gerber MA, Randolph MF, DeMeo KK. Liposome immunoassay for rapid identification of group A Streptococci directly from throat swabs. J Clin Microbiol 1990;28:1463–1464.

[j]Ehrlich TP, Schwartz RH, Wientzen R, Thorne MM. Comparison of an immunochromatographic method for rapid identification of group A streptococcal antigen with culture method. Arch Fam Med 1993;2:866–869.

[k]Centor RM, Meier FA, Dalton HP. Throat cultures and rapid tests for diagnosis of group A streptococcal pharyngitis. Ann Intern Med 1986;105:892–899.

[l]Ho-Yen DO, Martin KW. The relationship between atypical lymphocytosis and serological tests in infectious mononucleosis. J Infect 1981;3:324–331.

[m]Fleischer GR, Collins M, Fager S. Limitations of available tests for diagnosis of infectious mononucleosis. J Clin Microbiol 1983;17:619–624.

[n]Evans AS, Niederman JC, Cenabre LC, et al. A prospective evaluation of heterophile and Epstein-Barr virus-specific IgM antibody tests in clinical and subclinical infectious mononucleosis: specificity and sensitivity of the tests and persistence of the antibody. J Infect Dis 1975;132:546–554.

[o]Farber I, Wutzler P, Wohlrabe P, et al. Serological diagnosis of infectious mononucleosis using three anti-Epstein Barr virus-recombinant ELISAs. J Virol Met 1993;42:301–308.

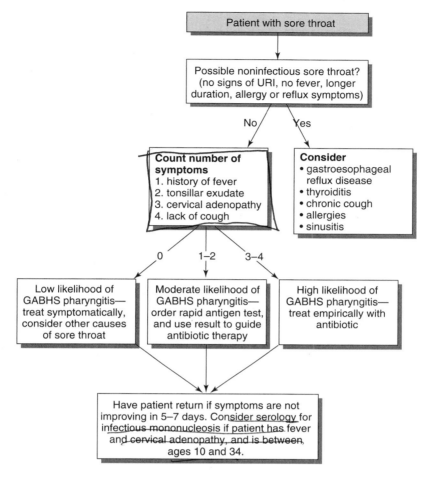

Figure 40.1. *General approach to the patient with sore throat.*

Gastroesophageal reflux disease responds well to antacids, H₂ antagonists, and proton pump inhibitors. Lifestyle changes, in particular weight loss and cessation or reduction of tobacco, alcohol, and/or caffeine use, are particularly important in this condition. Recommendations should be individualized to the patient's specific risk factors and response to changes and should also include elevating of the head of the bed by several inches and avoiding tight-fitting clothing.

Treatment of other bacterial causes of pharyngitis (i.e., *Chlamydia, Mycoplasma pneumoniae*, gonorrhea) may be somewhat less important than treatment of streptococcal pharyngitis because of the absence of risk of rheumatic fever. There is also no evidence that treatment of these infections reduces the duration of symptoms or

decreases the likelihood that the disease will be spread to others.

Group A β-Hemolytic Streptococcal Pharyngitis

Patients at very low risk for GABHS pharyngitis (<5%) based on their demographics, history, and physical examination should be reassured that they do not appear to have a bacterial cause for their sore throat. Patients with none of the cardinal symptoms of GABHS pharyngitis summarized in Table 40.6 fall into this category. Although many patients have come to expect an antibiotic, a simple explanation of why they are very unlikely to have GABHS pharyngitis and why that is the only type of sore throat to benefit

Table 40.6.
Clinical Prediction Rule for the Diagnosis of Group A β-Hemolytic Streptococcal (GABHS) Pharyngitis

1. Count how many of the following characteristics your patient has
   - History of fever
   - Cervical adenopathy
   - Tonsillar exudates
   - Lack of cough
2. Find the row with your patient's age and clinical setting.
3. Find the column with the number of clinical characteristics that your patient has.
4. The percentage for that row and column is the likelihood that your patient has GABHS pharyngitis as a cause of his or her sore throat.

| Age | Setting | All Patients | Probability of GABHS Pharyngitis (%) | | | | |
| | | | Number of Clinical Characteristics | | | | |
			0	1	2	3	4
0–4	Office or ER	15	2	5	12	27	53
5–9	Office	25	5	9	20	41	68
10–19	Office	15	2	5	12	27	53
Adult	Office	8	1.5	3	7	17	36
Adult	ER	20	3	7	16	34	61

Adapted from Centor RM, Meier FA, Dalton HP. Throat cultures and rapid tests for diagnosis of group A streptococcal pharyngitis. Ann Intern Med 1986;105:892–899; Poses RM, Cebul RD, Collins M, Fager SS. The importance of disease prevalence in transporting clinical prediction rules. Ann Intern Med 1986;105:586–591; Wigton RS, Connor JL, Centor RM. Transportability of a decision rule for the diagnosis of streptococcal pharyngitis. Arch Intern Med 1986;146:81–83.

from antibiotics is usually satisfying to the patient. Studies have shown that although many patients expect antibiotics, physicians are not good at guessing which patients want an antibiotic, and the patient's ultimate satisfaction with the encounter depends on the quality of the explanation and the length of time spent with the physician, rather than whether they got an antibiotic prescription (24).

Patients with a very high probability of GABHS pharyngitis (>30%) based on the history and physical examination should be treated empirically without further laboratory testing, since the likelihood of disease even in the presence of a negative rapid antigen test remains over 5% due to the number of false-negative results. Patients with three or four cardinal symptoms (see Table 40.6) fall into this category. Patients with an intermediate probability (5 to 30%) should be evaluated using a rapid antigen test and only receive an antibiotic if that test is positive (6). All patients should have adequate follow-up to assure that they are responding to therapy; at a minimum they should be told to return if their symptoms are worsening or changing.

Clearly, an accurate estimate of the risk of GABHS pharyngitis is especially important when using the above strategy. Each patient should therefore receive a careful, focused history and physical examination. Use of a clinical prediction rule will help you quantify the likelihood of GABHS pharyngitis using a few key signs and symptoms. In an objective comparison of three such rules, the one with the greatest ability to distinguish between patients with streptococcal and nonstreptococcal pharyngitis was that of Centor and colleagues (10). This score assigns one point for each of the following characteristics: tonsillar exudate, anterior cervical adenopathy, lack of a cough, and a history of fever. In the original population of 234 emergency room patients, patients with all four characteristics had a 56% probability of streptococcal pharyngitis; those with three variables had a 32% probability; those with two variables had a 15% probability; those with one variable had a 6.5% probability; and those with none had a 2.5% probability.

When the pretest probability was taken into account, Centor's clinical prediction rule was found to be equally effective in other groups of patients

(10). However, you have to consider the age and setting of the patient in order to use the score most effectively. The likelihood of GABHS pharyngitis based on the score, patient age, and setting has been calculated and is shown in Table 40.6.

The symptomatic benefit of antibiotic therapy in GABHS pharyngitis is actually quite modest. Randomized controlled trials have shown that patients given penicillin experience one fewer day of sore throat than patients given placebo (approximately 4 days of symptoms with antibiotic versus 5 days without) and have a 20% rate of antibiotic-related adverse effects compared with 5% for patients given placebo (25). The levels of evidence for therapeutic interventions in GABHS pharyngitis are summarized in Table 40.7.

The traditional antibiotic recommendation is for penicillin V, 250 mg given 4 times a day for 10 days. The risk of serious allergic reaction is quite small when the drug is give orally, approximately 0.025% compared with a risk of 0.64% when given intramuscularly (26). Compliance is important because the treatment failure rate has been shown to be only 12% in compliant patients and 34% in those who are noncompliant (27). It is therefore not surprising that several studies have attempted to identify alternate antibiotic regimens that involve fewer doses per day, a shorter course of treatment, or both. These alternatives are summarized in Table 40.8. However, many involve second-line and third-line antibiotics that are associated with more adverse effects (especially diarrhea), are very expensive, and may increase the risk of antibiotic resistance

in the community. An effective regimen (as long as patients do not have infectious mononucleosis) is amoxicillin 1, given twice daily for 6 days. This was shown to be just as effective as penicillin V 500 mg, given 3 times a day for 10 days in a randomized controlled trial, and is no more expensive (28).

Patients with exudative pharyngitis and severe pain may benefit from intramuscular corticosteroids. Dexamethasone given in a single 10-mg injection halved the time to relief of symptoms from 33 to 15 hours. This therapy should be reserved for patients without any immuno-compromising conditions and with no evidence of peritonsillar abscess (29). Patients with suspected peritonsillar abscess should be evaluated on the same day by an otorhinolaryngologist for possible incision and drainage.

Parents will often ask when their child can return to school. Studies of throat cultures show that patients become "culture-negative" within 24 hours of initiating antibiotic therapy. It is therefore reasonable to recommend that children spend the day following the office visit at home, but if feeling better and afebrile should be allowed to return to school on the second day following the office or emergency department visit (30).

Infectious Mononucleosis

Identification of patients with infectious mononucleosis is important because of the more protracted course of the disease (typically 1 to 2 months) and the possibility of serious complica-

Table 40.7.
Therapeutic Options Available for the Treatment of Sore Throat

Treatment	Level of Evidence for Effectiveness[a]	Comment
Antibiotics for GABHS pharyngitis	A	Reduces symptoms by about 1 day but reduces risk of rheumatic and suppurative complications significantly
Dexamethasone (IM) for severe pain and tonsillar enlargement	A	Not in immunocompromised patients or those with peritonsillar abscess
2% viscous Xylocaine gargle or salt water gargle or throat lozenges for throat pain	C	
Nonsteroidal anti-inflammatory drugs or acetaminophen for pain and fever relief	C	

[a]Level of evidence for effectiveness: A, strong or moderate research-based evidence (consistent across several studies, including at least two randomized controlled trials); B, limited research-based evidence (less consistent or extensive evidence, but preponderance of evidence supports use of treatment); C, common practice with little or no research-based evidence.

Table 40.8.
Drugs Recommended for the Treatment of Group A β-Hemolytic Streptococcal (GABHS) Pharyngitis

Drug	Dosing Range	Adverse Effects	Comment
First-line Drugs			
Amoxicillin[a]	500 mg PO tid × 10 d or 1 g PO bid × 6 d	Rash in patients with infectious mononucleosis	Check for allergy
Penicillin G[b]	250 mg PO qid × 10 d or 500 mg PO tid × 10 d		Compliance may be problematic Check for allergy
Erythromycin ethyl succinate	400 mg PO tid × 10 d	Nausea	For penicillin- and amoxicillin-allergic patients
Alternate drugs			
Azithromycin	250 mg (adults) or 10 mg/kg (children) PO qd × 3 d		
Cefixime	8 mg/kg (children) PO qd × 5 d		
Dexamethasone[c]	10 mg IM once		For severe sore throat only

[a]Peyramond, D, et al. Six-day amoxicillin vs. 10-day penicillin V for group A β-hemolytic streptococcal acute tonsillitis in adults: a French multicentre, open-label randomized study. Scand J Infect Dis 1996;28:497–501.

[b]McWhinney I. A Textbook of Family Medicine, 2nd ed. Oxford: Oxford University Press, 1997:261.

[c]O'Brien JF, Meade JI, Falk JL. Dexamethasone as adjuvant therapy for severe acute pharyngitis. Ann Emerg Med 1993;22:212–215.

tions in approximately 1% of patients. Such complications include splenic rupture and respiratory compromise due to pharyngeal edema and tonsillar swelling.

You should have a high index of suspicion for infectious mononucleosis in younger patients, particularly those aged 15 to 24 years, and in patients with posterior cervical adenopathy. Patients without anterior or posterior cervical adenopathy and fever are extremely unlikely to have the diagnosis, as are those over age 35, which will help rule it out in many patients. Diagnostic tests are relatively insensitive during the first week of illness when many patients present. A reasonable strategy is to evaluate for noninfectious causes and GABHS pharyngitis at the initial visit as described above and withhold laboratory evaluation for infectious mononucleosis for those patients who do not respond and return during the second week of their illness.

Patients with infectious mononucleosis should be treated symptomatically with rest, oral fluids, and nonsteroidal anti-inflammatory agents or acetaminophen for fever and myalgias. Aspirin should be avoided because Reye's syndrome has been reported in association with infectious mononucleosis (23). No contact sports should be allowed for at least the first 2 to 3 weeks of the ill-

ness and until the spleen is no longer palpable and the patient has no abdominal pain.

Patients with coexisting streptococcal pharyngitis or those at high risk for streptococcal pharyngitis based on their signs and symptoms (see Table 40.6) should be started on an antibiotic. Use an antibiotic other than amoxicillin, though, because it causes a rash in approximately 80% of patients with infectious mononucleosis. The mechanism of this reaction is not well understood. The level of evidence for treatment recommendations in infectious mononucleosis is shown in Table 40.7.

Patient Education

Education of the patient with sore throat has several goals. First, patients should understand that only a minority of "sore throats" are caused by streptococcal pharyngitis or other bacteria and that symptomatic treatment is usually sufficient. They should also be told how to relieve the symptoms of sore throat, using salt water gargles, NSAIDs, over-the-counter throat sprays, and lozenges. Finally, patients should know the symptoms of bacterial or complicated sore throat, such as fever, chills, sweats, swollen glands, and respiratory impairment, that require physician evaluation.

CASE STUDY

A 12-year-old boy and his mother present to your family practice office with a complaint of 2 days of fever, sore throat, and headache. He denies a cough. On examination he has tonsillar exudates and significant cervical lymphadenopathy. His mother wonders whether he might have "mono" because his best friend has this disease, and she demands a blood test for infectious mononucleosis.

QUESTIONS

1. Which tests, if any, should you order for streptococcal pharyngitis and infectious mononucleosis?
2. What is your management plan for this patient?

DISCUSSION

Based on his symptoms and age, you refer to Table 40.6 and find that his pretest probability of GABHS pharyngitis is 53%. You decide to treat empirically with penicillin V because even if one of the confirmatory tests was negative, he would still have an unacceptably high chance of disease. You avoid amoxicillin because of the recent exposure to infectious mononucleosis.

Regarding the blood test for infectious mononucleosis, you should explain to the mother that you will certainly order the blood test if he is still experiencing symptoms next week, but that the test is not very accurate this early in the course of the illness. In addition, a positive test would not change your management of the patient during the next week. You arrange a follow-up visit for the boy to assure that he is improving and to check a Monospot or VCA-IgM if he is still symptomatic.

REFERENCES

1. National Ambulatory Medical Care Survey. Hyattsville, MD: National Center for Health Statistics, 1993.
2. Randolph MF, Gerber MA, DeMeo KK, Wright L. Effect of antibiotic therapy on the clinical course of streptococcal pharyngitis. J Pediatr 1985;106:870–875.
3. Bennike T, Brochner-Mortensen K, Kjaer E, Skadhange K, Trolle E. Penicillin therapy in acute tonsillitis, phlegmonous tonsillitis, and ulcerative tonsillitis. Acta Med Scand 1951;139:253–274.
4. Poskanzer DC, Feldman HA, Beadenkopf WG, Kuroda K, Drislane A, Diamond EL. Epidemiology of civilian streptococcal outbreaks before and after penicillin prophylaxis. Am J Public Health 1956;46: 1513–1524.
5. Centor RM, Meier FA, Dalton HP. Throat cultures and rapid tests for diagnosis of group A streptococcal pharyngitis. Ann Intern Med 1986;105:892–899.
6. McWhinney I. A Textbook of Family Medicine, 2nd ed. Oxford: Oxford University Press, 1997:261.
7. Williams WC, Williamson HA Jr, LeFevre ML. The prevalence of *Mycoplasma pneumoniae* in ambulatory patients with nonstreptococcal sore throat. Fam Med 1991;23:117–121.
8. Del Mar C. Managing sore throat: a literature review. I. Making the diagnosis. Med J Aust 1992;156:572–575.
9. Hoagland RJ. Infectious mononucleosis. Primary Care 1975;2:295–307.
10. Poses RM, Cebul RD, Collins M, Fager SS. The importance of disease prevalence in transporting clinical prediction rules. Ann Intern Med 1986;105:586–591.
11. Ehrlich TP, Schwartz RH, Wientzen R, Thorne MM. Comparison of an immunochromatographic method for rapid identification of group A streptococcal antigen with culture method. Arch Fam Med 1993;2: 866–869.
12. Holmberg SD, Faich GA. Streptococcal pharyngitis and acute rheumatic fever in Rhode Island. JAMA 1983;250:2307–2312.
13. Wigton RS, Connor JL, Centor RM. Transportability of a decision rule for the diagnosis of streptococcal pharyngitis. Arch Intern Med 1986;146:81–83.
14. Komaroff AL, Pass TM, Aronson MD, et al. The prediction of streptococcal pharyngitis in adults. J Gen Intern Med 1986;1:1–7.
15. Hoffman S. An algorithm for a selective use of throat swabs in the diagnosis of group A streptococcal pharyngo-tonsillitis in general practice. Scand J Prim Health Care 1992;10:295–300.
16. Axelrod P, Finestone AJ. Infectious mononucleosis in older adults. Am Fam Physician 1990;42:1599–1606.
17. Fry J. Infectious mononucleosis: some new observations from a 15-year study. J Fam Pract 1980;10: 1087–1089.
18. Everett MT. The cause of tonsillitis. The Practitioner 1979;223:253–259.
19. Hanson CJ, Higbee JW, Lednar WM, Garrison MJ. The epidemiology of acute pharyngitis among soldiers at Ford Lewis, Washington. Mil Med 1986;7: 389–394.
20. Walsh T, Bookheim WW, Tompkins RK. Recognition of streptococcal pharyngitis in adults. Arch Intern Med 1975;135:1493–1497.
21. Hickner J, Barry H, Kreher N. Diagnosis of streptococcal pharyngitis: An UPRNet study. J Fam Pract 1997; in press.
22. Ho-Yen DO, Martin KW. The relationship between atypical lymphocytosis and serological tests in infectious mononucleosis. J Infect 1981;3:324–331.

23. Bailey RE. Diagnosis and treatment of infectious mono-nucleosis. Am Fam Physician 1994;49:881–885.

24. Hamm RM, Hicks RJ, Bemben DA. Antibiotics and respiratory infections: are patients more satisfied when expectations are met? J Fam Pract 1996;43:56–62.

25. DeMeyere M, Mervielde Y, Verschraegen G, Bogaert M. Effect of penicillin on the clinical course of streptococcal pharyngitis in general practice. Eur J Clin Pharmacol 1992;43:581–585.

26. Tompkins RK, Burnes DC, Cable WE. An analysis of the cost-effectiveness of pharyngitis management and acute rheumatic fever preventions. Ann Intern Med 1977;86:481–489.

27. Shulman ST, Gerber MA, Tanz RR, Markowitz M. Streptococcal pharyngitis: the case for penicillin therapy. Pediatr Infect Dis J 1994;13:1–7.

28. Peyramond D, et al. 6-day amoxicillin vs. 10-day penicillin V for group A β-hemolytic streptococcal acute tonsillitis in adults: a French Multicentre, open-label randomized study. Scand J Infect Dis 1996;28:497–501.

29. O'Brien JF, Meade JI, Falk JL. Dexamethasone as adjuvant therapy for severe acute pharyngitis. Ann Emerg Med 1993;22:212–215.

30. Snellman LW, Stang HJ, Stang JM, et al. Duration of positive throat culture for group A streptococci after initiation of antibiotic therapy. Pediatrics 1993;91:1166–1170.

41. Thyroid Disease

MINDY SMITH AND M. DEAN HAVRON, JR.

Key Clinical Questions

1. Is a solitary thyroid nodule likely to be cancer?
2. How does the etiology of hyperthyroidism alter treatment choices?
3. Should you routinely screen for thyroid disease?
4. Should patients with subclinical hypothyroidism or hyperthyroidism be treated?

Thyroid hormones influence the growth and maturation of tissues, cell respiration, total energy expenditure, and the turnover of various substrates, vitamins, and hormones. The primary action of the hormone is exerted through binding to intracellular receptor complexes, which in turn bind to specific regulatory sites in the chromosomes to influence gene expression. The majority of thyroid hormone is secreted as thyroxin (T_4), which is later converted (primarily in the liver and kidneys) to triiodothyronine (T_3), the biologically active hormone, or to the inactive reverse T_3. About 80% of circulating T_3 is derived from deiodination of T_4.

Thyroid function is regulated both by thyroid-stimulating hormone (TSH or thyrotropin) that is secreted by cells in the anterior pituitary and by changes in thyroid organic iodine content. TSH stimulates thyroid hypertrophy and hyperplasia, accelerates thyroid metabolism, and stimulates the synthesis and secretion of thyroid hormones. TSH is regulated by two opposing influences: thyrotropin-releasing hormone (TRH) from the hypothalamus and thyroid hormones themselves. The former stimulates TSH synthesis and secretion while the latter both directly inhibits TSH and antagonizes the action of TRH. Fluctuations in the body's iodine content also affect thyroid function by causing changes in thyroid iodide transport and modifying the response to TSH.

Conditions termed thyroid disease include alterations in thyroid hormone secretion (either insufficient secretion causing hypothyroidism or excessive secretion causing hyperthyroidism),

enlargement of the thyroid gland (generalized or focal), or both. If left untreated, these conditions may result in significant morbidity and mortality. Hypothyroidism may lead to infertility, miscarriage, fetal or newborn abnormalities, depression, and in severe cases, obtundation (myxedema coma). Untreated hyperthyroidism can cause increased bone mineral loss and fracture, arrhythmias, tachycardia, and cardiac enlargement. Nodules may represent areas of hyperfunction or cancer, and diffuse enlargement (goiter) can compress adjacent structures in the neck or mediastinum. In this chapter, we will discuss the approach to patients with four common thyroid conditions: a solitary thyroid nodule, goiter, hypothyroidism, and hyperthyroidism.

SOLITARY THYROID NODULE

Pathophysiology

The major causes of benign solitary thyroid nodules include adenoma, Hashimoto's thyroiditis, cysts, macrofollicular (colloid) nodules, and focal nonspecific thyroiditis (1). Adenomas, the most common nodule, are usually solitary and less than 3 to 4 cm in diameter; they sometimes enlarge and become painful as a result of intranodular hemorrhage. They rarely become active (i.e., inducing hyperthyroidism) or compress nearby vital structures. Cysts usually result from degeneration of an adenoma or may arise in a multinodular goiter.

Clinically recognized thyroid cancer is rare (0.004% per year), and the death rate from thyroid cancer has been reported as 6 per million population. However, small thyroid cancers have been reported at autopsy in 13 to 24% of individuals from various ethnic groups. The likelihood that a solitary nodule is cancer depends on the patient's age and exposure history; about 5% of individuals exposed to low doses of therapeutic head and neck radiation eventually develop thyroid cancer. Environmental radiation also plays a role in increasing rates of thyroid cancer. The incidence of thyroid cancer among the Belarus children rose 32-fold in the 5 years after the Chernobyl nuclear power plant accident in 1986, from 0.5% to 16.1% (2). These cancers appear to be of the same type as nonradiation-induced tumors (listed below), but they are more often multifocal and associated with benign thyroid conditions.

Differential Diagnosis

Clinically palpable nodules are found in up to 5% of the population; more than 95% are benign (Table 41.1). Nodules are more common in women (4:1 female/male ratio) and occur more commonly in the middle-aged or elderly. The differential diagnosis of neck masses in the region of the thyroid gland includes branchial cyst (child), thyroglossal duct cyst (child), cystic hygroma (child), lymphoma, infectious or inflammatory adenopathy, nasopharyngeal tumor,

metastasis (laryngeal, pulmonary, gastrointestinal), aneurysm of the aorta or great vessels, cellulitis, neurofibroma. Differentiating features of infectious masses include warmth, tenderness, and fever. Cancerous masses are often hard and on palpation appear fixed to adjacent tissues.

Only approximately 5% of solitary nodules and 1% of multinodular glands prove to be malignant. Thyroid cancers fall into two main categories: well-differentiated and poorly differentiated. Of the well-differentiated cancers, papillary adenocarcinoma (60 to 70%) and follicular carcinoma (20 to 25%) are the major types. The poorly differentiated malignancies generally have a poor prognosis. They include medullary carcinoma (5 to 10%) and undifferentiated carcinoma (10 to 15%). Rare causes of malignant thyroid tumors include lymphoma, sarcoma, and metastatic tumors.

Table 41.1.
Differential Diagnosis of Thyroid Disease

Diagnosis	Frequency in Primary Care; US Prevalence (Female:Male Ratio)
Solitary thyroid nodules	Very common; 1–5% (4:1)
Benign	Very common
Malignant	Rare; 0.004%
Thyroid enlargement with normal or abnormal function	Very common; 2–5% (3:1)
Simple or multinodular	Common
Acute thyroiditis (infectious)	Rare
Invasive fibrous thyroiditis (Riedel's)	Rare
Neoplasia	Extremely rare
Goitrous hypothyroidism	
Chronic lymphocytic (Hashimoto's)	Common[a] (6:1)
Pharmacologic inhibition	Uncommon
Genetic[b]	Rare
Goitrous hyperthyroidism	
Graves' disease	Common (7:1)
Toxic nodular goiter (Plummer's)	Uncommon[c]
Transient goitrous hyperthyroidism and/or hypothyroidism	
Postpartum thyroiditis (within 3–6 mo)[d]	Very common; 2–16%
Subacute granulomatous thyroiditis	Uncommon (5:1)
Subacute lymphocytic thyroiditis (painless)	Uncommon (4:1)
Nongoitrous hypothyroidism	
Radioactive iodine therapy (RAI)	Common
Surgical hypothyroidism	Uncommon
External irradiation	Rare
Pituitary/hypothalamic disease	Rare

[a]The presence of subclinical disease is reported in 4 to 8%; thyroid autoantibodies are present in about 10% of unselected populations.

[b]Due to inborn errors of thyroid hormone biosynthesis, pituitary thyroid hormone receptor defect or peripheral resistance and usually accompanied by hypothyroidism.

[c]More common than Graves' disease in the elderly with thyrotoxicosis.

[d]Likely a heterogeneous condition characterized by transient hyperthyroidism followed by hypothyroidism, which may become permanent in up to 40% of women.

Clinical Evaluation

History

The key clinical question in the evaluation of a thyroid nodule is: could it be cancer? As noted earlier, less than 5% of solitary nodules and 1% of multinodular glands are malignant. Risk factors from the history are shown in Table 41.2. Especially high rates of malignancy are found in children with a thyroid nodule (40%) and among patients who present with a nodule and report a significant history of exposure to radiation (40%). A report of dysphagia in a patient with a nodule makes malignancy somewhat more likely (LR+ 1.4) (1).

Physical Examination

The physical findings of a hard, fixed mass significantly increase the likelihood of malignancy (LR+ 5.2 for fixed mass, LR+ 3.8 for hard mass). Tracheal deviation and unilateral cervical adenopathy also increase the likelihood of malignancy but to a much smaller degree (see Table 41.2).

Laboratory Tests

Fine-needle aspiration biopsy (FNAB) is the preferred initial step in the workup of thyroid nodules in the euthyroid patient. It has proven to be accurate, safe, and cost-effective. FNAB provides conclusive cytologic evidence for whether the nodule is benign, malignant, or suspicious in 60 to 80% of biopsies. If a positive result is defined as cytopathologically suspicious or definite for malignancy, the LR+ is 3.5 and the LR− is 0.17 (using a gold standard of histopathologic diagnosis following surgical excision) (Table 41.3). If the aspirate is judged to be malignant, then it is very likely that the surgeon will find a cancer on excisional biopsy (LR+ 74) (1). Where the cytopathology is deemed benign (typically a colloid nodule or thyroiditis), malignancy is very unlikely (LR− < 0.1). Thus, if the likelihood of malignancy is 5% before the FNAB, a benign result reduces the likelihood to below 0.5%. Using FNAB cytology, the proportion of surgically excised nodules that prove to be malignant now approaches 30 to 50%, and the number of surgeries for thyroid nodules has dropped by 25 to 50%.

An estimated 20 to 40% of FNAB attempts yield samples that are inadequate (too few cells) or otherwise nondiagnostic. Experience with the procedure may lessen the percentage of inadequate or indeterminate results. Even at high-volume centers, however, 10 to 20% of smears will be inadequate or indeterminate. Although cysts are often responsible for inadequate smears, about

Table 41.2.
Risk Factors Associated with Thyroid Disease

Disease State	Risk Factor
Thyroid cancer	Family history of thyroid disease Nodule in patient <40 years Prior head or neck irradiation Living in iodine-deficient area, endemic goiter area, or near a volcano Exposure to carcinogens
Hypothyroidism	Family or personal history of thyroid disease Prior thyroid surgery or radioactive iodine treatment (RAI) Nonthyroid autoimmune disease Hypercholesterolemia Medication exposure[a] Recent pregnancy
Hyperthyroidism	Family or personal history of Graves' disease or goiter Nonthyroid autoimmune disease Use of thyroid hormone Anterior neck pain
Postpartum thyroiditis	Family or personal history of thyroid disease Delivery within the past 3–6 months (can be up to 1 year) Cigarette smoking Detection of thyroid microsomal antibodies at delivery

[a]Exposure to lithium carbonate, amiodarone, glucocorticoids, dopamine, furosemide, phenytoin.

Table 41.3.

Characteristics of Diagnostic Tests Useful in Patients with Thyroid Disease

Condition To Be Confirmed	Test	Result	Sensitivity[a]	Specificity[a]	LR+	LR−
Benign nodule	FNAB	Benign	—	—	—	0.1
Malignant nodule	FNAB	Suspicious/ positive	87	75	3.5	0.17
	Physical examination	Hard mass	42	89	3.8	0.65
		Fixed mass	31	94	5.2	0.73
		Tracheal deviation	37	67	1.1	0.94
		Unilateral cervical node	5	96	1.2	0.99
	Scan	Cold	(87)			
Simple goiter	TSH	0.5–6	—	—	—	—
Primary hypothyroidism	sTSH	>10	99	99	99	0.01
	FT₄	<4	90	90	9	0.11
Hashimoto's or postpartum thyroiditis	TMAb	Positive	(90)	—	—	—
Primary hyperthyroidism	sTSH	<0.1	99	99	99	0.01
	FT₄	>11	90	91	10	0.11
Thyroiditis (acute)	FNAB	Purulent	(100)			
Thyroiditis (subacute)	Gram stain	Positive[b]				
Granulomatous (painful)	ESR	>50	(95)	(99)	95	0.05
Granulomatous or lymphocytic	RAIU	Suppressed	(100)	—	—	—

Adapted from Dolan JG. Thyroid nodules. In: Panzer RJ, Black ER, Griner PF, eds. Diagnostic Strategies for Common Medical Problems, 2nd ed. American College of Physicians, 1991:385–393; Oppenheimer JH, Braverman LE, Toft A, et al. A therapeutic controversy. Thyroid hormone treatment: when and what? J Clin Endocrinol Metab 1995;80(10):2873–2876; de los Santos ET, Mazzaferri EL. Thyroid function tests. Postgrad Med 1989;85(5):333–352.

FNAB, fine-needle aspiration biopsy; Scan, scintiscan using either radioactive iodine or technetium-99m pertechnetate; TSH, thyrotropin (thyroid-stimulating hormone); sTSH, ultrasensitive TSH (an immunometric assay 10 to 100 times as sensitive as the older radioimmunoassays and capable of discriminating very low TSH values); FT₄, free T₄; TMAb, thyroid microsomal antibody; RAIU, radioactive iodine uptake (suppressed generally at <5%).

[a]Parentheses indicate estimates that are midrange from those provided in the literature; when only one estimate was found, the figures stand alone and the reference is cited.

[b]Gram stain may be positive for bacteria or fungi; if tuberculosis is suspected, an acid-fast stain should be performed.

25% of nodules with indeterminate or suspicious findings prove to be malignant at surgery.

For many years, the scintiscan ("thyroid scan") using radioactive iodine (RAI) or technetium was the initial screening test for thyroid nodules. Although the sensitivity for the detection of "cold" nodules (loss of functional ability) is high, specificity and diagnostic accuracy are poor; only about 20% of "cold" nodules prove to be malignant. Looking for a solid or mixed lesion using ultrasonography also has high sensitivity and poor specificity. These tests have a limited role in the evaluation of the solitary nodule (see Table 41.3).

Management

With benign cytology on FNAB, a solitary nodule may be observed and FNAB repeated after a year. Malignant or suspicious aspirates are an in-dication for thyroid resection. Cysts that resolve with aspiration should be resected if they recur, since the likelihood of malignancy is higher. If the sample contains too few cells, FNAB should be repeated; a diagnostic smear is obtained in up to 50% of repeat attempts.

Various algorithms have been devised to deal with the problem of nondiagnostic or indeterminate FNAB results. One is shown in Figure 41.1. Because FNAB in this scenario has a high false-negative rate, some thyroidologists recommend resection. Another valid approach suggested is to determine the patient's thyrotropin level using a highly sensitive assay, e.g., sTSH (3). Because neoplastic nodules are rarely hyperfunctional, a depressed sTSH suggests a toxic goiter, and a scintiscan with RAI would be the next step in the evaluation. If the patient is euthyroid or hypothyroid, however, the nodule should be resected. Surgery is recommended when there is a

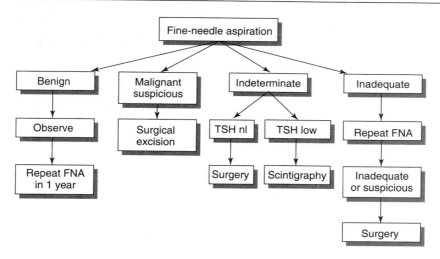

Figure 41.1. *General approach to the patient with thyroid nodule.* *nl,* normal. (Adapted from Woever KA. Cost-effective evaluation of the patient with a thyroid nodule. Surg Clin North Am 1995;25(3):357–363.)

high pretest likelihood of cancer (e.g., children or patients with a positive radiation history) or in the workup of a dominant nodule in a patient with Graves' disease. Several randomized trials have failed to support the strategy of suppressing a solitary nodule with thyroid hormone (4). These studies demonstrate that thyroid hormone, administered for 6 months to 3 years, does not reduce the size of solitary thyroid nodules; about one-third of nodules regressed in both treatment and placebo groups.

GOITER

Goiter is diffuse enlargement of the thyroid. It is the most common endocrine disorder worldwide, with a prevalence of nearly 90% in areas of dietary iodine deficiency and 4 to 6% even in areas with adequate iodine intake such as the United States (5). It is believed to be a spectrum of progressive change in the gland, from diffuse enlargement to nodular enlargement. The nodules in a goiter appear to arise from clones of cells representing newly generated follicles, which may retain function (i.e., "hot" nodules), lose functional ability (i.e., "cold" nodules), or become fibrotic from loss of blood supply, further accentuating remaining nodules.

Pathophysiology

Multiple factors contribute to the development of goiter including iodine deficiency, TSH stimu-lation or other circulating growth factors, drugs, autoimmunity, heredity, infection, and cancer (5). Worldwide, iodine deficiency is still a devastating problem, affecting 800 million people (6). The consequences include endemic goiter (190 million people), hypothyroidism, decreased fertility, increased perinatal and infant mortality rates, and growth and mental retardation (cretinism). Even today, despite the widespread availability of iodinated salt in the United States, endemic goiter (defined as goiter in ≥10% of the population) persists in certain areas, likely as a result of exposure to certain natural and pollutant environmental agents (7).

Regardless of the cause of nodular goiter, the thyroid gland may expand enormously (up to 2 kg in weight) and encroach upon surrounding vital structures, causing disorders such as dysphagia, stridor, and superior vena cava syndrome. Although most patients with multinodular goiter (MNG) remain euthyroid, hyperfunction within the nodules may lead to hyperthyroidism (toxic MNG).

Thyroiditis, an inflammatory disease of the thyroid, is a heterogeneous group of disorders that usually present with the clinical finding of goiter. This group includes two forms that are infectious in etiology. Subacute granulomatous (De Quervain's) thyroiditis is self-limited and believed to be caused by a virus. It has been associated with a number of viral syndromes, including mumps, influenza, and infectious mononucleosis; symptoms usually follow an upper respiratory infection (8). Mild thyrotoxicosis (due to leakage of hormone from the thyroid gland) followed by hypothyroidism may occur before returning to normal thyroid function over a period of several months. It is the most common cause of an anterior neck mass and pain in the thyroid gland in this country.

In acute (pyogenic/suppurative) thyroiditis, bacteria are the most common agents, although parasites and fungi also have been implicated. The infection usually arises from a pyogenic infection elsewhere. The most common pathogens are *Staphylococcus aureus, Streptococcus pyogenes* and *Streptococcus pneumoniae.* Unusual pathogens, such as *Pneumocystis carinii,* may be found in patients with AIDS. Half of the patients have preexisting thyroid disease (including anatomic defects such as a thyroglossal duct). Permanent sequelae are rare.

Differential Diagnosis

The differential diagnosis of goiter is largely based on the clinical evaluation and associated thyroid hormonal function (see Table 41.1). In clinical practice in the United States, the most common presentation of goiter with euthyroidism or transient hormonal dysfunction is thyroiditis; etiologies range from acute bacterial infections to autoimmune disease. The differential diagnosis of a painful, anterior neck mass includes subacute granulomatous thyroiditis, acute hemorrhage into a thyroid cyst or adenoma, painful Hashimoto's thyroiditis, an infected thyroglossal duct or branchial cleft cyst, acute suppurative thyroiditis, cellulitis, or a carcinoma with rapid enlargement and/or hemorrhage. The first two conditions listed comprise over 90% of cases (8). Patients with nontender goiters may have any of the remaining conditions in Table 41.1. Goitrous hypothyroidism and hyperthyroidism will be addressed in the section on thyroid hormonal disorders.

Clinical Evaluation

History

Patients with goiter from a noninflammatory cause may report painless enlargement of the neck or symptoms of compression including voice change, dysphagia, or a sense of obstruction, particularly on looking downward or raising their arms above their head (Pemberton's sign) (5). You should ask specifically about:

- Area of residence (to rule out iodine deficiency or excess and environmental exposure to pollutant goitrogens)
- Possible radiation exposure
- Use of drugs including inorganic or organic iodide (i.e., amiodarone), lithium, thiocyanate, and sulfonamides
- Exposure to food goitrogens (e.g., cassava, cabbage, soybeans)
- A family history of goiter
- An acute enlargement of a dominant area in the gland or a solitary nodule (consider malignancy)

In addition, signs of hyper- and hypothyroidism should be sought (Table 41.4).

Patients with acute and subacute thyroiditis will often report the abrupt onset of unilateral, anterior neck pain and fever. Symptoms of hypermetabolism (diaphoresis, palpitations, tachycardia, and weight loss) may be present when there is coexistent hyperthyroidism caused by release of thyroid hormone; this is true in about 50% of patients with subacute granulomatous thyroiditis. Other symptoms include pharyngitis, dysphagia, or pain radiating to the jaw or ear on the affected side. Subacute thyroiditis is usually preceded by viral upper respiratory symptoms.

Physical Examination

The presence of goiter is extremely helpful in determining the causes of the thyroid disorder and subsequent management. Several maneuvers help you detect goiter during the physical examination (9):

- Have the patient fully extend her neck for inspection.
- Observe the neck from the side.
- Palpate the gland by locating the isthmus first (between the cricoid cartilage and suprasternal notch).
- Have the patient swallow.

In addition to size assessment, the gland should be examined for texture, mobility, and nodularity. In the examination of a multinodular goiter, if the nodules are diffusely spread and of relatively long duration, there is little likelihood of cancer. However, if a single nodule enlarges more rapidly than others, a workup for thyroid malignancy is in order. The thyroid gland is very tender in patients

Table 41.4.

Key Elements of the History and Physical Examination for Thyroid Hormone Disorders

System	Signs and Symptoms		Differential Diagnosis
	Hypothyroidism	Hyperthyroidism	
Cardiovascular	Bradycardia	Tachycardia/palpitations	Cardiac causes
	Increased size	Atrial fibrillation	Congestive heart failure
	Poor contractility	Angina[a]	Ischemia[a]
Gastrointestinal	Constipation	Hyperdefecation	GI dysmotility
	Poor appetite	Change in appetite	Anorexia
General	Cold intolerance	Heat intolerance	
	Weight gain	Weight loss	
Hematologic anemia		Anemia/leukopenia	Malignancy
Musculoskeletal	Joint ache/myalgia	Muscle weakness	Myopathy
	Fine motor weakness	Osteoporosis	
	Carpal tunnel syndrome	Pretibial myxedema	
Nervous system	Lethargy	Nervous or fatigued	Depression
	Slow movements	Tremor, hyperkinesis[a]	Pheochromocytoma[a]
	Abnormal temperature	Insomnia, irritability	Anxiety disorder
	Paresthesia	Sudden paralysis[b]	Neuropathy
	Slow DTR relaxation	Hyperreflexia	
Ophthalmologic	Periorbital edema	Infrequent blinking[c]	
		Lid lag	
		Widened palpebral fissures	
Pulmonary	Shallow, slow breaths	Exertional dyspnea[a]	Cardiac causes[a]
	Sleep apnea		Chronic obstructive pulmonary disease
	Hypoxia		
	CO_2 retention		
Renal	Hyponatremia		Nephrotic syndrome
	Hyposmolarity		
	Poor bladder emptying		
Reproductive	Galactorrhea	Irregular menses	Pituitary adenoma
	Menorrhagia	Hypomenorrhea	
	Infertility	Infertility	
	Miscarriage		
Skin/hair	Dry, scaly skin	Warm, moist skin	
	Pale, cool skin	Smooth skin	
	Alopecia	Alopecia	
		Onycholysis	
Thyroid gland	Goiter	Goiter	
		Bruit	

DTR, deep tendon reflex; GI, gastrointestinal.

[a]Differential diagnosis associated with a particular sign or symptom.

[b]Occurs almost entirely in Asians.

[c]Eye findings of hyperthyroidism should be distinguished from ophthalmopathy of Graves' disease, as the former are reversible.

with thyroiditis; most have unilateral swelling, although the opposite lobe may be thickened. The overlying skin may also be erythematous.

Laboratory Tests

A complete blood count and sedimentation rate may be useful in the diagnosis of thyroiditis; both are usually elevated. In contrast to patients with subacute granulomatous thyroiditis whose sedimentation rates are usually above 50 mm/hour, patients with subacute lymphocytic thyroiditis will have normal or slightly elevated levels. Patients with the former condition may have a mild normochromic, normocytic anemia.

A TSH with or without free thyroxine (T_4)

should be performed for all patients with a goiter. Patients with acute thyroiditis will usually be euthyroid (normal TSH and free T$_4$), and when this is the case, a fine-needle aspiration of the lesion should be performed. The diagnosis is confirmed by the presence of purulent material; this material should be Gram stained and cultured.

Patients with subacute granulomatous hyperthyroidism will be either hyperthyroid with a low TSH and elevated free T$_4$ (approximately 50% of cases) or euthyroid. These patients—patients with painless goiter and euthyroidism and those with acute thyroiditis with laboratory evidence of hyperthyroidism—should undergo a thyroid scan with RAI. This test will be either normal (in patients with acute thyroiditis) or suppressed (less than 2% in 24 hours, found in patients with acute thyroiditis with diffuse inflammation or subacute granulomatous thyroiditis). Patients with the other conditions in the differential diagnosis will have normal scans, and scans of patients with Graves' disease will reveal elevated uptake.

Thyroid scans with technetium may also be useful to delineate functioning ("hot") or nonfunctioning ("cold") nodules for patients with acute thyroiditis or MNG. In acute thyroiditis, a cold defect will be seen in the affected lobe; in MNG, hot nodules are often benign adenomas, whereas cold nodules, if dominant or solitary, may be malignant.

Management

The level of evidence for therapeutic options in the management of thyroid disorders is summarized in Table 41.5.

Endemic Goiter

The treatment for endemic goiter (presentation in a population in which ≥10% of the population displays goiter) is to provide iodine and eliminate goitrogens. Iodine may be added to the diet as iodized salt, by adding iodine to drinking water, or by administering iodized oil by the oral or intramuscular routes. Large goiters require surgery, particularly if they are compressing other structures in the neck.

Nonendemic Goiter

For individuals with nonendemic goiter, the options include (a) removing goitrogens, when present; (b) TSH suppression with levothyroxine; (c) radioactive iodine (RAI); and (d) surgery (5). Sup-

pression of TSH with levothyroxine (2.2 μg/kg) is effective in reducing the diffuse goiter of Hashimoto's thyroiditis. The efficacy of levothyroxine for reducing the thyroid volume in multinodular goiter (MNG) is less clear; a recent comparison of placebo with levothyroxine alone or with carbimazole for treatment of sporadic MNG found a response to treatment (measured by ultrasonography) in 58% of the levothyroxine group, 35% of the combined treatment group, and 5% of the placebo group (10).

Radioactive iodine (^{131}I) ablative therapy is traditionally reserved for patients with toxic uninodular goiter or MNG, but it may be useful for patients with nontoxic MNG if enough functioning tissue can be destroyed to relieve obstructive symptoms. Total thyroidectomy is the treatment of choice for large MNG-producing obstructive symptoms because there is a high incidence of goiter recurrence in remaining tissue (11). In a small (N=60) prospective, randomized, double-blind study of the effectiveness of levothyroxine suppressive therapy in preventing postoperative recurrence of MNG, investigators observed a significantly lower rate of recurrence with suppressive therapy after a 3-year follow-up (6 of 28 versus 25 of 32) (12).

Thyroiditis

For patients with thyroiditis, pain should be treated with nonsteroidal anti-inflammatory drugs (NSAIDs). Hypothyroid symptoms are treated with levothyroxine, and hyperthyroid symptoms are managed with a β blocker or calcium channel blocker until the symptoms resolve (2 to 16 weeks). Sodium ipodate, which inhibits hormonal release from the thyroid gland and blocks extra-thyroidal conversion of T$_4$ to T$_3$, may be considered as an alternative treatment (Table 41.6). Treatment of acute thyroiditis also includes antibiotics against the most common pathogens, and drainage is occasionally necessary. Acceptable alternatives for antibiotics include oral amoxicillin/clavulanate (Augmentin 500 mg three times a day for 7 to 10 days), a first- or second-generation cephalosporin (e.g., ceph-alexin 500 mg four times a day for 7 to 10 days), a penicillinase-resistant penicillin (e.g., dicloxacillin 500 mg four times a day for 7 to 10 days), or intravenous equivalents when symptoms are severe. Although the majority of patients with subacute or granulomatous thyroiditis will recover by 6 months, permanent hypothyroidism may occur in 5% of patients; follow-up testing in these patients may be warranted (8).

Table 41.5.

Therapeutic Options Available for the Management of Thyroid Disorders

Treatment Strategy (Endpoint)	Level of Evidence for Effectiveness[a]	Comments
Solitary nodule: benign		
Observation	C	
Hormone suppression	X	
Solitary nodule: malignant		
Surgery	A	
Simple goiter (reduce size)		
Hormone suppression	A	Also effective in reducing size of MNG.
Surgery (subtotal thyroidectomy)	A	Used to relieve obstruction. May be more effective when combined with suppressive T_4.
RAI	C	Effective if enough functioning tissue is present.
Hypothyroidism (euthyroidism)		
Thyroid hormone replacement	A	Over age 50 or in presence of cardiac disease, replace with lower initial doses. Reevaluate at 6- to 8-week intervals using TSH.
Myxedema coma		
Intravenous thyroid hormone	A	Treatment in ICU recommended with endocrinologist consultant.
Corticosteroids	C	
Treat precipitating cause(s)	C	
Thyrotoxicosis (alleviate symptoms)		
β-Adrenergic blockers	B	May not be useful when combined with ATDs.
Calcium channel blockers	B	
Thyroid storm (resolve crisis)		
Antithyroid drugs (ATDs)	A	PTU is the preferred agent as it also inhibits peripheral conversion of T_4s.
Cholestyramine	B	Binds iodothyronines.
Supportive therapy	C	Treatment in ICU recommended with endocrinologist consultant.
Treat precipitating cause(s)	C	
Drugs to inhibit hormone release (iodine, lithium carbonate)	C	Used as adjunctive agents. Iodine seems preferred due to fewer side effects.
Corticosteroids	C	Adrenal-insufficiency may coexist.
Graves' or toxic nodular goiter (resolve hyperthyroidism)		
ATDs (inhibit hormone synthesis)	A	Used for 6 months to 2 years. High relapse rate on discontinuing therapy. The most serious reaction is agranulocytosis (0.3%). Preferred for children and during pregnancy.
Radioactive iodine therapy	A	Most commonly used therapy. Contraindicated in pregnancy or if breast-feeding. Pretreatment of the elderly or those at risk of cardiac problems with ATDs is suggested.
Surgery	A	Indicated for very large goiter, allergy to ATDs, or suspected malignancy. Major complications are hypoparathyroidism and injury to the recurrent laryngeal nerve (<4%).
Thyroiditis, acute (resolve condition)		
Antibiotics; drainage	B	
Supportive therapy	C	Hospitalization is recommended, as abscess rupture may occur with resultant sepsis.
Thyroiditis, subacute painful (resolve condition)		
Oral corticosteroids	A	Dramatic reduction in pain and swelling.

continued

Table 41.5. *(continued)*
Therapeutic Options Available for the Management of Thyroid Disorders

Treatment Strategy (Endpoint)	Level of Evidence for Effectiveness[a]	Comments
β Blockers; levothyroxine (L-T$_4$)	B	Useful for symptomatic treatment.
Salicylates, NSAIDs	C	Pain control, only effective if mild.
Thyroiditis, subacute painless (resolve condition)		
β Blockers	B	Useful for symptomatic hyperthyroidism.
Oral corticosteroids	X	
Thyroiditis, chronic/Hashimoto's		
L-T$_4$ if hypothyroid or large goiter	A	
L-T$_4$ if subclinical or euthyroid	C	Left untreated, 5%/year become hypothyroid.

[a]Level of evidence for effectiveness: A, strong or moderate research-based evidence (consistent across several studies, including at least two randomized controlled trials); B, limited research-based evidence (less consistent or extensive evidence, but preponderance of evidence supports use of treatment); C, common practice with little or no research-based evidence; X, moderate or strong evidence suggesting that this treatment is not effective.

HYPOTHYRODISM

Pathophysiology

Hypothyroidism is common, with a prevalence from population studies of 0.35 to 3%, and is more common in women. It is found in 1 in every 5,000 newborns. Chronic autoimmune thyroiditis, a frequent cause of hypothyroidism, is divided into two clinical forms based on whether a goiter is present (Hashimoto's disease) or absent (atrophic thyroiditis).
    Hypothyroidism is a common problem in elderly patients; frank hypothyroidism has been reported in 0.9 to 10% of elderly populations and subclinical hypothyroidism (elevated TSH with normal T$_4$) in up to 14% (13). An increase with age in the titers of thyroid antibodies is also associated with subsequent development of hypothyroidism.

Differential Diagnosis

Possible causes of hypothyroidism include loss of thyroid tissue from radiation exposure, idiopathic goitrous conditions (iodine deficiency, genetic, Hashimoto's, drug-induced), self-limited causes such as thyroiditis, and rare pituitary and hypothalamic disorders (see Table 41.1). The majority of cases are due to Hashimoto's thyroiditis, RAI therapy for hyperthyroidism, and surgery (14).

Table 41.6.
Drugs Recommended for Use in the Management of Thyroid Disorders

Drug	Indications	Common Dosing Range	Comments
Levothyroxine (Synthroid)	Hypothyroidism	100–200 μg/day	
β-Adrenergic blockers			
Propranolol (Inderal)	Hyperthyroidism	10–40 mg bid to qid	
Atenolol (Tenormin)	Hyperthyroidism	50–200 mg/day	
Calcium channel blockers			
Diltiazem (Cardizem)	Hyperthyroidism	30–90 mg bid	
Verapamil (Calan)	Hyperthyroidism	240–360 mg/day	
Antithyroid drugs (ATDs)			
Propylthiouracil	Hyperthyroidism	100–600 mg q8h	Initial dose 100–200 mg q8h
Methimazole	Hyperthyroidism	10–40 mg/day	Initial dose 20–40 mg/day
Ipodate sodium	Hyperthyroidism	0.5–3.0 g/day	
Radioactive iodine (^{131}I)	Hyperthyroidism	5–15 mCi	

Clinical Evaluation

History

Key elements of the history and physical examination of a patient with a suspected thyroid hormonal disorder are presented in Table 41.4. The spectrum of disease is quite wide, ranging from subclinical disease to life-threatening conditions.

Lack of thyroid hormone can affect multiple organ systems. Patients commonly report lethargy, slowness of movement, dry skin, cold intolerance, poor appetite, and constipation. Younger women may report menstrual complaints such as menorrhagia (heavy periods) or infertility. Over 20 years ago, Billewicz developed an index for the detection of hypothyroidism that achieved a sensitivity of nearly 100%, specificity of 50%, positive likelihood ratio (LR+) of 1.98 and a negative likelihood ratio (LR−) of 0.02 (Table 41.7) (15). Similar results were obtained when the index was used more recently in a study from India (16).

The most serious form of hypothyroidism is myxedema coma due to severe long-standing hypothyroidism. This condition, most often seen in

Table 41.7.

Clinical Scoring Systems for Hypothyroidism and Hyperthyroidism

Billewicz Index[a] for Hypothyroidism
Weights for Individual Items of the Diagnostic Index Based on the Full Sample

Symptoms	Present	Absent	Signs	Present	Absent
Physical tiredness	0	+2	Slow movements[b]	+11	−3
Slow cerebration	−3	+1	Coarse skin	+7	−7
Diminished sweating[b]	+6	−2	Cold skin	+3	−2
Dry skin	+3	−6	Periorbital puffiness	+4	−6
Cold intolerance[b]	+4	−5	Pulse rate[b]	+4	−4
Dry hair	−2	+2	Ankle jerk[b]	+15	−6
Weight increase	+1	−1			
Constipation	+2	−1			
Hoarseness	+5	−6			
Paraesthesiae	+5	−4			
Deafness	+2	0			

Crooks Index[c] for Hyperthyroidism
Weighting Factors Allocated to the Symptoms and Signs of Thyrotoxicosis

Symptoms	Present	Absent	Signs	Present	Absent
Dyspnea on effort	+1		Palpable thyroid	+3	−3
Palpitations	+2		Bruit over thyroid	+2	−2
Tiredness	+2		Exophthalmos	+2	
Preference for heat		−5	Lid retraction	+2	
(irrespective of duration)			Lid lag	+1	
Indifferent to temperature	0		Hyperkinetic movements	+4	−2
Excessive sweating	+3		Fine finger termor	+1	
Nervousness	+2		Hands hot	+2	−2
Appetite increased	+3		Hands moist	+2	−2
Appetite decreased		−3	Casual pulse rate:	+4	
Weight increased		−3	auricular fibrillation		
Weight decreased	+3		Regular rate:		
			Under 80		−3
			80–90	0	
			Over 90	+3	

[a]Euthyroid of 30 or less; hypothyroid if more than 30. (From Billewicz WZ, Chapman RS, Crooks J, et al. Statistical methods applied to the diagnosis of hypothyroidism. Q J Med 1969;38:255–266.)

[b]Items used in the first stage procedure because they had the largest discriminate factor.

[c]Euthyroid if 10 or less; hyperthyroid if more than 10. (From Bayer MF. Effective laboratory evaluation of thyroid status. Med Clin North Am 1991;75(1):1–26.)

elderly women with chronic hypothyroidism, is characterized by stupor, respiratory depression, cardiac dysfunction, and hypothermia (<90°F). It carries a mortality of 50% despite optimal therapy and is often precipitated by surgery, trauma, or infection.

Risk factors for hypothyroidism are listed in Table 41.2. In addition to questions about current symptoms, patients should be asked about the following:

- A personal or family history of thyroid disease;
- A personal history of autoimmune disease such as diabetes or collagen vascular disease;
- Current medication use (see the footnote, Table 41.2); and
- Recent pregnancy.

Physical Examination

Signs of hypothyroidism are summarized in Table 41.4. Typical features include bradycardia, goiter, periorbital edema, hoarseness, delayed relaxation of the deep tendon reflexes, slow speech, and cool, dry skin (14).

Laboratory Tests

With suspected hypothyroidism, the diagnostic algorithm in Figure 41.2 should be followed (17). Initial laboratory testing includes a TSH and an estimate or direct measurement of free T_4. Often a high serum TSH is sufficient for the diagnosis of primary hypothyroidism, especially using the ultrasensitive "third-generation" TSH assays (sTSH) (18). This would be the preferred strategy if the pretest probability of hypothyroidism is low. An elevated sTSH and a subnormal free thyroxine (FT_4) unequivocally confirm primary hypothyroidism. Because treatment is not based on a specific cause, further testing is unnecessary.

In patients without a history of previous radiation, thyroid ablation, or thyroid removal, thyroid autoimmune disease (Hashimoto's disease) is likely. The presence of thyroid microsomal antibodies (TMAb) and/or thyroglobulin antibodies (TgAb) establishes the diagnosis but is unnecessary for treatment purposes. Although antibodies may be negative in 5% of patients with Hashimoto's, an alternate etiology should be considered (i.e., drug-induced hypothyroidism or iodine deficiency). In patients with subclinical hypothyroidism (an elevated sTSH with a normal FT_4), antibody tests could be considered because the presence of a high

antibody titer predicts subsequent development of clinical hypothyroidism. Many physicians consider treatment rather than follow-up testing in these cases, although evidence to support this approach is lacking.

In secondary hypothyroidism (caused by pituitary or hypothalamic disease), the sTSH is usually normal but FT_4 is low. A TRH test can distinguish between a pituitary disorder (a blunted response) and a hypothalamic lesion (normal response). This test is performed by injecting TRH intravenously and measuring serial serum TSH concentrations. The peak serum TSH increment (2 to 20 μU/mL) should occur in 10 to 45 minutes. TSH fails to rise in thyrotoxic subjects; the response is exaggerated (>30 μU/mL) in patients with primary hypothyroidism. This test is expensive and time-consuming and often causes side effects (headache, nausea, urinary urgency, and rarely hypertension).

Management

Initial Management

The levels of evidence for therapeutic options in the management of thyroid disorders are summarized in Table 41.5. Consensus panels from the American Thyroid Association and the American Association of Clinical Endocrinologists in conjunction with the American College of Endocrinology recommend levothyroxine as the treatment of choice in the management of hypothyroidism (14, 19). Other thyroid preparations are available that contain combinations of thyroxine and triiodothyronine. These preparations have been shown to produce a supraphysiologic rise in T_3 several hours after ingestion and may result in cardiac adverse effects (20).

Dosing can be determined by ideal body weight, with younger adults requiring approximately 1.7 μg/kg/day, older adults approximately 1 μg/kg/day, and children up to 4 μg/kg/day. In practice, an initial dose of 50 to 100 μg per day is started for most adults with gradual increases (25 to 50 μg/day) at 6-week intervals until the TSH is normalized. Individuals who are under age 50, who have been recently treated for hyperthyroidism, or who have only been hypothyroid for a few months may be treated with full-replacement doses of levothyroxine. Older individuals should be started with 25 μg/day and advanced slowly.

Patients who are taking drugs that interfere with levothyroxine absorption (i.e., cholestyramine, ferrous sulfate, sucralfate, and aluminum

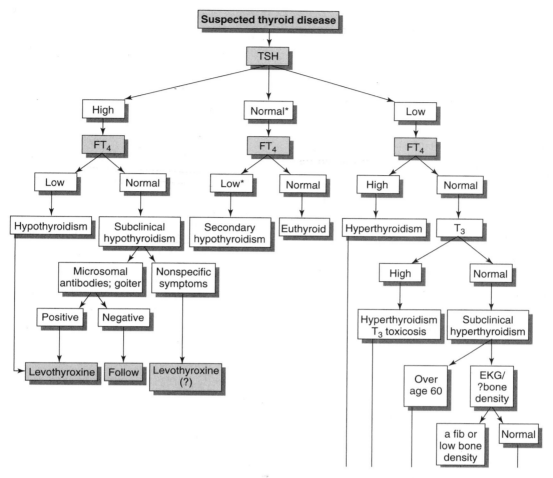

Figure 41.2. *Algorithm for evaluation of thyroid status in ambulatory patients.* *Asterisk* indicates serum TSH may be in the normal range in patients with hypothyroidism secondary to hypothalamic or pituitary disease; *a fib*, atrial fibrillation; *TSH*, thyrotropin; *FT₄*, free T_4; *T_3*, triiodothyronine.

hydroxide-containing antacids) or accelerate its metabolism (i.e., anticonvulsants and rifampin) may require higher replacement doses. Levothyroxine should be taken at least 4 hours apart from medications that interfere with its absorption. Generic levothyroxine products appear to be bioequivalent to brand-name products and may be substituted in most patients without adverse effects (21). Patients may become symptomatic, however, when changing from one generic preparation to another (22).

Long-Term Management

Patients with stable hypothyroidism should be re-examined annually, including a measurement of their sTSH level (14). If a patient's dose requires readjusting, his or her clinical and biochemical response should be reassessed in 2 to 3 months. Patients who become pregnant or are started on medications that may alter absorption or metabolism of levothyroxine should be rechecked. It is unclear whether thyroid hormone replacement should continue indefinitely and whether levothyroxine doses should be adjusted for asymptomatic patients with either mildly elevated or mildly suppressed sTSH levels.

With respect to indefinite need for replacement, investigators in one study withdrew 79 patients with Hashimoto's thyroiditis (diagnosed according to suggestive cytologic features and/or the presence of thyroid antibodies) from levothyroxine therapy after 1 year to assess the further need for treatment (23). After withdrawal of treatment, nine patients (11.4%) showed normalization of the thyroid blood tests. The presence of a large goiter (≥ 35 g), TSH levels > 10 mU/L, and a family history of thyroid disease was associated with an increased incidence of recovery of normal thyroid function (odds ratio, 5.4; 95% CI 2.8 to 10.7).

Concern about deviations in the TSH value is justified only if the change observed on a single test is truly indicative of the average TSH and if there is an effect of subclinical hyper- or hypothyroidism on long-term health (20, 24). Considerable variation in TSH levels was demonstrated in five patients on a constant dose of levothyroxine (25). It therefore seems prudent to repeat the TSH level in an otherwise stable patient before making a decision on dosage adjustment.

Although doses of thyroxine that suppress TSH may have subtle multisystem effects, most studies show no increases in morbidity or mortality. In addition, study findings conflict about decreasing bone mineral density, and there is no evidence of an increased rate of bone fracture. One author suggests widening the acceptable range for sTSH to reduce the number of dose changes (24).

HYPERTHYROIDISM

Pathophysiology

Hyperthyroidism occurs commonly in women (2% prevalence) with a female-to-male ratio of 10:1. Graves' disease, a type of autoimmune thyroid disease, is the cause of the majority of cases. The thyroid receptor antibodies (TRAb) associated with this disease fall into several categories, including those directed against the receptor for TSH and others that stimulate the receptor. This results in high levels of thyroid hormone in the bloodstream and the accompanying systemic effects. The reasons for the development of TRAb are not well delineated, but there is clearly a genetic component: identical twin studies show a 50% chance of the second twin developing Graves' disease if one sibling is affected.

Besides thyrotoxicosis, Graves' disease can cause an infiltrative ophthalmopathy in over 80% of patients within 18 months of diagnosis, although ophthalmic signs such as proptosis, inflammation, and swelling may be seen in the absence of hyperthyroidism.

Differential Diagnosis

Hyperthyroidism may result from abnormal thyroid stimulation as in Graves' disease, adenoma, toxic multinodular goiter (MNG or Plummer's disease), or rarely from pituitary disease. Hyperthyroidism may also arise from the release of existing thyroid hormone (thyroiditis) or from extrathyroidal hormone sources (exogenous or ectopic) without thyroid hyper-function (Table 41.1) Graves' disease is the most common condition resulting in hyperthyroidism in younger patients, and toxic MNG is the most common disorder in the elderly (14).

Distinguishing Graves' ophthalmopathy can be challenging because eye findings may precede the onset of hyperthyroidism. The differential diagnosis include metastases to the extraocular muscles and pseudotumor. The eye findings in Graves' disease are usually gradual in onset and associated with only mild discomfort compared to orbital pseudotumors, which present with an abrupt, painful onset. Consultation with an ophthalmologist may be helpful to evaluate for neoplastic or other conditions associated with lid retraction and proptosis.

Clinical Evaluation

History

Hyperthyroidism typically affects multiple organ systems (see Table 41.4). Patients report fatigue, palpitations, nervousness, and excessive sweating. In patients with hyperthyroidism, thyrotoxic crisis or storm may occur. This is a decompensated state of thyrotoxicosis characterized by extreme irritability, delirium or coma, fever (>104°F), tachycardia and tachyarrhythmia, vomiting, and diarrhea. Although most patients have a wide pulse pressure and an elevated systolic blood pressure, marked cardiac decompensation can occur that results in hypotension. Hepatic necrosis may also occur, resulting in jaundice. Atypical thyrotoxicosis may occur, especially among elderly patients with toxic MNG. This condition is characterized by few symptoms, with patients progressing quietly into coma and death. Thyroid storm is often precipitated by surgery, trauma, or infection.

Age also influences the clinical presentation of less-serious forms of hyperthyroidism. Young patients with Graves' disease are more likely to have goiter (99% vs. 73%), irritability, heat intolerance, perspiration, and increased appetite, whereas older patients have higher rates of atrial fibrillation, decreased appetite, and weight loss (26).

The Crooks index for the diagnosis of hyperthyroidism may be useful in evaluating a patient with possible hyperthyroidism (see Table 41.7) (27). Use of this index in an independent population produced a sensitivity of 95% and specificity of 68% (LR+ 2.9, LR− 0.07) (28). The index can be used to establish the likelihood of hyperthyroidism prior to laboratory testing (29).

Risk factors for hyperthyroidism are listed in Table 41.2. For patients with suspected hyperthyroidism you should ask about:

- A personal or family history of thyroid disease;

- A personal history of autoimmune disease such as diabetes or collagen vascular disease;

- Use of thyroid hormone; and

- Anterior neck pain.

Physical Examination

Signs of hyperthyroidism are also listed in Table 41.4. The examination should focus on the patient's weight (weight loss), blood pressure (elevated systolic pressure), thyroid (goiter), cardiac examination (tachycardia or tachyarrhythmia), muscle (proximal muscle weakness and tremor), skin (pretibial edema) and eyes (as below). Distinguishing between Graves' disease and other forms of hyperthyroidism, particularly subacute painless thyroiditis, is aided by the presence in Graves' disease of the following eye signs (30):

- Lid retraction (drawing back of the eyelid, allowing more of the sclera to be visible above the iris)

- Lid lag (upper eyelid is delayed in descending, especially on downward gaze)

- Frank proptosis (displacement of the eye in the anterior direction)

Proptosis can be measured by placing a ruler at the corner of the eye and measuring the distance from the lateral orbital ridge to the anterior projection of the cornea (true proptosis may be over 20 mm).

Laboratory Tests

Hyperthyroidism is confirmed by a clearly subnormal (≤0.1 μU/mL) or undetectable sTSH and an elevated FT_4 (see Fig. 41.1) (26). As with testing for hypothyroidism, some authors believe that a low sTSH is sufficient to make the diagnosis. A subnormal sTSH, however, is not entirely specific for hyperthyroidism. A retrospective review of patients with suppressed sTSH levels found 17% of cases caused by conditions other than intrinsic hyperthyroidism or excessive hormone replacement (31). Likewise, elevated sTSH levels may be seen on recovery from severe illness and in hyperthyroid patients with inappropriate TSH secretion.

A subnormal or undetectable sTSH and a normal FT_4 should be followed with a T_3/FT_3 assay. This will differentiate T_3 toxicosis (elevated T_3) from subclinical hyperthyroidism. Low T_3 levels may result from malnutrition, chronic renal failure, and cirrhosis caused by decreased peripheral conversion of T_4 to T_3.

Individuals with either an undetectable (or very low) sTSH and elevated FT_4 or a low sTSH and a normal FT_4 can be further tested for thyroid autoantibodies (TMAb, TgAb) to differentiate autoimmune diseases from other causes. Often the clinical appearance, along with the sTSH and FT_4, is sufficient to diagnose Graves' disease. If the clinical picture is uncertain, a radioactive iodine (RAI) uptake test may be useful. This test of thyroid function, measured at 24 hours after administration of the radioactive iodine (^{123}I), helps to distinguish between the numerous causes of thyrotoxicosis. An elevated RAI uptake result (>30%) is compatible with Graves' disease, nodular hyperthyroidism (toxic MNG or solitary hyperfunctioning nodule), human chorionic gonadotropin (HCG)-mediated thyrotoxicosis (i.e., molar pregnancy), or TSH-mediated (i.e., pituitary tumor) thyrotoxicosis.

A scan of the thyroid gland using technetium (^{99m}Tc) usually immediately follows RAI uptake. Graves' disease, toxic MNG, and toxic adenoma can often be distinguished by the pattern of technetium uptake; a homogenous pattern is seen in Graves' disease, a patchy pattern in MNG, and a single focus of intense uptake surrounded by areas of suppressed uptake is seen in toxic adenoma. If the RAI uptake is subnormal (<8 to 10%), the differential diagnosis includes transient forms of hyperthyroidism (subacute thyroiditis, postpartum thyroiditis, lymphocytic thyroiditis), ectopic hormone production (lingual goiter, struma ovarii, metastatic thyroid cancer [postoperative]), or iodine-associated or factitious thyrotoxicosis. Patients who do not fit into the above categories require consultation with an endocrinologist.

Management

Initial Management

Recommendations for management and their level of evidence are summarized in Table 41.5. Either β blockers or calcium channel blockers may be used to control acute symptoms of hyperthyroidism (see Table 41.6). These medications may offer no additional benefit to patients already on antithyroid drugs (ATDs) (32).

For patients with thyrotoxicosis, the three primary forms of therapy include ATDs, radioactive iodine (RAI) administration, and surgery. None of these therapies is indicated in patients with hyperthyroidism and a low RAI uptake, which usually represents thyroiditis, a self-limited condition.

The ATDs methimazole (MMI) and propylthiouracil (PTU) inhibit the biosynthesis of thyroid hormone and can be used as primary or adjunctive therapy. When used as primary therapy, they are given for 6 months to 2 years (14); dosage ranges and possible adverse effects are shown in Table 41.6. A recent small, randomized clinical trial found that a single daily dose of MMI (15 mg) is as effective as the multiple-dose regimen; within 8 weeks, almost 80% of the patients in both groups became euthyroid (33).

The main concern with ATDs is the variable rate of remission (9 to 80%) following discontinuation of therapy. Higher thyrotropin-releasing antibody (TRAb) levels at the time of diagnosis and at the end of treatment as well as shorter courses of therapy are associated with lower remission rates. Conversely, absence of these antibodies is associated with a low likelihood of relapse of Graves' disease after ATD treatment (34, 35). It is still unknown whether treatment should be continued until antibodies are undetectable. Patients can be continued indefinitely on ATDs because maintenance doses are usually small and side effects are uncommon. The most serious adverse effect of either drug is agranulocytosis (0.3% of patients); hepatitis is rarely seen with PTU. Some clinicians obtain a white blood cell (WBC) count prior to initiating therapy because a mild leukocytosis can be seen in Graves' disease. Patients developing rash, fever, jaundice, arthralgia, or oropharyngitis should discontinue the medication and be reevaluated (14).

Levothyroxine can be given in conjunction with ATDs to avoid the need for frequent adjustments in dosing. Such treatment, however, does not appear to alter the recurrence rate of hyperthyroidism (38). Drugs that inhibit the release of thyroid hormone (lithium carbonate, inorganic iodine, and ipodate sodium) can be used after initiation of ATDs for patients who require immediate improvement such as patients with thyroid storm. A small recent double-blind placebo-controlled trial found that cholestyramine (an anion exchange resin that binds iodothyronines) used adjunctively with an ATD and a β blocker lowered thyroid hormone levels faster than standard therapy alone.

In the United States, radioactive iodine is the most commonly prescribed treatment for Graves' disease, toxic MNG, and toxic adenoma. Iodine-131 (^{131}I) is selectively absorbed by thyroid tissue, where it destroys some or all of the hyperfunctioning thyroid follicles by emitting β-particles over a range of a few millimeters. It is a simple and cost-effective treatment. Patients must stop the use of ATDs and iodine for at least several weeks prior to receiving RAI, because these agents reduce uptake of the ^{131}I.

The effects of RAI treatment are apparent within a few weeks. Maximum effects occur at 5 to 8 weeks, when 50 to 75% of treated patients will be euthyroid; 50 to 90% of patients with Graves' disease treated this way eventually become hypothyroid. Long-term follow-up of 754 patients treated with ^{131}I found that thyroid supplementation was taken by 178 (93%) of the treated patients with Graves' disease, compared with 21 (47%) of the treated patients with toxic MNG. RAI treatment also reduces thyroid gland size in a dose-dependent manner, regardless of initial gland size (37).

Transient hypothyroidism occurs in a significant proportion of RAI-treated patients, and patients should be monitored every 6 to 8 weeks until they achieve normal T_4 levels. The first symptom of hypothyroidism arising in this setting is usually muscle cramps (38). Short-term complications of therapy include acute transient tenderness and swelling of the thyroid gland (treated with NSAIDs) and rare transient exacerbation of hyperthyroidism due to release of stored hormone (occurring within days to weeks after treatment). Contraindications to the use of RAI are pregnancy (^{131}I crosses the placenta and can ablate fetal thyroid tissue) and breast-feeding. Because of the risk of hyperthyroidism, patients at risk of developing cardiac complications may be pretreated for up to several months with ATDs to decrease their T_4 stores to near-normal.

Surgery, primarily subtotal thyroidectomy, is infrequently used to treat Graves' disease. Specific indications include patients with a very large goiter who may be resistant to RAI, those with allergy to ATDs, and those with nodules suspicious for malignancy. The recurrence rate of hyperthyroidism following surgery is small (3.4% in one large study) and about half the patients become hypothyroid. Surgical complications occur in less than 4% of patients but may be serious, including hemorrhage, hypoparathyroidism, and damage to the recurrent laryngeal nerve resulting in vocal cord paralysis.

To analyze the benefits and risks of common treatments, a group of 179 patients with Graves' hyperthyroidism were randomly assigned to medical or surgical therapy for young patients (age 20 to 34; N=60) and medical, surgical, or RAI (^{131}I) treatment for older adults (age 35 to 55; N=119) (39). They were followed for at least 48 months. All treatments normalized the mean serum hormone levels within 6 weeks. The risk of relapse was highest in the medically treated young and old adults (42% vs. 34%, respectively), followed by RAI treatment (21% among older adults) and surgical treatment (3% among young adults and 8% among older adults). Elevated TSH receptor antibodies at the end of medical therapy or increasing TSH receptor antibody values after medical or surgical treatment increased the probability of relapse. Ninety percent of the subjects in all groups were satisfied with their treatment.

Management of Graves' ophthalmopathy depends on the visual status, rapidity, and severity of the eye symptoms. In general, the eye findings (except proptosis) are ameliorated with control of the hyperthyroidism, and only a minority of patients will progress after thyroid ablation. The development of overt hypothyroidism appears to be an important factor associated with the development or exacerbation of Graves' ophthalmopathy (40). Supportive measures include hourly use of artificial tears, propping the head of the bed to minimize orbital edema, taping the eyelids closed at night, and using sunglasses for outdoor activity. The use of 2% guanethidine eye drops can be useful for control of dryness, redness, and tearing (30). For severe eye involvement (subluxation of the globe, new-onset ophthalmoplegia, moderate or severe inflammation, progressive proptosis, or compressive optic neuropathy), anti-inflammatory therapies, radiation, or surgery should be considered (30).

Long-Term Management

ATD = Antrthyroid Drug

Patients treated with ATDs should be seen at 4 to 12-week intervals until they become euthyroid (14). At this time, the ATD dose can often be decreased with follow-up intervals increased to 3 to 4 months while continuing treatment. The interval examination should include weight, pulse, blood pressure, thyroid, and eye examinations (14). A FT$_4$ should also be obtained; FT$_3$ may be indicated if the patient appears clinically hyperthyroid. TSH levels are less useful in early follow-up because TSH may remain suppressed for several months after thyroid hormones normalize. On discontinuing the medication, patients should be seen every 4 to 6 weeks for the first 3 to 4 months and at least yearly for the next 2 to 3 years (14).

The recommended follow-up interval for patients treated with radioactive iodine is every 4 to 6 weeks for the first 3 months and then as determined by the clinical outcome. Hypothyroidism usually develops within the first 6 to 12 months and is treated with levothyroxine.

Visits for patients after thyroidectomy are determined by the clinical needs of the patient, with thyroid tests performed initially at 2 months. Further follow-up is then based on whether treatment is needed for hypothyroidism or hyperthyroidism. Patients who are euthyroid may be followed yearly.

SPECIAL CONSIDERATIONS

Screening for Thyroid Hormonal Disease

Several evidence-based groups including the U.S. Preventive Services Task Force recommend against screening asymptomatic adults for thyroid disease. This recommendation is based on the low risk of overt disease, the lack of evidence of benefit in treating patients with subclinical disease, the cost of screening, and the potential adverse effects of screening. There is much disagreement about this; the American Association of Clinical Endocrinologists recommends screening older patients, particularly women (19), and a recent cost-effectiveness analysis concluded that screening for mild thyroid failure compares favorably with other accepted preventive medicine practices (41). The latter conclusions were based on potential health benefits including preventing progression to overt thyroid failure, reversing the accompanying hypercholesterolemia that may occur, and improving unrecognized symptoms. Although varying rates of progression to overt disease have been reported, patients with high antibody titers are more likely to progress to overt hypothyroidism and may benefit from treatment. In a prospective study of 258 healthy, elderly subjects, 13.2% (N=34) were found to have subclinical hypothyroidism, and 8 of 24 subjects followed for 4 years developed thyroid failure; all of these subjects had high-titer ($\geq$1:1600) antimicrosomal antibodies (42). Finally, although the term subclinical implies lack of symptoms, many patients do have mild symptoms that improve with treatment (43).

Patients with type I diabetes mellitus and those who have undergone radiation therapy to the head and neck should be considered for screening because of the high incidence of associated hypothyroidism.

Effects on the Thyroid of Nonthyroid Systemic Disease

The most common thyroid abnormality found in patients with systemic illness is a low serum T_3 concentration, a result of inhibition of the enzyme conversion from T_4, and more reverse T_3 from decreased clearance by the same enzyme. The normal TSH and free serum T_4 (FT_4) in most patients and the transient nature of these findings has led to the classification of this disorder as the "euthyroid sick syndrome." In severe disease, there can be reductions in TSH, thyroxine-binding globulin (TBG), and T_4 and FT_4 concentrations. Some medications also may impair hormone synthesis, alter metabolism, or reduce the secretion of TSH, including glucocorticoids, dopamine, furosemide, and phenytoin.

Thyroid Changes in Pregnancy

Changes in thyroid function in pregnancy are the result of (a) increased renal clearance of iodide; (b) transfer of iodide and iodothyronine to the fetus; (c) increased serum concentration of TBG (first trimester); (d) increased human chorionic gonadotropin (HCG), which has some TSH-like bioactivity; and (e) increased T_4 utilization by 25 to 50% (44).When iodine intake is poor, goiter can develop more readily during pregnancy. Under normal conditions, the increased TBG is accompanied by increases in serum total T_3 and T_4 concentrations so that TSH remains normal.

Postpartum thyroiditis, affecting approximately 5% of women during the 12 months after delivery, is likely part of a spectrum of autoimmune disorders. A wide range in the incidence of this condition has been reported (2% to 16%) depending on whether the diagnosis is based on the detection of thyroid microsomal antibodies (TMAb) or on the development of overt disease (45). During late pregnancy, thyroid autoimmune disorders such as Graves' disease and Hashimoto's thyroiditis tend to improve, only to relapse in the postpartum period. This is probably due to a rebound in immune surveillance following pregnancy. Risk factors for postpartum thyroiditis are shown in Table 41.2. The detection of TMAb during pregnancy or immediately postpartum increases the risk of thyroid dysfunction. In a follow-up study of 55 women with positive TMAb titers at delivery, 40 women (73%) developed early disease (goiter and/or hormonal dysfunction within the first 11 months after delivery), and treatment was required in 21 women (46). The detection of higher antibody titers resulted in higher percentages of women developing disease and requiring treatment (odds ratio for requiring treatment = 23.0 when titers were >6400; 95% CI = 1.2 to 412). Although postpartum thyroiditis is considered a transient disease, up to 50% of patients have a recurrence in a subsequent pregnancy, and up to 48% have permanent goiter and/or hormonal dysfunction at 3-year follow-up (47).

CASE STUDY

Ms. W., a 28-year-old woman, complains that for several days her neck has been tender and swollen, swallowing is painful, and she's had a low-grade fever. She has not been around anyone with a sore throat and denies a cough, runny nose, anxiety, irritability, irregular menses, weight loss, or hyperdefecation. Her health is generally good, and she receives Depo-Provera injections every 3 months for contraception. A sister was diagnosed with "a thyroid disorder" at age 35 and is on a chronic medication, type unknown.

On examination, Ms. W. is of average build and appears comfortable. Except for a resting pulse of 104, her vital signs are normal. You can easily see a moderate symmetric enlargement of the anterior base of her neck. On palpation the mass is smooth, firm, and slightly tender, without nodules. There is no tracheal deviation or palpable neck adenopathy. Her skin is warm and dry and there is no proptosis, lid lag, or hyperreflexia.

QUESTIONS

1. What should you tell Ms. W. about the cause of her neck soreness?
2. What more serious causes are unlikely based on the history and physical?
3. What laboratory tests should be ordered?
4. What is the best course of treatment for Ms. W., and what is the prognosis?

DISCUSSION

The patient's goiter is obvious, and the history and physical examination suggest acute but mild hyperthyroidism. Thyroid cancer is unlikely because no nodules are felt, the trachea is midline without adenopathy, and the patient is symptomatic. At this point, the differential diagnosis includes subacute granulomatous (De Quervain's) thyroiditis, subacute lymphocytic (Hashimoto's) thyroiditis, Graves' disease, acute suppurative thyroiditis, and toxic multinodular goiter.

The pretest likelihood of thyroid disease is high and you should order a thyroid panel including sTSH and free T_4; a stat CBC with differential to rule out infection; and a sedimentation rate. If the TSH is depressed, hyperthyroidism is confirmed. A markedly elevated sedimentation rate (>50) points toward De Quervain's thyroiditis or infection. If acute infection seems likely, consider fine-needle aspiration and send the aspirate for Gram stain and culture.

If the patient is hyperthyroid, your next step should be a radioactive iodine uptake study (RAI) with scintigraphy (scan). An elevated uptake (>30%) can help rule in Graves' disease or toxic MNG, and the scan pattern can help differentiate be-

tween them. Thyroid receptor antibodies (TRAb), if positive, point toward Graves' disease. Thyroid microsomal antibodies (TMAb) or thyroglobulin antibodies (TgAb) are seen in autoimmune thyroiditis. If the hyperthyroid patient's TSH is mildly depressed, some authorities advise a head computed tomography (CT) scan to rule out a pituitary tumor. However, the tumors are rare, and the use of iodine for imaging may delay the start of ablative radioactive iodine therapy.

Because the patient's main initial complaint is pain, she should be started on nonsteroidal anti-inflammatory agents. One also may consider adding a β blocker or calcium channel blocker to help control hyperthyroid symptoms. Radioactive iodine (^{131}I) ablative therapy is the most commonly used treatment for patients with multinodular goiter or Graves' disease. The ATDs propylthiouracil or methimazole may be preferred in milder cases of Graves' disease, but patients may relapse when medication is stopped.

Ms. W's prognosis will vary, of course, with the nature of her disease. Autoimmune thyroiditis is usually self-limited and resolves spontaneously within 6 months, although permanent hypothyroidism may result in 5% of patients. If the patient receives radioactive ablative therapy for MNG or Graves' disease, there is a substantial risk (50% or greater) of subsequent hypothyroidism requiring lifetime treatment with levothyroxine.

REFERENCES

1. Dolan JG. Thyroid nodules. In: Panzer RJ, Black ER, Griner PF, eds. Diagnostic Strategies for Common Medical Problems, 2nd ed. Philadelphia: American College of Physicians, 1991:385–393.
2. Astakhova LN, Vorontsova TV, Drozd VM. Thyroid nodule pathology in children of the Republic of Belarus following the Chernobyl accident. In: Robbins J, ed. Treatment of Thyroid Cancer in Childhood. Proceedings of a Workshop at NIH, Sept. 10–11, 1992. Bethesda, MD: National Institute of Health, 1994: 35–39.
3. Woeber KA. Cost-effective evaluation of the patient with a thyroid nodule. Surg Clin North America 1995; 75(3):357–363.

4. Smith SA, Gharib H. Thyroid nodule suppression. In: Mazzaferri EL, Bar RS, Kreisberg RA, eds. Advances in Endocrinology and Metabolism, vol. 2. St. Louis: Mosby-Year Book, 1991:107–124.

5. Greenspan FS. The problem of the nodular goiter. Med Clin North Am 1991;75(1):195–209.

6. Delange F, Ermans A-M. Iodine deficiency. In: Braverman LE, Utiger RD, eds. The Thyroid: A Fundamental and Clinical Text., 6th ed. Philadelphia: JB Lippincott, 1991:367–390.

7. Gaiton E. Environmental goitrogens. In: Van Middlesworth L, Givens JR, eds. The Thyroid Gland: Practical Clinical Treatise. Chicago: Mosby-Year Book, 1986:263–280.

8. Singer PA. Thyroiditis. Acute, subacute, and chronic. Med Clin North Am 1991;75(1):61–77.

9. Siminoski K. Does this patient have a goiter? JAMA 1995;273(10):813–819.

10. Berghout A, Wiersinga WM, Drexhage HA, et al. Comparison of placebo with L-thyroxine alone or with carbimazole for treatment of sporadic nontoxic goiter. Lancet 1990;336(8709):193–197.

11. Berghout A, Wiersinga WM, Drexhage HA, et al. The long-term outcome of thyroidectomy for sporadic non-toxic goiter. Clin Endocrinol 1989;31:193–199.

12. Miccoli P, Antonelli A, Iacconi P, et al. Prospective, randomized, double-blind study about effectiveness of levothyroxine suppressive therapy in prevention of recurrence after operation: result at the third year of follow-up. Surgery 1993;114(6):1097–1102.

13. Levy EG. Thyroid disease in the elderly. Med Clin North Am 1991;75(1):151–167.

14. Singer PA, Cooper DS, Levy EG, et al. Treatment guidelines for patients with hyperthyroidism and hypothyroidism. JAMA 1995;273:808–812.

15. Billewicz WZ, Chapman RS, Crooks J, et al. Statistical methods applied to the diagnosis of hypothyroidism. Q J Med 1969;38:255–266.

16. Sexhadri MS, Samuel BU, Kanagasabapathy AS, et al. Clinical scoring system for hypothyroidism: is it useful? J Gen Intern Med 1989;4:490–492.

17. Pittman JG. Evaluation of patients with mildly abnormal thyroid function tests. Am Fam Physician 1996; 54(3):961–966.

18. Bayer MF. Effective laboratory evaluation of thyroid status. Med Clin North Am 1991;75(1):1–26.

19. American Association of Clinical Endocrinologists and the American College of Endocrinology: AACE clinical practice guidelines for the evaluation and treatment of hyperthyroidism and hypothyroidism. Endocrine Pract 1995;1:56–62.

20. Toft AD. Thyroxine therapy. N Engl J Med 1994;331 (30):174–180.

21. Dong BJ, Hauck WW, Gambertoglio JG, et al. Bioequivalence of generic and brand-name levothyroxine products in the treatment of hypothyroidism. JAMA 1997;277:1205–1213.

22. Copeland PM. Two cases of therapeutic failure associated with levothyroxine brand interchange. Ann Pharmacother 1995;29(5):482–485.

23. Comtois R, Faucher L, Lafleche L. Outcome of hypothyroidism caused by Hashimoto's thyroiditis. Arch Intern Med 1995;155(13):1404–1408.

24. Oppenheimer JH, Braverman LE, Toft A, et al. A therapeutic controversy. Thyroid hormone treatment: when and what? J Clin Endocrinol Metab 1995;80(10): 2873–2876.

25. Fish LH, Schwartz HL, Cavanaugh J, et al. Replacement dose, metabolism, and bioavailability of levothyroxine in the treatment of hypothyroidism. Role of triiodothyronine in pituitary feedback in humans. N Engl J Med 1987;316:764–770.

26. Nordyke RA, Gilbert FI Jr, Harada AS. Graves' disease. Influence of age on clinical findings. Arch Intern Med 1988;148:626–631.

27. Crooks J, Murray IPC, Wayne EJ. Statistical methods applied to the clinical diagnosis of thyrotoxicosis. Q J Med 1959;28:211–234.

28. Gurney C, Hall R, Harper M, et al. Newcastle thyrotoxicosis index. Lancet 1970;2:1275–1278.

29. Dolan JG. Hyperthyroidism and hypothyroidism. In: Panzer RJ, Black ER, Griner PF, eds. Diagnostic Strategies for Common Medical Problems, 2nd ed. Philadelphia: American College of Physicians, 1991: 375–384.

30. Char DH. The ophthalmopathy of Graves' disease. Med Clin North Am 1991;75(1):97–119.

31. Ehrmann DA, Sarne DH. Serum thyrotropin and assessment of thyroid status. Ann Intern Med 1989;10: 179–181.

32. Kvetny J, Frederikesen PK, Jacobsen JG, et al. Propranolol in the treatment of thyrotoxicosis. A randomized double-blind study. Acta Med Scand 1981;209(5): 389–392.

33. Mashio Y, Beniko M, Ikota A, et al. Treatment of hyperthyroidism with a small single daily dose of methimazole. Acta Endocrinol (Copenh) 1988;119(1):139–144.

34. Allannic H, Fauchet R, Orgiazzi J, et al. Antithyroid drugs and Graves' disease: a prospective randomized evaluation of the efficacy of treatment duration. J Clin Endocrinol Metab 1990;70(3):675–679.

35. Feldt-Rasmussen U, Schleusener H, Carayon P. Meta-analysis evaluation of the impact of thyrotropin receptor antibodies on long-term remission after medical therapy of Graves' disease. J Clin Endocrinol Metab 1994;78(1):98–102.

36. McIver B, Rae P, Beckett G, et al. Lack of effect of thyroxine in patients with Graves' hyperthyroidism who are treated with an antithyroid drug. N Engl J Med 1996;334(4):220–224.

37. Peters H, Fischer C, Bogner U, et al. Reduction in thyroid volume after radioiodine therapy of Graves' hyperthyroidism: results of a prospective, randomized, multicentre study. Eur J Clin Invest 1996;26(1): 59–63.

38. McDougall IR. Graves' disease. Current concepts. Med Clin North Am 1991;75(1):79–95.

39. Torring O, Tallstedt L, Wallin G, et al. Graves' hyperthyroidism: treatment with antithyroid drugs, surgery, or radioiodine—a prospective, randomized study. Thyroid Study Group. J Clin Endocrinol Metab 1996;81(8): 2986–2993.

40. Kung AW, Yau CC, Cheng A. The incidence of ophthalmopathy after radioiodine therapy for Graves' disease: prognostic factors and the role of methimazole. J Clin Endocrinol Metab 1994;79(2):542–546.

41. Danese MD, Powe NR, Sawin CT, Ladenson PW. Screening for mild thyroid failure at the periodic

health examination. A decision and cost-effectiveness analysis.

42. Rosenthal MJ, Hunt WC, Garry PJ, Goodwin JS. Thyroid failure in the elderly. Microsomal antibodies as discriminant for therapy. JAMA 1987;258:209–213.

43. Cooper DS, Halpern R, Wood LC, et al. *l*-Thyroxine therapy in subclinical hypothyroidism. A double-blind, placebo-controlled trial. Ann Intern Med 1984;101(1):18–24.

44. Fisher DA. Physiologic variations in thyroid hormones: physiological and pathophysiological considerations. Clin Chem 1996;42(10):135–139.

45. Becks GP, Burrow GN. Thyroid disease and pregnancy. Med Clin North Am 1991;75(1):121–147.

46. Solomon BL, Fein HG, Smallridge RC. Usefulness of antimicrosomal antibody titers in the diagnosis and treatment of postpartum thyroiditis. J Fam Pract 1993;36:177–182.

47. Nikolai TF, Turney SL, Roberts RC. Postpartum lymphocytic thyroiditis: prevalence, clinical course, and long-term follow-up. Arch Intern Med 1987;147:221–224.

48. de los Santos ET, Mazzaferri EL. Thyroid function tests. Postgrad Med 1989;85(5):333–352.

42. Vaginitis

BARBARA D. REED

Key Clinical Questions

1. Can the diagnosis of *Candida* vulvovaginitis be made accurately by women themselves or by their physician after a telephone consultation?
2. What symptoms, signs, and laboratory tests best identify women with bacterial vaginosis, *Candida* vulvovaginitis, or *Trichomonas* vaginitis?
3. Other than vaginitis, what are three additional potential diagnoses in a woman complaining of vulvar discomfort?

Vaginal symptoms are very common among postpubertal women seeing their family physicians. These symptoms, although rarely progressive or life-threatening in the acute, symptomatic phase, lead to large health-related costs due to the resulting morbidity, medical expenses, and time taken from work for evaluation and treatment. Data in the past decade indicate that two of the most common vaginal syndromes—bacterial vaginosis (BV) and *Trichomonas* vaginitis (TV)—are associated with adverse pregnancy outcomes and that prompt diagnosis and treatment of these disorders, even in the asymptomatic phase, decreases these complications (1). For the women affected, the associated symptoms are distressing; however, their concerns are often met with insufficient evaluation (historical, physical, or laboratory) to correctly identify the diagnosis and risk factors and to rule out more serious disease.

Nonprescription medication for the self-treatment of *Candida* vulvovaginitis (CVV) has led to self-diagnosis and misdiagnosis. Women presenting to the medical office with vaginal symptoms are now more likely to have already self-diagnosed and possibly self-treated prior to being seen for their symptoms. Therefore, the probability of vaginal symptoms representing a less-common diagnostic entity has increased. The diagnosis of vaginal symptoms has always required a diligent look at differentiating the causal agent(s); it requires this conscientious look now more than ever, with a broad differential diagnostic armamentarium by the physician, to assure appropriate care to the women with these symptoms.

PATHOPHYSIOLOGY AND DIFFERENTIAL DIAGNOSIS

Pathophysiology

Vaginal symptoms such as increased discharge, itching, odor, swelling, or irritation, may present in any woman—partnered or single, sexually active or not, premenopausal or postmenopausal. Although children can present with similar symptoms, these symptoms are less common prior to menarche, and symptoms in the pediatric age groups will not be addressed here.

The normal vaginal milieu consists of clear or white vaginal fluid that on microscopic examination demonstrates desquamated vaginal nonkeratinized epithelial cells. The bacterial flora of the vagina consists predominantly of *Lactobacillus acidophilus*—a gram-positive, facultative long rod—although also present are diphtheroids, *Staphylococcus epidermidis*, γ-hemolytic streptococci, and coliforms. The normal pH is 4.5 or less. White blood cells are not part of the normal vaginal fluid contents; when present, they commonly reflect vaginal or cervical inflammation, although a specific cause cannot always be determined. The presence of copious discharge or discharge that is curd-like, foamy, or discolored suggests vaginal infection, as does a fishy odor of the discharge or swelling of the genital tissues (often identified as shiny, smoother skin in the vestibule or vagina). Erythema of the tissues suggests inflammation or an allergic reaction, and lesions (ulcers, papules, warts, pigmentary changes, dystrophic changes) suggest a nonvaginitis etiology (see below).

Symptoms of vaginal infection reflect alterations in the normal protective vaginal flora, overgrowth of organisms not typically predominant in the vagina (*Gardnerella vaginalis*, *Mobiluncus* anaerobes, *Trichomonas vaginalis*) and/or overgrowth or reactions to organisms occasionally found in the vagina in an asymptomatic state (*Candida* vulvovaginitis). Vaginal symptoms may also be unrelated to vaginal infection, as is the case in entities stemming from neuropathic, dermatologic, or allergic origins, discussed later. Symptoms may be related to an inflammatory reaction, the altered acidity of the vaginal contents, an invasion of organisms into the vaginal lining, or the response of the tissues to toxic byproducts of altered flora or pathologic organisms.

Bacterial Vaginosis

Bacterial vaginosis (BV), the most common infection-causing vaginal syndrome, is present in approximately one-third of women with vaginal symptoms and in 21% or more of all women (regardless of symptoms) (2, 3). The "etiology" of BV is not clearly understood, but women with this entity are more likely to have one or more of the following in the vaginal discharge: *Gardnerella vaginalis* (a facultative gram-variable coccobacillary, or short-rod organism), *Mobiluncus* (an anaerobic, curved gram-variable, motile short rod), *Mycoplasma hominis*, and one or more types of anaerobes such as *Bacteroides* and *Peptostreptococcus*. Furthermore, women with BV have an "abnormal" background flora observed on normal saline microscopic examination, characterized by a lack of long rods typical of lactobacilli and a predominance of short rods, curved rods, or coccobacilli. Data suggest that women lacking lactobacilli in the vagina, or those with H_2O_2-negative lactobacilli, are prone to developing BV (but not *Candida* vulvovaginitis or *Trichomonas* vaginitis) over a 2-year period (4).

Whether BV is sexually transmitted remains controversial, and research is hampered by the lack of a clinical correlate of BV in the male. Treatment trials of women with BV and their male sexual partners show conflicting results (5, 6). However, a study on lesbian women suggests BV concordance among monogamous women partners is high (72.7%) (7). Furthermore, studies suggest BV is associated with an increased risk of other STDs, including *Chlamydia*, *Neisseria gonorrhoeae* (GC), herpes, and syphilis, and with having a new partner.

BV is associated with pregnancy risk as described below. The mechanism is unclear, but data suggest that BV is associated with intraamniotic fluid infection, with infection of the chorioamnion, with elevations in endotoxin, mucinase, sialidase, and interleukin-1α, and

with a decrease in lactobacilli, which is also associated with preterm delivery (8).

Candida Vulvovaginitis

Candida vulvovaginitis (CVV) is present in roughly one-quarter of women with vaginal symptoms. Approximately 20% of women without vaginal symptoms also culture positive for *Candida* species in the vagina, suggesting that not all women respond with symptoms and/or signs when *Candida* is present.

A number of factors are associated with *Candida* vulvovaginitis, such as use of oral contraceptives, use of the contraceptive sponge, use of the IUD or barrier methods, recent use of antibiotics, gastrointestinal carriage of *Candida*, a diet rich in sugars or yeasts, and the presence of diabetes (9). Unfortunately, careful study of the value of these as risk factors suggests that none is consistently associated with symptomatic *Candida* vulvovaginitis (9–12). Information about other risk factors is similarly unclear; data clearly support an association between the presence of *Candida* species in the vagina and presence in the rectum and oral cavity of the woman and in the penis, semen, rectum, and oral cavity of her sexual partner (13, 14), with an association between cunnilingus and *Candida* vulvovaginitis in women as well (15, 16). However, data are lacking to indicate that this colonization or eradication of these other sources of *Candida* is imperative or effective in decreasing recurrences of symptomatic *Candida* vulvovaginitis in the woman (17, 18).

The significance of asymptomatic *Candida* colonization of the vagina, recognized in approximately 20% of women, is unknown; no recommendations for screening or treatment in asymptomatic cases are proposed (12, 19).

Trichomonas Vaginitis

Trichomonas vaginitis (TV) is caused by a flagellated protozoan and is the only cause of vaginitis that is clearly identified as being sexually transmitted. It is more common in women who have had multiple sexual partners or who have recently had a new partner. However, the presence of *Trichomonas vaginalis* may be overlooked for years—by both the patient and her medical provider—and hence this diagnosis does not necessarily imply a recent exposure. Approximately 30% or more of women with *Trichomonas* vaginitis have other STDs (20), and this coinfection may increase the risk of upper genital tract disease (21). Thus, women with *Trichomonas* vaginitis should be routinely tested for STDs that are easily missed (*Chlamydia trachomatis*, cervical changes associated with human papillomavirus [HPV], and *Neisseria gonorrhoeae* in particular).

Differential Diagnosis of Vaginal Symptoms

The most common diagnoses in women with vulvovaginal complaints are

- Bacterial vaginosis, previously called Non-specific vaginitis and *Gardnerella vaginitis*, among other names (33 to 52% of cases)

- *Candida* vulvovaginitis (20 to 25%)

- *Trichomonas* vaginitis (7 to 14%)

Roughly one-third of cases are not caused by any of these three (12, 22). Other diagnoses, including entities not yet characterized, comprise this group.

Less commonly identified, and less often considered, are other possible diagnoses associated with symptoms of "vaginitis," listed in Table 42.1. Although less common in prevalence and incidence, these other entities, described below, may be associated with long-term complications, symptoms, pregnancy risk, or progression that would negatively affect the health and well-being of the woman involved. Treatment is also specific to the diagnosis, so a shotgun approach, although sometimes effective in decreasing the

Table 42.1.

Differential Diagnoses in Women with Vaginal Symptoms

1. Bacterial vaginosis
2. *Candida* vulvovaginitis
3. *Trichomonas* vaginitis
4. Cervicitis
5. Allergic vaginosis
6. Atrophic vaginitis
7. Genital ulcers: herpes simplex, syphilis, and chancroid
8. Lichen sclerosis
9. Lichen planus
10. Lichen chronicus simplex
11. Vulvar intraepithelial neoplasia
12. Pelvic inflammatory disease (PID)
13. Lactobacillosis
14. Vulvodynia or vestibulitis

symptoms, is unlikely to adequately address the problem if the diagnosis is unclear or erroneous.

- **Cervicitis** is often asymptomatic in women, but may result in increased cervical mucous discharge that is described by the woman as "vaginal discharge." This finding should alert the clinician to the possibility of *Chlamydia trachomatis* or *Neisseria gonorrhoeae*. The potential sequelae of cervicitis are reviewed elsewhere (Chapter 36, Sexually Transmitted Diseases), but they include severe pelvic infections (PID), pelvic organ scarring, infertility, and an increased risk of ectopic pregnancy.

- **Vulvodynia** and **vestibulitis** are important vulvar pain syndromes that are often misdiagnosed as recurrent *Candida* vulvovaginitis infections or dermatitis. Important differences include either lack of *Candida* present or lack of response to *Candida* treatment; chronic or recurring vulvar pain (burning, stinging, or rawness) that is associated with touch, tampon insertion, and intercourse; and lack of physical findings other than occasional mild erythema. Scratching does not help these symptoms—evidence of skin changes secondary to scratch suggest other diagnoses such as *Candida* vulvovaginitis or lichen simplex chronicus.

- **Lichen sclerosis et atrophicus** is a chronic dermatologic disease of women of any age; it presents as ivory-white atrophic macules on the vulva with associated atrophy. Biopsy is diagnostic.

- **Lichen planus** is a papular dermatosis consisting of flat, angular, violaceous and scaly papules, associated with itching. Biopsy again makes the diagnosis. This is often self-limited and may heal with hyperpigmentation and atrophy.

- **Lichen simplex chronicus,** or localized neurodermatitis, is characterized by chronic itching and thickened, scaly or dry skin caused by development of a chronic cycle of itching and scratching—often after the initial inciting reason for itching is gone. Excoriations, lichenification, and pigmentary changes may result.

- **Lactobacillosis** is a vaginal syndrome characterized by vaginal discharge and discomfort prior to menses. It is identified by a background flora on normal saline preparation marked by very long filaments, which are lactobacilli that have organized into chains. The reason for this atypical chaining is unknown, but treatment of this disorder with antimicrobials such as amoxicillin/clavulanate results in symptom resolution and clearing of the chaining lactobacilli (23).

- Genital ulcers are usually caused by herpes simplex, syphilis (primary infection), or chancroid. In the case of herpes and chancroid, these are painful and are often mistaken by the woman for a vaginal infection. Any woman with an identified genital ulcer, or in whom a history of a genital ulcer is elicited, should be evaluated for these infections, and directed treatment given.

- **Vulvar intraepithelial neoplasia** may be associated with vulvar itching. Any suspicious lesion of the vulva should be biopsied to rule out malignant or premalignant lesions. Vaginitis per se is not associated with vulvar lesions.

- Allergic vaginosis presents as vaginal itching, discharge, or edema in response to an allergic reaction to a local or systemic allergen. Douches and other topical preparations are common causes. A detailed exposure history is needed for patients with these symptoms who do not have identifiable pathogens suggesting the more common types of vaginitis.

- **Atrophic vaginitis** is typically found in menopausal women who have lower estrogen levels; it may be associated with itching and discharge. White blood cells and parabasal cells are evident on the normal saline microscopic examination. Treatment consists of topical or oral estrogen.

CLINICAL EVALUATION

The clinical evaluation includes taking a careful history and focusing on risk factors for vaginitis and symptoms of other genital problems; performing a physical examination with a pelvic evaluation; performing office laboratory assessment and determining if central laboratory tests are indicated; making a diagnosis, and discussing treatment options. Figure 42.1 summarizes the evaluation of the history and physical examination, which is discussed in more detail in the next section.

History and Physical Examination

Historical and physical examination findings associated with the most common causes of vaginal symptoms are listed in Tables 42.2 and 42.3, along with an estimate of the strength of the factor and the scientific level of the data from which

this was estimated. In general, risk factors may identify a group of women at increased risk for a specific infection and may be useful in implicating the need for studies. However, no factor is pathognomonic of a specific infection, so in caring for individual patients, overreliance on a "risk-factor" may lead to misdiagnosis.

Bacterial Vaginosis (BV)

Women with BV often complain of noticing a "fishy" odor from the vaginal area, and this odor may become accentuated after exposure to semen during intercourse. Although not typical of BV, itching may occur, but it is usually not at as severe as seen in women with *Candida* vulvovaginitis or even *Trichomonas* vaginitis. Approximately one-half of women with BV do not complain of symptoms at all.

On your examination of the patient with BV, you will often note an increased quantity of discharge, which may be creamy white, yellow, green, or gray. Signs of inflammation (marked erythema, swelling of the labia or vagina, or excoriations from scratching) will typically be absent. You also may be aware of a fishy odor, but although this is a common complaint in the history, it is not typically appreciable during the examination.

Candida Vulvovaginitis (CVV)

The classic history of CVV consists of a thick, curd-like, white vaginal discharge with a normal vaginal pH, accompanied by itching and no odor. The majority of women with this diagnosis do not present with these characteristics, however, and women with CVV often have NO discharge obvious on examination or only mild itching. Many women report similar episodes in the past that may or may not have resolved.

The signs of CVV on physical examination range from florid, thick, curd-like white discharge clinging to the vaginal and cervical mucosa with marked erythema of the vaginal and/or vulvar lining and edema of the tissues to a fairly normal-appearing genital examination with minimal discharge in women complaining of vaginal itch. Small sensitive mucosal tears, with a "paper-cut" appearance, occasionally occur on the vulva.

Trichomonas Vaginitis

Women with this diagnosis may complain of increased vaginal discharge, often thin or foamy in texture, and discolored (yellow or gray). Other

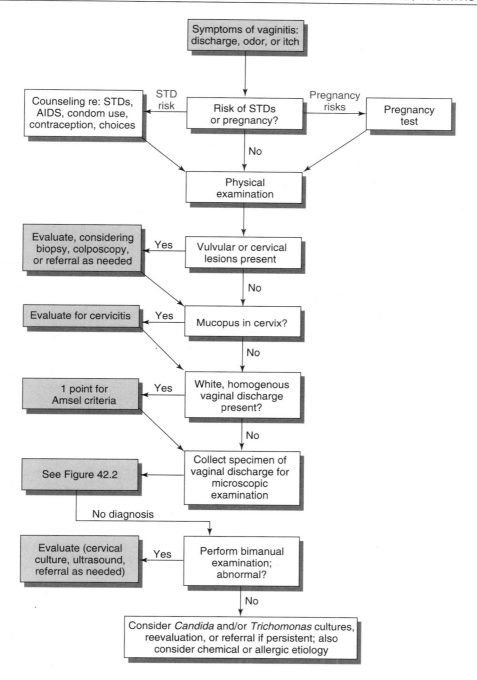

Figure 42.1. *Evaluation of vaginal symptoms: history and physical examination.*

symptoms overlap with the other causes of vaginitis—including itching that may be mild to severe and odor. In severe cases, lower abdominal pain and occasionally fever may be present.

Classically, the discharge of *Trichomonas* vaginitis is copious, thin, discolored (green, gray, tan), and occasionally foamy in consistency. A fishy odor may be appreciated but is not typically

Table 42.2.

Historical Factors Associated with Common Types of Vaginal Infections

Diagnosis	Risk Factor	Strength of Association	Level of Evidence[a]	Limitations and/or References
Bacterial vaginosis	Ever sexually active	Strong	A	100% of BV patients vs. 94% in those without. Limited value clinically.[a]
	Complaints of genital symptoms	Low (<50%)	A	Presence of odor or discolored discharge helpful; absence not useful.[a–c]
	Complaints of odor	Moderate	B	Often noticed after intercourse.
	Has IUD	Moderate	B	19% in BV patients vs. 5% in non-BV patients.[a]
	New sexual partner	Moderate	C	Increased risk with new partner in past 30 days.[d]
	H/O *Trichomonas* infection	Moderate	C	24% in BV vs. 8% in those without.[a]
Candida vulvovaginitis (CVV)	Taking oral contraceptives	Low	A	Not predictive of diagnosis.[b, e, f]
	Recent use of antibiotics	Low	A	Not predictive of diagnosis.[b, e, f]
	Gastrointestinal carriage	Moderate	A	Relationship of treatment to outcome unclear. Oral nystatin had little effect.[h–k]
	Sexual transmission	Moderate	A	Same strain carriage is common.[l–n] Conflicting data on significance.[o–r] Therapy not associated with outcome.
	Genital itching	Moderate	A	Seen in 22% of those without CVV.[e, t, u]
	Receptive oral sex	Moderate	B	Significance unclear.[p, s]
	Pregnancy	Low	B	Low power of study.[e]
	Diabetes	Low	B	Diabetics have increased risk, but few women with CVV have diabetes mellitus (DM).[e]
	Previous H/O CVV in past year	Moderate	B	Rate 17% in controls, 50% in cases.[f]
	Dietary sugars, milk, or yeasts	Low	C	May be a factor in selected women.[g]
	Tight clothes	Low	C	Reported in one study[w]
Trichomonas vaginitis	Presence of other STDs	Moderate	A	30% of women with this had other STDs.[v]
	Multiple sexual partners	Moderate	A	

[a]Level of evidence: A, strong or moderate research-based evidence, consistent across studies; B, limited research-based evidence (less consistent or extensive evidence, but preponderance of evidence supports use of treatment); C, common practice with little or no research-based evidence.

REFERENCES

a. Amsel R, Totten PA, Spiegel CA, Chen KC, Eschenbach D, Holmes KK. Nonspecific vaginitis. Diagnostic criteria and microbial and epidemiologic associations. Am J Med 1983;74(1):14–22.

b. Reed BD, Huck W, Zazove P. Differentiation of *Gardnerella vaginalis, Candida albicans,* and *Trichomonas vaginalis* infections of the vagina. J Fam Pract 1989;28(6):673–680.

c. Eschenbach DA, Hillier S, Critchlow C, Stevens C, DeRouen T, Holmes KK. Diagnosis and clinical manifestations of bacterial vaginosis. Am J Obstet Gynecol 1988;158(4):819–828.

d. Hawes SE, Hillier SL, Benedetti J, et al. Hydrogen peroxide-producing lactobacilli and acquisition of vaginal infections. J Infect Dis 1996;174(5):1058–1063.

e. Abbott J. Clinical and microscopic diagnosis of vaginal yeast infection: a prospective analysis. Ann Emerg Med 1995;25(5):587–591.

f. Geiger AM, Foxman B. Risk factors for vulvovaginal candidiasis: A case-control study among university students. Epidemiology 1996;7:182–187.

continued

Table 42.2. *(continued)*
Historical Factors Associated with Common Types of Vaginal Infections

g. Horowitz BJ, Edelstein SW, Lippman L. Sugar chromatography studies in recurrent *Candida* vulvovaginitis. J Reprod Med 1984;29(7): 441–443.

h. Group NMS. Therapy of candidal vaginitis: The effect of eliminating intestinal *Candida*. Am J Obstet Gynecol 1986;155(3):651–655.

i. Hilton AL, Warnock DW. Vaginal candidiasis and the role of the digestive tract as a source of infection. Br J Obstet Gynaecol 1975;82(11):922–926.

j. Miles MR, Olsen L, Rogers A. Recurrent vaginal candidiasis. Importance of an intestinal reservoir. JAMA 1977;238(17):1836–1837.

k. Davidson F, Mould RF. Recurrent genital candidosis in women and the effect of intermittent prophylactic treatment. Br J Vener Dis 1978;54(3):176–183.

l. Schmid J, Rotman M, Reed B, Pierson CL, Soll DR. Genetic similarity of *Candida albicans* strains from vaginitis patients and their partners. J Clin Microbiol 1993;31(1):39–46.

m. Lockhart SR, Reed BD, Pierson CL, Soll DR. Most frequent scenario for recurrent *Candida* vaginitis is strain maintenance with "substrain shuffling:" demonstration by sequential DNA fingerprinting with probes Ca3, C1, and CARE2. J Clin Microbiol 1996;34(4):767–777.

n. Warnock DW, Speller CD, Milne JD, Hilton AL, Kershaw PI. Epidemiological investigation of patients with vulvovaginal candidosis. Application of a resistogram method for strain differentiation of *Candida albicans*. Br J Vener Dis 1979;55(5):357–361.

o. Horowitz BJ, Edelstein SW, Lippman L. Sexual transmission of *Candida*. Obstet Gynecol 1987;69(6):883–886.

p. Buch A, Christensen ES. Treatment of vaginal candidosis with natamycin and effect of treating the partner at the same time. Acta Obstet Gynecol Scand 1982;61:393–396.

q. Bisschop MP, Merkus JM, Scheygrond H, van Cutsem J. Cotreatment of the male partner in vaginal candidosis: a double- blind randomized control study. Br J Obstet Gynaecol 1986;93(1):79–81.

r. Davidson F. Yeasts and circumcision in the male. Br J Vener Dis 1977;53:121–122.

s. Markos AR, Wade AA, Walzman M. Oral sex and recurrent vulvo-vaginal candidiasis [letter]. Genitourin Med 1992;68(1):61–62.

t. Bertholf ME. Symptom diagnosis of *Candida* vaginitis [letter]. J Fam Pract 1983;17(5):775, 777.

u. McCormack WM, Starko KM, Zinner SH. Symptoms associated with vaginal colonization with yeast. Am J Obstet Gynecol 1988;158(1): 31–33.

v. Reynolds M, Wilson J. Is *Trichomonas* vaginalis still a marker for other sexually transmitted infections in women? Int J STD AIDS 1996;7(2):131–132.

w. Elegbe IA, Elegbe I. Quantitative relationships of *Candida albicans* infections and dressing patterns in Nigerian women. Am J Public Health 1983;73(4):450–452.

noted. In practice, however, the majority of women with *Trichomonas* infection have a nondescript discharge that is white and homogenous, not unlike that characteristic of BV. A "strawberry" cervix is suggestive of *Trichomonas* infection but is an unusual finding.

Diagnostic Criteria

The diagnostic criteria used for bacterial vaginosis, *Candida* vulvovaginitis, and *Trichomonas* vaginitis vary in their dependence on physical examination findings and laboratory testing results.

Table 42.3.
Physical Examination Findings Associated with Common Types of Vaginal Infections

Clinical Entity	Physical Findings	Sensitivity	Specificity	LR+[a]	LR−[a]	References
Bacterial vaginosis	Homogenous discharge	Low (50%)	Moderate (74%)	1.92	0.66	a
	Grey discharge	Low (22%)	High (99%)	22.0	0.78	a
Candida vulvovaginitis	"Typical" discharge	Moderate (61%)	Moderate (62%)	1.6	0.63	b
	Vaginal itching	Moderate (61–75%)	High (78–82%)	2.8–4.2	0.3–0.5	b, c
Trichomonas vaginitis	"Typical" discharge	Low (35%)	Low (50%)	0.7	1.3	a
	Strawberry cervix	Low (2–44%)	High (99%)	2–43	.57–.99	d–f

[a]LR+ is the relative odds of having the infection versus odds of not having the infection if the characteristic is positive; LR− is the relative odds of having the infection versus odds of not having the infection if the characteristic is negative.

REFERENCES
a. Reed BD, Huck W, Zazove P. Differentiation of *Gardnerella vaginalis, Candida albicans,* and *Trichomonas vaginalis* infections of the vagina. J Fam Pract 1989;28(6):673–680.

b. Hopwood V, Crowley T, Horrocks CT, Milne JD, Taylor PK, Warnock DW. Vaginal candidosis: relation between yeast counts and symptoms and clinical signs in nonpregnant women. Genitourin Med 1988;64(5):331–334.

c. McCormack WM, Starko KM, Zinner SH. Symptoms associated with vaginal colonization with yeast. Am J Obstet Gynecol 1988;158 (1):31–33.

d. McLellan R, Spence MR, Brockman M, Raffel L, Smith JL. The clinical diagnosis of trichomoniasis. Obstet Gynecol 1982;60(1):30–34.

e. Fouts AC, Kraus SJ. *Trichomonas vaginalis:* reevaluation of its clinical presentation and laboratory diagnosis. J Infect Dis 1980;141(2): 137–143.

f. Wolner-Hanssen P, Krieger JN, Stevens CE, et al. Clinical manifestations of vaginal trichomoniasis. JAMA 1989;261(4):571–576.

The diagnosis of bacterial vaginosis is made clinically during the office visit and does not require central laboratory confirmation. No culture result, including that of *Gardnerella vaginalis*, is diagnostic of bacterial vaginosis. The Amsel criteria have been used routinely to make this diagnosis over the past decade and correlate well with symptomatology and response to treatment (24). More recent data on the accuracy of the Gram stain diagnosis of BV suggest this may be used as well (25). Table 42.4 summarizes these criteria.

The diagnosis of *Candida* vulvovaginitis in a symptomatic woman is made by identifying the organism—either on the KOH microscopic preparation in the office, by culture (in the office or at a referral laboratory), or by DNA or antigen detection methods. Presence or absence of risk factors and other clinical findings may be suggestive but is inaccurate and can be misleading.

Diagnosing *Trichomonas* vaginitis depends on identifying the organism—either on the normal saline microscopic examination, on culture, or on molecular DNA testing. Identifying *Trichomonas* on a cytology smear (Papanicolaou test) is inaccurate; such a report should prompt reevaluation, not diagnosis and treatment.

Laboratory Tests

Office testing occurs first; if the diagnosis is unclear, central laboratory identification is needed. Data indicate that although office tests exist for diagnosing BV, *Candida* vulvovaginitis, and *Trichomonas* vaginitis, only the minority of cases have a clear diagnosis made by these methods alone (2, 12). Table 42.5 lists the available laboratory tests and their use as first- or second-line evaluations when the diagnosis is uncertain or the patient has persistent symptoms or prompt recurrences. Statistical characteristics are included as are the relative costs.

Office Testing

Figure 42.2 discusses the laboratory assessment of vaginal symptoms.

- pH assessment: To conduct this test, apply a drop or two of vaginal discharge to a small piece of pH paper that changes color in the desired pH range (4.0 to 5.5 is adequate). The pH of vaginal secretions is increased (>4.5) in most cases of bacterial vaginosis and *Trichomonas* vaginitis compared to cases with *Candida* vulvovaginitis, in which the pH is usually normal (≤4.5.)

- Amine test (whiff test): Place a small amount of vaginal discharge on a microscope slide and add a drop or two of 10% KOH (potassium hydroxide) solution. The release of aromatic amines (described as a "fishy" odor) indicates the increased presence of anaerobes. This finding is associated with bacterial vaginosis and *Trichomonas* vaginitis.

- Normal saline (NS) microscopic evaluation: Mix a drop of vaginal discharge with a small amount of nonbacteriostatic normal saline and place the solution on a microscope slide at the time of microscopic evaluation (not at the time of collection). First look for motile *Trichomonas vaginalis*. If at low power you notice motile organisms that are approximately the size of white blood cells (as opposed to sperm,

Table 42.4.
Clinical Criteria Used for Office Diagnosis of Bacterial Vaginosis

Amsel Criteria (Score of 3 or More Considered Positive)[a]	Nugent Criteria: (Score of 7 or More Considered Positive)[b]		
	Lactobacillus Morphotypes	*Gardnerella* and *Bacteroides* spp.	Curved Gram-Variable Rods
1. Homogenous vaginal discharge	4+	0	0
2. Elevated pH of vaginal secretions (>4.5)	3+	1+	1+ or 2+
3. Positive amine (whiff) test	2+	2+	3+ or 4+
4. Clue cells	1+	3+	
	0	4+	

[a]Amsel R, Totten PA, Spiegel CA, Chen KC, Eschenbach D, Holmes KK. Nonspecific vaginitis. Diagnostic criteria and microbial and epidemiologic associations. Am J Med 1983;74(1):14–22.

[b]Wolner-Hanssen P, Krieger JN, Stevens CE, et al. Clinical manifestations of vaginal trichomoniasis. JAMA 1989;261(4):571–576.

Table 42.5.
Diagnostic Tests Used to Diagnose Vaginitis

Clinical Entity	Diagnostic Test	1st Line	2nd Line	Sensitivity	Specificity	LR+[a]	LR−[a]	Relative Cost	References
Bacterial vaginosis	Whiff test	X		Low (29%)	High (95%)	5.8	.75	+	a
	pH > 4.5	X		Moderate to high (72–89%)	Low-moderate (49–73%)	1.4–3.3	.15–.57	+	a (using pH 5), b
	Clue cells present	X		Variable (37–97%)	High (79–92%)	1.8–48.0	.03–.79	+	a–c
	3 or 4 Amsel criteria	X		Moderate 70%	High (94%)	11.7	.32	+	Compared to Gram stain, b
	Abnormal background flora on Gram stain	X	X	High (89–100%)	High (83–97%)	5.2–33	0.1–.13	+	Compared to Amsel criteria; b, c
	Culture—*Gardnerella*		—	Moderate (88%)	Moderate (86%)	6.3	.14	++	d
	PCR—*Gardnerella*		—	High (91–95%)	Low (60–63%)	2.3	.15	+++	e, f
	Proline amino-peptidase assay		X	High (93%)	High (91–93%)	10.3–13.3	.08	++	g
	Cytology—clue cells		X	High (88%)	High (99%)	88	.12	++	c
Candida vulvovaginitis	pH of secretions ≤ 4.5	X		High (82%)	Low (9%)	.90	2	+	h
	KOH prep	X		Low-moderate (22–61%)	Moderate-high (77–94%)	.96–10.2	.41–1.1	+	a, b, i–k
	Candida culture		X	High (93–100%)	High in symptomatic (83%)	5.4	0.1	++	Is the current gold standard; l, m
	Slide latex agglutination		—	Moderate (65–81%)	Moderate-high (59–98%)	1.6–40.4	0.2–0.6	++	j, m–o
	Molecular testing—immunologic or PCR		X	High (75%)	High in symptomatics (96%)	18.8	0.3	++	e
	Cytology		—	Moderate (80%)	High (99+ %)	80.0	0.2	Moderate	p
Trichomonas vaginitis	Normal saline prep	X	—	Low-moderate (37–80%)	High (96–98%)	9.3–40	0.7	+	e, q–t
	Trichomonas culture		X	High (80%)	High (100%)	80.0	0.2	++	u
	Enzyme-linked immunosorbent		X	Moderate (77–93%)	High (98–100%)	38.5–46.5	0.1–0.2	++	s, t

continued

Table 42.5. *(continued)*
Diagnostic Tests Used to Diagnose Vaginitis

Clinical Entity	Diagnostic Test	1st Line	2nd Line	Sensitivity	Specificity	LR+[a]	LR−[a]	Relative Cost	References
	Molecular testing (immunologic, PCR)	—	X	High (90%)	High (94–99%)	15.0–90	0.1	++	e, q, u
	Cytology	—	—	Moderate (64%)	Low (55%)	1.4	0.7	++	v

[a]LR+ is the relative odds of having the infection versus odds of not having the infection if the characteristic/test is positive; LR− is the relative odds of having the infection versus odds of not having the infection if the characteristic/test is negative.

REFERENCES

a. Reed BD, Huck W, Zazove P. Differentiation of *Gardnerella vaginalis*, *Candida albicans*, and *Trichomonas vaginalis* infections of the vagina. J Fam Pract 1989;28(6):673–680.
b. Schwebke JR, Hillier SL, Sobel JD, McGregor JA, Sweet RL. Validity of the vaginal Gram stain for the diagnosis of bacterial vaginosis. Obstet Gynecol 1996;88(4 pt 1):573–576.
c. Platz-Christensen JJ, Larsson PG, Sundstrom E, Wiqvist N. Detection of bacterial vaginosis in wet mount, Papanicolaou-stained vaginal smears and in Gram-stained smears. Acta Obstet Gynecol Scand 1995;74(1):67–70.
d. Cristiano L, Coffetti N, Dalvai G, Lorusso L, Lorenzi M. Bacterial vaginosis: prevalence in outpatients, association with some micro-organisms and laboratory indices. Genitourin Med 1989;65(6):382–387.
e. Ferris DG, Hendrich J, Payne PM, et al. Office laboratory diagnosis of vaginitis. Clinician-performed tests compared with a rapid nucleic acid hybridization test. J Fam Pract 1995;41(6):575–581.
f. van Belkum A, Koeken A, Vandamme P, et al. Development of a species-specific polymerase chain reaction assay for *Gardnerella vaginalis*. Mol Cell Probes 1995;9(3):167–174.
g. Schoonmaker JN, Lunt BD, Lawellin DW, French JI, Hillier SL, McGregor JA. A new proline aminopeptidase assay for diagnosis of bacterial vaginosis. Am J Obstet Gynecol 1991;165(3):737–742.
h. Geiger AM, Foxman B, Sobel JD. Chronic vulvovaginal candidiasis: characteristics of women with *Candida albicans*, *C. glabrata* and no *Candida*. Genitourin Med 1995;71(5):304–307.
i. McCormack WM, Starko KM, Zinner SH. Symptoms associated with vaginal colonization with yeast. Am J Obstet Gynecol 1988;158(1):31–33.
j. Rajakumar R, Lacey CJ, Evans EG, Carney JA. Use of slide latex agglutination test for rapid diagnosis of vaginal candidosis. Genitourin Med 1987;63(3):192–195.
k. Oriel JD, Partridge BM, Denny MJ, Coleman JC. Genital yeast infections. Br Med J 1972;4(843):761–764.
l. Mendel EB, Haberman S, Hall DK. Isolation of *Candida* from clinical specimens Comparative study of Pagano-Levin and Nickerson's culture media. Obstet Gynecol 1960;16(2):180–184.
m. Hopwood V, Warnock DW, Milne JD, Crowley T, Horrocks CT, Taylor PK. Evaluation of a new slide latex agglutination test for diagnosis of vaginal candidosis. Eur J Clin Microbiol 1987;6(4):392–394.
n. Abbott J. Clinical and microscopic diagnosis of vaginal yeast infection: a prospective analysis. Ann Emerg Med 1995;25(5):587–591.
o. Reed BD, Pierson CL. Evaluation of a latex agglutination test for the identification of *Candida* species in vaginal discharge. J Am Board Fam Pract 1992;5(4):375–380.
p. Siapco BJ, Kaplan BJ, Bernstein GS, Moyer DL. Cytodiagnosis of *Candida* organisms in cervical smears. Acta Cytol 1986;30(5):477–480.
q. DeMeo LR, Draper DL, McGregor JA, et al. Evaluation of a deoxyribonucleic acid probe for the detection of *Trichomonas vaginalis* in vaginal secretions. Am J Obstet Gynecol 1996;174(4):1339–1342.
r. Rubino S, Muresu R, Rappelli P, et al. Molecular probe for identification of *Trichomonas vaginalis* DNA. J Clin Microbiol 1991;29(4):702–706.
s. Yule A, Gellan MC, Oriel JD, Ackers JP. Detection of *Trichomonas vaginalis* antigen in women by enzyme immunoassay. J Clin Pathol 1987;40(5):566–568.
t. Watt RM, Philip A, Wos SM, Sam GJ. Rapid assay for immunological detection of *Trichomonas vaginalis* and *Gardnerella vaginalis*. J Clin Microbiol 1986;24(4):551–555.
u. Briselden AM, Hillier SL. Evaluation of affirm VP Microbial Identification Test for *Gardnerella vaginalis* and *Trichomonas vaginalis*. J Clin Microbiol 1994;32(1):148–152.
v. Perl G. Errors in the diagnosis of *Trichomonas vaginalis* infections as observed among 1199 patients. Obstet Gynecol 1972;39(1):7–9.

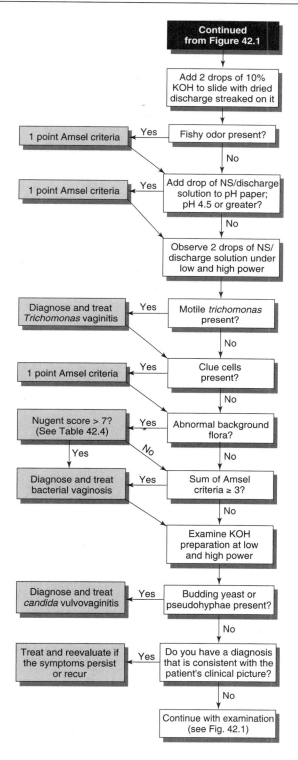

Figure 42.2. *Evaluation of vaginal symptoms: laboratory assessment.*

which are much smaller), use high power to confirm the presence of beating flagella and the typical teardrop yet fluctuating shape of motile *Trichomonas vaginalis.*

Next, assess this NS specimen for the presence of clue cells (epithelial cells covered with bacteria that obscure the typical smooth border of normal epithelial cells), white blood cells, and atypical background flora. Typical background flora consist of epithelial cells with the majority of the cytoplasm appearing clear, with few or no surrounding white blood cells, and with most of the surrounding bacterial flora consisting of long rods. Lack of a long-rod predominance and/or the presence of a large proportion of short rods, cocci, or curved rods suggests an "abnormal background flora," which is independently associated with bacterial vaginosis (see Table 42.5). In women with *Candida* vulvovaginitis or *Trichomonas vaginitis,* white blood cells may be abundant; however, in many (milder) cases they may be present only in low numbers.

- Potassium hydroxide (KOH) microscopic preparation: Perform this test with the same slide used for the amine ("whiff") test—a sample of undiluted vaginal discharge (or swabbing of the moist vaginal walls if no discharge is observed) that you apply directly to a microscope slide. After adding one to two drops of 10% KOH to the slide, perform the whiff test and allow the slide to sit (during examination of the NS prep) for several minutes, after which the slide should be scanned at low power looking for hyphal or budding yeast components, with confirmation by high power. Although budding yeast may occur singly, diagnosis based on single yeast forms is less accurate than that based on the identification of budding yeast forms (two or more forms still connected together while budding) or of pseudohyphae (consisting of branching filaments with budding yeast forms attached along the edge). Although the majority of *Candida* strains causing vulvovaginitis are *C. albicans,* 7 to 16% of cases are associated with *Torulopsis glabrata*—a non-hyphae-forming fungus (26).

Central Laboratory Testing

If your physical examination and office testing fails to clarify the diagnosis, further laboratory information may be required. This will be true in

a sizable proportion of cases. Office tests for *Candida* and *Trichomonas* have low sensitivity (12, 22). The following are useful tests conducted by a central laboratory:

- If cervicitis is suspected, test for *Chlamydia trachomatis* and *Neisseria gonorrhoeae* by culture or by molecular means, including immunologic or DNA identification techniques. The molecular means have the advantage of not requiring viable organisms for diagnosis, hence resulting in easier specimen handling and transport. A specimen taken from the cervical os, including discharge and cells, should be inoculated into specific transport media for these tests. See Chapter 36, Sexually Transmitted Diseases (STDs).

- *Gardnerella* or *Mobiluncus* evaluation: The diagnosis of bacterial vaginosis is based on clinical criteria, such as the Amsel criteria or the abnormal Gram stain (described previously), and no central laboratory confirmation is recommended.

- *Candida* culture: Because 50% of cases of *Candida* vulvovaginitis will have a positive KOH preparation, clearly indicating pseudohyphae or budding yeast forms, an accurate diagnosis may require *Candida* culture. *Candida* culture can be performed by transporting the vaginal specimen in a transport medium used for bacterial specimens, or it may be directly inoculated onto a fungal growth media such as Sabouraud CG or Nickerson's media or placed in Diamond's Media Modified and incubated up to 48 hours. Typical white domed-shaped colonies (2- to 3-mm diameter) on solid agar suggest yeast growth, which can be confirmed by microscopic evaluation of a sample of the growth. Liquid Diamond's Media Modified also can be examined microscopically to determine yeast (or trichomonal) growth (27).

- *Trichomonas* culture: Only half of women with *Trichomonas* infection will have vaginal discharge with enough *Trichomonas* actively swimming on the normal saline preparation to allow an accurate diagnosis. Therefore, a *Trichomonas* culture may be beneficial in women with persistent symptoms. Liquid Diamond's Media Modified can be used for these organisms (28). A small sample of vaginal discharge is inoculated into the liquid (at room temperature), and the medium is incubated at approximately 35°C for 3 to 10 days. A drop from deep in the tube (a more "anaerobic" environment) can be removed for microscopic evaluation daily or every few days.

- Molecular testing for *Candida* species or *Trichomonas vaginalis:* Molecular tests are becoming available for identifying *Trichomonas vaginalis, Gardnerella vaginalis,* and *Candida* species, including immunologic tests such as direct immunofluorescence or enzyme immunoassay and DNA identification using DNA probes. All suggest a higher sensitivity than obtained with wet smear alone. A DNA-probe test for *Trichomonas vaginalis* (Affirm VP Microbial Identification Test) suggests 80 to 90% sensitivity and 99.8 to 100% specificity compared to culture in women with high numbers of organisms present (29, 30). *Gardnerella vaginalis* can also be identified by this test. This closely reflects the data obtained by clue cell evaluation microscopically, suggesting this might serve as a surrogate test for clue cell evaluation (30).

- Cytology smear (Papanicolaou) diagnosis of genital infections: Diagnoses reported on cytology examinations can be helpful in some cases (*Candida* infection) but are less accurate with others (*Trichomonas vaginalis* or *Chlamydia trachomatis* infection). The presence of budding yeast forms or pseudohyphae on cytology indicates yeast, but the absence of such findings cannot rule out this infection, owing to a sensitivity of only 80% (31).

Self-Diagnosis of *Candida* Vulvovaginitis by Women

Over-the-counter antifungal medication is now available for the treatment of *Candida* vulvovaginitis. This availability implies to women that they should be able to self-diagnose for this disorder and treat themselves without risk. As indicated previously, the diagnosis of *Candida* vulvovaginitis is often unclear, and even the "classic" symptoms are not always predictive of this entity. Data clearly indicate that women with and without a previous history of *Candida* vulvovaginitis are inaccurate in diagnosing a "classic case" of *Candida* vulvovaginitis (34% and 11% accurate, respectively), and that women with a prior history of CVV are more likely to diagnose CVV in cases of PID, BV, UTI, and *Trichomonas* vaginitis than were those without such a history. This suggests that inappropriate self-treatment is likely to occur

should those symptoms arise (32). This poor diagnostic accuracy is expected in light of the high proportion of cases of *Candida* vulvovaginitis that are not "classic" in symptoms and presentation and is congruent with the data indicating that physicians cannot make the diagnosis in the majority of cases using history alone (2).

MANAGEMENT

Protocols for treating acute bacterial vaginosis, *Candida* vulvovaginitis, and *Trichomonas* vaginitis are listed in Table 42.6, and adverse effects noted from these therapies (Table 42.7) are listed in the following sections.

Treatment for Bacterial Vaginosis

Treatment for acute bacterial vaginosis consists primarily of metronidazole or clindamycin, either intravaginally or orally. Several other regimens have also been suggested (see Table 42.6). The efficacy of treatment for these entities is good ($\geq$ 80%) when an accurate diagnosis is made. Meta-analysis of the data on oral metronidazole regimens for the treatment of BV suggests that a 2-g stat dose is as effective as the 500-mg twice-daily dose for 7 days, although recurrences may be slightly higher (33, 34).

Recurrent infection and persistence of BV can occur with any of the regimens and has been noted in as many as one-third of women within 1 to 3 months of therapy (35). All cases of recurrent or persistent infection should be evaluated for other diagnoses (such as *Candida* vulvovaginitis), because multiple diagnoses occur commonly in women with recurrent disease. *Mobiluncus* species, recognized as curved rods on the normal saline preparation in some women with BV, may be less susceptible to metronidazole than to clindamycin; hence, this may direct original therapy or therapy for recurrences. Other recommendations for treatment of recurrent BV have been made, including prolonged courses (14 days minimum) of the oral or intravaginal metronidazole or clindamycin regimens or of amoxicillin/clavulanate 500 mg by mouth three times daily, with continuation until the microscopic examination normalizes (lack of clue cells and curved rods) (36). This prolonged course is based on data suggesting relapse is related to a failure of the normalization of the vaginal ecosystem as reflected in a persistently abnormal background flora (37). The reestablishment of a lactobacilli-predominant

Table 42.6.
Treatment for Bacterial Vaginosis, Candida Vulvovaginitis, and Trichomonas Vaginitis

Clinical Entity	Medication	Strength	Dosage	Efficacy	OTC	Cost to the Patient ($)[a]
Bacterial vaginosis	Metronidazole	500-mg tablet	1 PO bid × 7 days, or 2 g PO stat	87–97%	No	6.33
	Clindamycin	2% vaginal cream	1 applicatorful in vagina q hs × 7 days	72–94%	No	33.85
	Metronidazole	0.75% vaginal gel	5 g in vagina bid × 5 days	79% at 2 weeks	No	31.74
	Clindamycin	300-mg tablets	1 PO bid × 7–14 days	94%	No	36.99–73.98
Resistant or recurrent cases	Acute regimens above	See above	Extend the course to 14 days	Little data available	No	—
	Povidone-iodine gel or suppositories	5 g	In vagina bid × 14–28 days	No data found	No	27.22
Candida vulvovaginitis	Miconazole	200-mg suppository	1 q hs × 3 days		Yes	28.83
		2% vaginal cream	1 applicatorful in vagina q hs × 7 days	66%	Yes	13.92
		100-mg vaginal suppository	1 in vagina q hs × 7 days		Yes	13.92
	Clotrimazole	100-mg suppository	1 in vagina q hs × 7 days	52–72% long-term clinical or microbiologic	Yes	13.00
		1% vaginal cream	1 applicatorful in vagina q hs × 7 days		Yes	13.00
		500-mg suppository	1 in vagina once	72–77% short term and 50–65% long term	No	13.88
	Butoconazole	2% vaginal cream	1 applicatorful in vagina q hs × 3 days	81–92%; may be useful in non-*C. albicans* species	Yes	15.57
	Terconazole	80-mg suppository	1 in vagina q hs × 3 days	See below	No	27.88
		0.8% vaginal cream	1 applicatorful in vagina q hs × 3 days	In vitro, less effective in non-*C. albicans*	No	27.88
		0.4% vaginal cream	1 applicatorful in vagina q hs × 7 days	See above	No	27.88
	Tioconazole	6.5% vaginal ointment	1 applicatorful in vagina once	Note: ointment base will melt or dissolve condoms! Avoid intercourse with condoms for 3 days after use.	Yes	27.00

	Drug	Formulation/Dose	Regimen	Efficacy	Generic/OTC	Cost
	Fluconazole	150-mg tablet	1 tablet orally once	56%–98%	No	27.00
	Itraconazole	100-mg tablet	2 tablets PO qd × 3 days	74–85% short term and 51–85% long term	No	36.83
Persistent or recurrent cases	Topical treatments above	See above	Prolong the course to 14–21 days	—	Varies	See above
	Oral regimens above	See above	Extended dosing regimens are being studied	No data available	No	See above
	Boric acid	600 mg in vaginal suppository	1 intravaginally bid for 14 days	Limited data, but anecdotal reports common	No	14.00
Maintenance regimens for recurrent disease	Miconazole	100-mg suppository	2 times/week	No data found	No	84.99/month (9 suppositories)
	Terconazole	0.8% vaginal cream	Weekly applicatorful intravaginally	Decreased to 4 episodes per 10 women over 6 months	No	41.85/month
	Fluconazole or itraconazole	No data available	—	No data available	No	—
	Oral yogurt	Culture positive (10⁸/mL) for H₂O₂-producing lactobacilli	240 g (8 oz) daily	0.38 episodes/6 months compared to 2.54 for placebo	Yes	30/month
Trichomonas vaginitis	Metronidazole	500 mg	4 tablets PO once for patient and partner(s)	80–96%	No	3.95/person
	Metronidazole	500 mg	1 tablet PO bid × 7 days	May add intravaginal gel as adjunct	No	6.33
Resistant or recurrent cases	Metronidazole	500 mg	Prolong the course to bid 14 or 21 days, and/or increase the dosage to as high as 1500 mg bid	Unknown	No	12.88–18.99
	Adjuncts to metronidazole above	Acetic acid vaginal wash 3% or 10% solution povidone-iodine douche	2 times/week. Twice a day for 4 days repeated in 2 weeks or 28 day course	92% response to a 28-day course of povidone-iodine suppositories	Yes	11.71

[a]Data on prices as of May, 1997 provided by Gary Brion, R.Ph., at Seaway Foodtown Pharmacy, Milan, MI.

Table 42.7.
Adverse Effects of Commonly Used Medications for Vaginitis

Medication	Adverse Effect	Miscellaneous
Metronidazole—oral[a, b]	Antabuse effect with alcohol	Common if exposed to alcohol; preventable
	Gastrointestinal upset	Moderately common (10–20%)
	Metallic taste	Moderately common
	Neurologic symptoms, including headache	Rare (<10%)
	Allergic reactions	Rare (<5%)
	Candida vulvovaginitis	17–25% within 1 month
Metronidazole—intravaginal[c]	Gastrointestinal upset	Up to 30% with intravaginal application
	Candida vulvovaginitis	In 3–15%
Clindamycin—oral[b]	Gastrointestinal upset	Approximately 10%
	Rash	Rare (<5%)
Clindamycin—intravaginal[d, e]	*Candida* vulvovaginitis	Approximately 10%
	Gastrointestinal symptoms	Approximately 10%
Intravaginal antimycotics[f–h]	Contact irritation or allergy	Unclear—low (3–7%)
	Headache	Low (9%)
	Abdominal pain	Low (3%)
	Pain on insertion	Low (2%)
Oral antimycotics[i]	Liver toxicity	Low with ketoconazole (1–10%) but serious in 1 of 15,000 women; less common with fluconazole (5% when treated for skin disease) and itraconazole (0.9%), and with short courses of therapy
	Gastrointestinal upset	5% with fluconazole; 7–10% with itraconazole
	Headache	1.5–12% for fluconazole
	Abdominal pain	7% for fluconazole
	Nausea	4% for fluconazole
	Anaphylaxis	Rare
	Interaction with other medications: Alterations in serum levels of other drugs taken concomitantly	Moderate: warfarin, oral hypoglycemics, cyclosporine, phenytoin, rifampin, theophylline
	Cardiac arrhythmias	Rare, but serious with terfenadine or astemizole

[a]Borin MT, Powley GW, Tackwell KR, Batts DH. Absorption of clindamycin after intravaginal application of clindamycin phosphate 2% cream. J Antimicrob Chemother 1995;35(6):833–841.

[b]Greaves WL, Chungafung J, Morris B, Haile A, Townsend JL. Clindamycin versus metronidazole in the treatment of bacterial vaginosis. Obstet Gynecol 1988;72(5):799–802.

[c]Sobel JD, Walter C, Thomason J, et al. Comparative study of intravaginal metronidazole and triple-sulfa therapy for bacterial vaginosis. Infect Dis Obstet Gynecol 1996;4:66–70.

[d]Schmitt C, Sobel JD, Meriwether C. Bacterial vaginosis: treatment with clindamycin cream versus oral metronidazole. Obstet Gynecol 1992;79(6):1020–1023.

[e]Hillier S, Krohn MA, Watts DH, Wolner-Hanssen P, Eschenbach D. Microbiologic efficacy of intravaginal clindamycin cream for the treatment of bacterial vaginosis. Obstet Gynecol 1990;76(3 pt 1):407–413.

[f]Sobel JD, Brooker D, Stein GE, et al. Single oral dose fluconazole compared with conventional clotrimazole topical therapy of *Candida* vaginitis. Am J Obstet Gynecol 1995;172(4 pt 1):1263–1268.

[g]Anonymous. A comparison of single-dose oral fluconazole with 3-day intravaginal clotrimazole in the treatment of vaginal candidiasis. Report of an international multicentre trial. Br J Obstet Gynaecol 1989;96(2):226–232.

[h]Adamson GD. Three-day treatment of vulvovaginal candidiasis. Am J Obstet Gynecol 1988;158(4):1002–1005.

[i]Faro S. Systemic vs. topical therapy for the treatment of vulvovaginal candidiasis [review article]. Infect Dis Obstet Gynecol 1994;1:202–208.

vaginal milieu may be delayed following treatment due to the potential effect of clindamycin or amoxicillin/clavulanate on this organism. Whether direct attempts to recolonize H_2O_2-producing *Lactobacillus acidophilus* in the vagina (by douching with yogurt or sweet acidophilus milk) will help prevent recurrent BV is unknown at this time, although preliminary studies suggest this may be a useful adjunct to antimicrobial therapy (38).

Treatment of sexual partners of women with BV is controversial and has not been consistently shown to reduce recurrences. You may wish to consider this in cases of recurrent BV (6, 39).

Treatment of BV in pregnancy is recommended, to reduce the risk of spontaneous abortion prior to 22 weeks of gestation (RR 3.1), preterm birth (RR 1.9) and premature rupture of membranes (RR 3.5) associated with this infection (1). The use of oral clindamycin, 300 mg by mouth twice daily for 7 days early in pregnancy, or of metronidazole, 250 mg by mouth three times daily for 7 days (40), or a combination of metronidazole and erythromycin has been associated with a 50% decrease in the risk of preterm birth (40, 41) and premature rupture of membranes (40). Intravaginal clindamycin during pregnancy resolves vaginal findings of BV, but it does not decrease rates of preterm birth or low birth weight (42). Concerns regarding the safety of metronidazole during early pregnancy may have resulted in less use of this medication for treating BV (or trichomonas infection) during pregnancy; however, a recent meta-analysis revealed no increased teratogenic risk when used in the first trimester (43), and human studies have failed to suggest increased rates of cancer or mutagenesis (44). Because BV is associated with a history of second-trimester pregnancy loss, treatment prior to pregnancy or in the early first trimester may have additional benefits, and women should be screened at their first prenatal visits and treated for BV regardless of the presence of symptoms. Women should then be reevaluated for cure and re-treated if needed. The value of screening and treating nonpregnant women with BV is unproven but may be considered during pelvic examinations of women of childbearing potential.

Adverse effects of metronidazole and clindamycin given orally and intravaginally are listed in Table 42.7. Intravaginal use of metronidazole and clindamycin is associated with low amounts of systemic absorption (2 to 5% bioavailability of clindamycin) (45), but it increases the risk of *Candida* vulvovaginitis following treatment.

Treatment of *Candida* Vulvovaginitis

Treatment options for acute Candida vulvovaginitis are numerous; several of these medications are now available over-the-counter, with all oral medications and a few intravaginal preparations requiring prescription (see Table 42.6). Clinical improvement and microbiologic response to topical and oral agents are comparable.

Treatment of *Candida* vulvovaginitis in pregnancy is often provided to decrease symptoms. Data on the use of topical antifungal agents in pregnant patients with *Candida* vulvovaginitis are available for miconazole and clotrimazole, with 6- to 7-day protocols resulting in high cure rates without a demonstrated risk to the pregnancy (46). Data on butoconazole and terconazole use in pregnancy are lacking.

Resistant or recurrent cases (be sure the diagnosis is correct!), such as those seen with *Torulopsis glabrata* and *Candida tropicalis* infection as well as many with *Candida albicans*, may respond to boric acid suppositories (47) or to the less commonly used oral antimycotics such as itraconazole (48) or flucytosine orally or topically (26, 49). The role of *Candida* allergy in recurrent *Candida* vulvovaginitis remains incompletely studied, and at this time immunotherapy for women with recurrent disease is experimental.

Maintenance therapy with antifungal topical and oral regimens for recurrent *Candida* vulvovaginitis decreases the frequency of recurrence. Monthly maintenance treatment with clotrimazole suppositories and cream on days 5 through 11 of the menstrual cycle resulted in decreased symptomatic recurrences, although recolonization with *Candida* species was not prevented (46, 50). Monthly use of a clotrimazole 500-mg suppository on the last day of menses or the use of the suppository at the outset of any symptoms have been used, with fewer recurrences (2.2 versus 3.7 episodes per patient in 6 months) but more medication used (7.3 versus 3.6 suppositories/patient) when compared to symptomatic treatment (51). The women enrolled preferred use when symptomatic, however, which was also most cost-effective. Weekly use of 0.8% terconazole cream intravaginally resulted in a low rate of recurrent CVV (14% over 6 months), but the rate of recurrence following discontinuation was high (78%) (52). Sobel et al. evaluated the use *prophylaxis*

of 400 mg oral ketoconazole 5 days per month starting at the time of menses or ketoconazole 100 mg daily for 6 months and found recurrence rates were decreased during prophylaxis (38 to 42%) compared to women given placebo (72%) (53). The value of oral ingestion of yogurt containing H_2O_2-producing *Lactobacillus acidophilus* in decreasing *Candida* vulvovaginitis recurrences is unclear. One study suggests a marked reduction in recurrences when eating 8 oz. of such yogurt daily (54); however, another study suggested little benefit (55). Studies on maintenance regimens of other oral agents, such as fluconazole, for the prevention of recurrent *Candida* vulvovaginitis are underway.

Patient preference regarding treatment options for *Candida* vulvovaginitis suggests that women with a previous history of CVV select oral treatment preferentially to topical (47%), as do those without such a history (65%), but physicians prefer topical treatment (77%) (56). Women with a history of CVV prefer short courses of treatment (1 day) compared to longer treatments, whereas physicians (56) and women without a history of CVV (57) preferred longer therapies.

Adverse effects of topical antifungal agents (Table 42.7) include contact irritation or allergic reactions (3% in one study) (58)—sometimes misdiagnosed as recurrent CVV owing to similarity to the vaginitis symptoms—and less commonly headache (9%), abdominal pain (3%), and pain on insertion (2%) (59). Terconazole has occasionally been associated with a flu-like illness. Early oral agents, including ketoconazole, were associated with liver toxicity; however, this is less likely with fluconazole (60) and itraconazole (48). Common adverse effects in patients treated with fluconazole are headache (1.5 to 12%), abdominal pain (4 to 7%), and nausea (1 to 4%) (58 to 60). In addition, drug interactions exist between fluconazole and a number of other medications, including but not limited to astemizole, caffeine, Coumadin, cyclosporine, oral hypoglycemics, phenytoin, rifampin, terfenadine, and theophylline, making the necessity of appropriate use and avoidance of concomitant use of these drugs imperative (61). Itraconazole has been associated with a low rate of adverse reactions (1.9 to 15%) (48, 62) and hepatic injury (48).

"Risk factor" modification in women with *Candida* vulvovaginitis may be of value in individual women but has not been shown to be efficacious in general; hence, it is not generally recommended. In women with recurrent disease not responsive to other measures or women who are interested in alternatives to medication, you can try dietary changes (decreasing intake of dairy products, artificial sweeteners, and sucrose), oral contraception discontinuation, or periodic intravaginal yogurt ingestion. Only clear reduction in recurrence should result in regimen continuation beyond a 3- to 4-month trial.

Treatment of *Trichomonas* Vaginitis

The treatment of *Trichomonas* vaginitis consists of one option: oral metronidazole—the only antimicrobial found to be effective in eradicating the organism. Management of persistent or recurrent *Trichomonas* vaginitis consists of higher doses of this medication for prolonged periods of time or combines topical and oral delivery. For patients allergic to this medication, in-hospital desensitization has been performed with good results and should be considered in symptomatic women and those who may become pregnant. Case reports of women successfully treated with povidone-iodine douches or pessaries suggest this may be tried in nonpregnant women who are nonresponsive to metronidazole regimens. Treatment of all sexual partners of women with *Trichomonas* vaginitis is clearly indicated because *Trichomonas* is sexually transmitted in the majority of cases. Adverse effects of oral metronidazole are listed in Table 42.7. Pregnant women with *Trichomonas* vaginitis can be treated with metronidazole (see previous discussion of treatment of BV with metronidazole during pregnancy). Lactating women should take 2 g of metronidazole for *Trichomonas* vaginitis and discontinue breast-feeding for 24 hours.

Patient Education

Your patients with vaginal symptoms need to know the limitations of diagnosis without examination and laboratory assessment so that if they find that their symptoms persist or recur soon after treatment, they will return for a follow-up evaluation. The risks and benefits of a treatment trial (OTC or prescription) should be discussed if the patient is opting to self-treat or if you have seen the patient and cannot microscopically confirm a suspected diagnosis.

No telephone diagnosis or prescription therapy should be given unless there have been previous documentation of **recurrent** *Candida* vulvovaginitis by laboratory (KOH and/or culture) and clear discussion of the limitations of this diagnostic method (even in the case of recurrent symptoms). Recurrent bacterial vaginosis and *Trichomonas* vaginitis should be reevaluated in the office to rule out coexistent infection or CVV (which is a recognized adverse effect of the treatments used).

In women with recurrent vaginal symptoms, you should review the following:

- Symptoms that are NOT associated with *Candida* vulvovaginitis: discolored discharge, pelvic pain, abnormal bleeding, and vaginal odor.
- Symptoms that are more suggestive of *Candida* vulvovaginitis: genital itching, vulvar swelling or redness, and a white, nonodorous discharge.

CASE STUDY

Mrs. Conrad is a 25-year-old woman, married for 6 months, who calls in to request treatment for her "yeast infection." She has noted increased discharge for the past 2 weeks that is white with a faint yellow tinge, and she has mild vulvar itching. She had a yeast infection 2 years earlier that she self-treated and her symptoms resolved, but she wants to get a prescription medication this time so that it will be covered by her insurance. Mrs. Conrad is on oral contraceptives, smokes 1/2 pack per day, and is not diabetic.

QUESTIONS

1. How likely is the diagnosis of *Candida* vulvovaginitis in this woman?
2. Does her use of oral contraceptives and her previous response to OTC antifungals make you more certain of her current diagnosis?
3. Should she be encouraged to try OTC antifungals and come into the office if her symptoms persist?

DISCUSSION

Women and medical providers are quick to make the diagnosis of *Candida* vulvo-

vaginitis when vaginal discharge is present. However, more common in sexually active women is the diagnosis of bacterial vaginosis. This is the case even in the presence of commonly perceived "risk factors" for *Candida* infection, including the use of oral contraceptives or being pregnant. Nevertheless, women can obtain treatment for CVV over-the-counter, and many will self-treat for presumed CVV when a discharge occurs. Our responsibility as their health professionals is to be sure the woman is aware of the inaccuracy of diagnosing vaginitis based on symptoms alone and that symptoms may improve with antifungal creams even when the diagnosis is something other than CVV. We should reiterate that the patient is welcome and encouraged to come to the office for a more definitive evaluation and discussion. If, however, the woman chooses to self-treat with OTC antifungals for a presumed *Candida* infection, she should be encouraged to come in if the symptoms persist or recur (within the next 2 months or so). If she has pelvic pain, fever, discolored discharge, vaginal odor, or any visible lesions, she should be informed of the likelihood of another diagnosis and should be cautioned against self-treatment.

REFERENCES

1. McGregor JA, French JI, Parker R, et al. Prevention of premature birth by screening and treatment for common genital tract infections: results of a prospective controlled evaluation. Am J Obstet Gynecol 1995;173 (1):157–167.
2. Berg AO, Heidrich FE, Fihn SD, et al. Establishing the cause of genitourinary symptoms in women in a family practice. Comparison of clinical examination and comprehensive microbiology. JAMA 1984;251(5):620–625.
3. Hillier SL, Krohn MA, Nugent RP, Gibbs RS. Characteristics of three vaginal flora patterns assessed by Gram stain among pregnant women. Vaginal Infections and Prematurity Study Group. Am J Obstet Gynecol 1992;166(3):938–944.
4. Hawes SE, Hillier SL, Benedetti J, et al. Hydrogen peroxide-producing lactobacilli and acquisition of vaginal infections. J Infect Dis 1996;174(5):1058–1063.
5. Vejtorp M, Bollerup AC, Vejtorp L, et al. Bacterial vaginosis: a double-blind randomized trial of the effect of treatment of the sexual partner. Br J Obstet Gynaecol 1988;95(9):920–926.

6. Mengel MB, Berg AO, Weaver CH, et al. The effectiveness of single-dose metronidazole therapy for patients and their partners with bacterial vaginosis. J Fam Pract 1989;28(2):163–171.

7. Berger BJ, Kolton S, Zenilman JM, Cummings MC, Feldman J, McCormack WM. Bacterial vaginosis in lesbians: a sexually transmitted disease. Clin Infect Dis 1995;21(6):1402–1405.

8. Hillier SL, Nugent RP, Eschenbach DA, et al. Association between bacterial vaginosis and preterm delivery of a low-birth-weight infant. The Vaginal Infections and Prematurity Study Group. N Engl J Med 1995;333 (26):1737–1742.

9. Reed BD. Risk factors for *Candida* vulvovaginitis. Obstet Gynecol Surv 1992;47(8):551–560.

10. Abbott J. Clinical and microscopic diagnosis of vaginal yeast infection: a prospective analysis. Ann Emerg Med 1995;25(5):587–591.

11. Leegaard M. The incidence of *Candida albicans* in the vagina of "healthy young women." How often do they have symptoms? Possible etiologic factors. Acta Obstet Gynecol Scand 1984;63(1):85–89.

12. Reed BD, Huck W, Zazove P. Differentiation of *Gardnerella vaginalis*, *Candida albicans*, and *Trichomonas vaginalis* infections of the vagina. J Fam Pract 1989;28(6): 673–680.

13. Horowitz BJ, Edelstein SW, Lippman L. Sexual transmission of *Candida*. Obstet Gynecol 1987;69(6): 883–886.

14. O'Connor MI, Sobel JD. Epidemiology of recurrent vulvovaginal candidiasis: identification and strain differentiation of *Candida albicans*. J Infect Dis 1986;154(2): 358–363.

15. Hellberg D, Zdolsek B, Nilsson S, Mardh PA. Sexual behavior of women with repeated episodes of vulvovaginal candidiasis. Eur J Epidemiol 1995;11(5): 575–579.

16. Geiger AM, Foxman B. Risk factors for vulvovaginal candidiasis: A case-control study among university students. Epidemiology 1996;7:182–187.

17. Buch A, Christensen ES. Treatment of vaginal candidosis with natamycin and effect of treating the partner at the same time. Acta Obstet Gynecol Scand 1982;61: 393–396.

18. Bisschop MP, Merkus JM, Scheygrond H, van Cutsem J. Co-treatment of the male partner in vaginal candidosis: a double-blind randomized control study. Br J Obstet Gynaecol 1986;93(1):79–81.

19. Bro F. The diagnosis of *Candida* vaginitis in general practice. Scand J Prim Health Care 1989;7(1):19–22.

20. Reynolds M, Wilson J. Is *Trichomonas vaginalis* still a marker for other sexually transmitted infections in women? Int J STD AIDS 1996;7(2):131–132.

21. Paisarntantiwong R, Brockmann S, Clarke L, Landesman S, Feldman J, Minkoff H. The relationship of vaginal trichomoniasis and pelvic inflammatory disease among women colonized with *Chlamydia trachomatis*. Sex Transm Dis 1995;22(6):344–347.

22. Ferris DG, Hendrich J, Payne PM, et al. Office laboratory diagnosis of vaginitis. Clinician-performed tests compared with a rapid nucleic acid hybridization test. J Fam Pract 1995;41(6):575–581.

23. Horowitz BJ, Mardh PA, Nagy E, Rank EL. Vaginal lactobacillosis. Am J Obstet Gynecol 1994;170(3):857–861.

24. Amsel R, Totten PA, Spiegel CA, Chen KC, Eschenbach D, Holmes KK. Nonspecific vaginitis. Diagnostic criteria and microbial and epidemiologic associations. Am J Med 1983;74(1):14–22.

25. Nugent RP, Krohn MA, Hiller SL. Reliability of diagnosing bacterial vaginosis is improved by a standardized method of Gram stain interpretation. J Clin Microbiol 1991;29(2):297–301.

26. Redondo-Lopez V, Lynch M, Schmitt C, Cook R, Sobel J. *Torulopsis glabrata* vaginitis: clinical aspects and susceptibility to antifungal agents. Obstet Gynecol 1990; 76(4):651–655.

27. Eyler A PC, Reed BD. Improved diagnosis of *Candida* vulvovaginitis using Diamond's Media Modified. J Womens Health 1996;5(1):79–84.

28. Gelbart SM, Thomason JL, Osypowski PJ, Kellett AV, James JA, Broekhuizen FF. Growth of *Trichomonas vaginalis* in commercial culture media. J Clin Microbiol 1990;28(5):962–964.

29. DeMeo LR, Draper DL, McGregor JA, et al. Evaluation of a deoxyribonucleic acid probe for the detection of *Trichomonas vaginalis* in vaginal secretions. Am J Obstet Gynecol 1996;174(4):1339–1342.

30. Briselden AM, Hillier SL. Evaluation of affirm VP Microbial Identification Test for *Gardnerella vaginalis* and *Trichomonas vaginalis*. J Clin Microbiol 1994;32(1): 148–152.

31. Siapco BJ, Kaplan BJ, Bernstein GS, Moyer DL. Cytodiagnosis of *Candida* organisms in cervical smears. Acta Cytol 1986;30(5):477–480.

32. Ferris DG, Dekle C, Litaker MS. Women's use of over-the-counter antifungal medications for gynecologic symptoms. J Fam Pract 1996;42(6):595–600.

33. Lugo-Miro VI, Green M, Mazur L. Comparison of different metronidazole therapeutic regimens for bacterial vaginosis. A meta-analysis. JAMA 1992;268(1):92–95.

34. Lossick JG. Treatment of sexually transmitted vaginosis/ vaginitis. Rev Infect Dis 1990;12 Suppl 6:S665–S681.

35. Sobel JD, Schmitt C, Meriwether C. Long-term follow-up of patients with bacterial vaginosis treated with oral metronidazole and topical clindamycin [letter]. J Infect Dis 1993;167(3):783–784.

36. Soper DE. Bacterial vaginosis and trichomoniasis: epidemiology and management of recurrent disease. Infect Dis Obstet Gynecol 1995;2:242–247.

37. Cook RL, Redondo-Lopez V, Schmitt C, Meriwether C, Sobel JD. Clinical, microbiologic, and biochemical factors in recurrent bacterial vaginosis. J Clin Microbiol 1992;30(4):870–877.

38. Hallen A, Jarstrand C, Pahlson C. Treatment of bacterial vaginosis with lactobacilli. Sex Transm Dis 1992; 19(3):146–148.

39. Piot P. Bacterial vaginosis. An evaluation of treatment. Scand J Urol Nephrol Suppl 1984;86:229–235.

40. Morales WJ, Schorr S, Albritton J. Effect of metronidazole in patients with preterm birth in preceding pregnancy and bacterial vaginosis: a placebo-controlled, double-blind study. Am J Obstet Gynecol 1994;171(2): 345–347; discussion 348–349.

41. Hauth JC, Goldenberg RL, Andrews WW, DuBard MB, Copper RL. Reduced incidence of preterm delivery with metronidazole and erythromycin in women with bacterial vaginosis. N Engl J Med 1995;333(26): 1732–1736.

42. Joesoef MR, Hillier SL, Wiknjosastro G, et al. Intra-

vaginal clindamycin treatment for bacterial vaginosis: effects on preterm delivery and low birth weight. Am J Obstet Gynecol 1995;173(5):1527–1531.

43. Burtin P, Taddio A, Ariburnu O, Einarson TR, Koren G. Safety of metronidazole in pregnancy: a meta-analysis. Am J Obstet Gynecol 1995;172(2 Pt 1):525–529.

44. Schwebke JR. Metronidazole: utilization in the obstetrics and gynecologic patient. Sex Transm Dis 1995;22: 370–376.

45. Borin MT, Powley GW, Tackwell KR, Batts DH. Absorption of clindamycin after intravaginal application of clindamycin phosphate 2% cream. J Antimicrob Chemother 1995;35(6):833–841.

46. Doering PL, Santiago TM. Drugs for treatment of vulvovaginal candidiasis: comparative efficacy of agents and regimens. Drug Intell Clin Pharm 1990;24(11): 1078–1083.

47. Nyirjesy P, Seeney SM, Grody MH, Jordan CA, Buckley HR. Chronic fungal vaginitis: the value of cultures. Am J Obstet Gynecol 1995;173(3 Pt 1):820–823.

48. Cauwenbergh G, De Doncker P, Stoops K, De Dier AM, Goyvaerts H, Schuermans V. Itraconazole in the treatment of human mycoses: review of three years of clinical experience. Rev Infect Dis 1987;9 suppl 1: S146–S152.

49. Horowitz BJ. Topical flucytosine therapy for chronic recurrent *Candida tropicalis* infections. J Reprod Med 1986;31(9):821–824.

50. Davidson F, Mould RF. Recurrent genital candidosis in women and the effect of intermittent prophylactic treatment. Br J Vener Dis 1978;54(3):176–183.

51. Fong IW. The value of prophylactic (monthly) clotrimazole versus empiric self-treatment in recurrent vaginal candidiasis. Genitourin Med 1994;70(2):124–126.

52. Stein GE, Mummaw NL, Schooley SL. Prevention of recurrent vaginal candidiasis with weekly terconazole cream. Ann Pharmacother 1996;30(10):1080–1083.

53. Sobel JD. Recurrent vulvovaginal candidiasis. A prospective study of the efficacy of maintenance ketoconazole therapy. N Engl J Med 1986;315(23):1455–1458.

54. Tooley PJ. Patient and doctor preferences in the treatment of vaginal candidosis. Practitioner 1985;229(1405): 655–660.

55. Tooley PJ. Treatment of vaginal candidosis—a UK patient survey, 1989. Br J Clin Pract Symp Suppl 1990;71: 73–76.

56. Feczko JM. Fluconazole: an overview. In: Richardson RG, ed. Fluconazole and Its Role in Vaginal Candidiasis. No. 160. London: Royal Society of Medicine Services Limited, 1989.

57. Zervos M, Meunier F. Fluconazole (Diflucan): a review. Int J Antimicrob Agents 1993;3:147–170.

58. Anonymous. A comparison of single-dose oral fluconazole with 3-day intravaginal clotrimazole in the treatment of vaginal candidiasis. Report of an international multicentre trial. Br J Obstet Gynaecol 1989;96 (2):226–232.

59. Sobel JD, Brooker D, Stein GE, et al. Single oral dose fluconazole compared with conventional clotrimazole topical therapy of *Candida* vaginitis. Am J Obstet Gynecol 1995;172(4, part 1):1263–1268.

60. Sanz Sanz F, del Palacio Hernanz A. Randomized comparative trial of three regimens of itraconazole for treatment of vaginal mycoses. Rev Infect Dis 1987;9 Suppl 1:S139–S142.

61. Hilton E, Isenberg HD, Alperstein P, France K, Borenstein MT. Ingestion of yogurt containing *Lactobacillus acidophilus* as prophylaxis for candidal vaginitis. Ann Intern Med 1992;116:353–357.

62. Shalev E, Battino S, Weiner E, Colodner R, Keness Y. Ingestion of yogurt containing *Lactobacillus acidophilus* compared with pasteurized yogurt as prophylaxis for recurrent candidal vaginitis and bacterial vaginosis. Arch Fam Med 1996;5:593–596.

43. Weight Management and Obesity

PAUL F. DUNN

Key Clinical Questions

1. What is the definition of obesity, and how is it best measured?
2. What evidence exists that being obese is a health risk?
3. Who is the best candidate for aggressive treatment?
4. What are the best treatments for obesity?
5. What are the successes, risks, or advantages of the various treatments available?

A substantial portion of your patients may be enrolled in managed care programs that strongly emphasize preventive services as part of their marketing strategy. Lifestyle problems associated with weight control are classic examples of the linkage between prevention, the marketing of quick and easy commercial programs to manage obesity, and the need for physicians to stay on top of the latest treatment fads.

In the past century, people identified as "overweight" have suffered from negative perceptions in our society. Current attitudes in western cultures differ from times when being "big" was often a sign of affluence and attractiveness.

There is good evidence that obesity produces adverse psychosocial effects in children (1), reduced acceptance to major colleges (2), active employment discrimination (3), and disrespectful treatment by the medical profession (4). Despite these hardships, people who are "obese" do not have more serious psychopathology than the general population (5).

Weight management services in the United States are a multibillion dollar industry. Your patients may be purchasing vitamins and special foods or attending one or more of the hundreds of available programs. They may have obtained exercise equipment that promises to transform their bodies into sleek machines worthy of admiration. Some of your patients will come to you saying they want to lose just a few pounds. Others may need to lose weight for medical reasons because of extreme obesity and high risk of disease or sudden death.

These are management issues that continue to be difficult for all clinicians. This chapter is intended to provide you with a practical and evidence-based approach to the management of obesity and will help you navigate the medical, cultural, and social needs of your patient.

In 1990, 44 million Americans were engaged in weight loss either personally or in organized programs (6). Since the 1970s, the prevalence of obesity throughout diverse populations in the United States has increased dramatically (7). Although more than 30% of Americans are now obese, obesity is highest among African-American and Hispanic women. Fourteen percent of U.S. children, 12% of adolescents, 33% of men, and 36% of women in the general U.S. population are obese by body mass index (BMI) data (NHANES III) (8). Adolescent obesity is a better predictor of adult obesity than obesity identified at younger ages (9).

DIAGNOSIS

Obesity is excess body fat. The majority of overweight people are also obese (10). The terms "obesity and overweight" are used interchangeably in medical literature. When we discuss being overweight, we usually refer to individuals who are too heavy for their height and fall outside the Metropolitan Life Insurance Company table definitions for "desirable weight." Although the Metropolitan tables are still the most commonly used reference in medical offices, they do not specifically address adiposity, which is the principal medical risk in terms of morbidity as well as mortality (11). Currently there is no inexpensive, simple-to-use, accurate, and reproducible measure to determine the total body-fat-mass to fat-mass ratio. There is a developing office-based instrument for measuring these parameters through impedance techniques. On comparison with water immersion and DEXA testing (the new gold standard for determining fat and lean mass), these impedance machines maintain a .92 correlation in both men and women. For now, you should use the BMI as the office-based standard.

In all of its large cross-sectional studies (NHANES I-II-III studies), the National Center for Health Statistics (NCHS) used BMI as the measure of adiposity (12). Table 43.1 shows the BMI scoring system. It is easy to use and has a correlation of 0.7 to 0.8 with body fat content in both adults and adolescents (9, 13–15). Obesity is defined as a BMI > 27.8 for men and > 27.3 for women (16).

Instructions for calculating a patient's BMI are found in Figure 43.1. The BMI should be placed in the patient's chart for future reference. Patients are always interested to find out where they are on the scale.

Other measures of adiposity include the waist-to-hip ratio (WHR), the waist-to-thigh ratio, and the waist-to-height ratio. All have some measure of reliability when addressing some aspect of morbidity, e.g., hypertension, insulin resistance, or coronary artery disease. A WHR > 1.0 in men and > 0.8 in women has been shown to predict coronary artery disease independent of BMI (14). The WHR, however, has not been evaluated in all ethnic groups (16).

PATHOPHYSIOLOGY

There are several theories about why people accumulate excess body fat and why they maintain it despite their efforts to lose. Contrary to popular belief, there are no studies supporting the claim that "hypo" thyroid humans tend to gain weight faster or that "hyper" thyroid patients lose weight faster. Weight cycling (losing weight repetitively and regaining fat mass repetitively) results in lower metabolic rates and an increased risk of all the diseases associated with obesity, e.g., hypertension, glucose intolerance, early coronary artery disease, sudden

death (especially when associated with sleep apnea), and cataract formation (16, 17).

Studies of twins have demonstrated that within and outside of genetic families (adoption), weight has a strong genetic link (18). Environmental factors also clearly play an important role; however, there may be limits to the amount of weight that can actually be lost in any given individual. One's adipose volume or thermogenic "set-point" may inhibit a person from losing and/ or maintaining a markedly reduced weight. Recent research shows that removal of "brown fat" vs. "white fat" in rats results in the production of greatly increased hunger and resultant adiposity in rats not previously obese (19). Brown fat is more metabolically active and hence more thermogenically active. We currently have no simple way of determining the percentage of high-thermogenic brown fat mass in humans.

There may be other factors influencing the expression of genetic characteristics that induce weight gain or allow weight loss. Leptin is a hormone that is produced by adipocytes. It seems to provide the brain with needed feedback concerned with the dynamic stability of body fat mass (20). A loss of body fat leads to a decrease in leptin, which in turn leads to a state of positive energy-balance. In other words, low leptin levels lead to a state in which food intake exceeds energy expenditure, and other adaptive changes are also seen. Conversely, an increase in adiposity leads to an increase in the levels of leptin and a state of negative energy-balance. In this case, energy expenditure exceeds food intake. The question is whether this knowledge will allow us to safely modulate weight in humans. Whatever the mechanism of weight gain and loss, total weight is supported by energy expenditure balanced by caloric intake and resting metabolic rate.

There is evidence that reducing weight in obese individuals reduces their risk of developing disease (21). Excess mortality is associated with "morbid obesity" (BMI > 45.4 in men and > 44.8 in women), and reduction of weight reduces risk factors for related disorders. There is good evidence showing that weight loss will increase longevity. A 16-year study of 115,195 nurses reveals a linear correlation with weight gain and coronary disease (22), the major cause of death in the United States in the 30 to 55 year age range (Fig. 43.2). Obesity increases the risk of systolic hypertension in both men and women (23). Data on the most common disorders associated with obesity are included in the Table 43.2.

Table 43.1.
Body Mass Index (BMI)

BMI Nomenclature	BMI Score Men	BMI Score Women
Underweight	20.7	<19.1
Average or acceptable	20.7–27.8	10.1–27.3
Overweight (20–30% overweight)	27.8–31.1	27.3–32.3
Severe overweight (moderately obese)	31.1–45.4	32.3–44.8
Clinically severe overweight (morbidly obese)	>45.4	>44.8

To calculate your own BMI, use your accurate body weight and your standing height without shoes.

Weigh Your Risk With BMI

How to use this chart:
1. Look down the left column to find your height *(measured in feet and inches)*.
2. Look across that row and find the weight nearest your own.
3. Look to the number at the top of the column to identify your BMI.
4. If your number is 27 or greater, you may be at risk.

BMI ▶	25	26	27	28	29	30	31	32	33	34	35	36	37	38	39	40
						WEIGHT *(In Pounds)*										
4'10"	119	124	129	134	138	143	148	153	158	162	167	172	177	181	186	191
4'11"	124	128	133	138	143	148	153	158	163	168	173	178	183	188	193	198
5'	128	133	138	143	148	153	158	164	169	174	179	184	189	194	199	204
5'1"	132	137	143	148	153	158	164	169	174	180	185	190	195	201	206	211
5'2"	136	142	147	153	158	164	169	175	180	186	191	196	202	207	213	218
5'3"	141	146	152	158	163	169	175	180	186	192	197	203	208	214	220	225
5'4"	145	151	157	163	169	174	180	186	192	198	203	209	215	221	227	233
5'5"	150	156	162	168	174	180	186	192	198	204	210	216	222	228	234	240
5'6"	155	161	167	173	179	185	192	198	204	210	216	223	229	235	241	247
5'7"	159	166	172	178	185	191	198	204	210	217	223	229	236	242	248	255
5'8"	164	171	177	184	190	197	203	210	217	223	230	236	243	249	256	263
5'9"	169	176	182	189	196	203	209	216	223	230	237	243	250	257	264	270
5'10"	174	181	188	195	202	209	216	223	230	236	243	250	257	264	271	278
5'11"	179	186	193	200	207	215	222	229	236	243	250	258	265	272	279	286
6'	184	191	199	206	213	221	228	235	243	250	258	265	272	280	287	294
6'1"	189	197	204	212	219	227	234	242	250	257	265	272	280	287	295	303
6'2"	194	202	210	218	225	233	241	249	256	264	272	280	288	295	303	311
6'3"	200	208	216	224	232	240	247	255	263	271	279	287	295	303	311	319
6'4"	205	213	221	230	238	246	254	262	271	279	287	295	303	312	320	328

(The left-side vertical label reads "HEIGHT"; the band between the 26 and 27 columns reads "AT RISK".)

Used by Knoll Pharmaceutical Company with permission from George Bray, M.D.

Figure 43.1. *Body mass index.*

CLINICAL EVALUATION

History

The history should include a complete review of systems with particular attention to issues of high medical risk, including a frank discussion of mental fitness, sleep habits, and the possibility of apneic spells as well as the ingestion of over-the-counter (OTC) medications, e.g., laxatives and chromium supplements. Because family and friends are essential to the success of a weight control program, identify and record the support people in the chart for future reference. Ask the patient the following questions to get a sense for the scope of the problem as perceived by the patient:

1. Do you think your weight interferes with your health? If yes, then, in what way(s)?
2. Does your weight ever stop you from doing something you need to do (i.e., not feel like doing it)?
3. Have other people told you your weight is a problem?
4. Have you ever tried to lose weight? If yes, did you do it by yourself, or through some weight control program?

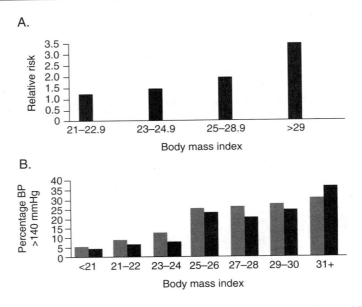

Figure 43.2. *Relationship between obesity and cardiovascular problems.*

5. Were you successful in losing weight? If yes, then,
   - How long ago was that?
   - How did you feel during the program?
   - How long did it take you to lose ___ pounds?
   - Did you have any "golden rules" to live by regarding your weight program?
6. What were the good aspects of your weight loss?
7. What obstacles did you encounter during the program (from friends, spouse, children, etc.)?
8. Did you regain any of the weight? If yes, what do you think is the reason for regaining?
9. Are you willing to set goals and begin again?
10. Do you have any goals for the next month or two?

Remember that individuals who have lost and gained in programs in the past may have a history of failure with weight control. Being positive when asking your questions is essential to get honest responses.

Physical Examination

The physical examination of the person who is obese should be directed at those pertinent positives from the review of systems. They also in-clude an assessment of respiratory capacity and functioning of all weight-bearing joints.

It would seem quite reasonable to "eyeball" the patient and then just label him or her as obese. This may work well for some of your patients, but is based on a personal selection bias. Consequently, you may not identify some patients needing interventions to prevent or treat obesity. Remember that obesity is associated with some specific diseases, e.g., Cushing's syndrome, that must be first ruled out before obesity management begins. Table 43.3 lists the methods used for quantification of adipose tissue and their reliability under testing.

An interesting way to have both adolescents and adults identify what size they are and whether they connect their perceived size as problematic is to use body image silhouettes (Fig. 43.3) (24). Have the patient circle the size they think they are now and what size they would like to achieve.

Laboratory Tests

Because we know that lipid, respiratory, and car-diovascular abnormalities are associated with obe-sity, you should get the following tests dependent on the relative size and risk level of the patient:

- A fasting fractionated lipid panel to determine the ratio of high-density lipoprotein (HDL) to low-density lipoprotein (LDL) and

Table 43.2.
Common Disorders Associated with Obesity

Disease	Associated BMI Increase and Risk	Level of Evidence for Effectiveness[a]
Hypertension[b]	Each 10-kg increase increases systolic and diastolic BP 3 mm	B
High lipids[c]	>27.8 men, >27.3 women: 1.5× risk	B
Coronary artery disease[d]	Higher BMI = more CAD	B
Diabetes[e]	Type II: 2× to 5× to 10×	B
Gallbladder disease[f, g]	>27.8 men, >27.3 women: stones 3–4× more common	B
Respiratory compromise[h]	>27.8 men, >27.3 women: decreased lung volume and vital capacity, sleep apnea syndrome	B
Sleep apnea[i]	>27.8 men, >27.3 women: linear relation to BMI increase; risk 10× for sudden death	B
Colorectal and prostate cancers[j]	40% overweight (BMI 31–34), men: risk 1.33×	B
Breast, cervical, endometrial/ gallbladder cancers[j, k]	40% overweight (BMI 31–34), women: risk 1.55×	B
Gout[l]	BMI increase from 21 to 31: gout increased 7–31%	B
Cataracts[m]	BMI 29–34 = 12% increase in cataracts	
Osteoarthritis[n]	Increased prevalence: men 0.75–1.45%, women 0.4–1.45%	B

[a]Level of evidence for effectiveness: A, strong or moderate research-based evidence (consistent across several studies, including at least two randomized controlled trials); B, limited research-based evidence (less consistent or extensive evidence, but preponderance of evidence supports use of treatment); C, common practice with little or no research-based evidence; X, moderate or strong evidence suggesting that this treatment is not effective.

[b]Boe J, Humerfelt S, Wedervang G. The blood pressure in a population: blood pressure readings and height and weight determinations in the adult population of the city of Bergen. Acta Med Scand 1957;157(suppl 321):1–336.

[c]Glueck CJ, Taylor HL, Jacobs D, Morrison JA, Beaglehole R, Williams OD. Plasma high-density lipoprotein cholesterol: associations with measurement of body mass. The Lipid Research Clinics Program Prevalence Study. Circulation 1980;62(IV):62–69.

[d]Feinleib M. Epidemiology of obesity in relation to health hazards. Ann Intern Med 1985;103:1019–1024.

[e]National Commission on Diabetes, United States. Report to the Congress of the United States. Publication no. 76–1021, Vol 1. Bethesda, MD: US Department of Health, Education, and Welfare, 1975.

[f]Maclure KM, Hayes KC, Colditz GA, Stampfer MJ, Speizer FE, Willett WC. Weight, diet, and the risk of gallstones in middle-aged women. N Engl J Med 1989;321:563–569.

[g]Friedman GD, Kannel WB, Dawber TR. The epidemiology of gallstones: observations in the Framingham study. J Chronic Dis 1966;19: 273–292.

[h]Waltemath CL, Bergman NA. Respiratory compromise in obese patients. Anesthesiology 1974;41:84–85.

[i]Kopelman PG, Apps MC, Cope T, Ingram DA, Empey DW, Evans SJ. Nocturnal hypoxia and sleep apnea in asymptomatic obese men. Int J Obes 1986;10:211–217.

[j]Garfinkel L. Overweight and cancer. Ann Intern Med 1985;103:1034–1036.

[k]Lubin F, Ruder AM, Wax Y, Modan B. Overweight and changes in weight throughout adult life in breast cancer etiology. A case-control study. Am J Epidemiol 1985;122:579–588.

[l]Rimm AA, Werner LH, Yserloo BV, Bernstein RA. Relationship of obesity and disease in 73,532 weight-conscious women. Public Health Rep 1975;90:44–54.

[m]Glynn RJ, Christen WG, Manson JE, Bernheimer J, Hennekens CH. Body mass index: an independent predictor of cataract. BMJ 1995;113:1131–1137.

[n]Leach RE, Baumgard S, Broom J. Obesity: its relationship to osteoarthritis of the knee. Clin Orthop 1973;93:271–273.

the triglyceride levels. Triglyceride levels are a sensitive indicator for glucose intolerance and insulin resistance in those having a WHR > 1:0 or a BMI > 28;

- A sleep study to determine whether sleep apnea exists, especially if a family member verifies the history; and

- An exercise treadmill to determine safe fitness as a prelude to an exercise prescription.

MANAGEMENT

The data clearly show that excess adiposity is bad for our health. The problem is usually not in the ability to lose weight. The problem is how fast the weight is lost and in maintaining that lower weight. In January 1996, the U.S. Department of Agriculture and the U.S. Department of Health and Human Services published the updated *Dietary Guidelines for Americans* (25). In

Table 43.3.
Techniques Used to Measure Adipose Tissue

Technique	Rating/Comments	Level of Evidence for Effectiveness[a]
Skin caliper[b]	Tested at three anatomic landmarks; $20–50; does not measure central obesity	B
Infrared densitometry[c]	Determination of time in adults and adolescents; $100–180; appears to be excellent validity over time in children and adults	A
Body mass index (scale)[d–g]	Easy to use in the office; free; high correlation with fat mass	A
Waist-to-hip ratio[h]	More specifically associated with CAD and insulin resistance; free; not validated in ethnic groups	B

[a]Level of evidence for effectiveness: A, strong or moderate research-based evidence (consistent across several studies, including at least two randomized controlled trials); B, limited research-based evidence (less consistent or extensive evidence, but preponderance of evidence supports use of treatment); C, common practice with little or no research-based evidence; X, moderate or strong evidence suggesting that this treatment is not effective.

[b]Bellisari A, Roche AF, Siervogel RM. Reliability of B-mode ultrasonic measurements of subcutaneous adipose tissue and intra-abdominal depth: comparisons with skinfold thickness. Int J Obes Rel Metabol Disorders 1993;17(8)475–480.

[c]Cassady SL, Nielson DH, Janz KF, Wu YT, Cook JS, Hansen JR. Validity of near-infrared body composition analysis in children and adolescents. Med Sci Sports Exercise 1993;25(10):1185–1191.

[d]Centers for Disease Control and Prevention. Update: prevalence of overweight among children, adolescents, and adults—United States, 1988–1994. MMWR 1997;46(9).

[e]Guo SS, Roche AF, Chumlea WC, et al. The predictive value of childhood body mass values for overweight at age 35 years. Am J Clin Nutr 1994;39:810–819.

[f]US Preventive Services Task Force. Guide to Clinical Preventive Services. Report of the US Preventive Services Task Force, 2nd ed. Baltimore: William & Wilkins, 1996:219.

[g]Dietary Guidelines Advisory Committee, 1995. Report to the Secretary of Health and Human Services and the Secretary of Agriculture. US Department of Agriculture, Agricultural Research Service. Springfield, VA: National Technical Information Service, 1995.

[h]Cox BD, Whichelow MJ. Ratio of waist circumference to height is better predictor of death than body mass index. BMJ 1996;313:1487.

this document, the guidelines call for 30 minutes or more of exercise at a "moderate" physical activity level on *all* days of the week. For the first time, the guidelines call for the attainment of *weight maintenance* rather than weight reduction for those in a "single healthy weight range," emphasizing prevention rather than weight reduction later. There is a clear warning against "crash" diets, suggesting slow steady weight loss of 1/2 pound a week over time. The data clearly support the need for a multidimensional approach to obesity. Medical, personal-psychologic, and community support from family and friends are essential to success over the long term. Those programs that include all of the above have the longest success rates (26, 27). There are management strategies that have been proven to work in long-term, controlled studies. No one treatment regimen works sufficiently by itself to keep the weight off in the maintenance phase. The "successful" programs in which patients have succeeded in

maintaining their weight loss for more than 1 year included both medical and behavioral approaches. Table 43.4 lists commercial groups that specialize in weight control. Not all groups can be found in all areas.

Many authorities are now suggesting that success in weight control should be defined as *maintenance* of at least 50% of the loss of excess weight at 1 year to be successful. Maintenance of at least 50% of the loss of excess weight maintained at 5 years is an accepted standard following obesity surgery (28).

Table 43.5 lists the nonpharmacotherapies with proven efficacy in weight reduction and their associated benefits.

Pharmacotherapies

Medications in weight control have always been controversial. In recent years we have witnessed the reemergence and disappearance of combination drugs such as phentermine (Ionamin) and

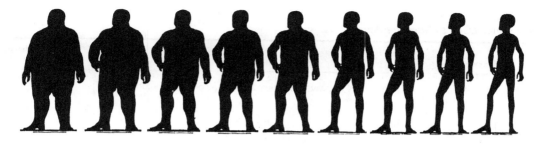

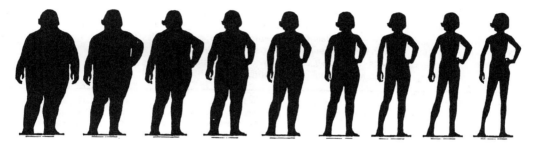

Figure 43.3. *Body silhouettes.*

Table 43.4.
Commerical Weight Control Programs

Program	Fee	Foods	Exercise	Comments
Weight Watchers	Monthly or each meeting fee	Diet recommended; some "name-brand" foods are available	No formal exercise component	Group support is vital part of treatment; relatively standardized approach between cities and towns
Taking Off Pounds Sensibly (TOPS)	Monthly or meeting fee; often not lead by professional	No special diet foods to purchase	No formal exercise component	Group support is vital; groups vary greatly in how they operate
Nutri-System	Visit fee or standard contract for pounds lost	Special foods and vitamins sold as part of package	No formal exercise component	Although some have groups, others are one-on-one only
Spas and clubs	Often expensive; great variability	Usually no specific foods but may have individual counselors or trainers; more scientific in approach to weight loss	Formalized exercise component	Due to high volume, individualized support is episodic; some have group sessions; great variability
Severe caloric restriction; doctor supervised	Expensive due to testing	400–800 kcal/day: very specific foods	No exercise during the program	Often behavior modification strategies

Table 43.5.
Efficacy of Weight Reduction Modalities

Modality	Associated Benefit	Level of Evidence for Effectiveness[a]
Cardiac rehabilitation exercise training in obese individuals with CAD	Dramatically improved physical and behavioral/psychologic parameters[b]	A
	Decreased BMI, $p < 0.0001$	
	Decreased body fat, $p < 0.0001$	
	Increased exercise capacity, $p < 0.0001$	
	Decreased total cholesterol, $p < 0.01$	
	Decreased HDL:LDL ratio, $p < 0.01$	
	Decreased depression, anxiety, and somatization, $p < 0.0001$	
Increasing perceived self-efficacy (women)	Those with more "self-assuredness" lost significantly more weight than low-self-esteem women[c]	B
Hypnosis[d]	With hypnosis, patients lost twice as much weight as subjects with no hypnosis; meta-analysis.	A
Caloric restriction with behavior modification[e]	1200-kcal diet with behavior modification; kept weight off for 1 yr	B
Surgery	BMI > 40 with failure at other modalities; overall mortality 1.7% with minimal revisional surgery[f, g]	A
	Bypass: Roux-en-Y with behavior modification	B
	Restrictive: vertical gastric banding (VGB)	B

[a]Level of evidence for effectiveness: A, strong or moderate research-based evidence (consistent across several studies, including at least two randomized controlled trials); B, limited research-based evidence (less consistent or extensive evidence, but preponderance of evidence supports use of treatment); C, common practice with little or no research-based evidence; X, moderate or strong evidence suggesting that this treatment is not effective.

[b]Lavie CJ, Milani RV. Effects of cardiac rehabilitation, exercise training, and weight reduction on exercise capacity, coronary risk factors, behavioral characteristics, and quality of life in obese coronary patients. Am J Cardiol 1997;79(4):397–401.

[c]Dennis KE, Goldberg AP. Weight control self-efficacy types and transitions affect weight loss outcomes in obese women. Addict Behav 1996;21(1):103–116.

[d]Kirsch I. Hypnotic enhancement of cognitive-behavioral weight loss treatments—another meta-reanalysis. J Consult Clin Psychol 1996;64(3):517–519.

[e]Wadden TA. Treatment of obesity by moderate and severe caloric restriction: results of clinical research trials. Ann Intern Med 1993;119(7):1:688–693.

[f]Benotti PN, Forse RA. The role of gastric surgery in the multidisciplinary management of severe obesity. Am J Surg 1995;169(3):361–367.

[g]Benotti PN, Forse RA. Safety and long-term efficacy of revisional surgery in severe obesity. Am J Surg 1996;172(3):232–235.

fenfluramine (Pondimin) and the marketing of "new" drugs, e.g., dexfenfluramine (Redux). In August 1997, following a letter sent to prescribers by the makers of fenfluramine not to prescribe phen/fen together, Wal-Mart Corporation began refusing to fill prescriptions for these two agents if they were to be used together. This action was taken due to reports of increases in primary pulmonary hypertension (PPH), ischemic colitis, stroke (29), mitral valve dysfunction, psychotic mania (30), and occasionally fatal serotonin syndrome (31). Redux used by itself appeared to be safe and was the only weight reduction drug approved by the Food and Drug Administration for up to 1 year; however, on September 21, 1997, the FDA asked the manufacturers to remove dexfen-fluramine (Redux) and fenfluramine (Pondimin) from the market (Table 43.6) (32).

Medications must be taken regularly for at least 1 year, although weight loss tends to plateau at 6 months. Patients should be seen every month and given specific targets for weight loss, nutrition, etc. Combined with behavioral therapies, weight loss maintenance at 1 year was the same or greater than with just medications alone (33).

Weight loss management should be systematized as well as multifaceted. Because most patients can lose weight, but few maintain the weight they have lost, it is imperative that you see the patient on a regular basis—at least bi-weekly. Contract with the patient at the first

Table 43.6.
Currently FDA-Approved Antiobesity Medications

DEA Schedule	Catecholaminergic	Serotonergic	Dosages
III	Phendimetrazine (Bontril)		35 mg bid-tid 1hr before meals
IV	Benzphetamine (Didrex)	Dexfenfluramine (Redux) (removed from market 9/21/97)	25–50 mg qd 15 mg bid
	Diethylpropion (Tenuate)		25 mg tid or 75 mg (sr) qd
	Mazindol (Mazanor)		1mg tid, 1 hr before meals
	Phentermine (Ionamin, Fastin)		15–37.5 mg po qd before breakfast
OTC	Phenylpropanolamine		25 mg tid, 30 min before meals, or 75 mg (sr) qd
		Fenfluramine (Pondimin)	20 mg tid, 1 hr before meals

Adapted from Pi-Sunyer FX. Current Approaches to the Management of Obesity. San Antonio, TX: Dannemiller Memorial Education Foundation, 1996:33.

visit to set realistic goals. The act of contracting is essential to success and is born out in the literature. Patients need NOT stand on the scale at each visit.

Reducing adipose tissue and adding lean mass changes the way clothes fit long before the patient sees weight change on a scale. Praise the patient for even small reductions in BMI. Use every laboratory parameter to reinforce the connection between the change in body composition and health (e.g., lower blood glucoses, better hypertension control, lower triglycerides, higher HDL). If necessary, refer the patient to a psychiatric counselor who understands the issues surrounding family systems, support, and weight control and get the patient's permission to confer with the counselor. Consulting with such a counselor in your community will help you provide more comprehensive care to your patients.

The rate of weight loss should be no greater than 2 to 3 lbs. in a week (8 to 12 lbs./month). Use these estimates for determining short- and long-range goals. The patient should not skip any meals, as this can lead to overeating. The perfect recipe for weight gain is skipping a meal, followed by overeating at supper, followed by inactivity and sleep.

When a patient achieves a goal (e.g., a reduction of the BMI by 1% from 33 to 32) then a celebration is in order. Food is not an appropriate reward. Encourage the patient to use other rewards such as buying a new article of clothing or

a book or going to the movies. Achieving the next goal could be tied to a newly-defined reward. Take time to discuss psychosocial issues and reinforce the patient for any successes.

Surgery

Gastric surgery to control obesity is reserved for patients whose BMIs are >35 and/or patients who have repeatedly tried and failed to achieve sustained weight loss and suffer from substantial health risks due to obesity. The person contemplating surgery must have a counseling session with the surgeon or her or his team to review the benefits and adverse effects of the procedure.

Depending on the type of surgery and the resolve and skill of the patient to follow a regular exercise program, the success rate of either vertical gastric banding or gastric bypass approaches 50 to 70% of excess weight. The weight loss is sustained over time in most cases. It's important to emphasize to the patient that failure to control food portion sizes and failure to maintain a substantial aerobic (walking) program after surgery decreases the chances for success. Despite surgery, some patients regain weight due to overeating and insufficient energy output.

Vertical Gastric Banding

This procedure involves banding or stapling a vertical segment of the stomach or implanting a band around the upper segment of the stomach. This decreases the stomach size where food enters and causes the food to stay longer; thus, satiation occurs much more quickly. If the patient overeats, nausea can occur. Nutritional deficiencies are usually rare and are usually the result of poor food choices combined with a smaller capacity to fill (less total food sources).

Roux-en-Y and Extensive Bypass of the Stomach

The Roux-en-Y gastric bypass (RGB) is the most common form of gastric bypass done today. A restrictive gastric pouch is created first; then, the distal stomach is attached from the pouch to the latter aspect of the jejunum. Because most nutrients are digested and absorbed in the duodenum and proximal jejunum, much of the food does not get absorbed. Although this procedure is successful in reducing weight, it carries the highest complication rates. Malabsorption can cause anemia because B_{12} is decreased and iron is absorbed in the duodenum. Calcium deficiency often occurs for the same reason. Dumping syndrome with symptoms of nausea, diarrhea, weakness, and sweating following a meal are common. Pancreatic and bile salts often need replacement as well. Thirty percent of patients will have gallbladder problems if bile salt replacement is not made.

Surgery is not for everyone, but it does carry high success rates. Because a loss of 10 to 20% of body weight results in much better diabetes and hypertension control, patients must make every effort to loose weight using traditional methods before surgery is considered. This includes proper nutrition sources and timing of foods combined with daily exercise and often weekly psychiatric counseling.

Patient Education

Patient education is a vital aspect of weight control management with or without concomitant medication. Ideally, all patients should see a dietitian when beginning a weight management program and then again about 4 to 6 months in the process. At each visit, the patient should bring a completed 3-day dietary (food and drink) record. This record should include the times any item is consumed as this is a very important issue. If your patient sees a dietitian, ask permission to speak with the dietitian and get a copy of her or his notes.

If a dietitian is not available, you can perform a substantial amount of dietary counseling yourself. Using the "Daily Food Pyramid" (Fig. 43.4) and knowledge of portion sizes (1/2 cup is one exchange of most vegetables, a small apple or 1/2 banana is one exchange of fruit) you can use the same 3-day record to convert the patient's food and drink choices into exchanges (e.g., one piece of bread = 1 mark on the bread, starches, and gains line at the bottom of the pyramid). For example, if a patient drinks one can of a regular soft drink, this equals 10 teaspoons of sugar; thus 10 marks go on the fat/oils/sweets line at the top of the pyramid. This process gets much easier each time you do it. You can convert the first page of the record and the patient can convert the rest of the record.

Through this process, the patient will learn that eating from the bottom of the pyramid is better. A graphical representation of a diet shows where the problems lie. If you are nonjudgmental and avoid using words like "should" or "must," patients will learn to change their diet on their own over time. Review the food and drink records at each visit. Data shows that the more people are

DAILY FOOD CHOICES

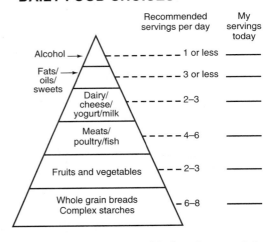

Figure 43.4. Food pyramid. Complete your 3-day food and drink record. Put a mark next to each category of serving from your list for the complete 3 days. What did you learn? Do this at weekly or monthly intervals. Seek the dietitian's help if it is a problem. The goal is to eat primarily from the bottom of the pyramid.

conscious of what they eat, the more they will change to a desired meal plan.

Keep the following points in mind when educating your patients about weight management:

- "Medical" success in weight control is maintenance of reduced weight at 1 year. The patient may consider success as the first 5 lbs. lost! However, make sure the patient's goal is always a long-term one.

- Knowledge of the normal course of weight control is essential if the patient is to be protected from unrealistic goals. Let the patient know he or she will plateau in weight after 10 to 20 lbs. are lost.

- Have the patient make positive self-affirmations each day, e.g., "I am looking better, I feel energetic today, I can do anything I set my mind to."

- Get the patient to subscribe to the 11 rules for successful weight control:

  1. Eat throughout the day. Do not skip meals. Skipping leads to overeating later in the day, often with foods higher in simple sugars and fat.

  2. Get some physical activity during the day—preferably in the morning for 15 to 30 minutes. Eating without exercising encourages fat storage and increasing weight.

  3. Never eat a large meal and then go to bed.

  4. Reduce your portion sizes first—especially at the largest meal of the day.

  5. Always try to eat soluble fibers (lentils, green peas, pinto or kidney or butter beans) with a large meal—especially if the meal is high in fat content.

  6. If you eat simple sweets, always eat them as part of a meal, not as a snack. Simple sugars are not metabolized in the same manner when consumed with a meal mixed with proteins and fats.

  7. Make one change at a time. It takes about 21 days to establish a new habit. Once the new habit is established, then change something else.

  8. Look at yourself in the mirror each evening or morning and give yourself a positive message—even if it seems untrue. Your mind listens and believes in your messages.

  9. When you encounter problems or roadblocks, share them with your family or doctor. Others have probably encountered the same problems—you're not alone.

  10. Do not start a "popular diet" or food supplement without counsel. Some may be bad for you.

  11. Be frank with your health provider and expect and demand his or her support.

Make encouraging statements to the patient in the examination room, no matter how small the success may seem to be.

Weight Control Strategies in the Office

The weight management strategies (Figs. 43.5–43.8) are a series of tasks that should be done with patients over at least five different visits. The tasks for each meeting are outlined in the figures. These outlines should help organize your efforts with patients. Weight management, when done in the primary care office, requires the following:

- Patience with the process of weight loss and maintenance over time

- A provider that has available, regularly scheduled hours

- Access to a dietitian

- Knowledge and skills in determining the stage of change a patient is in, determining his or her self-efficacy, and setting realistic goals

In their book *Changing for Good*, Drs. Prochaska and DiClemente discuss predictable stages of change (34) (see Chapter 6, Helping Your Patients Stay Healthy). The frustration that physicians often feel is that change does not happen fast enough or in the way they think it should. This leads to complaints that the patient is noncompliant when in fact the clinician is knowledge-deficient and probably lacks the skills to help patients who want to lose weight.

Behaviors begin in the realms of subtle cognition (precontemplative stage). Your job is to move the patient to "consider" a change. What usually happens is the "scare tactic" (e.g., "You're going to have a stroke if you don't . . . "). This tactic is often an excellent short-term motivation, but then the patient gets scared and rebels. Once the patient achieves some level of understanding and education about his or her condition, he or she can think about making a change (contem-

Cognitive

1. Determine BMI

2. Assess patient's reason for the visit

3. Assess daily activity and work patterns

4. Assess previous experience with weight control programs, OTC medications and "alternative" methods of losing weight he/she might have tried

5. Assess potential or real supports—family, friends, coworkers, ect.

6. Assess body image—with pictures and discuss (then put in chart)

7. Assess self-efficacy

8. Assess medical risks and discuss, e.g.:
   - genetic predisposition
   - elevation in lipids
   - arthritis/joint problems
   - sleep apnea
   - orthopnea
   - hypertension
   - glucose intolerance
   - restrictive lung disease
   - cancers
   - hiatal hernia
   - CAD/chest pain or past MI
   - gallbladder problems

9. Perform physical examination including heart, lungs and extremities

10. Get baseline clinical data including BP, triglycerides, weight, and TSH (HgbA1c if diabetic)

Behavioral

11. Make behavioral goal contract, i.e., agree to meet weekly for first month and for patient to do homework; have patient sign contract in chart

12. Patient homework complete a 3-day prospective food and drink record with annotations of times and amounts of consumption

13. Assess self-efficacy again now

14. Schedule visits weekly for next 4 weeks

15. Document reasons for frequent visits and plans for next meeting

16. Consider medication/surgery if BMI > 40 and medical risk severe

Figure 43.5. Weight control strategies: first visit (45–60 minutes).

Cognitive

1. Discuss in retrospect how patient felt and what patient thought after last visit.

2. Assess 3-day food and drink record for obvious pattern problems and/or large fat intake—use food pyramid

3. Discuss previous clinical data and labs

4. Give praise for any forward progress no matter how small; do not concentrate on failures—only omissions

5. Assess whether patient mustered support of friends, ect. for program

Musculo-skeletal examination, BP, lungs

Behavioral

6. Make new behavioral goal contract with specific attention to realistic goals—no more than 2–3 lbs/week and beginning exercise only after your assessment of cardiac and musculoskeletal risk; sign in chart

7. Reassess self-efficacy again now

8. Consider need for medication to get immediate weight loss if the patient has low self-efficacy but *does* exercise; do not offer medication unless patient agrees to visits and agrees to exercise under pre-scription; consider making appointment with dietitian

9. Patient perform another 3-day prospective food and drink record with annotations of times of consumption

10. Document successes and plans for this meeting and plan to discuss exercise and possibly drug tolerance at next meeting

Figure 43.6. *Weight control strategies: second visit (30 minutes).*

Cognitive

1. Discuss in retrospect how patient felt and what patient thought after last visit

2. Assess exercise pattern, time, distance, and number of days completed

3. Give praise for any forward progress no matter how small; do not concentrate on failures—only omissions

4. Assess 3-day food and drink record for obvious pattern problems and/or large fat intake—use food pyramid

5. Assess any new strengths the patient brings—supports and experiences

6. Reassess self-efficacy

Behavioral

7. Make new behavioral goal contract with specific focus on realistic goals with realistic exercise prescription

8. Consider need for medication to get immediate weight loss if the patient has low self-efficacy but *does* exercise

9. Perform another 3-day prospective food and drink record with annotation of times of consumption; consider dietitian revisit

10. Document physical examination including heart and lung examination, weight and patient successes (food, drink, exercise) and omissions from contract; plan for the next meeting to review all above

Figure 43.7. Weight control strategies: third and fourth visits (30 minutes).

Cognitive

1. Discuss in retrospect how patient felt and what patient thought after last visit

2. Assess exercise pattern, time, distance, and number of days completed

3. Give praise for any forward progress no matter how small; do not concentrate on failures—only omissions

4. Assess 3-day food and drink record for obvious pattern problems and/or large fat intake—use food pyramid

5. Assess any new strengths the patient brings—supports and experiences

6. Reassess self-efficacy

Musculo-skeletal examination, BP, lungs

May choose to review fasting triglycerides

Behavioral

7. Make new behavioral goal contract with specific focus on realistic goals with realistic exercise prescription; set visits at 1–3 weeks apart until 3 months; also consider group class referral if low supports

8. Reassess self-efficacy

9. Consider need for medication to get immediate weight loss if the patient has low self-efficacy but *does* exercise. If no changes and patient demoralized and BMI > 40, consider surgical intervention

10. Patient perform another 3-day prospective food and drink record with annotations of times of consumption

11. Document physical examination including heart and lung examination, weight and patient successes (food, drink, exercise) and omissions from contract; plan for the next meeting to review all above

Figure 43.8. *Weight control strategies: fifth and subsequent visits (30 minutes).*

plative stage). With your help, the patient can move on to the planning stage, during which realistic goals are set. The action stage moves from words to overt behavior. This might be walking a specified amount of time in a specific place with a specific person at a specific hour and some specific interval (e.g., daily). The patient should plan for obstacles such as rainy days or high heat-index days. The clearer the plan, the better both you and the patient will understand how to measure success and have ways to talk about corrective actions (not "failures"). The change stages go on to discuss helping patients with maintenance, the toughest stage. During this stage there is a real possibility of lapsing and reentering the cycle at some earlier point. People drop out of the cycle for many reasons. It is essential that you be nonjudgmental and that you maintain open communication with your patient so those reasons can be discussed.

Self-efficacy is what the patient believes he or she is capable of and whether the patient believes his or her actions will lead to positive outcomes. Research shows that with many types of groups (smoking cessation, diabetes control, and weight control), the self-efficacy of an individual is a vital and important variable in the "success" of engaging in, and sticking to, a behavior (35). Once the plan is made, ask the patient these two questions: "Do you think you can do that behavior (e.g., walk daily)?" and "If you do perform the behavior, do you believe you will attain your goal?" If the patient answers "yes" twice, he or she is ready to take action; if the patient answers "no" to either question, further discussion is warranted before action is taken. Data also show that in people who doubted they would attain their goals, a fair percentage increased their self-efficacy as they practiced the behavior.

Realistic goal setting means that the goal should be attainable with the level of effort desired and with all other constraints considered. The goal must be the patient's and not yours. The patient should write that goal in the chart and sign it. A goal of losing 50 pounds over the next 2 months is not realistic even under optimum conditions, but a goal of losing 10 pounds over 4 to 6 weeks, with an exercise program in place, is attainable. When it is reached, it should be celebrated and a new goal set. Goals should be short, attainable, and reset at every meeting in some way. There are long-term and short-term goals. These can be placed on a sheet of paper and followed at subsequent visits.

CASE STUDY 1

Mr. F. is a 44-year-old Caucasian man who has "been heavy" many years. He is a full-time college professor. He noticed a gradual weight gain over the past 10 years. He married about 12 years ago when he weighed 200 lbs. He now weighs 230 lbs. and is 5'11" tall (BMI: 31.5). He wants to lose about 20 to 30 lbs. In the past, he has lost as much as 10 lbs. just by "cutting back" his food portion sizes. He always regains the weight. He seems motivated to work on this problem.

His medical history is significant for hypertension, well controlled on an ACE inhibitor, Type II diabetes mellitus, well controlled on Glucophage (metformin), and an increasingly painful left knee for the past 2 years. He is a smoker (one pack/day × 20 years).

QUESTIONS

1. How would you approach this obviously well-educated and potentially motivated man?
2. How severe is his obesity?
3. What threats to his health does his obesity pose?
4. What is the possibility that, given his history with dieting, he will succeed?
5. What are the risks of weight cycling, and how can they be overcome?

DISCUSSION

This professionally successful man has been able to lose weight in the past. His chances of losing weight again are good. His challenge is lose weight and then maintain a lower level. If he has good continuity of care with you, he will probably succeed.

Remembering that 1 year is a goal for weight maintenance, it would be important to set realistic goals and make sure that regular exercise is a part of the management plan. He would greatly benefit from a dietitian's guidance both in the beginning and along the way. He would not be a candidate for surgery because his BMI does not exceed 40.

Reassessing his goals on a monthly basis would be most helpful, as would some tangible reward, e.g., a certificate of weight maintenance or treating himself to something he desires. He might celebrate those weight targets with family, friends, and coworkers.

It is important to investigate his beliefs about smoking cessation. It would be prudent to either wait and address this habit later after weight loss has begun in earnest or pursue it first and then address the weight in 3 to 6 months. It is difficult for any person to deal with more than one major lifestyle change at the same time.

CASE STUDY 2

Ms. C. is a 52-year-old Caucasian woman. She says she has been "overweight" since junior high school. When she was a teenager she secretly joined a popular weight control group. The program consisted of weekly meetings, special low-fat foods, and group interaction. Mandatory weighing in front of the group was evaluated by "boos" or "yeas"! She lost 30 lbs. despite, or because of, the "humiliation." She had gained back all 30 lbs. within 6 months, lost her motivation to deal with the problem, and admits she just gave up the diet.

In the past 12 to 14 years, she has attended five different programs and lost weight in all of them. Each time she regained her weight. On her visit today she is requesting weight control pills. She wants to lose 100 or more pounds. She is sick and tired of being told her weight is a major problem—she knows that. She is married. Her husband has a BMI of 24.

Her medical history is significant for a sedentary job, depression, BMI of 43.6, hy-

pertension, incapacitating osteoarthritis of both knees, a cholesterol of 280 mg/dL with an LDL of 190 mg/dL and an HDL of 26 mg/dL. She has persistent monilial infections in skin folds but no evidence of diabetes.

QUESTIONS

1. Given the socialization this woman has experienced in her life, how would you approach her evaluation and treatment?
2. What are this woman's risks given her weight and history?
3. What is the likelihood she will reduce her weight by diet, exercise, and possibly medications?
4. In the presence of hypertension, could pharmacologic therapies be considered?
5. Would you consider surgical intervention in this person?

DISCUSSION

This woman has experienced many disappointments and embarrassments in her life, including poor self-esteem, ridicule, work embarrassment, self-loathing, expensive "large woman's" clothing, and a husband who would prefer she stay her current size.

Upon questioning the husband, he claims that she snores terribly and has such severe sleep apnea that he wonders why she hasn't died yet! This one fact increases her chances of sudden death tenfold.

Upon questioning her, you discover that she lost the weight by starving herself and then inevitably overeating. She gets up at night to eat. She is convinced that the "weight pill" is the only way out for her. She is not interested in exercise because her knees are so painful. You recommend water exercise and she says she's afraid of water.

Ask the patient whether she is interested in a program you have that involves diet, exercise, and regular visits. The patient may be willing to "consider another program," or you might determine that because she has never had sustained weight loss, self-efficacy might be a major problem. Once this is determined, you can plan for the right course of action. Decide what you, as a physician, are willing to do and then talk with the patient about it. Do not be judgmental; respond in an empathic way so that the patient knows that you are listening to her concerns. Do not be afraid to send the patient on to someone else if you are uncomfortable.

Careful attention to lipids and the possibility of developing acute cholecystitis and heart dysrhythmias during a rapid drop in weight are important. Psychologic counsel is also essential for her to address her body image and adjust her perceptions over time. Keep in mind that reductions of 10% of body weight often improve blood pressure and glucose tolerance/triglyceride profiles.

Constant realistic praise and nonjudgmental follow-up will cement your relationship and facilitate success. Remember that maintenance of reduced weight at 1 year is the goal.

REFERENCES

1. Staffieri JR. A student of social stereotype of body image in children. J Pers Soc Psychol 1967;7:101–104.
2. Canning H, Mayer J. Obesity—its possible effects on college admissions. N Engl J Med 1966;275:1172–1174.
3. Larkin JE, Pines HA. No fat persons need apply. Soc Work Occup 1979;6:312–327.
4. Rand CS, Macgregor AM. Successful weight loss following obesity surgery and the perceived liability of morbid obesity. Int J Obes 1991;15:577–579.
5. Stunkard AJ, Wadden TA. Psychological aspects of severe obesity. Am J Clin Nutr 1992;55:524S–532S.
6. Horm J, Anderson K. Who in America is trying to lose weight? (NHIS annual study of 45,000 U.S. households). Ann Intern Med 1993;119(7 pt 2):672–676.
7. Kuczmarski RJ, Flegal KM, Campbell SM, et al. Increasing prevalence of overweight among U.S. adults. JAMA 1994;272:205–211.
8. Centers for Disease Control and Prevention. Update: prevalence of overweight among children, adolescents, and adults—United States, 1988–1994. MMWR 1997; 46(9).
9. Guo SS, Roche AF, Chumlea WC, et al. The predictive value of childhood body mass values for overweight at age 35 years. Am J Clin Nutr 1994;39:810–819.
10. US Preventive Services Task Force. Guide to Clinical Preventive Services. Report of the US Preventive Services Task Force, 2nd ed. Baltimore: William & Wilkins, 1996:219.
11. Metropolitan Life Insurance Company. Metropolitan height and weight tables. Stat Bull Metrop Insur Co 1983;64:2–9.
12. Najjar MF, Rowland M. Anthropometric reference data and prevalence of overweight—United States 1976–1980. Vital and Health Statistics. DHHS publication no. (PHS) 87–1688. Washington, DC: Government Printing Office, 1987;11(238).
13. Deleted in proof.
14. Gray DS, Fujioka K. Use of relative weight and body mass for the determination of adiposity. Am J Epidemiol 1991;44:545–550.
15. Schey HM, Michieluttie R, Corbett WT, et al. Weight-for-height indices as measures of adiposity in children. J Chronic Dis 1984;37:397–400.
16. Rowland ML. A nomogram for computing body mass index. Diet Currents 1989;16(2):1–12.
17. Lissner L, Odell PM, D'Agostino RB, et al. Variability of body weight and health outcomes in the Framingham population. N Engl J Med 1991;324:1839–1844.
18. Brownell KD. Dieting and the search for the perfect body: where physiology and culture collide. Behav Ther 1991;22:1–12.
19. Bray GA. Progress in understanding the genetics of obesity. J Nutr 1997;127(5 suppl):940S–942S.
20. Friedman JM. The alphabet of weight control. Nature 1997;385(6612):119–120.
21. Kushi LH, Kaye SA, Folsum AR, et al. Accuracy and reliability of self-measurement of body girth. Am J Epidemiol 1988;128:740–748.
22. Manson JE, Willett WC, Stampler MJ, et al. Body weight and mortality among women. N Engl J Med 1995;333:677–685.
23. Expert Group, Minister of National Health and Welfare. Report: Canadian Guidelines for Healthy Weights, 1988. Catalog no. H39–134/1989E. Ottawa, Canada: Minister of National Health and Welfare, 1988:69.
24. Anderson LA, Janes GR, Ziemer DC, Phillips LS. Diabetes in urban African-Americans. Body image, satisfaction with size, and weight-change attempts. Diabetes Educ 1997;23.
25. Dietary Guidelines Advisory Committee, 1995. Report to the Secretary of Health and Human Services and the Secretary of Agriculture. US Department of Agriculture, Agricultural Research Service. Springfield, VA: National Technical Information Service, 1995.
26. Lavie CJ, Milani RV. Effects of cardiac rehabilitation, exercise training, and weight reduction on exercise capacity, coronary risk factors, behavioral characteristics, and quality of life in obese coronary patients. Am J Cardiol 1997;79(4):397–401.
27. Parham ES. Enhancing social support in weight loss management groups. J Am Diet Assoc 1994;94(7):715–716.
28. Benotti PN, Forse RA. Safety and long-term efficacy of revisional surgery in severe obesity. Am J Surg 1996;172(3):232–235.
29. Schembre DB, Boynton KK. Appetite-suppressant drugs and primary pulmonary hypertension. N Engl J Med 1997;336(7):510–513.
30. Raison CL, Klein HM. Psychotic mania associated with

fenfluramine and phentermine use. Am J Psychol 1997; 154(5):711.

31. Brown TM, Skop BP, Mareth TR. Pathophysiology and management of the serotonin syndrome. Ann Pharmacother 1996;30(5):527–533.

32. Davis R, Faulds D. Dexfenfluramine: an updated review of its therapeutic use in the management of obesity. Drugs 1996;52(5):696–724.

33. National Task Force on the Prevention and Treatment of Obesity. Long-term pharmacotherapy in the management of obesity. JAMA 1996;276(23): 1907–1915.

34. Prochaska JO, Norcross JC, DiClemente CC. Changing for Good. New York: William Morrow, 1994.

35. Bandura A. Self-efficacy mechanism in human agency. Am Psychol 1982;37:122–127.

Index

Page references in *italics* denote figures; those followed by "t" denote tables

AA (*see* Alcoholics Anonymous)
Abdominal examinations, 83
Abdominal pain
    case studies of, 240–241
    in children, 240
    clinical conditions that present as
        appendicitis, 233, 239
        biliary tract disease, 227, 228t–230t, 235–236
        bowel obstruction, 232–233, 238
        diverticulitis, 233–234, 239
        dyspepsia, 227, 229, 231–232, 236–238
        ectopic pregnancy, 234–235, 239
        endometriosis, 235, 239
        gastric cancer, 231–232
        irritable bowel syndrome, 234, 239
        pancreatic cancer, 232, 238
        pancreatic disease, 232, 238
        pancreatitis (*see* Pancreatitis)
        pelvic inflammatory disease, 235, 239
        peptic ulcer disease, 228, 230t, 231
    clinical evaluation of
        algorithm, 225
        history, 224, 226
        laboratory tests, 226
        physical examination, 226
        red flags, 224, 224t
    considerations for, 221, 239–240
    differential diagnosis, 222t, 223–224, 224t
    in elderly, 240
    environmentally induced, 54t
    nonspecific, 224
    pathophysiology of
        extra-abdominal, 222–223
        intra-abdominal, 221–222, 222
        psychologic conditions, 223
    prevalence of, 221
    recurrent, 240
Abnormal uterine bleeding (*see* Uterine bleeding, abnormal)
Abortion, 105t
Abrasions, 614–615
Abscess
    peritonsillar, 625
    skin, 602–603
Abstinence, 105t
Acarbose, 392–393
Accolate (*see* Zafirlukast)
Acetaminophen, clinical uses of
    ankle pain, 269t
    fever in infants and preschool children, *442*, 444t
    headaches, 457t
    knee pain, 269t
    low back pain, 494t
Acetohexamide, 390t
Achilles tendonitis
    description of, 263
    management of, 270

ACL (*see* Anterior cruciate ligament)
Acne
    contraceptive formulations for patients with, 116t
    contraceptive-induced, 118t
    description of, 607
    treatment of, 608t
Acromioclavicular joint
    anatomy of, 581, *582*
    degenerative disease, 590t, 593
    separations of, 590t, 593
Actinic keratosis, 607
Acupuncture, 195
Acute calculous cholecystitis, 227, 230t
Acute cardiac ischemia, chest pain caused by
    description of, 349–350
    drug therapy, 363t
    electrocardiographic evaluation of, 356
    gender-based differences, 353
    management of, 358–361, 359t
    time-insensitive predictive instrument for diagnosing, 352, 353t
Acute cholangitis, 227
Acute cholecystitis
    diagnosis of, 228t
    management of, 235–236
Acute neurolabyrinthitis, 407
Acyclovir, 604
ADA (*see* Americans With Disabilities Act)
Addiction (*see also* Substance abuse)
    case studies of, 258–261
    differential diagnosis, 245
    DSM-IV definitions of, 243–244
    education regarding, 257–258
    etiology of, 244
    family education regarding, 257–258
    pathophysiology of, 245, 247t
    patient education regarding, 257–258
    prevalence of, 243–245
    prevalent age of onset, 244
    treatment for
        aversion therapy, 255
        cognitive-behavioral techniques, 254
        considerations, 251, 253
        drug-based approaches, 255–256
        interventions, 256
        long term, 256–257
        Minnesota model, 254
        self-help groups, 253–254, 254t
        success rates, 256
Adenosine, 371t
Adhesive capsulitis, 590t, 594
Adipose tissue, 682, 684t
Adolescents
    bedside manner, 7
    case study of, 17–18
    counseling
        contraception, 104, 106
        topics for, 150t
    health needs, 16
    needs of, 16

699

Adolescents—*Continued*
  pregnancy risks, 100–101
  rearing of, 31–32
  screening of, for well care
    cervical dysplasia, 145–146
    congenital heart disease, 145
    growth and development, 144–145
    hypertension, 145
    sexually transmitted diseases, 146
    substance abuse, 146
    suicide, 146
    tuberculosis, 145
    venereal disease, 145–146
    youth violence, 146
  treatment approaches for, 16–17
β-Adrenergic blockers, 644t
Adults
  abdominal pain in, 240
  headaches in, 458
  middle aged
    case study of, 18–20
    needs, 18
  older
    approaching, 20–21
    bedside manner, 8–9
    case study of, 22–23
    developmental tasks, 32
    treating, 20
    transitions, 19t
  urinary tract infections in, 420–421
  well care for
    chemoprophylaxis, 163–164
    description of, 159
    education
      description of, 174
      for men, 172t–173t
      for women, 168t–169t
    immunizations
      description of, 159, 162–164
      for women, 165t–166t
    morbidity and mortality causes, 157, 158t
    overview, 157–158
    preventive care (*see also* Preventive medicine)
      case studies, 176
      challenges associated with, 175–176
      considerations for, 174
      description of, 157–158
      implementation of, 175
    risk assessment
      depression, 159, *162*
      diet history, 159, *160–161*
      for men, 170t
      sexual history taking, 158, 159t
      for women, 165t
    screening for asymptomatic disease
      description of, 164
      medical coverage for, 164, 174
      in men, 170t–172t
      in women, 166t–168t
    travel considerations, 159–160
    women, 165t–170t
AFDC (*see* Aid to Families with Dependent Children)
Agency for Toxic Substances and Disease Registry, 59t
Aging, systemic changes associated with, 21t
β$_2$-Agonists, for asthma, 318t–319t, 321

Aid to Families with Dependent Children, 100
AK (*see* Actinic keratosis)
Albuterol
  for asthma, 319t, 321
  for chronic obstructive pulmonary disease, 327t
Alcohol
  abuse of (*see also* Addiction; Substance abuse)
    detoxification regimen, 251t
    parental counseling for, 153
    systemic effects, 247t
    Withdrawal Assessment Scale, 252t–253t
    withdrawal symptoms, 249
  death rates, 81t
Alcoholics Anonymous, 253–254, 254t
Aleve (*see* Naproxen sodium)
Alexander technique, 195
Allergic vaginosis, 660
Allopathic medicine, comparison with complementary therapies, 192
Allopurinol, 302
Alprazolam, 363t
Alternative medicine (*see* Complementary therapies)
Alzheimer's disease, 191
Amenorrhea, 510
American Academy of Family Physicians, 63
American College of Occupational and Environmental Medicine, 59t
American Heart Association, diet history advocated by, 159, *160–161*
American Medical Association, 79
Americans With Disabilities Act, 67
Amiodarone, 371t
Amitriptyline, 457t
Amniocentesis, 135
Amoxicillin
  for fever in infants and preschool children, 444t
  for group A β-hemolytic streptococcal pharyngitis, 632t
Amoxicillin/clavulanate, for urinary tract infections, 417t
Anaprox (*see* Naproxen sodium)
Anemia
  aplastic, 55t
  iron deficiency, in first trimester of pregnancy, 131
Angina pectoris
  description of, 369
  environmentally induced, 54t
  management of, 369–370
  mechanical interventions, 370
  medications for, 370, 371t
  pathophysiology of, 369
  risk factors, 369
Angiotensin-converting enzyme inhibitors, clinical uses of
  acute cardiac ischemia, 363t
  heart failure
    from diastolic dysfunction, 374
    from systolic dysfunction, 373
  hypertension, 478t
Ankle
  anatomy of, *264*
  fracture of, 269–270
  ligaments of, 263, *264*
Ankle pain
  case study of, 277–278
  clinical evaluation of

history, 265, 268t
overview, 263, 265
physical examination, 265–266, *267*, 268t
radiologic tests, *266*, 266–268
"red flags," 265t
stress test, *267*
description of, 263
differential diagnosis, 263, 264t
management of
from Achilles tendonitis, 270
from fracture, 269–270
from sprain, 268–269
pathophysiology of, 263
Ankle sprain
classification of, 265
management of, 268t, 268–269
Anovulation, persistent, 116t
Antabuse (*see* Disulfiram)
Anterior cruciate ligament
anatomy of, *271*
injuries
description of, 270
imaging of, 275
management of, 276t, 277
Antiarrhythmic agents, 371t
Antibiotics
for chronic obstructive pulmonary disease, 327t
for fever in infants and preschool children, 441–442, 444t
for group A β-hemolytic streptococcal pharyngitis, 631t
for urinary tract infections, 417
Antidepressants (*see* Tricyclic antidepressants)
Antigens
prostate-specific (*see* Prostate-specific antigen test)
Rh testing, 131
Antihypertensive medications
characteristics of, 478t
costs of, 479
dosing of, 479
effect on coexisting medical conditions, 479
normal activity effects, 479
patient population considerations, 478–479
Antimycotics, 672t, 673
Antiretroviral therapy, for human immunodeficiency virus
agent selection, 466
agents used in, 465t
algorithmic approach, *468*
changes in, 466
costs of, 463
goal of, 463
initiation of, 463
monitoring of, 466
nonnucleoside reverse transcriptase inhibitors, 465t
nucleoside reverse transcriptase inhibitors, 465t
protease inhibitors, 465t
Antithyroid drugs, 644t, 650
Antitrust, 72
α_1-Antitrypsin deficiency
in chronic obstructive pulmonary disease, 324
treatment of, 325–326
Anxiety
case study of, 289–290
clinical evaluation
associated medical condition, 283–284
diagnostic criteria, 283
primary diagnosis, 284–285
psychiatric in nature, 284
description of, 281
differential diagnosis, 282–283
generalized anxiety disorder
characteristics of, 283
diagnostic criteria, 285t
pharmacologic treatment, 286–288
management of
counseling and education, 286
overview, 285
pharmacologic, 286–288
psychotherapy, 288–289
symptom control, 286
panic disorder without agoraphobia
characteristics of, 283
diagnostic criteria, 285t
pharmacologic treatment, 286–287
pathophysiology of, 281–282
prevalence of, 282t
referral indications, 289
Apnea, obesity and, 683t
Appendicitis
abdominal pain associated with, 233
diagnosis of, 228t
progression of, 222
treatment for, 239
Appendix, 233
Applied kinesiology, 194–195
ARC (*see* Hidden agenda)
Aromatherapy, 196
Arrhythmias (*see also* Cardiac disease; Heart disease)
classification of, 374
description of, 374
environmentally induced, 54t
etiology of, 374
medications for, 370, 371t
types of
atrial fibrillation, 375–376
bradycardia, 375
premature atrial contractions, 374–375
premature ventricular contractions, 374–375
supraventricular tachycardia, 375
wide complex tachycardia, 376–377
Arsenic, in drinking water, 55
Arthritis
alternative therapies, 296
case study of, 307
clinical evaluation of
history, 291
joint fluid, 294, 295t
physical examination, 291–292
radiology, 294
fatigue associated with, 426
general management of
description of, 294–295
medication, 295–296
osteoarthritis (*see* Osteoarthritis)
rheumatoid (*see* Rheumatoid arthritis)
Ascorbic acid (*see* Vitamin C)
Aspirin
for ankle pain, 269t
for diabetes mellitus complications, 396
for knee pain, 269t
for low back pain, 494t

Association of Occupational and Environmental
  Clinics, 59t
Asthma
  acute exacerbations, 322
  case study of, 328–329
  chronic obstructive pulmonary disease and, 324
  classification of, 316t
  clinical evaluation of
    history, 310–311, 311t
    physical examination, 311t, 311–312
  definition of, 309
  description of, 309
  differential diagnosis, 314
  environmentally induced, 54t
  family education regarding, 323
  laboratory evaluation of
    chest radiographs, 314
    pulmonary function tests, 312–314
    pulse oximetry, 314
    spirometry, *313*, 313–314
  management of
    anti-inflammatory medications, 321
    bronchodilators
      β₂ agonists, 321–322
      description of, 321
    corticosteroids, 317, 321
    exposure prevention, 314–315
    inhaled medications
      delivery of, 315
      metered-dose inhaler, *320*
    lung function measures for monitoring asthma
      status, 315, 316t
    NIH recommendations, 314
    pharmacotherapy, 315, 318t–320t
  pathophysiology of
    infection, 310
    inflammation, 309–310
  patient education regarding, 323
  during pregnancy, 323–324
  prevalence of, 309
  risk factors, 323t
  triggers
    exposure reduction, 314–315
    skin testing for, 315
    types of, 312t
Asymptomatic bacteriuria, 421
Atenolol, 363t, 371t, 644t
Atrial fibrillation, 375–376
Atrophic vaginitis, 660
Augmentin (*see* Amoxicillin/clavulanate)
Aventyl (*see* Nortriptyline)
Azathioprine, 304t
Azithromycin, for group A β-hemolytic streptococcal
  pharyngitis, 632t
Azmacort (*see* Triamcinolone acetonide)
AZT (*see* Zidovudine)

B vitamins, 93t
Back pain (*see* Low back pain)
Bacterial vaginitis
  diagnosis of, 664, 664t
  history findings, 660, 662t
  laboratory tests, 665t
  pathophysiology of, 658
  physical examination findings, 660, 663t
  treatment of, 669, 670t, 673

Barrier method, of contraception
  condoms, 121
  diaphragm, 122
  spermicides, 121–122
  sponge, 122
Basal cell carcinoma, 607 (*see color plate*)
Beclomethasone dipropionate, 319t, 321
Bedside manner, 6–9
Behavior
  changing of
    success rates, 89
    support groups, 89
  of parents, 129
Behavioral prescription slip, *88*
Benazepril, 371t
Benign prostatic hyperplasia
  case study of, 539–540
  clinical evaluation of
    history, 532–533
    laboratory tests, 533
    physical examination, 533
  differential diagnosis, 532
  management of
    algorithm, *535*
    outcomes, 536t
    patient education, 536–537
    pharmacologic, 534, 537t
    surgery, 535–536
  pathophysiology of, 532
  signs and symptoms of, 532–533, 533t
Benzodiazepines, 288
Benzphetamine, 687t
β Blockers
  for acute cardiac ischemia, 359–360, 363t
  for angina pectoris, 370, 371t
  for hypertension, 478t
Biaxin (*see* Clarithromycin)
Biceps
  pain in, 587
  tendonitis of, 590t, 592–593
Bicipital groove, 581
Bile duct stones, 227
Biliary tract disease
  gallstones, 227
  management of, 235–236
  types of, 227
Biofeedback, 193
Biopsychosocial model, of disease, 206
Bitolterol, 320t
Bladder cancer, 54t
α₁ Blockers, for hypertension, 478t
Blood pressure
  elevated levels (*see* Hypertension)
  evaluations during third trimester of pregnancy,
    135
  screening
    in men, 171t
    technique, 473
    in women, 166t
Blue Cross/Blue Shield, 65
Body mass index
  nomenclature, 680t
  ratio, *681*
Bodywork
  Alexander technique, 195
  applied kinesiology, 194–195

description of, 194
reflexology, 194
therapeutic massage, 194
therapeutic touch, 195
Bones (*see* Skeletal system)
Bontril (*see* Phendimetrazine)
Boundaries, of family, 30
Bowel habits, of infants and newborns, 151–152
Bowel obstruction
    abdominal pain associated with, 232–233
    diagnosis of, 228t
    treatment for, 238
BPH (*see* Benign prostatic hyperplasia)
Brachial plexus, 582
Bradycardia, 375
Breast cancer
    age-related increases in, 339
    contraceptive formulations for patients with, 116t–117t
    hormone replacement therapy and, 185–186
    oral contraceptives and, 113
    palpable breast mass and, 339
    "red flags" suggestive of, 342t
Breast-feeding
    advantages of, 149–150
    description of, 149–150
    for well child care, 149–150
Breasts
    pain associated with
        clinical evaluation of
            history, 332, 332t
            laboratory tests, 333
            overview, 331–332
            physical examination, 332t, 332–333
        cyclic mastalgia
            description of, 331–332
            nonpharmacotherapy for, 333
            pharmacotherapy for, 333t, 333–334, 335t
        description of, 331
        differential diagnosis, 331, 332t
        management of, 333–334, 334t–335t, 335
        noncyclic mastalgia
            description of, 331
            management of, 334, 335t
        pathophysiology of, 331
    palpable mass of
        case study of, 345
        clinical evaluation of
            biopsy, 343
            history, 339, 341t
            laboratory tests, 342–343
            physical examination, 339–342, 341t
        description of, 339
        differential diagnosis, 339, 341t
        malignant
            diagnostic tests, 342t
            physical findings of, 339–340
        management of, 343, *344*
        pathophysiology of, 339
    tenderness, contraceptive-induced, 118t
Brethaire (*see* Terbutaline)
Bromocriptine, for cyclic mastalgia, 333t, 334
Bronchiolitis, 436, 553–554
Bronchitis
    acute, 554
    chronic, 54t, 554

description of, 436
    pneumonia and, differential diagnosis of, 545
Budesonide turbuhaler, 319t
Bupropion, 287t
Bursae, of shoulder, 581–582
Bursitis
    description of, 297–298
    management of, 298
Buspirone, 363t
Butoconazole, 670t
Butorphanol, 457t
BV (*see* Bacterial vaginitis)

CABG (*see* Coronary artery bypass grafting)
CAD (*see* Coronary artery disease)
Calan (*see* Verapamil)
Calcium
    recommendations, 93t
    reductions for hypertension treatment, 477, 477t
Calcium channel blockers
    for cardiac disease, 371t
    for hypertension, 478t
    for left ventricular dysfunction, 360
    for thyroid disorders, 644t
Cancer (*see also* Carcinoma)
    bladder, 54t
    breast
        age-related increases in, 339
        contraceptive formulations, 116t–117t
        hormone replacement therapy and, 185–186
        oral contraceptives and, 113
        palpable breast mass and, 339
        "red flags" suggestive of, 342t
    gastric
        description of, 231–232
        diagnostic tests, 230t
        symptoms of, 231–232
    lung, 54t
    obesity and, 683t
    occupationally-induced, 49t
    ovarian, 116t
    pancreatic, 232, 238
    prostate (*see* Prostate cancer)
    skin (*see* Carcinoma, of skin)
Candida vulvovaginitis
    diagnosis of, 664
    history findings, 660, 662t
    laboratory tests, 665t, 668
    nonprescription medication, 657
    pathophysiology of, 658
    physical examination findings, 660, 663t
    self-diagnosis of, 669
    treatment of, 670t–671t, 673–674
Candidiasis, as cause of sore throat, 623–624
Captopril (Capoten), 371t
Carbamazepine, 494t
Carcinoma, of skin (*see also* Cancer; *color plates*)
    basal cell, 607 (*see color plate*)
    benign growths and, differential diagnosis, 607, 609
    description of, 607, 609
    melanoma, 607, 609t (*see color plate*)
    squamous cell, 607 (*see color plate*)
Cardiac arrhythmias (*see* Arrhythmias)
Cardiac disease (*see also* Heart disease)
    arrhythmias (*see* Arrhythmias)
    differential diagnosis, 367, 369

Cardiac disease—*Continued*
  general approach, *368*
  pathophysiology of, 367, 369
  prevalence of, 367
  risk factors, 369
Cardiovascular system
  age-related changes, 21t
  disease of
    contraceptive formulations for patients with,
      116t–117t
    occupational, 49t
    oral contraceptive use and, 113
Cardizem (*see* Diltiazem)
Cardura (*see* Doxazosin)
Care (*see* Health care; Well care)
Carpal tunnel syndrome, 297–298, 522
Cataracts, obesity and, 683t
CBE (*see* Clinical breast examination)
CBT (*see* Cognitive-behavioral therapy)
Cefixime, 632t
Cefotaxime, 444t
Ceftriaxone, 444t
Cellulitis, 602
Cephalexin, 417t
Cervical caps, 122
Cervical polyps, as cause of dysmenorrhea, 505–506
Cervical radiculopathy, 595
Cervicitis, 659
  description of, 569
  differential diagnosis, 573
  history, 573
  laboratory tests, 574, 668
  management of, 574, 575t
  pathophysiology of, 573
  physical examination, 573–574
Chamomile, 197t
Chancroid, 563, 571t, 576t
Chemoprophylaxis, 81t
Chest pain
  acute, 351–352
  acute cardiac ischemia time-insensitive predictive
    instrument, 352, 353t
  case study of, 362, 364
  description of, 349
  differential diagnosis, 351t, 351–352
  drug therapy for, 363t
  evaluation of
    complete approach
      history, 352t, 354–355
      laboratory testing, 356–358
      physical examination, 356
    rapid approach
      history, 352t, 352–354
      laboratory testing, 356
      physical examination, 356
  general approach to, 349
  management of, 358–362, 359t, *360*
  pathophysiology of
    acute cardiac ischemia (*see* Acute cardiac is-
      chemia)
    coronary artery disease (*see* Coronary artery dis-
      ease)
    description of, 349
    esophageal spasm, 350
    gastroesophageal reflux disease (*see* Gastroe-
      sophageal reflux disease, chest pain caused by)
  mitral valve prolapse, 350–351
  musculoskeletal pain, 350, 354
  panic disorder (*see* Panic disorder, chest pain
    caused by)
  pleural pain, 351
  pulmonary pain, 351
  stable angina, 350
  "red flags" for serious etiology, 354t
  in respiratory infections, 544–545
  symptoms associated with, 355
  temporal nature of, 355
Chickenpox, 604
Childbirth, companion support during, 130
Children
  abdominal pain in, 240
  bedside manner, 6–7
  counseling topics for, 150t
  development of
    adult roles, 15t
    milestones, 14t
  examining, 13–16
  headaches in, 458
  rearing of, 31
  school phobia, 30
  sinusitis in, 551
  skin disease in, 599
  urinary tract infections in, 419–420
  well care in
    case study of, 153–154
    counseling for parents
      alcohol use, 153
      bowel habits, 151–152
      crying, 151
      dental health, 152
      description of, 149
      diet, 153
      drug use, 153
      exercise, 153
      feeding, 149–150
      infant stimulation, 149
      injury prevention, 152
      preventive, principles of, 149
      sexual behavior, 153
      skin care, 151
      sleeping, 151
      sudden infant death syndrome, 152
      tobacco use, 153
      topics commonly discussed, 150t
      youth violence, 153
    description of, 141
    immunizations
      adverse reactions associated with, 148
      contraindications, 147t
      measles, mumps, rubella, 148
      oral polio vaccine, 148
      precautions, 147t
      schedule for, 148t
    parental involvement, 141
    screening, 146–147
      description of, 142
      growth and development, 144–145
      heart disease, 145
      hypertension, 145
      iron deficiency anemia, 143
      lead toxicity, 143–144
      for newborns, 143

recommended types based on age, 142t–143t
tuberculosis, 145
vision problems, 144
visits, 141
Chiropractics, 194
Chlamydia trachomatis
in adolescents, 145
characteristics of, 560–562
health effects of, 561t
screening tests for, 566t
treatment of, 570t
Chloasma, contraceptive-induced, 118t
Chlorpromazine, 457t
Chlorpropamide, 390t
Chlorzoxazone, 494t
Cholelithiasis
diagnostic tests, 230t
management of, 235
Cholesterol
reductions of, 369–370
screening
in men, 171t
in women, 166t
Chondrocalcinosis (*see* Pseudogout)
Chondromalacia patellae, 271
CHOP, 49
Chronic bronchitis, 324
Chronic fatigue syndrome
coping strategies for, 433
description of, 427
diagnostic criteria, 428t
management of, 432, 432t
patient education regarding, 433
Chronic obstructive pulmonary disease
α_1-antitrypsin deficiency in, 324
asthma and, 324
clinical evaluation of
history, 324
laboratory tests
arterial blood gases, 325
chest radiograph, 325
spirometry, 325
physical examination, 325
definition of, 324
description of, 309
etiology of, 309
exacerbations, 326, 328
incidence of, 309
management of
corticosteroids, 325
ipratropium bromide, 325
long term, 325–326
oxygen therapy, 326
regimens, 326t–327t
smoking cessation, 328
occupational exposure-induced, 324
pathophysiology of, 324
patient education regarding, 328
Cigarette smoking (*see* Tobacco)
Cimetidine, 363t
Ciprofloxacin (Cipro), 417t
CK (*see* Creatine kinase)
Claforan (*see* Cefotaxime)
Clarithromycin, 550–551
Clavicle fractures, 590t, 594–595
Clindamycin, 670t, 672t

Clinical breast examination
for adult women, 167t
clinical uses
breast pain, 332–333
nipple discharge, 338
palpable malignant breast mass, 342t
Clonazepam, 363t
Clonidine, 478t
Clotrimazole, 670t
Clunk test, 585
Cluster headaches
clinical evaluation of, 451–452
pathophysiology of, 447
treatment of, 456
Cocaine, systemic effects of, 247t
Codeine, 494t
Cognitive-behavioral therapy, 288–289
Colchicine, 302
Cold (*see* Common cold)
Colic
signs and symptoms of, 151
treatment approaches, 151
Colicky pain, 226
Colon cancer, screening of
in men, 171t
in women, 166t–167t
Common cold
description of, 547
history of, 547
physical examination of, 547
treatment of, 547
Community medicine
case study of, 44
cultural diversity of, 41–42
dimensions, 41
leadership in
advocacy for community, 42–44
case study of, 44
discussion, 42–44
primary care, 43–44
resources, 42
Community-oriented primary care, 43–44
Compazine (*see* Prochlorperazine)
Complementary therapies
acupuncture, 195
allopathic medicine and, comparisons, 192
aromatherapy, 196
bodywork
Alexander technique, 195
applied kinesiology, 194–195
description of, 194
reflexology, 194
therapeutic massage, 194
therapeutic touch, 195
chiropractic, 194
cultural context of, 192–193
definition of, 191
dietary, 195–196
education regarding, 192
herbal medicine, 196
homeopathy, 196, 199
for menopause, 186
mind-body
biofeedback, 193
description of, 193
hypnosis, 193

Complementary therapies—*Continued*
  meditation, 193–194
    mindful exercise, 194
  population groups that commonly use, 191
  prevalence of, 191–192
  principles of, 193
  religious beliefs and, 191
  types of, 191
Condoms (*see also* Contraception)
  description of, 121
  effectiveness, 105t
  female version, 121
  sexually transmitted disease prevention, 578
Conduction system, rhythm disturbances of, 369
Condylomata acuminata, 604
Condylomata lata, 562
Confidentiality
  contraception, 106
  medical records, 57–58
Congenital heart disease (*see also* Cardiac disease;
    Heart disease)
  in adolescents, 145
  in children, 145
Consultations
  advice, 70
  description, 64
  ethics, 70
  referrals *versus*, 69–70
Contraception
  clinical evaluation, 106–108
  condoms, 153
  confidentiality, 106
  consent, 106
  counseling
    algorithm, *109*
    components, 103–106
  for menopausal women, 186
  methods
    barriers
      condoms, 121
      diaphragm, 122
      spermicides, 121–122
      sponge, 122
    case history, 123–125
    choice factors, 108
    comparison, 105t
    condom, 105t
    failure rates, 104t
    fertility awareness, 122–123
    future of, 123
    implants, 105t
    injectables, 105t
    intrauterine devices, 119–121
    oral (*see* Oral contraceptives)
    postcoital, 122
    rhythm, 122–123
    sterilization, 123
  overview, 102–103
  prevalent methods of, *102*
  sexual abuse, 106
Contusions, 613–614
COPC (*see* Community-oriented primary care)
Cordarone (*see* Amiodarone)
Coronary artery bypass grafting, 370
Coronary artery disease
  chest pain caused by

description of, 350, 352
  earlobe evaluations, 356
  laboratory testing, 357–358
  management of, 359t, 361
  predictive algorithm, 354, *355*
  risk factors, 353–355
  obesity and, 683
Corticosteroids, clinical uses of
  asthma, 317, 321
  chronic obstructive pulmonary disease, 325, 327t
  rheumatoid arthritis, 304, 305t
  rhinitis, 552
  skin diseases
    adverse effects, 599–600
    dispensing of, 600, 601t
    duration of therapy, 601
    mechanism of action, 599
    selection of, 600, 600t
Costochondritis, 331
Cough, 54t, 548
Counseling (*see also* Education)
  contraception
    for adolescents, 104, 106
    algorithm, *109*
    components, 103–106
  of parents, for providing well care to children
    alcohol use, 153
    bowel habits, 151–152
    crying, 151
    dental health, 152
    description of, 149
    diet, 153
    drug use, 153
    exercise, 153
    feeding, 149–150
    infant stimulation, 149
    injury prevention, 152
    preventive, principles of, 149
    sexual behavior, 153
    skin care, 151
    sleeping, 151
    sudden infant death syndrome, 152
    tobacco use, 153
    topics commonly discussed, 150t
    youth violence, 153
  of patients
    aspects, 85–86
    expectations, 86–87
    importance, 85
    key steps, 85t
    model, 86
    strategies, 87, 89
      exercise, 89, 91
      healthy diet, 91
      injury prevention, 91
      mental health, 93–95
      tobacco use, 89
      violence, 92–93
Crank test, 585
C-reactive protein, 292
Creatine kinase, myocardial infarction and, 356–357
Crepitus, 292
Crixivan (*see* Indinavir)
Cromolyn, 318t–319t
Cross tolerance, 244
Croup, 553

Crying, of newborn, 151
Cryptorchidism, in adolescents, 147
Cyclobenzaprine, 494t
Cyclosporin A, 304t
Cyproheptadine, 457t

Danazol
  for cyclic mastalgia, 333t, 334
  for dysmenorrhea, 507t
Decision making
  algorithm, 206, *206*
  elements involved in
    assembling of information, 206–207
    gathering of information, 206
    organizing the patient encounter, 207
  types of decisions, 217
Degenerative arthritis, 519
Degenerative disc disease, 484
Delavirdine, 465t
Dental health, in children, counseling for, 152
Depakene (*see* Valproic acid)
Depakote (*see* Valproic acid)
Dependence, definition of, 244
Depomedroxyprogesterone acetate (Depo-Provera),
  118–119
Depression
  case study of, 289–290
  clinical evaluation
    associated medical condition, 283–284
    diagnostic criteria, 283
    primary diagnosis, 284–285
    psychiatric in nature, 284
  contraceptive use and, 116t, 118t
  differential diagnosis, 282–283
  drugs that exacerbate, 284t
  dysthymia
    characteristics of, 283
    pharmacologic treatment, 286–287
  major depressive disorder
    characteristics of, 282–283
    diagnostic criteria, 285t
    pharmacologic treatment, 286–288
  management of
    counseling and education, 286
    overview, 285
    pharmacologic, 286–288, 287t
    psychotherapy, 288–289
    symptom control, 286
  mood disorder secondary to medical condition, 283
  pathophysiology of, 281–282
  prevalence of, 282t
  referral indications, 289
  seasonal affective disorder, 283
  suicide risks, 286
  Zung self-rating scale, 159, *162*
Dermatitis
  atopic, 605–606 (*see color plate*)
  contact, 605
  definition of, 605
  seborrhea, 606 (*see color plate*)
Desipramine, 287t, 363t
Development
  adult roles, 15t
  family stages, 30–32
  milestones, 14t
Dexamethasone, 631, 631t–632t

Dexfenfluramine, 687t
Diabetes mellitus
  case study of, 399
  clinical evaluation of
    history, 382–383
    laboratory tests, 384–385
    physical examination, 383, *384*
  complications, 396
  contraceptive formulations for patients with, 116t
  description of, 381
  differential diagnosis, 385
  epidemiology of, 381–382
  gestational, 136
  glucose monitoring
    description of, 395
    fasting levels, 395
    home methods for, 395–396
    metabolic indices, 395t
  insulin-dependent
    characteristics of, 382
    clinical evaluation, 383
    description of, 382
    dietary guidelines, 389
    home blood glucose monitoring, 395–396
  long-term management of, 396–397
  management of
    behavior changes
      diet, 388–389, 389t
      exercise, 388
    initial steps, *387*
    overview, 385–386
    pharmacologic
      acarbose, 392–393
      α-glucosidase inhibitors, 392–393
      insulin, 393–395
      metformin, 391
      sulfonylurea drugs, 389–391, 390t
      troglitazone, 391–392
  mortality causes, 381
  non-insulin-dependent
    characteristics of, 382
    clinical evaluation, 382–383
    complications, 396
    description of, 382
    glucose monitoring, 395
    α-glucosidase inhibitors, 392–393
    management of, 385–386
    physical examination, 383
  obesity and, 683t
  office visit, 397–398, 398t
  pathophysiology of, 381–382
  renal function monitoring, *386*
  thyroid hormonal disease screening and, 652
  vascular complications
    description of, 381
    risk factors, 383
Diabetic ketoacidosis
  description of, 383
  differential diagnosis, 385
Diagnosis (*see also specific disease or condition*)
  common types of, 205
  methods of establishing
    clinical reasoning, 207–208
    epidemiology, 209
    judgment regarding further investigations, 209
  prescription writing after, 210, *211*

Diagnosis—*Continued*
　problem-oriented progress note, 210
　uncertainty regarding, 209–210
Diagnostic tests (*see also specific disease or condition*)
　clinical prediction rules, 214–215
　gold standard evaluations, 212–213
　likelihood ratios, 213–214, 214t
　predictive value, 213
　sensitivity, 213
　specificity, 213
　types of, 212
Diapers, 151–152
Diaphragm, 122
Diazepam, 363t, 494t
Diclofenac, 269t, 296t, 494t
Didanosine, 465t
Didrex (*see* Benzphetamine)
Diet
　complementary therapies, 195–196
　considerations for menopausal women, 186
　healthy
　　promoting, 91
　　tips, 92t
　history, American Heart Association provisions, 159, *160–161*
　for non-insulin-dependent diabetes, 388–389, 389t
　poor, death rates and, 81t
　vegan, 196
　vegetarian, 196
Diethylpropion, 687t
Diffuse peritonitis, 226
Digestive system, age-related changes in, 21t
Digital rectal examination, 83, 529
Digoxin, 371t, 373
Dihydroergotamine, 456, 457t
Diltiazem, 371t, 644t
Diphtheria, pertussis, tetanus vaccine, adverse reactions associated with, 148
Diseases (*see specific disease*)
Disequilibrium
　description of, 402–403
　history findings, 406
　physical examination, 407
Disulfiram, 255
Diuretics, 371t
Diverticulitis
　abdominal pain associated with, 233–234
　description of, 233–234
　management of, 236t–237t, 239
　signs and symptoms of, 233–234
Dizziness
　anxiety as cause (*see* Anxiety)
　case study of, 408–409
　chronic, 408
　clinical evaluation of
　　description of, 403–404
　　general approach, 404, *405*
　　history, 404
　　laboratory tests, 407
　depression as cause (*see* Depression)
　differential diagnosis, 403t, 403–404
　disequilibrium
　　description of, 402–403
　　history findings, 406
　　physical examination, 407
　general approach, 401

　management of, 407–408
　mixed component
　　description of, 403
　　history findings, 406
　presyncope
　　description of, 402
　　history findings, 406
　　physical examination, 407
　prevalence of, 401
　"red flags" that suggest progressive or life-threatening illness as cause of, 404t
　undiagnosed, 407–408
　vertigo
　　benign paroxysmal positional, 405, 407
　　case study of, 409
　　description of, 401–402
　　history findings, 405–406
　　physical examination, 405
DKA (*see* Diabetic ketoacidosis)
DMPA (*see* Depomedroxyprogesterone acetate)
Down syndrome, pregnancy screening for, 135
Doxazosin, 537t
DRE (*see* Digital rectal examination)
Drinking water, arsenic-laced, 55
Drop sign, 587
Drug testing, 248t, 248–249
Drugs (*see also* Prescriptions; *specific drug*)
　contraceptive-induced interactions, 118t
　illicit, 81t, 116t
　parental counseling for, 153
Dry cough, 54t
DUB (*see* Dysfunctional uterine bleeding)
Duct papilloma, 336
Dupuytren's tendonitis, 298
Dysfunctional uterine bleeding
　definition of, 510
　differential diagnosis, 512
　etiology of, 511
Dysmenorrhea
　age of onset, 501
　case study of, 514–516
　clinical evaluation of
　　history, 503t, 503–504
　　laboratory tests, 504, 505t
　　overview, 502–503
　　physical examination, 503t, 504
　contraceptive formulations for patients with, 116t
　contraceptive-induced, 118t
　definition of, 501
　differential diagnosis, 502
　general approach to, *506*
　human immunodeficiency virus testing and, 504
　management of
　　drug therapy, 507t
　　for primary causes, 505
　　for secondary causes, 505–506, 508
　primary
　　case study of, 514–516
　　differential diagnosis, 502
　　management of, 505
　　pathogenesis, 501
　"red flags" that suggest progressive or life-threatening disease associated with, 504t
　secondary
　　diagnosis of, 502

differential diagnosis, 502, 502t
endometriosis and, 502
management of, based on etiology
  cervical polyps, 505–506
  endometriosis, 508
  ovarian cysts, 505–506
  pelvic inflammatory disease, 506, 508
  tubo-ovarian abscess, 506
pathogenesis, 501
physical examination, 504
signs and symptoms of, 503–504
Dyspepsia
  description of, 227
  management of, 236–238, 237t
  prevalence of, 227
Dyspnea, 54t
Dysthymia, 283, 286–287
Dysuria, causes of
  prostate infection (*see* Prostatitis)
  sexually transmitted diseases (*see* Sexually transmitted diseases)
  urinary tract infections (*see* Urinary tract infections)
  vaginitis (*see* Vaginitis)

Earache, 544, 544t
EBM (*see* Evidence-based medicine)
Echinacea, 197t
Ectopic pregnancy
  abdominal pain associated with, 234–235
  clinical findings, 234
  diagnosis of, 229t, 234–235
  treatment for, 239
Eczema, 605 (*see color plate*)
EDC (*see* Expected date of confinement)
Education (*see also* Counseling)
  for health promotion, 87
    exercise, 89, 91
    healthy diet, 91
    injury prevention, 91
    mental health, 93–95
    tobacco use, 89
    violence, 92–93
  of patients (*see also specific disease or condition, patient education regarding*)
    aspects, 85–86
    expectations, 86–87
    importance, 85
    key steps, 85t
    model, 86
Elavil (*see* Amitriptyline)
Electrocardiogram
  for acute cardiac ischemia, 356, 357t
  for chest pain evaluations, 356, 357t
Emphysema, 54t
Empty can test, 586
Enalapril, 363t, 371t
Endometriosis
  characteristics of, 235
  contraceptive formulations for patients with, 116t
  diagnosis of, 229t
  management of, 236t–237t, 239, 508
  secondary dysmenorrhea and, 502, 508
  signs and symptoms of, 235
Entrapment syndrome (*see* Carpal tunnel syndrome)
Environmental hazards
  agencies for assistance, 59t

case studies of, 58, 60–62
criteria, 55
diagnostic investigations, 52t–53t
frequency, 48
history, 49, 51
  form, *50*
human immunodeficiency virus, 468–469, 469t
prevalent types of, 49t
recognition of, 49
related diseases, 54t
treatment plan, 57
Epicondylitis, 297–298
Epidemiology, 209
Epididymitis
  clinical evaluation of, 569
  complications of, 565
  differential diagnosis, 565, 569
  laboratory tests, 569
  management of, 569
  pathophysiology of, 565, 569
Epivir (*see* Lamivudine)
Ergotamine tartrate, 457t
ERT (*see* Estrogen replacement therapy)
Erythroblastosis fetalis, 131
Erythrocyte sedimentation rate
  description of, 292
  for headaches, 454
  for osteoarthritis, 299
Erythromycin ethyl succinate, 632t
Esmolol, 363t
Esophageal spasm, 350
ESR (*see* Erythrocyte sedimentation rate)
Estrogen
  function, 108
  natural form of, 183
  in oral contraceptives, 514t
  production of, 179
  types of, 109, 179
Estrogen replacement therapy
  description of, 183
  disease risk reduced using
    heart disease, 184
    osteoporosis, 184–185
  formulations for, 184t
  recommendations, 168t
Ethinyl estradiol, 109
  for dysmenorrhea, 507t
  estrogenic content, 514t
  progestogenic content, 514t
Etodolac, 269t
Evidence-based medicine
  approaches to
    description of, 210
    for prognosis, 215
    for therapy, 215–216
  diagnostic tests
    clinical prediction rules, 214–215
    gold standard evaluations, 212–213
    likelihood ratios, 213–214
    predictive value, 213
    sensitivity, 213
    specificity, 213
    types of, 212
  evidence evaluations, 211–212
  practice guidelines developed using, 216–217
  principles of, 210

Exercise
  for diabetes management, 388
  for hypertension, 476–477
  prescription for, 91t
  promotion, 89, 91
  recommendations
    for adult men, 172t
    for adult women, 168t
Expected date of confinement, 129
External rotation lag sign, 587
Extrapyramidal syndrome, 54t
Eyes
  age-related changes, 21t
  contraceptive effects on, 118t

Family
  belief systems of, 36–37
  cultural differences in, 35–36
  dispersion, 32
  effect on physician, 36–38
  life cycle
    case study of, 32–33
    stages
      childbearing, 31
      empty nest, 32
      older couple, 32
      overview, 30t
      preschool-age children, 31
      school-age children, 31
      teenagers, 31–32
    parenting, 31–32
Family conferences, 34–36, 35t
Family planning services
  contraceptive, 103–106
  description of, 101–102
Family practice (see also Health care)
  career selection, 63
  case study, 204–205
  clinical decisions in, 217
  clinical reasoning
    approaches
      algorithmic, 207
      exhaustive, 207
      heuristic, 207–208
      hypotheticodeductive, 208
    decision making (see Decision making)
    description of, 205–206
    differential diagnosis, 208
    styles, 207–208
  job hunting, 63–64
  office practices
    consultations, 69–70
    equipment, 67–68
    ethical considerations, 70
    finances, 68–69
    location and space considerations, 66–67
    managed care, 65
    medical records, 68
    personnel, 67
    referrals, 69–70
    supplies, 67–68
    types of, 64–65
    utilization review, 65
  range of problems addressed in, 203
  reasons for visits, 203
  residency training, 63–64

symptoms and diagnosis commonly seen, 203, 205t
Family systems theory
  boundaries, 30
  interaction patterns, 28–29
  roles, 28–29
  triangulation, 30
Family violence
  description of, 174
  prevention of, 92–93
  SAFE screening approach, 174, 175t
  victims of, 174
Family-of-origin, of physician
  effect on patient care provided, 38t
  issues, 36–38
Family-oriented care
  case study of, 28–29
  levels, 27–28
  physician, 26–27, 27t
  principle, 27
  tools, 28, 29t
Famotidine, 363t
Fastin (see Phentermine)
Fasting, 196
Fatigue
  case study of, 433–434
  clinical evaluation of
    history, 427–429, 429t–430t
    laboratory tests, 430
    overview, 427
    physical examination, 429t, 429–430
  differential diagnosis, 425, 426t
  management of
    algorithm, 431
    initial visit, 430
    second visit, 430–432
  pathophysiology of
    chronic fatigue syndrome (see Chronic fatigue
      syndrome)
    lifestyle, 426–427
    physical, 425–426, 430t
    psychologic, 425, 430t
  prevalence of, 425
  "red flags" suggestive of progressive or life-threat-
    ening illness as cause of, 429t
  resolution of, 425
Fecal occult blood test
  for adult women, 167t
  for men, 171t
Fee-for-service, 65
Fenfluramine, 684, 686
Fentanyl, 494t
Fertility awareness, 122–123
Fetal hydrops, 131
FEV₁ (see Forced expiratory volume in the first sec-
    ond)
Fever, in infants and preschool children
  case study of, 443
  clinical evaluation of
    history, 437, 438t
    laboratory tests, 439–441
    overview, 437
    physical examination, 437–439, 438t, 439
  definition of, 435
  differential diagnosis, 435–437, 437t
  management of
    age-based, 441, 442

antibiotics, 441–442, 444t
    fever reduction, 441, 443t–444t
    follow-up, 442–443
    measurement of, 435
    pathophysiology of
        bacteremia, 436–437
        bronchiolitis, 436
        bronchitis, 436
        otitis media, 436
        pneumonia, 436
        upper respiratory infection, 436
    serious bacterial infections as cause of
        definition of, 435
        diagnostic tests, 439–440, 440t
        risks of, based on patient age, 436t
        signs and symptoms of, 437–438
Feverfew, 197t
Fibromyalgia, 297, 426, 427t
Finasteride, 534, 5367t
Fine-needle aspiration, for palpable malignant breast
        mass, 342t, 343
Flea bites, 601 (see color plate)
Flesh-eating bacteria (see Necrotizing fasciitis)
Flovent (see Fluticasone propionate)
Flu (see Influenza virus)
Fluconazole, 671t
Flunisolide, 319t
Fluoride, 152t
Fluoxetine
    description of, 287t
    for dysmenorrhea, 507t
Flurbiprofen, 296t
Fluticasone propionate, 319t
Follicle-stimulating hormone, 108, 179
Folliculitis, 602
Food pyramid, 688
Forced expiratory volume in the first second, 313
Forced vital capacity, 313
FSH (see Follicle-stimulating hormone)
Fungal infections, of skin
    causes of, 604
    types of, 604–605
Furosemide, 371t
FVC (see Forced vital capacity)

GAD (see Generalized anxiety disorder)
Galactography, 338
Galactorrhea, 118t, 336
Gallbladder disease, 683t
Gallstones, 227
Garlic, 197t–198t
Gastric cancer
    description of, 231–232
    diagnostic tests, 230t
    symptoms of, 231–232
Gastroesophageal reflux disease
    chest pain caused by
        description of, 350, 354
        drug therapy, 363t
        laboratory testing, 358
        management of, 359t, 362
    sore throat caused by
        description of, 624
        treatment of, 629
GBS infection (see Group B streptococcal infection)
GC (see Neisseria gonorrhoeae)

Generalized anxiety disorder
    characteristics of, 283
    diagnostic criteria, 285t
    pharmacologic treatment, 286–288
Genital itching, 577–578
Genital ulcer disease
    clinical evaluation, 576
    differential diagnosis, 573
    management of, 576, 576t
    pathophysiology of, 573
    vaginitis and, 660
Genogram
    case study of, 33–34
    description of, 32
    symbols, 33
Gerber's test (see Lift off test)
GERD (see Gastroesophageal reflux disease)
Gestational diabetes, 136
Ginger, 197t–198t
Ginkgo, 197t–198t
Ginseng, 197t–198t
Glaucoma screening
    for adult men, 172t
    for adult women, 168t
Glenohumeral joint
    anatomy of, 581
    capsule, tears of, 587
    chronic instability of, 593–594
    dislocation, 594
    stability tests, 585
Glimepiride, 390t
Glipizide, 390t
Glucophage (see Metformin)
α-Glucosidase inhibitors, 392–393
Glyburide, 390t
Goiter
    clinical evaluation of, 640–642, 641t
    definition of, 639
    differential diagnosis, 640
    endemic, 642
    management of, 642, 643t
    nonendemic, 642
    pathophysiology of, 639–640
Goldenseal, 197t
Gonorrhea (see Neisseria gonorrhoeae)
Gout
    acute, 301
    chronic, 301–302
    clinical evaluation of
        history, 300
        laboratory tests, 301
        physical examination, 300–301
    description of, 300
    differential diagnosis, 300, 301t
    management of, 301–302
    obesity and, 683t
    pathophysiology of, 300
Graves' disease, 648
Graves' ophthalmopathy, 651
Greater tuberosity, 581
Group A β-hemolytic streptococcal pharyngitis
    clinical evaluation of
        history, 625
        laboratory tests, 627, 628t
        physical examination, 625–626
    management of, 629–631, 630t–632t

Group A β-hemolytic streptococcal pharyngitis—*Continued*
  prevalence of, 624, 624t
Group B streptococcal infection, during pregnancy, 136
Group practice, 64–65

H₂ antagonists, 363t
Haemophilus ducreyi, 563, 571t
Haemophilus influenzae, 436
Hair, age-related changes in, 21t
Hashimoto's thyroiditis, 646–647
Hawkins' test, 586, 586t
Hazards (*see* Environmental hazards)
Headaches
  case study of, 458–459
  characteristics of, 447
  in children, 458
  clinical evaluation of
    history, 450–451, 452t
    physical examination, 451, 452t
  computed tomographic imaging of, 453–454
  differential diagnosis, 449–450, 450t
  environmentally induced, 54t
  general approach, 447, *448*
  genetic factors, 451
  laboratory tests, 453–454
  magnetic resonance imaging of, 453–454
  management of, 454–458, 455t, 457t
  in menopause, complementary therapies for, 188t
  in older adults, 458
  prevalence of, 447
  primary
    cluster
      clinical evaluation of, 451–452
      pathophysiology of, 447
      treatment of, 456
    migraine
      clinical evaluation of, 451
      drug therapy, 456, 457t
      pathophysiology of, 447
    tension
      clinical evaluation of, 452
      pathophysiology of, 447, 449
      treatment of, 456–458, 457t
  "red flags" that suggest progressive or life-threatening cause of, 451t
  in respiratory tract infections symptomatology, 543
  secondary
    intracranial masses
      clinical evaluation of, 452–453
      pathophysiology of, 449
    management of, 458
    sinusitis
      clinical evaluation of, 452
      pathophysiology of, 449
    subarachnoid hemorrhage
      clinical evaluation of, 453
      diagnostic tests, 454t
      pathophysiology of, 449
    temporal arteritis, 449
    temporomandibular joint disorders
      clinical evaluation of, 453
      pathophysiology of, 449
    trauma, 449

Health, methods to promote
  cessation of tobacco use, 89
  healthy diet, 91, 92t
  injury prevention, 91–93
  mental health, 93–94
  physical activity, 89, 91
  spirituality, 94–95
  stress management, 94
Health care (*see also* Family practice)
  community-based (*see* Community medicine)
  financing of
    expenditures, 70
    insurance, 70–72
  home-based
    case study of, 48
    emergence of, 44–45
    equipment for, 47t
    patient in
      management of, 46–47
      selection of, 46–47
    physician's role in, 45t, 45–46
    technology, 44–45
  office-based (*see* Office practice)
  regulations
    antitrust, 72
    liability, 72–73
    practice, 73–74
  restructuring, 75
  spending allocations, *71*
Health maintenance organizations (*see* Managed care)
Hearing
  changes, age-related, 21t
  loss of, occupational causes, 49t
  screening of, 83
Heart disease
  case study of, 377–378
  congenital, 145
  estrogen use and, 184
  valvular, 377
Heart failure
  case study of, 377–378
  classification of, 367, 369
  clinical evaluation
    ancillary tests, 372–373
    history, 371–372
    laboratory tests, 372–373
    physical examination, 371–372
  description of, 371
  from diastolic dysfunction, management of, 374
  functional criteria, 372t
  medications for, 370, 371t
  from systolic dysfunction, management of, 373–374
Heart valves
  description of, 369
  disease of, 377
Helicobacter pylori infection
  diagnostic tests, 230t
  management of, 236–237
Heparin, for acute cardiac ischemia, 360
Hepatitis A
  for adult men, 170t
  for adult women, 166t
Hepatitis B
  health effects of, 561t
  in human immunodeficiency virus patients, prophylaxis treatment for, 467t

pregnancy screening, 131
Herbal medicine, 196, 197t–198t (*see also specific herb*)
Heroin, 247t
Herpes gingivostomatitis, 604 (*see color plate*)
Herpes simplex virus
  description of, 562
  genital ulcers and, 576t
  health effects of, 561t
  screening tests for, 567t–568t
  skin-related effects, 604
  treatment of, 570t
  type 1, 604
  type 2, 604
Herpes zoster, 604 (*see color plate*)
Hidden agenda, 203–204, 206–207
HIV (*see* Human immunodeficiency virus)
Hivid (*see* Zalcitabine)
Home care
  case study of, 48
  considerations for, 47–48
  emergence of, 44–45
  equipment for, 47t
  patient in
    management of, 46–47
    selection of, 46–47
  physician's role in, 45t, 45–46
  prevalence of, 46
  technology, 45
Homeopathy, 196, 199
Hormonal therapy
  cessation of, 183
  description of, 181, 183
  estrogen replacement
    description of, 183
    formulations for, 184t
  hormone replacement (*see* Hormone replacement therapy)
Hormone replacement therapy
  breast cancer risk and, 185–186
  formulations for, 184t
  principles of, 183
  systemic diseases reduced using, 183t
  therapy options, 183
Hot flashes
  complementary therapies, 187t
  description of, 180
HPV (*see* Human papillomavirus)
HRT (*see* Hormone replacement therapy)
HSV (*see* Herpes simplex virus)
Human immunodeficiency virus
  in adolescents, 146
  antiretroviral therapy for
    agent selection, 466
    agents used in, 465t
    algorithmic approach, *468*
    changes in, 466
    costs of, 463
    goal of, 463
    initiation of, 463
    monitoring of, 466
    nonnucleoside reverse transcriptase inhibitors, 465t
    nucleoside reverse transcriptase inhibitors, 465t
    protease inhibitors, 465t
  case study of, 469–471
  CD4 counts, 464, *465*

clinical evaluation of
  history, 461–462, 462t
  laboratory testing, 462–463
  physical examination, 462, 462t–463t
counseling, 469t
definition of, 461
diagnosis of, 461
dysmenorrhea and, 504
health effects of, 561t
management of, 463
occupational exposure to, 468–469, 469t
opportunistic infections
  early diagnosis of, 466–467
  prophylaxis for, 467t
  treatment of, 466–467
patient education, 467–468
in pregnancy, 131, 468–469
prognosis of, 463
quality of life considerations, 467
"red flags" that suggest life-threatening disease associated with, 462, 463t
risk factors, 461
signs and symptoms of, 461
transmission prevention of, 463
worldwide incidence of, 461
Human papillomavirus
  description of, 563
  health effects of, 561t
  screening tests for, 567t
  treatment of, 570t, 603t
Hydrochlorothiazide, 371t
Hyperprolactinemia, 336
Hyperpyrexia, 435
Hypertension
  in adolescents, 145
  case studies of, 480–481
  in children, 145
  clinical evaluation of
    history, 475
    laboratory tests, 475
    overview, 474t
    physical examination, 475
  in diabetes mellitus, management of, 396
  diagnosis of, 473–474
  differential diagnosis, 474–475
  isolated systolic, 474
  obesity and, 683t
  patient education, 475
  prevalence of, 473
  treatment of
    ambulatory monitoring, 480
    antihypertensive medications
      characteristics of, 478t
      costs of, 479
      dosing of, 479
      effect on coexisting medical conditions, 479
      normal activity effects, 479
      patient population considerations, 478–479
    clinical studies, 475–476
    general approach, 475–476, *476*
    lifestyle modifications
      alcohol intake reductions, 477
      biofeedback, 477
      calcium supplementation, 477
      effectiveness of, 477t
      exercise, 476–477

Hypertension—*Continued*
 potassium supplementation, 477
 sodium restriction, 477
 stress reduction, 477
 weight loss, 477
 long term, 480
 patient compliance with, 480
Hyperthyroidism
 clinical evaluation of, 641t, 648–649
 differential diagnosis, 648
 management of, 650–651
 pathophysiology of, 648
 risk factors, 637t
Hypnosis, 193
Hypothyroidism
 clinical evaluation of, 641t, 645–646
 differential diagnosis, 644
 fatigue associated with, 426
 management of, 643t
  algorithm for, 647
  initial approach, 646–647
  long term, 647–648
 pathophysiology of, 644
 risk factors, 637t
 secondary, 646
 transient, 650
Hytrin (*see* Terazosin)

Ibuprofen, 296t
 for ankle pain, 269t
 for dysmenorrhea, 507t
 for fever in infants and preschool children,
  444t
 for headaches, 457t
 for knee pain, 269t
 for low back pain, 494t
IDDM (*see* Insulin-dependent diabetes mellitus)
Imipramine, 287t, 363t
Immunizations
 for adults, 159, 162–164
 for children
  adverse reactions associated with, 148
  contraindications, 147t
  measles, mumps, rubella, 148
  oral polio vaccine, 148
  precautions, 147t
  schedule for, 148t
 death rates, 81t
 description, 81t
 importance, 79
Impetiginous flea bites, 601 (*see color plate*)
Impetigo, 601–602
Impingement syndrome (*see* Rotator cuff, tendonitis)
Impingement tests
 Neer's, 586
 overview, 586t
 Yocum's, 586, 586t
Independent practice association, description, 65
Inderal (*see* Propranolol)
Indinavir, 465t
Indomethacin, 269t, 494t
Infants (*see also* Children; Newborn)
 fever in (*see* Fever, in infants and preschool chil-
  dren)
 sleeping patterns, 151
Infections (*see specific infection*)

Infectious mononucleosis
 clinical evaluation of
  history, 625
  laboratory tests, 627
  physical examination, 626–627
 management of, 631–632
 prevalence of, 624, 624t
Infiltrative ophthalmopathy, 648
Influenza virus
 in human immunodeficiency virus patients, prophylaxis treatment for, 467t
 vaccine
  for adult men, 170t
  for adult women, 166t
Infrared densitometry, 684t
Injuries
 in children, preventive counseling for, 152
 musculoskeletal, 49t
 prevention of
  for adult men, 172t
  for adult women, 168t
 strategies, 91
Insomnia during menopause, complementary therapies for, 187t
Insulin
 lispro, 394, 394t
 pharmacokinetics of, 394t
Insulin-dependent diabetes mellitus
 characteristics of, 382
 clinical evaluation, 383
 description of, 382
 dietary guidelines, 389
 home blood glucose monitoring, 395–396
 insulin preparations, 393–395
Insurance
 Medigap coverage, 71–72
 preventive medicine and, 85
 professional liability, 72–73
 types, 65
Intermenstrual bleeding, 510
Internal rotation lag sign, 587
International Classification of Diseases and Related Health
  Problems, 68
Intracranial masses, headaches caused by
 clinical evaluation of, 452–453
 pathophysiology of, 449
Intrauterine devices
 costs, 121
 effectiveness, 105t, 119–120
 problems, 120–121
 types, 120
Invirase (*see* Saquinavir)
Ionamin (*see* Phentermine)
IPA (*see* Independent practice association)
Ipodate sodium, 644t
Ipratropium bromide, 318t, 322
Iron, 93t
Iron deficiency anemia
 in children, 143
 in first trimester of pregnancy, 131
Irritability during menopause, complementary therapies for, 188t
Irritable bowel syndrome
 abdominal pain associated with, 234
 characteristics of, 234
 clinical evaluation, 234

diagnosis of, 229t, 234
management of, 236t–237t, 239
Isoniazid, 145
Isosorbide dinitrate, 371t
Isosorbide mononitrate, 371t
Itraconazole, 671t
IUD (*see* Intrauterine devices)

Job hunting, 64
Jobe's maneuver (*see* Empty can test)
Joint line tenderness, 273
Joints (*see also specific joint*)
age-related changes, 21t
arthritic, 291
Juice, 196

Keflex (*see* Cephalexin)
Ketoacidosis (*see* Diabetic ketoacidosis)
Ketoprofen, 296t
Ketorolac, 457t
Knee joint
anatomy of, *271*
function of, 270
imaging of, 273, 275t, 275–276
joint line tenderness of, 273
ligaments of, 270, *271*
Knee pain
anterior
description of, 271, 273, 275
management of, 276t
anterior cruciate ligament
anatomy of, *271*
injuries
description of, 270
imaging of, 275
case study of, 278
chronic, 271
clinical evaluation
history, 272, 272t
McMurray test, 273, *274*
physical examination, 272–273
"red flags," 265t
differential diagnosis, 264t, 270–271
management of
based on cause, 276t
initial approach, 276–277
long term, 277
surgery referral, 276
pathophysiology of, 270–271
posterior cruciate ligament
anatomy of, *271*
injuries to, 271

Lacerations
case study of, 621
definition of, 615
management of
aftercare, 620, 620t
anesthesia, 615
area-specific considerations, 618, 620
inspection, 615
suture closure, 616t–617t, 616–618, *617–619*
Lactational amenorrhea method, of contraception,
105t
Lactobacillosis, 659–660
Lamivudine, 465t

Lanoxin (*see* Digoxin)
Laryngitis, 553
Lasix (*see* Furosemide)
Lassitude (*see* Fatigue)
LE test (*see* Leukocyte esterase test)
Lead exposure
in children, 143–144
signs and symptoms of, 143
treatment approaches, 144
Leukemia, 54t–55t
Leukocyte esterase test, 414
Leukotriene modifiers, 318t–319t, 321
Levothyroxine, 644t, 646–647, 650
Liability, 72–73
Libido, contraceptive effects on, 118t
Lice, 564, 571t
Lichen planus, 659
Lichen sclerosis et atrophicus, 659
Lichen simplex chronicus, 659 (*see color plate*)
Life cycle
case study of, 11–12
of family
case study of, 32–33
stages
childbearing, 31
empty nest, 32
older couple, 32
overview, 30t
preschool-age children, 31
school-age children, 31
teenagers, 31–32
seasons, 12–13
Lifestyle, of physician
home life, 9–10
office, 5–6
settling in, 4–5
starting out, 3–4
Lift off test, 586
Likelihood ratios, of diagnostic tests, 213–214, 214t
Lipase, 232
Lisinopril, 363t
Lispro insulin, 394, 394t
Literature
critical appraisal of, 211–212
sources of, 212t
Lopressor (*see* Metoprolol)
Lotensin (*see* Benazepril)
Low back pain
case study of, 498
classification of, 483
clinical evaluation of
guidelines for, 486–488
history, 486t, 488
laboratory tests, 489–492, 491t
physical examination, 486t, 488–489
complicated
description of, 484–485
general approach, *487*
differential diagnosis, 485–486
general approach, *487*
management of
acute, patient education, 497t
acute episodes, 492, 493t–494t, 494–495
chronic
approach to, 495
patient education, 497t

Low back pain—*Continued*
  pharmacologic therapy, 494t
  surgery, 495, 497
  treatment options, 496t
  neurologic examination, 489
  pathophysiology of, 483–485
  patient education, 497, 497t
  prevalence of, 483
  prognosis for, 492
  "red flags" suggesting progressive or life-threatening disease associated with, 489t
  referred, 485
  systemic causes of, 485
  uncomplicated
    classification of, 485t
    description of, 483
    pathophysiology of
      degenerative disc disease, 484
      malalignment, 484
      muscle and ligament injury, 483–484
      osteoarthritis, 484
Lung cancer, 54t
Lung diseases, occupationally induced, 49t
Luteinizing hormone, 108

Macrobiotics, 195
Magnesium, reductions for hypertension treatment, 477, 477t
Major depressive disorder
  characteristics of, 282–283
  diagnostic criteria, 285t
  pharmacologic treatment, 286–288
Malpractice, 72–73
Mammary duct ectasia, 337
Mammography
  clinical uses
    nipple discharge, 338
    palpable breast mass, 342, 342t
  recommendations, 167t
Managed care
  description, 65
  insurance, 65
  physicians in, 74t
  utilization review, 65, 66t
Marijuana, 247t
Massage (*see* Therapeutic massage)
Mastalgia (*see also* Breasts, pain associated with)
  cyclic
    description of, 331–332
    nonpharmacotherapy for, 333
    pharmacotherapy for, 333t, 333–334, 335t
  noncyclic
    description of, 331
    management of, 334, 335t
Mastitis
  definition of, 336, 343
  incidence of, 343
  in lactating breast, 343–344
  management of, 343–344
Material Safety Data Sheets, 51
Maternal serum α-fetoprotein testing, 135
Maxair (*see* Pirbuterol)
Mazindol (Mazanor), 687t
MDD (*see* Major depressive disorder)
Measles, mumps, rubella vaccine, 148

Medicaid
  coverage, 72t
  description, 72
Medical practice (*see* Family practice)
Medical records
  criteria, 68
  release, authorization, 57–58
Medicare
  coverage, 71–72, 72t
  description, 70
  part A, 70
  part B, 70
Medications (*see specific medication*)
Medigap coverage, 71–72
Meditation, 193–194
Medrol, 305t
Medroxyprogesterone acetate, 507t
Mefenamic acid, 507t
Melanoma, 607, 609t (*see color plate*)
Meningitis, drug therapy for, 444t
Meniscus tear
  description of, 272t
  management of, 276t, 277
Menometrorrhagia, 510
Menopause
  anticipatory guidance for, 186, 189
  average age of onset, 179
  case study of, 189–190
  clinical evaluation of
    algorithm, *182*
    differential diagnosis, 181
    history, 179–180, 180t–181t
    physical examination, 180–181
  description of, 179
  natural history of, 179
  patient education, 186, 189, 189t
  symptoms
    clinical evaluation of, 180, 180t–181t
    complementary therapy for, 187t–188t
  treatment of, 7
    algorithm, *182*
    complementary, 186, 187t–188t
    hormonal therapy (*see* Hormonal therapy)
    objectives, 181
Menorrhagia, 510
Menstrual syndromes
  abnormal uterine bleeding (*see* Uterine bleeding, abnormal)
  dysmenorrhea (*see* Dysmenorrhea)
  premenstrual (*see* Premenstrual syndrome)
Mental function, age-related changes in, 21t
Mental health (*see also specific illnesses*)
  environmentally induced, 54t
  occupational, 49t
  screenings, 93–94
  spirituality, 94–95
  stress management, 94
Mental status examination, 159, *163*
Mestranol, 109
Metformin, 390t, 391
Methadone, 255, 494t
Methimazole, 644t, 650
Methotrexate, 304t
Methylprednisolone, 305t, 319t
Methylxanthines
  for asthma, 318t–319t

removal of, for preventing cyclic mastalgia, 333
Methysergide, 457t
Metoclopramide, 457t
Metoprolol, 363t, 371t, 457t
Metronidazole, 670t–672t
Metrorrhagia, 510
Miconazole, 670t–671t
Microalbuminuria, 385
Migraines
    clinical evaluation of, 451
    contraceptive formulations for patients with, 116t
    drug therapy, 456, 457t
    pathophysiology of, 447
Milk thistle, 197t–198t
Mind-body therapies
    biofeedback, 193
    description of, 193
    hypnosis, 193
    meditation, 193–194
    mindful exercise, 194
Mindful exercise, 194
Minerals, recommendations for, 93t
Minipress (*see* Prazosin)
Minnesota model, of addiction treatment, 254
Mitral valve prolapse, 350–351
MMR vaccine (*see* Measles, mumps, rubella vaccine)
Moexipril, 371t
Molluscum contagiosum
    description of, 563
    health effects of, 561t
    treatment of, 571t
Mondor's disease, 331
Mood disorder, secondary to medical condition, 283
Motrin (*see* Ibuprofen)
MSAFP (*see* Maternal serum α-fetoprotein testing)
MSDS (*see* Material Safety Data Sheets)
Multiculturalism
    family and, 35–36
    identity, 41–42
Multispecialty groups, 64–65
Muscles, age-related changes in, 21t
Musculoskeletal pain, chest pain caused by, 350, 354, 362
MVP (*see* Mitral valve prolapse)
Mycobacterium avium complex, prophylaxis treatment for, 467t
Mycobacterium tuberculosis, prophylaxis treatment for, 467t
Mycoplasma pneumoniae, 555
Myocardial infarction
    creatine kinase levels and, 356–357
    definition of, 369
    epigastric pain associated with, 222
    management of, 359t
Myxedema coma, 643t, 645–646

Nabumetone, 269t, 296t
Naproxen sodium, 269t, 296t, 457t, 494t
Nardil (*see* Phenelzine)
National Institute for Occupational Safety and Health, 59t
National organizations, 43
Neck pain
    acute, 519
    case study of, 524–525
    causes of, 520, 520t
    chronic syndromes, 523–524
    clinical evaluation of
        history, 519–520
        laboratory tests, 521–522
        physical examination, 520–521
        psychologic features, 520
    common causes of, 519, 520t
    impairment assessments, 524
    management of
        exercises, 523, *524*
        initial, 522
        overview, 522t
        persistent, 523
    prevalence of, 519
Necrotizing fasciitis, 603
Nedocromil, 318t–319t, 321
Needle electromyography, for low back pain, 491
Neer's test, 586, 586t
Nefazodone, 287t
Neisseria gonorrhoeae
    in adolescents, 145
    description of, 145, 562
    health effects of, 561t
    screening tests for, 566t
    treatment of, 570t
    urethritis, 572t
Nelfinavir, 465t
Neonate (*see* Newborn)
Nervousness during menopause, complementary therapies for, 188t
Neuropathy, peripheral, 54t
Nevirapine, 465t
Newborn (*see also* Infants)
    counseling topics for, 150t
    screening
        description of, 143
        vision problems, 144
    urinary tract infections in, 420
Niacin, 93t
NIDDM (*see* Non-insulin-dependent diabetes mellitus)
Nipple discharge
    case study of, 345–346
    causes of, 334
    clinical evaluation of
        history, 336–337, 337t
        laboratory tests, 337
        malignancy, 338–339
        physical examination, 337
    differential diagnosis, 336, 337t
    ductal papillomas and, 336
    hyperprolactinemia and, 336
    management of, 338–339, *340*
    nonphysiologic, 334
    pathophysiology of, 336
    physiologic, 334
    prevalence of, 334
Nitrates, 371t
Nitrofurantoin, 417t
Nitroglycerin, 360, 363t
Nizatidine, 363t
Non-insulin-dependent diabetes mellitus
    characteristics of, 382
    clinical evaluation, 382–383
    complications, 396
    description of, 382

Non-insulin-dependent diabetes mellitus—*Continued*
  glucose monitoring, 395
  α-glucosidase inhibitors, 392–393
  management of, 385–386
  physical examination, 383
Nonspecific abdominal pain, 224
Nonsteroidal anti-inflammatory drugs, clinical uses of
  acute gout, 301
  acute low back pain, 492, 493t–494t
  ankle pain, 269t
  arthritis, 295–296
  dyspeptic patient use of, 238
  headaches, 455t
  knee pain, 269t
  neck pain, 522
  osteoarthritis, 299–300
  premenstrual syndrome, 510
  primary dysmenorrhea, 505, 507t
  rheumatoid arthritis, 295–296, 296t, 303–304
  shoulder pain, 589
  sore throat, 627
  thyroiditis, 642
Norplant, 119
Nortriptyline, 287t, 457t
Norvir (*see* Ritonavir)
NSAIDs (*see* Nonsteroidal anti-inflammatory drugs)
NSAP (*see* Nonspecific abdominal pain)
Nucleoside reverse transcriptase inhibitors, 465t

OAM (*see* Office of Alternative Medicine)
Obesity
  case studies of, 694–696
  clinical evaluation of
    history, 681–682
    laboratory tests, 682–683
    physical examination, 682
  contraceptive formulations and, 116t
  diagnosis of, 679–680
  disorders associated with, 683t
  management of
    description of, 683–684
    pharmacotherapies, 684, 686–687, 687t
    surgical
      description of, 687
      Roux-en-Y gastric bypass, 688
      vertical gastric banding, 687–688
    weight control programs, 685t
  pathophysiology of, 680
  patient education regarding, 688–689
  prevalence of, 679
Occupational health
  back-to-work form, 56
  ethical considerations, 57–58
  exposure-related disease and injury
    agencies for assistance, 59t
    case studies of, 58, 60–62
    criteria, 55
    diagnostic investigations, 52t–53t
    frequency, 48
    history, 49, 51
      form, 50
    human immunodeficiency virus, 468–469, 469t
    prevalent types of, 49t
    recognition of, 49
    related diseases, 54t
    treatment plan, 57

  regulation, 73
  resources, 58, 59t
  worker's compensation, 57
Occupational Safety and Health Administration
  description, 59t
  rule complexity, 67
  surveillance programs, 51
Office of Alternative Medicine, 192
Office practice
  consultations, 69–70
  equipment, 67–68
  ethical considerations, 70
  finances, 68–69
  location and space considerations, 66–67
  managed care, 65
  medical records, 68
  personnel, 67
  referrals, 69–70
  supplies, 67–68
  types of, 64–65
  utilization review, 65
Offices
  designing, 5–6
  location, 66–67
  space, 66–67
  test tracking systems, 84–85
Oligomenorrhea, 510
OM (*see* Otitis media)
Onychomycosis, 605 (*see color plate*)
Opiates
  detoxification regimen, 251t
  withdrawal symptoms, 249
Opportunistic infections, in human immuno-
    deficiency virus patients (*see also specific
    infection*)
  early diagnosis of, 466–467
  prophylaxis for, 467t
  treatment of, 466–467
Oral contraceptives, 112
  advantages, 110, 112
  algorithm, 111
  breast cancer and, 113
  cardiovascular effects, 113
  clinical uses
    abnormal uterine bleeding, 513
    cyclic mastalgia, 333t, 334
    metromenorrhagic women, 186
  composition of, 114t
  contraindications, 112–113
  dosage, 115
  for dysmenorrhea, 507t
  effectiveness, 105t
  estrogenic content of, 514t
  indications, 110, 112
  medical condition considerations, 116t7
  noncontraceptive benefits of, 110, 112
  prescribing of, 115, 117
  problems associated with, 118t
  progestogenic content of, 514t
  selection of, 113, 115
  types of
    biphasic, 114t, 115
    injectables, 118–119
    minipill, 117–118
    monophasic, 114t, 115
    subdermal progestins, 118–119

triphasic, 114t, 115
Oral glucose tolerance test, 384
Oral polio vaccine, 148
OSHA (*see* Occupational Safety and Health Administration)
Osteoarthritis
  case study of, 306
  clinical evaluation of
    history, 298
    laboratory tests, 299
    physical examination, 298–299
  description of, 298
  incidence of, 292t
  joint involvement in, *299*
  of knee joint
    imaging of, 275–276
    management of, 276t, 277
  low back pain associated with, 484
  management of, 299–300
  obesity and, 683t
  pathophysiology of, 298
  primary, 298
  secondary, 298
  signs and symptoms of, 299
Osteoporosis
  estrogen replacement therapy to reduce risk of, 184–185
  preventive therapy, 185t
  risk factors, 185t
  steroid-induced, 304
Otitis media
  antibiotic therapy, 444t
  clinical evaluation of, 552–553
  description of, 436, 552
  otitis externa, differential diagnosis of, 545
  treatment of, 553
Oto-ophthalmoscope, 47t
Otrivin (*see* Xylometazoline hydrochloride)
Ovarian cancer, 116t
Ovarian cysts, 505–506
Oxaprozin, 269t
Oxycodone, 494t

PAD (*see* Pelvic adhesive disease)
Pain
  abdominal (*see* Abdominal pain)
  biceps, tests of, 587
  breast (*see* Breasts, pain associated with)
  chest (*see* Chest pain)
  low back (*see* Low back pain)
  neck (*see* Neck pain)
  parietal, 221–222
  pelvic (*see* Pelvic pain)
  visceral, 221
Palpable breast mass
  case study of, 345
  clinical evaluation of
    biopsy, 343
    history, 339, 341t
    laboratory tests, 342–343
    physical examination, 339–342, 341t
  description of, 339
  differential diagnosis, 339, 341t
  malignant
    diagnostic tests, 342t
    physical findings of, 339–340

management of, 343, *344*
  pathophysiology of, 339
Pamelor (*see* Nortriptyline)
Pancreatic cancer
  abdominal pain associated with, 232
  treatment for, 238
Pancreatitis
  abdominal pain associated with, 232
  acute
    description of, 230t, 232
    management of, 238
  chronic
    description of, 230t, 232
    management of, 238
  diagnostic tests, 232
Panic disorder
  chest pain caused by
    description of, 350, 354
    management of, 361–362
  without agoraphobia
    characteristics of, 283
    diagnostic criteria, 285t
    pharmacologic treatment, 286–287
Pap smear
  for adult women, 167t
  for human immunodeficiency virus patients, 462
  during pregnancy, 131
  for vaginitis diagnosis, 669
Paroxetine, 287t
Patellar injuries
  management of, 277
  patella compression test for evaluating, 273
Patients
  adolescents (*see* Adolescents)
  adults (*see* Adults)
  bedside manner, 6–9
  care of
    case study of, 25–26
    coordination, 69–70
    family oriented
      case study of, 28–29
      levels, 27–28
      principle, 27
      tools, 28, 29t
    maximizing, 23–24
  children (*see* Children)
  counseling
    aspects, 85–86
    expectations, 86–87
    importance, 85
    key steps, 85t
    model, 86
    strategies, 87, 89
      exercise, 89, 91
      healthy diet, 91
      injury prevention, 91
      mental health, 93–95
      tobacco use, 89
      violence, 92–93
  home care (*see* Home care)
  medical history authorization, 57–58
  medications, 87t (*see also specific medication*)
Peak expiratory flow rate, 313
PEFR (*see* Peak expiratory flow rate)
Pelvic adhesive disease, 575t
Pelvic examination, for adult women, 167t

Pelvic inflammatory disease
  abdominal pain associated with, 235
  characteristics of, 506
  definition of, 235
  description of, 569
  diagnosis of, 229t, 235
  differential diagnosis, 573
  history, 573
  laboratory tests, 574
  management of, 236t–237t, 239, 506, 508, 574, 575t
  pathophysiology of, 573
  physical examination, 573–574
Pelvic pain
  chronic, 575t
  description of, 569
  differential diagnosis, 573
  history, 573
  laboratory tests, 574
  management of, 574, 575t
  pathophysiology of, 573
  physical examination, 573–574
Penicillin G, 632t
Peptic ulcer disease
  abdominal pain, 231
  description of, 231
  diagnosis of, 228t, 230t, 231
  treatment of, 238
Percutaneous transluminal coronary angioplasty, 370
Periactin (*see* Cyproheptadine)
Pericarditis, 353
Peritonitis, 228t
Personnel, 67
Pharyngitis
  diagnosis of, 548–549
  group A β-hemolytic streptococcal (*see* Group A β-hemolytic streptococcal pharyngitis)
  treatment of, 548–549
Phendimetrazine, 687t
Phenelzine, 457t
Phentermine, 684, 686, 687t
Phenylpropanolamine, 687t
Phosphorus, 93t
Physician
  community role of, 42–44
  demand, 74
  family-of-origin
    effect on patient care provided, 38t
    issues, 36–38
  family-oriented, 26–27
  finances of, 74t
  in home-based care, 45t, 45–46
  job hunting, 64
  liability
    case study of, 72–73
    insurance, 72–73
  lifestyle of
    home life, 9–10
    office, 5–6
    settling in, 4–5
    starting out, 3–4
  patient relations, 6–9
  practice of
    consultations, 69–70
    equipment, 67–68
    finances, 68–69
    medical records, 68
    office, 66–67
    referrals, 69–70
    staffing, 67
    supplies, 67–68
    tasks, 65–66
    types, 64–65
  qualifications of, 73–74
  residency, 63–64
  specialty choice, 63
  utilization review, 65
PID (*see* Pelvic inflammatory disease)
Pill (*see* Oral contraceptives)
Pirbuterol, 320t
Piroxicam, 269t
Plantar fasciitis, 298
Pneumococcal vaccine
  for adult men, 170t
  for adult women, 166t
Pneumocystis carinii, prophylaxis treatment for, 467t
Pneumonia
  atypical, 555t
  bacterial pathogens, 554–555
  bronchitis and, differential diagnosis of, 545
  clinical evaluation of, 555–556
  community-acquired, 555, 557t
  laboratory tests, 556
  management of, 556–557, 557t
  nonaspiration, 556
  treatment of, 555
  typical, 555t
Point of maximal impulse, 312
Polio vaccine, adverse reactions associated with, 148
Polymenorrhea, 510
Polyps
  cervical, 505–506
  nasal, 551–552
Postcoital contraception, 122
Posterior cruciate ligament
  anatomy of, *271*
  injuries to, 271
Postpartum thyroiditis
  description of, 652
  risk factors, 637t
Potassium, 93t
Povidone-iodine gel, 670t
PPO (*see* Preferred provider organizations)
Prazosin, 537t
Predictive value, of diagnostic tests, 213
Prednisolone, 319t
Prednisone, 305t, 319t, 322
Preferred provider organizations, 65
Pregnancy
  abnormal uterine bleeding and, 511
  bacterial vaginosis during, 658, 673
  diagnosis of, 129
  "due date" determinations, 129
  ectopic
    abdominal pain associated with, 234–235
    clinical findings, 234
    diagnosis of, 229t, 234–235
    treatment for, 239
  effects, 31
  family physician's approach, 136–137
  human immunodeficiency virus during, 468–469
  planning of, 128–129
  postdate, 136

sexual activity during, 134
tests for determining, 129
unintended
  causes of, 101
  contraception
    clinical evaluation, 106–108
    counseling, 103–106
    methods, 108–112
  costs associated with, 101
  definition of, 99
  family planing services, 101–102
  high-risk populations, 99–100
  prevalence of, 99, 101
  societal effects of, 101
Premature atrial contractions, 374–375
Premature ventricular contractions, 374–375
Premenstrual syndrome
  case study of, 516–517
  clinical evaluation of, 508
  differential diagnosis, 508
  management of, 508, 510
  pathophysiology of, 508
  signs and symptoms of, 508
  symptom chart for, 508, *509*
Prenatal care
  benefits of, 127–128
  case study of, 138–139
  description of, 127
  family physician's approach, 136–137
  first trimester
    description of, 130
    flowchart for recording findings, 132t
    history, 130
    laboratory testing, 131, 133t
    patient education, 131, 134
    physical examination, 130–131
    psychosocial support, 131, 134
    Rh-antigen screening, 131
    risk assessment, 130
    screening tests, 131
  genetic abnormality testing, 134–135
  goals of, 129–130
  infant mortality rate reductions and, relationship
    between, 127
  obstetric consultation, 137t, 137–138
  risk assessments, 128–129
  second trimester, 134
  third trimester, 135–136
  topics evaluated in, 128t
  ultrasound, 134
Prescriptions
  for exercise, 91t
  patient's awareness, 87t
  slip for, *88*
  writing of, 210, *211*
Presyncope, 402
  description of, 402
  history findings, 406
  physical examination, 407
Preventive medicine
  case study of, 95–96
  clinical history, 79
  criteria, 81–82
  description of, 157
  examinations, 84–85
  insurance, 85

intervention types, 81t
levels, 80–81
objectives, 80
patient counseling (*see* Counseling, of patients)
physicals
  AMA recommendations, 79
  extent of, 83
  practices, 79–80
  priorities, 83–84
  tools, frequency, 84T
  unintended pregnancies, 101–102
Primary care
  community-oriented, 43–44
  consultations, 69–70
  future, 74–75
  office-based (*see* Office practice)
  practice guidelines, 75
  regulations, 73–74
Primary care physicians
  finances, 68–69
  numbers, 74t
  referrals, 69–70
  workload, 75
Primrose oil, for cyclic mastalgia, 333t, 333–334
Problem patients, 217–218
Problem-oriented progress note, 210
Prochlorperazine, 457t
Professional qualifications, 73–74
Progesterone, 183–184, 510–511, 514t
Progestins
  function, 108–109
  subdermal, 118–119
  types, 109–110
Progestogens, in hormonal therapy, 184t
Prognosis, 215
Prolactin, drugs that affect serum levels of, 336–337
Propranolol, 371t
  for headaches, 457t
  for thyroid disorders, 644t
Propylthiouracil, 644t, 650
Proscar (*see* Finasteride)
Prostate, annual examination of, 83
Prostate cancer
  advanced, 532
  age of onset, 527
  localized, 531t, 531–532
  metastases, 528
  obesity and, 683t
  racial predilection of, 527
  risk of developing, 527
  screening for
    description of, 528–529
    digital rectal examination, 529
    limitations of, 530
    prostate-specific antigen, 529t, 529–530
    recommendations, 530–531
    transrectal ultrasound, 530
  staging of, 527, 528t
  treatment of, 531–532
Prostate screening test, 172t
Prostate-specific antigen test, 82, 529t, 529–530
Prostatitis
  acute bacterial, 537–539, 538t
  chronic bacterial, 538t, 539
  clinical findings, 413t
  description of, 537

Prostatitis—*Continued*
  nonbacterial, 538t, 539
Prostatodynia, 538t, 539
Protease inhibitors, 465t
Proventil (*see* Albuterol)
Prozac (*see* Fluoxetine)
PSA test (*see* Prostate-specific antigen test)
Pseudoephedrine, 547
Pseudogout, 302
Psoriasis, 606–607 (*see color plate*)
Psychiatric disorders
  prevalence of, 281
  underdiagnosis of, 281
Psychoses, acute, 54t
PTCA (*see* Percutaneous transluminal coronary angio-plasty)
Public Health Service Act, 101–102
Pulmonary function tests, 312–314
Put Prevention into Practice program, 85
Pyelonephritis
  acute, in younger women, 418–419
  clinical findings, 413t
  occult, 417

Radiculopathy (*see* Sciatica)
Radioactive iodine, 644t, 650
Radiofrequency catheter ablation, for wide complex tachycardia, 377
Radiographs
  for low back pain, 490, 491–492
  for neck pain, 521–522
  for pneumonia, 555
  for shoulder pain, 587–588, 588t
Ranitidine, 363t
Readiness to Change model, 86
Rectal examinations, 83, 529
Redux (*see* Dexfenfluramine)
Referrals
  advice, 70
  consultation *versus*, 69–70
  ethics, 70
Reflexology, 194
Refractive errors, 144
Reglan (*see* Metoclopramide)
Regulations
  health care
    antitrust, 72
    liability, 72–73
    practice, 73–74
    professional qualifications, 73–74
Reproductive system
  age-related changes, 21t
  disorders, occupationally induced, 49t
Rescriptor (*see* Delavirdine)
Reserpine, 478t
Residency programs, 63–64
Respiratory syncytial virus, 436
Respiratory system, age-related changes in, 21t
Respiratory tract infections
  anatomic considerations, 543
  case study of, 557–558
  clinical evaluation of
    history, 543–545, 544t
    physical examination, 545
  diagnostic tests, 546
  differential diagnosis, 545, 545t
  epidemics, 546–547

lower
  bacterial causes of, 553
  bronchiolitis, 553–554
  bronchitis (*see* Bronchitis)
  croup, 553
  description of, 553
  influenza, 554
  laryngitis, 553
  pneumonia (*see* Pneumonia)
  pathophysiology of, 543
  signs and symptoms of, 544t
  treatment of, 546–547
  upper
    common cold, 547–548
    otitis media (*see* Otitis media)
    pharyngitis, 548–549
    sinusitis (*see* Sinusitis)
Retrovir (*see* Zidovudine)
Reye's syndrome, 632
Rezulin (*see* Troglitazone)
Rh-antigen screening, during pregnancy, 131
Rheumatoid arthritis
  clinical evaluation of
    history, 303
    physical examination, 303
  description of, 302
  differential diagnosis, 303
  finger deformities in, 302
  laboratory tests, 303
  management of
    corticosteroids, 304, 305t
    medications, 303–304, 304t
    orthopedic, 305
    supportive, 305
  pathophysiology of, 302–303
  prognosis of, 306
Rheumatoid disorders
  alternative therapies, 296
  arthritis (*see* Rheumatoid arthritis)
  clinical evaluation of
    history, 291
    joint fluid, 294, 295t
    physical examination, 291–292
    radiology, 294
  general management of
    description of, 294–295
    medication, 295–296
  incidence of, 292t
  laboratory tests, 292–294
  nonarticular features of, 294t
  osteoarthritis
    clinical evaluation of
      history, 298
      laboratory tests, 299
      physical examination, 298–299
    description of, 298
    incidence of, 292t
    joint involvement in, 299
    management of, 299–300
    pathophysiology of, 298
    primary, 298
    secondary, 298
    signs and symptoms of, 299
  rheumatoid arthritis (*see* Rheumatoid arthritis)
Rheumatoid factor
  description of, 292–293
  rheumatoid arthritis, 293

sensitivity of, 293–294
Rhinitis
    allergic, 551–552
    costs associated with, 551
    history of, 551
    physical examination of, 551
    treatment of, 551–552
    vasomotor, 551–552
Rhinorrhea, 543
RhoGAM, 135
Ribavirin, 554
Risk assessment, for adults
    depression, 159, *162*
    diet history, 159, *160–161*
    for men, 170t
    sexual history taking, 158, 159t
    for women, 165t
Ritonavir, 465t
Rocephin (*see* Ceftriaxone)
Root work, 192
Rotator cuff
    anatomy of, 581, *583*
    tears
        physical examination of, 586t, 586–587
        treatment of, 590t, 592
    tendonitis, 590, 590t, 592
Roux-en-Y gastric bypass, 688
RSV (*see* Respiratory syncytial virus)
Rubella immunizations, for adult women, 165t

SAD (*see* Seasonal affective disorder)
Saint-John's-wort, 197t–198t
Salmeterol, 319t
Sansert (*see* Methysergide)
Saquinavir, 465t
Sarcoptes scabiei, 563
Saw palmetto, 197t
SBI (*see* Serious bacterial infections)
Scabies
    description of, 563
    health effects of, 561t
    treatment of, 571t
Scapulothoracic joint, 581, *582*
Sciatica, 484–485
Screening
    of sexually transmitted diseases, 565, 566t–568t
    tests
        description, 81t
        sensitivity, 82
    for thyroid hormonal disease, 651–652
    well care
        for adolescents
            cervical dysplasia, 145–146
            congenital heart disease, 145
            growth and development, 144–145
            hypertension, 145
            sexually transmitted diseases, 146
            substance abuse, 146
            suicide, 146
            tuberculosis, 145
            venereal disease, 145–146
            youth violence, 146
        for adults
            description of, 164
            medical coverage for, 164, 174
            in men, 170t–172t
            in women, 166t–168t

for children, 146–147
    description of, 142
    growth and development, 144–145
    heart disease, 145
    hypertension, 145
    iron deficiency anemia, 143
    lead toxicity, 143–144
    for newborns, 143
    recommended types based on age, 142t–143t
    tuberculosis, 145
    vision problems, 144
Seasonal affective disorder, 283
Sebaceous hyperplasia, 609
Seborrhea, 606 (*see color plate*)
Seborrheic keratosis, 609
Selective serotonin reuptake inhibitor, 286, 287t
Senna, 197t–198t
Sensitivity, of diagnostic tests, 213
Serevent (*see* Salmeterol)
Serious bacterial infections
    definition of, 435
    diagnostic tests, 439–440, 440t
    risks of, based on patient age, 436t
    signs and symptoms of, 437–438
Serpasil (*see* Reserpine)
Sexual abuse, 106
Sexual activity
    history of, 158, 159t
    parental counseling, 153
    during pregnancy, 134
Sexual development, 144–145
Sexually transmitted diseases
    abnormal uterine bleeding and, 511
    biologic factors associated with, 559
    case studies of, 578–580
    description of, 559
    evaluation of, 564–565
    exposure to, 576–577, 577t
    pathogens involved in
        Chlamydia trachomatis, 560–562, 561t, 566t, 570t
        Haemophilus ducreyi, 563, 571t
        herpes simplex virus, 561t, 562, 567t–568t, 570t
        human papillomavirus (*see* Human papillo-
            mavirus)
        lice, 564, 571t
        molluscum contagiosum, 561t, 563, 571t
        Neisseria gonorrhoeae, 561t, 562, 566t, 570t
        scabies, 561t, 563, 571t
        syphilis, 561t, 562–563, 571t
        Treponema pallidum, 561t, 562–563, 571t
        Trichomonas vaginalis, 561t, 562, 568t, 571t
    patient education, 578
    primary care problems associated with
        cervicitis
            description of, 569
            differential diagnosis, 573
            history, 573
            laboratory tests, 574
            management of, 574, 575t
            pathophysiology of, 573
            physical examination, 573–574
        epididymitis
            clinical evaluation of, 569
            complications of, 565
            differential diagnosis, 565, 569
            laboratory tests, 569
            management of, 569

Sexually transmitted diseases—*Continued*
    pathophysiology of, 565, 569
    treatment of, 572t
  genital itching, 577–578
  genital ulcer disease
    clinical evaluation, 576
    differential diagnosis, 573
    management of, 576, 576t
    pathophysiology of, 573
  pelvic inflammatory disease
    description of, 569
    differential diagnosis, 573
    history, 573
    laboratory tests, 574
    management of, 574, 575t
    pathophysiology of, 573
    physical examination, 573–574
  pelvic pain
    chronic, 575t
    description of, 569
    differential diagnosis, 573
    history, 573
    laboratory tests, 574
    management of, 574, 575t
    pathophysiology of, 573
    physical examination, 573–574
  urethritis
    clinical evaluation of, 569
    complications of, 565
    differential diagnosis, 565, 569
    laboratory tests, 569
    management of, 569
    pathophysiology of, 565, 569
    treatment of, 570t
  racial predilection, 564
  reporting card for, *560*
  risk of acquiring, epidemiologic factors that affect, 564t
  screening for
    description of, 565
    during pregnancy, 131, 136
    tests, 566t–568t
  social factors associated with, 559
  treatment of, 577t, 578
Shingles (*see* Herpes zoster)
Shoulder
  anatomy of, 581, *582*
  glenohumeral joint
    anatomy of, 581
    capsule, tears of, 587
    chronic instability of, 593–594
    dislocation, 594
    stability tests, 585
  range of motion
    description of, 584–585
    exercises for, 589
  subacromial bursa
    anatomy of, 582–583
    impingement tests of, 586
Shoulder pain
  case study of, 595–596
  causes of
    acromioclavicular degenerative joint disease, 590t, 593
    acromioclavicular joint, 587, 590t, 593
    adhesive capsulitis, 590t, 594

    algorithms for, *591*
    biceps tendonitis, 590t, 592–593
    cervical radiculopathy, 595
    clavicle fractures, 590t, 594–595
    glenohumeral joint
      dislocation, 594
      instability, 593–594
    rheumatologic disorders, 595
    rotator cuff
      tears, 590t, 592
      tendonitis, 590, 592
    treatment for, 590t
  classification of, 581
  clinical evaluation of
    history, 583–584
    physical examination, 584–589, 586t
  diagnostic tests
    computed tomography, 589
    magnetic resonance imaging, 589
    overview, 588t
    plain film arthrography, 588–589
    plain radiographs, 587–588
    ultrasound, 589
  differential diagnosis, 582–583, 584t
  general management of, 589
  pathophysiology of, 581–582
  prevalence of, 581
  "red flags" that suggest progressive or life-threatening disease associated with, 585t
Siberian ginseng, 197t, 199t
SIDS (*see* Sudden infant death syndrome)
Sigmoidoscopy
  for adult men, 171t
  for adult women, 167t
Sinus tachycardia, 356
Sinusitis
  in children, 551
  common cold, differential diagnosis of, 545
  definition of, 549
  headaches caused by
    clinical evaluation of, 452
    pathophysiology of, 449
  history of, 549
  laboratory tests, 549
  physical examination of, 549
  predisposing factors, 549
  treatment of, 549–551, *550*
Skeletal system, age-related changes in, 21t
Skin
  age-related changes, 21t
  care of, for infants and newborns, 151
  examination
    for adult men, 172t
    for adult women, 169t
Skin diseases (*see color plates*)
  acne, 607, 608t
  bacterial infections
    abscess, 602–603
    cellulitis, 602
    common sites for, 602t
    folliculitis, 602
    impetigo, 601–602
    necrotizing fasciitis, 603
  carcinoma
    basal cell, 607 (*see color plate*)
    benign growths and differential diagnosis, 607, 609

description of, 607, 609
squamous cell, 607 (*see color plate*)
case studies of, 609–611
clinical evaluation of
history, 597–598
laboratory tests, 599
physical examination, 597
prevention examination, 598–599
dermatitis
atopic, 605–606
contact, 605
definition of, 605
seborrhea, 606 (*see color plate*)
types of, 605–606
description of, 597
fungal infections
causes of, 604
types of, 604–605
heredity considerations, 599
lesions associated with, 598t
psoriasis, 606–607 (*see color plate*)
from sun damage, 607
topical corticosteroids for
adverse effects, 599–600
dispensing of, 600, 601t
duration of therapy, 601
mechanism of action, 599
selection of, 600, 600t
treatment of, 606
viral infections
herpesviruses, 604
warts, 603t, 603–604
Skin wounds
abrasions, 614–615
contusions, 613–614
diagnostic approach, 613
laceration
case study of, 621
definition of, 615
management of
aftercare, 620, 620t
anesthesia, 615
area-specific considerations, 618, 620
inspection, 615
suture closure, 616t–617t, 616–618, *617–619*
"red flags" regarding, 614t
Sleep
age-related changes, 21t
disorders, 426
infant patterns of, 151
mental health and, 94
Sleep apnea, obesity and, 683t
Small bowel obstruction
abdominal pain associated with, 232–233
diagnosis of, 228t
treatment for, 238
Smoking (*see* Tobacco)
Sodium
recommendations, 93t
reductions for hypertension treatment, 477, 477t
Soft tissue syndromes
bursitis, 297–298
description of, 296
distribution of, *297*
epicondylitis, 297–298
myofascial trigger points, 296–297

tendonitis, 297–298
Solitary thyroid nodule
clinical evaluation of, 637–638, 638t
differential diagnosis, 636, 636t
management of, 638–639, *639*, 643t
pathophysiology of, 635–636
Sore throat
case study of, 633
clinical evaluation of
history, 625, 626t
laboratory tests, 627, 628t
physical examination, 625–626, 626t
description of, 623
differential diagnosis, 624
group A β-hemolytic streptococcal pharyngitis
clinical evaluation of
history, 625
laboratory tests, 627, 628t
physical examination, 625–626
management of, 629–631, 630t–632t
prevalence of, 624
infectious mononucleosis
clinical evaluation of
history, 625
laboratory tests, 627
physical examination, 626–627
management of, 631–632
prevalence of, 624
management of, *629*, 629–632, 630t–632t
pathophysiology of, 623–624
patient education regarding, 632
"red flags" that suggest progressive or life-threatening disease, 625t
Specificity, of diagnostic tests, 213
Speed's test, 585
Spermicides, 105t, 121–122
Spinal cord compression, 521
Spirituality, 94–95
Squamous cell carcinoma, 607 (*see color plate*)
Stable angina
description of, 350
signs and symptoms of, 354–355
Stadol (*see* Butorphanol)
Staphylococcus epidermidis, 657
Stavudine, 465t
STDs (*see* Sexually transmitted diseases)
Sterilization, as form of contraception, 105t, 123
Sternoclavicular joint, 581, *582*
Streptococcus pneumoniae, 436, 467t, 555–556
Stress management, 94
Subacromial bursa
anatomy of, 581–582
impingement tests of, 586
Subarachnoid hemorrhage, headaches caused by
clinical evaluation of, 453
diagnostic tests, 454t
pathophysiology of, 449
Substance abuse (*see also* Addiction; Alcohol)
in adolescents, 146
annual costs of, 245
clinical evaluation
laboratory testing, 248t, 248–249
physical findings, 247t, 248
"red flags," 246, 246t, 248
screening, 245–246, 247t
differential diagnosis, 245

Substance abuse—*Continued*
  DSM-IV definitions of, 243–244
  etiology of, 244
  management of
    algorithm, *250*
    initial approaches, 249, 251
    psychiatric stability, 249, 251
    withdrawal syndrome, 249
  pathophysiology of, 245, 247t
  prevalence of, 243–245
  prevalent age of onset, 244
Sudden infant death syndrome, 152
Suicide, 146, 286
Sulcus sign, 585
Sulfasalazine, 304t
Sulfonylureas, 389–391, 390t
Sumatriptan, 457t
Supraventricular tachycardia, 375
Suturing, of skin lacerations, 616t–617t, 616–618,
    617–619
Symptoms (*see also specific disease or condition*)
  common types of, 205
  description of, 203, *204*
  psychosocial issues, 203–204
Syndesmosis sprain, 268
Synovial fluid, laboratory findings of
  in acute rheumatic fever, 295t
  in gout, 295t
  in osteoarthritis, 295t
  in pseudogout pyrophosphate, 295t
  in rheumatoid arthritis, 295t
  in septic arthritis, 295t
Synthroid (*see* Levothyroxine)
Syphilis
  description of, 562–563
  genital ulcers and, 576t
  health effects of, 561t
  screening tests, 566t–567t
  treatment of, 571t

T_3 (*see* Triiodothyronine)
T_4 (*see* Thyroxin)
Tachycardia
  reentry, 375
  supraventricular, 375
  wide complex, 376–377
Tamoxifen, for cyclic mastalgia, 333t, 334
TCA (*see* Tricyclic antidepressants)
Temporal association, 55
Temporomandibular joint disorders, headaches
    caused by
  clinical evaluation of, 453
  pathophysiology of, 449
Tendonitis
  biceps, 590t, 592–593
  description of, 297–298
  management of, 298
Tenormin (*see* Atenolol)
Tenosynovitis, 297
Tension headaches
  clinical evaluation of, 452
  pathophysiology of, 447, 449
  treatment of, 456–458, 457t
Tenuate (*see* Diethylpropion)
Terazosin, 537t
Terbutaline, 320t

Terconazole, 670t
Testosterone
  estrogen and, 184t
  in hormonal therapy, 184t
Tetanus, diphtheria boosters
  for adult men, 170t
  for adult women, 165t
Theophylline
  for asthma, 319t
  for chronic obstructive pulmonary disease,
    327t
Therapeutic massage, 194
Therapeutic touch, 195
Therapy
  definition of, 215–216
  evidence-based approach to, 215–216
Thiazide diuretics, for hypertension, 478t
Thoracic outlet syndrome, 521
Thorazine (*see* Chlorpromazine)
Thyroid
  functional changes during pregnancy, 652
  nonthyroid systemic disease effects, 652
  regulation of, 635
Thyroid cancer
  classification of, 636
  environmental causes of, 635
  incidence of, 635
  risk factors, 637t
Thyroid disease
  case study of, 652–653
  differential diagnosis, 636t
  hyperthyroidism
    clinical evaluation of, 641t, 648–649
    differential diagnosis, 648
    management of, 650–651
    pathophysiology of, 648
    risk factors, 637t
  hypothyroidism
    clinical evaluation of, 641t, 645–646
    differential diagnosis, 644
    fatigue associated with, 426
    management of, 643t
      algorithm for, *647*
      initial approach, 646–647
      long term, 647–648
    pathophysiology of, 644
    risk factors, 637t
    secondary, 646
    transient, 650
  risk factors, 637t
  solitary thyroid nodule
    clinical evaluation of, 637–638, 638t
    differential diagnosis, 636, 636t
    management of, 638–639, *639*, 643t
    pathophysiology of, 635–636
  thyroiditis (*see* Thyroiditis)
Thyroid hormonal disease, 651–652
Thyroid storm, 643t
Thyroidectomy, 651
Thyroiditis
  acute, 640
  diagnostic tests, 638t
  goiters associated with, 639
  management of, 642, 643t–644t
  postpartum
    description of, 652

risk factors, 637t
subacute granulomatous, 639–640
Thyroid-stimulating hormone, 635, 641–642, 648
Thyrotoxicosis, 643t
Thyrotropin-releasing hormone, 635
Thyroxin, 635
Ticonazole, 670t
Tietze's syndrome, 331
Tinea capitis, 605
Tinea corporis, 605 (*see color plate*)
Tinea cruris, 605
Tinea pedis, 605 (*see color plate*)
Tiredness (*see* Fatigue)
TMP/SMX (*see* Trimethoprim/sulfamethoxazole)
Tobacco use
    cessation of
        algorithm, *90*
        for coronary artery disease prevention, 361
    contraceptive formulations and, 116t–117t
    death rates, 81t
    parental counseling for, 153
    prevention strategies, 89
    systemic effects of, 247t
    transition products, 89
Tolazamide, 390t
Tolbutamide, 390t
Tolmetin, 269t
Toradol (*see* Ketorolac)
Tornalate (*see* Bitolterol)
Toxoplasma gondii, prophylaxis treatment for, 467t
Transrectal ultrasound, 530
Transvaginal ultrasound, for abnormal uterine bleeding, 512
Traveler's diarrhea, 164
Traveling, immunizations for, 159–160, 163–164
Trazodone, 287t
Treponema pallidum (*see* Syphilis)
TRH (*see* Thyrotropin-releasing hormone)
Triamcinolone acetonide, 305t, 319t
Triangulation, 30
Trichomonas vaginalis
    description of, 562
    health effects of, 561t
    screening tests, 568t
    treatment of, 571t
    urethritis, 572t
    vulvular findings, 573
Trichomonas vaginitis
    diagnosis of, 664
    history findings, 660–661, 663
    laboratory tests, 665t–666t, 668–669
    pathophysiology of, 658–659
    physical examination findings, 660–661, 663, 663t
    treatment of, 671t, 674
Tricyclic antidepressants
    costs of, 287
    indications, 288
    for panic disorder, 361–362
    therapy considerations, 287–288
    types of, 287t
Trigger points, myofascial
    description of, 296–297
    management of, 298
Triggers, of asthma
    exposure reduction, 314–315
    skin testing for, 315

types of, 312t
Triiodothyronine, 635
Trimethoprim/sulfamethoxazole
    for sinusitis, 550
    for urinary tract infections, 417t, 444t
Trisomy 21 (*see* Down syndrome)
Troglitazone, for diabetes mellitus, 390t, 391–392
TRUS (*see* Transrectal ultrasound)
TSH (*see* Thyroid-stimulating hormone)
Tuberculosis
    in adolescents, 145
    in children, 145
    environmentally induced, 54t
    incidence of, 145
    screening tests for, 145
Tubo-ovarian abscess, management of, 506

Ultrasound
    for palpable malignant breast mass, 342t
    for prenatal care, 134
    for shoulder pain, 589
    transvaginal, for abnormal uterine bleeding, 512
Unintended pregnancy
    causes of, 101
    contraception
        clinical evaluation, 106–108
        counseling, 103–106
        methods, 108–112
    costs associated with, 101
    definition of, 99
    family planing services, 101–102
    high-risk populations, 99–100
    prevalence of, 99, 101
    societal effects of, 101
Univasc (*see* Moexipril)
Unstable angina, 349–350
Upper respiratory infections, 436
Urethritis
    clinical evaluation of, 569
    clinical findings, 413t
    complications of, 565
    differential diagnosis, 565, 569
    laboratory tests, 569
    management of, 569
    pathophysiology of, 565, 569
    treatment of, 569
URI (*see* Upper respiratory infections)
Urinalysis, for urinary tract infection diagnosis, 414t, 414–415
Urinary system, age-related changes in, 21t
Urinary tract infections
    in adult men, 419
    asymptomatic bacteriuria, 421
    bacterial etiology of, 411
    case study of, 421–422
    catheter-associated, 420–421
    in children, 419–420, 444t
    clinical evaluation of
        history, 412, 413t
        laboratory tests
            specimen collection, 413
            urinalysis, 414t, 414–415
            urine culture, 415
        physical examination, 413
    differential diagnosis, 412, 412t

Urinary tract infections—*Continued*
  lower tract
    acute uncomplicated infection, 416–417
    complicated infection, "red flags" for, 413t
    history findings suggestive of, 412
  management of
    acute pyelonephritis, 418–419
    acute uncomplicated lower tract infection, 416–417
    algorithm, *416*
    drug therapy, 417t
    general approach, 415–416
    information gathering, 415–416
    recommendations, 415t
    recurrent infections, 417–418
  in older adults, 419
  pathophysiology of, 411–412
  predisposing factors, 412
  recurrent, 417–418
  route of infection, 411–412
  upper tract, 412
Urine culture, for urinary tract infection diagnosis, 415
U.S. Preventive Service Task Force
  age-specific charts, 83–84
  mental health screenings, 94
  recommendations, 82
U.S. Public Health Service, 85
Uterine bleeding, abnormal
  anovulatory, 513, *515*
  clinical evaluation of
    description of, 503t
    history, 511–512
    laboratory tests, 512
    physical examination, 512
  drug therapy, 507t
  general approach to, *513*
  hormonal dysfunctions associated with, 510–511
  intermenstrual, *516*
  management of, 512–514
  pathophysiology of, 510–511
  types of, 510
Uterus
  bleeding
    contraceptive formulations, 116t
    intrauterine device-induced, 120
    size of, and expected date of confinement estimations, 129
UTI (*see* Urinary tract infections)
Utilization review, 65

Vaccines
  diphtheria, pertussis, tetanus, 148
  influenza virus
    for adult men, 170t
    for adult women, 166t
  measles, mumps, rubella, 148
  oral polio, 148
  pneumococcal
    for adult men, 170t
    for adult women, 166t
Vaginitis
  atrophic, 660
  bacterial
    diagnosis of, 664, 664t
    history findings, 660, 662t

    laboratory tests, 665t
    pathophysiology of, 658
    physical examination findings, 660, 663t
    treatment of, 669, 670t, 673
  Candida vulvovaginitis
    diagnosis of, 664
    history findings, 660, 662t
    laboratory tests, 665t, 668
    nonprescription medication, 657
    pathophysiology of, 658
    physical examination findings, 660, 663t
    self-diagnosis of, 669
    treatment of, 670t–671t, 673–674
  case study of, 675
  clinical evaluation of
    algorithm, *661*
    history, 660–661, 662t, 663
    physical examination, 660–661, 663, 663t
  clinical findings, 413t
  differential diagnosis, 659t, 659–660
  laboratory tests, 664, 665t–666t, *667*, 668–669
  management of, 669–675 (*see also specific disease*)
  overview, 657
  pathophysiology of, 657–659
  patient education regarding, 674–675
  Trichomonas
    diagnosis of, 664
    history findings, 660–661, 663
    laboratory tests, 665t–666t, 668–669
    pathophysiology of, 658–659
    physical examination findings, 660–661, 663, 663t
    treatment of, 671t, 674
Valerian, 197t, 199t
Valproic acid, 457t
Valvular heart disease, 377
Varicella zoster virus, 604
Vasotec (*see* Enalapril)
Vegan diet, 195
Vegetarian diet, 195
Venereal disease (*see* Sexually transmitted diseases)
Venlafaxine, 287t
Ventolin (*see* Albuterol)
Verapamil, 371t, 457t, 644t
Vertical gastric banding, 686t, 687–688
Vertigo
  benign paroxysmal positional, 405, 407
  case study of, 409
  causes of, 401
  central, 402
  definition of, 401
  description of, 401–402
  history findings, 405–406
  peripheral, 402
  physical examination, 405
Vestibulitis, 659
VGB (*see* Vertical gastric banding)
Videx (*see* Didanosine)
Violence
  family, 92–93
  youth, 146, 153
Viracept (*see* Nelfinavir)
Viral infections (*see specific virus*)
Viramune (*see* Nevirapine)
Vision, screening of, 83, 144
Vitamin A, 93t
Vitamin C, 93t

Vitamin D, 93t
Vitamin E, 93t
Vitamin K, 93t
Vitamins, 93t, 186 (*see also specific vitamin*)
Vulvar intraepithelial neoplasia, 660
Vulvodynia, 659

Waist-to-hip ratio, 680, 684t
Warfarin, 376
Warts, 603t, 603–604
Weight
  gain, contraceptive-induced, 118t
  management of
    commercial programs, 685t
    goals, 694
    modalities, 686t
    services that provide, 679
    strategies, 689, 690t–693t
  screening of
    in men, 171t
    in women, 166t
Well care
  for adolescents, screening guidelines
    cervical dysplasia, 145–146
    congenital heart disease, 145
    growth and development, 144–145
    hypertension, 145
    sexually transmitted diseases, 146
    substance abuse, 146
    suicide, 146
    tuberculosis, 145
    venereal disease, 145–146
    youth violence, 146
  for adults
    chemoprophylaxis, 163–164
    description of, 159
    education
      description of, 174
      for men, 172t–173t
      for women, 168t–169t
    immunizations
      description of, 159, 162–164
      for women, 165t–166t
    morbidity and mortality causes, 157, 158t
    overview, 157–158
    preventive care
      case studies, 176
      challenges associated with, 175–176
      considerations for, 174
      description of, 157–158
      implementation of, 175
    risk assessment
      depression, 159, *162*
      diet history, 159, *160–161*
      for men, 170t
      sexual history taking, 158, 159t
      for women, 165t
    screening for asymptomatic disease
      description of, 164
      medical coverage for, 164, 174
      in men, 170t–172t
      in women, 166t–168t
    travel considerations, 159–160
    women, 165t–170t
  for children
    case study of, 153–154

  counseling for parents
    alcohol use, 153
    bowel habits, 151–152
    crying, 151
    dental health, 152
    description of, 149
    diet, 153
    drug use, 153
    exercise, 153
    feeding, 149–150
    infant stimulation, 149
    injury prevention, 152
    preventive, principles of, 149
    sexual behavior, 153
    skin care, 151
    sleeping, 151
    sudden infant death syndrome, 152
    tobacco use, 153
    topics commonly discussed, 150t
    youth violence, 153
  description of, 141
  immunizations
    adverse reactions associated with, 148
    contraindications, 147t
    measles, mumps, rubella, 148
    oral polio vaccine, 148
    precautions, 147t
    schedule for, 148t
  parental involvement, 141
  screening, 146–147
    description of, 142
    growth and development, 144–145
    heart disease, 145
    hypertension, 145
    iron deficiency anemia, 143
    lead toxicity, 143–144
    for newborns, 143
    recommended types based on age, 142t–143t
    tuberculosis, 145
    vision problems, 144
  visits, 141
Wheezing, in children, 310
Whiplash injuries, 520, 520t, 523t
White blood cell count, 440
WHR (*see* Waist-to-hip ratio)
Wide complex tachycardia, 376–377
Wigraine (*see* Ergotamine tartrate)
Worker's compensation, 57
World Health Organization, 68

X-rays (*see* Radiographs)
Xylometazoline hydrochloride, 548

Yergason's test, 585
Yocum's test, 586, 586t
Youth violence, 146, 153

Zafirlukast, 319t
Zalcitabine, 465t
Zerit (*see* Stavudine)
Zidovudine (ZDV), 465t
Zileuton (Zyflo), 319t, 321
Zinc, 547
Zovirax (*see* Acyclovir)